Oxford Textbook of

Respiratory Critical Care

OXFORD TEXTBOOKS IN CRITICAL CARE

Oxford Textbook of Advanced Critical Care Echocardiography
Edited by Anthony McLean, Stephen Huang, and Andrew Hilton

Oxford Textbook of Neurocritical Care
Edited by Martin M Smith, Giuseppe G Citerio, and W Andrew I Kofke

Oxford Textbook of Respiratory Critical Care
Edited by Suveer Singh, Paolo Pelosi, and Andrew Conway Morris

Oxford Textbook of

Respiratory Critical Care

EDITED BY

Suveer Singh BSc (hons), MBBS, PhD, EDIC, DICM, FHEA, FFICM, FRCP

Consultant Respiratory and Intensive Care Physician, Royal Brompton Hospital and Chelsea & Westminster Hospital; Professor of Practice, Imperial College London, United Kingdom

Paolo Pelosi MD, FERS, FESAIC

Full Professor in Anesthesiology and Critical Care, Department of Surgical Sciences and Integrated Diagnostics, University of Genoa; Director of Anesthesiology and Critical Care, San Martino Policlinico Hospital, IRCCS for Oncology and Neuosciences, Genoa, Italy

Andrew Conway Morris BSc (hons), MB ChB(hons), PhD, MRCP, FRCA, FFICM

MRC Clinician Scientist, Division of Anaesthesia, Department of Medicine, University of Cambridge; Division of Immunology, Department of Pathology, University of Cambridge; Honorary Consultant in Intensive Care Medicine, JVF Intensive Care Unit, Addenbrooke's Hospital, Cambridge, United Kingdom

Consultant Editor

Matthew P Wise MRCP, FFICM, D.Phil

Associate Medical Director for Research and Development, Cardiff & Vale University Health Board; Consultant Critical Care Physician, Adult Critical Care, University Hospital of Wales, Cardiff, United Kingdom

OXFORD
UNIVERSITY PRESS

OXFORD
UNIVERSITY PRESS

Great Clarendon Street, Oxford, OX2 6DP,
United Kingdom

Oxford University Press is a department of the University of Oxford.
It furthers the University's objective of excellence in research, scholarship,
and education by publishing worldwide. Oxford is a registered trade mark of
Oxford University Press in the UK and in certain other countries

First Edition published in 2023

Published in the United States of America by Oxford University Press
198 Madison Avenue, New York, NY 10016, United States of America

British Library Cataloguing in Publication Data
Data available

Library of Congress Control Number: 2022943454

ISBN 978–0–19–876643–8

DOI: 10.1093/med/9780198766438.001.0001

Printed in the UK by
Bell & Bain Ltd., Glasgow

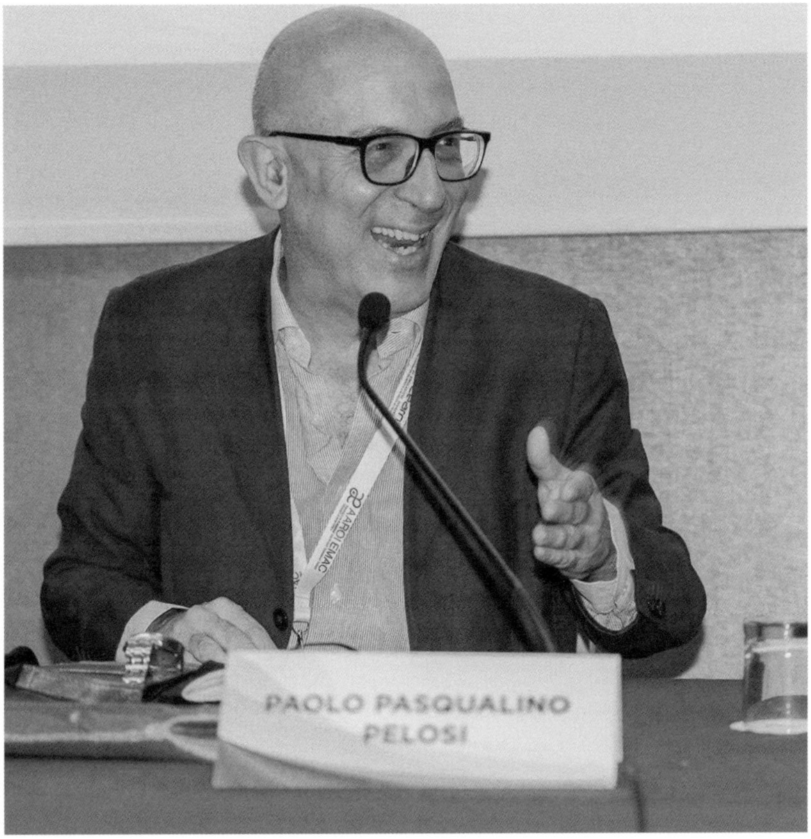

We dedicate this book to Professor Paolo Pelosi who passed before the final publication of this textbook. He was a great clinician, academic and educator locally, nationally and internationally with whom we have had the pleasure of working through the years.

Foreword

As a new entry to the Oxford University Press Medicine textbooks family, first edition of the *Oxford Textbook in Respiratory Critical Care* (OTRCC), edited by eminent respiratory and critical care physician colleagues Singh, Pelosi, and Conway Morris, provides a much-needed comprehensive up-to-date knowledge base on how to manage common and more importantly, unusual respiratory conditions within critical care settings.

The *Oxford Textbook in Respiratory Critical Care* will be relevant to a global readership, given the expert international contributors providing an engaging narrative with schematic illustrations on a wide range of respiratory disorders. The breadth of topics covered ranges from common respiratory conditions in critical care (such as COPD, Asthma) to less common respiratory diseases in critical care (such as ILD, Transplant related lung disease), and longer-term issues (such as Home Ventilation). Each chapter beings with a set of key messages, controversies, and areas for further research, which are useful summaries for the practicing senior clinicians, as well as physicians in training, and to researchers. This layout means that one can efficiently look up 'what should I do' for specific respiratory problems that arise in day-to-day practice in critical care.

I have no doubt that over time, the *Oxford Textbook in Respiratory Critical Care* will become a treasured practical guide to acute care clinicians across many specialities, from critical care, acute medicine, respiratory medicine, and emergency medicine. I have no hesitation in recommending *OTRCC* as an essential resource for all healthcare professionals involved in looking after critically ill patients.

Manu Shankar-Hari, PhD
Chair of Translational Care Medicine
University of Edinburgh

Preface

Respiratory critical care forms the central element of modern critical care medicine and demands a working knowledge of respiratory anatomy, physiology, and biology to provide effective support to the critically sick lungs. It has evolved from its origins in the polio epidemic of the 1950s, where positive-pressure mechanical ventilatory support led to substantial survival benefit over negative pressure strategies. It is now a rigorously studied discipline with increasing scientific knowledge of specific lung conditions, their pathophysiological basis, and evidence-based management strategies.

A better understanding of the molecular and physiological basis of conditions has been paralleled by the development of new therapeutic strategies (e.g. non-invasive ventilation) and greater understanding of the risk:benefit balance of interventions. These developments have led to standardization of care and, in many situations, better outcomes for patients.

Modern respiratory critical care requires knowledge of the complexity of lung-systemic organ and comorbid interactions in the critically ill patient, as well as an understanding of specific primary lung pathology, diagnosis, trajectories, and treatments. Further, respiratory critical care is truly multi-disciplinary. Thus, the critical care clinician requires skills taken from intensive care, anaesthesia, respiratory medicine, infectious diseases, cardiology, nephrology, radiology, pathology, and other disciplines. Excellent respiratory critical care dictates close working with specialists from multiple disciplines.

The *Oxford Textbook of Respiratory Critical Care* recognizes the essence of a common knowledge base and skills that are required for the management of critically ill patients with lung diseases and/or respiratory failure. Leading experts from across the world have contributed chapters to provide a comprehensive global overview of the specialty. Each chapter of this book highlights advances in the respective areas but also emphasizes the importance of getting the basics right. In this way, it will provide a framework for developing the meticulous attention to detail that underlies the clinical practice of respiratory critical care.

This text will equip the reader with detailed, evidence-based, up-to-date knowledge of clinical practice for the respiratory system, lung diseases within critical care medicine, and the impact of critical illness on lung biology. Each chapter offers key messages, controversies, and further research points as adjuncts to the authoritative text and key references.

The 10 sections cover (1) basic and historical concepts of the lung in critical illness; (2) organizational aspects of critical care and emergency planning; (3) practice of non-invasive ventilation, a major advance in respiratory disease over the last 30 years; (4) basis of invasive mechanical ventilation; (5) monitoring and investigation of the critically ill respiratory patient; (6) airway management and advanced respiratory support for respiratory failure; (7) bedside management of the ventilated patient; (8) respiratory infections in critical illness; (9) common and rare lung diseases associated with critical illness; and (10) weaning and long-term ventilation.

Each of the 65 chapters offers the reader options of key practice points and detailed reference, while providing a ready resource for educational delivery, grant, or paper writing.

As such, it should be useful as a stand-alone evidence-based clinical management reference and as an educational tool for consultants, postgraduate trainees, academic clinical staff, nurses, allied health professionals, and students.

The book will appeal to a global readership, while providing clinical practice points for respiratory disease presenting outside their usual sphere of practice and for less common respiratory disease manifestations. A chapter dedicated to COVID-19, as well as up-to-date individual chapters, makes reference to the impact of this novel virus in specific areas of respiratory critical care.

The editors are experienced in respiratory critical care through their disciplines of intensive care, anaesthesia, and respiratory medicine, while being active in research, education, and scientific writing. Their links with experts, international societies, and a broad network of medical and allied health professionals provide the basis for the book, which we hope will be valued by all who read it.

We would like to thank our colleagues who have contributed to this book, our families for their forbearance during its preparation, and of course our patients and staff colleagues from whom we learn every day.

Suveer Singh
Paolo Pelosi
Andrew Conway Morris

Contents

Abbreviations

ABCDE	Airway, breathing, circulation, decontamination, and elimination
ABLC	Lipid complex amphotericin B
ACE	Angiotensin converting enzyme
ACPO	Acute cardiogenic pulmonary oedema
AGE	Alveolar gas equation
AIDS	Acquired immune deficiency syndrome
APACHE II	Acute Physiology and Chronic Health Evaluation
APRV	Airway pressure release ventilation
ARDS	Acute respiratory distress syndrome
ARF	Acute respiratory failure
BAL	Bronchoalveolar lavage
BPA	Bronchopulmonary aspergillosis
BSI	Bloodstream infection
CA	*Candida albicans* spp.
CAO	Central airway obstruction
C_aO_2	Arterial oxygen content
CAPA	COVID-19-associated pulmonary aspergillosis
CarboxyHb	Carboxyhaemoglobin
C_CO_2	End capillary oxygen content
CDC	Centres for disease control
CFU	Colony-forming unit
CMV	Continuous mechanical ventilation
CNS	Central nervous system
CO	Carbon monoxide
CO_2	Carbon dioxide
COHb	Carboxyhaemoglobin
COPD	Chronic obstructive pulmonary disease
COT	Conventional oxygen therapy
CPIS	Clinical pulmonary infection score
CRP	C-reactive protein
CSV	Continuous spontaneous ventilation
CT (scan)	Computed tomography
CT	Computed tomography
CTPA	Computed tomography pulmonary angiogram
CUS	Compression ultrasound
C_vO_2	Venous oxygen content
CynHb	Cyanohaemoglobin
DLCO	Diffusion capacity of the lungs for carbon monoxide
DNI	Do-not-intubate
DO_2	Oxygen delivery
DVT	Deep vein thrombosis
EAdi	Electrical activity of the diaphragm
ECDC	European Centre for Disease Prevention and Control
ECMO	Extracorporeal membrane oxygenation
ETT	Endotracheal tube
F_EO_2	Fraction of expired oxygen
F_iO_2	Fraction of expired oxygen
FOB	Fibreoptic bronchoscopy
GBS	Guillain-Barrè syndrome
GCS	Glasgow coma scale
GI	Gastrointestinal
HAART	Highly active antiretroviral therapy
HAP	Hospital-acquired pneumonia
Hb	Haemoglobin
HCN	Hydrogen cyanide
HFOT	High-flow oxygen therapy through nasal cannula
HFPV	High-frequency percussive ventilation
HIT	Heparin-induced thrombocytopenia
HIV	Human immunodeficiency virus
HSCT	Haematopoietic stem cell transplant
H2RA	Histamine-2-receptor antagonist
ICU	Intensive care unit
IFIs	Invasive fungal infections
IL	Interleukin
IMV	Intermittent mandatory ventilation
iMV	Invasive mechanical ventilation
IPC	Indwelling pleural catheter
IVAC	Infection-related ventilator-associated condition
IVC	Inferior vena-cava
kPa	Kilopascal
L-AmB	Liposomal amphotericin B
LAO	Lower airway obstruction
LDH	Lactate dehydrogenase
LMWH	Low molecular weight heparin
MetHb	Methemoglobinemia
MG	Myasthenia gravis
mmHg	Millimetre of mercury
MMV	Mandatory minute ventilation
MV	Mechanical ventilation
NAC	*Candida* non-*albicans* spp.
NAVA	Neurally adjusted ventilatory assist
NBL	Non-directed bronchial lavage
nCPAP	Continuous positive airways pressure
NHSN	National Healthcare Safety Network
NICE	National Institute for Health and Care Excellence
NIV	Non-invasive ventilation
NMD	Neuromuscular disease
NPA	Nasopharyngeal aspirate

NIPPV	Non-invasive positive pressure ventilation
NSAIDs	Nonsteroidal anti-inflammatory drugs
O_2	Oxygen
OR	Odds ratio
P_A	Alveolar partial pressure
P_a	Arterial partial pressure
$PaCO_2$	Arterial carbon dioxide partial pressure
PAM	Pralidoxime
PaO_2	Partial pressure of oxygen
PAV	Proportional assist ventilation
P_B	Atmospheric partial pressure
PC	Pressure-controlled
PCR	Polymerase chain reaction
PCT	Procalcitonin
PE	Pulmonary embolism
PEEP	Positive end-expiratory pressure
PESI	Pulmonary embolism severity index
P_{eso}	Oesophageal pressure
PET (scan)	Positron emission tomography
PFT	Pulmonary function testing
pH	Potential of hydrogen
P_I	Inspired partial pressure
P_{insp}	Inspiratory pressure
PJP	Pneumocystis jiroveci pneumonia
P_{peak}	Peak inspiratory pressure
PPI	Proton pump inhibitor
P_{plat}	Inspiratory plateau pressure
PSB	Protected specimen brush
$P_{SVP\ Water}$	Saturated vapour pressure of water
Q_S	Shunted blood flow
Q_T	Total blood flow (cardiac output)
R	Resistance
RCT	Randomized controlled trial
REPE	Re-expansion pulmonary oedema
RR	Respiratory rate
RS	Respiratory system
RVD	Right ventricular dysfunction
SaO_2	Arterial oxygen saturation
SBP	Systolic blood pressure
SBT	Spontaneous breathing trial
SDD	Selective decontamination of the digestive tract
SOD	Selective oral decontamination
SOT	Solid organ transplant
SpO_2	Oxygen saturation measured by pulse oximeter
SUP	Stress ulcer prophylaxis
SVP	Saturate vapour pressure
TBA	Tracheobronchial aspirate
Ti-M	Inspiration time of the ventilator
Ti-N	Inspiration time of the patient
TLCO	Transfer factor of the lungs for carbon monoxide
TNF	Tumour necrosis factor
TOE	Transoesophageal echocardiography
TREM	Triggering receptor expressed on myeloid cells
TSA	Trial sequential analysis
TTE	Transthoracic echocardiography
UAO	Upper airway obstruction
UFH	Unfractionated heparin
V	Volume
V/Q	Ventilation–perfusion
V_A	Alveolar ventilation
VAC	Ventilator-associated condition
VAP	Ventilator-associated pneumonia
VAT	Ventilator-associated tracheobronchitis
VC	Volume-controlled
V_{CO2}	Carbon dioxide production
V_D	Dead space ventilation—takes no part in gas exchange
V_E	Minute ventilation
VILI	Ventilator-induced lung injury
VKA	Vitamin K antagonist
VO_2	Oxygen consumption
V_{O2}	Oxygen uptake
VRE	Vancomycin-resistant enterococcus
V_T	Tidal volume
VTE	Venous thromboembolism
WOB	Work of breathing

Contributors

Ahmed Al-Hindawi Intensive Care Medicine, University College London, London, UK; Magill Department of Anaesthesia, Intensive Care Medicine and Pain Management, Imperial College London Chelsea and Westminster Hospital, London, UK

Hollmann D Aya Adult Intensive Care Directorate, St George's University Hospitals NHS Foundation Trust, London, UK

Jonathan Ball General Intensive Care Unit, St George's University Hospital NHS Foundation Trust, London, UK

Lorenzo Ball Assistant Professor of Anesthesia and Intensive Care, Department of Surgical Sciences and Integrated Diagnostics (DISC), University of Genoa, Genoa, Italy; Anesthesia and Intensive Care, San Martino Policlinic Hospital, IRCCS for Oncology e le Neurosciences, Genoa, Italy

Matteo Bassetti Department of Health Sciences (DISSAL), University of Genoa, Genoa, Italy; Clinica Malattie Infettive, San Martino Policlinico Hospital—IRCCS for Oncology and Neurosciences, Genoa, Italy

Gianluigi Li Bassi Critical Care Research Group, The Prince Charles Hospital, Brisbane, Australia; University of Queensland, Brisbane, Australia; St Andrew's War Memorial Hospital, Brisbane, Australia; The Wesley Hospital, Brisbane, Australia; Queensland University of Technology, Brisbane, Australia; Institut d'Investigacions Biomèdiques August Pi i Sunyer, Barcelona, Spain

Philippe R Bauer Consultant, Division of Pulmonary and Critical Care Medicine; Associate Professor of Medicine, College of Medicine; Vice Chair Critical Care IMP Research Subcommittee, Mayo Clinic, Rochester, MN, USA

Simone Bazurro Resident Physician in Anesthesiology, Resuscitation and Intensive Care, Emergency Department, Anaesthesia and Intensive Care Unit, Ospedale San Paolo, ASL2, Sistema Sanitario Regione Liguria, Savona, Italy

Danielle E Bear Department of Nutrition and Dietetics, Critical Care, Guy's and St Thomas' NHS Foundation Trust, London, UK

Thomas Bein Department of Anesthesia and Operative Intensive Care, University Hospital Regensburg, Regensburg, Germany

Derek Bell Consultant Physician, Professor of Medicine, Faculty of Medicine, Imperial College, London, UK

Christoph Boesing Department of Anesthesiology and Critical Care Medicine, University Medical Centre Mannheim, Medical Faculty Mannheim of the University of Heidelberg, Mannheim, Germany

Fraser Brims Consultant Respiratory Physician, Curtin Medical School, Curtin University, Bentley, Western Australia, Australia; Department of Respiratory Medicine, Sir Charles Gairdner Hospital, Nedlands, Western Australia, Australia; Institute for Respiratory Health, Curtin University, Nedlands, Western Australia, Australia

Eleonora Bunsow Vall d'Hebron Institute of Research, Barcelona, Spain

Luigi Camporota Consultant Critical Care Physician, Director of Extracorporeal Support, Guy's and St Thomas' NHS Foundation Trust, UK

Alessia Carnelutti Infectious Diseases Division, Udine University Hospital, Udine, Italy

Alastair C Carr Clinical Director of Intensive Care Medicine, Consultant in Intensive Care Medicine and Anaesthesia, Honorary Senior Lecturer in Intensive Care Medicine and Anaesthesia, University of Otago, New Zealand; Chair, New Zealand ICU CNM and CD Network, New Zealand Regional Chair, Australia and New Zealand Intensive Care Society, New Zealand

Andrea Carsetti Associate Professor of Anaesthesiology, Department of Biomedical Sciences and Public Health, Università Politecnica delle Marche, Ancona, Italy; Anaesthesia and Intensive Care Unit, Azienda Ospedaliero Universitaria delle Marche, Ancona, Italy

Maurizio Cecconi Department of Biomedical Sciences, Humanitas University, Milan, Italy; Department of Anaesthesia and ICU, IRCCS Humanitas Research Hospital, Milan, Italy

Nirmala Mary Chakkalakal Clinical Fellow in International Emergency Medicine, Chelsea and Westminster Hospital, Chelsea and Westminster Hospital NHS Foundation Trust, London, UK

Dhruva Chaudhry Department of Pulmonary and Critical Care Medicine, Pt BD Sharma Postgraduate Institute of Medical Sciences, Rohtak, Haryana, India

Davide Chiumello Unità Operativa Complessa di Anestesia e Rianimazione, Ospedale San Paolo-Polo Universitario, ASST Santi Paolo e Carlo, Milan, Italy; Dipartimento di Scienze della Salute, Università degli Studi di Milano, Milan, Italy

Felix Chua Consultant Respiratory Physician, Interstitial Lung Disease Unit, Royal Brompton Hospital, Guy's and St Thomas' NHS Foundation Trust, London, UK; National Heart and Lung Institute, Imperial College London, London, UK

Bronwen Connolly Wellcome-Wolfson Institute for Experimental Medicine, Queen's University Belfast, UK; Department of Physiotherapy, The University of Melbourne, Victoria, Australia; Lane Fox Respiratory Unit, Guy's and St Thomas' NHS Foundation Trust, UK; Centre for Human & Applied Physiological Sciences, King's College London, London, UK

Andrea Cortegiani Department of Surgical, Oncological and Oral Science (Di.Chir.On.S.), University of Palermo, Italy

Timothy Crozier Consultant in Intensive Care, Intensive Care Unit, Monash Medical Centre, Monash Health, Victoria, Australia; Department of Intensive Care Services, Eastern Health, Victoria, Australia; Department of Obstetrics & Gynaecology, Monash University, Victoria, Australia

Andrew Cumpstey NIHR Clinical Lecturer in Anaesthesia and Intensive Care Medicine, Perioperative and Critical Care theme, NIHR Southampton Biomedical Research Centre, University Hospital Southampton/University of Southampton, UK

Rachel D'Oliveiro Consultant in Intensive Care and Respiratory Medicine, Royal Papworth Hospital NHS Foundation Trust, Cambridge, UK

Michael Davies Consultant Physician, Respiratory Support and Sleep Centre, Clinical Director for Thoracic and Ambulatory Services; Associate Lecturer, University of Cambridge, Royal Papworth Hospital NHS Foundation Trust, Cambridge, UK

Marcelo Gama de Abreu Professor of Anaesthesiology, Cleveland Clinic Lerner College of Medicine, Case Western Reserve University, Cleveland, OH, USA; Staff Physician, Department of Intensive Care and Resuscitation, and Department of Outcomes Research, Anesthesiology Institute, Cleveland Clinic, Cleveland, Ohio, USA; Professor of Translational Research in Anesthesiology and Intensive Care, Dresden University of Technology, Dresden, Germany

Audrey de Jong Consultant in Anaesthesia and Intensive Care, Unité de Réanimation et de Transplantation, Département d'Anesthésie-Réanimation Saint Eloi, CHU de Montpellier Hôpital Saint Eloi, Montpellier Cedex, France

Ivan Dell'atti Department of Anaesthesiology, Critical Care Medicine and Emergency, SS Annunziata Hospital, Chieti, Italy

Giorgio Della Rocca Full Professor of Anesthesiology, Department of Medicine University of Udine, Udine, Italy

Stephan Ehrmann CHRU Tours, Médecine Intensive Réanimation, CIC INSERM 1415, CRICS-Trigger SEP FCRIN Research Network, Tours, France; INSERM, Centre d'Etude des Pathologies Respiratoires, U1100, Université de Tours, Tours, France

Jonathon P Fanning Critical Care Research Group, The Prince Charles Hospital, Brisbane, Australia; University of Queensland, Brisbane, Australia; St Andrew's War Memorial Hospital, Brisbane, Australia; Nuffield Department of Population Health, University of Oxford, UK

Muriel Fartoukh Consultant in Intensive Care, Service de Médecine Intensive réanimation, Hôpital Tenon, Assistance Publique-Hôpitaux de Paris, Paris, France; Faculté de médecine Sorbonne Université, Paris, France

Simon J Finney Consultant in Anaesthesia and Intensive Care Medicine, St Bartholomew's Hospital West Smithfield, London, UK

Iacopo Firpo Resident Physician in Anesthesia and Intensive Care, Department of Surgical Sciences and Integrated Diagnostics (DISC), University of Genoa, Genoa, Italy

Paolo Formenti Operative unit for Anaesthesia and Critical Care, San Paolo-Polo University Hospital, ASST Santi Paolo e Carlo, Milan, Italy

Edward TH Fysh Adjunct Clinical Senior Lecturer, University of Western Australia, Western Australia, Australia; Respiratory and Intensive Care Consultant and National Health and Medical Research Council Early Career Fellow, Departments of Intensive Care and Respiratory Medicine, St John of God Midland Public and Private Hospitals, Midland, Western Australia, Australia; Faculty of Health and Medical Sciences, University of Western Australia, Curtin University Medical School, Curtin University, Western Australia, Australia

Rodney A Gabriel Department of Anesthesiology, University of California, San Diego, CA, USA

Vanya Gant Consultant in Infectious Disease and Microbiology, Director of Pathology, University College London Hospital, London, UK

Benjamin Garfield Intensive Care Unit, Royal Brompton Hospital, Royal Brompton and Harefield NHS Foundation Trust, London, UK; Division of Anaesthetics, Pain Medicine and Intensive Care, Department of Surgery and Cancer, Faculty of Medicine, Imperial College London, London, UK

Suneel Kumar Garg Consultant in Intensive Care Medicine, Institute of Critical Care Medicine, Max Super Speciality Hospital, Saket, India

Peter M George Consultant Respiratory Physician, Interstitial Lung Disease Unit, Royal Brompton Hospital, Guy's and St Thomas' NHS Foundation Trust, London, UK; National Heart and Lung Institute, Imperial College London, London, UK

Daniele Roberto Giacobbe Department of Health Sciences (DISSAL), University of Genoa, Genoa, Italy; Clinica Malattie Infettive, San Martino Policlinico Hospital—IRCCS for Oncology and Neurosciences, Genoa, Italy

Aude Gibelin Consultant in Intensive Care, Service de Médecine intensive réanimation, Hôpital Tenon, Assistance Publique-Hôpitaux de Paris, Paris, France; Faculté de médecine Sorbonne Université, Paris, France

Manjunath B Govindagoudar Department of Pulmonary and Critical Care Medicine, Pt BD Sharma Postgraduate Institute of Medical Sciences, Rohtak, Haryana, India

Maja M Green Metro Pain Research Institute, Clayton, VIC, Australia

Cesare Gregoretti Department of Surgical, Oncological and Oral Science (Di.Chir.On.S.), University of Palermo, Italy; Department of Anaesthesia, Intensive Care and Emergency, Policlinico Paolo Giaccone, Palermo, Italy; Fondazione 'Giglio', Cefalù, Italy

Mark Griffiths Professor of Critical Care Medicine, National Heart and Lung Institute, Imperial College London, London, UK; Consultant in Critical Care, Barts Heart Centre, Barts Health NHS Trust, London, UK

Mike Grocott Professor of Anaesthesia and Critical Care, Perioperative and Critical Care theme, NIHR Southampton Biomedical Research Centre, University Hospital Southampton/ University of Southampton, UK

Oliver Grottke Consultant in Anaesthesiology and Intensive Care, Department of Anaesthesiology, RWTH Aachen University Hospital, Aachen, Germany

Vimal Grover Consultant in Critical Care Medicine and Anaesthesia, Royal Marsden Hospital, London, UK

Emma Louise Hartley Consultant Intensive Care Medicine, Department of Adult Critical Care, Royal Infirmary of Edinburgh, Edinburgh, UK

Thomas Hellyer Faculty of Medical Sciences, Newcastle University, Newcastle upon Tyne, UK

Christopher D Hingston Consultant in Intensive Care Medicine, Adult Intensive Care, University Hospital of Wales, Cardiff, UK; Consultant in Pre-hospital Medicine, Emergency Medical Retrieval and Transfer Service (EMRTS) Cymru, Llanelli, UK

Markus Honickel Consultant in Anaesthesiology and Intensive Care, Department of Anaesthesiology, RWTH Aachen University Hospital, Aachen, Germany

Johannes M Huitink Anesthesiologist and Retrieval Specialist, Airway Management Academy, Amsterdam, The Netherlands

Giovanni Carmine Iovino Department of Anaesthesiology, Critical Care Medicine and Emergency, SS Annunziata Hospital, Chieti, Italy

Mariachiara Ippolito Department of Surgical, Oncological and Oral Science (Di.Chir.On.S.), University of Palermo, Palermo, Italy

Samir Jaber Consultant in Intensive Care, Département d'Anesthésie-Réanimation Saint Eloi, CHU de Montpellier Hôpital Saint Eloi, Montpellier Cedex, France

Hannah Jarvis Department of Respiratory Medicine, St Mary's Hospital, Imperial College Healthcare NHS Trust, London, UK

Andrew Jones Consultant Respiratory and Critical Care Physician, Guy's and St Thomas' NHS Foundation Trust, UK

Ricardo J José Consultant in Respiratory Medicine, Department of Host Defence, Royal Brompton Hospital, London, UK

Nicole P Juffermans Laboratory of Experimental Intensive Care and Anesthesiology, Amsterdam University Medical Center, Amsterdam, The Netherlands; Department of Intensive Care, OLVG Hospital, Amsterdam, The Netherlands

Deven Juneja Consultant in Intensive Care Medicine, Institute of Critical Care Medicine, Max Super Speciality Hospital, Saket, India

Richard Keays Director of Intensive Care, Chelsea and Westminster Hospital, London, UK

Thomas Kiss Head of Department, Department of Anaesthesiology, Intensive, Pain and Palliative Care Medicine, Radebeul Hospital, Germany; Academic Hospital of the Technische Universität Dresden, Germany

Onn Min Kon Department of Respiratory Medicine, St Mary's Hospital, Imperial College Healthcare NHS Trust, London, UK

Vasilis Kouranos Consultant Respiratory Physician, Interstitial Lung Disease Unit, Royal Brompton Hospital, Guy's and St Thomas' Hospital NHS Foundation Trust, London, UK

Mette Krag Associate Professor, Department of Anaesthesiology and Intensive Care, Holbæk Hospital, Denmark and Department of Clinical Medicine, University of Copenhagen, Copenhagen, Denmark

Joerg Krebs Department of Anesthesiology and Critical Care Medicine, University Medical Centre Mannheim, Medical Faculty Mannheim of the University of Heidelberg, Mannheim, Germany

Leonel Lagunes CIBERES, Barcelona, Spain

Loïc Lang-Lazdunski Division of Thoracic Surgery, Department of Surgery, Université Laval, Quebec, QC, Canada

Richard Leach Richard Leach Consultant Respiratory and Critical Care Physician and Medical Director, Guy's and St Thomas' Hospital Trust, UK; Honorary Professor of Medicine Kings College London, UK

Susannah Leaver General Intensive Care Unit, St George's University Hospital NHS Foundation Trust, London, UK

Matthieu Legrand Professor, Department of Anaesthesia and Perioperative Care, Division of Critical Care Medicine, University of California San Francisco, USA

Federico Longhini Anesthesia and Intensive Care, Department of Medical and Surgical Science, 'Magna Graecia' University, Catanzaro, Italy

Julien Lopinto Consultant in Intensive Care, AP-HP, Sorbonne Université, Hôpital Tenon, Pôle TVAR, Service de Médecine intensive réanimation, France; AP-HP, Hôpitaux Universitaires Henri Mondor, DHU A-TVB, Service de Réanimation Médicale, Créteil, France; Université Paris Est Créteil, Faculté de Médecine, Groupe de recherche clinique CARMAS, Créteil, France

Thomas Luecke Department of Anesthesiology and Critical Care Medicine, University Medical Centre Mannheim, Medical Faculty Mannheim of the University of Heidelberg, Mannheim, Germany

Salvatore Maurizio Maggiore Professor of Anaesthesiology and Intensive Care Medicine, "Gabriele d'Annunzio" University of Chieti-Pescara; Department of Anaesthesiology and Intensive Care Medicine, SS, Annunziata Hospital, Chieti, Italy

John J Marini Professor of Medicine, University of Minnesota, Minneapolis/St Paul, MN, USA

Greg McAnulty Consultant in Intensive Care Medicine and Thoracic Anaesthesia, Alice Springs Hospital, Central Australia Health Service, Minyerri, Australia

Steve McGoughlin Director Intensive Care, Alfred Health, Melbourne, Victoria, Australia

Armand Mekontso-Dessap Consultant in Intensive Care, AP-HP, Hôpitaux Universitaires Henri Mondor, DHU A-TVB, Service de Réanimation Médicale, Créteil, France; Université Paris Est Créteil, Faculté de Médecine, Groupe de recherche clinique CARMAS, Créteil, France

Antonio Messina Humanitas Clinical and Research Center—IRCCS, Milano, Italy; Department of Biomedical Sciences, Humanitas University, Pieve Emanuele, MI, Italy

Lucrezia Mincione Department of Anaesthesiology, Critical Care Medicine and Emergency, SS Annunziata Hospital, Chieti, Italy

Fiona Moghaddas Specialty Physician in Immunology and Allergy, North Bristol NHS Trust, Bristol, UK

Alex Molin Department of Surgical Sciences and Integrated Diagnostics, University of Studies of Genoa, Genoa, Italy; Clinical UOC Anesthesiology and Intensive Care, IRCCS San Martino Polyclinic Hospital, Genoa, Italy

Morten Hylander Møller Associate Professor, Department of Intensive Care, Copenhagen University Hospital Rigshospitalet, Copenhagen, Denmark

Philip L Molyneaux Consultant Respiratory Physician, Interstitial Lung Disease Unit, Royal Brompton Hospital, Guy's and St Thomas' Hospital NHS Foundation Trust, London, UK

Andrew Conway Morris MRC Clinician Scientist, Division of Anaesthesia, Department of Medicine, University of Cambridge; Division of Immunology, Department of Pathology, University of Cambridge; Honorary Consultant in Intensive Care Medicine, JVF Intensive Care Unit, Addenbrooke's Hospital, Cambridge

Patrick B Murphy Consultant Respiratory Physician, Director, Lane Fox Unit, Guy's and St Thomas' NHS Foundation Trust, UK

Sabine Nabecker Department of Anesthesia and Pain Management, Sinai Health System, University of Toronto, Toronto, Ontario, Canada

Arjun Nair Consultant Radiologist and Honorary Senior Lecturer, University College Hospital, London, UK

Paolo Navalesi Department of Medicine—DIMED, University of Padua, Padua, Italy; Anesthesia and Intensive Care, University Hospital of Padua, Padua, Italy

Gary Nieman Department of Surgery, SUNY Upstate Medical University, Syracuse, New York, USA

Judit Orosz Intensivist and Infectious Diseases Physician, Alfred Health, Melbourne, Victoria, Australia

Christopher Orton Consultant Respiratory Physician, Royal Brompton Hospital, Guy's and St Thomas' Hospital NHS Foundation Trust, London, UK

Marlies Ostermann Department of Critical Care, Guy's and St Thomas' NHS Foundation Trust, London, UK

Jack Parry-Jones Critical Care Consultant, University Hospital of Wales, Cardiff and Vale University Health Board, Wales, UK

Nilima Parry-Jones Consultant Haematologist, Aneurin Bevan University Health Board, Wales, UK

Sunil Patel Intensive Care Unit, Royal Brompton Hospital, Royal Brompton and Harefield NHS Foundation Trust, London, UK; Division of Anaesthetics, Pain Medicine and Intensive Care, Department of Surgery and Cancer, Faculty of Medicine, Imperial College London, London, UK

Nicolò Patroniti Science Department Surgical and Integrated Diagnostics, University of the Studies of Genoa, Genoa, Italy; COU Anesthesiological Clinic and Intensive Care, IRCCS San Martino Polyclinic Hospital, Genoa, Italy

Caroline Patterson Consultant Respiratory Physician, Transplant Unit, Royal Papworth Hospital, Cambridge, UK

Paolo Pelosi Professor of Anesthesia and Intensive Care, Department of Surgical Sciences and Integrated Diagnostics (DISC), University of Genoa, Genoa, Italy; Anesthesia and Intensive Care, IRCCS San Martino Policlinico Hospital, Genoa, Italy

Michael Pfeifer Professor of Respiratory Medicine, University Hospital Regensburg, Regensburg, Germany

Michael R Pinsky Department of Anesthesiology, Department of Critical Care Medicine, University of Pittsburgh, PA, USA

Lara Pisani Department of Specialistic, Diagnostic and Experimental Medicine (DIMES), Respiratory and Critical Care, Sant'Orsola Mal-pighi Hospital, Alma Mater Studiorum, University of Bologna, Italy

Michael I Polkey Consultant Respiratory Physician, Sleep and Ventilation Unit, Royal Brompton and Harefield Hospitals, Guy's and St Thomas' NHS Foundation Trust, London, UK

Imperial College London, London, UK

Laura C Price Consultant Respiratory Physician, National Pulmonary Hypertension Service, Royal Brompton and Harefield Hospitals, Guy's and St Thomas' NHS Foundation Trust, London, UK; Honorary Senior Clinical Lecturer, Imperial College, London, UK

Zudin Puthucheary William Harvey Research Institute, Barts and The London School of Medicine and Dentistry, Queen Mary University of London, London, UK; Adult Critical Care Unit, Royal London Hospital, Barts Health NHS Trust, London, UK

Jordi Rello Vall d'Hebron Institute of Research, Barcelona, Spain; CIBERES, Barcelona, Spain; Universitat Internacional de Catalunya, Barcelona, Spain

Andrew Retter Consultant Intensive Care Medicine and Haematology, Department of Adult Critical Care, St Thomas' Hospital, Guy's and St Thomas' NHS Foundation Trust, London, UK

Mara Ricci Department of Anaesthesiology, Critical Care Medicine and Emergency, SS Annunziata Hospital, Chieti, Italy

Patricia Rieken Laboratory of Pulmonary Investigation, Carlos Chagas Filho Biophysics Institute, Federal University of Rio de Janeiro, Rio de Janeiro, Brazil; COVID-19 Virus Network, Ministry of Science, Technology and Innovation, Brasília, Brazil

Elda Righi Department of Diagnostics and Public Health, University of Verona, Verona, Italy

Stephen M Robinson Consultant in Anaesthetics and Intensive Care Medicine, Southmead Hospital, North Bristol NHS Trust, Bristol, UK

Macedo Rocco Laboratory of Pulmonary Investigation, Carlos Chagas Filho Biophysics Institute, Federal University of Rio de Janeiro, Rio de Janeiro, Brazil; COVID-19 Virus Network, Ministry of Science, Technology and Innovation, Brasília, Brazil

Patricia RM Rocco Laboratory of Pulmonary Investigation, Carlos Chagas Filho Biophysics Institute, Federal University of Rio de Janeiro, Rio de Janeiro, Brazil; Member of the National Academy of Medicine in Brazil and Brazilian Academy of Science, Brazil

Eli Rogers Magill Department of Anaesthesia, Intensive Care Medicine and Pain Management, Imperial College London Chelsea and Westminster Hospital, London, UK

Rolf Rossaint Head in Anaesthesiology and Intensive Care, Department of Anaesthesiology, RWTH Aachen University Hospital, Aachen, Germany

Anthony Rostron Faculty of Medical Sciences, Newcastle University, Newcastle upon Tyne, UK; Sunderland Royal Hospital, Sunderland, UK

Vincenzo Russotto Department of Emergency and Intensive Care, University Hospital San Gerardo, University of Milano Bicocca, Monza, Italy

Christopher MR Satur Consultant Surgeon, University Hospitals of North Midlands, UK; Honorary Clinical Lecturer, Keele University, UK

Martin Scharffenberg Department of Anesthesiology and Intensive Care Medicine, University Hospital Carl Gustav Carus, Dresden, Germany

Marcus J Schultz Amsterdam UMC, location 'AMC', Department of Medicine, Amsterdam, The Netherlands Oxford University, Nuffield Department of Medicine, Oxford, UK; Mahidol University, Mahidol Oxford Tropical Medicine Research Unit, Bangkok, Thailand

Timothy E Scott Consultant in Intensive Care and Anaesthesia, Royal Stoke University Hospital, Staffordshire, UK

Yahya Shehabi Critical Care and Perioperative Medicine, School of Clinical Sciences, Monash University and Monash Health, Clayton, Victoria, Australia; Clinical School of Medicine, University of New South Wales, Randwick, New South Wales, Australia

Pedro Leme Silva Laboratory of Pulmonary Investigation, Carlos Chagas Filho Biophysics Institute, Federal University of Rio de Janeiro, Rio de Janeiro, Brazil

A John Simpson Faculty of Medical Sciences, Newcastle University, Newcastle upon Tyne, UK

Omender Singh Director, Institute of Critical Care Medicine, Max Super Speciality Hospital, Saket, India

Pawan Kumar Singh Department of Pulmonary and Critical Care Medicine, Pt BD Sharma Postgraduate Institute of Medical Sciences, Rohtak, Haryana, India

Suveer Singh Consultant Respiratory and Intensive Care Physician, Royal Brompton Hospital, London, UK; Consultant Respiratory and Intensive Care Physician Chelsea and Westminster Hospital, London, UK; Professor of Practice (Respiratory and Intensive Care), Imperial College London, London, UK

Jasmeet Soar Consultant in Anaesthesia and Intensive Care, Southmead Hospital, North Bristol NHS Trust, Bristol, UK

Sabri Soussi Department of Anesthesiology, Critical Care, Lariboisière—Saint-Louis Hospitals, DMU Parabol, AP-HP Nord, Inserm UMR-S 942, Cardiovascular Markers in Stress Conditions (MASCOT), University of Paris, Paris, France; Interdepartmental Division of Critical Care, Keenan Research Centre for Biomedical Science and Institute of Medical Sciences, Faculty of Medicine, University of Toronto, Toronto, ON, Canada

Francesco Tasso Resident Physician in Anesthesia and Intensive Care, Department of Surgical Sciences and Integrated Diagnostics (DISC), University of Genoa, Genoa, Italy

Lorenz G Theiler University Department of Anaesthesiology and Pain Therapy, University Hospital of Bern, Switzerland

Marco Tixi Resident Physician in Anesthesia and Intensive Care, Department of Surgical Sciences and Integrated Diagnostics (DISC), University of Genoa, Genoa, Italy

Paul Twose Critical Care, Cardiff and Vale University Health Board, Cardiff, UK; School of Healthcare Sciences Cardiff University, Cardiff, UK

Michele Umbrello Unità Operativa Complessa di Anestesia e Rianimazione, Ospedale San Paolo-Polo Universitario, ASST Santi Paolo e Carlo, Milan, Italy

Rosanna Vaschetto Anesthesia and Intensive Care, 'Maggiore Della Carità' Hospital, Novara, Italy; Department of Translational Medicine, Eastern Piedmont University 'A Avogadro', Novara, Italy

Veronica Vercesi Resident Physician in Anesthesia and Intensive Care, Department of Surgical Sciences and Integrated Diagnostics (DISC), University of Genoa, Genoa, Italy

Luigi Vetrugno Associate Professor of Anesthesiology Department of Medical, Oral and Biotechnological Sciences University of Chieti-Pescara, Chieti, Italy

Marcela P Vizcaychipi Magill Department of Anaesthesia, Intensive Care Medicine and Pain Management, Imperial College London Chelsea and Westminster Hospital, London, UK

Guillaume Voiriot Consultant in Intensive Care, Sorbonne Université, Assistance Publique—Hôpitaux de Paris, Service de Médecine Intensive Réanimation, Hôpital Tenon, Paris, France

Athol U Wells Consultant Respiratory Physician, Interstitial Lung Disease Unit, Royal Brompton Hospital, Guy's and St Thomas' Hospital NHS Foundation Trust, London, UK

Mary White Consultant in Cardiothoracic Critical Care Medicine and Cardiothoracic Anaesthesia, Barts Heart Centre, Barts Health NHS Trust, London, UK

Thomas S. Wilkinson Associate Professor in Microbiology and Infectious Disease, Institute of Life Science, Microbiology and Infectious Disease, Swansea University Medical School (SUMS), Swansea, Wales, UK

Matthew P Wise Associate Medical Director for Research and Development, Cardiff and Vale University Health Board, Consultant Critical Care Physician, Adult Critical Care, University Hospital of Wales, Cardiff, UK

David R Woods Speciality Registrar in Respiratory and Critical Care Medicine, Royal Brompton Hospital, London, UK

S John Wort Consultant Respiratory Physician, National Pulmonary Hypertension Service, Royal Brompton and Harefield Hospitals, Guy's and St Thomas' NHS Foundation Trust, London, UK; Reader, Imperial College, London, UK

Hemang Yadav Assistant Professor of Medicine, Consultant Physician, Department of Pulmonary and Critical Care Medicine, Mayo Clinic, Rochester, Minnesota, USA

PART 1
Basic Concepts—Lung and Critical Care

1

History of Mechanical Ventilation

Mark Griffiths, Mary White, and Nirmala Mary Chakkalakal

KEY MESSAGES

- The history of mechanical ventilation and respiratory critical care are intimately connected.
- Mechanical ventilation was originally developed for resuscitation and peri-operative care before becoming the founding technology of critical care in the 1950s.
- The technological development of mechanical ventilation has been paralleled by increased understanding of pulmonary biology and pathophysiology.

Introduction

The evolution of artificial mechanical ventilation has played an important role in the development of respiratory and critical care medicine. Mechanical ventilation is a mainstay of resuscitation, intensive care medicine, and anaesthesia. There has been movement from crude mechanically delivered support to evolved, patient-triggered, micro-processor-controlled systems. This path has been instrumental in achieving effective life support with reduced risk and increased comfort. There has been increased knowledge of disease and physiology, as well as new challenges that have been educational, ethical, technical, and economic.[1]

Historical Perspective

One may begin with the Theories of Respiration and Air as described in ancient Egyptian, Greek, and Chinese scripts. Then, there are descriptions of early principles of resuscitation in the Book of Kings in the Old Testament, including one instance where the Prophet Elisha breathed from his mouth into that of a dying child.[2,3]

The first known mention of endotracheal intubation was made by Hippocrates in his book *De aere, aquis et locis*. The treatise on Air, Water, and Places states that 'one should introduce a cannula into the trachea along the jawbone so that air can be drawn into the lung'. Further innovation can be attributed to Vesalius, who in *De Humani Corporis Fabrica Libri Septem* (1543) described performing a tracheostomy on a dog in order to carry out artificial respiration so that 'life may be restored to the animal'.[3]

> *'You will then blow into this so that the lung may rise again and the animal take in air…And also as I do this, and take care that the lung is inflated in intervals, the motion of the heart and arteries does not stop….'*

Having established a means of accessing the airway, the technique of assisted ventilation using 'Fire Bellows' to pump air into a connected tube in the patient's mouth is credited to the German physician and toxicologist Paracelsus in the early 1500s.[3] Robert Hooke, the brilliant British scientist and curator of the Royal Society of London, conducted experiments on dogs that had thoracotomies discovering that both chest movement and maintenance of phasic airflow in the lungs are important in preventing asphyxia. In 1744, John Fothergill from England reported on the first successful instance of mouth-to-mouth resuscitation. The Dutch 'Society for the Rescue of Drowned Persons' initially put these ideas into practice; however, the attempts were complicated by fatal lung injury due to over-vigorous use of the bellows. The popularization of the concept that externally supporting the lungs could allow the sustaining or prolongation of life led to the invention of mechanical devices to complete that task. In the 1800s, the prevailing view was that positive pressure ventilation should not be used because of associated lung damage, in a large part based on pioneering experiments of the Parisian surgeon, Jean-Jacques-Joseph Leroy d'Etoilles, who presented his findings to the French Academy of Sciences in 1829. The 19th and early 20th century therefore became the era of negative pressure ventilation.[1]

In 1838, the Scottish physician, John Dalziel, described a full-body 'tank-ventilator', which was an airtight box in which negative pressure was achieved by pumping air out. Alfred Jones of Kentucky patented his invention in 1864 in which the patient's body was enclosed in the tank from neck downwards. Variations were developed, including manually operated versions and a negative pressure operating chamber by Sauerbach in 1904.[4,5] Negative pressure ventilation was key in the management of poliomyelitis pandemics. The 'Iron Lung' (**Figure 1.1**), designed by Drinker and Shaw, consisted

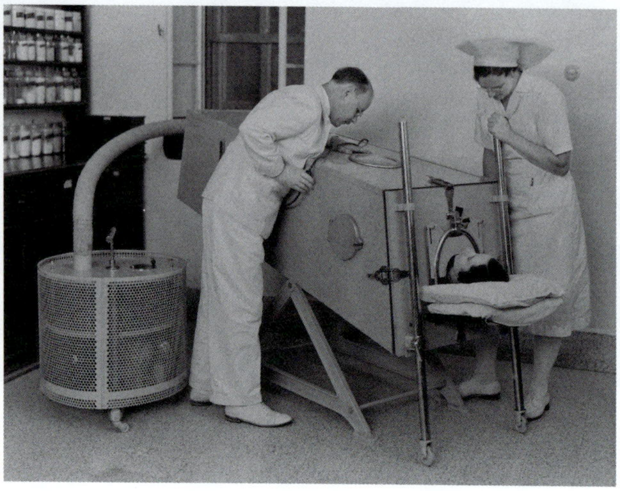

Figure 1.1 Iron lung negative pressure 'tank' ventilator.
© Everett Collection/Shutterstock.

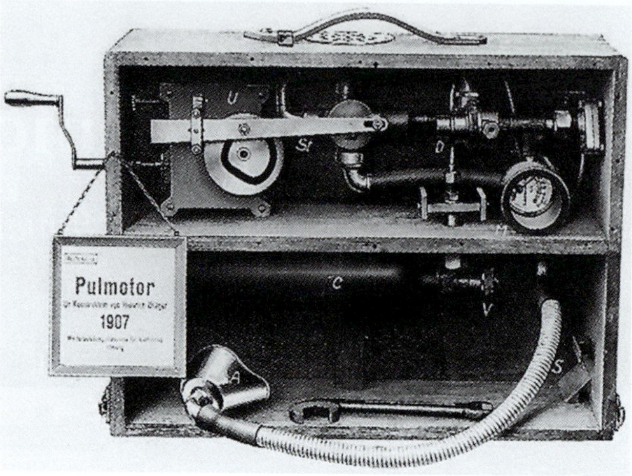

Figure 1.2 The original Pulmotor (1907). Protype of the first Pulmotor that Heinrich Dräger patented.
© Drägerwerk AG & Co. KGaA.

of a large metal cylinder, encasing the whole patient except for the head and neck. Negative pressure was created in the cylinder by an electric pump. The second successful design, the Cuirass, was a box or shell encasing just the thorax. Chronic paralytic disorders could be managed with home ventilation for periods of over 20 years using these devices.[4] The issues that came to light over time were that whilst useful in patients with respiratory muscle weakness, this form of ventilation was not sufficient to support patients with complex lung disease and was further limited by the need for the patient to be conscious and have upper airway integrity. The equipment was often large, cumbersome, and difficult to sterilize. Access to the patient and nursing care were also a challenge. There were also complications such as peripheral venous pooling known as 'tank shock'.[4]

The Scandinavian polio epidemic of 1952 was a turning point in this journey. The disease hit Copenhagen between July and December with 2722 patients being treated at the Blegdam Community Disease Hospital with 315 of these requiring ventilator support. As there was only one iron lung available in the city, patients were managed with over 1400 medical and dental students providing manual ventilation via tracheostomy tubes, which was established as a strategy by the pioneering anaesthetist Dr Bjorn Ibsen. These measures successfully reduced mortality from 80% to just over 20% at the end of the epidemic. This, in turn, drove research and design of positive pressure ventilation devices.[3]

Non-invasive positive pressure ventilation, provided through a mask, was used primarily in the field of resuscitation by the frontline emergency services of the time. Drager introduced the Pulmotor (Figures 1.2 and 1.3) in 1911,[6] which cycled both positive and negative pressures via oxygen under pressure in a gas cylinder.

The decades that followed witnessed the evolution from first- to fourth-generation ventilators. The early invasive ventilators (1900–1970s) were simple, allowed only one mode of ventilation and had either no monitoring or limited monitoring capability. The machines invented in the 1950s and 1960s were known as 'mechanical students'. They included the Engstrom and Radcliffe in the UK and the Bird Mark 7 in the USA.[6] By the late 1970s and early 1980s, second-generation ventilators integrated monitoring and allowed patient-triggered inspiration. The Bennet-MAI ventilator was revolutionary in incorporating alarms, sigh breaths, and positive end expiratory pressure, as well as Synchronised Intermittent Mandatory Ventilation.[6] Clinicians were faced with the new challenges of provision of partial support. Balancing mechanical and spontaneous ventilator workload and the concepts of respiratory muscle reconditioning were introduced. The most evolved machine of the time was the Servo 900C, which introduced pressure support and aided spontaneously breathing.[5,6]

The next-generation ventilators had microprocessors, were responsive to patients, and had extensive monitoring capabilities. Embedded waveforms of pressure, flow, and volume were present, which the clinician used to tailor individual ventilator strategy. They were less bulky than anaesthetic machines, durable, and had reusable circuits. The last 20 years has taken us into an era of sophisticated, versatile, electronic ventilators, which allow a wide variety of ventilator modes, including airway pressure release ventilation and neutrally adjusted ventilator assist.[3] Iatrogenic issues related to prolonged intubation and ventilation have risen in prominence in response to increasingly higher expectations. Hence, modern ventilators are expected to guarantee safety, minimize the risk of lung injury, enhance patient–ventilator synchrony, and expedite weaning.

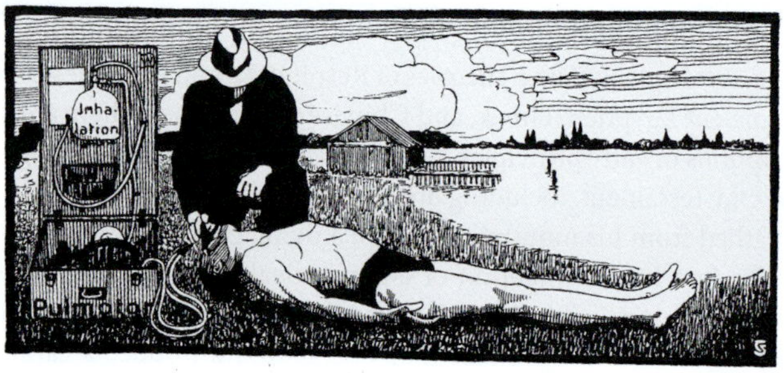

Figure 1.3 Use of the Pulmotor at a bathing accident—contemporary drawing from 1913.
© Drägerwerk AG & Co. KGaA.

Changing Patterns of Disease

Understanding the changing patterns of disease plays a significant role in understanding the history of mechanical ventilation. The earliest endeavours were associated with resuscitation whereas thereafter polio-related acute and chronic respiratory muscle failure presented a new challenge. The two world wars resulted in clinicians being exposed to larger numbers of casualties with traumatic lung injuries and oxygenation failure. Positive pressure ventilation was developed to meet this challenge and associated complications including inefficient clearance of airway debris and atelectasis. It was felt that large tidal volumes of 10–20 mL/kg and normal arterial blood gases were optimal, alongside breathing cycles that mimicked spontaneous breaths.

The following decades brought increased understanding of respiratory physiology as well as the iatrogenic issues related to prolonged intubation and mechanical ventilation. Acute respiratory distress syndrome (ARDS) was first described in 1967. There was no definition initially; however, the condition was thought to involve a widespread immune response within the lungs resulting in diffuse alveolar damage, inflammation, and surfactant dysfunction. Forms of lung injury, including barotrauma attributed to ventilation, as well as infection, were found to be precursors of ARDS. Paediatricians were the first to note this pathology, especially in neonates with surfactant deficiency. Their lung-protective strategies, such as limiting pressure damage via permissive hypercapnia and alveolar recruitment, were useful in managing adult ARDS. The 1990s saw intensive care units' trial, high-frequency oscillation, as well as inhaled nitric oxide to improve gas exchange, with varying results.[1]

More recently, the rapid and global dissemination of communicable diseases that cause acute respiratory failure has raised new challenges. The spread of severe acute respiratory syndrome and the H1N1 influenza and COVID-19 pandemics are pertinent examples. Management of ARDS associated with pandemic H1N1 2009 contributed to renewed interest in Extra-Corporeal Life Support and Extra-Corporeal Membrane Oxygenation (ECMO) in particular. Early extra-corporeal circulatory experiments were conducted by Dr John H Gibbon, Jr, in the 1930s, and these techniques eventually led to the development of the heart and lung machine. In the mid-1970s, Bartlett and colleagues successfully applied bedside cardiopulmonary bypass to treat a newborn with meconium aspiration, thereby introducing ECMO to critical care. Several clinical trials were published in the 1980s, demonstrating clear survival benefit in infants suffering from severe respiratory failure, but despite widespread uptake and national commissioning in the UK, the evidence supporting its use in adults remains equivocal. The extracorporeal life support organization (ELSO), an international organization comprised of programmes and institutions 'dedicated to the development and evaluation of novel therapies for support of failing organ systems', was established in 1989.[7]

Management of respiratory failure has also been influenced by increasing knowledge of the work of breathing as well as the effect of the ventilatory mode on respiratory effort. This led to developing modes of assisted ventilation and partial support in order to allow reconditioning of the respiratory muscles.

Development of Specialist Centres

Modern intensive care medicine has evolved to address many issues of multi-organ dysfunction over the last 50 years. These organ/system failures are increasingly managed in specialized care facilities. Having specialized knowledge and leadership dependent on the organ in focus has resulted in successful management. Examples of these include the development of long-term ventilation and weaning units, as well as ECMO centres.[1]

The future holds endless possibilities such as smart ventilators that offer goal-direct, self-adapting systems, allowing remote access to information and flexibility. The ongoing role of clinicians will be to ensure that infrastructure is defined, quality indicators are set up, and educational standards met to keep pace with these technological advances.[6]

REFERENCES

1. Kalezic N, Markovic D, Unic D, et al. History of mechanical ventilation. In: Randelovic D, Ed. *Fourth Annual Spring Scientific Symposium in Anaesthesiology and Intensive Care*. Nis: Galaksija; April 2012:23.
2. MacKenzie I. The history of mechanical ventilation. *Core Topics in Mechanical Ventilation*. 2008;**1**:388–403.
3. Kotur PF. Mechanical ventilation: Past, present and future. *Indian J. Anaesth*. 2004;**48**(6):430–432.
4. Marini JJ. Mechanical ventilation: Past lessons and near future. *Critical Care*. 2013;**17**:S1.
5. Kacmarek RM. The mechanical ventilator: Past, present and future. *Respiratory Care*. 2011;**56**(8):1170–1180.
6. Bahns E. It began with the Pulmotor: One hundred years of artificial ventilation. *Drager Technology*. 2007;1–113.
7. Morch ET. History of mechanical ventilation. In: *Clinical Applications of Ventilatory Support*. New York: Churchill-Livingstone Inc; 1990:1.

2

The Respiratory System

Richard Leach

KEY MESSAGES

- The respiratory system consists of the airways, lungs, pleura and thoracic cage and the blood, and lymphatic and neural supply to these tissues.
- The respiratory system is optimized to ensure gas exchange, allowing oxygenation of the blood and removal of carbon dioxide.
- The interactions between the lungs and the other major intrathoracic organ, the heart, are crucial to the understanding of pulmonary physiology.
- Although gas exchange is the major physiological role of the lungs, they also serve many other important roles, including endocrine, toxicological, and filtration and immunomodulatory functions, and are critical to the wider health of the entire body.

Introduction

The primary function of the respiratory system is gas exchange which ensures adequate oxygen uptake to maintain tissue metabolism and clearance of carbon dioxide, the by-product of respiration. Lung structure is the perfect biological example of the paradigm that 'function follows form and form follows function'. Understanding respiratory anatomy and physiology enables the clinician to effectively manage many respiratory disorders, optimize ventilatory performance, maintain airway patency, apply mechanical ventilatory support (both non-invasive and invasive), and undertake respiratory endoluminal procedures. Other respiratory system functions include chemical and drug clearance from the systemic circulation, microthrombi breakdown, hormone activation (e.g. conversion of angiotensin I to angiotensin II), speech generation, and immune protection (see Chapter 4).

This chapter reviews lung anatomy, including alveolar microanatomy, pulmonary mechanics, control of breathing/ventilation, gas exchange, pulmonary circulation, ventilation–perfusion mismatch, tissue oxygen transport, and the impact of low atmospheric pressure on gas exchange. Finally, heart–lung interactions and the consequences of respiratory disease on these relationships are briefly examined.

Gross Anatomy of the Lungs and Respiratory Tract

The respiratory system comprises the right and left lungs with their associated blood, nerve, and lymphatic supplies; upper (i.e. nose, nasal cavities, sinuses, pharynx, and upper larynx above the vocal cords) and lower (i.e. lower larynx, cricoid cartilage, trachea, bronchi, bronchioles, and alveoli) respiratory tracts; and the thoracic cage (i.e. sternum, ribs, vertebral column, intercostal muscles, and diaphragm) with their independent blood, nerve, and lymphatic supplies. The right and left pleural cavities, which are not interconnected, separate the thoracic cage and lungs.

Lung architecture is complex but optimizes its main function, gas exchange.[1,2] Lung tissue contains >40 cell types and a sophisticated connective tissue network. However, at end inspiration >80% of the lung volume is air, ~10% blood, and <10% tissue (a few hundred grams). The right lung is divided by the oblique and transverse fissures into three lobes: the upper, middle, and lower. The left lung has two principal lobes, the upper and lower separated by an oblique fissure, and a small 'residual middle' lingula lobe due to teleological displacement by the heart. Each lobe is divided into wedge-shaped bronchopulmonary segments with their apices at the hilum and bases at the lung surface. Vessels, nerves, and lymphatics enter each lung through the 'hilum' on the medial aspect of each lung. Each bronchopulmonary segment is supplied by its own segmental bronchus, artery, vein, and lymphatic supply, and is readily removed surgically from remaining lung with minimal bleeding or air leakage. Lung nerve supply originates as the pulmonary nerve plexus behind each hilum and includes vagal and the 2nd–4th sympathetic trunk ganglia nerve fibres. Vagal nerve supply includes sensory afferents from the lungs, parasympathetic secretory/motor, vasoconstrictor efferents, and non-adrenergic, non-cholinergic (NANC) fibres. Lung sympathetic nerve fibres are limited but widespread β_2-agonist receptors are activated by catecholamines released from adrenal glands. Lymph channels accompany blood vessels and convey lymph to the hilum and bronchopulmonary (±tracheobronchial) nodes. Some lymph directly drains into the posterior mediastinal nodes.

The tracheobronchial tree describes the branching airways of the lower respiratory tract (LRT). Intervals between divisions are referred to a branching 'generations' and in adults there are ~23. Airway numbers double with successive generations such that the LRT cross-sectional area is greater than that of the upper airways. About 50%–70% of airways resistance resides in the trachea, oropharynx, and nasal passages rather than in 'small' airways with their large 'total' cross-sectional area. Consequently, a tracheostomy that bypasses the upper respiratory tract substantially reduces resistance and work of breathing and aids weaning from mechanical ventilation (Chapter 64).

The trachea, bronchi, and bronchioles (generations (gen.) 0–16) are air passages that deliver air to the respiratory bronchioles, alveolar ducts, and alveoli (gen. 17–23) where gas exchange takes place. The trachea (diameter (dia.) 1.8 cm) divides into the two main bronchi (dia. 1–1.4 cm) at the level of the sternal angle (T4/5 vertebrae on CXR; lower when upright and after inspiration), which have U-shaped cartilages, and enter the lungs at each hilum. They divide into ~20 lobar bronchi (gen. 3; dia. ~6–9 mm; the limit of bronchoscope passage) suppling the main lobes and then into 'bronchopulmonary' segmental lobe bronchi (gen. 4–6; dia. 1–6 mm) and small bronchi (gen. 6–11; dia. <1 mm). Lobar, segmental, and small bronchi are supported by irregular plates of cartilage surrounded by helical smooth muscle bands. For bronchioles (gen. 12) and beyond, cartilage is absent, airways are embedded in 'elastic' lung tissue, and elastic recoil holds them open (i.e. like tent ropes). The terminal bronchiole (gen. 16) leads to respiratory bronchioles (gen. 16–19), alveolar ducts, and alveolar sacs (gen. 20–23). The alveoli appearance mimics three-dimensional 'bubble wrap' (i.e. 'interconnected' bubbles, a single air entry and exit tract; see the Alveolar Microstructure and Micromechanics section). This tracheobronchial system creates 'dead space' (i.e. ~150 mL of air that fills airways after exhalation and is breathed back into alveoli before 'fresh' air enters). Likewise, at end inspiration, airways contain air that is exhaled without ever making contact with gas exchanging surfaces.

The trachea to the respiratory bronchioles are lined with ciliated columnar or cuboidal epithelial cells. Goblet and submucosal glands secrete mucous. Synchronous beating of cilia moves mucous and other inhaled debris towards the mouth ('mucociliary escalator'). The trachea, bronchi, and terminal bronchioles receive their blood supply from their bronchial arteries arising from the descending aorta. In contrast, respiratory bronchioles, alveolar ducts, and alveoli receive their supplies from the pulmonary circulation (see below). The lung is covered by a thin connective tissue lining called the visceral pleura, which is continuous with the parietal pleura that lines the chest wall, diaphragm, and mediastinal contents. In health, the space between the two linings is small containing ~10–20 mL (protein concentration <1.5 g/dL) of lubricating pleural fluid. The chest wall parietal pleura is segmentally innervated by the intercostal nerves and the diaphragm by the phrenic nerve such that 'pleural' diaphragmatic pain is felt over the shoulder tip. The visceral pleura lacks sensory innervation[1,2] (see Chapter 52).

Pulmonary Mechanics

Lung Volumes

The lungs expand and contract during breathing (respiratory rate (RR) ~12/min), and the volumes of air moved in and out of the lungs (i.e. tidal volume (TV), ~500 mL; maximum inspiration/expiration) can be measured by spirometry (Figure 2.1). Forced vital capacity (FVC; ~5–6 L) and forced expiratory volume in one second (FEV_1; ~80% FVC) define obstructive (FEV_1/FVC ratio <75%) and restrictive (reduced FEV_1 and FVC, but FEV_1/FVC ratio is >75%) disease patterns. During expiration not all air can be expelled; this is the residual volume (RV; ~1.1 L). Functional residual capacity (FRC) is the 'resting mid-position' at which normal tidal inspiration starts and expiration finishes. Measurement of RV, FRC (~2.5–3 L), and total lung capacity (TLC; ~6 L) requires special techniques (i.e. body plethysmography and helium dilution) not always accessible in critical care settings. Ready availability of cheap, portable bedside spirometers aids rapid diagnosis. Minute ventilation (MV = TV × RR; ~6 L/min) is a useful measure in critical illness and reported by most modern-day ventilators. Alveolar ventilation (AV), which requires 'dead space' measurement (AV = TV – 'dead space' × RR) is more difficult to assess.

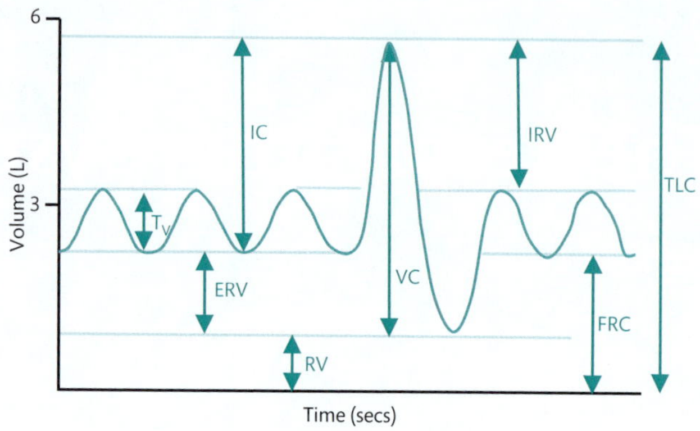

Figure 2.1 Spirometer trace and measurements.

Upward movement = inspiration of air, downwards movements = expiration of air. Background tidal ventilation with maximal inspiration and expiration.

T_V = Tidal volume ~0.5L; IC = Inspiratory capacity ~3.5L; IRV= inspiratory reserve volume ~3L; ERV = expiratory reserve volume ~1.5L, VC= vital capacity ~6L, RV = residual volume 1L; FRC = functional residual capacity ~2.5L; TLC = total lung capacity ~6L.

At end expiration, the airways contain ~150 mL of alveolar air, which is breathed back into the alveoli during inspiration, and is termed 'dead space ventilation'. As TV is 600 mL, only about 450 mL of fresh air enters the alveoli with each breath and is mixed with and diluted by the 2.5–3 L air that remains in the alveoli after expiration (i.e. FRC). Consequently, the composition of alveolar air changes very little during breathing and has a PaO_2 ~ 13.5 kPa (100 mmHg) and a $PaCO_2$ ~ 5.3 kPa (40 mmHg).

Mechanics of Breathing

The mechanisms controlling air movement in and out of gas exchanging alveoli is often referred to as 'respiratory mechanics'.[3–7] It is dependent on chest wall structure (e.g. respiratory muscles), RR, lung and chest wall compliance, impedance due to resistance in airways (RAW), and elastic resistance due to alveolar surface tension and stretching of lung/chest wall tissues. These factors create a negative intrathoracic pressure (ITP), which draws air into the lungs. Conversely, a reduction in lung volume increases ITP, which forces air out.

Chest wall compliance/structure: At rest, inspiration is mostly due to contraction and flattening of the diaphragm, pushing the abdominal wall outwards ('abdominal breathing'). Simultaneously, the intercostal muscles pull the ribs upwards and outwards (like a bucket handle), increasing the antero-posterior and transverse diameters, and enlarging the thoracic cavity. This enlargement reduces ITP and the elastic lungs expand to fill the increased space, drawing air into the lungs through the airways. As alveoli are open to environmental air, they are at atmospheric pressure (101 kPa at sea level), but the pressure causing air movement in and out of alveoli rarely exceeds 2–3 kPa. During exhalation, the diaphragm and intercostal muscles relax and the chest and abdomen return to their 'resting mid-position' at which point the lungs contain their FRC (2.5–3.0 L). Resting exhalation takes twice as long as inspiration as passive diaphragmatic relaxation is slower than active contraction.

During forced inspiration (e.g. exercise), 'accessory muscles' extending from the skull base and cervical vertebrae to the upper ribs and clavicles contract to enhance intercostal muscle action and increase the intrathoracic volume ('clavicular breathing'). Likewise, during forced exhalation, the abdominal muscles contact, elevating the diaphragm and lowering the ribs to reduce the intrathoracic volume below the 'resting mid-position FRC'. However, at least 1 L of air (RV) remains in the lungs after maximal expiration.

Respiratory rate adjusts to meet the needs of the body. As oxygen demand increases and carbon dioxide accumulates RR increases to facilitate gas transfer (see below).

Lung compliance or lung 'stretchiness' is the change in lung volume per unit change in distending pressure ($CL = \Delta V/\Delta P$), where P is the pressure difference across the lung (i.e. alveolar-intrapleural pressure).[3,4] It is normally about 200 mL/cmH_2O (1–1.5 L/kPa). It falls in fibrotic lung disease, pulmonary oedema, and pneumonia (i.e. stiff lungs have increased elastic recoil, with an increased tendency to shrink to their resting position if stretched) and increases with emphysema. Pleural pressure is determined by measuring oesophageal pressure. When air flow stops, alveolar pressure must become equal to mouth pressure (i.e. zero) and transmural pressure (P) is then equal to intrapleural pressure.

Static compliance is determined from pressure–volume curves (i.e. step breath increases with measurement whilst the breath is held). Inspiratory and expiratory plots differ due to hysteresis, a property of elastic bodies (Figure 2.2). Static lung compliance, the slope of the steepest part of the pressure–volume plot, is usually just above FRC. Accurate compliance measurements require total relaxation of inspiratory and expiratory muscles and are best performed in intensive care unit when the patient is ventilated and sedated (note: distensible ventilator tubing contributes to compliance, especially in those with stiff lungs). Techniques employed include rapid airways occlusion (Figure 2.3), super syringe method, or the pulse method.

Dynamic compliance is measured by plotting intrapleural pressure (i.e. oesophageal balloon) and volume (i.e. pneumotachograph or spirometer) during a normal breathing cycle. At end inspiration and expiration, flow and alveolar pressure will be zero. The slope joining these two points is dynamic compliance. It is best plotted in expiration due to hysteresis (this eliminates the pressure required to

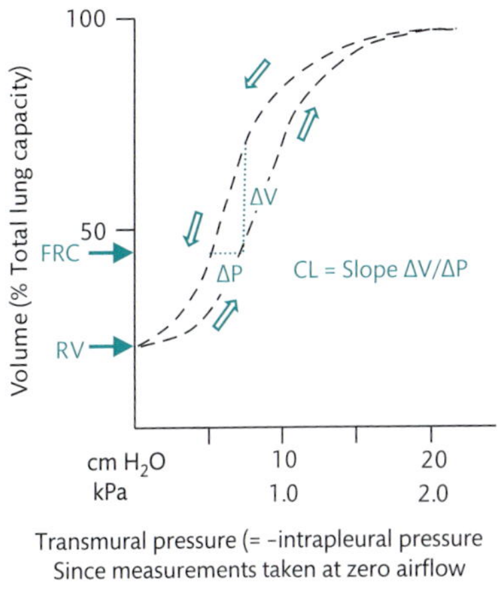

Figure 2.2 Static pressure-volume loop.
The subject breathes in steps and pressure is measured when there is no airflow (alveolar pressure then equals atmospheric pressure) and the transmural pressure is equal to intrapleural pressure (measured as oesophageal pressure using an oesophageal balloon). The pressure-volume curve of the lung during a respiratory cycle can then be plotted and shows hysteresis with a greater lung volume achieved for any given pressure during expiration than inspiration.
CL = Lung compliance, RV = residual volume, FRC = functional residual capacity.

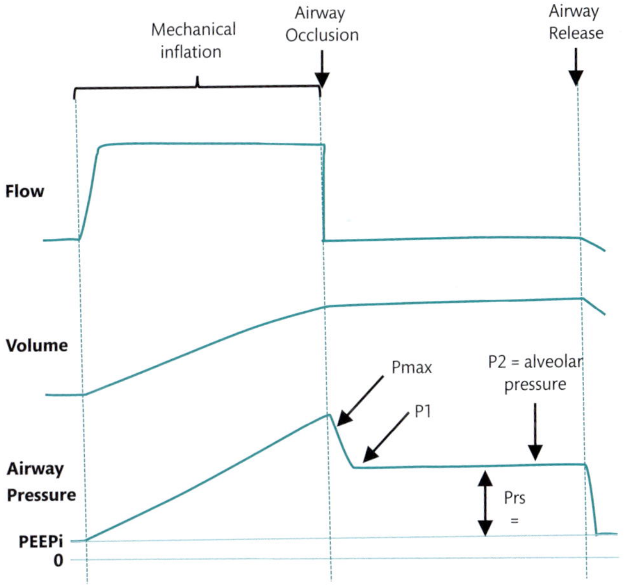

Figure 2.3 Use of the rapid airway occlusion technique to determine compliance in a mechanically ventilated patient.
Flow, volume and airways resistance (Pao) are illustrated during the procedure. Following a constant inspiratory flow, the airway is occluded at end-inspiration (by pressing the expiratory hold button on the ventilator). Pao falls rapidly from a peak (Pmax) to P1, and a more slowly to a plateau P2. The elastic recoil of the respiratory system is given by (P2-PEEP). Prs is the respiratory system pressure. A series of occlusions are performed at different inflation volumes and an inspiratory pressure-volume curve is constructed. Compliance is the gradient of the linear curve which tends to be just above FRC.
Adapted from: *Respiratory Critical Care*, C Davidson and D Treacher (eds), © 2002 Arnold. Reproduced by permission of Taylor & Francis Group through PLSclear.

overcome alveolar surface tension during inspiration) and is unreliable during airflow limitation.

Total respiratory system compliance comprises lung, chest wall, and abdominal components as respiratory muscle weakness and chest wall diseases (e.g. kyphoscoliosis) that affect chest wall elasticity or reductions in abdominal compliance (e.g. peritonitis) have profound effects on overall compliance.

Intrinsic positive end expiratory pressure (PEEPi, auto-PEEP) is the presence of positive alveolar pressure at end expiration.[5,6] It occurs when expiration is incomplete, before the next inspiration during spontaneous or positive pressure ventilation. Causes include (a) insufficient expiratory time to achieve the relaxed volume (resting mid-position/FRC) due to airflow obstruction and rapid ventilation or (b) dynamic airways collapse with flow limitation (e.g. emphysema). Continued expiratory muscle contraction at end expiration contributes to PEEPi but is not normally attributed as a cause. As greater inspiratory effort is required, PEEPi increases work of spontaneous breathing and reduces the ability to trigger a ventilator breath during assisted modes of ventilation (see Chapter 11). In asthma or chronic obstructive pulmonary disease (COPD), PEEPi can be up to 20 cmH_2O (see Chapters 41 and 42). Application of extrinsic PEEP may help overcome PEEPi and is used to improve ventilator synchrony and/or reduce work of breathing. Early recognition of PEEPi, and an understanding of its aetiology, is important in critical care. For example, a high PEEPi in a patient with airflow limitation (±hyperinflation) suggests the need for a prolonged expiratory time and application of extrinsic PEEP; in contrast, extrinsic PEEP in a patient with PEEPi due to expiratory muscle activation simply increases work of breathing further.

Static PEEPi is measured by occluding the airway at end expiration. The resulting plateau pressure is the average PEEPi in non-homogenous lung and can be measured on most commercial ventilators (expiratory effort causes a falsely high value).

Dynamic PEEPi is obtained by recording the pressure at which inspiratory flow begins (i.e. after the airway pressure has exceeded PEEPi). It reflects the lowest regional PEEP and may be less than static PEEPi in patients with airflow limitation or pulmonary inhomogeneity.

Resistance of the airways (RAW): Resistance to ventilation is due to chest wall factors, pulmonary causes (e.g. fibrosis and pulmonary oedema), and RAW (e.g. dynamic airways compression during expiration, increased flow rates, and turbulent (non-laminar) flow).[3–7] Pulmonary resistance is the important factor in most situations with 80% attributable to RAW and 20% to lung tissue resistance. During laminar flow (i.e. gas particles move parallel to the airway walls), the relationship between flow (F), pressure difference (ΔP; i.e. mouth—alveolar pressure), and RAW is $F = \Delta P/\text{RAW}$ or $\text{RAW} = \Delta P/F$, and applying Poiseuille's law: as resistance is related to air viscosity ($\acute{\eta}$), airway length (l), and airway radius (r): $F = \Delta P/\text{RAW} = \Delta P(\pi r^4/8l\acute{\eta})$ and therefore $\text{RAW} = 8l\acute{\eta}/\pi r^4$.

The inverse fourth-power relationship between airway radius and resistance means that small changes in radius substantially alter resistance. Halving the airway radius increases its resistance 16-fold. However, as the combined cross-sectional area of the small bronchioles is very large, the greatest resistance occurs in the larger airways. The nose and pharynx contribute substantially to resistance, which can be reduced by mouth breathing (e.g. during exercise). Airway resistance falls with increasing lung volume as at end inspiration there is greater traction on small airways as elastic recoil increases. Conversely, during forced expiration at low volumes, positive pleural pressure is transmitted to small airways, which are compressed or may even collapse (dynamic compression), increasing RAW. Finally, at higher velocities, airflow may become turbulent especially in larger airways or at branching points requiring greater pressures to drive the same flow (i.e. flow $\propto \sqrt{\Delta P}$ (not ΔP)). Increased RAW usually results from airflow limitation but is also increased in acute respiratory distress syndrome (ARDS) or pulmonary oedema due to airway wall oedema, lumen secretions, or fewer airways due to functional lung loss. In practice, although disease often affects peripheral airways, they are often referred to as the 'silent zone', as the effect has to be considerable to increase RAW (i.e. because small airways have a large cross-sectional area). In contrast, halving the radius of an endotracheal tube (ETT) increases resistance 16-fold, or doubling the length doubles the resistance, with significant impact on work of breathing.

In the ventilated patient, resistance is determined using the rapid occlusion technique as for the assessment of static compliance (Figure 2.3). Before completion of mechanical inflation at a constant flow (F), the airway is occluded until a plateau airway pressure is achieved (press expiratory hold button). The peak airways pressure (P_{max}) falls rapidly to P1 and then slowly to a plateau P2. The maximum respiratory resistance (Rtot_{max}) = (P_{max} − P2)/F and includes chest wall and elastic resistance, whereas the minimum respiratory resistance (Rtot_{min}) = (P_{max} − P1)/F mainly represents RAW (but respiratory tubing and ETT contribute to resistance).

Factors affecting RAW include parasympathetic bronchoconstriction and β-receptor-activated relaxation by epinephrine or salbutamol. Sympathetic nerves are sparse and have little effect on airways. Slowly adapting stretch receptors inhibit parasympathetic bronchoconstriction, and CO_2 has a direct bronchodilator effect. Pollutants, mucosal hypertrophy, mast cell degranulation, and eosinophils (e.g. asthma and COPD) increase RAW due to bronchoconstriction, mucous secretion, and airways inflammation. Likewise, increased transmural (airway-intrapleural) pressure gradients during forced expiration can cause airway collapse (dynamic compression) and increase RAW.

Alveolar Microstructure and Micromechanics

Gas exchange takes place in alveoli, which account for 90% of lung volume. Distal airways and clusters of alveoli form ~30,000 'blind-ending' parenchymal units called acini. Within an acinus, all airways (e.g. alveolar ducts and terminal bronchioles) have alveoli attached to their walls. The 'wall' of an alveolar duct is simply a lattice of alveolar openings. The inter-alveolar septum provides the structural basis for gas exchange and separates alveolar airspace from blood in capillary lumens. Septal requirements for efficient gas exchange include a large surface area (~140 m^2), thin diffusion barrier (~2 μm), stability (i.e. to prevent collapse and over-distension), and flexibility (i.e. movement during breathing). Lung alveoli are stabilized by pulmonary surfactant and a connective tissue backbone (see later). The inter-alveolar septal barrier separating air and blood has two continuous cell layers: the alveolar air facing 'alveolar epithelium' and the capillary blood facing endothelium. Between them is an interstitial space of varying thickness and composition.

The alveolar epithelium is a mosaic of type 1 alveolar epithelial cells covering ~95% of the alveolar surface, interspersed with cuboidal type 2 cells with characteristic surfactant-storing lamellar bodies, which aid renewal and repair. A thin aqueous hypophase (200 nm) containing surfactant (90% phospholipid and 10% surfactant proteins (SP A-D)) separates alveolar epithelium from air and constitutes the air–liquid interface.[8–12]

The interstitium contains fibroblasts and an extracellular network of elastic fibres, collagen bundles, and alveolar capillaries. The inter-alveolar septum has thin areas (~50% total area) that promote gas exchange where alveolar epithelium and capillary endothelium share a common basal lamina (diffusion barrier <1 μm) and a thick part containing cell nuclei and structural fibres.[9,10] The connective tissue network consists of the following components:

- *Axial fibres* to support airways from the hilum to the alveolar ducts (i.e. hilum to periphery) where they form a lattice of entrance rings into alveoli.
- *Peripheral fibres* extending from visceral pleura into interlobular septa demarcating bronchopulmonary segments (i.e. periphery to hilum).
- *Septal fibres* that are anchored to axial fibres at alveolar entrance rings and peripheral fibres at the distal acini boundary.

This continuous network of connective tissue provides the self-stabilizing and elastic structure of normal lung. At the alveolar entrance rings (i.e. alveolar duct walls), where connective tissue axial fibres meet the 'elastic' septal fibres, collagen density is greatest such that most breath-related deformation occurs in the distal alveolus. As gas exchange occurs through 'capillarized' alveolar septa and not in ductal air spaces, the ratio of alveolar to ductal airspace is important (see below).

Arteries follow conducting airways in bronchopulmonary units such that blood flows from the centre to the periphery, whereas veins run in the connective tissue septa separating these units. The alveolar capillary network is different from the systemic circulation. Individual segments form small loops (segment length equals capillary diameter), creating a dense meshwork with vertical tissue pillars between and allowing 'sheet flow' in alveolar capillaries. A single capillary sheet exchanges oxygen and carbon dioxide with two adjacent alveoli. During breath-related inter-alveolar septum stretching, the septal fibres interwoven with this 'capillary sheet' spread it in a zig-zag pattern over both alveolar surfaces maximizing air–blood contact with minimal connective tissue interference.

During breathing, distal airspaces are subject to volume changes that deform ('strain') ductal/alveolar airspaces and inter-alveolar septa. These are often described in terms of lung volumes (e.g. TV) in relation to baseline state (i.e. FRC) or in relation to lung volumes at a given PEEP in mechanically ventilated. These pressure-change relationships are also described at a microscopic level in alveolar ducts, alveolar airspaces, and inter-alveolar septa, which all have different stabilizing elements and mechanical properties. The alveolar duct does not have a 'wall of its own', and volume changes result in deformations and stretch of the axial fibre system in the entrance rings to the alveolar spaces. The alveolar walls (i.e. inter-alveolar septa) have less septal wall, mainly 'elastic' fibre, connective tissue connecting the axial and peripheral fibres (as described above), but it is most dense towards the alveolar entrance rings. Septal fibres, located between the basal lamina of the capillary endothelium and alveolar epithelium in the 'thick' alveolar wall sections, form the backbone of alveolar septa and transmit distending forces during alveolar expansion.[8,9]

The linear stress–strain relationship of elastic fibres allows a doubling of baseline length such that these fibres contribute to elastic recoil and stabilization of lung parenchyma at lower lung volumes (defined as 40%–80% of TLC). 'Curly' collagen fibres straighten as volumes increase at low lung volumes but then become rigid and have a non-linear stress–strain relationship. During breathing in healthy lungs, these stabilizing elements allow volume changes with minimal effort and without interfering with gas exchange in 'thin' air–blood barrier areas. In addition, the alveolar epithelium is subject to little stress or damage during TV alveolar deformation as the scaffold is stress bearing whilst surfactant reduces surface tension at low lung volumes. Although the basal lamina has some stabilizing properties, cellular components of the inter-alveolar septa contribute little to stiffness or elasticity. However, when lung volumes increase from ~40% to 100% TLC, the basal lamina surface area increases by ~35%, and at larger lung volumes, alveolar epithelial and endothelial cells, which are attached to the basal lamina, may be damaged (i.e. denudation and blebbing) as seen microscopically during high-volume ventilation in ventilator-induced lung injury (VILI). Type 2 alveolar epithelial cells are more resilient to stress-induced damage and promote repair. Mechanisms like alveolar wall 'pleating' and plasma cell membrane tear repair systems enable cells to manage damage, which may occur even under normal conditions (e.g. sighing).[10,11,12]

The pulmonary surfactant layer at the alveolar air–liquid interface also plays an important role in pulmonary micromechanics, especially at low lung/alveolar volumes, as it counteracts the high surface tension that promotes alveolar collapse and deformation shear stress. At end expiration, the alveoli are stabilized, and axial elastic fibres are only slightly stretched because surface tension is reduced to nearly zero by surfactant. In addition, the alveolar entrance axial fibre rings support the alveolar duct and counteract the alveolar air–liquid surface tension. Surfactant reduction due to type II alveolar epithelial cell injury results in alveolar duct enlargements (i.e. ductal to alveolar air space increases with reduced gas exchange), and inter-alveolar septa collapse (pleating) reduces alveolar surface area. The relationship between surface forces and the fibre system is important during normal breathing (40%–80% TLC) as the inter-alveolar septa and alveolar epithelium are protected from potentially harmful mechanical stresses. At higher lung volumes (>80% TLC), although surface tension increases, the connective tissue matrix become stress bearing (and this stress is transmitted to cells) such that surface tension, and therefore surfactant, plays a lesser role.[10,11]

During an average lifetime, alveolar structures experience 10^9 breaths. The alveoli, inter-alveolar septa, and epithelium are structurally well adapted to mechanical stress as described above. It is estimated that during tidal breathing (40%–80% TLC) alveolar surface area increases by 4%–10% and by as little as 20% during deep sighs or exercise. Only ~35% of TV results in alveolar volume increases during normal breathing with ~65% remaining in ductal/conducting airways. Microscopy has confirmed the small alveolar volume increases (~3%–4%) during tidal ventilation. However, at higher lung volumes, alveolar and alveolar duct volumes increased by 50%. Thus, during normal breathing, alveoli and alveolar walls are predicted to be very stable and stresses balanced as long as surface tension is reduced.[10,11,12] The potential mechanisms by which alveoli and inter-alveolar septa adapt to mechanical stress during normal breathing, physiological stresses (e.g. sighs, exercise), iatrogenic (e.g. mechanical ventilation), and pathological (ARDS) conditions include the following:

- *Recruitment and derecruitment* of complete alveolar units would partially explain the hysteresis in quasi-static pressure–volume loops. However, in healthy lungs, direct visualization and design-based stereology show no intra-tidal recruitment/derecruitment above functional RV.
- *Folding (pleating) and unfolding* (i.e. like an accordion) of alveolar septal walls is reported at low lung volumes both in vivo and ex vivo. During MV if PEEP is reduced (i.e. airway opening pressure), elastance increases and lungs are stiffer correlating with decreased alveolar size due to inter-alveolar septal pleat formation on electron microscopy during deflation. However, in healthy lungs this mechanism is rarely seen with airways pressures of 3–16 cmH_2O.
- *Change in alveolar shape* (e.g. from dodecahedral to spherical and back) increases alveolar size as reported on synchrotron refraction-enhanced computer tomography.
- *Isotopic stretching/destretching* with balloon-like changes in size occurring at high lung volumes (i.e. 30 cmH_2O transpulmonary pressure). Alveolar surface area (ASA) and the basal lamina increase by about 35% between 40% and 100% TLC, and 80% of this increase occurs between 80% and 100%. Between 40% and 80% TLC, ASA remains relatively stable. Increases in ASA of the magnitude demonstrated between 80% and 100% TLC can result in epithelial cell injury and suggest that lung volumes do not have to exceed TLC during ventilation to potentially damage the epithelium.

In summary, the microalveolar tissue components (e.g. connective tissue fibre system, epithelial lining, and capillary mesh) and the surfactant system are essential and interdependent components of alveolar micromechanics, forming a complex but elegant gas exchange system. Understanding this basic physiology is a perquisite to addressing many of the fundamental issues (e.g. VILI, shunt) in respiratory critical care.[12]

Gas Exchange and Control of Breathing

Alveolar Gas Exchange

Gas exchange is examined in detail in Chapter 3 and is reviewed briefly here. As described in previous sections, alveolar air has a semi-permanent volume of ~2.5–3 L (FRC) to which ~450 mL of 'fresh' air is added with each breath. Gas tensions in this air are relatively constant with a P_AO_2 of 13.5 kPa (~100 mmHg) and a P_ACO_2 of 5.3 kPa (40 mmHg). In comparison, the atmospheric air breathed in has a PO_2 of 21 kPa (160 mmHg) and a PCO_2 of 0.04 kPa (0.3 mmHg). Water vapour pressure, uptake of oxygen, and release of carbon dioxide in the alveolus account for the fall in P_AO_2 compared with PO_2, as calculated from the simplified alveolar gas equation: $P_AO_2 = PIO_2 - (1.25 \times PaCO_2)$, where $PIO_2 = FiO_2 \times$ [barometric − water vapour pressure] and FiO_2 is the inspired fraction of oxygen (i.e. 21% or 0.21). Thus, in breathing air: $PIO_2 = 0.21 \times (101 - 6.2) = 19.9$ kPa and $P_AO_2 = 19.9 - (1.25 \times 5.3) \sim 13.5$ kPa (101 mmHg). Oxygen transfer from alveolar gas to capillary blood is almost seamless. The alveolar-arterial oxygen tension difference is calculated as $P(A\text{-}a)O_2 = P_AO_2 - PaO_2 = 13.5 - 13 = 0.5$ kPa, and when breathing air the difference between P_AO_2 and P_aO_2 should be <1 kPa (<7.5mmHg).[1,2,13,14]

Alveolar gas tensions must equilibrate with those in pulmonary capillary blood. This occurs by diffusion across the thin (~2 μm) 'air–blood' membrane forming the 'thin' section of the inter-alveolar septal walls (see above). As pulmonary capillaries run through alveolar walls, they are in contact with air in two alveoli that share the same alveolar wall (i.e. gas exchange occurs all around the capillary). The 300 million alveoli (75–300 μm diameter) in adult lungs have a surface area of ~140 m^2 for gas exchange. Blood returning to pulmonary capillaries from body tissues has a PvO_2 ~6–7 kPa (45–53 mmHg) (~60%–70% saturation (SaO_2)), and there is net oxygen diffusion from alveolar air into capillary blood until it equilibrates with alveolar P_AO_2 at 13.5 kPa (101 mmHg) (SaO_2 100%). Blood needs to be in contact with alveolar air for ~0.25 s to achieve this equilibration. At rest, this contact time is ~0.75 s, and large increases (>300%) in pulmonary flow (i.e. cardiac output) are tolerated before this limits oxygenation at normal atmospheric pressure (see altitude in the Effect of Low Atmospheric Pressure section). Similarly, returning alveolar capillary blood $PvCO_2$ is 6 kPa (45 mmHg), and there is net diffusion of carbon dioxide into alveoli which have a P_ACO_2 of 5.3 kPa (40 mmHg).[13,14]

Control of Breathing

In health, $PaCO_2$ is remarkably constant, and ventilation is closely matched to metabolic CO_2 load. Chemical control of ventilation and gas exchange utilizes peripheral chemoreceptors, the aortic and carotid bodies (which monitor mainly PaO_2), and central chemoreceptors, a diffuse collection of neurons on the ventrolateral anterior surface of the medulla which monitor brain extracellular hydrogen ion concentration ($[H^+]$). The $[H^+]$ tracks arterial $PaCO_2$ changes almost instantaneously as CO_2 diffuses readily across the blood–brain barrier. At sea level, breathing rate and depth are determined primarily by $PaCO_2$ rather than PaO_2, and central chemoreceptors account for ~80% of the ventilation response to $PaCO_2$. Thus, a rise or fall in $PaCO_2$, and to a lesser extent PaO_2, causes reflex changes in rate (±depth) of breathing until blood gases return to baseline levels. However, many central (e.g. cough and swallowing) and peripheral sensors (e.g. chest wall 'mechanical' afferent sensory nerves) also modulate ventilation. Additional oxygen and carbon dioxide sensors in the lung alter bronchiole and capillary diameter, controlling air and blood flow in the lung.[1,2,15,16]

Ventilation (L/min) is linearly related to P_ACO_2. Minute ventilation increases by ~15–25 L/min per kPa rise in P_ACO_2 (2.7 L/min per mmHg). However, there is considerable variability (i.e. less response in athletes and chronic respiratory disease), and a P_ACO_2 >10 kPa (75 mmHg) reduces ventilation due to central chemoreceptor suppression. Metabolic acidosis shifts this linear response to the left (i.e. increasing ventilation) and a metabolic alkalosis to the right (i.e. reducing ventilation). If this homeostasis is compromised, a respiratory acidosis (i.e. reduced ventilation with increased $PaCO_2$) or respiratory alkalosis (i.e. increased ventilation with reduced $PaCO_2$) occurs. These changes are compensated by slow renal adjustments of H^+ and HCO_3 concentrations in the plasma. Ventilation increases during exercise to exhale additional CO_2 produced by increased muscle metabolism. Until P_AO_2 falls to <8 kPa (60 mmHg), ventilation is relatively unchanged, but the response is potentiated by a raised $PaCO_2$.[15,16]

The respiratory centres, located in the pons and medulla oblongata, generate periodic inspiration and expiration (central pattern generator). These respiratory brainstem neurons (e.g. medullary dorsal tract group (DGT) inspiratory neurons and pontine pneumotaxic centre) set the basic rhythm of ventilation and control the responsible respiratory muscles. They are modulated by inputs from peripheral and central chemoreceptors, sensory afferents (e.g. lung receptors via the vagus nerve), and higher function centres. These areas form a complex network reflecting the need to coordinate ventilation with functions such as coughing, speech, and swallowing.[1,15,16]

Many 'peripheral' lung receptors modify ventilation. Stretch receptors in bronchial wall smooth muscle (vagal nerve afferents) inhibit lung inflation (Hering–Breuerer inspiratory reflex) with shorter, shallower inspiration but stimulate inspiratory muscle activity during deflation. Although minimal during normal breathing, this effect is important with larger tidal volumes to protect against over-inflation. Juxtapulmonary (J) receptors (±afferent C-fibres and vagus nerve) in alveoli and bronchial walls are stimulated (e.g. pulmonary oedema and inflammation) to suppress ventilation, heart rate, blood pressure, and smooth muscle contraction. Irritant receptors, located throughout the airways, are stimulated (e.g. dust, smoke, rapid inflation, and inflammation) to cause cough if tracheal and hyperpnoea (±sighs/deep breaths that prevent lung collapse) are in the lower airways. Proprioceptors monitor respiratory muscle and joint position (but not diaphragm) and communicate by afferents nerves in the dorsal roots and spinal cord to optimize ventilation.

Effect of Low Atmospheric Pressure

The density and partial pressure of air decrease with altitude, halving every 5500 m. As composition is unchanged (i.e. 21% oxygen), the concentration of oxygen falls (i.e. $mmolO_2/L$) in proportion to the fall in atmospheric barometric pressure (ABP). Thus, more air must be inhaled at high altitude (i.e. deeper, faster breathing) to obtain the same amount of oxygen. In addition, a disproportionate fall in P_AO_2 occurs at altitude related to humidification of inhaled air. During passage through the nose/pharynx, inhaled air is 100% saturated. Partial pressure of water vapour (PH_2O) in 100% saturated air is only dependent on temperature and is 6.3 kPa (47 mmHg) even at high altitude. At sea level (ABP 101 kPa), PO_2 is ~21 kPa (157 mmHg) (21% of 101 kPa), but once air is saturated in upper airways, the PO_2 of air entering the trachea is $ABP - PH_2O \times 0.21 = 101 - 6.3 \times 0.21 = 19.9$ kPa (149 mmHg).

For comparison, at the summit of Everest, ABP is 34 kPa and PO_2 is 7.1 kPa (53 mmHg) (0.21% of 34 kPa). As PH_2O is unavoidably 6.3 kPa, the PO_2 of air entering the trachea is $APB - PH_2O \times 0.21 = 34 - 6.3 \times 0.21 = 5.8$ kPa (43 mmHg), a greater proportional fall in PO_2 than expected due to altitude alone. At sea level, $PaCO_2$ is maintained close to 5.3 kPa (40 mmHg) (whereas PaO_2 considerably varies before hypoxic ventilation is stimulated). However, if ABP falls below ~70% (~3000 m altitude), oxygen takes priority over carbon dioxide homeostasis. Hyperpnoea at high altitude causes the $PaCO_2$ to fall (and pH rises) and contributes to high-altitude sickness if too rapid. At Everest's summit, and assuming a large fall in $PaCO_2$ (e.g. 2.0 kPa), the P_AO_2 (using the alveolar gas equation) is $P_AO_2 = PIO_2 - (1.25 \times PaCO_2)$, where $PIO_2 = FiO_2 \times [ABP - PH_2O]$: $P_AO_2 = (0.21 \times [34 - 6.3]) - (1.25 \times 2.0) \sim 3.5$ kPa (~30 mmHg), a PaO_2 theoretically incompatible with life! As the atmospheric oxygen tension decreases the time taken to equilibrate with capillary blood increases, and oxygenation can become perfusion limited in settings of increased cardiac output (e.g. with exercise) at altitude.

Several mechanisms contribute to acclimatization to altitude including improved ventilation/perfusion matching. At sea level, due to gravity, the lung apices receive less blood than the bases, which are relatively over-perfused (see below). At altitude, low PaO_2 stimulates hypoxic pulmonary vasoconstriction (HPV), which increases PAP and distributes lung blood flow more evenly. Likewise, a chronically low blood oxygen content promotes oxygen-sensitive kidney cells to release erythropoietin (EPO), which stimulates bone marrow red cell production increasing haemoglobin and oxygen carriage. Consequently, high-altitude dwellers often have a higher haematocrit and better oxygen delivery (see below).[1,2,17]

Pulmonary Circulation

Pulmonary circulation and alveolar capillary unit structure are described above. Pulmonary and systemic circulations are in series, and ~5 L/min blood flows through both. Compared to the systemic circulation, pulmonary vascular resistance (PVR) is low (~15% of systemic resistance), and the right ventricle generates pulmonary artery pressures of 24/9 mmHg (mean ~15 mmHg) to propel cardiac output through the lungs. Capillary pressure falls from ~14 mmHg (arterial end) to ~8 mmHg (venous end), and left atrial pressure (LAP) is ~5 mmHg. Due to this even PVR distribution, pulmonary capillary flow remains pulsatile. Although sympathetic and parasympathetic nerves innervate pulmonary vessels, their influence is weak.[18,19]

Lung Zones, Effects of Gravity, and V/Q Mismatch/Shunt

Pulmonary arterioles constrict in response to hypoxia (hypoxic pulmonary vasoconstriction (HPV)), and this is potentiated by a high PCO_2. This aids gas exchange by diverting blood from under- to well-ventilated lung regions but is unhelpful with global hypoxia as it contributes to pulmonary hypertension and right ventricular failure. Autoregulation in systemic vascular beds (e.g. renal and cerebral) modulates perfusion pressure (by vasoconstriction/dilation) and maintains constant blood flow, but this does not occur in the pulmonary circulation. As venous return increases, PVR falls because vessels are recruited and distended, pulmonary blood flow increases, and pulmonary pressure rise is limited. As flow increases, alveolar gas contact time falls, but as blood requires ~0.25 s for full gas exchange and normal alveolar contact time is ~0.75 s, increases in flow have little impact on oxygenation or CO_2 clearance.[1,17,18,19]

Net filtration of pulmonary capillary fluid occurs despite the relatively low capillary hydrostatic pressure (~10 mmHg) compared to capillary oncotic pressure (~27 mmHg). This is because interstitial oncotic pressure is relatively high (~18 mmHg), and interstitial hydrostatic pressure is negative (~–4 mmHg). Pulmonary oedema develops when filtration is greater than pulmonary lymphatic clearance as can occur when pulmonary capillary pressure increases in mitral stenosis or left ventricular failure (i.e. LAP >25 mmHg).

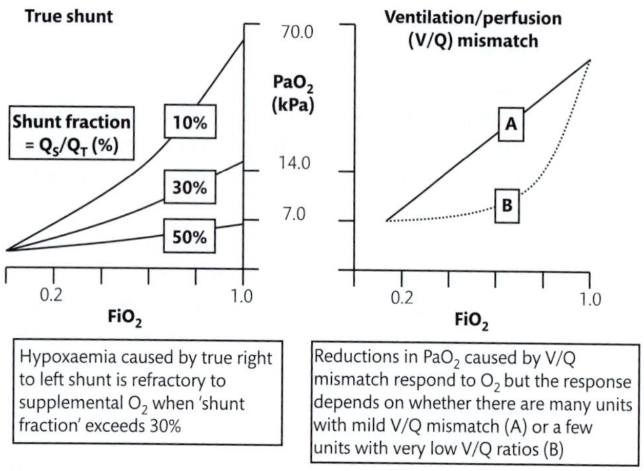

Figure 2.4 Effect of true shunt (Q_S/Q_T) and ventilation/perfusion mismatch on the arterial oxygen tension (PaO_2) and inspired oxygen fraction (FiO_2) relationship.

Republished with permission of Wiley from *Critical Care Medicine at a Glance* 3rd Edition, R Leach, © Wiley 2014; permission conveyed through Copyright Clearance Center, Inc.

Alveolar ventilation (VA) and perfusion vary in different lung regions but are best matched for optimal gas exchange (i.e. good perfusion and ventilation). Hydrostatic pressure in blood vessels varies with height above/below the heart due to the weight of blood. When standing, increased pressure at the lung bases distends vessels, increasing flow. At the apices, vascular pressure generated by the right heart may be so low that diastolic blood flow stops (i.e. falls below alveolar pressure). Consequently, blood flow per unit volume of lung increases from the lung apex to base. Gravity also has effects on intrapleural pressure (i.e. less negative at bases than apices) and therefore distribution of ventilation. At FRC, apical alveoli are more expanded with less capacity to expand during inspiration. Thus, ventilation is also greater at the bases than apices, but less so than for perfusion, such that VA/Q is greatest at the apices. Three lung zones are recognized: relatively over-perfused lung bases, mid-zones where ventilation and blood flow are well matched, and the apices which are relatively poorly perfused. In reality, the effect of this VA/Q mismatch is minor as regions with low VA/Q are still ventilated sufficiently for nearly all blood passing through them to be saturated with oxygen.[18,19]

Of the 5 L/min pulmonary blood flow, <2% is not fully oxygenated in young adults and is termed 'shunt fraction'. Ventilation/perfusion (VA/Q) mismatch occurs when poorly ventilated alveoli (e.g. consolidated and/or collapsed) are perfused, and the associated blood is not fully oxygenated contributing to an increase in the normal right to left shunt often termed 'venous admixture'. Blood passing through poorly ventilated areas will have undergone some gas exchange, but PaO_2 is lower and $PaCO_2$ is higher than normal. Alternatively, an under-perfused but well-ventilated alveolus contributes to dead space, and blood from these regions has a high PaO_2 but relatively low $PaCO_2$.[18,19] In practice, increased VA/Q mismatch with venous admixture is the commonest cause of gas exchange failure in respiratory diseases (e.g. COPD, pulmonary oedema, infection, and inflammation). HPV reduces VA/Q mismatch severity by diverting blood from poorly to well-ventilated regions. In addition, because 'ventilation defects' tend to be partial (i.e. poorly rather than unventilated alveoli), PaO_2 response to oxygen therapy is better in these conditions than those with 'pure' shunt (e.g. direct right to left heart shunts) but depends on the proportion of alveoli affected and degree of VA/Q mismatch as illustrated in Figure 2.4. In 'true' anatomical shunts (e.g. right to left heart defects), oxygen is never in contact with, and cannot affect oxygenation of, shunted blood. Calculation of venous admixture and the equivalent 'true' shunt fraction is illustrated in Figure 2.5.

Oxygen Transfer

The respiratory physician is increasingly, and appropriately, involved in the care of critically ill patients and is therefore concerned with systemic as well as pulmonary oxygen transport.[1,2,20] Since tissues have no oxygen storage system, a continuous supply, matched to the changing metabolic requirements, is necessary to maintain aerobic metabolism and normal cellular function. Failure of oxygen supply to meet metabolic needs is the feature common to all forms of circulatory failure or 'shock'. Prevention, early identification, and correction of tissue hypoxia are essential skills for managing critically ill patients, and this requires an understanding of oxygen transport, delivery, and consumption.

Oxygen transport describes the processes by which atmospheric oxygen is delivered to the tissues. These process are either convective

$$Q_S/Q_T = (Cc O_2 - CaO_2) / (Cc O_2 - CvO_2)$$

Where C denotes oxygen content and c, a and v denote end capillary, arterial or venous (end capillary and calculated alveolar oxygen tensions are assumed to be equivalent)

$$Cc,a,vO_2 = [(Hb \times SaO_2 \times k) + (PaO_2 \times 0.023)]$$

Where: Hb = haemoglobin (g/l); k = coefficient of Hb oxygen binding capacity (1.36 mlO_2/g Hb); $PaO_2 \times 0.023$ = oxygen dissolved in plasma

Venous admixture in a man breathing air with a Hb 95g/L, SaO_2 83% and SvO_2 50% is:

$$Q_S/Q_T = ([95\times0.98\times1.36]-[95\times0.83\times1.36])/([95\times0.98\times1.36]-[95\times0.5\times1.36]) = (127-107)/(127-65) = 0.32 = 32\% \text{ venous admixture}$$

The 'true shunt' (i.e. corrected for partial V/Q mismatch) is calculated using 100% O_2.
In this case on 100% O_2 the SaO_2 was 96% and SvO_2 = 63%

$$Q_S/Q_T = ([95\times1\times1.36]-[95\times0.96\times1.36])/([95\times1\times1.36]-[95\times0.63\times1.36]) = (129-124)/(129-81) = 0.07 = 7\% \text{ shunt}$$

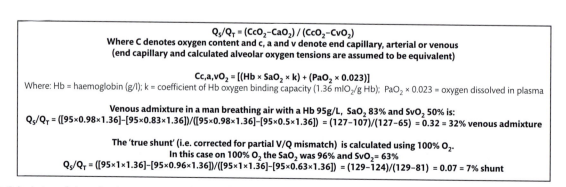

Figure 2.5 Calculation of shunt fraction or venous admixture (Q_S/Q_T).

Q_S/Q_T = shunt fraction; Cc,a,vO_2 = Oxygen content (ml/L); PaO_2 = arterial O_2 tension SaO_2 = arterial oxygen saturation, SvO_2 = mixed venous oxygen saturation, Hb = haemoglobin, V/Q = ventilation / perfusion ratio, $PaCO_2$ = arterial CO_2 tension.

Adapted with permission of Wiley from *Critical Care Medicine at a Glance* 3rd Edition, R Leach, © Wiley 2014; permission conveyed through Copyright Clearance Center, Inc.

or diffusive: (1) the convective or 'bulk flow' phases are alveolar ventilation and transport in blood from the pulmonary to systemic microcirculation: these are energy requiring stages that rely on work performed by the cardiac and respiratory 'pumps'; (2) the diffusive phases include the movement of oxygen from alveolus to pulmonary capillary and from systemic capillary to cell: these stages are passive and depend on oxygen partial pressures gradients, the tissue capillary density (i.e. diffusion distance), and the cells ability to take up and use oxygen.

Oxygen Delivery

Global oxygen delivery (DO_2) is the total amount of oxygen delivered to tissues per minute irrespective of blood flow distribution. Under resting conditions, it is normally more than adequate to meet the total oxygen requirements of the tissues (VO_2) and maintain aerobic metabolism. Inadequate DO_2 causes progressive metabolic acidosis, hyperlactataemia, and reduced mixed venous oxygen saturations (SvO_2), as well as organ-specific features such as oliguria and impaired consciousness. Serial lactate measurements monitor progression of the underlying problem and/or the response to treatment. Raised lactate levels (>2 mmol/l) are due to increased production or reduced hepatic metabolism, and both occur in critical illness, as reduced DO_2 produces tissue ischaemia and impaired liver function, although mitochondrial dysfunction and catecholamine-driven glycolysis are also major contributors to the lactataemia seen in critical illness.

DO_2 is calculated from the oxygen content of arterial blood (CaO_2) and cardiac output (Qt): $DO_2 = Qt \times CaO_2 \sim 1000$ mL/min, where $CaO_2 = [Hb \times SaO_2 \times k + (PaO2 \times 0.023)] \sim 200$ mLO_2/L, where Hb is haemoglobin (g/L); k is the coefficient of Hb oxygen binding capacity (1.36 mLO2/g Hb); and $PaO_2 \times 0.023$ = oxygen dissolved in plasma. DO_2 is compromised by anaemia, desaturation, and low cardiac output, either singly or in combination. In addition, DO_2 depends on arterial oxygen saturation (SaO_2) rather than PaO_2, and increasing PaO_2 above 9 kPa (68 mmHg) is of little benefit due to the sigmoid shape of the oxyhaemoglobin dissociation curve (i.e. >90% Hb is saturated at PaO_2 9 kPa). This does not apply to the diffusive component of oxygen transport that is dependent on the PaO_2 gradient.

Although blood transfusion seems the most effective way to increase DO_2, blood viscosity markedly increases above 100 g/L. This impairs blood flow, especially in small vessels, and if perfusion pressure falls it exacerbates tissue hypoxia. Ideally, Hb should be maintained at 70–90 g/L. In patients with coronary artery disease, higher concentrations (~100 g/L) may improve outcomes, although the evidence for this remains contested.

Oxygen Consumption

Global oxygen consumption (VO_2) measures the total oxygen consumed by the tissues per minute. It can be directly measured from expired minute volume and inspired and mixed expired oxygen concentrations, or derived from cardiac output (Qt) and arterial and venous oxygen contents: $VO_2 = Qt - (CaO_2 - CvO_2) \sim 250$ mL/min. The amount of oxygen consumed (VO_2) as a fraction of oxygen delivered (DO_2) is the oxygen extraction ratio (OER): $OER = VO_2/DO_2 = \sim 25\%$ (~75% during maximal exercise). Oxygen not extracted by tissues returns to the lungs where the 'mixed' venous saturation (SvO_2) measured in the pulmonary artery represents pooled SvO_2 from all organs (e.g. hepatic SvO_2 <50%, renal SvO_2 >80%, and hence the need for a mixed sample). Mixed SvO_2 depends on both DO_2 and VO_2; a value >70% is normal, although values of >80% may indicate cytotoxic dysoxia, microcirculatory shunts due to vasodilation or elevated PaO_2. By contrast values of <55% suggests inadequate DO_2.

Cellular metabolic rate determines VO_2 and increases during physical activity, shivering, hyperthermia, and sympathetic drive (e.g. pain). Certain drugs (e.g. adrenaline) and feeding regimens (i.e. excessive glucose) also increase VO_2. MV eliminates the metabolic cost of breathing which, although normally <5% of total VO_2, may rise to ~30% in catabolic critically ill patients with respiratory distress. MV also facilitates sedation, analgesia, and/or paralysis, further reducing VO_2.[20]

Regional and Tissue Oxygen Delivery

Organ hypoxia often results from disordered regional blood flow to and within organs rather than from inadequate DO_2. During increased metabolic demand (e.g. exercise), local vascular tone determines regional blood flow and ensures 'consumption drives delivery'. During sepsis, loss of normal autoregulation may cause 'shunting' and tissue hypoxia even if global DO_2 (±SvO_2) is raised. In this situation, improving peripheral distribution is more effective than increasing global DO_2.

Microcirculatory distribution is determined by complex endothelial, neural, metabolic, and pharmacological interactions. Endothelium, a dynamic interface between tissue and flowing blood components, promotes vascular homeostasis. It not only maintains a physical barrier between blood and body tissues but modulates leucocyte migration, angiogenesis, coagulation, and distribution of regional blood flow (i.e. vasomotor tone by releasing vasoconstrictor (e.g. endothelin) and relaxing factors (e.g. prostacyclin)). In sepsis, inflammatory mediators activate nitric oxide synthase with vasodilation.[8,10,20]

Underlying pathology often determines regional blood flow. In critical illness, endogenous vasoconstrictors can reduce splanchnic perfusion and failure to maintain enteral nutrition compromises gut mucosa. Splanchnic ischaemia renders the gut mucosa 'leaky', allowing translocation of endotoxins and bacteria into the circulation causing widespread endothelial damage. Attempts to maintain splanchnic perfusion by increasing global DO_2 are often inefficient and may have adverse effects. In sepsis, norepinephrine (noradrenaline) counteracts hypotension and improves vital organ perfusion but may further compromise splanchnic blood flow. Strategies that aim to modulate regional DO_2 by exploiting different receptor populations remain controversial. For example, dopexamine (β-adrenergic, dopaminergic, but not α-adrenergic effects) may selectively increase splanchnic blood flow.[20]

Oxygen delivery from capillary blood to the cell depends on capillary DO_2, cellular oxygen use/uptake (VO_2), oxygen–haemoglobin dissociation relationships, and factors affecting diffusion (i.e. partial pressure gradient). The oxygen–haemoglobin dissociation relationship is illustrated in Figure 2.6. It is defined by the PaO_2 at which 50% of Hb is saturated (P50; normally ~3.5 kPa (26 mmHg)). An increase in P50 or rightward shift in this relationship (e.g. with pyrexia, acidosis, and increased 2,3-diphosphoglycerate) reduces Hb saturation (SaO_2) for a given PaO_2, increasing tissue oxygen availability. Diffusion is modified by inter-capillary distance (e.g. peripheral oedema), especially during 'hypoxia' due to a reduced partial pressure gradient between capillary and cell and increased diffusion distance (but is less of a factor if tissue hypoxia is due to anaemia or reduced flow).

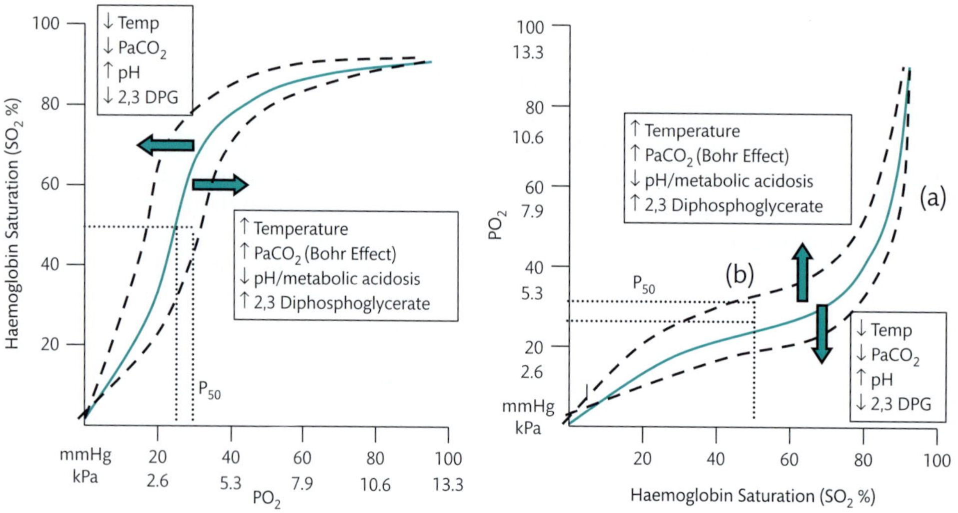

Figure 2.6 Relationship between oxygen tension (PO_2) and haemoglobin saturation (SO_2).

Left: traditional oxyhaemoglobin curve showing effect of temperature, pH and 2,3 diphosphoglycerate. Right religned to show its two key features (a) haemoglobin maintains high levels of saturation despite falling oxygen tension (i.e. pick up of oxygen in the lung is maintained despite reduced oxygen tension) (b) oxygen tension remains fairly stable as oxyhaemoglobin saturation falls (i.e. oxygen delivery to tissues maintained despite falling oxyhaemoglobin saturation).

Republished with permission of Wiley from *Critical Care Medicine at a Glance* 3rd Edition, R Leach, © Wiley 2014; permission conveyed through Copyright Clearance Center, Inc.

Individual organs and cells vary in their sensitivity to hypoxia. Neurons and cardiac and renal tubular cells are very sensitive to sustained hypoxaemia. Irreversible damage occurs within 3 min of stopping brain perfusion. Renal cortex and hepatocytes tolerate ~20 min and skeletal muscle ~90 min, whereas vascular smooth muscle tolerates >24 h hypoxia. Maintaining blood flow to susceptible organs is a primary goal during cardiac arrest (e.g. to limit the profound consequences of hypoxic brain injury). Tolerance to hypoxia may develop with repeated exposure (ischaemic preconditioning) as it does during altitude acclimatization. The answer to when hypoxic tissue damage occurs is dependent on circumstances (e.g. pathology), comorbid factors (e.g. atheroma), and hypoxia duration.

Heart–Lung Interactions

The heart and lungs coexist within the sealed thoracic cavity and are highly interdependent[1,20,21,22] as discussed in Chapter 17. They are well adapted to deliver the additional cardiac output (CO), DO_2, and ventilation/gas exchange required by increased metabolic activity (i.e. oxygen/substrate needs and waste clearance). However, complex heart–lung interactions often modify cardiovascular function. Firstly, to deliver extra metabolic activity requires additional ventilation (i.e. 'work of breathing'), which increases overall CO and DO_2 requirements and generates waste (e.g. CO_2) that must be removed. Secondly, increased lung volumes (i.e. above resting end expiratory volume) alter autonomic tone and PVR and 'compress' the heart with profound haemodynamic consequences. Finally, intrathoracic pressure (ITP) changes during spontaneous and positive pressure ventilation (PPV; e.g. MV, CPAP) affect right atrial (RA) venous return and left ventricular (LV) afterload. Reduced ITP during spontaneous inspiration promotes RA venous return whilst impeding LV ejection. In contrast, increased ITP during PPV reduces venous return whilst off-loading the left ventricle (which increases CO). Although, ITP changes account for most cardiovascular differences to spontaneous ventilation and PPV, the response is also influenced by lung volume, myocardial reserve, circulating blood volume, blood flow distribution, and extra-thoracic pressures.[21,22]

Intrathoracic Pressure Effects on Cardiac Function

As the heart is 'enclosed' within the thoracic cavity, ITP changes alter RA venous return and LV afterload independently of the heart. Increased ITP reduces the pressure gradient for venous return (i.e. by raising right atrial pressure), increases LV ejection (i.e. by reducing transmural LV systolic pressure), and reduces intrathoracic blood volume. Conversely, decreased ITP augments venous return, impedes LV ejection, and increases intrathoracic blood volume. Right atrial pressure (RAP) determines RA venous return from systemic venous reservoirs, and the cardiovascular effects of ventilation are mainly due to RAP (±venous reservoir pressure) effects. Mean systemic pressure, the driving pressure for RA venous return, is relatively constant throughout ventilation, and RAP is the main factor affecting RA venous return (and its cyclical pattern). During PPV, positive inspiratory pressure increases RAP reducing RA venous return. In contrast, during spontaneous ventilation, negative inspiratory pressure increases RA venous return due to a reduction in RAP and an increase in intraabdominal pressure associated with diaphragmatic descent (see below). However, this potential increase in RA venous return is limited by collapse of the great veins as they enter the thorax when ITP (and hence central venous pressure) falls below atmospheric pressure.[21,22]

ITP changes also modulate LV afterload due to its effects on LV ejection pressure (i.e. arterial pressure relative to ITP) and end-diastolic volumes. If arterial pressure remains constant as ITP increases, transmural LV pressure and consequently afterload decrease. Conversely, if ITP decreases, LV wall tension and afterload increase. Thus, increases and decreases in ITP reduce and increase LV afterload, respectively. During PPV (e.g. MV), sequential analysis of the ITP-related cyclical changes in arterial pulse pressure and systolic pressure variation can be used to identify volume responsive critically ill patient who require further fluid resuscitation.

During weaning, increased afterload (i.e. reduced ITP with spontaneous inspiration) is an important factor in weaning-induced LV ischemia (i.e. as myocardial O_2 consumption increases) and subsequent LV failure. Consequently, weaning to spontaneous ventilation increases not only the 'work of breathing' (i.e. DO_2 requirements) but also myocardial O_2 consumption. In obstructive airway disease (e.g. acute bronchospasm and asthma) or in patients with stiff lungs (e.g. interstitial lung disease and acute lung injury), forced spontaneous inspiratory effort results in profound negative ITP swings, which also increase LV afterload. This may precipitate acute heart failure and pulmonary oedema, especially in those with pre-existing impaired LV systolic function.[20,21,22]

PPV effectively treats heart failure and improves LV function by reducing LV afterload. Unfortunately, reductions in venous return (±intrathoracic blood volume) limit the benefit. Reducing negative ITP swings also reduces LV afterload, improving LV performance, but without changing venous return which remains constant until ITP is positive. Consequently, preventing 'negative' ITP swings reduces LV afterload without impeding venous return. This mechanism also contributes to the value of continuous positive airway pressure (CPAP) in the management of acute cardiogenic pulmonary oedema (i.e. reduced negative inspiratory ITP swings, decreased intrathoracic volume, and improved oxygenation by maintaining airways/alveolar patency). Furthermore, night-time CPAP selectively improves respiratory muscle strength, reduces serum catecholamine levels, and improves LV contraction in patients with obstructive airway disease (±pre-existent heart failure).

The CO reductions associated with PPV (e.g. MV) can be corrected by fluid resuscitation, increasing mean systemic pressures and/or by limiting ITP and lung volume changes. Thus, reducing tidal volumes and positive end expiratory pressures or prolonging expiratory time improves RA venous return. However, if PPV requires increased lung volumes, the fall in CO that might occur due to increased RAP is mitigated by the enhanced RA venous return, due to the increased intraabdominal pressure as the diaphragm descends, on the large volume of systemic venous blood in the intraabdominal compartment.[20,21,22]

Other Lung Functions

The lungs have other important roles.[1,2,10,20] Irritant receptors induce coughing or sneezing to expel irritant particles or mucous, mucosa-associated lymphoid tissue mediates immunity, and the respiratory epithelium excretes many factors that act as antimicrobials (e.g. immunoglobulins (IgA), collectins, defensins, and anti-oxidants), promote immune cell recruitment (e.g. cytokines and chemokines), and are anti-inflammatory agents (e.g. surfactant, proteases, and anti-oxidants) (see Chapter 4). It has a fibrinolytic system that breaks down blood clot emboli from the systemic circulation and clears many chemicals (e.g. prostaglandins, serotonin, bradykinin, and norepinephrine) and/or drugs (e.g. propranolol) from the circulation. Finally, angiotensin converting enzyme on the surface of pulmonary capillary endothelial cell converts ~70% of angiotensin I in blood passing through the lungs to aldosterone-releasing angiotensin II, which also causes vasoconstriction and increases blood pressure.

REFERENCES

1. Hsia CC, Hyde DM, Weibel ER. Lung structure and the intrinsic challenges of gas exchange. *Compr Physiol.* 2016;**6**:827–895.
2. Pocock G, Richards CD. Human Physiology: The Basis of Medicine. 3rd ed. Oxford: Oxford University Press;2006:315–317.
3. Nickol AH, Polkey MI. Respiratory muscles, Pulmonary mechanics and ventilator control. In: Davidson C, Treacher D, Ed. *Respiratory Critical Care.* Arnold; 2002:4–21.
4. Adler D, Janssens J-P. The pathophysiology of respiratory failure: Control of breathing, respiratory load, and muscle capacity. *Respiration.* 2019;**97**:93–104.
5. Grinnan DC, Truwit JD. Clinical review: Respiratory mechanics in spontaneous and assisted ventilation. *Crit Care.* 2005;**9**(5):472–484.
6. Marini JJ. Dynamic hyperinflation and auto-positive end-expiratory pressure: Lessons learned over 30 years. *Am J Respir Crit Care Med.* 2011;**184**(7):756–762.
7. Mitzner W. Mechanics of the lung in the 20th century. *Compr Physiol.* 2011;**1**: 2009–2027.
8. Weibel ER. Lung morphometry: The link between structure and function. *Cell Tissue Res.* 2017;**367**:413–426.
9. Ochs M, Knudsen L, Hegermann J, et al. Using electron microscopes to look into the lung. *Histochem Cell Biol.* 2016;**146**:695–707.
10. Knudsen L, Ochs M. The micromechanics of lung alveoli: Structure and function of surfactant and tissue components. *Histochem Cell Biol.* 2018;**150**(6):661–676.
11. Loring SH, Topulos GP, Hubmayr RD. Transpulmonary pressure: The importance of precise definitions and limiting assumptions. *Am J Respir Crit Care Med.* 2016;**194**:1452–1457.
12. Knudsen L, Lopez-Rodriguez E, Berndt L, et al. Alveolar micromechanics in bleomycin-induced lung injury *Am J Respir Cell Mol Biol.* 2018;**59**(6):757–769.
13. Wagner PD. The physiological basis of pulmonary gas exchange: Implications for clinical interpretation of arterial blood gases. *European Resp J.* 2015;**45**:227–243.
14. Petersson J, Glenny RW. Gas exchange and ventilation–perfusion relationships in the lung. *European Resp J.* 2014;**44**:1023–1041.
15. Dempsey JA, Smith CA. Pathophysiology of human ventilatory control. *European Resp J.* 2014;**44**:495–512.
16. Chowdhuri S, Badr MS. Control of ventilation in health and disease. *Chest.* 2017;**151**:917–929.

17. Prisk GK. Microgravity and the respiratory system. *European Resp J.* 2014;**43**:1459–1471;
18. West JB, Dollery CT, Naimark A. Distribution of blood flow in isolated lung: Relation to vascular and alveolar pressures. *J Appl Physiol.* 1964;**19**:713–724.
19. Townsley MI. Structure and composition of pulmonary arteries, capillaries and veins. *Compr Physiol.* 2012;**2**: 675–709.
20. Leach, RM, Treacher DF. The pulmonary physician in critical care 2: Oxygen delivery and consumption in the critically ill. *Thorax.* 2002;**57**:170–177.
21. Cheyne WS, Harper MI, Gelinas JC, et al. Mechanical cardiopulmonary interactions during exercise in health and disease. *J Appl Physiol.* 2020;**128**:1271–1279.
22. Pinsky MR. Cardiopulmonary interactions: Physiologic basis and clinical applications. *Ann Am Thorac Soc.* 2018;**15**:S45–S48.

3

Gas Exchange

Andrew Cumpstey and Mike Grocott

KEY MESSAGES

- Gas exchange refers to the movement of both oxygen and carbon dioxide between the lung alveolar air spaces and blood in the pulmonary capillaries.
- Respiratory failure (i.e. inadequate oxygenation) can be either normocapnic (sometime called 'Type 1') or hypercapnic ('Type 2').
- Alveolar ventilation is inversely proportional to P_aCO_2.
- Cooperative binding between oxygen and haemoglobin facilitates oxygen uptake in the lungs and oxygen extraction at the tissues.
- Hypoxaemia can only be caused by either inadequate FiO_2, hypoventilation, diffusion impairment, *V*/*Q* mismatch, or shunting.
- Arterial blood gases should be analyzed using a systematic approach, starting with the pH before considering the carbon dioxide levels and only looking at the base excess or bicarbonate values last.

Introduction

Gas exchange refers to the movement of gases between the alveoli and the pulmonary capillaries. We are most interested in the uptake of oxygen (O_2) and the removal of carbon dioxide (CO_2), but the principles could theoretically equally be applied to other gases as well. These processes constitute one of the primary roles of the lungs and are essential for life.[1,2]

In health, the respiratory system is exceptionally well adapted to performing efficient gas exchange and able to closely match O_2 uptake and CO_2 elimination to the body's constantly changing metabolic demands. However, disease can quickly impair these processes and result in harmfully low levels of O_2, high levels of CO_2, or both. Inadequate gas exchange (respiratory failure) is the most common reason for admission to critical care, associated with higher sickness severity scores and a poorer prognosis. In 2012, more than 44,500 patients suffered acute respiratory events in American hospitals, with an in-hospital mortality rate approaching 40%, rising to over 80% if deterioration resulted in cardiac arrest.[3] A thorough understanding of the underlying physiology is therefore essential in managing the critically ill with respiratory failure.

This chapter addresses normal gas exchange processes before examining how these can be impaired, resulting in hypoxaemia and/or hypercapnia. We then look at how these processes can be investigated (for example with arterial blood gases) and briefly discuss what results we might expect to see both in health, in some common critical illnesses, and also under extreme physiology conditions (such as at high altitude).

The Principles of Normal Gas Exchange

Pulmonary gas exchange can broadly be considered to occur in three separate but related processes (see Figure 3.1):

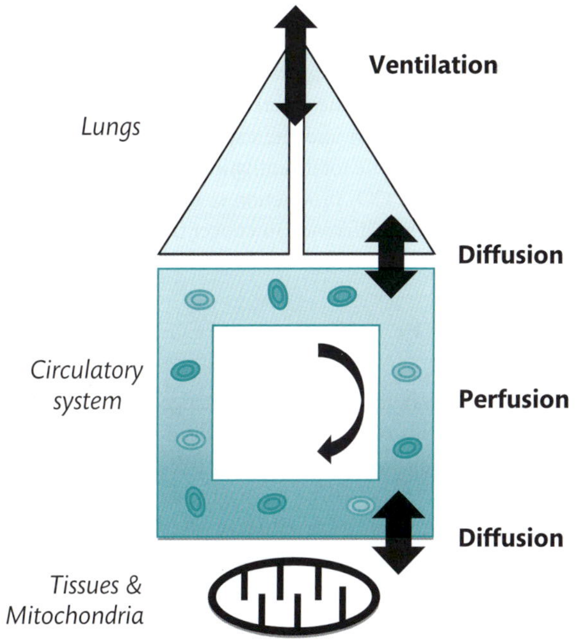

Figure 3.1 The stages of normal gas exchange.

Adapted with permission of the © ERS 2021: *European Respiratory Journal* 45 (1) 227–243; doi:10.1183/09031936.00039214 Published 31 December 2014. Figure can be downloaded at https://erj.ersjournals.com/content/45/1/227.figures-only

1. Ventilation
2. Diffusion
3. Perfusion

Ventilation

Ventilation refers to the movement of air into and out of the lungs and is normally described in terms of volume of gas moved per unit time, typically as litres of air moved per minute—or minute ventilation.

The different lung structures are well adapted to optimize this process. Initially, large-diameter airways (e.g. the trachea and bronchi) allow large volumes of gas to move via mass transport against minimal resistance. Traversing the smaller airways, diffusion becomes the dominant process until gases reach the approximately 300 million alveolar spaces. These alveoli are structured to facilitate maximal diffusion into the pulmonary capillaries (see Chapter 2).[1,2]

Minute ventilation (V_E, typically 5–8 L/min in a normal adult) is comprised of alveolar ventilation (V_A)—the volume of gas that reaches the alveolar spaces and takes part in gas exchange with the capillaries—and dead space ventilation (V_D)—the remaining volume of inhaled air which does not take part in gas exchange, either because it is in the large conducting airways (e.g. trachea) or in alveoli that are poorly perfused. These are known as 'anatomical' and 'alveolar' dead spaces, respectively, and together they comprise the 'physiological dead space'.

Equation 3.1: Minute ventilation is equal to alveolar ventilation + dead space ventilation

$$V_E = V_A + V_D$$

We can further quantify ventilation for each gas we are interested in. For example, if we first consider CO_2 and assume that CO_2 diffuses out of the pulmonary capillaries into every alveolar space equally, then the amount of CO_2 being produced by the body and leaving the lungs (V_{CO_2}) is equal to the difference between the inspired concentration of CO_2 (F_iCO_2) and the expired concentration of CO_2 (F_ECO_2), multiplied by the total ventilation (V_E)—see Equation 3.2:

Equation 3.2: Total CO_2 production is equal to minute ventilation multiplied by the difference in concentration of inspired and expired CO_2.

$$V_{CO_2} = V_E \times (F_ECO_2 - F_iCO_2)$$

However, since no significant gas exchange occurs within dead space ventilation (this is the definition of dead space) or $V_D \approx 0$, we can assume from Equation 3.1 that $V_E \approx V_A$. We can also ignore F_iCO_2 as inspired CO_2 is so close to 0, i.e. it is negligible. However, it is clinically more useful to use partial pressures of gases rather than fractions or concentrations of gases as this corrects for changes in atmospheric pressure (see below).[4] The alveolar fraction of CO_2 is also an approximation for the alveolar partial pressure of CO_2 (P_ACO_2), and at equilibrium, P_ACO_2 and P_aCO_2 will be identical because of passive diffusion (see below). This means that Equation 3.2 can be simplified further to show that the partial pressure of CO_2 is inversely proportional to alveolar ventilation (see Equation 3.3 and Figure 3.2).

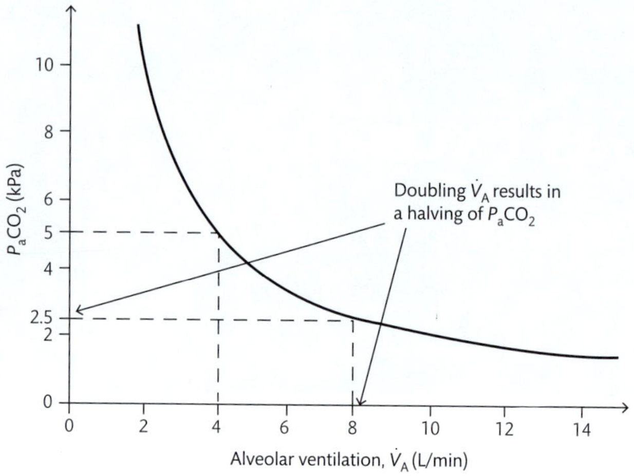

Figure 3.2 Alveolar ventilation (V_A) is inversely proportional to P_aCO_2.
Reproduced from Chambers D, et al., *Basic Physiology for Anaesthetists*. © Cambridge University Press 2015.

i.e.

$$V_{CO_2} = V_E \times (F_ECO_2 - F_iCO_2)$$

But as $V_E = V_A + V_D$ and V_D has no gas exchange:

$$V_{CO_2} = V_A \times (F_ACO_2 - F_iCO_2)$$

And as $F_iCO_2 = 0$:

$$V_{CO_2} = V_A \times F_ACO_2$$

Assuming $F_ACO_2 = P_ACO_2$ and rearranging gives

$$V_A = V_{CO_2} / P_ACO_2$$

And as P_ACO_2 is equal to P_aCO_2 at equilibrium:

Equation 3.3: Alveolar ventilation is inversely proportional to the arterial partial pressure of CO_2:

$$V_A = \frac{V_{CO_2}}{P_aCO_2}$$

Another way to think about this is to consider what would happen to gas exchange if minute ventilation increased. Initially, alveolar gas would be exchanged with atmospheric air more rapidly, and the composition of alveolar gas would therefore tend towards the composition of atmospheric air (where the CO_2 concentration is almost zero). Consequently, the alveolar concentration of CO_2 will fall as alveolar ventilation increases—resulting in an inverse relationship between V_A and P_aCO_2. This is a key concept that we will return to.

O_2 uptake can also be considered in a similar way to CO_2 production and Equation 3.2 can be re-written but with the inspired and expired concentrations reversed to show that oxygen is being absorbed and not eliminated net (see Equation 3.4).

Equation 3.4: Total O_2 uptake is equal to minute ventilation multiplied by the difference in concentration of inspired and expired O_2:

$$V_{O_2} = V_E \times (F_iO_2 - F_EO_2)$$

Again, increasing minute ventilation will cause the alveolar partial pressure of oxygen (P_AO_2) to tend towards P_iO_2 and cause it to increase—however P_AO_2 will never actually reach P_iO_2 for two reasons:

Firstly, atmospheric air is dry and gets humidified in the large airways during inspiration until it becomes fully saturated with water vapour (i.e. the saturated vapour pressure of water or $P_{\text{SVP water}}$ is reached). At body temperature, SVP remains constant at 6.3 kPa (47 mmHg) regardless of the ambient pressure or altitude.

Secondly, the O_2 concentration in the alveolus is always being reduced both by O_2 uptake and CO_2 elimination due to cellular respiration. This ratio of CO_2 elimination to O_2 production is known as the respiratory quotient (R) and is normally approximately 0.8 for a typical Western diet composed of mixed amounts of protein, carbohydrate, and fats. R is calculated by dividing V_{CO2} by V_{O2}—and dividing Equation 3.2 by Equation 3.4 and then simplifying and rearranging the terms will generate the alveolar gas equation (AGE), see Equation 3.5. This important equation relates the levels of alveolar O_2 and alveolar CO_2 and lets us estimate the P_AO_2 from the P_iO_2 and P_aCO_2 alone—again an essential concept that we will come back to.[1,2]

Equation 3.5: The simple AGE:

$$P_AO_2 = F_iO_2(P_B - P_{\text{SVP water}}) - \frac{P_aCO_2}{R}$$

Passive Diffusion

As previously stated, all gas exchange occurs through passive diffusion, but the rate of this diffusion is dependent on a number of different factors.

Firstly, Graham's law states that the rate of diffusion of a gas in a liquid is proportional to the solubility of the gas in that liquid (sometimes called the solubility coefficient) and inversely proportional to the square root of the gas's molecular weight (see Equation 3.6).

Equation 3.6: Graham's law of diffusion

$$\text{Rate of diffusion} = \frac{\text{Solubility coefficient}}{\sqrt{\text{Molecular weight}}}$$

Both CO_2 and O_2 are small molecules with low molecular weights, helping them to diffuse rapidly according to Graham's law. CO_2 is 20× more soluble than O_2 and consequently diffuses much faster than O_2 does.

Secondly, Fick's law states that the rate at which a particular gas can diffuse across a membrane is proportional to the difference in partial pressures of the gas on either side of the membrane (i.e. the pressure gradient), proportional to the surface area of the membrane, and inversely proportional to the thickness of the membrane (see Equation 3.7). Christian Bohr first applied this law to pulmonary gas exchange in 1909.[5]

Equation 3.7: Fick's law of diffusion

$$\text{Rate of diffusion} \propto \frac{(\text{Pressure gradient} \times \text{Surface area})}{\text{Membrane thickness}}$$

The alveolar membrane (i.e., the blood gas barrier) is exceptionally well adapted for gas exchange according to Fick's law as it is <0.3 μm thick, and the total surface area of all of the alveoli membranes is around 100 m^2. This is approximately the size of a tennis court—exceptionally large given the relatively small volume the lungs occupy. In total, the cross-sectional area increases 64 times from the terminal bronchiole supplying each acinus (a group of 8000–9000 alveoli) to the periphery of each alveolar sac where gas exchange occurs.[2,4]

The pulmonary surface area available for gas exchange can be measured indirectly using carbon monoxide (CO), which is a diffusion-dependent gas, and this is one of the ways we can assess the efficiency of pulmonary gas exchange. This measurement, known in Europe as the Transfer factor of the Lungs for Carbon Monoxide (TLCO) and in North America/Australasia as the Diffusion capacity of the Lungs for Carbon Monoxide (DLCO) is performed by asking the subject to inhale a single breath of the test gas mixture through a spirometer, hold their breath for 10 s, and then completely exhale.[4]

Fick's law also explains the importance of maintaining an adequate P_AO_2 (through appropriate F_iO_2 and consequently P_iO_2 levels) as a higher P_AO_2 will create a higher diffusion pressure and drive more oxygen uptake across the alveolar–capillary membrane.[1,2] However, maintenance of a diffusion gradient is also dependent on O_2 being moved away effectively after it has diffused into the blood stream—showing again the importance of perfusion to gas exchange. Approximately 98% of the O_2 in the bloodstream is transported bound to haemoglobin (Hb) molecules inside red blood cells, with each molecule of Hb able to bind, carry, and transport up to four O_2 molecules. Using Hb as an O_2 carrier molecule has a number of physiological advantages: at normal atmospheric pressure and body temperature, 100 mL of blood can only carry around 0.3 mL of dissolved O_2, but an Hb concentration of 15 g/dL allows a further 19.5 mL of O_2 to be transported (see Equation 3.8).

Equation 3.8: Arterial oxygen content (CaO_2) calculation, where 1.39 = Hüfner's constant, or the amount of O_2 in mL that 1 g of fully saturated Hb can bind.[6]

$$C_aO_2 = (1.39 \times [Hb] \times S_aO_2) + (0.023 \times P_aO_2)$$

Secondly, binding O_2 to Hb essentially 'removes it' from the alveolar-arterial gradient (A-a) pressure gradient, allowing more O_2 to diffuse into the bloodstream. And finally, because Hb binds O_2 in a cooperative way (i.e. the second O_2 molecule binds more easily than the first, the third O_2 molecule then binds more easily than the second, etc.), the oxyhaemoglobin curve is sigmoid shaped rather than linear. This allows oxygen uptake in the pulmonary circulation and tissue oxygen extraction to *both* be optimized with the former occurring on the flatter part at the top of the curve and the latter occurring on the steeper section, which means large amounts of oxygen are offloaded for relatively small changes in oxygen tension. Cooperative binding also links gas exchange to metabolism through alterations in the Hb–O_2 binding affinity (see Figure 3.3).

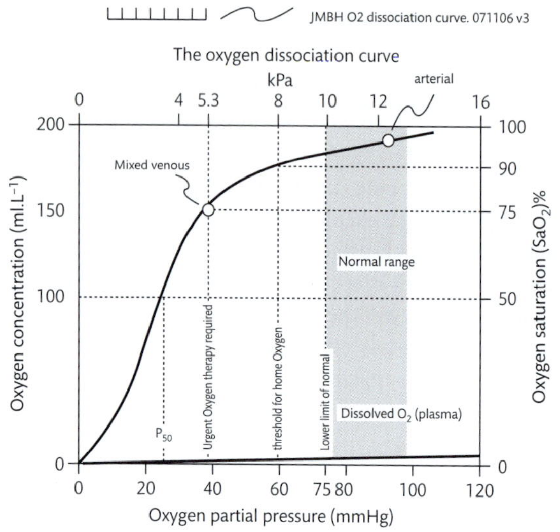

Figure 3.3 The oxyhaemoglobin dissociation curve describes the relationship between S_aO_2 and P_aO_2. The p50 describes the point where Hb is 50% saturated and is used to describe the position of the curve. For example, this moves to the right under acidotic conditions, increasing tissue extraction.

Reproduced from Hughes JMB. Review Series: Lung function made easy: Assessing gas exchange. *Chronic Respiratory Disease*. Nov 1;4(4):205–14. © SAGE Publications 2007.

Given Fick's law above, we might expect the A-a gradient to be large, but it is actually normally very small—less than 1.5 kPa in healthy adults. This is because, although the pulmonary arterial oxygen tension will always be slightly less than that in the alveoli, gas exchange is normally so efficient that an equilibrium is almost reached between the two compartments—so long as pulmonary ventilation remains matched to pulmonary perfusion.[7] However, if perfusion is reduced, then diffusion and gas exchange will also be impaired.

Perfusion

Once O_2 uptake has occurred, adequate pulmonary blood flow is essential to move O_2 away from the pulmonary circulation, maintain the alveolar–capillary diffusion gradient, and enable O_2 to be delivered to the tissues by the systemic circulation. Equally adequate perfusion is required to deliver CO_2 back to the lungs so that it can diffuse from pulmonary blood and then be exhaled. Blood flow is classically dependent on arterial pressure and vascular resistance, with the ratio of these determining the cardiac output, and consequently these factors will all also influence the lung's diffusion capacity. Similarly, factors that affect the blood's ability to carry gases, such as the haemoglobin concentration and the blood's bicarbonate pH buffer system, will also influence the diffusion capacity and be the dominant determinants of O_2 and CO_2 transport, respectively.[2,7]

And yet, good convective flow around the systemic circulation is not enough on its own to provide adequate tissue oxygen delivery—indeed, studies in septic patients have shown that significant areas of regional tissue hypoxia remain even after systemic haemodynamic parameters have been normalized with treatment.[8] Hence, ongoing study of the microcirculation in different physiological and pathophysiological states is proposed. The microcirculation comprises the very smallest vessels in the circulatory system—the arterioles, capillaries, and venules that measure less than 100 μm in diameter. It is the part of the circulation where tissue gas exchange occurs through passive diffusion.[9] Microcirculatory dysfunction is well recognized in many critical illnesses including sepsis and multi-organ dysfunction syndrome.[8,10] It has also been demonstrated in physiological conditions associated with hypoxic stress such as at high altitude.[11,12] It follows that good microcirculatory function is likely to be just as important to gas exchange as a well-functioning systemic haemodynamic system. Indeed, the persistence of microcirculatory dysfunction when the systemic 'macrocirculatory' parameters are adequate has led to the term 'haemodynamic incoherence'.

Whilst thinking of gas exchange in separate stages (such as ventilation, diffusion, and perfusion) may initially seem very simple, there are number of clinically important caveats to highlight.

Firstly, whilst diffusion is a passive process, ventilation and perfusion are active processes and energy is required to power respiratory and cardiac muscular activity, respectively. This means that although different disease processes can affect each of these three stages independently, ventilation and perfusion can be impaired by processes such as cardiac failure and pulmonary muscular pathology, and gas exchange may deteriorate further if patients are allowed to fatigue.[1]

Secondly, the lung's 300 million alveoli are not ventilated and perfused equally. The actual ventilation to perfusion ratio of a particular alveolar/capillary unit is affected by gravity, age, different disease states, and even different levels of oxygenation among other factors we will discuss below.[1,2,13] This ventilation/perfusion ratio (V/Q) has been shown to directly affect both O_2 and CO_2 diffusion independently because of the difference in the shapes of their respective dissociation curves, with O_2 transfer being affected more at normal V/Q ratios and CO_2 being affected most at high V/Q ratios.[5]

Ultimately, impairments in one or more of ventilation, passive diffusion, or perfusion will reduce overall gas exchange and cause hypoxaemia. Whether or not hypercapnia also results will depend on whether or not V_A is also reduced.

Hypoxaemia

Hypoxaemia is defined as a lower-than-normal PaO_2 (typically <8 kPa (60 mm|Hg)) and should not be confused with the term 'hypoxia', which refers to low levels of oxygen at the tissue or cellular level. These two terms are often incorrectly used interchangeably, and it is not unusual to hear hypoxaemic patients being inaccurately described as 'hypoxic'—this should be avoided to prevent confusion as the lists of possible causes for hypoxia and hypoxaemia are not the same.

Considering hypoxaemia first, there are only five possible causes of hypoxaemia, which we now consider in turn:[14]

1. Low levels of inspired O_2 (e.g. at altitude)
2. Diffusion impairment (e.g. pulmonary fibrosis)
3. Hypoventilation (e.g. opiate toxicity)

4. An imbalance between alveolar ventilation and pulmonary capillary perfusion or 'V/Q mismatch' (e.g. acute respiratory distress syndrome (ARDS))
5. Shunting (e.g. pulmonary oedema or atelectasis)

Low Levels of Inspired Oxygen

The partial pressure of oxygen in the air (P_BO_2) is determined by the fraction of oxygen in the air (F_iO_2) and the total atmospheric pressure (P_B). At sea level, atmospheric pressure is typically 101.3 kPa (760 mmHg), and the air we breathe is composed of 20.9% O_2. The partial pressure of oxygen available for inspiration (P_iO_2) is therefore equal to 101.3 × 20.9/100 or 21.2 kPa (159 mmHg).

P_B decreases with increasing height above sea level resulting in a reduction in P_iO_2 even though the F_iO_2 of air at altitude remains unchanged. For example, at 5300 m—the height of Everest base camp—the air is still composed of 20.9% O_2, but the barometric pressure has dropped to only 53.8 kPa (approximately half that at sea level). Consequently, the PO_2 available for inspiration (P_iO_2) is only 53.8 × 20.9/100 = 11.2 kPa (88 mmHg).[6]

If the P_iO_2 is reduced, we would expect less oxygen to diffuse down to the alveoli and diffuse across into the pulmonary capillaries. The converse is also true—if the F_iO_2 or P_iO_2 increased, then we would expect more oxygen to reach the capillary bed and the arterial partial pressure of oxygen (P_aO_2) to increase. However, knowing the P_iO_2 does not in itself tell us how much oxygen is available in the alveolus to diffuse into the capillary or what P_aO_2 to expect, we need to use the AGE to calculate this.

For example, the normal P_AO_2 at sea level is

$$\begin{aligned} P_AO_2 &= F_iO_2\left(P_B - P_{\text{SVP water}}\right) - PaCO_2 / R \\ &= 20.9\%\left(101.3 - 6.3\right) - 5.3 / 0.8 \\ &= 13.3\ \text{kPa} \end{aligned}$$

However, if at Everest base camp (without any acclimatization/hyperventilation so $PaCO_2$ remains unchanged), the P_AO_2 would be

$$\begin{aligned} P_AO_2 &= F_iO_2\left(P_B - P_{\text{SVP water}}\right) - PaCO_2 / R \\ &= 20.9\%\left(53.8 - 6.3\right) - 5.3 / 0.8 \\ &= 3.3\ \text{kPa}\ \ (25\ \text{mmHg}) \end{aligned}$$

In other words, reducing P_iO_2 by approximately 50% (i.e. reducing P_BO_2 from 21.2 kPa to 11.2 kPa (159 mmHg to 84 mmHg) causes a larger relative reduction in P_AO_2 of roughly 75% (from 13.3 kPa to 3.3 kPa (100 mmHg to 25 mmHg) even though the absolute reduction in P_AO_2 is the same as the reduction in P_iO_2 (both reduced by 10 kPa (75 mmHg).

Fortunately, this situation rarely occurs. On arrival at altitude, stimulation of the hypoxic ventilatory drive increases minute ventilation and reduces P_aCO_2 as part of the acclimatization response.[15] In clinical practice, ward patients either breathe air or higher concentrations of oxygen, and in operating rooms anaesthetic machines have a number of safety mechanisms to prevent the delivery of gas flows containing less than 21% O_2.

Diffusion Impairment

All gases move between the alveolar spaces and the pulmonary capillaries through passive diffusion as stated above. Consequently, any impairment to diffusion will lead to a reduction in gas exchange and may cause hypoxaemia.

A number of different physiological variables can potentially influence diffusion limitation as discussed above. Piper and Scheid simplified these into one mathematical model, which allows the extent of diffusion limitation for oxygen under hypoxic conditions to be predicted using a ratio of just three components: the ratio of the diffusing capacity (D), to the product of the blood flow (Q) and the effective solubility in blood (β), i.e. $D/(Q \times \beta)$.[1,16]

Fortunately, diffusion impairment is a very rare cause of clinical hypoxaemia. Each red blood cell takes approximately 0.75 s to completely transit the pulmonary capillary in each alveolar–capillary unit. However, it only takes approximately 0.25 s for the oxygen tension in the capillary red cell to equilibrate with the alveolar oxygen tension in healthy adults at rest at sea level. This means there is a three-fold reserve that needs to be lost before clinically significant diffusion impairment is seen.[1,5]

This reserve is so large that it is rarely exceeded at sea level except during extreme exercise and is sufficient to insulate many patients with chronic respiratory conditions from diffusion impairment. Consequently, diffusion limitation is rarely clinically significant in patients with conditions such as COPD,[17] asthma,[18] and even pulmonary embolic disease.[19] The exception to this rule is those patients who have fibrotic interstitial lung disease, e.g. idiopathic pulmonary fibrosis. This group may demonstrate diffusion limitation during exercise or even at rest—particularly if their condition is very advanced or their baseline pulmonary function is less than 50%.

However, it is more controversial whether or not critical illness impairs overall diffusion, with some sources suggesting it is not limited,[1] whilst others have shown that diffusion capacity remains limited in patients with ARDS throughout a 12-month follow-up period.[20]

The one situation where diffusion seems to be almost universally impaired is in subjects exercising at high altitude where P_iO_2, and hence the driving pressure for diffusion, and red cell transit time are both reduced.

Hypoventilation

Hypoventilation refers not just to a decrease in the minute ventilation (V_E) but more specifically to a decrease in alveolar ventilation (V_A). Unlike all other causes of hypoxaemia, patients without underlying pulmonary disease but who are hypoxaemic due to isolated hypoventilation will have a normal A-a gradient—so long as their hypoxaemia is due to hypoventilation alone and not compounded by any additional cause of hypoxaemia listed above. This is because hypoventilation has no effect on the lung's diffusion capacity (DLCO).[21] Importantly though, hypoventilation must also be associated with an increase in P_aCO_2 as well as a decrease in P_aO_2 because of the inverse relationship between V_A and P_aCO_2 defined by Equation 3.3 earlier.

Table 3.1 Possible causes of hypoventilation

Site of impairment	Diagnosis	Pathogenesis
Brain stem	• Over-analgised/over-sedated • Monge's disease (chronic mountain sickness)	Loss of ventilator drive Decreased chemoreceptor sensitivity
Spinal cord	• Motor neurone disease • Polyneuropathy (e.g. Guillain Barré)	Impaired neuronal conduction (anterior horn/motor neurone loss) Impaired neuronal conduction (demyelination)
Neuromuscular junction	• Myasthenia Gravis	Impaired synaptic signal transmission
Respiratory muscles	• Myopathy • Tiring	Inadequate ventilation Weakening ventilation
Chest wall deformity	• Kyphosis • Ankylosing spondylitis	Decreased tidal volumes (especially at night) Decreased tidal volumes
Intrinsic lung disease	• COPD • Obstructive sleep apnoea	*V/Q* mismatch + loss of central drive *V/Q* mismatch + hypoventilation

Source: Adapted from Hughes JMB. Review Series: Lung function made easy: Assessing gas exchange. *Chronic Respiratory Disease*. Nov 1;4(4):205–14. © SAGE Publications 2007.

Hypoventilation can broadly be classified into two separate categories—either a decreased neurological drive to breathe or a mechanical problem making it physically more difficult to breathe.[4] A problem with the respiratory control centre in the medulla, the brain stem, or the spinal cord may reduce the neurological drive to breathe, meanwhile any problem with the airways, respiratory muscles, chest wall, or the alveolar-interstitial tissue of the lung parenchyma may cause a physical impairment to ventilation. Certain diseases can be thought of as affecting either or both of these categories, e.g. COPD where airway disease physically impairs ventilation, but excess oxygen might reduce the hypoxic ventilatory drive in patients who are chronic CO_2 retainers (sometimes previously referred to as 'blue bloaters'). However, all of these causes will ultimately reduce V_A, causing both hypercapnia and hypoxaemia (see Table 3.1).

Ventilation/Perfusion Inequality–*V/Q* Mismatch

Ventilation and perfusion are not equally matched across the lungs. Both ventilation and perfusion are greater at the lung bases because of the effect of gravity. Gravity pulls blood downwards increasing perfusion lower down in the lung. Basal alveoli are more compressed than apical alveoli because of the weight of lung above them with the result that the smaller alveoli at the bases open proportionately more with each inspiration than those at the apices. Consequently, ventilation is increased towards the bases. In fact, both ventilation and perfusion increase lower down the lung, although perfusion increases proportionately more than ventilation (see Figure 3.4).[2,5]

West described this effect in the 1960s in a classic paper using the relationship between pulmonary arterial and venous and alveolar pressures to separate the lung into different zones. At the apices (where blood flow is least), alveolar pressure is larger than both pulmonary arterial and pulmonary venous pressures representing what West called 'zone 1'. However, at the bases both pulmonary arterial and pulmonary venous pressures are greater than alveolar pressure (hence the alveoli are relatively compressed), and West called this area zone 3. West zone 2 refers to the transition between these two extremes where alveolar pressure is still greater than pulmonary venous pressure but less than pulmonary arterial pressure[22,23] (see Figure 3.5).

This relationship means that even in health, there is always a disparity between the amount of ventilation (*V*) and perfusion (*Q*) occurring in each part of the lungs—the so-called *V/Q* mismatch. Any inequality between ventilation and perfusion will impair gas exchange. At the apex where alveolar pressure is greater

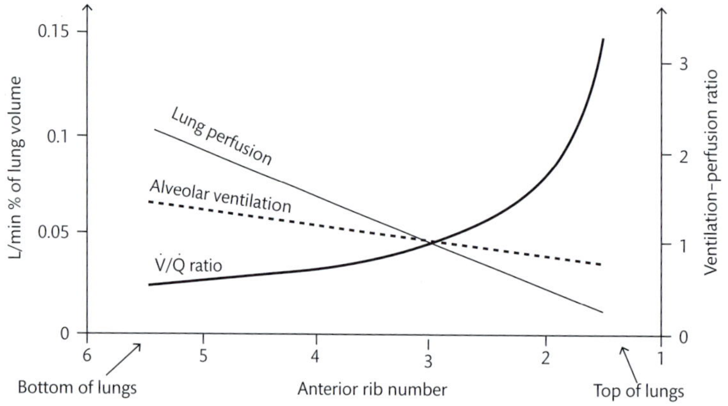

Figure 3.4 Ventilation, perfusion, and *V/Q* ratio across the lungs.
Reproduced from Chambers D, et al., *Basic Physiology for Anaesthetists*. © Cambridge University Press 2015.

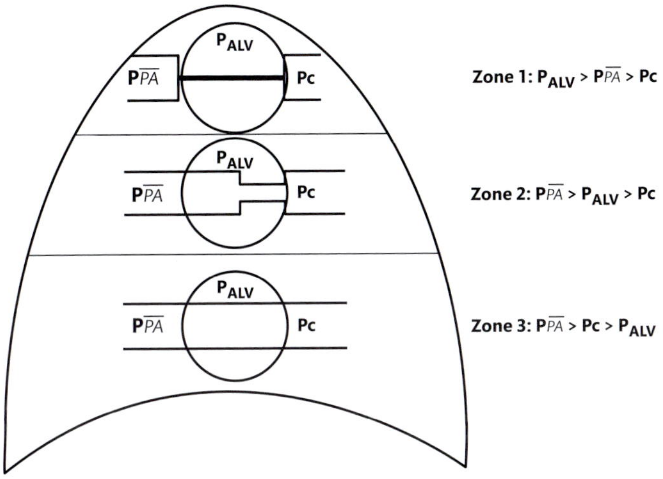

Figure 3.5 West zones of the lung.

Reproduced from: *Mechanical Ventilation: Physiology and Practice* (2 ed.), John W. Kreit, © 2017 Oxford University Press. Data from West JB, et al., Distribution of blood flow in isolated lung: relation to vascular and alveolar pressures. *J Appl Physiol.* 1964 Jul;19:713–24.

than perfusion pressure (West zone 1), the lung can be considered as tending towards dead space with *V*/*Q* ratios above 1 as the capillaries remain collapsed and closed. This situation never occurs in healthy lungs but can develop if hypotension occurs or during intermittent positive pressure ventilation. Meanwhile at the bases where perfusion pressure is greatest (West zone 3), gas exchange tends towards shunting (see below) with *V*/*Q* ratios less than 1.[1]

In health, the effect of this *V*/*Q* inequality on arterial oxygenation is minimal. However, increased *V*/*Q* mismatching is the most common cause of hypoxaemia with essentially all acute lung diseases and most cardiovascular conditions increasing the degree of *V*/*Q* mismatch occurring, and any increase in *V*/*Q* mismatch resulting in decreased arterial oxygenation. Importantly though, hypoxaemia due to increased *V*/*Q* mismatch normally responds well to increased F_iO_2; even poorly ventilated alveoli will be able to increase the P_AO_2 enough to normalize P_aO_2 if given enough time as diffusion is not impaired in healthy lungs.

Shunting

Shunting is defined as blood flow that does not take part in gas exchange. Although shunting could be considered as one extreme of *V*/*Q* mismatching (the opposite extreme to dead space), it is normally considered separately as it behaves very differently. In contrast to the response in hypoxaemia secondary to *V*/*Q* mismatch or diffusion limitation, increasing the F_iO_2 does not significantly reverse hypoxaemia secondary to shunting. This is because the increased F_iO_2 will not reach the shunted blood flow, and the Hb in the non-shunted blood flow is already maximally saturated so increasing the F_iO_2 has no further effect on the arterial oxygen tension. Consequently, shunting is normally assessed clinically using 100% F_iO_2 to remove any confounding cause of hypoxaemia such as *V*/*Q* mismatching or diffusion limitation.[1]

Theoretically, shunting might be expected to cause hypercapnia as CO_2 in the shunted flow will also not be able to be exchanged and will start to accumulate. In practice though, this increase in CO_2 stimulates peripheral and central chemoreceptor reflexes resulting in hyperventilation and adequate compensation for this effect—particularly at lower levels of shunt. This response is not linear with compensation being increasingly likely to be overwhelmed with larger shunt fractions. Consequently, P_aCO_2 will often remain almost normal with shunts as high as 20%, so long as higher minute ventilation can be maintained and the patient does not tire, but significant hypercapnia may develop with shunt fractions of nearer 40%–50%.[1]

Not all shunting is pathological, and physiological shunting occurs even in healthy patients. The venous drainage from the large airways drains directly into the left side of the heart bypassing the lungs, as does blood draining from the coronary circulation via the Thesbian veins, causing an anatomical shunt. Equally, a degree of functional shunting due to *V*/*Q* mismatching (see above) is also normal.[5]

Pathological shunting is seen in a number of different conditions, and one way of classifying this is by the location of the shunt. Intrapulmonary shunts are the most common type of pathological shunts and can be very severe. For example, in ARDS, pneumonia or pulmonary oedema, fluid or pus in the alveolar space will impair gas diffusion in otherwise well perfused alveoli.[1,5] Pathological shunts can also occur through large communicating vessels—typified by abnormal pulmonary arterio-venous connections (or pulmonary AV malformations), e.g. in hepato-pulmonary syndrome secondary to severe cirrhosis, or hereditary haemorrhagic telangiectasia.

Intra-cardiac shunts, such as in an atrial or ventricular septal defect, allow blood to flow directly from the right side of the circulation into the left without passing through the lungs.[1,7] Although more commonly associated with cyanotic neonates, intra-cardiac shunting may actually be relatively common in the adult population, with some reports suggesting that over a third of adults may have an undiagnosed patent foramen ovale.[24] Interestingly, obstructive airways conditions (such as COPD and asthma) are not associated with significant shunting.[17,18]

And finally, although historically shunting has usually been considered to be a systemic circulatory phenomenon, increasing evidence is suggesting that microcirculatory shunting may be important in both the development and progression of critical illnesses and shock, particularly in the context of sepsis.[8]

The amount of shunting can be estimated using the shunt equation (see Equation 3.9), where Q_S is the flow of blood through the shunt, Q_T is the total blood flow or cardiac output, C_aO_2 is the O_2 content of arterial blood, C_VO_2 is the O_2 content of venous blood and C_CO_2 is the O_2 content of end capillary blood, i.e. the amount of O_2 in the blood leaving the alveolus.

Equation 3.9: The shunt equation

$$\frac{Q_S}{Q_T} = \frac{C_CO_2 - C_aO_2}{C_CO_2 - C_vO_2}$$

C_aO_2 and C_vO_2 can both be calculated from Equation 3.8 by using S_aO_2/P_aO_2 and S_vO_2/P_vO_2 measurements, respectively. And although C_CO_2 cannot be measured directly, it can also be estimated with Equation 3.8 by assuming that blood leaving the alveolus will be 100% saturated and the partial pressure will be equivalent to

P_AO_2, which can in turn be calculated from the AGE (Equation 3.5). In other words, all that is required to calculate the shunt fraction (Q_S/Q_T) is a paired set of arterial and venous blood gases (which will also usually contain the Hb concentration) at a known F_IO_2.[2,5]

Hypoxia

All of the above conditions will result in hypoxaemia (low arterial oxygen tension) or 'hypoxic hypoxia'. However, it is an oversimplification to assume that cellular hypoxia only results from hypoxic hypoxia or the failure of gas exchange.

Almost 100 years ago, Barcroft stated that oxygen delivery failure could be due to any combination of inadequate cardiac output ('circulatory hypoxia'), insufficient haemoglobin ('anaemic hypoxia'), and/or decreased arterial oxygen levels ('hypoxic hypoxia').

Even if global oxygen delivery is maintained, tissue hypoxia may still be present and causing tissue damage. Microcirculatory dysfunction may disrupt regional oxygen delivery, increased cellular oxygen demand could outstrip the available supply, or cellular dysfunction may prevent delivered oxygen being utilized by the mitochondria (e.g. sepsis and carbon monoxide poisoning).[25,26] Hypoxia affects different tissue types in different ways, with some tissues very prone to harm from hypoxia, whilst others are remarkably resistant to hypoxic injury. For example brain tissue cannot survive more than 3 min under conditions of absolute hypoxia (i.e. no flow), whilst smooth muscle can survive 24–72 h and hair and nails can survive many days of hypoxia without sustaining irreversible tissue damage.[27] Meanwhile, many malignant cells actually undergo biochemical transformations to allow them to thrive in profoundly hypoxic conditions as part of the process of becoming cancerous.[28]

Ultimately, tissue hypoxia is exceptionally common among hospital patients and underlies most critical illness.[14] However, increasing the F_iO_2 to try and improve tissue oxygenation also has its own risks.

Hyperoxia

High flow oxygen has the potential to reverse hypoxaemia caused by diffusion limitation, low levels of F_iO_2, or even V/Q mismatching. Moreover, a high concentration F_iO_2 is routinely used in anaesthetic practice for short periods to pre-oxygenate patients or more correctly to de-nitrogenate patients, by washing nitrogen out of the alveoli and replacing it with oxygen. This builds a small oxygen reservoir in the lungs that can be used even if ventilation has ceased, buying the anaesthetist time in the event of an unexpected difficult airway.[29]

However, prolonged periods of inspiring 100% oxygen may paradoxically worsen gas exchange through the development of atelectasis. Alveoli filled with 100% oxygen rather than 79% nitrogen will slowly reduce in volume as this oxygen diffuses across into the bloodstream, eventually collapsing completely. This hyperoxic atelectasis will increase shunting and worsen V/Q mismatching.[30]

Harm from hyperbaric oxygen therapy was first documented in the 19th century and is still known eponymously. The Paul Bert effect refers to the symptoms of hyperbaric oxygen toxicity on central nervous system causing seizures and unconsciousness.[31] The James Lorrain Smith effect describes the pulmonary complications of hyperbaric oxygen toxicity, including bronchopulmonary dysplasia and atelectasis.[32]

More recently, evidence has suggested that even short periods of normobaric hyperoxia may also cause harmful cellular changes and structural remodelling of tissues. In the early 1980s, Davis et al. showed that prolonged hyperoxia was associated with increased alveolar–capillary leak and pulmonary macrophage activation.[33] Hyperoxia also seems to result in considerable vascular remodelling, including microcirculatory dysfunction and functional shunting such that hyperoxia appears to decrease oxygen uptake at the tissues.[34] Hyperoxia also appears to increase coronary vascular resistance and decrease coronary blood flow, likely secondary to increased production of reactive nitrogen species and other free radicals.[34]

A large clinical trial has recently taken these findings further to show that supplemental oxygen therapy in normoxic patients with ST elevation myocardial infarction is associated with larger infarct sizes at six months.[35] Similar trials have shown that hyperoxia is associated with no benefit or increased harm, when compared to normoxia, in the perioperative setting as well as in adult resuscitation.[36,37]

Based on all this evidence, tighter oxygen targets are now more routinely used in critical care. Whilst both high and low P_aO_2 values at 24 h are associated with increased mortality rates in observational studies, randomized controlled trials in patients with acute respiratory failure or ARDS have demonstrated that conservative oxygen strategies appear not to show benefit, and in the more severe patients, i.e. ARDS, targets too low (e.g. 88%–92%) could cause harm. Thus, lower P_aO_2 targets of 8 kPa (60 mmHg) do not produce higher mortality than higher targets,[38] but conservatively targeting SpO_2 88%–92% may result in higher mortality.[39]

Respiratory Failure

Respiratory failure means a failure of gas exchange and it is one of the most common reasons for a patient being referred to the critical care team. There are two different types depending on which type of gas exchange is affected. 'Type 1' respiratory failure refers to patients in whom O_2 uptake alone is affected. In 'Type 2' respiratory failure, CO_2 elimination is also impaired, and hypercapnia is present as well as hypoxaemia. Arguably, however, it is less confusing and therefore better practice to refer to Type 1 and Type 2 respiratory failures as normocapnic and hypercapnic respiratory failures, respectively.[21]

Normocapnic respiratory failure is caused by conditions that only impair gas diffusion and do not affect ventilation (e.g. pneumonia, pulmonary oedema, etc.)—hence CO_2 remains normal. Any disease process that causes hypoventilation (see Table 3.1) may result in hypercapnic respiratory failure.

Conventionally, respiratory failure is a laboratory diagnosis based on blood gas measurements, with normocapnic respiratory failure being defined as $P_aO_2 < 8$ kPa (60 mmHg) and $PaCO_2 < 6$ kPa (45 mmHg) (i.e. normal or low) and hypercapnic respiratory failure being defined as $P_aO_2 < 8$ kPa and $P_aCO_2 > 6$ kPa. These criteria refer to patients breathing air (i.e. $F_iO_2 = 21\%$)—at higher F_iO_2 values we need to use the AGE (Equation 3.5) to predict what P_AO_2 and therefore what P_aO_2 value we should expect to determine whether or not gas exchange is adequate or respiratory failure is present (see the Arterial Blood Gas Analysis section below).[21]

It is also important to remember that these are arbitrary numbers and an individual patient's gas exchange may be normal for them even with numbers outside of these ranges.[21] For example, a patient with severe COPD may 'chronically retain' and function normally with a P_aCO_2 of 6.5 kPa (49 mmHg) or higher, and fit and healthy climbers summiting Mount Everest typically have P_aO_2 values of only around 3 kPa (23 mmHg).[7]

Equally—and perhaps more importantly—a patient may not appear to have respiratory failure biochemically but actually be extremely unwell. For example, a 'normal' P_aCO_2 level in a young asthmatic may be a sign of near-life threatening disease.

Arterial Blood Gas Analysis

In terms of gas exchange, arterial blood gas analysis needs to focus on two particular questions—is oxygenation adequate and is ventilation adequate?

Adequate oxygenation is determined through use of the AGE (Equation 3.5). For example, if we were administering 50% oxygen at sea level, then we would expect P_AO_2 to be approximately 41 kPa (308 mmHg) according to the AGE:

$$P_AO_2 = F_iO_2\left(P_B - P_{\text{svp water}}\right) - \frac{P_aCO_2}{R}$$

$$P_AO_2 = 0.5 \times (101 - 6.3) - 5.3/0.8$$

$$P_AO_2 = 47.35 - 6.625$$

$$P_AO_2 = 40.725\,\text{kPa}$$

Given that the A-a gradient is normally <1.5 kPa, we would expect a P_aO_2 of around 40 kPa (300 mmHg) with normal gas exchange and any value significantly less than this would suggest hypoxaemic respiratory failure. As a rule of thumb, P_aO_2 is about 10 kPa (75 mmHg) lower than P_iO_2.

However, if the patient is hypoxaemic but the A-a gradient is normal, then either the P_iO_2 must be low (e.g. altitude and hypoxic inspiratory gas mixture) or hypoventilation must be present.

Ventilation can be assessed through evaluating the pH status, which is tightly controlled through ventilatory and metabolic (renal) compensation within a normal physiological pH range between 7.35 and 7.45. Hypoventilation will induce hypercapnia as explained above, and as CO_2 is acidic this will decrease the pH below 7.35 causing a respiratory acidosis. Equally, the opposite changes will be seen in hyperventilation resulting in a respiratory alkalosis.

If these pH alterations are allowed to persist for more than few hours, renal compensation will start to develop through altered excretion of alkaline bicarbonate ions (HCO_3), with either decreased excretion in the event of an initial acidosis or increased excretion in an alkalosis, allowing the pH to tend back towards normal. Compensatory processes will never fully normalize the pH. Often blood gases will also give a 'base excess' (BE), which is a calculated value to show how much metabolic change has occurred. A more negative BE value shows a greater magnitude of metabolic acidosis (e.g. in compensation for a respiratory alkalosis) is occurring.

Even though a lower pH would suggest respiratory acidosis and the need to assess the adequacy of ventilation, it is not possible to simply look at the pH value—good metabolic compensation may mean this is almost normal even if severe hypoventilation is present. Instead, the pH, P_aCO_2, and either the BE or HCO_3 values all need to be viewed together. A suggested approach is as follows:

1. Look at the pH and decide if it is normal, acidotic or alkalotic.
2. Look at the P_aCO_2 value next (respiratory changes occur immediately, metabolic changes take hours to develop), and see if this fits the pH disturbance. For example, a high P_aCO_2 (high respiratory 'acid') together with a pH drop (acidosis) would suggest a primary respiratory acidosis.
3. Look at the BE or HCO_3 value—is this normal or not? And if not, is this change in the appropriate direction for a compensatory change (e.g. increased HCO_3 in the event of a respiratory acidosis) or not? If not, then there might be a mixed picture.

Other ions—such as sodium and chloride—and proteins such as albumin will also affect acid–base status, but this is out of the scope of this section. For further detail readers are referred to recent reviews on applying the so-called Stewart approach to acid–base disturbance.[40]

REFERENCES

1. Wagner PD. The physiological basis of pulmonary gas exchange: Implications for clinical interpretation of arterial blood gases. *Eur Respir J*. 2015 Jan 1;**45**(1):227–243.
2. West JB, Luks AM. *Respiratory Physiology—The Essentials*, 10th ed. Alphen aan den Rijn: Wolters Kluwer; 2016.
3. Andersen LW, Berg KM, Chase M, et al. Acute respiratory compromise on inpatient wards in the United States: Incidence, outcomes, and factors associated with in-hospital mortality. *Resuscitation*. 2016 Aug;**105**:123–129.
4. Hughes JMB. Review Series: Lung function made easy: Assessing gas exchange. *Chron Respir Dis*. 2007 Nov 1;**4**(4):205–214.
5. Wagner PD, West JB. Effects of diffusion impairment on O_2 and CO_2 time courses in pulmonary capillaries. *J Appl Physiol*. 1972 Jul 1;**33**(1):62–71.
6. Grocott MPW, Martin DS, Levett DZH, et al. Arterial Blood Gases and Oxygen Content in Climbers on Mount Everest. *N Engl J Med*. 2009 Jan 8;**360**(2):140–149.
7. Chambers D, Huang C, Matthews G. *Basic Physiology for Anaesthetists*. First. Cambridge Medicine; 2015.
8. Ince C, Sinaasappel M. Microcirculatory oxygenation and shunting in sepsis and shock. *Crit Care Med*. 1999 Jul;**27**(7):1369–1377.
9. Martin DS, Ince C, Goedhart P, et al. Abnormal blood flow in the sublingual microcirculation at high altitude. *Eur J Appl Physiol*. 2009 Jun;**106**(3):473–478.
10. Østergaard L, Granfeldt A, Secher N, et al. Microcirculatory dysfunction and tissue oxygenation in critical illness. *Acta Anaesthesiol Scand*. 2015 Nov;**59**(10):1246–1259.
11. Martin DS, Goedhart P, Vercueil A, et al. Changes in sublingual microcirculatory flow index and vessel density on ascent to altitude. *Exp Physiol*. 2010 Aug 1;**95**(8):880–91.

12. Martin DS, Ince C, Goedhart P, et al. Abnormal blood flow in the sublingual microcirculation at high altitude. *Eur J Appl Physiol.* 2009 Jun;**106**(3):473–478.
13. Wagner PD, Laravuso RB, Uhi RR, et al. Continuous Distributions of Ventilation-Perfusion Ratios in Normal Subjects Breathing Air and 100% O_2. *J Clin Invest.* 1974 Jul;**54**(1):54–68.
14. Grocott M, Montgomery H, Vercueil A. High-altitude physiology and pathophysiology: Implications and relevance for intensive care medicine. *Crit Care.* 2007;**11**(1):203.
15. Cumpstey A. High altitude respiratory physiology and pathophysiology. Shortness Breath [Internet]. 2015 [cited 2016 Jun 12]; Available from: http://www.shortnessofbreath.it/common/php/portiere.php?ID=12fe7ead1dc1eaa888ce1ee0fc8069b8
16. Piiper J, Scheid P. Model for capillary-alveolar equilibration with special reference to O_2 uptake in hypoxia. *Respir Physiol.* 1981 Dec 1;**46**(3):193–208.
17. Wagner PD, Dantzker DR, Dueck R, et al. Ventilation-perfusion inequality in chronic obstructive pulmonary disease. *J Clin Invest.* 1977 Feb 1;**59**(2):203–216.
18. Wagner PD, Dantzker DR, Iacovoni VE, et al. Ventilation-perfusion inequality in asymptomatic asthma. *Am Rev Respir Dis.* 1978 Sep 1;**118**(3):511–524.
19. Kapitän KS, Buchbinder M, Wagner PD, et al. Mechanisms of hypoxemia in chronic thromboembolic pulmonary hypertension. *Am Rev Respir Dis.* 1989 May 1;**139**(5):1149–1154.
20. Herridge MS, Cheung AM, Tansey CM, et al. One-year outcomes in survivors of the acute respiratory distress syndrome. *N Engl J Med.* 2003 Feb 20;**348**(8):683–693.
21. Roussos C, Koutsoukou A. Respiratory failure. Eur Respir J. 2003 Nov 16;**22**(47 suppl):3s–14s.
22. West JB, Dollery CT, Naimark A. Distribution of blood flow in isolated lung; relation to vascular and alveolar pressures. *J Appl Physiol.* 1964 Jul;**19**:713–724.
23. Levitzky MG. Teaching the effects of gravity and intravascular and alveolar pressures on the distribution of pulmonary blood flow using a classic paper by West et al. *Adv Physiol Educ.* 2006 Mar 1;**30**(1):5–8.
24. Kayser B. The International Hypoxia Symposium 2015 in Lake Louise: A report. *High Alt Med Biol.* 2015 May 8;**16**(3): 261–266.
25. Brealey D, Brand M, Hargreaves I, et al. Association between mitochondrial dysfunction and severity and outcome of septic shock. *Lancet Lond Engl.* 2002 Jul 20;**360**(9328):219–223.
26. Santis VD, Singer M. Tissue oxygen tension monitoring of organ perfusion: Rationale, methodologies, and literature review. *Br J Anaesth.* 2015 Sep 1;**115**(3):357–365.
27. Leach RM, Treacher DF. Oxygen transport—2. Tissue hypoxia. *BMJ.* 1998 Nov 14;**317**(7169):1370–1373.
28. Semenza GL. Hypoxia-inducible factors in physiology and medicine. *Cell.* 2012 Feb 3;**148**(3):399–408.
29. Martin DS, Grocott MPW. III. Oxygen therapy in anaesthesia: The yin and yang of O_2. *Br J Anaesth.* 2013 Dec 1;**111**(6):867–871.
30. Martin DSBs, Grocott MPWM. Oxygen therapy in critical illness: Precise control of arterial oxygenation and permissive hypoxemia. *Crit Care Med.* 2013 Feb;**41**(2):423–432.
31. La pression barométrique. Recherches de physiologie expérimentale. Paris, G. Masson, 1878. [Internet]. Open Library. [cited 2022 Nov 23]. Available from: https://openlibrary.org/books/OL6933470M/La_pression_barométrique.
32. Smith JL. The influence of pathological conditions on active absorption of oxygen by the lungs. *J Physiol.* 1898 Feb 17;**22**(4):307–318.
33. Davis WB, Rennard SI, Bitterman PB, et al. Pulmonary oxygen toxicity. *N Engl J Med.* 1983 Oct 13;**309**(15):878–883.
34. Reinhart K, Bloos F, König F, et al. Reversible decrease of oxygen consumption by hyperoxia. *Chest.* 1991 Mar;**99**(3):690–4.
35. Stub D, Smith K, Bernard S, et al. Air Versus Oxygen in ST-Segment-Elevation Myocardial Infarction. *Circulation.* 2015 Jun 16;**131**(24):2143–50.
36. Meyhoff CS, Jorgensen LN, Wetterslev J, et al. Increased long-term mortality after a high perioperative inspiratory oxygen fraction during abdominal surgery: Follow-up of a randomized clinical trial. *Anesth Analg.* 2012 Oct;**115**(4):849–854.
37. Kilgannon J, Jones AE, Shapiro NI, et al. Association between arterial hyperoxia following resuscitation from cardiac arrest and in-hospital mortality. *JAMA.* 2010 Jun 2;**303**(21):2165–2171.
38. Schjørring OL, Klitgaard TL, Perner A, et al. HOT-ICU investigators. Lower or higher oxygenation targets for acute hypoxemic respiratory failure. *N Engl J Med.* 2021 Apr 8;**384**(14):1301–1311.
39. Barrot L, Asfar P, Mauny F, et al. LOCO2 Investigators and REVA research network. Liberal or conservative oxygen therapy for acute respiratory distress syndrome. *N Engl J Med.* 2020 Mar 12;**382**(11):999–1008.
40. Story DAM. Stewart acid–base: A simplified bedside approach. *Anesth Analg.* 2016 Aug;**123**(2):511–515.

4

Airway Defences

Thomas S. Wilkinson

KEY MESSAGES

- The lungs have a range of defences against microbial and other harmful agents, including mucosal, immune cell, and physical protections.
- Expelling foreign or dangerous material via explosive air movements from the lower and upper airways leads to coughing and sneezing respectively.
- Mucous secretion and ciliary movement in an outwards direction ('mucociliary escalator') are critical to the removal of infectious and harmful particles.
- Pulmonary immunity is provided by resident and recruited immune cells, with significant roles played by associated lymphoid tissues as well as mucosal space immune cells such as macrophages.
- The recently described microbiome, consisting of symbiotic microorganisms that exist in the healthy lung, plays a key role in pulmonary health. Its disruption is associated with pathological changes and alterations in resistance to infection.

Introduction

Inside the lung, the air–liquid interface is an access route for foreign particles and pathogens. Thus, despite its primary function providing efficient gas exchange, the respiratory system has also developed an intricate series of mechanisms for sensing foreign or dangerous matter.[1] Strategically placed throughout the respiratory tract are respiratory epithelial cells where gradual changes in morphology from tall, pseudostratified columnar, ciliated forms in the larynx and trachea to a simple, cuboidal, non-ciliated form in the smallest airways are mirrored by similar progressive changes in host defence. In the upper airway nasal, pharyngeal and tracheal epithelial cells assist the mucociliary apparatus, along with the reflexes of sneeze and cough, together with the dendritic cell (DC) network and lymphoid structures. Similarly, in making the transition down the airway, bronchial and alveolar epithelial cells aid both interstitial and alveolar macrophages to produce opsonins and anti-microbial proteins essential for host defence. This chapter summarises current knowledge on pulmonary defence mechanisms.

The Nose and Oropharynx

Pulmonary defence begins in the nose[2]—the gateway to inspired air and a very effective 'scrubbing tower', filtering air where the dual passageways generate turbulence in the inspired air and enhance particle deposition with the walls of the cavity. Just inside the nares, in the vestibule, there are numerous hairs or vibrissae that remove large particles (>10 μm). The nasal cavity is lined by a mucosal layer, composed of at least four types of epithelial cell, including squamous epithelium, which is primarily restricted to the nasal vestibule; ciliated pseudostratified cuboidal/columnar epithelium (respiratory epithelium) in the main chamber and nasopharynx; non-ciliated cuboidal/columnar epithelium (transitional epithelium) lying between squamous epithelium and the respiratory epithelium in the proximal or anterior aspect of the main chamber; and olfactory epithelium, located in the dorsal or dorsoposterior aspect of the nasal cavity. Particles bound to whole areas of ciliated epithelium can synchronize their 'beat', termed the mucociliary apparatus (see later), thrusting particles towards the nasopharynx and oropharynx where they may be swallowed and cleared through digestion.

Sneeze

Sneezing[3] is a reflex activated by trigeminal nerve stimulation in the nose and oropharynx. External irritants can stimulate sensory nerve endings directly or release endogenous agonists (e.g. histamine). Once stimulated, the trigeminal nerves transmit signals to the sneeze centre, in the medulla to activate parasympathetic neurones supplying the lacrimal glands and motor neurons supplying the facial and the respiratory muscles. The transient receptor potential (TRP) family of ion channels is important here and includes the vanilloid receptor (VR-1) activated by capsaicin and temperatures exceeding 43 °C and the VR-like receptor (VRL-1) activated by temperatures in excess of 52 °C while the cold and menthol receptor (CMR-1) is activated by cool/cold (8–28 °C) and menthol. Specialized chemosensory epithelial cells express receptors for certain irritants and transduce signals to the trigeminal nerve. These cells express T2R 'bitter-taste' receptors and the chemosensory G-protein, α-gustducin, and the application of bitter substances results in trigeminal nerve stimulation and increased respiratory rate.

Conducting Zone

Cough

The process of cough[4] is classically described as a deep inspiration proceeded by a forced expiration against a closed glottis, which suddenly opens to produce a powerful expulsive phase where air is forced from the bronchi, mouth, and nose. Unlike sneeze, mechanisms of cough may also be voluntary and are transmitted by the vagus nerve to the cough centre in the medulla. Motor neurons from the medulla then innervate the respiratory muscles that mediate the expulsive contraction. The TRP family of ion channels also plays a vital role in cough mechanisms. In particular, the ankyrin 1 receptor (TRPA1) has been shown to be activated by many irritant stimuli known to cause injury and inflammation by activating sensory neurons. Indeed, TRPA1-deficient mice show markedly reduced irritation responses to toluene diisocyanate, a known tussive agent in humans, compared to their wild-type counterparts.

Mucociliary Escalator

The respiratory mucociliary epithelium is one of the major mechanical barriers defending the lung from microorganisms.[5] Composed of tiny hair-like projections called cilia, which are covered in a low-viscosity pericilial fluid and then an upper mucus layer, the mucociliary system is synchronized to direct mucus-associated particles to the oropharynx for swallowing. The system is present in both the nasal and bronchial epithelium, moving in opposite directions and towards the oropharynx. The ability of the mucociliary system to thrust particles along this escalator depends on the ciliary beat frequency where MgATP, calcium, and cyclic nucleotides are critical to this process. The physiological importance of the mucociliary escalator is highlighted in the rare autosomal recessive disorder primary ciliary dyskinesia where cilia are immotile or unable to synchronize resulting in recurrent chronic infections and inflammation of the respiratory tract

Mucins

Discussions of the mucociliary escalator cannot be complete without a reference to its integral glycoproteins, the mucins.[6] These form a heterogeneous group of high molecular weight, polydisperse, and richly glycosylated proteins, transcribed from the MUC genes. The mucociliary escalator of the lung has been shown to express five main mucins, including the membrane-associated MUC-1, 4, and 16 and the secreted mucins MUC-5B and MUC-5AC. The main functions of mucins are in hydration, lubrication, and protection (from host proteases), as well as in host defence. Infection models subtly change this view as MUC-1-deficient mice clear *Pseudomonas aeruginosa* lung infection more efficiently than wild-type mice suggesting a 'peacemaker' role for this mucin.[7]

Epithelial Cells

The respiratory tract is lined almost continuously from nostril to alveoli in epithelial cells.[8] Thus, nasal, tracheal, pharyngeal, bronchial, and alveolar types have been identified and studied. Within each of these anatomical locations, there are specialized cells (such as olfactory epithelium in the nose) and a gradual transition from proximal to distal airway. Epithelial cells have numerous functions in host defence. In particular, they are a physical barrier due to claudin-associated tight junctions[9] (Figure 4.1), and they possess the synthetic machinery necessary to respond to a pathogenic insult often referred to as 'inducible innate resistance' (Figure 4.2), where they can sense pathogens, recruit appropriate leukocytes, and generate anti-microbial responses.[8]

Sensing and Recruitment

Sensing of the extracellular environment is mediated by toll-like receptors (TLRs), whereas that of the intracellular environment is mediated through both TLRs and nucleotide-binding oligomerisation domain (NOD)-like receptors (NLRs)[10] (Figure 4.3). Both TLRs and NLRs are germ-line-encoded receptors that recognize conserved molecular patterns in the structures of foreign, dangerous, and even endogenous substances. These receptors are strictly compartmentalized with TLR-1, TLR-2, TLR-4, TLR-5, and TLR-6 expressed externally and TLR-3, TLR-7, TLR-8, and TLR-9 expressed intracellularly on endosomes. Nasal, bronchial, and small airway primary alveolar epithelial cell TLR expression appears to be space and stimulus specific. TLRs have relatively low constitutive expression in epithelial cells but are quickly and efficiently upregulated in response to lung pathogens, such as *Klebsiella pneumonia* and *P. aeruginosa*. Thus, TLRs of the respiratory epithelium are shuttled into the place of greatest threat to sense and respond to lung pathogens.

Recruitment

Epithelial cells recruit neutrophils and monocytes from the circulation through production of chemokines. These small proteins (~10 kDa) are grouped into four related families designated: CXC, CC, C, and CX_3C depending on their conserved cysteine residues.[11] The CXC chemokines can be divided further by their Glu-Leu-Arg (ELR) motif that precedes the first cysteine. Chemokines transmit their activity through seven transmembrane spanning G-protein-coupled receptors expressed on the recruited leukocyte surface and include receptors for CXC chemokines (CXCR) and CC chemokines (CCR).[11] Both CXCL1 and CXCL2 act through CXCR2 expressed on neutrophils. This *CXC2–CXCR2* axis is essential for neutrophil recruitment and antibody neutralization of CXCR2, and the equivalent knockout mice have confirmed the need for neutrophil recruitment in models of *P. aeruginosa* and in *Aspergillus fumigatus* pneumonia. The importance of monocytes is observed through the *CCL2–CCR2* axis[12], and transgenic mice overexpressing CCL2 in epithelial cells have improved bacterial clearance and mortality following pneumococcal and *Mycobacterium bovis* challenge compared to their wild-type counterparts. In contrast, CCL2 knockout mice had greater lung burden and more severe sepsis than their wild-type counterparts due to attenuated recruitment of monocytes and dendritic cells.

Anti-microbial Responses

Two types of molecules mediate anti-microbial responses. They are the large and small anti-microbial peptides, which contribute to the antibacterial activity of lining fluid.[13]

Large Anti-microbial Peptides

Numerous proteins have been identified that form a collection of large anti-microbial peptides whose molecular weights are ~14 kDa or greater. These include Lactoferrin, Lysozyme, Collectins

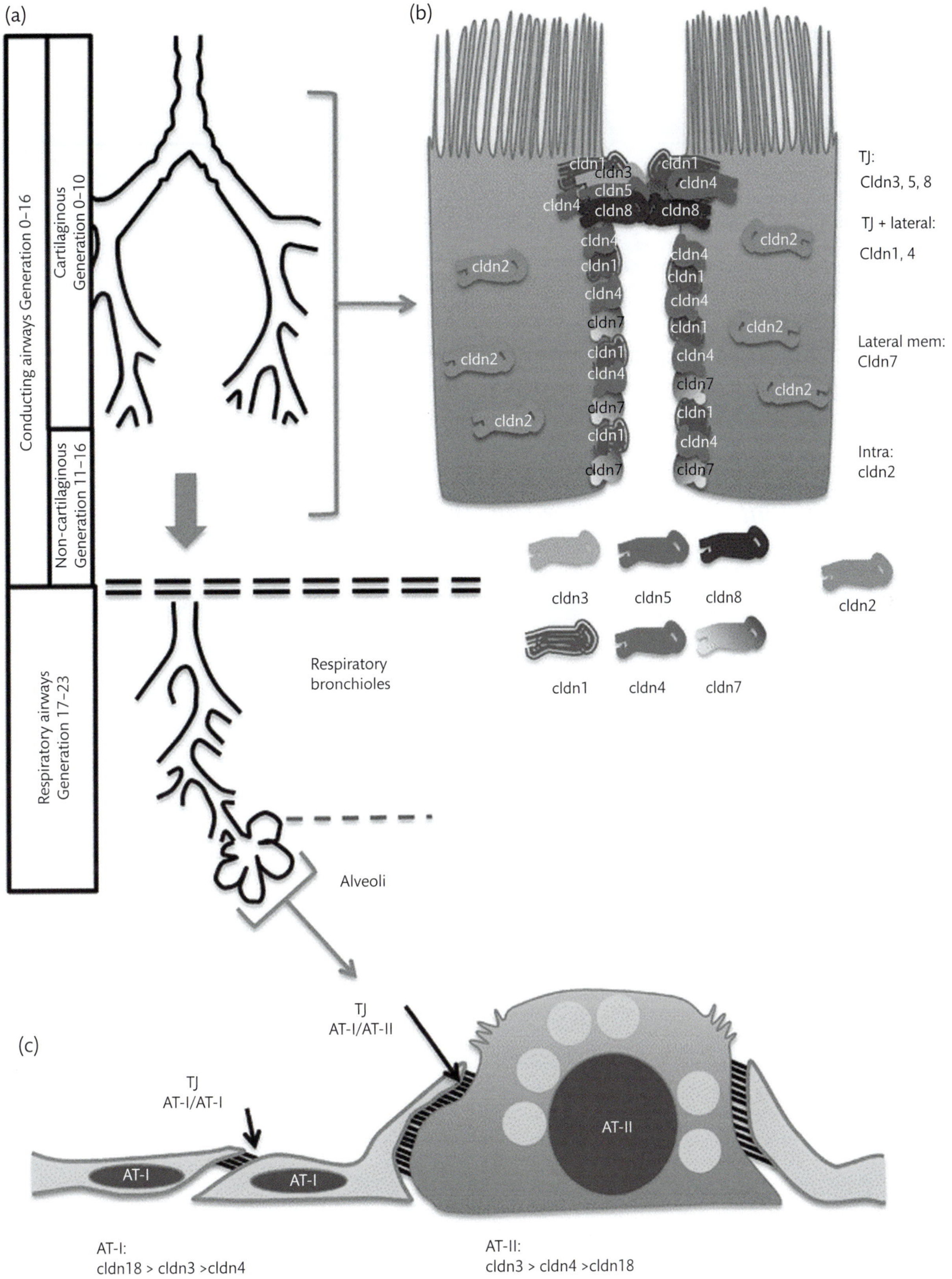

Figure 4.1 Function of epithelial cells: physical barrier and tight junctions. Organization of the airways and the airway epithelium. (a) The airways are subdivided into conductive and respiratory sections. The conductive airways contain cartilaginous and non-cartilaginous airways. The respiratory section constitutes the respiratory airways and the alveoli. (b) Scheme gives an overview of intracellular claudin (cldn) distribution in airway epithelial cells. The claudins predominantly localized at the tight junctions (TJ) (cldn3, 5, and 8), localized at the tight junctions and the lateral membrane (cldn1, 4), predominantly localized basolateral from the TJ (cldn7), and localized intracellular (cldn2) are depicted. (c) Scheme of the alveolar epithelium. The alveolar epithelium constitutes alveolar type I (AT-I) and type II (AT-II) cells. The tight junctions between adjacent AT-I cells are narrower than those between AT-I and AT-II cells. The most abundantly expressed claudins in AT-I and AT-II cells are cldn3, 4, and 18. See plate section.

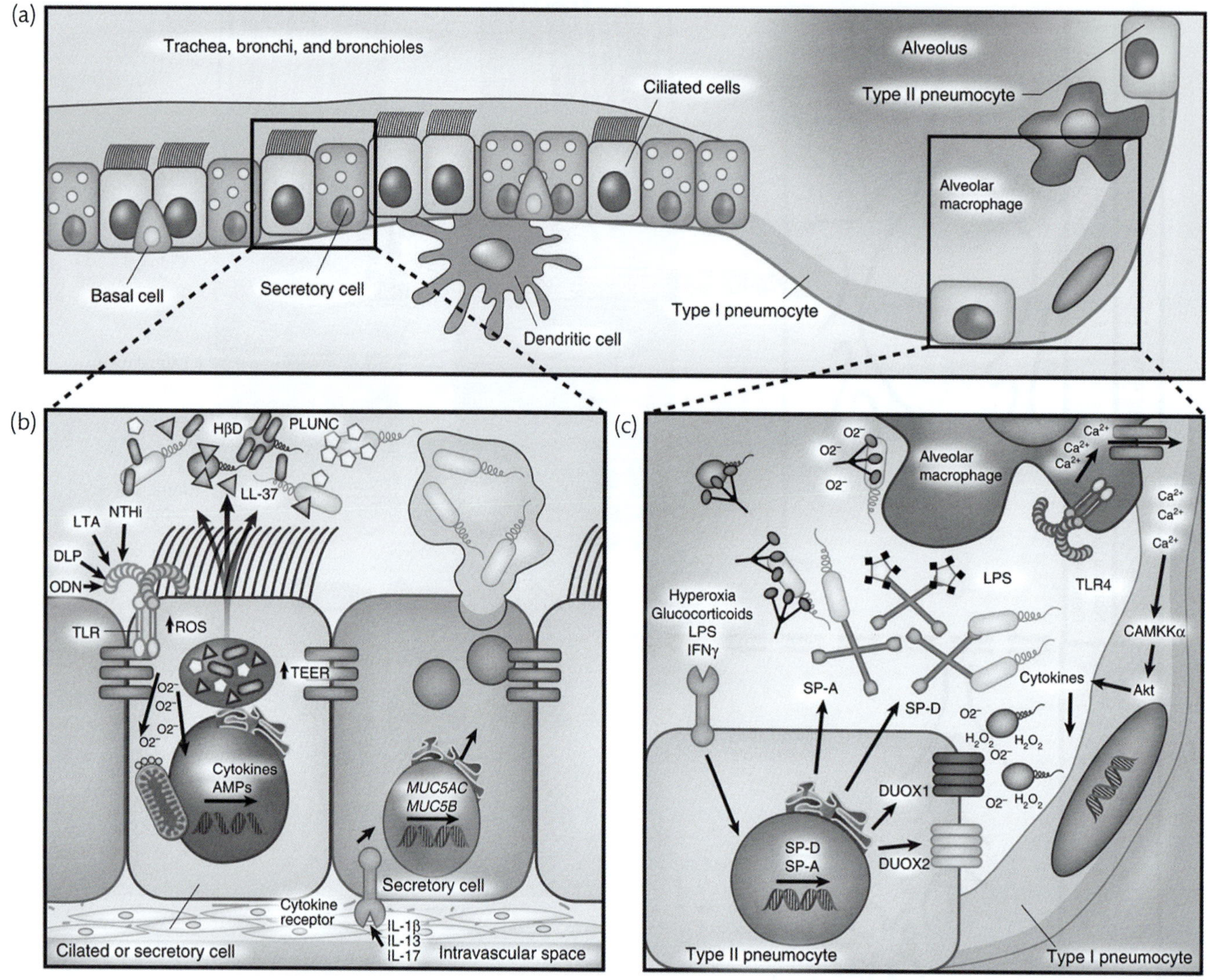

Figure 4.2 Epithelial cell function: inducible innate resistance.
Inducible antimicrobial resistance mechanisms of lung epithelial cells. (a) Cells contributing to inducible epithelial airspace defence. (b) Inducible responses in the conducting airways. Pattern-recognition and cytokine receptors detect local danger signals in the conducting airways, responding with enhanced barrier and mucociliary functions to improve pathogen exclusion, increased production of microbicidal antimicrobial peptides and volatile species, and secretion of mediators of leucocyte recruitment and activation. (c) Inducible responses in the alveolar compartment. Epithelial cells in the gas exchange units of the lungs detect pathogen-associated molecular patterns, perceive stress signals and communicate with lung resident leukocytes, and respond through inducible modulation of barrier function, enhanced production of antimicrobial peptides, collectins and volatile species, and secretion of leucocyte-active cytokines. LTA, lipotechtoic acid; DLP, diacylated lipopeptides; HβD, human β-defensin; NTHi, non-typeable *Haemophillus influenza*; ODN, oligodeoxynucleotide; ROS, reactive oxygen species; SP, surfactant protein; TLR, Toll-like receptor; TEER, transepithelial electrical resistance. See plate section.

Reproduced from Leiva-Juarez MM, et al., Lung epithelial cells: therapeutically inducible effectors of antimicrobial defense. *Mucosal Immunology*, 11(1): p. 21–34. © Springer Nature 2018.

(see the Surfactant Proteins section), and Lipocalin-2. Lactoferrin is a monomeric 80 kDa protein that forms part of the transferrin family of iron carriers and chelators and inhibits the formation of *P. aeruginosa* biofilms by an iron sequestration mechanism. Lipocalin-2 was originally implicated in lung infection, as part of a pulmonary transcriptome analysis, as a gene induced by interferon gamma in a model of *Chlamydia pneumoniae* infection, but exerts protection to other pathogens such as *M. tuberculosis* and *K. pneumoniae*. Lysozyme is a cationic protein of ~14 kDa, which damages the cell walls of bacteria and fungi by hydrolyzing the β1–4 glycosidic bond between N-acetylmuramic acid and N-acetylglucosamine, which are present in bacterial peptidoglycan and fungal chitin, respectively. The importance of lysozyme is confirmed during *K. pneumoniae* or *P. aeruginosa* infection where lysozyme deficient mice have a reduced clearance of bacteria compared to their wild-type controls.

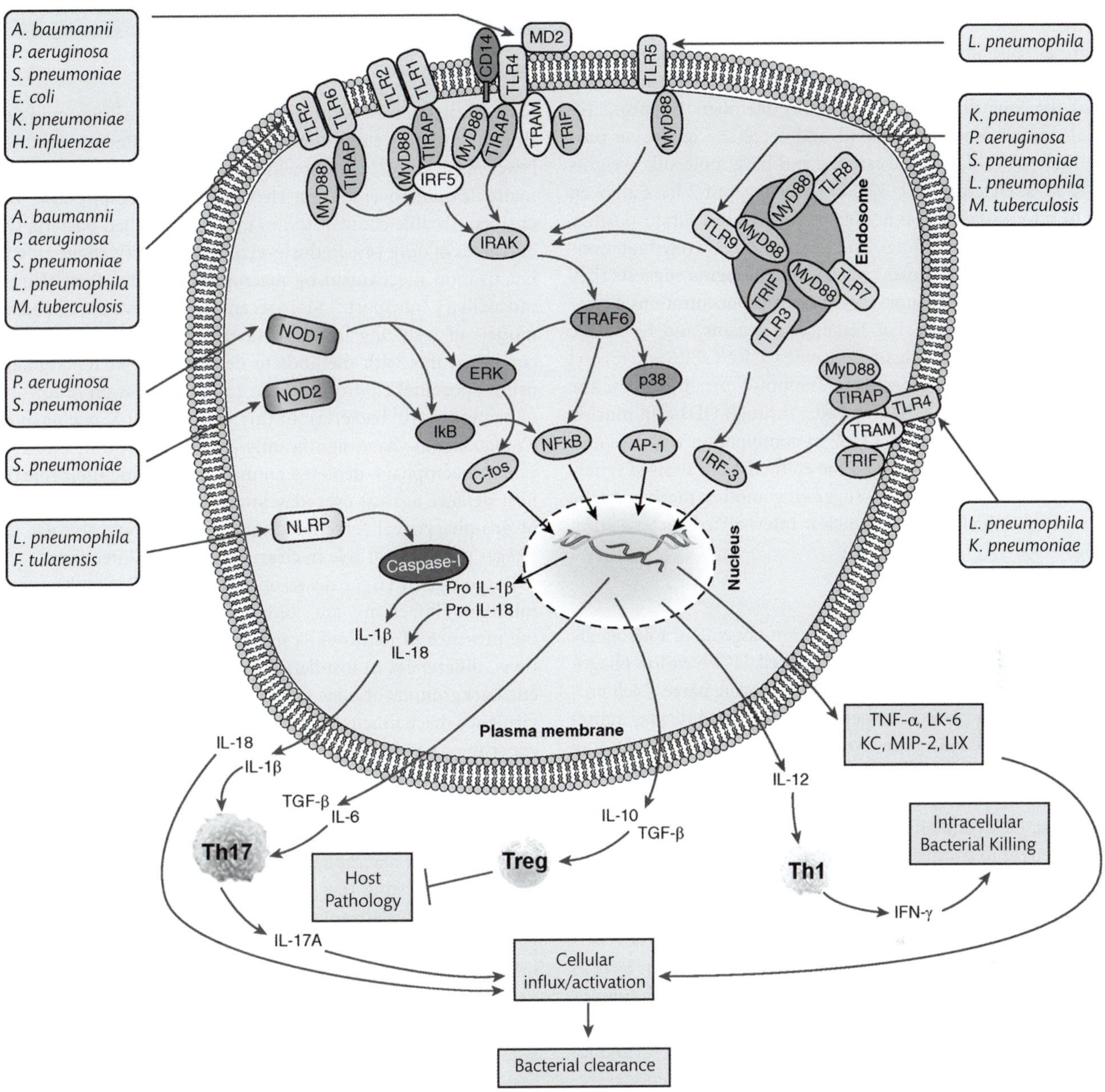

Figure 4.3 Signalling cascades on activation of pattern-recognition receptors by pulmonary pathogens. Plasma membrane–bound Toll-like receptors (TLRs) (TLR1, 2, 4, and 5) and endosome membrane–bound TLRs (TLR9) recognize bacteria in the lungs. After bacterial recognition, TLR2 (with TLR1 or 6), TLR4 (in association with MD-2 and CD14), TLR5, and TLR9 recruit MyD88, whereas TLR2 and TLR4 recruit both MyD88 and Toll-IL-1R domain-containing adapter protein (TIRAP). All of these TLRs activate IL-1 receptor-associated kinase (IRAK) after MyD88 recruitment, followed by recruitment of tumour necrosis factor receptor–associated factor 6 (TRAF6), ultimately resulting in activation of the transcription factor nuclear factor-kB (NF-kB) and mitogen-activated protein kinases (MAPKs). MAPK activation, in turn, results in the induction of transcription factors AP-1 and c-fos. In addition, TLR3 and TLR4 recruit the adaptor TIR-domain-containing adapter-inducing IFN-β (TRIF), ultimately leading to IRF3-mediated IFN-a/b and inducible nitric oxide synthase (iNOS) production through the intermediate signalling molecule TRAM, which is the bridging adaptor for TRIF-mediated signalling. In addition, pulmonary bacterial pathogens release ligands during infection that are recognized by nucleotide-binding oligomerization domains (NODs) and activate subsequent signalling pathways leading to NF-κB activation. Furthermore, when stimulated by ligands, the NOD-like receptor proteins (NLRP) induce activation of effector caspase-1, which cleaves the pro forms of IL-1β and IL-18. In turn, cytokine activation results in differentiation of naive T cells into Th1, Th17, or regulatory T cells (Tregs), thereby leading to pulmonary host defence or, in the case of Treg accumulation, resulting in host pathology. *A. baumannii, Acinetobacter baumannii; E. coli, Escherichia coli; F. tularensis, Francisella tularensis; H. influenzae, Haemophilus influenzae; K. pneumoniae, Klebsiella pneumoniae; L. pneumophila, Legionella pneumophila; M. tuberculosis, Mycobacterium tuberculosis; P. aeruginosa, Pseudomonas aeruginosa; S. pneumoniae, Streptococcus pneumoniae*. See plate section.

Small Anti-microbial Peptides

There are at least three families of small anti-microbial peptides, including (i) defensins; (ii) the one human cathelicidin, LL-37; and (iii) the four disulphide core family members trappin-2 (c-terminal domain known as elafin) and secretory leukocyte protease inhibitor (SLPI). All are cationic and have molecular weights below 12 kDa. Defensins, LL-37, SLPI, and trappin-2 have all been shown to have broad anti-microbial action against Gram positive and negative organisms, fungi, and viruses at relatively high concentrations in the micromolar range. Current dogma suggests they also have immunomodulatory activities at concentrations below their antimicrobial action. For instance, defensins and LL-37 are chemotactic through binding of monocyte CCR2/CCR6 and formyl peptide receptor-like-1, respectively. Trappin-2 can up-regulate the neutrophil chemokines, MIP-2 and KC, through CD14, in murine *P. aeruginosa* lung infection.[14] LL-37 in combination with live cultures of *P. aeruginosa* that invaded the epithelial cell showed synergistic increases in cell apoptosis, suggesting another mechanism by which anti-microbial peptides can clear internalized bacteria from the lung.[15]

Dendritic Cells

The ability of the lung to differentiate immunogenic or tolerogenic responses is the major role of the dendritic cell. DCs have low phagocytic capacity, high antigen presentation, stimulate naive T cell proliferation given the correct antigenic response, and display subset and tissue-specific maturation dynamics over human life. DCs of the respiratory system sample material within the airway, migrate to regional lymph nodes, and present antigen to rare antigen-specific T cells. Thus, DCs reside in the lung mucosa and parenchyma, and they are thought to comprise at least three different subsets termed 'myeloid DC' (mDC) type 1 (BDCA-1 (CD1c) +/HLA-DR+), myeloid DC type 2 (BDCA-3+/HLA-DR+), and plasmacytoid DC (BDCA-2+/CD123+). Functionally, mDC1 and mDC2 cell surface expression of TLR-2 is the most significant at protein level as stimulation produces pro-inflammatory cytokines such as tumour necrosis factor (TNF), IL-1, IL-8, and IL-6. In contrast, pDCs express TLR-7 and TLR-9 and release pro-inflammatory cytokines and IFN in response to imiquimod and CpG oligonucleotides, respectively. Interestingly, mDCs produce robust T cell proliferation responses, whereas pDCs have virtually none (with mDC2 having intermediate activity)[16], leading to the suggestion that mDCs are involved in a full adaptive immune response to bacteria and viruses whereas pDCs may be involved in maintaining tolerance to less dangerous inhaled antigens. It is also clear that resolution of primary lung infection leads to DCs that are functionally impaired in their ability to activate the correct T cell subsets, resulting in long-term immunosuppression and susceptibility to secondary invasive infections.[17] Recent research has addressed the issue of how DCs submerged underneath an epithelial monolayer defined by tight junctions gain access to antigen. Novel mechanisms in rat trachea show that intraepithelial DCs extend their processes ('snorkelling' or 'periscoping') between epithelial cells into the airway lumen for antigen sampling.[18] These observations were confirmed in an air–liquid interface model using both alveolar and bronchial epithelial cells showing that penetration of the epithelial cell monolayer was at the tight junction.

Alveolar/Respiratory Zone

Macrophages

Early studies of host pathogen interaction in the lung could demonstrate the presence of human pathogens (e.g. Pneumococci) in the lower respiratory tract following aerosolization together with a dramatic clearance over the first 4 h of infection.[19] Despite 80%–90% decreases in viable counts, studies using ^{32}P-labelled bacteria showed decreases of only 14% in the level of radioactivity, suggesting a local inactivation mechanism by macrophages rather than removal by mucociliary transport.[20] More recent studies have developed animal models of resolving infection in the absence of neutrophils and combined this with methods to deplete alveolar macrophages by using liposomal clodronate prior to administration of low inocula of bacteria ($<10^4$ bacteria). In this setting, both *S. pneumoniae* and *K. pneumoniae* have significantly attenuated clearance rates in alveolar macrophage-depleted animals, confirming their role in lung host defence against everyday low-grade infections and aspiration of oro-pharyngeal secretions during sleep. Thus, alveolar macrophages play a major role in clearing low-grade infections.

Responses to larger doses of bacteria ($>10^5$), resulting in more fulminant infections, are complicated by many factors not least the presence of neutrophils in both resolving and terminal infections, differences in instillation technique, and differences in genetic backgrounds of mice not to mention differences in pathogenic virulence mechanisms. It is clear that alveolar macrophage ablation experiments yield inconsistent findings as plenty of studies suggest positive and negative outcomes, respectively. Clarity may be offered in the ability of alveolar macrophages to undergo apoptosis. Dockrell and co-workers showed that caspase inhibition could decrease alveolar macrophage apoptosis resulting in increased bacteraemia suggesting that apoptosis is vital for microbiologic host defence.[21] But the advantage of macrophage apoptosis to the host is pathogen dependent as *Shigela flexneri* induces macrophage apoptosis to evade capture,[22] whereas *M. tuberculosis* inhibit apoptosis to prolong their time within their niche environment.[23] Further to this, macrophages, unlike neutrophils and monocytes, are relatively resistant to apoptosis suggesting that only robust stimuli like infection may be suitable to induce cell death.

In the lung, resident macrophages are reported to be either 'interstitial' (IM) or 'alveolar' (AM) confirming that they are anatomically and functionally distinct. When constitutive cytokine profiles and TLR stimulation are considered, AMs produce significantly more pro-inflammatory cytokines, such as TNF, IL-1β, and IL-12p70. In contrast, IM produce significantly more anti-inflammatory cytokines such as IL-10, and IL-1ra suggesting an immunoregulatory role. This is supported by an elegant study in a mouse allergy model where IM were found to be distinct from AM and produce high levels of IL-10, inhibit lipopolysaccharide (LPS)-induced maturation and migration of DC loaded with airborne antigen, and protect against asthmatic symptoms,[24] suggesting a role in lung homeostasis.

Mast Cells

Mast cells (MCs)[25] are long-lived tissue granulocytes originally derived from bone marrow CD34+ progenitor cells. MCs have great heterogeneity throughout the bronchial tree but can be characterized based on their granule contents, namely tryptase only (MC_T), chymase only (MC_C), or tryptase and chymase (MC_{CT}). In addition, MCs can be characterized based on production of soluble mediators and chemokine receptors, such as FcRεIα, IL-9R, histidine decarboxylase, 5-lipoxygenase, LTC4 synthase, rennin VEGF, and FGF. MCs have numerous functions in host defence which include the recruitment of inflammatory cell types, such as neutrophils, through secretion of cytokines, chemokines, lipid mediators, and proteases (e.g. TNF, leukotrienes, mMCP6, and CXCL1/2). MCs can also promote the migration of DCs and T cells to the draining lymph nodes and present bacterial antigens through major histocompatibility complex class I molecules. MCs may confer direct antibacterial activity by secreting anti-microbial peptides and by forming extracellular traps (MCETs). In contrast, MCs have a long-established role in asthma and anaphylactic reactions where chronic and hypersecretion of cellular contents result in excessive inflammation on a broncho-constrictive background.[25]

Opsonins

Surfactant Proteins

To date four surfactant proteins (SPs)[26] have been identified: SP-A, SP-B, SP-C, and SP-D. They are often termed the hydrophobic proteins, SP-B and SP-C, and the hydrophilic collectins, SP-A and SP-D, that play a greater role in host defence. Collectins have a distinctive four-domain structure comprising (i) a cysteine containing N-terminal domain, (ii) a collagen-like domain with Gly-X-Y repeats, (iii) a short hydrophobic neck domain, and (iv) a C-type lectin domain involved in carbohydrate recognition (CRD). Both SP-A an SP-D bind lung pathogens and enhance macrophage phagocytosis and killing through complement, antibody- and/or scavenger-associated receptor phagocytosis. SP-A and SP-D-deficient mice showed decreased uptake of bacteria, but respiratory burst was significantly decreased in SP-A deficiency alone suggesting subtly different roles.

Secretory Immunoglobulin A

Effective sampling of the antigenic load in the airspace takes place through DC uptake and processing leading to B-cell activation and immunoglobulin (Ig) production.[27] The major antibody molecule in lung secretions is IgA (secretory IgA, sIgA), which is composed of two IgA molecules, a joining region and a secretory component (SC). However, sIgA is produced in the lung lamina propria and transported into the lung lumen across the epithelial cell barrier. This mechanism of 'transcytosis' involves the binding of sIgA to the polymeric IgA receptor (pIgAR) expressed on the basolateral membrane of the respiratory epithelium. Once bound in this manner, the IgA–pIgAR complex is transported through the epithelial cell to the apical cell membrane. Here, the pIgAR is cleaved and its extracellular domain, termed SC, is released into the lumen. Binding of SC to IgA helps stabilize the antibody and protects it from proteolytic degradation. Phalipon and colleagues demonstrated that a dimeric/polymeric IgA is more efficient when bound to SC in protecting mice against bacterial infection of the respiratory tract.

Pulmonary LPS Binding Protein (LBP) and LBP-like Molecules

Lipopolysaccharide (LPS) signals through a complex of cell surface MD-2, CD14 (LPS receptor/binding site), and TLR-4. Bacterial-derived LPS monomers form aggregates, due to their amphipathic nature, and are transferred to CD14 by LBP. The ability of LBP to transfer monomeric LPS gives it a dual role to amplify the immune response to LPS up to 1000-fold and to neutralize LPS through transfer to molecules other than CD14 (e.g. lipoproteins). Production of LBP by lung epithelial cells suggests a role in local pulmonary defence. Specifically, LBP is needed to produce a protective response against Gram negative *K. pneumoniae* but not for pneumococcal pneumonia or mycobacterial infection. Furthermore, Knapp et al. showed that LBP enables the generation of a protective immune response to low LPS doses (<100 ng) while preventing an overwhelming, potentially harmful immune response to higher doses of LPS (>10 μg).[28] Indeed, cationic host defence peptides, such as trappin-2 and SLPI, have been likened to LBP and may complement LBP during early infection or in response to low inocula of bacteria.[14]

Cellular Interplay and Lung Axes

Cellular Interplay and Lung Axes Define Our Models of Pulmonary Host Defence in the 21st Century

The days of the one 'key player' in host defence are gone. Our current understanding focuses on synergistic relationships between cell types to protect the lung. The role of the CXCL2-CXCR2 and CCL2-CCR2 chemokine axes where the ligands are secreted by epithelial cells to attract receptor bound neutrophils and monocytes respectively has already been discussed. Beneficial interactions between luminal alveolar macrophages and basolaterally situated DCs, where their cellular processes have been shown to be entwined for the sharing and processing of antigen, have been noted. This mechanism allows constant and rapid sampling of lung antigens for decisions on tolerogenic or immunogenic responses. Recently, Snelgrove et al. studied the maintenance of a lower immunogenic 'tone' in an environment of heavy antigen load and suggested that the high threshold of 'ignorance' maintained in the lung may be due to the regulatory CD200-CD200R axis.[29] Here, the negative regulator receptor (CD200R) expressed on alveolar macrophages is 'restrained' by epithelial cells expressing CD200. Indeed, in mice lacking CD200, macrophages were especially sensitive to influenza resulting in delayed resolution of infection and death.

Adaptive Immunity Encourages Cellular Interplay in Respiratory Lymphoid Tissues

Mucosal-associated lymphoid tissue (MALT) is distributed throughout the whole respiratory tree (Figure 4.4). The unpaired nasopharyngeal tonsils (adenoids) and the paired palatine tonsils are the important site for nasopharynx-associated lymphoid tissues (NALTs)[30] and contain four specialized sections: (i) the reticular crypt epithelium, (ii) the extrafollicular area, (iii) the mantle zones of lymphoid follicles, and (iv) the follicular germinal centres. The tissue is constructed with a lymphoepithelium containing microfold (M) cells separating apical and basolateral compartments. Specialized M-cells express a dramatic phenotype with a basolateral invagination forming an intraepithelial 'pocket' where DCs and lymphocytes can gain better access for antigen sampling and cell activation. M-cells express a variety of immunosensing

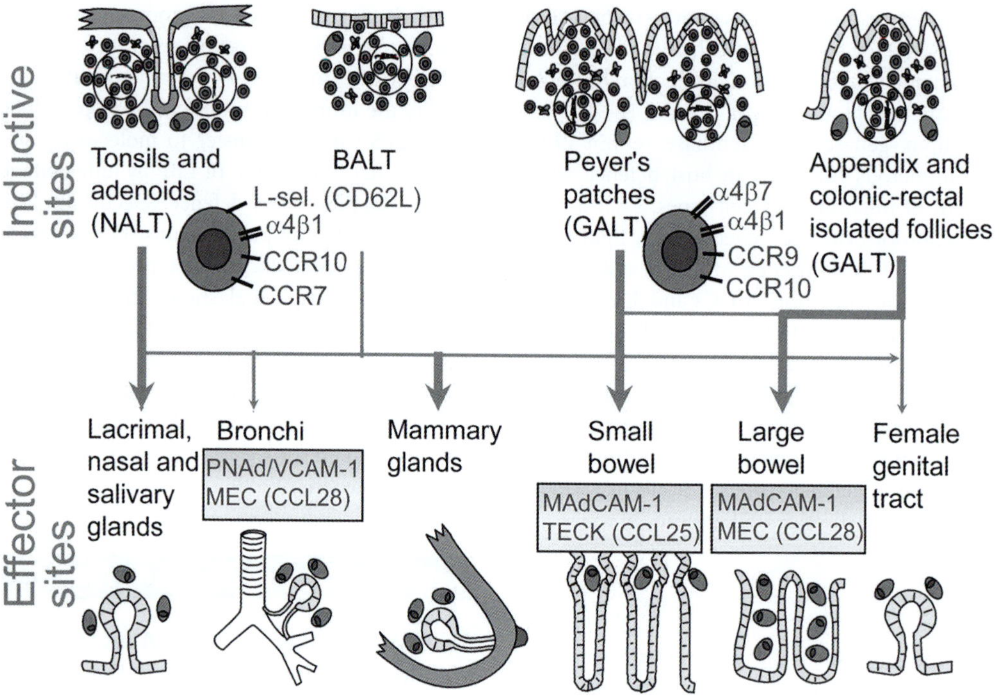

Figure 4.4 Mucosal associated lymphoid tissue in the lung: NALT, BALT, and GALT. Putative scheme for compartmentalized mucosal B-cell homing from inductive (top) to effector (bottom) sites in humans. Depicted are more or less preferred pathways (graded arrows) presumably followed by mucosal B cells of any isotype activated in nasopharynx-associated lymphoid tissue (NALT) represented by Waldeyer's lymphoid ring (including palatine tonsils and adenoids), and bronchus-associated lymphoid tissue (BALT), versus gut-associated lymphoid tissue (GALT) represented by Peyer's patches, appendix, and colonic-rectal isolated lymphoid follicles. The principal homing receptor profiles of the respective B-cell populations, and compartmentalized adhesion and chemokine cues directing their extravasation at different effector sites, are indicated (pink and blue panels). The gland-associated distribution of plasma cells (green), after terminal differentiation of extravasated mucosal B cells, is schematically depicted at the bottom.

Reproduced from Brandtzaeg P, Potential of nasopharynx-associated lymphoid tissue for vaccine responses in the airways. *American Journal of Respiratory Critical Care Medicine*, 183(12): p. 1595–604. © American Thoracic Society 2011.

molecules on their apical surface, including Glycoprotein-2 (GP-2), Tnfaip-2, CCL9, and Spi-B, where binding results in transcytosis and delivery of unprocessed antigen to DCs on the basolateral side. The MALT tissues of the conducting and respiratory zones are often referred to as bronchial-associated lymphoid tissue (BALT). BALT is rich in B-cell follicles with surrounding parafollicular zones rich in T cells, DCs, and HEVs. The B-cell follicles contain tight clusters of IgD+ B cells in a network of stromal follicular DCs expressing CD21, CXCL13, and lymphotoxin-β receptor. MALT tissues in the lung are often termed iBALT to emphasize their inductive nature. Thus, iBALT is often observed in inflammatory and infectious lung diseases, such as COPD, asthma, and pulmonary fibrosis.

Lung Microbiome Interactions: The Gut/Lung Axis

Historically, the lungs of healthy humans were believed to be sterile, based on results of classical, culture-based studies.[31] However, recent culture-independent methods demonstrate that the lungs of healthy never-smokers are inhabited by very low numbers of incredibly diverse bacterial communities (Figure 4.5). While results from published studies differ, *Proteobacteria*, *Firmicutes*, and *Bacteroidetes* are most commonly identified at the phylum level. At the genus level, *Pseudomonas*, *Streptococcus*, *Prevotella*, *Fusobacteria*, and *Veillonella* predominate, with lesser contributions from potential pathogens including *Haemophilus* and *Neisseria*. The biomass of the lung microbiome as detected by BAL or PSB remains greater than controls but less than the upper respiratory tract. The community resembles those in the mouth rather than those of the nose despite the lung having approximately half the number of species as the mouth. It is also clear that intra-subject variation is considerably less than inter-subject variation. While these generalizations give a good basic foundation, it is only over the last few years that it has become clear that respiratory commensals may regulate susceptibility to lung infections through interaction with host immune system.

There is an underlying paradigm that a certain proportion of inhaled antigen, including particles and microorganisms (10^4–10^6/m^3 of air), passing through the airways reaches the gut through microaspiration. In turn, PAMPs such as LPS released in the gut enter the portal circulation where the liver can release them into the systemic circulation and reach the lung. The mechanisms influencing gut-mediated lung immunity or vice versa are only now being established but involve (i) TLR activation. Ichinohe and colleagues showed that a single dose of LPS delivered intra-rectally, restored an immune response in the lung of influenza infected mice[32]; (ii) NLR activation. Potent NLR-stimulating bacteria in the upper airway (e.g. *S. aureus* and *S. epidermidis*) and intestinal microbiota (e.g. *Lactobacillus reuteri* and *Enterococcus faecalis*) promote resistance to lung infection through Nod2 and GM-CSF. (iii) T and B lymphocyte homing. Lung DCs can specifically up-regulate the expression of the gut-homing integrin α4β7 on T cells, which guide migration to the GI tract. In addition, intra-nasal immunization

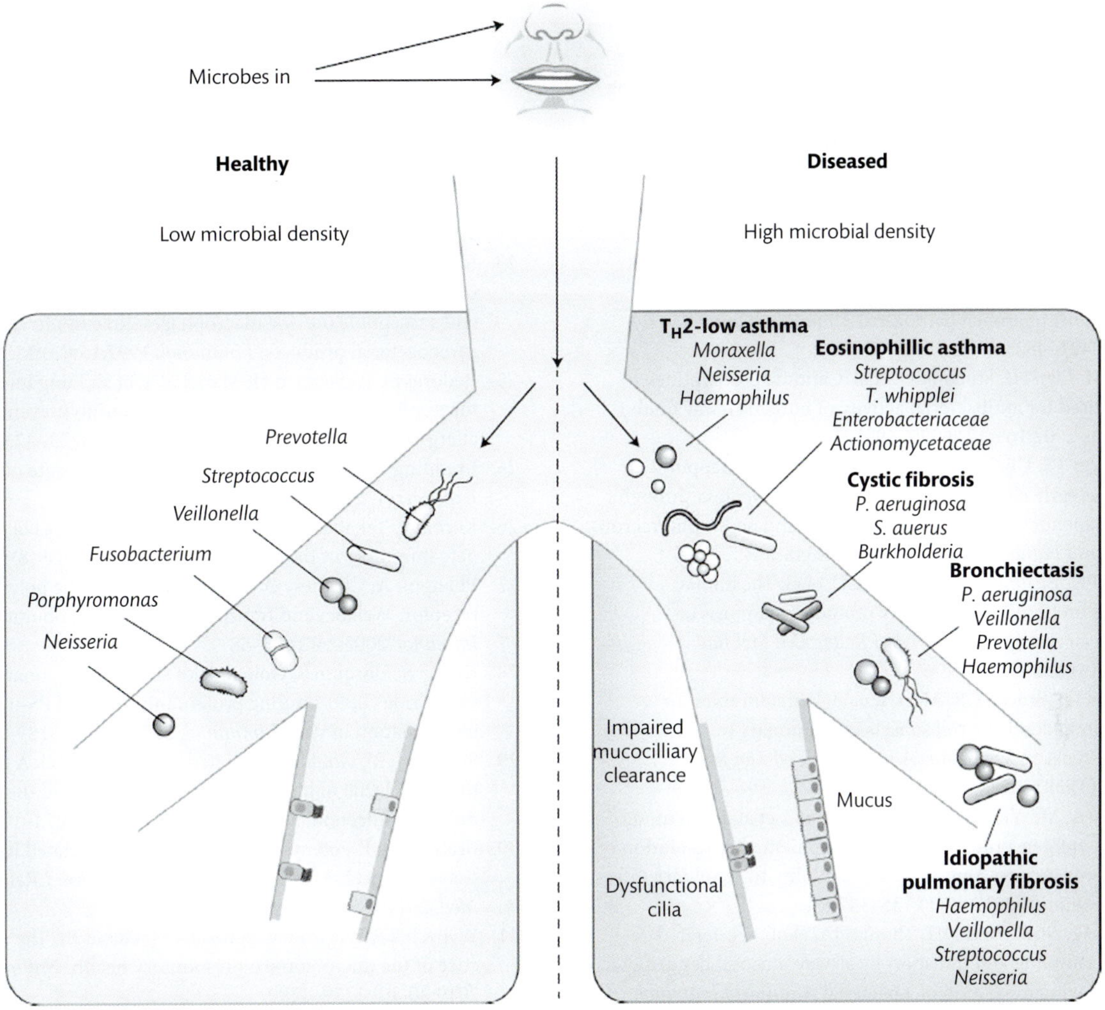

Figure 4.5 Lung microbiome and cell interplays. Lung microbiota in healthy versus diseased settings. Six major genera colonize the airways of the healthy lung (left; blue lobe): *Prevotella, Streptococcus, Veillonella, Fusobacterium, Porphyromonas,* and *Neisseria*. At steady state, the microbial density in the lung is low. It has been proposed that a balance between immigration of bacteria from the upper respiratory tract (e.g. via microaspiration) and elimination of bacteria by host defence mechanisms (e.g. mucociliary transport) determines the transient nature of the lung microbiota. Enhanced bacterial propagation in the diseased lung (right; red lobe) outpaces the capacity of the airways to clear the microbes, which results in increased microbial density. Dysfunctional cilia and enhanced mucus production may contribute to reduced clearance and trapping of microbes within airways. Different respiratory conditions are characterized by dominant bacterial species (right); for example, CF is often characterized by outgrowth of *P. aeruginosa, S. aureus,* and *Burkholderia* spp.; TH2-low asthma by *Moraxella, Haemophilus,* and *Neisseria*; eosinophilic asthma by *Streptococcus, T. whipplei, Actinomycetaceae,* and *Enterobacteriaceae*; and idiopathic pulmonary fibrosis by *Haemophilus, Veillonella, Streptococcus,* and *Neisseria*.

with *Salmonella* induced protective immunity against enteric challenge with *Salmonella* and was dependent on lung DCs. Such dramatic responses have profound implications for future vaccination strategies.

Understanding the networks and cellular interplay that exist in the lung to differentiate between inhaled 'pathogens' and innocuous materials is the goal to understanding lung immunity in the 21st century.

REFERENCES

1. Wilkinson TS, Sallanave J-M, Simpson AJ. Pulmonary defence mechanisms. *Curr Res Med Rev*. 2012;**8**:149–162.
2. Doorly DJ, Taylor DJ, Gambaruto AM, et al. Nasal architecture: Form and flow. *Philos Transact A Math Phys Eng Sci*. 2008;**366**(1879):3225–3246.
3. Geppetti P, Patacchini R, Nassini R, et al. Cough: The emerging role of the TRPA1 channel. *Lung*. 2010;**188**(Suppl 1): S63–68.
4. Bonvini SJ, Belvisi MG. Cough and airway disease: The role of ion channels. *Pulm Pharmacol Ther*. 2017;**47**:21–28.
5. Bustamante-Marin XM, Ostrowski LE. Cilia and mucociliary clearance. *Cold Spring Harb Perspect Biol*. 2017;**9**(4):a028241.
6. Ridley C, Thornton DJ. Mucins: The frontline defence of the lung. *Biochem Soc Trans*. 2018;**46**(5):1099–1106.
7. Kim KC, Lillehoj EP. MUC1 mucin: A peacemaker in the lung. *Am J Respir Cell Mol Biol*. 2008;**39**(6):644–647.

8. Leiva-Juarez MM, Kolls JK, Evans SE. Lung epithelial cells: Therapeutically inducible effectors of antimicrobial defense. *Mucosal Immunol.* 2018;**11**(1):21–34.
9. Wittekindt OH. Tight junctions in pulmonary epithelia during lung inflammation. *Pflugers Arch.* 2017;**469**(1):135–147.
10. Baral P, Batra S, Zemans RL, et al. Divergent functions of Toll-like receptors during bacterial lung infections. *Am J Respir Crit Care Med.* 2014;**190**(7):722–732.
11. Strieter RM, Belperio JA, Keane MP. Cytokines in innate host defense in the lung. *J Clin Invest.* 2002;**109**(6):699–705.
12. Serbina NV, Jia T, Hohl TM, et al. Monocyte-mediated defense against microbial pathogens. *Annu Rev Immunol.* 2008;**26**:421–452.
13. Cole AM, Liao HI, Stuchlik O, et al. Cationic polypeptides are required for antibacterial activity of human airway fluid. *J Immunol.* 2002;**169**(12):6985–6991.
14. Wilkinson TS, Dhaliwal K, Hamilton TW, et al. Trappin-2 promotes early clearance of *Pseudomonas aeruginosa* through CD14-dependent macrophage activation and neutrophil recruitment. *Am J Pathol.* 2009;**174**(4):1338–1346.
15. Barlow PG, Beaumont PE, Cosseau C, et al. The human cathelicidin LL-37 preferentially promotes apoptosis of infected airway epithelium. *Am J Respir Cell Mol Biol.* 2010;**43**(6):692–702.
16. Demedts IK, Bracke KR, Maes T, et al. Different roles for human lung dendritic cell subsets in pulmonary immune defense mechanisms. *Am J Respir Cell Mol Biol.* 2006;**35**(3):387–393.
17. Roquilly A, McWilliam HEG, Jacqueline C, et al. Local modulation of antigen-presenting cell development after resolution of pneumonia induces long-term susceptibility to secondary infections. *Immunity.* 2017;**47**(1):135–147 e5.
18. Jahnsen FL, Strickland DH, Thomas JA, et al. Accelerated antigen sampling and transport by airway mucosal dendritic cells following inhalation of a bacterial stimulus. *J Immunol.* 2006;**177**(9):5861–5867.
19. Stillman EG. The presence of bacteria in the lungs of mice following inhalation. *J Exp Med.* 1923;**38**(2):117–126.
20. Green GM, Kass EH. The role of the alveolar macrophage in the clearance of bacteria from the lung. *J Exp Med.* 1964;**119**:167–176.
21. Dockrell DH, Marriott HM, Prince LR, et al. Alveolar macrophage apoptosis contributes to pneumococcal clearance in a resolving model of pulmonary infection. *J Immunol.* 2003;**171**(10):5380–5388.
22. Zychlinsky A, Prevost MC, Sansonetti PJ. Shigella flexneri induces apoptosis in infected macrophages. *Nature.* 1992;**358**(6382):167–169.
23. Rojas Lopez M, Barrera L, Puzo G, et al. Differential induction of apoptosis by virulent Mycobacterium tuberculosis in resistant and susceptible murine macrophages: Role of nitric oxide and mycobacterial products. *J Immunol.* 1997;**159**(3):1352–1361.
24. Bedoret D, Wallemacq H, Marichal T, et al. Lung interstitial macrophages alter dendritic cell functions to prevent airway allergy in mice. *J Clin Invest.* 2009;**119**(12):3723–3738.
25. Bradding P, Arthur G. Mast cells in asthma—state of the art. *Clin Exp Allergy.* 2016;**46**(2):194–263.
26. Kuroki Y, Takahashi M, Nishitani C. Pulmonary collectins in innate immunity of the lung. *Cell Microbiol.* 2007;**9**(8):1871–1879.
27. Phalipon A, Corthesy B. Novel functions of the polymeric Ig receptor: Well beyond transport of immunoglobulins. *Trends Immunol.* 2003;**24**(2):55–58.
28. Knapp S, Florquin S, Golenbock DT, et al. Pulmonary lipopolysaccharide (LPS)-binding protein inhibits the LPS-induced lung inflammation in vivo. *J Immunol.* 2006;**176**(5):3189–3195.
29. Snelgrove RJ, Goulding J, Didierlaurent AM, et al. A critical function for CD200 in lung immune homeostasis and the severity of influenza infection. *Nat Immunol.* 2008;**9**(9): 1074–1083.
30. Brandtzaeg P. Potential of nasopharynx-associated lymphoid tissue for vaccine responses in the airways. *Am J Respir Crit Care Med.* 2011;**183**(12):1595–1604.
31. Wypych TP, Wickramasinghe LC, Marsland BJ. The influence of the microbiome on respiratory health. *Nat Immunol.* 2019;**20**(10):1279–1290.
32. Ichinohe T, Pang IK, Iwasaki A. Influenza virus activates inflammasomes via its intracellular M2 ion channel. *Nat Immunol.* 2010;**11**(5):404–410.

PART 2

The Critical Care Unit

5 Organization

Judit Orosz and Steve McGoughlin

KEY MESSAGES

- The care of critically ill patients in an intensive care unit requires a specifically trained, multi-disciplinary team.
- The organization of the patients and the team will impact on patient outcomes and the sustainability and satisfaction of skilled staff providing the care.

Introduction

Intensive care units (ICUs) care for critically ill patients and function with specialized infrastructure, equipment, and staffing models using a distinct system of care. Intensive care has recently been defined as 'a multi-disciplinary and interprofessional speciality dedicated to the comprehensive management of patients who have or at risk of developing, acute, life-threatening organ dysfunction. The primary goal of intensive care is to prevent further physiological deterioration while the underlying disease is treated and resolves'.[1] However, what is provided in a hospital when a patient is cared for in an ICU varies widely around the world and is influenced by available healthcare resources, staff availability and training, jurisdictional regulations, and available infrastructure and equipment.

Patient outcomes from critical illness have improved dramatically over recent decades due to advances in clinical care and continued improvements in the training and skills of critical care healthcare providers. In addition, a substantial body of evidence now suggests that organizational factors in relation to both the hospital and the ICU may significantly influence the outcomes of critically ill patients. An example of an organizational factor that may influence the outcomes of patients is the intensity of ICU staffing with nursing and medical staff across a 24 h period.[2]

The respiratory care and ventilatory support of the critically ill patient is a core component of intensive care, and therefore, it is likely that the impact of organizational factors on the outcomes of patients requiring respiratory support is even more pronounced, particularly given the invasive nature of mechanical ventilation. In addition to the wide global variation in the delivery of intensive care, there are also significant differences in intensive care capability at the local or jurisdictional level.

Variation in the delivery of intensive care makes summarizing an optimal way of organizing the delivery of intensive care challenging. This variation also makes it problematic to compare data on critically ill patients from different systems and then be able to extrapolate which methods of intensive care organization are superior.[3] Given this heterogeneity, the literature must be interpreted with caution when providing recommendations for what is the optimal organization of an ICU. Summaries of national or geographically proximal ICU structures have been increasingly published.

Physical Infrastructure and Organization

The physical environment and equipment available to provide intensive care will significantly influence how the ICU is organized. A discrete area to provide care to critically ill patients is essential to enable the centralization of highly trained staff and technologically advanced equipment. Ideally, the physical environment of an ICU enables each patient to be cared for in their own room, although this is not always possible in older infrastructure. Jurisdictional guidelines will provide a framework for a minimum standard for a critical care bedspace, but this will include access to oxygen, suction, electricity, ventilators, and monitoring with significant inbuilt redundancy. Particularly relevant to the respiratory care of patients is access to non-invasive and invasive ventilation as well as other forms of respiratory support such as high-flow nasal oxygen and extracorporeal membrane oxygenation.[1]

Intensive care is an expensive component of the healthcare system. The cost is determined both during the care of the patient in the ICU and the increasingly recognized cost extending into the care of the patient after intensive care as they recover from their critical illness. Despite what appears a high cost, recent evidence suggests that the care provided in intensive care is cost effective.[4] It is important that the organization of ICUs needs to also include preparation and planning for the extensive care required of patients after they are discharged from ICU, including the need for rehabilitation, particularly if the patient has had a long intensive care admission or even the need for readmission to hospital. A Finnish study found that 60% of ICU survivors required readmission to hospital within the first year.[4]

Of particular importance to the respiratory care of critically ill patients is determining the appropriate method of cohorting such patients. Simplistically, ICU can be specialized or mixed. A mixed ICU cares for patients regardless of the admission diagnosis or underlying condition of the patient. Specialist ICUs have a particular clinical focus; this may remain broad such as a medical or surgical intensive care or be even more subspecialized—examples include cardiothoracic, trauma, or neurosurgical ICUs. There have been variable results from studies investigating whether there are superior outcomes from mixed or specialized ICUs. Many of these studies have apparent limitations including the use of retrospective data and significant differences in the organization of the hospital or jurisdictional healthcare systems. So, it is emphasized that intensive care is just a component of an acute healthcare system.[5–8] It is likely that the mixed results demonstrate that while there may be some improvements gained from the development of subspecialized units and teams caring for patients, the wholistic care of critically ill patients may be best provided by a team with a general skill set.

There is evidence to suggest that critically ill patients benefit from care in high-volume centres, with increasing clinical benefits in the highest-risk conditions.[9] This finding was recently demonstrated in the UK National Health Service in patients with sepsis, the major cause of primary respiratory presentations.[10] While case volume is important, the organization of ICUs is obviously dependent on the size or the number of beds available. Less than 6–8 ICU beds will lead to a low case volume and inefficiencies in terms of cost and staffing, so it is often more effective to re-arrange smaller units into one larger department. Larger units will often divide the unit into more manageable patient numbers with smaller subunits of 8–12 beds each.[11] There is limited evidence for the maximum number of patients per subunit and supervising intensive care physician, but there is reasonable data that more than 14 leads to an increase in mortality.[12]

Increasingly ICUs are taking responsibility for the care of deteriorating patients outside of the ICU either in the form of referral for admission to ICU, a rapid response team (RRT), or follow-up of discharged ICU patients.[1] RRTs are used in most hospitals in Australasia, North America, UK, and increasingly in other parts of the world. They use 'track and trigger systems' identifying abnormal observations and vital signs as calling criteria to identify deteriorating patients but also respond to staff concerns.[13] The introduction of RRTs in hospitals is associated with a decreased rate of in-hospital cardiac arrest rates and a reduction in all-cause in-hospital mortality. They have changed our approach to patient safety outside intensive care and should now be considered standard practice in hospitals.[14]

Critical Care Staff

Within each ICU there should be a multi-disciplinary team to care for the patients, which will include nursing, allied health, and medical staff in addition to multiple ancillary staff (Figure 5.1). ICUs will also rely on the input from subspecialized medical and surgical teams whenever particular clinical expertise or interventions are required.

The levels of staffing provided are based on available resources, jurisdictional guidelines, and patient acuity. For medical staffing, ICUs in many countries now utilize clinical staff specifically trained in intensive care to manage the critically ill patients. We believe it is important, as much as possible, that healthcare systems ensure their intensive care medical staff have access to specific intensive care training programs. Various models of medical staffing of ICUs have been utilized to optimize the care of critically ill patients. This has included '*closed* ICUs' where the care of the patient is the responsibility of the treating intensive care specialist and '*open*' ICUs where the care of the patient remains the responsibility of the doctor caring for the patient outside of ICU, with or without the assistance of an intensive care trained specialist while the patient is in ICU. The literature does not provide evidence to definitively support one of closed or open models of care over another; however, there is a suggestion of improved outcomes in patients with acute lung injury, who are managed in closed ICUs.[15,16] A similar outcome was also demonstrated as a cardiac ICU transitioned from an open to a closed model of care.[17] Therefore, to provide care for patients requiring invasive or non-invasive support of their respiratory system, we would strongly recommend that the care of the patient be the primary responsibility of a clinical team that has specific training in mechanical ventilation support and therefore remains under the care of an intensive care trained specialist with close collaboration with other relevant specialists—this can be termed a 'closed collaborative model'.[11,18]

Medical Staffing Pattern

The optimal medical staffing roster pattern of an ICU is uncertain. A number of studies have investigated whether in-house intensive care specialist staffing overnight improves patient mortality, with no positive effect found, although there is significant heterogeneity among the studies and the ICUs included in the research.[19–21] It is probable that looking at medical staffing in isolation is unlikely to be informative as the intensity of medical staffing during day shift is likely to influence work out of hours and overnight. In addition, and most importantly, the multi-disciplinary nature of intensive care deems it unlikely that one component of clinical care and their staffing roster will influence patient outcomes significantly, outside of the effect of the team in its entirety. Increasing the density of staffing of ICUs will increase the operational costs; however, it is important that ICUs work towards providing a staffing pattern that ensures patient safety whilst also being responsible for cost effectiveness. A recent Dutch study has suggested an increase in efficiency with increased ratio of intensivists per bed.[22] In addition, as a demonstration of the importance of the multi-disciplinary team, an international cohort study demonstrated a benefit with 24/7 intensivist cover particularly when combined with a dedicated ICU pharmacist and higher nursing autonomy.[23]

Low-intensity ICU daytime staffing can be defined as optional consultation with an intensive care specialist. In comparison, high-intensity staffing is the involvement of specialist intensive care staff trained in the care of critically ill patients.

When caring for patients requiring respiratory system organ support, we would advocate for a model that enables high-intensity daytime staffing as a minimum, with primary responsibility for patient care moved to an intensive care physician or if this is not possible then mandatory consultation with an intensive care specialist.[24]

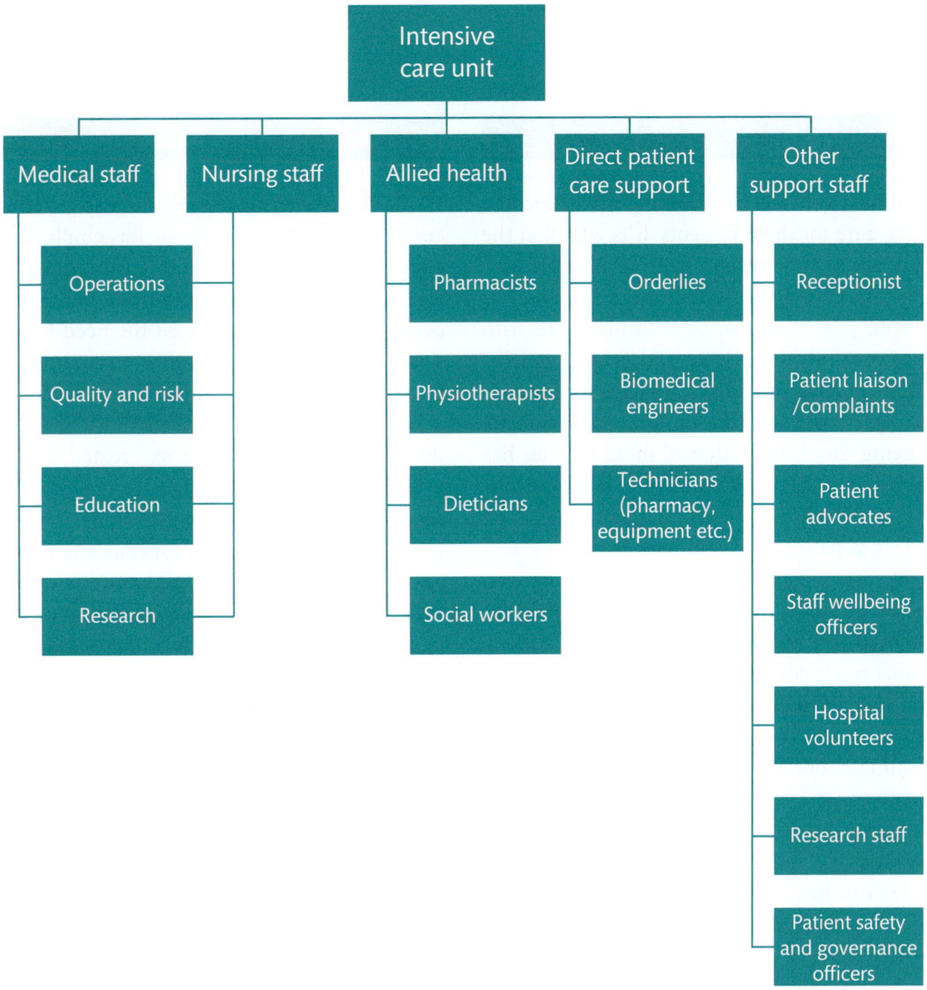

Figure 5.1 Multidisciplinary structure of intensive care.

Nurse Staffing

Specialized intensive care nursing care is a key component of the delivery of intensive care. There is international variation of the accepted ratio of nursing to patient ratios in intensive care. In Australia and the UK, ventilated patients are allocated their own critical care nurse although this is not the case in other healthcare systems either due to resource limitations or alternate healthcare policy. A review of Asian ICUs demonstrated significant heterogeneity, but the majority of ICUs functioned as closed units with a 1:1 or 1:2 nurse to patient ratio.[25] In Latin America, a large multinational study demonstrated a lack of appropriate technology for monitoring patients and a lack of appropriate specialists in medicine and nursing, particularly out of hours.[26]

Evidence suggests that improving the ratio of nurses to critical care patients improves patient outcomes[27,28] and that higher patient-to-nurse ratios lead to an increase in complications for patients and an increase in mortality.[3,12] Specific, post-graduate, training for nurses in the management of critically ill patients is vital, especially developing expertise in the management of mechanically ventilated patients. This remains a challenge in resource-poor environments where nursing training has limited availability. The utilization of trained physician assistants and advanced care practitioners, who are specifically trained in intensive care, from diverse base specialities such as nursing, physiotherapy, or other healthcare disciplines is gaining traction in the UK at least.

Processes of Care

It is not surprising that differences in the method or model of clinical care will impact patient outcomes. Processes that drive improvements of care have been demonstrated to impact the outcomes for critically ill patients. Examples include improving team communication either via a daily meeting of relevant clinical staff or a checklist of vital components of care.[27]

Regardless of the organization of the ICU, standardized protocols including care bundles and order sets to facilitate processes in the ICU are strongly recommended. This needs to include measuring outcomes; traditionally, this has involved measuring mortality, which often requires large samples to demonstrate any significant change.[29,30] Clinical protocols, pathways, and checklists are all best practice strategies for increasing the likelihood of the provision of better evidence-based and standardized care. This also enables and supports the autonomy of the ICU multidisciplinary team.[18] As an example, several studies have demonstrated an improvement in patient mortality with the addition of dedicated pharmacists to the intensive care multi-disciplinary team.[30]

Patient and Staff Well-being

Despite the severity of illness suffered by patients in ICU and the reliance on technology to care for these patients, it is vital that the human and emotional needs of patients and their families are also met.[31] In organizing and developing an ICU team, a key component, is ensuring the ability for the team to communicate with families and patients respectfully, effectively and empathetically. Examples of interventions include open door policies for families of ICU patients, humanized infrastructure design, and a holistic focus on patient well-being. Implementation of these policies has clearly been impacted by the COVID-19 pandemic; however, improved use of technology such as video communication has been used to mitigate the effect of patient and family isolation as much as possible.[31]

In addition to empathy and effective communication with patients and their families, a focus must be care of healthcare workers to ensure sustainable quality clinical care and prevent burnout of staff, which is common in critical care environments. A focus on 'displaying kindness and concern for all individuals who are part of the healthcare environment, not only patients and their families, is a necessity and the path toward building an excellent healthcare system'.[32] It is well recognized that ICU is a stressful working environment with a high prevalence of mental health issues for staff. The ongoing COVID-19 pandemic has emphasized this with increasing rates of anxiety, depression, and post-traumatic stress among ICU staff.[33] Unfortunately, there is a lack of quality evidence to assist in selecting interventions that are beneficial to the mental health or resilience of intensive care staff. It is likely that organizational factors are extremely important in the well-being of staff as this has been demonstrated in studies on other workforces in high stress environments. When determining the organization of an ICU, particularly given the current COVID-19 pandemic and the risk of ongoing strain, consideration of several basic staff needs is warranted. Thus, promoting affirmation within the team, moderating work hours, and providing targeted mental health support are important.

ICU Collaboration and Regionalization

Increasingly there is recognition that single, potentially isolated ICUs will vary widely in their clinical capability and that this poses a risk for patients, particularly in relation to volume capability and safety relationships. Therefore, there has been a move to regionalize critical care services so that ICUs can work together to develop areas of specialization and then ensure each patient receives the care they require. This is particularly relevant in complex diseases that are rare or those that require a high level of resourcing to care for the patient.[18] How this is operationalized in local regions will vary considerably based on funding, geography, and healthcare jurisdictions. For example, critical care networks are well established in the UK. Surveillance and tracking of bed availability, patient acuity status, and staffing between hospitals within and more broadly across networks can enable timely matching and transfer of patients to resource availability. This has developed during the COVID pandemic as discussed below.

ICU Organization and COVID-19

While emergency planning is discussed in the following chapter, the current COVID-19 pandemic has emphasized the need for the organization of an ICU to both ensure the quality care of patients as well as ensuring the safety and well-being of staff. The COVID pandemic has also demonstrated the need for high numbers of intensive care trained staff, and this 'surge capacity' needs to be factored into the organization and planning of ICUs.

Many if not all ICUs globally have had their capacity tested with the increase of ICU patients created by COVID-19. Units have needed to implement previously unplanned surge capacity to ensure access to ICU. In a large Belgian study, it was found that the 'proportion of supplementary beds specifically created for COVID-19 care to the previously existing total number of ICU beds was associated with increased in-hospital mortality among invasively ventilated patients'.[34] A Brazilian study found that hospital level structural factors, such as funding model and hospital occupancy strain, were more influential on patient mortality than a patient's individual comorbidities.[35] Further, in a multi-centre US study it was found that patients with COVID-19 who were treated in ICUs during periods of increased COVID-19 ICU demand had increased mortality as opposed to those treated during periods of low demand.[36]

We would suggest, most importantly, that this data emphasizes the need for public health measures, such as COVID-19 vaccination, to reduce the need for patients to require intensive care from COVID-19. In addition, health services need to work towards providing the safest care possible for critically ill patients in ICU by ensuring that individual ICUs, as much as possible, are able to maintain their usual model of care and avoid periods of excessive strain. Therefore, it is vital that health services and jurisdictions collaborate to ensure that where there is strain on intensive care systems the clinical load is balanced between services as much as possible. Ideally, this would be done before patients require intensive care.

It is essential that local and regional ICU pandemic plans are developed and resourced. While ensuring adequate equipment is available to provide critical care for patients is clearly vital, the global experience is that providing trained staff to care for patients is even more challenging. Methods to ensure appropriate staffing provision to ICUs require careful consideration, especially as there is a significant risk of staff furlough or even COVID-19 infection in ICU and this needs to be taken into account.

Maintaining the general skills of intensive care clinicians, particularly nursing and medical staff, even in specialized ICUs needs to be a priority given the recent strain on intensive care services. This coupled with pre-emptive planning and adaptability to rapidly changing scenarios is vital for ICUs managing patients in the current pandemic and also preparing for future events.[37]

The infrastructure and staffing organization of ICUs is also vital in relation to the implementation and maintenance of high infection control standards, to ensure staff safety, particularly relevant with management of COVID-19 patients. The physical environment of the unit must be such as to enable all intensive care staff to maintain rigorous infection control standards. The use of telemedicine capabilities has been enhanced in certain ICUs and broader healthcare systems during the pandemic. Thus, remote interprofessional clinical meetings with healthcare providers at the bedside have been enabled. The potential benefits are clear, although a more formal evaluation of outcomes is awaited. The current COVID-19 pandemic has also emphasized the need for the constant training and education of staff to ensure a high standard of infection control practices.

REFERENCES

1. Marshall JC, Bosco L, Adhikari NK, et al. What is an intensive care unit? A report of the task force of the World Federation of Societies of Intensive and Critical Care Medicine. *J Crit Care.* 2017;**37**:270–276.
2. Frankel SK, Moss M. The effect of organizational structure and processes of care on ICU mortality as revealed by the United States critical illness and injury trials group critical illness outcomes study. *Crit Care Med.* 2014;**42**(2):463–464.
3. Prin M, Wunsch H. International comparisons of intensive care: Informing outcomes and improving standards. *Curr Opin Crit Care.* 2012;**18**(6):700–706.
4. Jukarainen S, Mildh H, Pettila V, et al. Costs and cost-utility of critical care and subsequent health care: A multicenter prospective study. *Crit Care Med.* 2020;**48**(5):e345–e55.
5. Bukur M, Habib F, Catino J, et al. Does unit designation matter? A dedicated trauma intensive care unit is associated with lower postinjury complication rates and death after major complication. *J Trauma Acute Care Surg.* 2015;**78**(5):920–927; discussion 7–9.
6. Lombardo S, Scalea T, Sperry J, et al. Neuro, trauma, or med/surg intensive care unit: Does it matter where multiple injuries patients with traumatic brain injury are admitted? Secondary analysis of the American Association for the Surgery of Trauma Multi-Institutional Trials Committee decompressive craniectomy study. *J Trauma Acute Care Surg.* 2017;**82**(3):489–496.
7. Lott JP, Iwashyna TJ, Christie JD, et al. Critical illness outcomes in specialty versus general intensive care units. *Am J Respir Crit Care Med.* 2009;**179**(8):676–683.
8. Mielke D, Malinova V, Moerer O, et al. Does the subspecialty of an intensive care unit (ICU) has an impact on outcome in patients suffering from aneurysmal subarachnoid hemorrhage? *Neurosurg Rev.* 2019;**42**(1):147–153.
9. Nguyen YL, Wallace DJ, Yordanov Y, et al. The volume-outcome relationship in critical care: A systematic review and meta-analysis. *Chest.* 2015;**148**(1):79–92.
10. Maharaj R, McGuire A, Street A. Association of annual intensive care unit sepsis caseload with hospital mortality from sepsis in the United Kingdom, 2010–2016. *JAMA Netw Open.* 2021;**4**(6):e2115305.
11. Valentin A, Ferdinande P. Improvement EWGoQ. Recommendations on basic requirements for intensive care units: Structural and organizational aspects. *Intensive Care Med.* 2011;**37**(10):1575–1587.
12. Neuraz A, Guerin C, Payet C, et al. Patient mortality is associated with staff resources and workload in the ICU: A multicenter observational study. *Crit Care Med.* 2015;**43**(8):1587–1594.
13. Hillman KM, Chen J, Jones D. Rapid response systems. *Med J Aust.* 2014;**201**(9):519–521.
14. Solomon RS, Corwin GS, Barclay DC, et al. Effectiveness of rapid response teams on rates of in-hospital cardiopulmonary arrest and mortality: A systematic review and meta-analysis. *J Hosp Med.* 2016;**11**(6):438–445.
15. Costa DK, Wallace DJ, Kahn JM. The association between daytime intensivist physician staffing and mortality in the context of other ICU organizational practices: A multicenter cohort study. *Crit Care Med.* 2015;**43**(11):2275–82.
16. Treggiari MM, Martin DP, Yanez ND, et al. Effect of intensive care unit organizational model and structure on outcomes in patients with acute lung injury. *Am J Respir Crit Care Med.* 2007;**176**(7):685–690.
17. Miller PE, Chouairi F, Thomas A, et al. Transition from an Open to Closed Staffing Model in the Cardiac Intensive Care Unit Improves Clinical Outcomes. *J Am Heart Assoc.* 2021;**10**(3):e018182.
18. Kerlin MP, Costa DK, Kahn JM. The Society of Critical Care Medicine at 50 years: ICU organization and management. *Crit Care Med.* 2021;**49**(3):391–405.
19. Kerlin MP, Adhikari NK, Rose L, et al. An official American Thoracic Society systematic review: The effect of nighttime intensivist staffing on mortality and length of stay among intensive care unit patients. *Am J Respir Crit Care Med.* 2017;**195**(3):383–393.
20. Kerlin MP, Small DS, Cooney E, et al. A randomized trial of nighttime physician staffing in an intensive care unit. *N Engl J Med.* 2013;**368**(23):2201–2209.
21. Wilcox ME, Harrison DA, Short A, et al. Comparing mortality among adult, general intensive care units in England with varying intensivist cover patterns: A retrospective cohort study. *Critical Care.* 2014;**18**(4):491.
22. Wortel SA, de Keizer NF, Abu-Hanna A, et al. Number of intensivists per bed is associated with efficiency of Dutch intensive care units. *J Crit Care.* 2021;**62**:223–229.
23. Zampieri FG, Salluh JIF, Azevedo LCP, et al. ICU staffing feature phenotypes and their relationship with patients' outcomes: An unsupervised machine learning analysis. *Intensive Care Med.* 2019;**45**(11):1599–1607.
24. Wallace DJ, Angus DC, Barnato AE, et al. Nighttime intensivist staffing and mortality among critically ill patients. *N Engl J Med.* 2012;**366**(22):2093–2101.
25. Arabi YM, Phua J, Koh Y, et al. Structure, organization, and delivery of critical care in Asian ICUs. *Crit Care Med.* 2016;**44**(10):e940–948.
26. Estenssoro E, Alegria L, Murias G, et al. Organizational issues, structure, and processes of care in 257 ICUs in Latin America: A study from the Latin America Intensive Care Network. *Crit Care Med.* 2017;**45**(8):1325–1336.
27. Checkley W, Martin GS, Brown SM, et al. Structure, process, and annual ICU mortality across 69 centers: United States Critical Illness and Injury Trials Group Critical Illness Outcomes Study. *Crit Care Med.* 2014;**42**(2):344–356.
28. Sakr Y, Moreira CL, Rhodes A, et al. The impact of hospital and ICU organizational factors on outcome in critically ill patients: Results from the Extended Prevalence of Infection in Intensive Care study. *Crit Care Med.* 2015;**43**(3):519–526.
29. Weled BJ, Adzhigirey LA, Hodgman TM, et al. Critical care delivery: The importance of process of care and ICU structure to improved outcomes: An update from the American College of Critical Care Medicine Task Force on Models of Critical Care. *Crit Care Med.* 2015;**43**(7):1520–1525.
30. Soares M, Bozza FA, Azevedo LC, et al. Effects of organizational characteristics on outcomes and resource use in patients

with cancer admitted to intensive care units. *J Clin Oncol.* 2016;**34**(27):3315–3324.

31. Heras La Calle G, Ovies AA, Tello VG. A plan for improving the humanisation of intensive care units. *Intensive Care Med.* 2017;**43**(4):547–549.
32. Nin Vaeza N, Martin Delgado MC, Heras La Calle G. Humanizing intensive care: Toward a human-centered care ICU model. *Crit Care Med.* 2020;**48**(3):385–390.
33. Wozniak H, Benzakour L, Moullec G, et al. Mental health outcomes of ICU and non-ICU healthcare workers during the COVID-19 outbreak: A cross-sectional study. *Ann Intensive Care.* 2021;**11**(1):106.
34. Taccone FS, Van Goethem N, De Pauw R, et al. The role of organizational characteristics on the outcome of COVID-19 patients admitted to the ICU in Belgium. *The Lancet Regional Health—Europe.* 2020;**2**:100019.
35. Baqui P, Marra V, Alaa AM, et al. Comparing COVID-19 risk factors in Brazil using machine learning: The importance of socioeconomic, demographic and structural factors. *Sci Rep.* 2021;**11**(1):15591.
36. Bravata DM, Perkins AJ, Myers LJ, et al. Association of intensive care unit patient load and demand with mortality rates in US Department of Veterans Affairs Hospitals during the COVID-19 pandemic. *JAMA Netw Open.* 2021; **4**(1):e2034266.
37. Harris G, Adalja A. ICU preparedness in pandemics: Lessons learned from the coronavirus disease-2019 outbreak. *Curr Opin Pulm Med.* 2021;**27**(2):73–78.

6

Emergency Planning and Disaster Management

Richard Keays

KEY MESSAGES

- Templates exist for how to conceptualize the entire disaster management cycle.
- Each large-scale emergency is a learning opportunity and should be built into an adaptive process where lessons learned are fed back into future disaster management planning.

Introduction

This chapter describes emergency situations where more than one individual is affected by the same event—the more people affected, the more it is likely to be termed a 'disaster'. Here, the term disaster is used as the exemplar of emergencies, and these terms will be used interchangeably. From a hospital perspective, it is important to plan for different scenarios that consider whether the disaster involves affected patients alone, whether the hospital is also affected by the disaster, or whether the whole locality is impacted. This will alter the scope of which actions are possible. Definitions are such that if the local government can manage the situation, it is termed a 'local disaster'; if national government intervention is required, it becomes a 'national disaster'; if the national government is overwhelmed and other nations or transnational organisations' assistance is required, it is termed an 'international disaster'. Emergency management of specific respiratory situations is dealt with in other chapters.

Discussion around the management of disasters dates back to the 1930s, but the real focus only emerged in the 1970s when there was an increasing intolerance of the number of deaths, casualties, and economic losses associated with disaster events than previously. The focus shifted from reactive provision of relief to include proactive pre-disaster planning. What emerged was the concept of the disaster management cycle (Figure 6.1) with which governments and civil society could plan for disasters, attempt mitigation, relief response, and longer-term recovery. There have been many permutations of the cycle but, in general, they all contain a pre-disaster phase (prevention, mitigation, and preparedness) and a post-disaster phase (response, recovery, and development).

Preliminary study of the societal impact of disasters was initiated by the seminal work of Samuel Prince in 1920 after the catastrophic collision in the harbour at Halifax, Nova Scotia, of the French ship *Mont Blanc* with the Norwegian ship *SS Imo*, resulting in the former exploding and killing 2000 people and injuring a further 9000.[1] He described the initial panic and confusion, followed by emerging leaders and groups beginning to organize (military, police, etc.) to provide relief. It is noteworthy that there was sympathy and praise contained in this report—and clear identification of what was effective. He was also critical: 'There was also at times a lack of co-operation among the official committees themselves'. Friction and crises arose from time to time, which were only stopped short of scandal. They were the consequence of either assumption of authority upon the part of the subcommittees, of ineffectiveness of leadership, or of unfamiliarity with the principles of relief.

Subsequent work has tried to delineate the phases a community will go through from pre-disaster to recovery.

Powell described eight phases[2]:

1. Identification
2. Warning
3. Threat
4. Impact
5. Inventory
6. Rescue
7. Remedy
8. Recovery

A pre-disaster phase encompasses a community's identification and understanding of a specific hazard that threatens them. This is followed by a warning precautionary stage of community activity to address the potential threat. Conceiving of the threat leads to the community focusing on surviving the disaster. An assessment of the risk a hazard presents is really a calculation of the likelihood of a specific threat combined with an estimate of what consequences that might ensue. Reduction of either likelihood or consequences reduces risk and vice versa. When the disaster impacts it results in destruction and injury/death. The next stage is the inventory stage when the community takes stock of the scale of destruction and gets

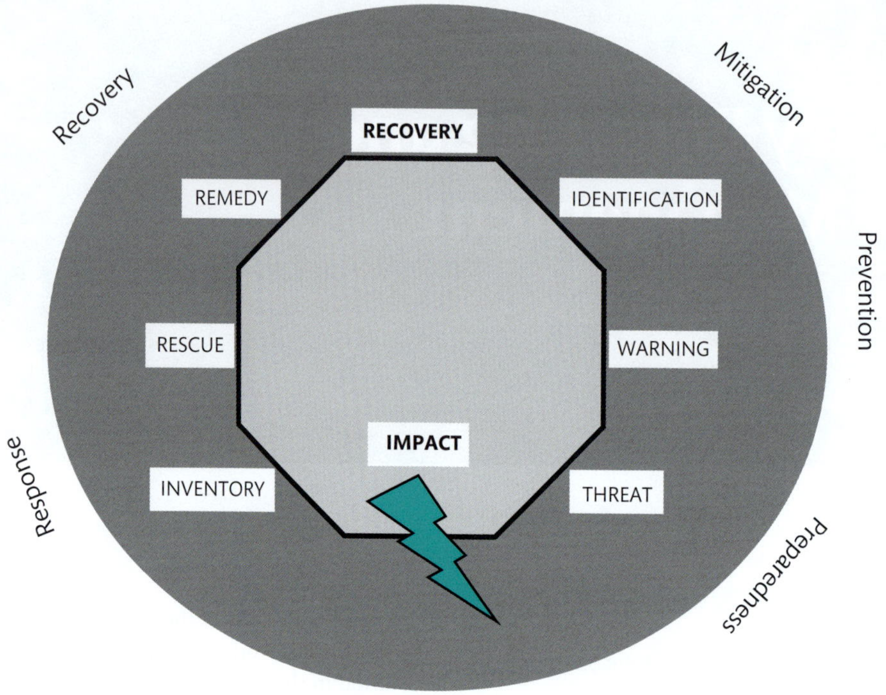

Figure 6.1 The disaster management cycle.
Data from Powell, J.W., 1954, *An introduction to the natural history of disaster*. College Park: University of Maryland Disaster Research Project.

some idea of the steps required to deal with the disaster event. The rescue phase follows, usually spontaneous efforts by the survivors at aid, search and rescue. Remedy occurs when more organised professional help arrives, in the shape of trained emergency providers. Finally, recovery begins when the community seeks to re-establish normal operations.

Subsequently, work has suggested that the impact phase could be much improved with specific pre-disaster training.

Disaster risk reduction (DRR) as a concept grew out of the Cold War organization of Civil Defence as a centrally led response to threats with civilian protection the core focus. In 1999, the United Nations created an International Strategy for Disaster Reduction at the end of the declared *Disaster Reduction Decade* (1990–1999), now named as the United Nations Office for Disaster Risk Reduction. The mandate was to coordinate disaster reduction strategies and to ensure synergies among the disaster reduction activities of the UN system and regional organizations and activities in socio-economic and humanitarian field. In 2005, the five Hyogo Framework for Action guiding principles were articulated and agreed[3]:

- Ensure that DRR is a national and a local priority with a strong institutional basis for implementation
- Identify, assess, and monitor disaster risks and enhance early warning
- Use knowledge, innovation, and education to build a culture of safety and resilience at all levels
- Reduce the underlying risk factors
- Strengthen disaster preparedness for effective response at all levels

This has now been superseded by the Sendai Framework for Disaster Risk Reduction that additionally seeks to assist developing countries and to build back better when disaster does strike.[4] Ambitious targets have been set to be achieved by 2030.

Disasters are accompanied by terminology that needs defining. The etymology of the word 'disaster' literally means 'bad star', which reflects the pre-enlightenment, superstitious belief that certain astrological events could portend crises. A 'hazard' is an event, phenomenon, or human activity that may cause loss of life, injury, property damage, social and economic disruption, or environmental degradation. 'Risk' can never be truly eliminated, but it can be reduced—it is defined as the likelihood of an adverse event coupled with the consequences of that event. 'Risk reduction' is merely the effort to reduce either the likelihood or the consequences of these hazards. 'Vulnerability' is formed of conditions that increase the susceptibility of a community to the impact of hazards; these can be physical, social, environmental, etc. 'Resilience' is the ability of a community to avoid losses in the event of a disaster and continue functioning—adopting structural, social, and organizational measures, together with learned experience from previous events.

A hazard can be considered in two broad categories: natural or anthropogenic. Natural hazards fall into three categories: geophysical—earthquakes, landslides, avalanche, etc.; hydro-meteorological—flood, drought, wildfires, storms, etc.; and finally biological—epidemics, infestations, stampede, etc. Anthropogenic hazards can be technological—engineering failures, transport disasters, etc.—or sociological—wars, riots, terrorism, etc. Large-scale or severe hazards are described as disasters. Around 94% of natural disasters are caused by earthquakes, tropical cyclones, floods, and droughts. The remainder of this chapter focuses on each facet of the disaster cycle and highlights instances where there were problems in the pre- or post-disaster activities.

Pre-disaster

Identification

This might appear to be the hardest part of the disaster planning cycle. Specific threats are often hard to identify, but broad concepts can still be brought to bear. Sadly, there is a tendency to ignore the lessons of the past.

A fire occurred at King's Cross Underground Station, London, UK, in 1987. A lit match falling through the gaps in a wooden escalator igniting the grease and accumulated rubbish underneath led to the death of 31 individuals, with many more seriously injured.[5] The event signified a failure to identify, heed the warning, and then respond to the threat. A fire three years previously at Oxford Circus Station, London, UK, had highlighted inadequacies. This was a warning which was not fully appreciated at the time—after all, only one person had died from fire on the underground since the Second World War. An investigation into this event noted that it was only luck that had prevented any serious injury—a comment revived after the King's Cross fire as 'the night when London Underground's luck ran out'. The Oxford Circus fire investigation concluded that it was most likely started by a discarded, lit cigarette at platform level. Smoking had been banned on tube trains a few months before the fire, and the investigation recommended extending the ban to the entirety of the underground system—which, apart from ground level platforms, it was. However, it was widely flouted. One of the main recommendations of the Fennell report was that improvements should be made to the communications systems: station staff did not have enough radios, underground reception, and transmission was hampered and the line controller phone was engaged.[6] This was finally addressed after the terrorist bombings in London on 7 July 2005 when a common emergency radio (Airwave) for emergency services was introduced—the contract expired in 2019 and was superseded by Emergency Services Network (ESN). A certain astonishment that this had not been prioritised for 17 years was expressed by the latter incident review.

That would seem to be a straightforward simple message of investigating, making recommendations and completing them or not. It gets a little more intriguing when one digs deeper. In 1903, a fire on a wooden escalator on the Paris Metro resulted in 83 deaths. As a result, the Board of Trade recommended wood should be removed from underground stations, but metal escalators were not available until the 1960s. From 1956 to 1988, there had been 400 fires on underground escalators. Staff had had minimal safety training. The only fire hydrant in King's Cross station was behind temporary hoarding, as was the station layout plans. A water-fog system over the escalators could have been activated, but the switch was behind a locked door and none of the staff knew it existed. There were no smoke detectors to pinpoint the fire location. The Oxford Circus fire had concluded that the best way to evacuate in a fire was by train—but trains were told not to stop at the station. And finally, a last tragedy was the failure to appreciate the gravity of a situation as it develops. There was 20 min from the start of the fire until the flashover fireball emerged from the trench of the elevator with catastrophic consequences—a quicker reaction to the first report of a fire may have saved many more lives. As the Fennell enquiry commented—until the fireball 20 min after the first alert of a fire not a single drop of water had been applied.

Warning

Severe Acute Respiratory syndrome due to a coronavirus-1 (SARS-1), the influenza viral strain H1NI causing Swine Flu, and the middle eastern respiratory syndrome (MERS), also due to a pathogenic coronavirus MERS-CoV, with respiratory predilection, were warnings that thankfully did not materialize into a global pandemic. This was not the case in SARS CoV-2, and we are still living through it at the time of writing. Lessons from history pointed to the inevitability of a pandemic—Spanish 'Flu had claimed 20 million victims a century ago.

In October 2016, the UK war-gamed the country's pandemic preparedness. *Exercise Cygnus* involved 950 officials from central and local government, NHS organizations, prisons, and local emergency response.[7] A fictitious, highly infectious influenza 'Swan Flu' was imagined that would cause 400,000 deaths. It was specifically designed to cause services to collapse and identified a number of vulnerabilities. The exercise predicted a shortage of ventilators, personal protective equipment, health workers, and bed capacity. The report was finally published in October 2020. Specifically, it noted that there was no central oversight of all the numerous preparedness plans in different organizations—perhaps a legacy of the 'pandemic' that the 2009 H1N1 scare had occasioned. It also identified that the privately run care home sector had unknown capacity but was likely already under significant strain with limited capability to support the NHS.

Exercise Alice was a one-day table-top exercise conducted in the same year and was more specifically relevant to a coronavirus outbreak of a MERS-CoV-type infection commencing in London and Birmingham. Commissioned by the Chief Medical Officer at the time it involved health and government officials, including officials from the cabinet office, and resulted in a 23-page report. The exercise predicted a shortage of personal protective equipment (PPE) and the need to stockpile it. It also highlighted the need to develop a proper isolation and test and trace strategy. The report was finally released under freedom of information laws in October 2021.

At the time of writing, the death toll from COVID-19 worldwide is >~6 million. Preparedness does require the preparedness to read, and act on, reports on preparedness.

Threat

Planning for a disaster involves a proper assessment of the nature of the threat. This is probably best exemplified during the Cuban missile crisis. President Kennedy's Generals could not seem to recognize any intermediate positions between conventional warfare and a fully committed nuclear war when tensions in Berlin increased. When it was suggested that 'We should plan for a war of nerve, of demonstration and of bargaining, not of tactical target destruction', it seemed like the driver who throws his steering wheel out the window during a game of 'chicken', but it impressed Kennedy. Crisis gaming followed adopting this strategy, with the result that there were no scenarios that emerged where protagonists would initiate a nuclear conflict. Kruschev, and Kennedy, eventually backed down during the actual crisis.[8]

Impact

It is required to assess whether the impact is natural or anthropogenic.

Post-disaster Response

A major incident is defined as 'An event or situation with a range of serious consequences which requires special arrangements to be implemented by one or more emergency responder agency'. The multi-agency emergency response in the UK is based around a model described as Gold, Silver, and Bronze commands. This delineates a separation between strategic, tactical, and operational commands. Most incident management systems mirror this arrangement to a greater or lesser degree, including the Federal Emergency Management Agency (FEMA) in the USA.[9] The Gold commander is not necessarily on site but is in control of the available resources. Silver commander is expected to formulate actions based on the strategic priorities of Gold and is also not on site. Bronze commander is located at the scene and controls the resources on site.

The Joint Emergency Services Interoperability Principles has developed five core principles:

Co-locate
Communicate
Coordinate
Jointly understand risk
Share situational awareness

- **Co-locate**: Various service commanders can fail to make rapid enough contact with each other and co-locating them can speed identification. If this is not possible, then telecom contact should be established.
- **Communicate**: A dedicated ESN exists for such situations. Service jargon is to be avoided and plain language should be used, with factual information. There is a cabinet office lexicon of civil protection terminology available here.[10] The commonly used framework for communicating between services and scenes is the M/ETHANE acronym—which stands for Major incident declared, Exact location, Type of incident, Hazards present or suspected, Access routes that are safe and available rendezvous points, Number, type, and severity of casualties, and emergency services required or present on site.
- **Coordinate:** Category 1 responders are relevant local authority and governmental bodies, who have a requirement to prepare for emergencies, and emergency service providers and the wider health service. One of the conclusions of the London Assembly report of the 7 July Review Committee was that detailed emergency plans existed, were robust, and were drilled and practised to a commendable level, but they were service-specific. They met the needs of the service but 'lacked an outward focus that took into account the needs of their client groups'.[11]

Understanding the risk and sharing situational awareness develops as events unfold. The Civil Contingencies Act 2004 declared that Category 1 responders must collectively learn and implement lessons from exercises, share lessons learned from emergencies and exercises in other parts of the UK, and make sure that those lessons are acted on to improve local arrangements. There is an obligation to share learning across multiple agencies, including counter terrorism. It also includes the devolved administrations. This Joint Organizational Learning model was created to focus more on the 'what' and the 'why' of incidents and exercises rather than assigning blame. This forms part of the modern approach to disaster management where *Adaptive Management* is the concept that all aspects of a disaster event be treated like an experiment, with areas where planning and subsequent response went well and other areas where it did not. The aim is to be nimble and flexible in disaster response as each event will be unique and nuanced.

Inventory

Taking into account the resources available to treat affected individuals has sometimes been an area where weaknesses have manifested. A frequent mistake is to direct casualties to one or two hospitals that rapidly become overwhelmed while other nearby hospitals are standing idly by. Numerous UK examples exist: The 1988 Clapham (London) Rail disaster where 35 people died and over 400 were injured—the patients were directed to St George's Hospital that was barely able to cope and urgent treatments on victims were postponed as the backlog increased. The casualties from the bombing of the Admiral Duncan Public House in 1999 where 3 people were killed and 79 were injured were mostly directed to ONE London Teaching Hospital. This has now been addressed and all receiving hospitals are notified to be on standby—the NHS in London managed to clear 1200 beds in the first three hours after the major incident was declared on 7 July 2005 following the London bombings.

Another problem encountered in the immediate aftermath of a disaster is the information overload that emergency responders have to deal with. A lot of it is speculative, unverifiable, and in such volume emergency telephone and radio systems are jammed. This hampered efforts in both the terrorist attacks in the major urban conurbations of New York and London. Reliance on mobile phones has become widespread among emergency responders, but networks can be quickly become overburdened—Vodafone experienced a 250% increase demand in the first hour of the London bombings. There are systems to restrict mobile phone access to networks within specific areas, but it is expensive and could lead to greater public panic.

The FEMA outline of resource management during an incident is summarized in Figure 6.2.

Rescue

9/11 emergency responders: The World Trade Centre actually consisted of seven buildings connected through an underground mall, the most iconic of which were the North and South Towers. At 110 storeys high (411 m) and 63.5 m^2, each tower contained 3 central stairwells, which ran essentially from top to bottom, and 99 elevators. Generally, elevators originating in the lobby ran to 'sky lobbies' on higher floors, where additional elevators carried passengers to the tops of the buildings.[12]

Stairwells A and C ran from the 110th floor to the mezzanine level of the lobby. Stairwell B ran from the 107th floor to level B6, six floors below ground, and was accessible from the West Street lobby level, just below the mezzanine. All three stairwells ran essentially straight up and down, except for two deviations in stairwells A and C where the staircases ended, a transfer hallway with closed smoke doors then had to be crossed to reach the continuation of the staircases. Doors leading from tenant space into the stairwells were never kept locked; re-entry from the stairwells was generally possible on at least every fourth floor.

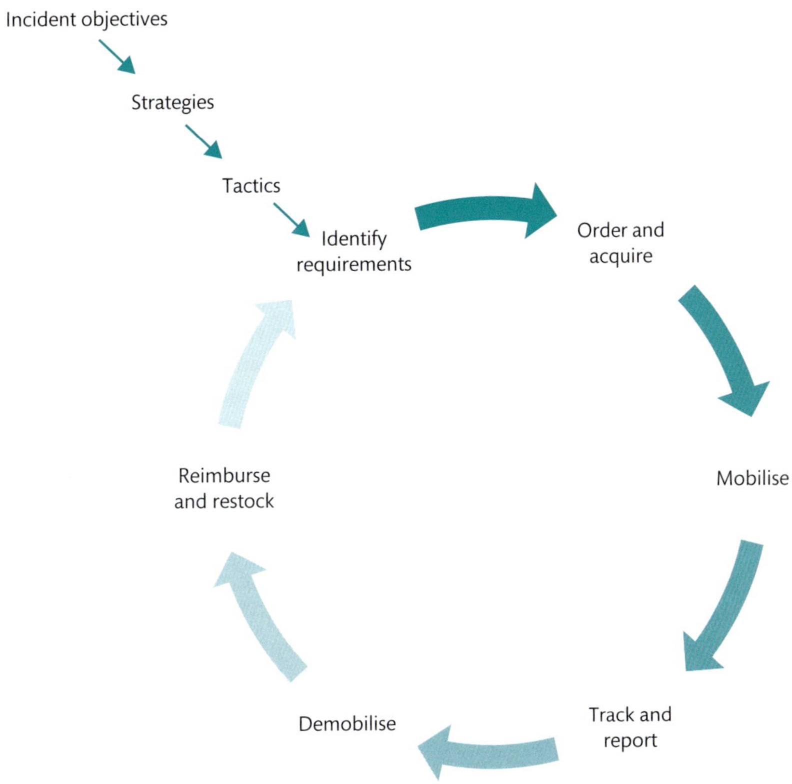

Figure 6.2 Incident resource management.

Data from National Incident Management System. Third edition. October 2017. FEMA. Department of Homeland Security. (pp 12) https://www.fema.gov/sites/default/files/2020-07/fema_nims_doctrine-2017.pdf

Doors leading to the roof were locked. There was no rooftop evacuation plan. The roofs of both the North Tower and the South Tower were sloped and cluttered surfaces with radiation hazards, making them impractical for helicopter landings and as staging areas for civilians. Although the South Tower roof had a helipad, it did not meet 1994 Federal Aviation Administration guidelines.

In 1993, a terrorist bomb had been detonated in the basement garage beneath the building. Six people died, hundreds were injured, and the evacuation via the stairwells of the building took four hours. A few people were evacuated from the roof by helicopter. After the exposure of considerable vulnerabilities, $100 million was spent on improving the safety of the building, including better power systems, communications, lighting, constant presence of fire wardens, regular fire drills and, crucially, glow strips on the staircase handrails. The drills did not include direction to escape stairwells, nor was full or partial building evacuation practised. Civilians were not told that evacuation could not be achieved if they headed to the roof. There was no plan to rescue people caught above a building-wide fire below them.

The first responders were Port Authority Police, New York City Police, New York Fire Department, and the Mayor's Office of Emergency Management in a facilitating role. Despite this, the police and fire department had not determined the mechanism with which they would coordinate their response efforts by the time of the September 11 attacks. The radio channel used by the fire department had a weak signal, and a repeater had been installed inside the towers to improve signal penetration through the concrete and steel in such a tall building—this repeater had to be activated at the lobby fire-safety desk.

At 8.46 am, the North Tower was hit by American Airlines Flight 11, cutting through floors 93 to 99. Descent was impossible for anyone above floor 92. The fire department response was rapid, and one ladder and one engine company began ascending North Tower stairwell C to try and reach the impact zone to assess the situation. Other fire department units gathered in the lobby and awaited instructions. Some of these units would later also climb stairs to reach and rescue where they could. It was speedily concluded that it was a rescue operation as there was no possibility of extinguishing the fire. The intention was to evacuate as many people as possible and then vacate the building.

Some people in the South Tower decided to commence evacuation before the impact of the second plane into their building—the order to evacuate, by the fire department, came seconds before the second impact at 9.03 am. Because of the communication with commanders was hampered, there was an uneven deployment of firemen—with teams being concentrated in the North Tower or the nearby Marriott Hotel with fewer teams being directed to the South Tower.

Advice from senior fire chiefs suggested that partial collapse of the affected floors was possible but not imminent—total collapse was not anticipated at all. Despite a message from an NYPD helicopter that large chunks of debris looked about to fall from the South Tower just prior to its collapse, this was not communicated to the teams on the ground.

Because the airliner that hit the South Tower was banking at the time of impact, the whole of floors 77–85 were not completely damaged. One stairwell from above the impact zone remained passable all the way from the top to the bottom of the building.

NYPD had a better radio communication system, but the Fire Departments radios were either too weak in signal or channels were overloaded with message traffic that made it incomprehensible. After the collapse of the South Tower, the order to evacuate the North Tower was given, but it was uncertain who had received it. The Fire Chief on the 23rd floor who got the message had a megaphone and went into all the stairwells, shouting 'All FDNY, get *** out!'

Miraculously, only 110 of the 2152 civilians who died were below the impact zones—a testament to the huge evacuation effort, in under an hour, getting out a large proportion of the estimated 18,000 individuals believed to be present in both buildings at 8.46 am. Sadly, 344 Firemen, 60 Police officers, and 8 Medical Technicians died in the tragedy—a huge loss of life among emergency responders—which underlines the heroism of those involved but cannot avoid the conclusion that the scale of loss could have been avoided.

In 2005, Police Commissioner Ray Kelly and Fire Commissioner Nicholas Scoppetta promised to improve the way they deploy officers and firefighters in disasters. 'We've revised our mobilization procedures, controlling the number of personnel who respond at any one time to an event'.

A heavy proportion of the senior fire department commanders lost their lives due to the location of command centres on the World Trade Centre complex. A more distant overall command centre was recommended if future destructive mass casualty events occurred again.

Remedy

The 2004 Boxing Day Tsunami was caused by an undersea earthquake releasing total energy $\sim 1.1 \times 10^{17}$ joules, greater than 1500 Hiroshima atomic bombs. As a tsunami reaches shallower water, the height of the wave increases, and the wave front slows. The fault line was in a north–south direction with most of the energy dispersed sideways in an east–west direction, which explains why Bangladesh was less affected than Somalia even though the latter was considerably further away. There were no tsunami warning systems in the Indian Ocean, unlike the Pacific Ocean despite the known risk of tectonic activity in the area. Proximity to the epicentre does offer one small advantage—the awareness that an earthquake has occurred and thus may allow timely evacuation. More distant regions may be adversely affected by the tsunami without the population having any warning of what is to occur. Most of the populations affected were taken completely by surprise despite the tsunami taking sometimes several hours to arrive. It is estimated that in excess of 250,000 people died, mostly in Indonesia, Sri Lanka, India, and Thailand.

Detailed planning for recovery did not take place in Indonesia until March 2005. Early fears that unburied bodies would lead to a health crisis meant that initial efforts were directed towards this as one of the priorities—to the detriment of other efforts. The concern over water supply and the emergence of waterborne diseases was successfully mitigated. However, the imposition of Martial Law a year before the tsunami due to a pre-existing secessionist conflict led to a paucity of non-governmental organizations able to assist. Local government was immediately overwhelmed, and 'competition' became acute between aid organizations for local implementers. The biggest hurdle in the recovery planning was the lack of people, trained or untrained, to help in coordinated efforts. UNICEF's report on its efforts in Indonesia recommended 'Develop better guidance on how to work with partners in emergencies, especially depleted local governments. Global agreements for personnel, both standby and private, should also be developed'. Among many other organizations, UN, WHO, etc., nearly $14 billion was made available to help with aid efforts in affected areas. As nearly 40% of funds were donated by private individuals (normally this is around 15%), there was a greater prominence of NGOs, such as the Red Cross, in the relief efforts which complicated the coordination.[13] Most coastal industries (predominantly tourism and fishing) were substantially destroyed. The separatist war in Aceh was brought to an end, which was a good outcome—but corruption and siphoning of aid monies was complicated by jealousy between poor communities who received financial assistance and poor communities that were deemed unaffected, and thereby undeserving.[14] An unusual problem also emerged in that, for once, fund-raising exceeded the need—but there was no ready mechanism to re-allocate these excess monies to other causes.[15]

In the UK, the Local Resilience Forum will have a Mass Fatalities Plan. This is required to deal with the identification and forensic examination of fatalities that exceed any local resource implementation. Silver command is tasked with establishing a victim holding area, usually within the inner cordon of the incident. Comprehensive documentation of victims is a priority, as determining what are complete humans and what are human remains can become extremely difficult in certain types of disasters. Appropriate storage of the deceased and human remains is the responsibility of the Scene Evidence Recovery Manager, usually a police officer. Potentially contaminated remains may be left in situ until advice has been sought from the Health Protection Agency, the Fire Service or Porton Down, and Department of Defence. The Home Office has produced a publication entitled 'The safe handling of contaminated fatalities'. The Scene Evidence Recovery Manager will take control of the inner cordon once the fire and rescue services have completed all possible attempts at rescue.

Requirement for mortuary facilities in such circumstances have been assigned four levels of need. Level 1 mortuary response indicates extant facilities within the national health service, NHS which are able to cope with some extra demand. At Level 2, enhanced arrangements are required with the provision of extra body storage units within the existing mortuary provision. Level 3 is Local Emergency Mortuary Arrangements, like the refrigeration containers that were seen recently during the first and second waves of the coronavirus pandemic, or other requisitioned land, premises, or other demountable structures. When the victim numbers exceed the hundreds to thousands, Level 4 National Emergency Mortuary Arrangements are required within the geography of the event.

This chapter has attempted to categorize how our current understanding has evolved to deal with cataclysm. Each event is different, uniquely testing human forethought and resilience. Each provides an opportunity to learn, improve, and react. While we may have escaped superstitious attributions to angered Gods, we have replaced it with conspiracy theorists. As health professionals, our job is ultimately simple—but a disaster is never simple and, for some, full recovery is never possible.

A final word from the 7 July 2005 bombing review: The London Underground Managing Director stated in his response to the committee 'The big lesson for us is to invest in your staff, rely on them; invest in technology but do not rely on it'.

REFERENCES

1. Prince SH. *Catastrophe and Social Change.* New York: Columbia University; 1920. https://archive.org/stream/catastrophesocia00prinuoft/catastrophesocia00prinuoft_djvu.txt
2. Powell JW. *An Introduction to the Natural History of Disaster.* College Park: University of Maryland Disaster Research Project; 1954.
3. Hyogo Framework for Action 2005–2015. Building the resilience of nations and communities to disasters. 2007. https://www.preventionweb.net/files/1217_HFAbrochureEnglish.pdf
4. Sendai framework for disaster risk reduction 2015–2030. 2015. https://www.preventionweb.net/files/43291_sendaiframeworkfordrren.pdf
5. McNulty D, Rielly P. King's Cross Fire in the London Underground November 18, 1987: A Report for Dr A. Buchanan, Dept. of Civil Engineering Canterbury University; 1992. https://www.railwaysarchive.co.uk/documents/LRT_OxfordCircus1984.pdf
6. Fennell D. Investigation into the King's Cross Underground Fire. HMSO; 1988.https://www.railwaysarchive.co.uk/documents/DoT_KX1987.pdf
7. Exercise Cygnus Report. 2016 (Redacted) https://assets.publishing.service.gov.uk/government/uploads/system/uploads/attachment_data/file/927770/exercise-cygnus-report.pdf
8. Freedman, Sir Lawrence. *Strategy.* Oxford University Press; 2013:172–173.
9. *National Incident Management System.* 3rd ed. FEMA. Department of Homeland Security; October 2017:12. https://www.fema.gov/sites/default/files/2020-07/fema_nims_doctrine-2017.pdf
10. UK Civil Protection Lexicon. Version 2.1.1 (February 2013) Cabinet Office https://www.gov.uk/government/publications/emergency-responder-interoperability-lexicon
11. London Assembly Report of the 7 July Review Committee. Greater London Authority. June 2006 https://www.london.gov.uk/sites/default/files/gla_migrate_files_destination/archives/assembly-reports-7july-report.pdf
12. National Commission on Terrorist Attacks Upon the United States. 2004. https://govinfo.library.unt.edu/911/report/911Report_Ch9.htm
13. The 2004 Indian Ocean Tsunami Disaster: Evaluation of UNICEF's response (emergency and initial recovery phase) Indonesia Report 2006. 2006.
14. Aceh redux—the tsunami that helped stop a war. *The New Humanitarian.* 23rd December 2014. https://www.thenewhumanitarian.org/analysis/2014/12/23/aceh-redux-tsunami-helped-stop-war
15. Flint M, Goyder H. *Funding the Tsunami Response.* London: Tsunami Evaluation Coalition; 2006.

PART 3
Non-invasive Ventilation

7

High-flow Nasal Oxygen Therapy

Federico Longhini, Paolo Navalesi, Mariachiara Ippolito, and Cesare Gregoretti

KEY MESSAGES

- High-flow oxygen therapy through nasal cannula (HFNC) has some advantageous physiological mechanisms over conventional oxygen therapy (COT) for patients with acute respiratory failure (ARF).
- Hypoxaemic ARF represents the main indication for HFNC. In these patients, HFNC reduces the risk of the need for intubation and the escalation of the respiratory support, compared to COT. However, caution should be taken not to delay intubation when required.
- In patients with exacerbations of chronic obstructive pulmonary disease (COPD), HFNC can be considered as an alternative to non-invasive ventilation (NIV), when NIV fails due to intolerance. HFNC should also be considered in preference to COT after extubation or during breaks from NIV.
- After extubation, HFNC reduces the onset of post-extubation ARF and need for reintubation, compared to COT. However, NIV should be preferred to HFNC in patients considered at risk of post-extubation ARF.
- In high-risk and/or obese patients undergoing cardiac or thoracic surgery, HFNC should be used in preference to COT after extubation. In all other surgical settings, CPAP and NIV are preferable to COT and HFNC.

CONTROVERSIES

- The literature remains inconclusive regarding the application of HFNC in the peri-intubation period, although continuation during intubation seems prudent in patients already in receipt of HFNC.

FURTHER RESEARCH

- Assessing the role of HFNC in the post-extubation period in patients undergoing non-cardiothoracic surgery and in patients with COPD.
- Assessing the role for peri-procedural HFNC during intubation in patients with different aetiologies and severities of ARF.

Introduction

Until the advent of humidified high-flow oxygen therapy through nasal cannula (HFNC), patients with acute respiratory failure (ARF) were managed with conventional oxygen therapy (COT) via nasal prongs or mask. If COT could not sufficiently correct gas exchange and relieve work of breathing, then non-invasive ventilation (NIV) or intubation for invasive mechanical could be used.

High-flow oxygen therapy through nasal cannula is an innovative system that delivers an heated humidified air–oxygen mixture, able to deliver an inspired fraction of oxygen (FiO_2) ranging from 21% to 100%, at flows of up to 60-70 L/min. The flow is generated by an air–oxygen blender or a turbine; the gases pass through an active heated humidifier and are delivered to the patient through a single-limb circuit with a large bore nasal cannula at its distal end. Since its introduction in the early part of the 21st century, evidence has accumulated regarding its clinical utility.[1]

Potential Advantageous Mechanisms

HFNC has some potentially advantageous mechanisms for patients affected by both hypoxaemic and hypoxaemic–hypercapnic ARF[2] (Figure 7.1). The administration of inadequately warmed and humidified medical gases, such as during by COT or NIV, shifts the isothermic saturation boundary farther down the bronchial tree, affecting the ciliary motion, damaging the respiratory tract epithelial cells, and reducing the water content of the bronchial secretions. Active heated humidification, which HFNC achieves with high efficiency, preserves cellular structure and function relative to exposure to dry conditions over 8 h. This translates into a reduction of the inflammatory responses associated with epithelial cell cilia damage and airway water loss.

HFNC also facilitates a washout effect of carbon dioxide (CO_2) from the pharyngeal dead space. In healthy adults, dead space is typically estimated at 2 mL/kg of body weight, constituting 30% of the tidal volume. Clearance from CO_2 of the nasal cavity (40–50 mL in healthy adults) therefore comprises at least 30% of the anatomical dead space in adults. This CO_2 washout effect is potentially relevant for patients with an increased dead space to tidal volume ratio, such those with chronic obstructive pulmonary disease (COPD) and

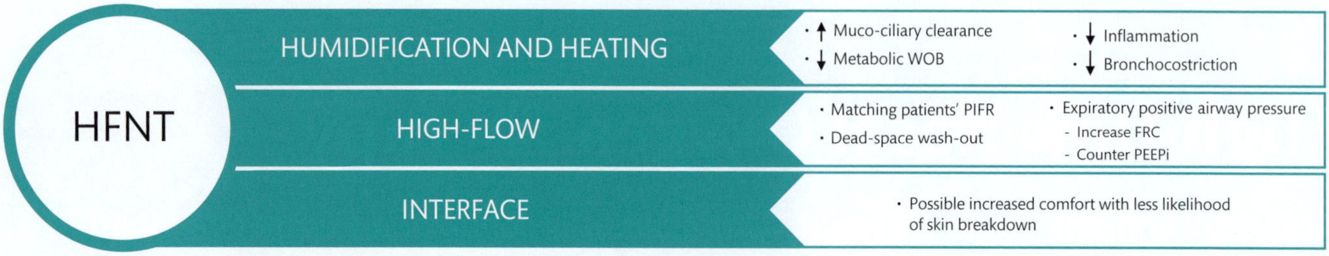

Figure 7.1 Potential advantageous mechanisms in high-flow nasal oxygen therapy (HFNT). WOB, work of breathing; PIFR, peak inspiratory flow rate; FRC, functional residual capacity; PEEPi, intrinsic positive end-expiratory pressure.

exercise intolerance. The washout effect by HFNC is dependent on the amount of flow delivered and the respiratory rate. This effect is directly proportional to the administered flow and inversely proportional to the respiratory rate.

A third advantage, compared to unassisted spontaneous breathing, comes from HFNC increasing expiratory resistances so generating greater end-expiratory pharyngeal pressure. During inspiration, pharyngeal pressure then drops to zero. Whilst healthy subjects can generate an end-expiratory pharyngeal pressure of 0.3–0.8 cmH_2O, depending on whether the mouth is open or closed, HFNC generates an expiratory positive airway pressure of up to 8 cmH_2O with a closed mouth, providing the airway stabilizing benefit of positive expiration pressure. This HFNC-derived pressure is dependent on the flow delivered to the patient and the size of the nasal prongs relative to the nostrils. HFNC, by delivering high flow and by splinting nasal boundaries, may decrease inspiratory airway resistance, thus reducing the work of breathing. Furthermore, nasal delivery of heated gases has anti-muscarinic effects, further reducing pulmonary resistances.

Delivery of a stable fraction of inspired oxygen (FiO_2) is important both for a reliable assessment of gas exchange by the PaO_2/FiO_2 ratio and to avoid hyperoxic hypercarbia in susceptible patients. Neither nasal prongs nor simple oxygen mask therapy is able to provide a stable FiO_2, and even a venturi mask may not provide the nominal fraction. Vents in venturi mask designed to prevent CO_2 rebreathing allow the entrainment of atmospheric air, especially if peak inspiratory flow exceeds that supplied to the mask. In patients with ARF, the mean inspiratory peak flow can reach values around 60 L/min. Therefore, HFNC guarantees a more stable FiO_2, as compared to COT through nasal prongs, oxygen, or venturi mask. Finally, HFNC minimizes the pain and discomfort associated with drying the mouth, throat, and airways, and is therefore better tolerated than COT and NIV, leading to better success rates for therapy.

Role of HFNC in Acute Respiratory Failure

HFNC has been used both in hypoxaemic and hypoxaemic–hypercarbic ARF, although the strongest evidence currently is for its use in the former situation. A summary of the recommendations for the use of HFNC is provided in Table 7.1.

Hypoxaemic Acute Respiratory Failure

The strongest evidence for, and predominant use of, HFNC is in patients experiencing hypoxaemic ARF.[1,3] HFNC has been successfully applied in the intensive care unit (ICU), monitored ward, and emergency department (ED) settings. In patients with hypoxaemic ARF, the mechanisms noted above of generation of low positive expiratory airway pressure, dead space washout, and reduction in inspiratory resistance all help reduce the work of breathing.

Recent guidelines released by the European Society of Intensive Care Medicine strongly recommend the use of HFNC in hypoxaemic ARF.[1] This advice is based on findings that, compared to COT, HFNC reduces the risk of escalation of respiratory support and intubation, although not major clinical outcomes including mortality, or ICU and hospital length of stay (LOS). An important issue is early detection of those patients failing HFNC treatment, in order to avoid delay of intubation. Retrospective studies have shown association between delayed intubation (>48 h of HFNC treatment) and mortality, with a large study indicating double the mortality risk (67% vs. 39%).[2] Avoidance of delayed intubation requires close monitoring of parameters including oxygenation, thoracoabdominal asynchrony, need for vasopressors, SOFA score, or disease severity and progression. Those with moderate to severe ARF (i.e. $PaO_2/FiO_2 < 200$ mmHg) are at greatest risk of failure. Recently, the ROX index, the ratio of SpO_2/FiO_2 to the respiratory rate, has been described and prospectively validated to predict success and failure of HFNC in patients with hypoxaemic ARF due to pneumonia.[2] When the ROX index is greater or equal to 4.88 at 2, 6, or 12 h after HFNC initiation, the risk of intubation is low. However, if the ROX index is below 2.85, 3.47, and 3.85 at 2, 6, and 12 h, respectively, the risk of HFNC failure and intubation is high. Calculation of the ROX index requires a minimum flow of 30 L/min and FiO_2 adjusted to maintain a peripheral oxygen saturation (SpO_2) greater than 92%.[4]

Hypoxaemic–Hypercapnic Acute Respiratory Failure

Although the majority of evidence for HFNC comes from its use in type I/hypoxaemic respiratory failure, it has also been used in patients with hypoxaemic–hypercapnic ARF, in particular in exacerbations of COPD[5,6] (see Chapter 40). Exacerbations of COPD are complex events typically associated with increased airway inflammation, increased mucus production, and marked gas trapping. These features manifest clinically as worsening dyspnoea, increased sputum purulence and volume, cough, and wheeze. Hypercapnic ARF develops in approximately 20% of hospitalized COPD patients and is associated with an increased risk of death. Hypercapnic ARF develops when respiratory workload exceeds respiratory muscles pump capacity and a rapid shallow breathing pattern develops. Dynamic hyperinflation also contributes to increase

Table 7.1. Summary of the available evidence on the role of high-flow nasal cannulae (HFNC) in different clinical settings and patient populations

Population/setting	Intervention	Comparison	Recommendation and certainty	Pro	Contra
Patients with acute hypoxaemic respiratory failure	HFNC	COT	• Strong recommendation to use HFNC • Moderate certainty	• Decreased the need for intubation • Decreased escalation of respiratory support	• May delay intubation • Not enough evidence on mortality, ICU LOS, hospital LOS, dyspnoea and comfort
Patients at high risk of post-extubation respiratory failure	HFNC	COT	• Conditional recommendation • Moderate certainty • Both treatments acceptable and feasible	• Reduced reintubation • Reduced post-extubation respiratory failure	• No effects of HFNC vs COT on mortality, need for escalation to NIPPV or ICU and hospital LOS
Patients at high risk of post-extubation respiratory failure	HFNC HFNC + NIPPV alternating >24 h (HIGH WEAN)	NIPPV/CPAP HFNC or NIPPV alone	• Conditional recommendation • Low certainty • Both treatments acceptable and feasible In high risk of reintubation patients (COPD, Heart dysfunction, obesity)	• No effect on the rates of reintubation or post-extubation respiratory failure • No effects of HFNC vs NIPPV/CPAP on mortality or ICU and hospital LOS • Reduced Reintubation rates from ~19%–11%	
Peri-intubation	HFNC	COT or NIPPV	• No recommendations for the peri-intubation period • For patients already receiving HFNC, conditional recommendation to continue HFNC during intubation • Moderate certainty	• No effect on the incidence of peri-intubation hypoxaemia, 28-day mortality, serious complications (composite of severe hypoxia, significant hypotension, use of vasopressors and cardiac arrest, or ICU LOS) • No effect on apnoeic time, PaO_2 after preoxygenation, PaO_2 after intubation or $PaCO_2$ after intubation	
Post-operative (high-risk and/or obese patients who underwent cardiac or thoracic surgery)	HFNC	COT	• Conditional recommendation to use HFNC • Moderate certainty	• Reduction in the rates of reintubation and escalation of respiratory support	• No effect on mortality, ICU LOS, hospital LOS or the incidence of post-operative hypoxia
Post-operative (other)	HFNC	COT	• Evidence insufficient to recommend prophylactic HFNC use	• Small absolute effects, mostly driven by obese patients and patients at high risk of post-operative respiratory complications	
Post-operative	HFNC	NIPPV	• Neither favoured or disfavoured HFNC use compared to NIPPV	• Skin breakdown more common with NIPPV	• No effect on reintubation rate, need for respiratory support, or ICU LOS

Source: The table shows the current summary of available evidence according to data from Rochwerg, B., Einav, S., Chaudhuri, D. et al. The role for high flow nasal cannula as a respiratory support strategy in adults: a clinical practice guideline. *Intensive Care Med* 46, 2226–2237 (2020). [1].

COT, conventional oxygen therapy; CPAP, continuous positive airway pressure; HFNC, high-flow nasal cannulae for humdified oxygen; ICU, intensive care unit; LOS, length of stay; NIPPV, non-invasive positive pressure ventilation.

the respiratory workload through the generation of intrinsic positive end-expiratory pressure.

Current guidelines strongly recommend the use of NIV with high evidential certainty, for hypercapnic ARF with acidosis. However, there is an increasing literature describing the potential for HFNC in exacerbated COPD patients with established hypercapnic ARF, as an alternative to NIV. HFNC has been successfully applied after NIV treatment failure due to poor tolerance of the interface or unmanageable air leak. Compared to COT, HFNC as first-line treatment decreases $PaCO_2$ at 1 h after its initiation without significant and clinically relevant modifications of respiratory and heart rate and SpO_2 in exacerbated COPD.[6]

A recent multicentre randomized controlled trial[5] has compared HFNC to NIV as first-line treatment in patients with exacerbation of COPD with mild respiratory acidosis (arterial pH 7.25–7.35). Although not inferior to NIV in mean $PaCO_2$ reduction, one-third of patients randomized to HFNC crossed over to NIV within 6 h of treatment initiation. Therefore, we suggest that HFNC can be considered as an alternative to NIV, especially when this latter fails due to poor comfort or patient tolerance to the interface.

In addition, HFNC has a role after extubation or at NIV discontinuation in patients with exacerbations of COPD. A few studies have shown that HFNC maintains good gas exchange, whilst decreasing discomfort, grade of dyspnoea, work of breathing, respiratory drive, and the amount of time spent on mechanical ventilation, compared to COT.

HFNC Following Extubation

Weaning is the entire process of liberation from mechanical ventilation, from reduction in ventilatory support to successful and enduring extubation. It is not necessarily a unidirectional process, and failed extubation (defined as need for reintubation within 48 h, or 72 h, of extubation) is an adverse event associated with worsened outcomes. Therefore, strategies that reduce the occurrence of post-extubation respiratory failure or avert reintubation would be predicted to improve patient outcomes.

In the context of patients deemed 'at risk' of post-extubation failure, trials have compared HFNC to both COT and NIV.[7]

Compared to COT, HFNC significantly reduces the onset of post-extubation ARF and need for reintubation. However, despite being better tolerated, HFNC had no such ameliorative when compared to NIV. Recent guidelines therefore suggest the use of HFNC following extubation in patients who required invasive mechanical ventilation for more than 24 h and considered at risk, as compared to COT.[1] However, NIV should be preferred to HFNC where this is already established practice.

HFNC in the Post-operative Period

Within 48 h of surgery, up to 55% of patients may experience hypoxaemia, as defined by a PaO_2/FiO_2 <300 mmHg. Hypoxaemia may be secondary to pathologies, including lung atelectasis and pneumonia; and several strategies have been proposed to reduce this risk.[8]

The prophylactic use of HFNC has been examined in 10 trials compared to COT and one versus NIV. Almost all of these trials were conducted in cardiac or thoracic surgery patients,[9,10] with only one in abdominal surgery.[11]

In cardiac surgery patients with, or at risk of, respiratory failure, a multicentre trial demonstrated that HFNC was characterized by a similar treatment failure rate (defined as reintubation, crossover or premature treatment discontinuation, skin breakdown, and mortality) when compared to NIV.[9] Mortality, ICU, and hospital LOS were similar between treatments. In another trial comparing HFNC with COT in cardiac surgery patients with a BMI >30 kg/m^2, HFNC failed to improve the radiological appearance of lung atelectasis, and no significant differences were found with regard to the ICU LOS. Similar findings were seen in a single-centre comparison of HFNC and COT in patients undergoing surgery for type-A aortic dissections.

In the OPERA trial, 220 patients undergoing major abdominal surgery were randomized to receive HFNC or COT after elective extubation. The two treatments showed similar effects on post-operative hypoxaemia 1 h after extubation, the need for supplemental oxygen therapy for persistent hypoxaemia after treatment discontinuation, the occurrence and severity of post-operative pulmonary complications, the need for any form of ventilatory assistance for ARF within 7 days after surgery, ICU, and hospital lengths of stay.[11]

Both a recent metanalysis[10] and the pooled data analysis for the recent ESICM guidelines[1] indicate that the use of HFNC after surgery is associated with a lower risk for reintubation and decreased escalation of respiratory support, as compared to COT. However, the low rate of reported events led the ESICM expert panel to record this as a low-certainty finding. These guidelines carry a recommendation to use HFNC in preference to COT in high-risk and/or obese patients undergoing cardiac or thoracic surgery. The recent ESA/ESICM guidelines[12] advise against the routine use of HFNC for the prevention post-operative hypoxaemia in all other setting and indicate that CPAP or NIV is preferable for the management of post-operative and peri-procedural hypoxaemia in non-cardiothoracic settings. The French REVA group have published the HIGH WEAN study, suggesting a combination of alternating HFNC and NIV for at least 24 h post extubation reduces reintubation rates more so than either alone in those at higher risk, i.e. Obese, COPD, or reduced left ventricular function. These findings require ratification in further trials.

HFNC in the Peri-intubation Period

HFNC's ability to generate a low PEEP and washout of the nasopharyngeal dead space has led to its proposed use during intubation to deliver apnoeic oxygenation and reduce the episodes of severe desaturation during the peri-intubation period.[13] Randomized trials in this area have produced contradictory results. A recent meta-analysis by Jhou et al.[14] found that HFNC was non-inferior to the standard of care during intubation with regard to the incidence of severe hypoxaemia and nadir oxygen saturation. Of note, the authors reported a borderline significant benefit of HFNC with respect to the incidence of severe hypoxaemia, although only in patients with a PaO_2/FiO_2 >200 mmHg, when compared to the standard of care. The recent ESICM guidelines[1] make no recommendation regarding the use of HFNC in the peri-intubation period. However, where it is in use prior to intubation, it is suggested that it should be continued during the peri-intubation period.

REFERENCES

1. Rochwerg B, Einav S, Chaudhuri D, et al. The role for high flow nasal cannula as a respiratory support strategy in adults: A clinical practice guideline. *Intensive Care Med.* 2020;**46**:2226–2237.
2. Spoletini G, Cortegiani A, Gregoretti C. Physiopathological rationale of using high-flow nasal therapy in the acute and chronic setting: A narrative review. *Trends Anaesth Crit Care.* 2019;26–27:22–29.
3. Ricard JD, Roca O, Lemiale V, et al. Use of nasal high flow oxygen during acute respiratory failure. *Intensive Care Med.* 2020;**46**:2238–2247.
4. Roca, O, Caralt, B, Messika, J, et al. An index combining respiratory rate and oxygenation to predict outcome of nasal high-flow therapy. *Am J Respir Crit Care Med.* 2019;**199**(11):1368–1376.
5. Cortegiani A, Longhini F, Madotto F, et al. High flow nasal therapy versus noninvasive ventilation as initial ventilatory strategy in COPD exacerbation: A multicenter non-inferiority randomized trial. *Crit Care.* 2020;**24**:692.
6. Pisani L, Astuto M, Prediletto I, et al. High flow through nasal cannula in exacerbated COPD patients: A systematic review. *Pulmonology.* 2019;**25**:348–354.
7. Granton D, Chaudhuri D, Wang D, et al. High-flow nasal cannula compared with conventional oxygen therapy or noninvasive ventilation immediately postextubation: A systematic review and meta-analysis. *Crit Care Med.* 2020;**48**:e1129–e1136.
8. Cortegiani A, Accurso G, Mercadante S, et al. High flow nasal therapy in perioperative medicine: From operating room to general ward. *BMC Anesthesiol.* 2018;**18**:166.
9. Stephan F, Barrucand B, Petit P, et al. High-flow nasal oxygen vs noninvasive positive airway pressure in hypoxemic patients after cardiothoracic surgery: A randomized clinical trial. *JAMA.* 2015;**313**:2331–2339.
10. Chaudhuri D, Granton D, Wang DX, et al. High-flow nasal cannula in the immediate postoperative period: A systematic review and meta-analysis. *Chest.* 2020;**158**:1934–1946.
11. Futier E, Paugam-Burtz C, Godet T, et al. Effect of early postextubation high-flow nasal cannula vs conventional oxygen

therapy on hypoxaemia in patients after major abdominal surgery: A French multicentre randomised controlled trial (OPERA). *Intensive Care Med.* 2016;**42**:1888–1898.
12. Leone M, Einav S, Chiumello D, et al. Noninvasive respiratory support in the hypoxaemic peri-operative/periprocedural patient: A joint ESA/ESICM guideline. *Intensive Care Med.* 2020;**46**:697–713.
13. Frat JP, Ricard JD, Quenot JP, et al. Non-invasive ventilation versus high-flow nasal cannula oxygen therapy with apnoeic oxygenation for preoxygenation before intubation of patients with acute hypoxaemic respiratory failure: A randomised, multicentre, open-label trial. *Lancet Respir Med.* 2019;**7**: 303–312.
14. Jhou HJ, Chen PH, Lin C, et al. High-flow nasal cannula therapy as apneic oxygenation during endotracheal intubation in critically ill patients in the intensive care unit: A systematic review and meta-analysis. *Sci Rep.* 2020;**10**:3541.

8

Non-invasive Ventilation in Critical Care

Cesare Gregoretti, Andrea Cortegiani, Vincenzo Russotto, and Lara Pisani

KEY MESSAGES

- Non-invasive ventilation (NIV) plays a key role in the management of acute respiratory failure (ARF), especially in the context of cardiogenic pulmonary oedema and exacerbated chronic obstructive airways disease
- Various devices can be used to NIV, with a variety of ventilator-patient interfaces, including masks and helmets
- Understanding the advantages and disadvantages of each type of ventilator and interface and how to troubleshoot is key to successful use of NIV

CONTROVERSIES

- The timing and role of NIV in acute respiratory distress syndrome (ARDS) and COVID-19 remains uncertain

FURTHER RESEARCH

- Optimal use of NIV during ARDS and COVID-19 pneumonitis, and timing of intubation
- Use of awake prone positioning as an adjunct to NIV and outcome studies

Introduction

Acute respiratory failure (ARF) is characterized by impaired gas exchange and increased work of breathing (WOB), secondary to an acute lung and/or respiratory pump failure (see Chapters 3, 16, and 21). Ventilatory assistance to respiratory function can be applied either invasively through an endotracheal tube or by means of external interfaces, such as masks, mouthpieces, prongs, and helmets, referred to as non-invasive ventilation (NIV). Whilst both invasive ventilation and NIV improve gas exchange and reduce patient's effort, only NIV preserves the ability to swallow, cough, and speak.[1,2] It also offers the advantage of averting complications associated with endotracheal intubation (see Chapter 20).[2,3] NIV involves the application of positive pressure to the airway, either intermittently during the inspiratory phase, often referred to as non-invasive positive pressure ventilation (NIPPV), or continuously throughout the whole breath, so-called non-invasive continuous positive airway pressure (CPAP), or, most commonly, both. Since the first reports decades ago,[4] NIV has been increasingly used in patients with mild forms of ARF[2] and then extended over the years to critically ill patients with more severe grade of ARF.[5]

The ideal environment for starting NIV should have expert staff (clinicians, nurses, respiratory therapists, etc.), rapid access to endotracheal intubation and invasive ventilation, and facilities for adequate monitoring. The intensive care unit (ICU) is the most appropriate location for the sickest patients on NIV, offering low nurse:patient ratios and access to other therapeutic and monitoring modalities. Intermediate units between ICU and wards, with higher nurse:patient ratios, can offer NIV safely to those less sick patients; however, many health systems have a shortage of such units. Close liaison is required between ICU and intermediate NIV units to reduce the risks of delayed transition to invasive ventilation when required.

NIV is well established in many emergency departments (EDs), with the potential to fully manage rapidly resolving causes of ARF such as acute cardiogenic pulmonary oedema in that environment. However, those likely to need longer term ventilatory support (i.e. pneumonia and acute respiratory distress syndrome, ARDS) should ideally be rapidly transferred to ICU. The early application of NIV in appropriate patients is likely to benefit patients with reversible conditions, and this has driven the steady increase in the ED use of NIV in recent decades (see Chapter 9).

In this chapter, we provide an overview on NIV focusing on its physiological effects, different types of interfaces and ventilators, ventilatory modes and triggers, and ventilator circuits.

Physiological Effects and Pathophysiological Rationale of Using NIV in Critically Ill Patients

NIV uses the patient's own upper airway. For efficient pressure delivery and transmission to the airways, the interface should provide a seal to limit leaks. The glottis dilates and constricts in phase with inspiration and expiration, respectively (see Chapter 2), and glottic constriction can be induced by high levels of non-invasively delivered positive airway pressure. In patients with hypercapnic acidosis, the pressure applied during inspiration can increase tidal volume (VT) either by augmenting the transpulmonary pressure (Ptp) or decreasing the extent of Ptp generated by the respiratory muscles, thereby reducing patient's WOB. In a series of 11 patients with acute exacerbation of chronic obstructive pulmonary disease (COPD), Brochard et al. first showed NIV enhances VT, reduces respiratory rate, decreases diaphragm activation and effort, and improves gas exchange.[4] It has also been shown to reduce the electrical activity of the diaphragm (EAdi) (i.e. the respiratory drive) at increasing levels of support, when compared to spontaneous breathing. Moreover, at the highest support levels, the respiratory drive was almost abolished. These features may help explain the beneficial effects of NIV when compared to simple face mask oxygen in various settings.[6–10]

In COPD patients with dynamic pulmonary hyperinflation and intrinsic positive end-expiratory pressure (PEEPi) undergoing NIV, Appendini et al. showed that an effective diaphragmatic effort reduction was only achieved by combining inspiratory and expiratory pressures, the latter by reducing the threshold load imposed by PEEPi on the respiratory muscles[11] and improving triggering function, as had previously been described during invasive ventilation.

Non-invasive airway pressure is also effective in other causes of ARF through a variety of mechanisms (see Chapter 9). In patients with acute lung volume reduction resulting from pulmonary oedema or atelectasis, CPAP increases functional residual capacity by opening collapsed alveoli, which improves oxygenation by decreasing the intrapulmonary shunt and reduces WOB by shifting VT to a more compliant portion of the pressure–volume relationship. In patients with cardiogenic pulmonary oedema, the increase in intrathoracic pressure also produces hemodynamic benefits, predominantly by reducing left ventricular (LV) afterload by limiting the inspiratory negative swing in intrathoracic pressure and thereby LV transmural pressure (i.e. the difference between systolic arterial pressure and intrathoracic pressure).[12]

Principles of Ventilator Functioning

Basic knowledge of the principles of ventilator functioning is helpful when choosing a ventilator for NIV, enabling matching of available devices to patient characteristics. Briefly, a mechanical ventilator can be considered as a series of consecutive functions that turn an input (energy) into an output (ventilatory variable), such as pressure, flow, or volume (see also Chapter 12).

Pneumatic System

Beside transport/emergency ventilators that may be pneumatically driven, all mechanical ventilators require electricity (AC external power or DC internal battery).

The gas source can be the following:

(a) an external high-pressure gas (centralized gas system or tanks),
(b) an internal compressor,
(c) a turbine or piston, and
(d) a combination of (a) and (c).

Dependent on the gas source, the ventilators for critically ill patients work either (1) with both oxygen and air at high pressure (4 atm, 400 kPa) or (2) with oxygen at high pressure and atmospheric air driven by a turbine, allowing variation in fraction of inspired oxygen (FiO_2) from 21% to 100%. High-pressure-driven ICU ventilators commonly achieve inspiratory flow rates exceeding 120 L/min and allow fast pressure rise time (PRT), the time taken to reach the preset inspiratory airway pressure. In the recent years, these devices have embedded NIV algorithms able to detect and compensate for air leaks. These ventilators always use a double-limb circuit with separated inspiratory and expiratory limbs and a built-in expiratory valve[13] (Figure 8.1).

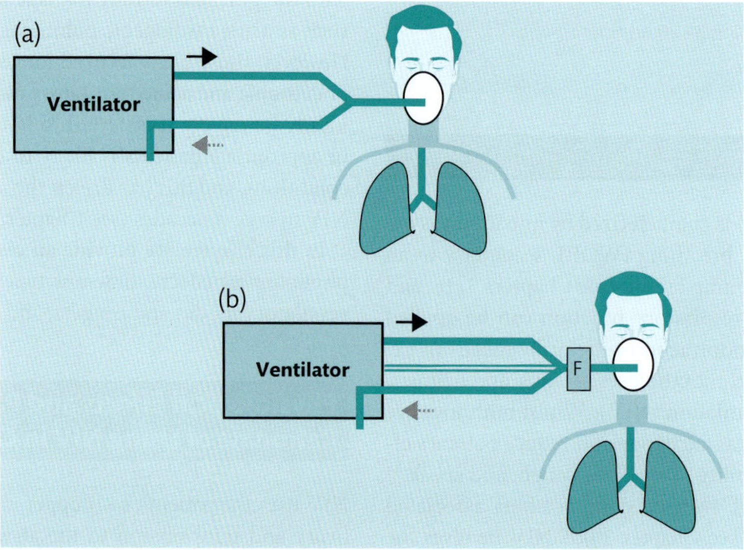

Figure 8.1 Double limb respiratory circuit: (a) without and (b) with a flow sensor (F) sited distal to the Y-piece. The solid and dotted arrows indicate the direction of inspiratory and expiratory flows, respectively. See the main text for further explanation.

Control Variable and Phase Variables

The principles of mechanical breathing apply to both invasive and non-invasive ventilation. It is characterized by (1) a *control variable*, corresponding to the ventilator target (e.g. flow and volume or airway pressure), and (2) some *phase variables*, including the following (see Chapter 12):

- Trigger variable—initiating mechanical inspiration.
- Cycle variable—terminating inspiration.
- Limit variable—limiting magnitude of any parameter (pressure, flow, and volume) during inspiration.
- Baseline variable—the pressure set during expiration (typically termed 'PEEP pressure').

Control Variable

Ventilators can control either flow/volume or pressure, with the other variable being dependent on respiratory system impedance (Chapter 10b); however, the pressure control is the dominant mode of NIV, especially in critically ill patients.

Triggering and Cycling Variables

As NIV requires the patient's own airway to be patent and maintained, non-invasive support should be initiated and terminated to cycle in unison with the patient's natural breathing activity to minimize asynchrony.[8] Response times of ≤100 ms are required to minimize asynchrony, and modern ventilators perform to this standard in bench tests.[13,14] 'Cycling on' is regulated by the 'inspiratory trigger', traditionally airway pressure deflection or inspiratory flow (or volume) generated by patient's inspiratory effort. More recently, some ventilators have incorporated more than one signal or have adopted complex calculations to improve ventilatory efficiency. In particular, these algorithms aim to ensure ventilator function in the presence of air leaks, which are unavoidable during prolonged NIV. One mode, available in both invasive and non-invasive ventilation, is neurally adjusted ventilatory assist (NAVA) that utilizes the EAdi, acquired by means of a dedicated catheter to drive the ventilatory support. During NAVA, the ventilator can cycle on based on either EAdi or the pneumatic signals, according to a hierarchy following the principle that 'first-serves-first'.

Whilst pressure triggering allows the detection of a pressure drop within the circuit due to the patient's inspiratory effort, flow triggering is achieved by measuring a flow variation using a flow sensor, either built-in ventilator or externally positioned at the airway opening (Figure 8.1). Some flow triggers work with the 'flow-by system', where air continuously flows through the ventilator double-limb circuit and triggering occurs when the difference between the flow getting in and out the circuit equals a preset trigger sensitivity, which is expressed in L/min. This so-called flow-by system reduces the intensity and duration of the effort required to trigger a breath leading to better patient–ventilator interaction compared to pressure triggering.

During NIV, the interaction between the patient and the ventilator is complex. Air leaks around the mask are likely to occur, and they affect patient–ventilator synchrony.[13] The aforementioned newer trigger algorithms, allowing air-leak compensation, improve patient–ventilator interaction and prevent ineffective triggering with pressure triggers and auto-triggering with flow triggers.

A breath may be pressure-, time-, volume-, or flow-cycled. Whilst volume and pressure cycling is no longer used, a breath can be defined as time-cycled when it is terminated after a given preset inspiratory time (i.e. pressure- or volume-controlled time-cycled breaths) or as a flow-cycled when the ventilator detects the very end of a patient's inspiration through inspiratory flow measurement and terminates the breath (e.g. pressure support mode, PSV). Until the advent of modern software-driven ventilators, which allow for leak detection and compensation, time cycling was the only possible approach. Flow cycling 'off' threshold is often termed the *expiratory trigger*. Air leaks, however, make flow cycling off problematic and often impossible, with major alterations in patient–ventilator interaction and synchrony, increasing WOB and discomfort. The threshold is generally set as an adjustable percentage of peak inspiratory flow, with absolute flows (L/min) and fixed triggers now less commonly used. With NAVA, the ventilator cycles off when the EAdi falls at 70% of its peak inspiratory value.

Limit Variable

A limit variable is the maximum value that a variable (pressure, flow, and volume) can attain. It limits the magnitude of a specific parameter during inspiration but does not affect the end of the inspiratory phase, distinguishing it from a 'cycle variable' that always ends inspiration. Theoretically, we could also include the variable *time* in a pressure-controlled flow-cycled breath (e.g. PSV). Although this concept seems trivial, it is of particular importance during NIV where the whole system including the patient, the interface, and the ventilator is 'not closed', unlike invasive ventilation. In PSV, the inspiratory time depends, by definition, on the interaction between patient's mechanics, pressure rise time (PRT), and expiratory trigger threshold. Because the system is 'not closed', the inspiratory to expiratory flow criteria (expiratory trigger) cannot be reached by prolonging the mechanical breath. This explains why most non-invasive ventilators have a maximal inspiratory time that can be set in a pressure-controlled flow-cycled breath.

Baseline Variable

It is usually zero PEEP (ZEEP) or set according to the clinician choice. Turbine-driven ventilators in intentional leaks configuration (see the section 'NIV Ventilators') always have a given amount of default expiratory positive airway pressure (EPAP) that may vary, depending on the manufacturer, from 2 to 4 cmH_2O.

NIV Ventilators

In the past decade, the performance of the turbine-driven ventilators has improved considerably, the most recent models achieving inspiratory flow rates and pressurization indices similar to those of high-pressure gas-driven ICU ventilators. In addition, these devices may outperform a traditional ICU ventilator in managing air leaks, ensuring satisfactory patient–ventilator interaction during NIV. Turbine-driven ventilators often adopt single-limb circuit. In this configuration, an expiratory valve is replaced by an intentional leak built in the interface or in the circuit proximal to the airway opening, or in an externally applied swivel connector (Figures 8.2 and 8.3). Because NIV can be delivered by ICU ventilators using dedicated NIV software or by a dedicated NIV ventilator, it is

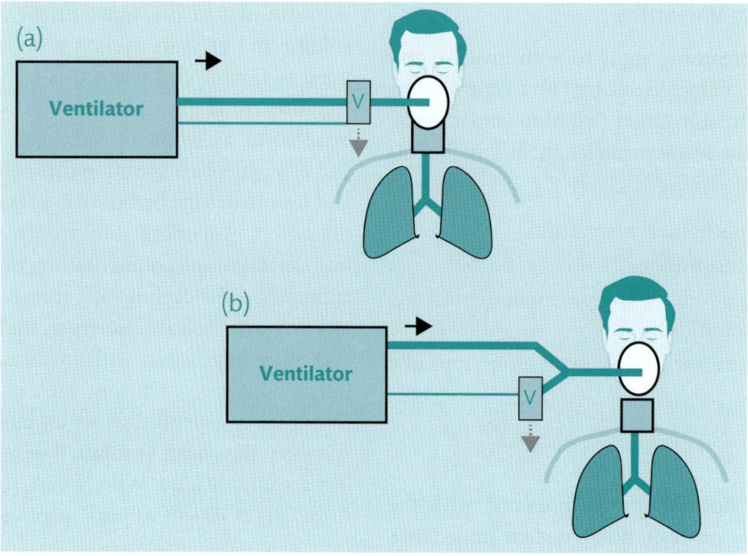

Figure 8.2 Single limb 'non-vented' respiratory circuit with an exhalation valve (V) sited at (a) the distal end of the inspiratory circuit or (b) at the end of a short expiratory limb. In both cases, the exhalation valve is driven by the ventilator pressure (green line). The solid and dotted arrows indicate the direction of inspiratory and expiratory flows, respectively.

Reproduced with permission of the European Respiratory Society ©: *Breathe* Sep 2013, 9 (5) 394–409; doi:10.1183/20734735.042312

essential to understand the principles governing the inspiratory and expiratory valves.

The inspiratory valve controls the respiratory cycle phases, along with the expiratory valve. The expiratory valve can be a simple valve that is closed in counter-phase with the inspiratory one (e.g. the mushroom or diaphragm valve of most turbine-driven ventilators) or a microprocessor-controlled proportional aperture valve. In the former case, the inspiratory valve only has an on–off function: pressure and flow both depend on the mechanical system (e.g. the rotational speed of the turbine). However, all expiratory valves also control the baseline variable, namely the expiratory pressure. This pressure can be ZEEP or a given level of positive end-expiratory

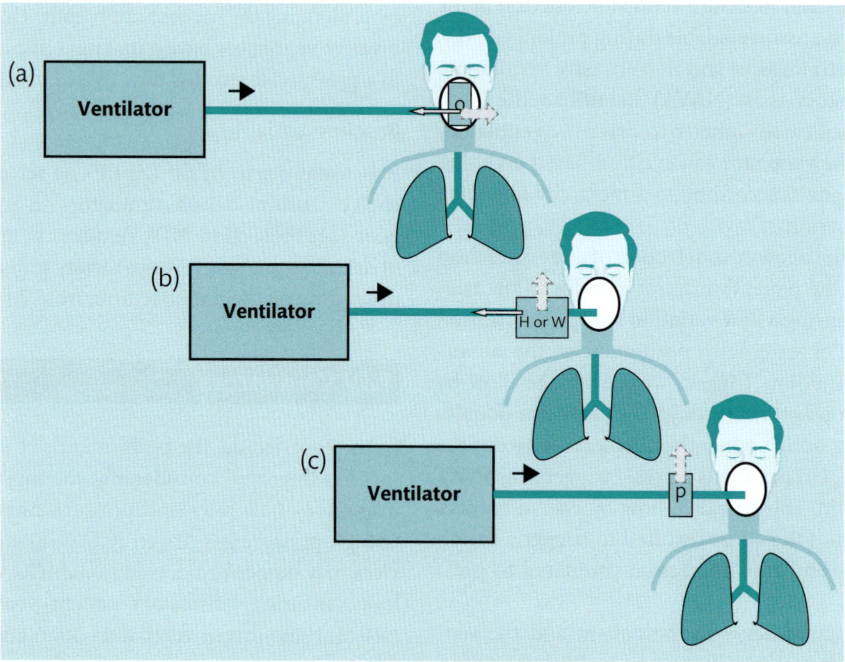

Figure 8.3 Examples of single limb 'vented' circuits. Exhalation occurs through single or multiple orifices sited either in (a) the mask shell or in the swivel connector (O), (b) a whisper swivel (W) or a hole orifice at the distal end of the circuit (H), or (c) a 'Plateau Valve'® Philips-Respironics (P) positioned between the circuit and the mask. The solid and dotted arrows indicate the direction of inspiratory and expiratory flows, respectively. See the main text for further explanation.

Reproduced with permission of the European Respiratory Society ©: *Breathe* Sep 2013, 9 (5) 394–409; doi:10.1183/20734735.042312.

pressure labelled as PEEP or EPAP dependent on the manufacturer. In gas-driven ventilators, the baseline variable (PEEP/EPAP) is always controlled by a microprocessor-driven proportional valve, whilst in most of the turbine-driven ventilators this variable is controlled mechanically using the mushroom expiratory valve and modulating the expiratory flow. Although one of the major advantages of NIV is the avoidance of tracheal intubation with tube-related inspiratory and respiratory resistance, expiratory valves may increase expiratory resistance. These can generate air trapping, especially in a patient breathing at high respiratory rate, and are to some extent dependent on the valve type.[13] Turbine-driven ventilators in an intentional leak configuration are not equipped with active expiratory valves, thus theoretically avoiding the aforementioned drawbacks. Studies that have compared ICU (high-pressure gas-driven) ventilators in the NIV mode and dedicated turbine-driven NIV ventilators have not convincingly demonstrated the superiority of one over the other when looking at patient-focused outcomes.

Respiratory Circuits

Ventilators can deliver non-invasive positive pressure to the patient's airway by using the respiratory circuit (RC). Although RC is not strictly part of the ventilator, its configuration plays in important role in the decision of 'what to use' during NIV in different settings (i.e. ICU vs step-down unit). The distal part of RC is connected to the patient via the non-invasive interface. There are three main types of circuits that can be used with NIV turbine-driven ventilators (Figures 8.1–8.3):

(a) Double-limb RCs composed of inspiratory and expiratory limbs whose proximal ends are connected respectively to the inspiratory and expiratory ports (where the inspiratory and expiratory non-rebreathing valves are positioned), whilst the distal parts are connected to the so-called Y-piece and then to the interface. This is the typical RC of high-pressure gas-driven ICU ventilators, but it can also be found in turbine-driven ventilators. The double-limb RC can also be provided with a proximal flow sensor flow that can be used either as simple monitoring tools or to control some ventilator functions.

(b) Single-limb circuits are directly attached to patient's non-invasive interface. This configuration is restricted to turbine-driven ventilators. As a single tube is used for inspiration and expiration, it could lead to a carbon dioxide rebreathing. Two different systems are available to avoid this problem:

   (i) A single RC with a non-rebreathing expiratory valve (e.g. a mushroom valve driven by ventilator pressure) usually labelled as 'non-vented' RC. This valve has an on–off function and often works as a PEEP valve.

   The single-limb RC can also be provided with a proximal flow sensor.

   (ii) A single RC without an active non-rebreathing valve usually labelled as 'vented' or intentional leak RC. CO_2 is vented out through a vented system embedded in the interface (some slots or holes on the frame or on the swivel elbow) or through a vented system placed into the RC proximally to the interface (see also the section 'Interfaces in the Acute Setting').

NIV Modes

NIV may be delivered for ARF as NIPPV or CPAP. Manufacturers often produce new ventilatory modes; however, scientific evidence demonstrating their effectiveness and clinical benefit is often lacking.

Non invasive CPAP

CPAP is the application of PEEP throughout the whole breath in a spontaneously breathing patient. Therefore, during CPAP, WOB is entirely delivered by the patient's respiratory muscles. Based on the pathophysiology, CPAP is primarily indicated for patients affected by hypoxaemic ARF. CPAP is aimed at improving oxygenation through an amelioration of ventilation–perfusion mismatch by promoting alveolar recruitment and maintaining open alveoli. In critically ill patients, CPAP requires driving gas achieving high and predetermined FiO_2. In ICU setting, CPAP can be delivered through different devices.

The presence of a reservoir bag is not required in the case of high gas flow delivery or when CPAP is applied with a helmet that works as a reservoir bag (see the section 'Interfaces in the Acute Setting'). In simulated respiratory settings, low flow is associated with a drop in P_{aw} during mask ventilation compared to helmet, but not during high-flow CPAP delivery.

Several types of flow generators are widely available: (a) O_2 at high pressure with entrainment of atmospheric air, employing the Venturi principle—this system rarely achieves O_2 higher than 60% or lower than 30%; (b) O_2 and air both at high pressure, achieving a wider range of FiO_2; and (c) ventilators generating a flow with the full range of FiO_2 (from 21% up to 100%). Despite the apparent advantage of a full-scale FiO_2 range, traditional high-pressure gas-driven ICU ventilators do not achieve an adequate air flow, compared to turbine-driven ventilators, which are more commonly used for domiciliary CPAP. However, these domiciliary devices cannot ensure a predetermined and stable FiO_2, limiting their use in critically ill patients. When CPAP is delivered by bi-level turbine-driven ventilator, an equal level of inspiratory pressure and EPAP/PEEP generates CPAP.

Venturi systems ((a) above) generate CPAP via a CPAP valve with an overpressure safety system. Using two oxygen sources, and proximal air entrainment to alter FiO_2, a differential pressure is generated between the inner and outer compartments of the circuit. Manufacturer-specific tables indicate the oxygen flows required to generate the desired FiO_2 for a given CPAP level. In the CPAP system defined as (a) and (b), a PEEP valve is usually positioned at the end of the expiratory circuit or directly on the interface. CPAP valves are available with various conformations: pre-calibrated valves (increasing levels of PEEP in steps of 2.5/5 cmH_2O up to 20 cmH_2O) or an adjustable gear with a wide range of pressure (usually from 2 up to 15 cmH_2O).

A different non-invasive CPAP valve is the Boussignac CPAP valve that can be fit in a standard face mask. Four micro-channels in the wall of the valve transform the gas flow in high-velocity micro-jets, which in turn generate a positive pressure resulting from the entrained air, like a 'virtual valve'. The Boussignac valve is a validated device in hypoxaemic respiratory failure. Within the Boussignac valve, the CPAP level depends on the delivered oxygen flow. Whilst the Boussignac valve device seems to be adequate during normal breathing with low air flow, during forced breathing (high air flow) it struggles to maintain a stable airway pressure, which could increase the WOB and cause respiratory fatigue. A now obsolete system, termed Twinpap (Starmed Intersurgical, Mirandola, Italy), periodically shifted between two levels of PEEP delivering a superimposed non-synchronized positive pressure breath during helmet CPAP,[15] which demonstrated benefits even at only 2 'breaths' per minute. However, this system is no longer commercially available.

NIPPV

NIPPV is usually applied in the acute settings in the pressure-controlled mode with both flow-cycled (e.g. PSV or labelled as bi-level ventilation in most of the turbine-driven ventilators) and time-cycled (assisted pressure-controlled ventilation, APCV, or the ST/T mode of turbine-driven ventilators). Although the volume-controlled mode has been used during home care ventilation setting, it is seldom used in the acute setting because with this mode air leaks are poorly compensated.

In an assisted pressure-controlled flow-cycled breath (e.g. PSV or bi-level ventilation of turbine-driven ventilators), the ventilator detects the patient's inspiratory effort and delivers inspiratory pressure. Inspiration ends when the patient's inspiratory flow decay reaches a preset percentage of inspiratory flow. This threshold, as noted above, is also labelled expiratory trigger and is usually set at 25% of inspiratory flow decay but can be adjusted in most ventilators. At this threshold, inspiratory pressure is discontinued and drops to the baseline variable, namely ZEEP, or at a given set level of PEEP/EPAP. Criteria for a flow-cycled breath to cycle to baseline variable pressure are the following:

- Flow reaches a predetermined percentage threshold of inspiratory peak flow (usually 25%).
- Flow reaches a preset percentage of inspiratory peak flow (e.g. from 1% to 80%) or labelled as number (e.g. from 1 to 5). The wider the range, the greater the chance of matching the patient's neural inspiratory time.
- According to particular algorithms linked to flow value or waveform.

The rationale behind expiratory trigger adjustability (see also the section 'Triggering and Cycling Variables') is to cope with different respiratory mechanics and possible air leaks, thus improving patient–ventilator synchrony.[14,16] It has been demonstrated in intubated patients that the higher the value (e.g. 50%) the lower the mechanical inspiratory time and vice versa. Usually, COPD patients benefit from values around 40%, whilst restrictive conditions benefit from lower values (i.e. 5%–25%).[17] PRT settings can also interfere with the expiratory trigger in mechanical inspiratory time. Restrictive conditions usually benefit from a medium range pressure rise time (PRT); the opposite is for obstructive conditions such as COPD. Air leak can hinder the correct measurement of inspiratory flow threshold, prolonging inspiratory time and cause patient–ventilator asynchrony.

Non-invasive PSV increases the tidal volume whilst unloading[18] the inspiratory muscles. Furthermore, EPAP/PEEP added to PSV may counteract the effects of PEEPi in COPD patients improving gas exchanges and inspiratory muscle effort. The majority of NIV studies in ARF use PSV, and it is the most commonly used mode in acute hypercapnic exacerbations of COPD (see Chapter 41).[10] In patients with COPD, different levels of PSV may induce different respiratory patterns and gas exchanges. PSV levels capable of obtaining satisfactory arterial blood gases (ABGs) may result in ineffective respiratory efforts if external PEEP is not applied. The addition of PEEP, not exceeding dynamic intrinsic PEEP, may also reduce the metabolic work of the diaphragm without altering gas exchange. Modification of PRT can result in the modification of tidal volume and time of the mechanical breath in pressure-controlled flow-cycled breath.

APCV is an assisted pressure-controlled time-cycled mode where the operator sets a preset respiratory rate and inspiratory time. Its use during NIV may be helpful in the presence of large leaks hindering expiratory cycling in the pressure-controlled flow-cycled mode, under very restrictive conditions not supporting flow-cycled breaths or when a backup rate is required.

Although the pressure-controlled time-cycled mode is usually labelled as AC-PCV in ICU ventilators, a time-cycled breath can cycle to baseline variable pressure (EPAP/PEEP or ZEEP) when

- a given preset time is chosen in the APCV mode,
- a given preset time is chosen in a pressure-controlled flow-cycled mandatory breaths when the patient breaths at a respiratory rate that is below the set backup rate in the so-called 'ST mode' of a turbine-driven bi-level ventilator. This time can be chosen by (1) setting a given inspiratory time (T_i) or an 'inspiratory to expiratory ratio' for the 'backup' breaths and by (2) setting a so-called T_{min} or T_{max}. Both can either work as the inspiratory time of the 'backup' breaths according to manufacturer's algorithm or (3) automatically as 1:2, i.e. the 'inspiratory to expiratory ratio' of the set 'backup' rate.

New Mode: Dual Modes

Several tidal-volume-guaranteed (V_{TG}) modes fall under the umbrella term 'dual mode'. The rationale behind their use is to guarantee a constant tidal volume in pressure-controlled modes despite changes in respiratory impedance. Dual modes have been implemented, using different algorithms, during pressure-controlled time or flow-cycled ventilation in most ICU and bi-level turbine-driven ventilators both in double- and single-limb circuits.

V_{TG} modes guarantee a preset volume independently from circuit configuration; however, there are differences between V_{TG} delivered by 'vented' vs 'non-vented' RCs in the presence of unintentional leaks. In the absence of unintentional leaks in 'vented' or 'non-vented' RC configuration, all ventilators measuring or making an estimation of inspiratory tidal volume increase the inspiratory pressure to guarantee the V_{TG}. Conversely, in a 'non-vented' RC configuration, all tested ventilators show a drop in the inspiratory pressure in the presence of leaks, resulting in a concomitant reduction in V_{Texp}. This difference must be taken into account as a possible risk when a V_{TG} mode is used in the presence of unintentional linear or non-linear leaks. In addition, when a patient's ventilatory demand produces a V_T higher than the preset one, the patient will no longer be supported. For this reason, a minimum value of preset pressure should be carefully set by the operator.

New Mode: Proportional-assisted Ventilation

Proportional-assisted ventilation (PAV) delivers positive airway pressure 'proportional' to the patient's effort by monitoring lung elastance and resistance. Simplistically, during PAV, the ventilator assistance is delivered in proportion to the patient's instantaneous flow and volume, compensating patient's resistive and elastic loads, thus amplifying the patient's own effort breath by breath. Non-invasive PAV is more comfortable than PSV and can improve patient–ventilator synchrony in acute setting. However, data from invasive ventilation studies show that whilst PAV improves patient–ventilator synchrony at the start of inspiration this is not necessarily the case at the end of inspiration. This type of asynchrony may be worsened in the presence of air leaks explaining some mixed results with this mode when used non-invasively. More recently, new software that is able to adapt ventilator assistance to the respiratory system mechanics (elastance and resistance are measured automatically and semi-continuously every 300 ms) has been developed (PAV+, Covidien), although data on patient outcomes with this mode are scarce.

New Mode: Neurally Adjusted Ventilatory Assist

With PAV, NAVA is the only mode of ventilation delivering assistance in proportion to a patient's demand, aiming to the enhancement of patient–ventilator synchrony. NAVA is a form of partial ventilatory support wherein the machine applies positive pressure to the airway opening in proportion to the EAdi, which is the best available signal to estimate the respiratory drive. EAdi is used to trigger on and cycle off the delivery of the mechanical assistance and regulate its amount and intra-breath profile; therefore, the patient retains full control of the breathing pattern. EAdi is detected by means of a dedicated nasogastric feeding tube, mounting a distal array of multiple electrodes, and is processed to provide the highest possible quality of signal. Compared to PSV, NAVA has been shown to improve patient–ventilator interaction and synchrony, either in invasive ventilation or NIPPV. Although NAVA may not produce improvements in the respiratory rate or blood gas profile, it does improve patient–ventilator interaction and synchrony. Notably, the application of leak-compensating software significantly improved patient–ventilator synchrony with pressure support during NIPPV but produced little or no benefit with NAVA.

Approaches to ventilator troubleshooting during NIV are shown in Table 8.1.

Monitoring

Close monitoring of the patient on NIV is strongly recommended. According to some authorities, patients on NIV should be monitored to detect the use of accessory muscles, thoraco-abdominal paradoxical breathing movements, patient–ventilator interaction, and respiratory muscle fatigue. Direct visualization and analysis of flow–time and pressure–time waveforms provides valuable information about the quality of ventilator–patient interaction (e.g. ineffective respiratory efforts, ventilator auto-triggering, dyssynchrony between a spontaneously breathing patient and the ventilator, dyssynchrony due to air leaks in the PSV mode, or to avoid inadequate inspiration or expiration times during pressure- or volume-controlled time-cycled breath). The analysis of flow and pressure waveforms generated by ventilators can be useful in the optimization of patient–ventilator interactions and can improve both physiological and patient-centred outcomes.

Interfaces in the Acute Setting

The choice of the interface for NIV is a key factor in NIV success.[14,19,20] The perfect NIV interface does not exist, but the choice of an adequate interface should be tailored to the patient's characteristics and influenced by ventilator setting and patient' type of respiratory failure. Patient comfort, with the prevention or minimization of complications such as leaks, claustrophobia, eye irritation, skin breakdown due to tissue hypoxia, facial skin erythema, and acneiform rash, should be the major goals for clinicians. The bridge of the nose, the upper lip, and the armpits (only with the helmet use) are the most common sites of friction at risk of skin breakdown.[21]

Types of Interfaces

In the acute setting, the oronasal masks (covering the surface around the nose and the mouth) are the most frequently used interface in the adults, followed by total face masks (TFMs) (covering the entire anterior surface of the face, including the mouth, eyes, and nose), nasal masks (covering the nose only), and helmets (a transparent hood and soft polyvinyl chloride or silicon collar that includes the neck and the whole head).

Nasal, oronasal, and TFM are available in vented and non-vented versions (see the section 'Dead Space and Mask Volume'). The vented configuration has some holes or slots on the frame or on the swivel elbow, which allow carbon dioxide diffusion during ventilation with 'intentional leak' RC. The vented configuration of oronasal and TFM is always equipped with an anti-asphyxia valve with automatic opening to prevent rebreathing in the case of a pressure failure or when the airway pressure falls below 2–3 cmH_2O. The 'non-vented' configuration is completely closed and requires the use of a double- or a single-limb circuit with an active expiratory valve (see the section 'Dead Space and Mask Volume').[22] Possible indication for interfaces in ARF and related troubleshooting are shown in Tables 8.2 and 8.3.

Oronasal and TFM, compared to nasal masks, have the potential advantage of smaller air leaks and greater stability in the delivered mean airway pressure, especially in the acute setting or during sleep. For these reasons, their use is preferred to nasal interfaces during the acute phase of respiratory failure when patients are intensively dyspnoeic and, generally, opened-mouth breathers. The TFM limits the risk of deleterious cutaneous side effects, avoiding the nasal bridge and creating an effective seal around the less pressure-sensitive perimeter of the face. The TFM also has the advantage of rapid and easy application, and is a useful alternative for patients who are unable to obtain a good seal with other masks. It can be used in the case of nasal bridge skin breakdown and facial irregularities. Its use has

Table 8.1 Ventilator troubleshooting during NIV

Type	Definition	Aetiology	Adjustments
Delayed pressurization	Pressurization and the dependent flow rate are not synchronized with the patient's neural Ti	Too long PRT; poor ventilator performance in some old turbine-driven ventilator: patient's inspiratory time too low compared to the ventilator performance (i.e. Ti below 400 ms); large intentional (vented mask) or non-intentional leaks hindering pressure to rise; too high elastic recoil of the interface as with helmet	Shorten PRT and eventually use a more performant ventilator; reduce the amount of intentional leaks; if necessary, change the vented mask with anyone with less intentional leak; change the interface; change ventilator settings with the helmet (i.e. shorten PRT, adjust PEEP, pressure, shorten the RC with the helmet or switch to NAVA)
Auto-triggering	Inadvertent positive pressure breaths delivered by the ventilator not according to the patient's effort; monitored breaths on the ventilator higher than those made by the patient	Cycle inappropriately triggered by an external signal such as air leak or heart rate or water in the RC; too sensitive inspiratory triggers (if sensitivity is adjustable on the ventilator)	Optimize interface to minimize air leak; decrease level of pressure support to minimize leaks; decrease ventilator trigger sensitivity; remove water from the RC
Ineffective triggering/ waste of effort	Patient's effort not followed by a ventilator positive pressure breath; monitored breaths on the ventilator lower than those made by the patient	Inspiratory trigger sensitivity set too low; increased resistances in the circuit (i.e. HME); COPD: PEEPi not countered by PEEP; too high inspiratory pressure generating too high V_T in COPD patients; too low ETT in PSV; too long Ti in a time-cycled breath	Adjust trigger sensitivity if allowed on the ventilator; remove HME; COPD: reduce inspiratory pressure, increase EPAP/PEEP to counter PEEPi; use a higher ETT; shorten Ti in a time-cycled breath; if insufficient patient effort (i.e. DMD) to initiate a positive pressure breath, try to use a ventilator mode with a backup rate
Double triggering	Double triggering is defined as two cycles separated by a very short expiratory time possibly resulting in breath stacking	High patient ventilatory demand causing two breaths with a limited expiratory phase due to a too short mechanical Ti compared to the patient's neural time; too high ETT in the PSV mode	Increase Ti in time-cycled mode; optimize flow in the volume-controlled mode; adjust the PSV level, PRT, and ETT to modify inspiratory to expiratory time in PSV
Premature cycling	Ventilator cycle before the end of patient's neural inspiration time	Improper ETT or improper NIV software	Adjust ETT to regulate inspiratory to expiratory time in PSV; decrease rise time in patients with high drive and restrictive lung disease
Delayed cycling	Ventilator cycle later than patient's neural inspiratory time	Inappropriate ETT or NIV software in the PSV mode; too long Ti in a time-cycled breath	Reduce air leaks in PSV; adjust PSV, ETT, and PRT to regulate inspiratory to expiratory time in the PSV mode (e.g. increase rise time in patients with tachypnoea or obstructive lung disease); decrease inspiratory time in the time-cycled mode

EPAP/PEEP, end positive expiratory airway pressure; COPD, chronic obstructive pulmonary disease; PRT, pressure rise time; DMD, neuromuscular disease; PEEPi, intrinsic positive end-expiratory pressure; T_i, inspiratory time; PRT, pressure rise time; V_T, tidal volume; NAVA, neurally adjusted ventilatory assist; ETT, expiratory trigger threshold; PSV, pressure support ventilation; RC, respiratory circuit; HME, heat-and-moisture exchanger.

some limitations in claustrophobic patients and in the presence of large leaks in the vented configuration. TFM allows a clear and unrestricted view as with the helmet. Nevertheless, there is no clear evidence of any real advantage in terms of effectiveness and compliance compared to oronasal masks.[20] A new type of full-face mask, provided with nasal and oral ports that can be used in ongoing endoscopic procedures in the case of respiratory failure without interrupting the procedure, has recently been introduced as prototype. This mask is able to support ventilation in a few seconds as it is made of two symmetrical parts that can be divided in order to place it on the patient during the procedure, even if an endoscopic probe is already inserted.

The helmet interface, which includes all the neck and the head, was originally used to deliver a precise oxygen concentration during hyperbaric oxygen therapy. Recent engineering improvements gave helmets more comfortable seals, better seal against leak, and better patient–ventilator interaction. Compared to the mask, the helmet has the advantages of ensuring longer periods of continuous application of respiratory support and better tolerance by the patient, whilst reducing side effects related to the interface (i.e. skin breakdown, gastric distension, and eye irritation).[23] Whilst the helmet has some advantages, there is the risk of CO_2 rebreathing, especially when the gas flow is below 60 L/min.[21]

Intentional and Unintentional Leaks

Intentional leaks, as mentioned above, are deliberately generated in 'vented' mask when NIV is administered using single RC without an active non-rebreathing valve usually labelled as an 'intentional leak RC'. Intentional leak ports in the interface are designed to avoid rebreathing. Even if intended by the manufacturer, intentional leaks can affect patient/ventilator synchrony. In 'vented' masks, intentional leaks can impair efficacy (pressurization) of ventilation, especially when leaks are >40 L/min. The clinical consequence is that trigger sensitivity and rebreathing should be checked when switching to a mask with different intentional leaks.

Table 8.2 Possible indication for interfaces in ARF

Type of interface	Mode of fitting	Advantages and indications	Drawbacks
Mouthpiece	Kept in place by teeth or lips	No skin breakdown; selected use in the critical care area in the weaning phases of patients who were already using it in the chronic setting (e.g. neuromuscular patients and quadriplegics)	Increased salivation; dry mouth; leaks and patient–ventilator asynchrony; increased likelihood of alarms
Nasal mask/nasal pillows	Covers the nose or inserted in the nostrils; kept in place by a head strap	Possible more comfortable than an oronasal mask; easier speech and clearance of secretions; less claustrophobia; the absence of skin breakdown on the nasal bridge (only pillows)	Air leak from an open mouth, especially in edentulous patients; reduces seal at high pressure (>15 cmH_2O); less effective with loss of nasal patency; skin breakdown on the nasal bridge (only nasal)
Oronasal mask and hybrid mask	Covers the nose and mouth and kept in place by a head strap; the hybrid skips the nasal bridge covering only the nose tip	Less leaks in the acute setting; more effective in mouth breather patients	Claustrophobia; increased risk of aspiration; difficulty in speaking, eating, and clearing secretions; pressure sore on the nasal bridge
Total face mask	Covers the full face including the mouth, nose, and eyes; kept in place by a head strap	Less leaks in the acute setting; possible better comfort and better patient's view; the absence of skin breakdown on the nasal bridge; possible easier fitting in patients with difficult face contour	Claustrophobia; increased risk of aspiration; difficulty in speaking, eating, and clearing secretions; increased risk of aspiration
Helmet	A transparent hood and soft polyvinyl chloride or silicon collar that includes the neck and/the whole head; it is kept in place with different systems according to the manufacturer	Minimum air leaks in the acute setting; possible better comfort; the absence of skin breakdown on the nasal bridge; possible easier fitting in patients with difficult face contour	Possible CO_2 rebreathing if CPAP system does not allow a flow >40 L/min or if CPAP is delivered with conventional double-limb high-pressure ventilators; poor patient–ventilator synchrony using NIPPV; noisy; less respiratory muscle unloading in the PSV mode; risk of asphyxiation with ventilator or CPAP system malfunctioning; possible armpits decubitus when kept in place by armpits slings

CO_2, carbon dioxide; NIPPV, non-invasive positive positive airway pressure; CPAP, continuous positive airway pressure; PSV, pressure support ventilation.

Unintentional leaks can occur between the mask and the face or between the helmet and the neck, and through the open mouth with nasal ventilation. Leaks are one of the most important factors affecting patient–ventilator synchrony.[14] The sealing ability of an interface is largely dependent on the pressure by which the mask is applied to the face in relation to the inspiratory pressure. Problems with discomfort, gastric insufflation, skin ulceration, and leaks are likely to increase as the inspiratory pressure increases. This, in turn, requires application of the mask to the face with higher pressure to maintain the seal. Unintentional leaks may impair the efficiency of NIV, in particular during the first hours of ventilation when the patient needs to adapt to NIV and during sleep due to the loss of voluntary muscle control and decreased muscle tone. Patient–ventilator asynchrony is generated by unintentional leaks, and it increases with increasing severity of leak.

Table 8.3 Troubleshooting related to the interface

Type	Aetiology	Adjustments
Skin breakdown	Too tight head strap or securing system; too tight helmet sling causing friction in the armpit region; bad skin hygiene; improper size	Improve skin hygiene; adjust head strap and minimize strap tension; change the mask; use a wound-care dressing or softer silicone patch seals on the nasal bridge; use some cotton patch under the armpits with helmet
Air leaks	Too loose strap tension; wrong size; too high inspiratory pressure or PEEP; moustache or beard	Reduce pressure if possible; optimize the type and fit of the interface; trim moustache or beard; try a TFM
Claustrophobia	Use of an oronasal/TFM or helmet	Try to use nasal masks/pillows (hybrid masks if possible)
Rebreathing	Increased level of inspiratory CO_2 with vented mask or helmet	Optimize interface to minimize rebreathing; use a vented mask with large intentional air leak; increase inspiratory pressure of 2–3 cmH_2O; increase EPAP inspiratory pressure of 2.3 cmH_2O; check if the bias flow with helmet in the CPAP mode is >40 L/m or whether CPAP is delivered with a high-pressure gas-driven ICU ventilator; CPAP alone cannot be used with high-pressure ICU ventilator

CO_2, carbon dioxide; EPAP, end positive airway pressure; CPAP, continuous positive airway pressure; TFM, total face mask; ICU, intensive care unit.

Dead Space and Mask Volume

Non-vented Mask

In normal human beings, alveolar ventilation decreases as dynamic dead space volume (VD) increases. During NIV, dynamic VD can be the sum of the physiological VD and the apparatus VD. The physiological VD depends on the tidal volume and respiratory rate, whereas the interface VD depends on the internal volume of the interface. Although measured device dead space may vary markedly (e.g. full-face mask 205 mL vs nasal mask 120 mL), the in vivo effects, accounting for anatomical structures, are closer (full-face mask 118 mL vs nasal mask 97 mL). Indeed, the use of computational fluid dynamics to model streaming of gas effects demonstrates that the effective dead space is usually much smaller than that measured in the interface and is critically dependent on patient's tidal volume.[24] Practically speaking, the measured dead space of mask interfaces has little impact on patient-centred or physiological outcomes.

Helmets, which have much larger volumes than any of the other NIV interfaces and always exceed V_T, are used in a semi-closed environment in which the increase in the inspired partial pressure of CO_2 ($PiCO_2$) is an important issue and depends on the following factors:

(1) the amount of CO_2 produced by the subject (VCO_2);
(2) the flow of fresh gas that flushes the environment.

When using helmet with CPAP generators, a flow of at least 40 L/min, and preferably ≥60 L/min, is required to avoid carbon dioxide rebreathing. For this reason, CPAP alone should not be used with ICU ventilators in non-vented configuration as a very low flow is generated. When turbine-driven ventilators are used with an intentional leak RC, using a vent at the helmet expiratory port, lower flows may still prevent CO_2 rebreathing. Of all available interfaces, the helmet has a higher amount of asynchronies because of its soft, compliant wall, the elevated internal compressible volume, and increased likelihood of swings during ventilation rising the elastic recoil of the system.

Vented Mask

In vented masks, different ventilator settings may influence dynamic V_D; notably, the addition of PEEP can decrease dynamic V_D to close to physiological levels. In vented masks, the site of the exhalation ports can influence carbon dioxide rebreathing. Carbon dioxide clearance is better with exhalation ports built into the mask.

In conclusion, the ability to provide better patient comfort whilst reducing adverse effects, such as skin lesions, might enable mask ventilation to be used successfully in a larger patient population. There is no perfect NIV interface for all patients in all situations. The choice of NIV interface requires a careful evaluation of the patient, the ventilation mode, and the clinical setting. Fitting the mask to the patient rather than trying to make the patient fit the mask is mandatory, but this is only possible when a large range of interfaces and sizes are available. Individualization is key to making the right choice of an NIV interface. The larger the availability of interfaces and sizes, the higher the probability of successfully fitting the interface to the patient.

Humidification

Although upper airways are not bypassed during NIV, humidification and warming of the inspired gas are often needed to prevent the adverse effects of cool, dry gases on the airway epithelium. Unidirectional inspiratory nasal air flow, such as during mouth air leak, breathing only through the mouth and gas having lower humidity than the ambient air, such as those delivered from ICU ventilators, can dry the nasal mucosa. If the nasal mucosa receives little or none of the moisture it would ordinarily receive from the exhaled gas, it can lose the capacity to heat and humidify inspired air progressively drying and releasing inflammatory mediators, such as leukotrienes, with an associated increased vascularity (see Chapter 4). Humidification can prevent these adverse effects. There are two types of humidification devices: heated humidifier and heat-and-moisture exchanger (HME) (see Chapter 10). They are used for both short- and long-term NIV. However, an HME, which is usually placed between the Y-piece and the interface, can add a significant amount of dead space, compared to a heated humidifier, which is placed in the inspiratory limb. As HMEs are associated with increased $PaCO_2$ and inspiratory effort, alveolar ventilation can only be maintained at the expense of greater WOB, compared to a heated humidifier. Despite this, the impact of different types of humidification systems on the success rate of NIV delivered for ARF with ICU ventilators is not strongly influenced by the humidification system used.[25] Based on the physiologic and available clinical data, although HMEs may have some undesirable physiologic effects, there are no recommendations reporting the need for using heated humidification during NIV.

Patient Selection and Beginning of NIV

General Inclusion and Exclusion Criteria

NIV should be considered in all patients having bedside alteration in respiratory pattern and alteration of ABGs due to lung and/or ventilatory pump failure.[22] The former should include increased dyspnoea (moderate to severe), tachypnoea (with respiratory rate>24 breaths/min), and use of accessory muscles or paradoxical abdominal movements. The latter should include hypercapnia and respiratory acidosis ($PaCO_2$ > 45 mmHg and pH < 735) and/or hypoxaemia PaO_2/FiO_2 ratio <200.[2] Absolute and relative contraindications and a possible algorithm on how to apply NIV in the first hours are shown in Table 8.4 and Box 8.1. NIV has been used at multiple stages in the patient journey,[22] including early to prevent intubation,[6] as a peri-intubation technique[7] (see Chapters 9 and 20), and to facilitate ventilator weaning,[26] with guidelines developed to aid in the selection and monitoring of patients

Table 8.4 Absolute and relative contraindications to use NIV in the acute setting

Absolute	Relative
• Inability to fit mask • Risk of respiratory arrest • Instability—hypotensive shock, uncontrolled cardiac ischaemia or arrhythmia, uncontrolled copious upper gastrointestinal bleeding • Inability to protect airway	• Excessive secretions not managed by secretion clearance techniques • Swallowing impairment or ongoing vomiting • Agitated, uncooperative patient • Multiple (i.e. two or more) organ failure • Recent upper airway or upper gastrointestinal surgery

Source: Adapted from *The Lancet*, 374(9685), Nava S, Hill N. Noninvasive ventilation in acute respiratory failure, pp. 250–259. Copyright 2009, with permission from Elsevier.

Box 8.1 Algorithm on how to apply NIV during first few hours

- Explain technique to patients reassuring them whenever possible
- Choose the proper interface and size trying it first on patient's face/neck
- Decide ventilatory mode/support
  - with PSV mode start from low levels (i.e. pressure support about 8 cmH_2O) and add, if needed, PEEP 4–5 cmH_2O according to patient's underlying disease; set PRT, inspiratory trigger, and ETT whenever allowed
  - with CPAP check pressure and bias flow, especially with helmet (e.g. with the helmet set CPAP not less than 6–8 cmH_2O and bias flow no less than 40 L/min)
  - with NAVA set the NAVA gain and PEEP
- Set FiO_2 on ventilator or add low-flow oxygen into the circuit using the dedicated oxygen adapter
- Place interface gently over face, holding it in place and gently securing it. Protect the skin if needed (e.g. wound-care dressing)
- Start ventilation
- Gently tighten straps just enough to optimize patent's comfort and to avoid major leaks
- Adjust FiO_2 on ventilator or low-flow oxygen into the circuit, aiming at $SO_2 > 90\%$
- Set alarms according to the patient's severity
- Adjust PSV and PEEP values according to the patient underlying disease (e.g. in hypoxemic patients, increase PEEP to get oxygen saturation ≥90%)
- Monitor SO_2, respiratory rate, and dyspnoea (e.g. VAS scale) every 30 min for 6–12 h and then within 1 h
- Measure ABGs at baseline and within 1 h from start
- Humidification advised for applications longer than 6 h
- Consider use of mild sedation in agitated patients

Source: Adapted from *The Lancet*, 374(9685), Nava S, Hill N. Noninvasive ventilation in acute respiratory failure, pp. 250–259. Copyright 2009, with permission from Elsevier.

NIV, non-invasive ventilation; PSV, pressure support ventilation; PEEP, positive end-expiratory pressure; PRT, pressure rise time; FiO_2, fraction of inspired oxygen; SO_2, oxygen saturation; ABGs, arterial blood gases; VAS, visual analogic scale; NAVA, neurally adjusted ventilatory assist; ETT, expiratory trigger threshold.

for this modality.[27] During the COVID-19 pandemic (see Chapter 35), it has been used in the management of acute hypoxic respiratory failure secondary to viral pneumonitis when adjuncted by awake prone positioning.[28–30] The need to manage extraordinary numbers of patients with COVID-19 related ARF, with the hope of avoiding invasive ventilation has led to a significantly increased use of NIV. Initial justification for this was in part due to an established role in at least mild-to-moderate ARF prior to the pandemic.[31] Although there are theoretical reasons to suggest that NIV may improve outcomes, and when combined with prone positioning may reduce ventilator-induced and self-induced lung injury,[16] the translation of this into improved patient-related outcomes has not been shown, and concerns related to possible barotrauma or delayed introduction of invasive ventilation have necessitated caution, without recommendation thus far in ARF due to COVID-19.

REFERENCES

1. Brochard L, Mancebo J, Wysocki M, et al. Noninvasive ventilation for acute exacerbations of chronic obstructive pulmonary disease. *N Engl J Med.* 1995 28;**333**:817–822.
2. Nava S, Hill N. Noninvasive ventilation in acute respiratory failure. *Lancet.* 2009;**374**:250–259.
3. Russotto V, Myatra SN, Laffey JG, et al. Intubation Practices and Adverse Peri-intubation Events in Critically Ill Patients From 29 Countries. *JAMA.* 2021;**325**(12):1164–1172.
4. Brochard L, Isabey D, Piquet J, et al. Reversal of acute exacerbations of chronic obstructive lung disease by inspiratory assistance with a face mask. *N Engl J Med.* 1990;**323**:1523–1530.
5. Gregoretti C, Burbi L, Biolino P, et al. Treatment of acute respiratory failure with pressure support ventilation by facial mask. *Acta Anaesthesiologica Italica.* 1990;**41**:65–68.
6. Ferrer M, Esquinas A, Leon M, et al. Noninvasive ventilation in severe hypoxemic respiratory failure: A randomized clinical trial. *Am J Respir Crit Care Med.* 2003;**168**:1438–1444.
7. Russotto V, Cortegiani A, Raineri SM, et al. Respiratory support techniques to avoid desaturation in critically ill patients requiring endotracheal intubation: A systematic review and meta-analysis. *J Crit Care.* 2017;**41**:98–106.
8. Cortegiani A, Russotto V, Antonelli M, et al. Ten important articles on noninvasive ventilation in critically ill patients and insights for the future: A report of expert opinions. *BMC Anesthesiol.* 2017 Sep 4;**17**(1):122.
9. Beltrame F, Lucangelo U, Gregori D, et al. Noninvasive positive pressure ventilation in trauma patients with acute respiratory failure. *Monaldi Arch Chest Dis.* 1999;**2**:109–114.
10. Ferreyro BL, Angriman F, Munshi L, et al. Association of noninvasive oxygenation strategies with all-cause mortality in adults with acute hypoxemic respiratory failure: A systematic review and meta-analysis. *JAMA.* 2020;**324**(1):57–67.
11. Appendini L, Patessio A, Zanaboni S, et al. Physiologic effects of positive end-expiratory pressure and mask pressure support during exacerbations of chronic obstructive pulmonary disease. *Am J Respir Crit Care Med.* 1994;**149**:1069–1076.
12. Chadda K, Annane D, Hart N, et al. Cardiac and respiratory effects of continuous positive airway pressure and noninvasive ventilation in acute cardiac pulmonary edema. *Crit Care Med.* 2002;**30**:2457–2461.
13. Thille AW, Lyazidi A, Richard JC, et al. A bench study of intensive-care-unit ventilators: New versus old and turbine-based versus compressed gas-based ventilators. *Intensive Care Med.* 2009;**35**:1368–1376.
14. Vignaux L, Vargas F, Roeseler J, et al. Patient–ventilator asynchrony during non-invasive ventilation for acute respiratory failure: A multicenter study. *Intensive Care Med.* 2009;**35**:840–846.
15. Cammarota G, Vaschetto R, Turucz E, et al. Influence of lung collapse distribution on the physiologic response to recruitment maneuvers during noninvasive continuous positive airway pressure. *Intensive Care Med.* 2011 Jul;**37**(7):1095–1102.
16. Russotto V, Bellani G, Foti G. Respiratory mechanics in patients with acute respiratory distress syndrome. *Ann Transl Med.* 2018;**19**:382.
17. Stell IM, Paul G, Lee KC, et al. Noninvasive ventilator triggering in chronic obstructive pulmonary disease. A test lung comparison. *Am J Respir Crit Care Med.* 2001;**164**:2092–2097.
18. L'Her E, Deye N, Lellouche F, et al. Physiologic effects of noninvasive ventilation during acute lung injury. *Am J Respir Crit Care Med.* 2005 Nov 1;**172**(9):1112–1118.
19. Nava S, Navalesi P, Gregoretti C. Interfaces and humidification for noninvasive mechanic ventilation. *Respir Care.* 2009;**54**:71–82.

20. Girault C, Briel A, Benichou J, et al. Interface strategy during noninvasive positive pressure ventilation for hypercapnic acute respiratory failure. *Crit Care Med.* 2009;**37**:124–131.
21. Racca F, Appendini L, Berta G, et al. Helmet ventilation for acute respiratory failure and nasal skin breakdown in neuromuscular disorders. *Anesth Analg.* 2009;**109**:164–167.
22. Nava S, Navalesi P, Conti G. Time of non-invasive ventilation *Intensive Care Med.* 2006;**32**:361–370.
23. Patel BK, Wolfe KS, Pohlman AS, et al. Effect of noninvasive ventilation delivered by helmet vs face mask on the rate of endotracheal intubation in patients with acute respiratory distress syndrome: A randomized clinical trial. *JAMA.* **2016;315**(22):2435–2441.
24. Fodil R, Lellouche F, Mancebo J, et al. Comparison of patient–ventilator interfaces based on their computerized effective dead space. *Intensive Care Med.* 2011;**37**:257–262.
25. Lellouche F, L'Her E, Abroug F, et al. Impact of the humidification device on intubation rate during noninvasive ventilation with ICU ventilators: Results of a multicenter randomized controlled trial. *Intensive Care Med.* 2014;40:211–219.
26. Vaschetto R. Early extubation followed by immediate noninvasive ventilation vs. standard extubation in hypoxemic patients: A randomized clinical trial. *Intensive Care Med.* 2019;**45**:62–71.
27. Rochwerg B, Brochard L, Elliott MW, et al. Official ERS/ATS clinical practice guidelines: Noninvasive ventilation for acute respiratory failure. *Eur Resp J.* 2017;**50**:1602426.
28. Foti G, Giannini A, Bottino N, et al. Management of critically ill patients with COVID-19: Suggestions and instructions from the coordination of intensive care units of Lombardy. *Minerva Anestesiol.* 2020;**86**:1234–1245.
29. Longhini F, Bruni A, Garofalo E, et al. Helmet continuous positive airway pressure and prone positioning: A proposal for an early management of COVID-19 patients. *Pulmonology.* 2020;**26**:186–191.
30. Coppo A, Bellani G, Winterton D, et al. Feasibility and physiological effects of prone positioning in non-intubated patients with acute respiratory failure due to COVID-19 (PRON-COVID): A prospective cohort study. *Lancet Respir Med.* 2020;**8**:765–774.
31. Bellani G, Laffey JG, Pham T, et al. Noninvasive ventilation of patients with acute respiratory distress syndrome. Insights from the LUNG SAFE Study. *Am J Resp Crit Care Med.* 2017;**195**:67–77.
32. Gregoretti C, Navalesi P, Ghannadian S, et al. Choosing a ventilator for home mechanical ventilation. *Breathe.* 2013;**9**(5): 394–409.

9

Clinical Applications of Non-invasive Ventilation in Critical Care

Federico Longhini, Rosanna Vaschetto, and Paolo Navalesi

KEY MESSAGES

- Acute respiratory failure (ARF) secondary to exacerbations of chronic obstructive pulmonary disease (COPD) represents the main indication for non-invasive ventilation (NIV). In these patients, NIV reduces the need for intubation and in-hospital mortality.
- In acute cardiogenic pulmonary oedema (ACPO), non-invasive continuous positive airway pressure (CPAP) speeds up the process of recovery, relieving dyspnoea and improving gas exchange. Non-invasive positive pressure ventilation (NIPPV) does not provide additional benefit, even in hypercapnic patients.
- For patients with de novo hypoxemic ARF, the indication for NIV remains controversial. While some patients might benefit, others could be seriously harmed. Various factors, such as severity, type and distribution of lung damage, and timing of NIV application, can affect NIV outcome. Immunosuppressed patients are more likely to benefit from NIV.
- NIV may be a valuable weaning strategy for some patients with hypercapnic ARF, primarily those with COPD.
- In patients at increased risk of extubation failure, NIV may prevent post-extubation respiratory failure and the consequent need for re-intubation. However, when post-extubation failure is established, NIV is not indicated.

CONTROVERSIES

- Recent RCTs suggest caution about using NIV in pneumonia and acute respiratory distress syndrome (ARDS), regarding outcomes.

FURTHER RESEARCH

- Assessing the role of NIV in weaning patients with resolving hypoxaemic, non-hypercapnic ARF.
- Comparing NIV and humidified high-flow oxygen therapy through nasal cannula in patients with ARF of different aetiologies as part of large trials.

Introduction

Non-invasive ventilation (NIV) is an effective treatment for patients with acute respiratory failure (ARF) of different aetiologies. The indications to NIV vary depending on the different forms of ARF and the characteristic of the patient. Its primary advantage is avoidance of endotracheal intubation, which is associated with increased risk of ventilator-associated pneumonia. In this chapter, with the term 'non-invasive ventilation' (or 'NIV'), we refer to both non-invasive continuous positive airway pressure (CPAP), where airway pressure is maintained above atmospheric pressure throughout the whole respiratory cycle by pressurization of the ventilatory circuit, and non-invasive positive pressure ventilation (NIPPV), where the positive pressure rises during the inspiratory phase and actively supports the inspiratory muscles (see Chapter 8 for details of non-invasive ventilators, circuits, and interfaces).

In this chapter, we systematically consider NIV application in ARF of different aetiologies.

NIV in COPD Exacerbation

Chronic obstructive pulmonary disease (COPD) (see Chapter 41) is characterized by an increased chronic inflammatory response of the airways to noxious particles causing persistent airflow limitation. During an acute exacerbation, inflammation leads to increased sputum production, worsening hyperinflation, increased work of breathing, and dyspnoea. If the workload exceeds the muscular pump force, respiratory acidosis may ensue. In this situation, NIV plays an important role in patient treatment.

In patients with exacerbated COPD, NIV may be considered with three different goals in mind: (a) to prevent respiratory acidosis, (b) to avoid invasive mechanical ventilation (iMV) in patients with mild-to-moderate respiratory acidosis, and (c) as an alternative to iMV in the case of severe respiratory acidosis and distress. NIV indications and effects on clinical outcomes, depending on the severity of the respiratory acidosis, are reported in Table 9.1.

Table 9.1 NIV indications and effects on the outcomes in COPD exacerbation

Respiratory acidosis	Aim of NIV treatment	NIV indications	Outcome effects of NIV reported
Absent (pH > 7.35)	To prevent further deterioration	Not indicated	Uneven reduction of intubation rate No difference in survival
Mild-to moderate (7.25 ≤ pH < 7.35)	To prevent iMV	Strongly recommended	Survival improvement Reduction in iMV need Reduction of hospital length of stay
Severe (pH < 7.25)	As an alternative to iMV	To be considered	Reduction of septic complications Reduction of time spent under ventilatory assistance

NIV to Prevent the Development of Respiratory Acidosis

Several studies have investigated the use of NIV in exacerbations of COPD without respiratory acidosis. Randomized trials in this situation find that NIV offers little benefit over conventional oxygen therapy (COT) in terms of reducing intubation or mortality. A large randomized controlled trial (RCT) included 342 COPD patients with a mean pH at randomization of 7.35, to receive within 24–48 h from admission either NIPPV or COT. When compared to COT, NIPPV decreased the number of patients meeting criteria for intubation but did not modify mortality.[1]

Recent guidelines suggest NIV not to be used in patients with hypercapnia without respiratory acidosis in the setting of a COPD exacerbation.[2] In these cases, physicians should administer medical therapy only, targeting the arterial oxygen saturation (SaO_2) between 88 and 92%, which has been associated with better survival.[2]

NIV to Prevent Endotracheal Intubation

Prior to the advent of NIV, medical management, consisting of oxygen, antibiotics, steroids, and bronchodilators, was the mainstay of COPD therapy. However, medical therapy fails in a high proportion of patients, and reports of failure range from around 25% to 75%. Patients with exacerbations of COPD and respiratory acidosis are those who benefit most from NIPPV, with favourable effects on gas exchange and dyspnoea, reductions of endotracheal intubation, length of the hospital stay, and mortality.

A meta-analysis including 14 studies assessed the impact of NIPPV in acute hypercapnic respiratory failure due to an exacerbation of COPD, on different outcomes.[3] Compared to medical therapy, NIPPV reduced the overall treatment failure by 50% and the risk of mortality by 48%. In a subgroup analysis, the mortality risk reduction was 49% with pH values <7.30 on admission, while 55% when pH ranged between 7.30 and 7.35. Notably, the survival effect not modified when NIPPV was used in intensive care units (ICUs) or medical wards.[3] NIPPV also shortened hospital length of stay by approximately 3 days, with a trend towards the decrease in ICU length of stay and in the number of complications.[3] Given this robust evidence, NIPPV is strongly recommended in patients with a pH of 7.25–7.35.[2]

NIV as an Alternative to Invasive Mechanical Ventilation

In patients with more severe COPD exacerbation, NIPPV has been compared to endotracheal intubation. Although iMV may induce more rapid improvements in gas exchange, NIPPV is associated with fewer septic complications and duration of ventilation without an increase in mortality. Interestingly, delayed intubation following a trial of NIV does not appear to be associated with increased mortality. Therefore, as per evidence based recommendations an NIPPV trial in patients with a severe exacerbation of COPD should be attempted, with consideration of early endotracheal intubation should there be no improvement or with further deterioration.[2] It is worth remarking, however, that the greater the severity of exacerbation (i.e. lower pH), the higher the rate of NIPPV failure.

Acute Cardiogenic Pulmonary Oedema

Acute cardiogenic pulmonary oedema (ACPO) is one of the most severe manifestations of acute heart failure. In ACPO, cardiac failure results in increased backpressure on the pulmonary circulation, which in turn precipitates extravasation of fluid into the alveoli. Consequently, the lungs become less compliant and the respiratory effort increases.

The medical treatment of this condition includes supplemental oxygen, diuretics, and treatments targeting the aetiology of ACPO. Patients with ACPO may require ventilatory support. The application of positive pressure to the airway increases the intrathoracic pressure, influencing the complex interplay between heart and lung. In particular, positive end expiratory pressure (PEEP) reduces the cardiac filling pressure and left-ventricular afterload by lowering left-ventricular transmural pressure, and recruits non-aerated lung areas ameliorating pulmonary mechanics and gas exchange (Chapter 17).

Several studies investigated the application of CPAP or NIPPV, in patients with ACPO. In 1991, Bersten et al. demonstrated that the application of CPAP through mask reduced the need for iMV from 35% to 0%, compared to medical therapy alone, with no significant difference in hospital length of stay and mortality.[4] Although early concerns were raised about an increase in myocardial infarction among patients treated with NIPPV, this has not been borne out as data have accumulated.[5] While the role of NIV for the in-hospital management of ACPO is clear, investigations have extended to the pre-hospital setting. Although the heterogenous settings and severity present challenges for researchers, data suggests that early application of NIV can limit mortality and need for intubation.[2] In light of the results emerging from clinical trials and from meta-analysis providing a moderate certainty of evidence, recent guidelines strongly recommend the use of NIV in patients with ARF due to ACPO in the hospital settings.[2] However, they also reflect less certain evidence for its pre-hospital use, where appropriate skills and infrastructure are present.

Hypoxaemic Acute Respiratory Failure

Differentiation of the patient presenting with hypoxaemic ARF into those suffering fluid overload (i.e. ACPO) and those with inflammatory lung injury due to pneumonia or acute respiratory distress syndrome (ARDS) is critical. While in the first case NIV can be a vital adjunct to medical management, in the case of pneumonia or ARDS, NIV should be approached with appropriate caution. The cornerstone of the ventilatory treatment of hypoxaemic respiratory failure, and in particular of ARDS, is protective iMV with assured low tidal volumes, limited airway plateau and driving pressures (see Chapter 21). However, iMV can be complicated by several conditions, such as mucus retention (Chapter 28) and ventilator-associated pneumonia (Chapter 32), leading to increased morbidity. A number of studies have investigated the role of NIV in avoiding intubation in hypoxaemic ARF. Here, we describe the use of NIV in hypoxaemic ARF in the following subpopulations: patients with de novo ARF, immunocompromised patients, pandemic viral illness, post-surgical ARF, and chest trauma. Figure 9.1 depicts a schematic representation for NIV indications in hypoxaemic ARF.

De Novo Hypoxaemic ARF

De novo ARF is defined as respiratory failure in the absence of prior chronic respiratory disease; frequently, it is characterized by hypoxaemia (defined by a ratio between arterial partial pressure to inspiratory fraction of oxygen (PaO_2/FiO_2) <200 mmHg), tachypnoea (i.e. respiratory rate >30 breaths/min), and the absence of a diagnosis of COPD. Pneumonia or ARDS are the commonest conditions causing de novo ARF.

NIV is commonly applied in de novo ARF in order to improve gas exchange while reducing work of breathing. NIV may or may not reduce the inspiratory effort in such patients. Nonetheless, when elevated inspiratory support is necessary or high tidal volumes are generated, one risks lung injury. High inspiratory pressures, more often than not, drive significant air leaks and patient intolerance, making NIPPV ineffective.

Several studies have examined this area and have produced contrasting results with some indicating reductions in need for ventilation, while others show no benefit.[6] The heterogenous nature of the patients included and the ventilator settings used may explain some of these divergent results. The lack of consistent evidence means that recent guidelines have avoided strong recommendations in this area.[2] However, they suggest that NIV can be trialled in community-acquired pneumonia or ARDS with careful patient selection by an experienced team in a closely monitored environment. Furthermore, these patients require early reassessment after NIV initiation and, in the case of no rapid improvement, intubation should not be delayed.[2]

ARF in Immunocompromised Patients

The use of immunosuppressive strategies in organ transplantation or disease treatments and the number of patients affected by immune deficiency is gradually increasing. These patients are at increased risk of developing hypoxaemic ARF and requiring ICU admission for ventilatory support. While endotracheal intubation is, in general, a predisposing factor for nosocomial pneumonia, immunodeficiency is a major predisposing factor for this complication, which in these patients can be severe and associated with particularly unfavourable outcomes. Several studies have investigated the potential of NIV in immunocompromised patients with hypoxaemic ARF and show that compared to COT, NIV is able to reduce need for intubation, complications of mechanical ventilation, sepsis and mortality.[7] Predictors of failure of NIV include

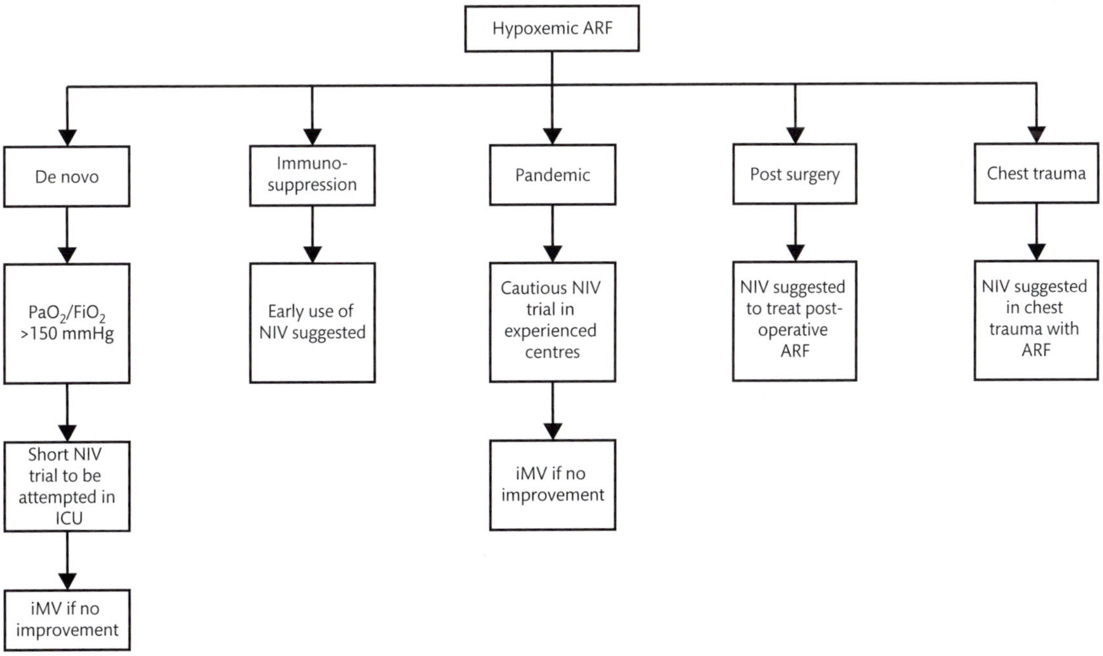

Figure 9.1 Schematic indications for NIV in hypoxemic acute respiratory failure.

delay in institution of this therapy, need for vasopressor and renal replacement support, and higher respiratory rate while on NIV. Notwithstanding these initial positive results, a multicentre French RCT by Lemiale et al., who randomized 374 immunocompromised patients with hypoxaemic ARF to receive either NIPPV or COT, found no difference in 28-day mortality (primary endpoint) between the two groups; intubation rate, ICU and hospital length of stay, and duration of mechanical ventilation were also similar.[8] A recent subgroup analysis of the FLORALI study[6] suggested that high-flow nasal oxygen (see Chapter 7) may lead to fewer intubations than NIPPV in this patient population. In spite of these apparently contradictory results, current guidelines suggest, with a moderate certainty of evidence, early NIV for immunocompromised patients with hypoxemic ARF.[2]

Pandemic Viral Illness

The use of NIV for severe ARDS due to pandemic viral illness has been evaluated in a few observational studies, showing a highly variable rate of failure ranging from 13% to 77%. While some studies show reductions in the use of iMV and no increase in mortality for those intubated later, others show converse results with higher hospital mortality among those who fail on this modality. During the recent COVID-19 pandemic (see Chapter 35), NIV has again found widespread use, although definitive studies showing its superiority to COT and iMV are currently lacking. There are studies suggesting a benefit of CPAP over High flow nasal oxygen therapy (RECOVERY-RS) but this is an area of uncertainty.

Given the low quality of evidence, recent guidelines do not provide any recommendation for NIV in patients with ARF due to pandemic viral illness, although a cautious NIV trial in carefully selected patients treated in a protected environment at experienced centres is not considered a contraindication.[2]

Post-surgical ARF

Post-operative pulmonary complications may occur up to 7 days after surgery in 20%–30% of patients. General anaesthesia, problematic pain control, and surgical procedures near the diaphragm increase the probability of developing impaired respiratory function, characterized by reduction in lung volume and hypoxaemia. Predisposing co-morbidities for post-operative ARF include obesity, obstructive sleep apnoea, and COPD.

NIV has been investigated as a preventive strategy in patients considered at increased risk of post-operative ARF, as well as means to reverse respiratory dysfunction, reducing atelectasis and increasing lung aeration, and improving arterial oxygenation.

The use of NIV to avert the occurrence of post-operative complications and prevent ARF after abdominal surgery was investigated by several studies whose results had been pooled in a meta-analysis.[9] The authors concluded that very low-quality evidence suggests NIV might reduce post-operative pneumonia and atelectasis, but its effects on mortality are unclear. Specific patient populations have been examined, including those following lung resection, and cardiac and abdominal surgery. A recent Cochrane review of NIV following lung resection did not find evidence of benefit from NIV, although the authors noted that the confidence intervals for effect size were wide and quality of studies was low to moderate.[10] Recent findings in cardiac surgery demonstrated both high-flow nasal oxygen and NIPPV equivalent in managing post-operative respiratory failure.[11] Jaber and colleagues have reported on the use of NIPPV in patients following abdominal surgery in several studies, finding reduced need for re-intubation, duration of ventilation, and secondary infections, although these benefits neither altered mortality nor the length of stay in ICU or hospital.[12] Notwithstanding the moderate certainty of evidence, recent guidelines provide a conditional recommendation in favour of NIV in patients with post-operative ARF.[2]

Chest Trauma

Chest trauma (see Chapter 55) is an acute physical injury to the chest involving one or more of the anatomical thoracic structures (rib cage, airways, lung, heart, vessels, oesophagus, and diaphragm). These injuries alter the mechanical properties of the respiratory system. In addition, lung contusion and atelectasis cause ventilation–perfusion mismatch or even frank right-to-left shunting. Therefore, ARF may develop, requiring ventilatory assistance. Studies in this area have tended to be small, either as subgroups of larger studies or stand-alone trials. Compared to COT, NIV reduces need for intubation and ICU length of stay in this patient group. When used in place of iMV, CPAP is associated with reduced length of stay and time spent on mechanical ventilation with consequent reduction infection. However, it is important that analgesia is well managed in these patients to maximize the benefits of NIV. Pooled analysis of these data indicates, notwithstanding the heterogeneity of the studies, that NIV decreases mortality, need for intubation, rate of nosocomial pneumonia, and ICU length of stay, making NIV advisable for chest trauma without a clear-cut recommendation.[2]

NIV to Facilitate Discontinuation of Mechanical Ventilation

Weaning is the entire process aimed at liberating patients from mechanical ventilation; it includes a series of stages from intubation and institution of iMV, to liberation from ventilatory support and extubation (see Chapter 64). The decision to extubate a patient is generally based on the results of the spontaneous breathing trial (SBT). However, in selected patients, NIV may substitute iMV, in order to avoid complications related to intubation and speed up the weaning process.

Weaning in Hypercapnic ARF

Nava et al. evaluated the effectiveness of NIPPV as weaning strategy in 50 patients with a severe exacerbation of COPD invasively ventilated and failing to pass a SBT within the first 48 h after ventilatory support initiation.[13] Patients were randomized to receive either conventional weaning through the endotracheal tube, with progressive reduction of pressure support level and SBTs twice a day, or NIPPV through a face mask after early extubation. Compared to conventional weaning, NIPPV shortened the ICU length of stay, reduced the rate of pneumonia, and improved 60-day survival.[13] Subsequent studies have confirmed the finding that NIPPV can shorten the duration of weaning and iMV, with significant impact on subsequent ICU and hospital length of stay. NIPPV is also associated with

Table 9.2 NIV for weaning in hypercapnic ARF

NIV for weaning in hypercapnic ARF*	
Criteria to proceed	**Effects on outcome**
✓ Blood gas normalization ✓ Good neurological status ✓ No fever ✓ Haemodynamic stability ✓ SaO_2 >88% with FiO_2 ≤40%	✓ Lower duration of iMV and related complications ✓ Lower rate of tracheostomy ✓ Shorter ICU length of stay ✓ Improved survival rate

*Procedure advisable in ICUs with experience with NIV (data confirmed by multiple studies).

higher probability of weaning success and a reduction in the need for tracheostomy. However, it is important to consider the patients included in such trials, as high rates of co-morbid conditions such as COPD and heart failure may influence their results, and findings may not be generalizable to all causes of ARF.

More recently, a multicentre RCT from 13 French ICUs compared NIPPV with conventional weaning and extubation followed by standard oxygen therapy (VENISE trial), in 208 patients with acute-on-chronic respiratory failure who failed an SBT after a minimum of 48 h of iMV.[14] The trial did not show any difference in probability of re-intubation between the three groups. However, NIPPV significantly decreased the occurrence of post-extubation ARF, compared to both other groups. Though the time spent under iMV was shortened, the overall time spent under ventilatory support, i.e. iMV and NIPPV, dedicated to weaning was found to be slightly increased in patients undergoing NIPPV. The time to rescue therapy was similar between the two non-NIPPV groups, for which rescue post-extubation NIPPV avoided re-intubation or death in 52% of patients.[14] Table 9.2 summarizes criteria for proceeding with using NIV to aid weaning in hypercapnic ARF and its impact on clinical outcomes.

Weaning in Hypoxaemic ARF

While several trials have been carried out in either hypercapnic subjects or mixed populations of patients, only one pilot study has investigated the feasibility of NIPPV application as a tool for weaning in patients recovering from hypoxaemic ARF.[15] This study enrolled 20 patients with a PaO_2/FiO_2 ratio ranging from 200 to 300 mmHg, undergoing iMV for at least 48 h, implemented through a pressure support ventilation modality, with a total applied pressure (i.e. PEEP + inspiratory support) ≤25 cmH_2O, and a PEEP between 8 and 13 cmH_2O. Patients were randomized to receive either conventional weaning based on iMV or to be extubated and to receive NIPPV with similar settings to those used during iMV.[15] Blood gases and vital parameters did not differ between groups. The study reported only one patient failing discontinuation of mechanical ventilation within 48 h in the NIPPV group, compared to five patients in the control group. In comparison with controls, patients randomized to NIPPV experienced more iMV free days after enrolment and after 28 days. A trend towards a reduction of tracheostomies was also observed in the NIPPV group, whereas no differences were detected with regard to septic complications, weaning, sedation, ICU length of stay, and mortality.[15] It should be pointed out that this is only a feasibility study, and a proper powered trial is required to assess the real effectiveness of NIPPV as a weaning strategy for patients with hypoxaemic ARF.

Evidence and Recommendations

Burns et al. conducted a meta-analysis[16] identifying 16 RCTs dealing with NIPPV as a weaning strategy, including a total number of 994 patients. Of these studies, nine included only patients with exacerbations of COPD, six referred to mixed populations (predominantly hypercapnic), while one small pilot trial recruited only pure hypoxemic subject. Compared to conventional weaning through endotracheal tube, weaning through NIPPV was associated with a decreased mortality, reduction of weaning failures, and lower incidence of ventilator-associated pneumonia.[16] Furthermore, ICU and hospital lengths of stay, the total duration of mechanical ventilation and iMV, and the rate of tracheostomy resulted to be also significantly reduced in the NIPPV cohort.[16] Subgroup analyses suggested greater benefits from weaning approach through NIPPV in trials enrolling exclusively COPD participants rather than in those including mixed populations.[16]

Since the use of NIV to wean patients from iMV is considered more difficult as compared to other indications, the recent guidelines only suggest rather than recommend its use in patients with hypercapnic ARF, with no indication for hypoaxemic ARF.[2]

Post-extubation Respiratory Failure

Despite fulfilling the criteria for weaning and successfully passing the SBT, some patients experience post-extubation respiratory failure leading to re-intubation. Extubation failure is an episode of respiratory failure requiring ventilatory support, occurring within 48–72 h. The need for re-intubation following extubation failure is a major clinical problem characterized by worsened outcomes including higher risk of pneumonia, longer duration of iMV, prolonged ICU and hospital length of stay, and increased mortality. Therefore, strategies able to lower the occurrence of post-extubation ARF or to avoid the need for re-intubation should, in principle, improve the patient's outcome. Several studies have investigated the role of NIV in this sense. Some studies applied NIV to treat overt post-extubation respiratory failure, while others used NIV to prevent it.

NIV to Treat Post-extubation ARF

One of the first studies, conducted by Hilbert et al., suggested a promising role of NIPPV to treat overt post-extubation ARF in COPD patients with respiratory acidosis within 72 h after extubation.[17] In this case-control study, NIPPV reduced the need for re-intubation and the duration of both ventilatory assistance and ICU stay, when compared with COT applied in an historical control group.[17] However, subsequent studies have not supported this early promise. Esteban et al. performed a large RCT in 37 centres, enrolling 221 patients who developed post-extubation respiratory failure in the 48 h following extubation and were randomized to receive either NIV or standard treatment.[18] The trial confirmed the lack of benefit of NIPPV, when compared with standard treatment, with regard to both rate of re-intubation and ICU length of stay. Of note, ICU mortality was higher in the NIPPV group, thus suggesting potential harm from NIPPV due to delayed intubation. Of note, the median time elapsed between respiratory failure and re-intubation was longer in the NIPPV group.[18]

Based on these findings, NIV is presently not advised for the prevention of re-intubation in patients with overt post-extubation respiratory failure.[2]

NIV to Prevent Post-extubation ARF

While NIV does not have a role in established post-extubation respiratory failure, several investigators have examined its prophylactic ability to prevent this situation arising. Early studies which were non-selective did not appear to show benefit; however, when trials were enriched for 'at-risk' patients, improvements in post-extubation respiratory function were found. Nava and colleagues found prophylactic NIPPV effective in averting failure after deliberate extubation.[19] Nava et al. enrolled 97 patients, randomized 1 h after extubation to receive either NIPPV (minimum 8 h/day for 2 days) or COT. Patients receiving NIPPV had lower rates of re-intubation, which resulted in a reduced risk of ICU mortality when compared to COT. Subsequent studies have supported these findings, although the optimal duration of NIV is uncertain as it differed between protocols. Interestingly, the benefit of NIV for the prophylaxis of post-extubation ARF appears to be greatest among those who develop hypercapnia during SBTs and this effect is not restricted to those with underlying COPD. Patients with morbid obesity (see Chapter 54) and pre-existing neuromuscular disorders (NMDs) (see Chapter 51) also show benefit from post-extubation NIV, although much of the data in this area comes from observational studies with historical control groups. Based on these studies, recent guidelines suggest the use of NIPPV after extubation to prevent post-extubation ARF in high-risk patients only.[2] Criteria to consider a patient 'at risk' for post-extubation ARF are listed in Box 9.1.

NIV in Asthma

Acute asthma is a sudden episode of bronchoconstriction, leading to a huge increase of airway resistance causing hyperinflation (see Chapter 42). It is characterized by accessory muscle recruitment and dyspnoea. The excessive load imposed on the respiratory muscles and hyperinflation may lead to failure of the respiratory muscle pump, which ultimately becomes exhausted, developing hypercapnia.

In principle, NIV might decrease the work of breathing, thus preventing respiratory muscle failure and need for intubation. Only a few studies are presently available. CPAP significantly reduced the work of breathing in patients with an acute episode of asthma as compared to routine care. Despite some physiological benefits, meta-analyses did not highlight any improvement in clinically relevant outcomes in favour of NIV as compared to the sole medical therapy.

Recently, a large multicentre retrospective cohort study reported data from 97 hospitals over a 4-year period on the use of NIV in adult patients with an acute episode of asthma.[20] A total of 668 patients received immediate iMV with no prior NIV trial, while NIV was attempted in 559 patients. Among the latter, 26 patients (4.7%) failed NIV and required intubation. The hospital mortality rate was 14.5% in patients receiving immediate iMV, 15.4% for patients failing NIV, and 2.3% for those succeeding NIV.[20] Due to the uncertainty of evidence, recent guidelines did not produce any recommendation on the use of NIV in patients with an acute episode of asthma.[2]

Box 9.1 Criteria to consider patients 'at risk' for post-extubation ARF

Risk factors for post-extubation ARF in the literature

Presence of more than one increases the risk of failure of weaning or extubation
- Chronic heart failure
- Hypercapnia at extubation or chronic respiratory disease
- More than one co-morbidity
- Weak cough
- Stridor after extubation
- >65 years/old
- Heart failure as reason for intubation
- APACHE II >12 at extubation
- ARF requiring >72 h of iMV
- Obesity (BMI ≥ 35)
- Swallowing impairment
- Neuromuscular disease

NIV in Neuromuscular Disorders

Neuromuscular disorders include a heterogeneous group of diseases, affecting the muscles and/or the nervous system (see Chapters 16 and 51). Although quite rare, NMDs often cause respiratory failure because of inspiratory, expiratory, and glottic muscle involvement, leading to respiratory pump failure. The deterioration of the respiratory function can be either progressive, acute, or acute-on-chronic. Although respiratory failure in patients with NMDs is most commonly chronic and progressive, here we focus on acute and acute-on-chronic episodes, which are the most common life-threatening complications of these pathologies (long-term home ventilation is covered in Chapter 65).

Guillain-Barrè syndrome (GBS) and myasthenia gravis (MG) with rapid-onset are the two most frequent causes of ARF due to NMDs. GBS is an inflammatory polyradiculoneuropathy caused by the immune system, damaging the peripheral nerves and leading to a rapid (from few hours to few days) onset of muscular weakness. GBS may also involve the phrenic nerve, leading to diaphragm dysfunction and ARF in up to 30% of patients. It is associated to dysautonomia, hemodynamic instability, and cardiac arrhythmias. In these patients, NIPPV can be instituted to initially support patients with ARF. However, it is crucial to identify patients at risk for NIPPV failure early in order to avoid delayed or emergency intubation. Such patients are characterized by a rapid onset of the disease (<7 days), inability to lift the head from the bed, ineffective cough, worsening of forced vital capacity >30% over 24 h, autonomic or bulbar dysfunction, and severe respiratory muscle weakness (as defined by a vital capacity <60% predicted, a maximal inspiratory pressure <–30 cmH_2O, or a maximal expiratory pressure <40 mmHg). In the presence of one or more of the aforementioned predictors, it is preferable to proceed with elective intubation and iMV rather than NIPPV.

MG is an autoimmune disease leading to a variable degree of skeletal muscle weakness. MG can be characterized by a very rapid onset with ARF or by intervening myasthenic crisis leading to acute-on-chronic respiratory failure. As these patients often require ventilatory assistance and iMV, early NIPPV has been proposed. Small retrospective case series indicate the ability of NIPPV to prevent the need for iMV. In a retrospective cohort, Seneviratne and colleagues found that NIPPV was found to reduce duration of mechanical ventilation and consequently ICU and hospital lengths of stay.[21] Wu et al. retrospectively analyzed 41 patients with myasthenic crisis, 14 of whom received NIPPV.[22] NIPPV failed in six (43%) patients characterized by higher baseline arterial carbon dioxide partial pressure ($PaCO_2$), who had longer ICU and hospital lengths of stay, as opposed to seven patients succeeding NIPPV. The role of bedside pulmonary function tests in predicting NIPPV failure is unclear, and the decision to start NIPPV is based on clinical judgement and should be taken as early as possible. NIPPV has also been proposed to facilitate weaning from iMV in patients recovering from myasthenic crisis. Notwithstanding the reported benefits, the use of NIPPV in MG should be limited to highly experienced centres, because of the potential rapid evolution of the disease, with potential for disastrous consequences.

Several other causes of neuromuscular weakness exist, the majority of which are characterized by a progressive course with episodes of acute-on-chronic respiratory failure. NIV may play a role in the management of these patients. Vianello et al. compared 14 neuromuscular patients receiving NIPPV because of ARF with 14 matched historical control patients receiving iMV.[23] Of note, 6 of 14 patients receiving NIPPV also underwent cricothyroid 'mini-tracheostomy', in order to facilitate the elimination of tracheabronchial secretions and to avoid mucus plugging and atelectasis.[23] Although the number of patients was small, NIPPV significantly reduced mortality, treatment failures, and ICU length of stay, as opposed to iMV. Another study by Servera et al. assessed the effectiveness of NIPPV, in association with the use of mechanical cough assistance, in 24 episodes of acute-on-chronic respiratory failure in 17 patients with NMDs of different aetiology.[24] NIPPV avoided endotracheal intubation in 79.2% of the analyzed episodes; of note, all patients with NMDs other than amyotrophic lateral sclerosis were successfully treated with NIV.[24] The combined use of cough assistance and NIPPV is indeed strongly advised in patients with ARF due to NMD. Recent guidelines suggest that NIPPV (1) should almost always be applied in the patients with ARF affected by NMD or (2) should be considered in acute illness when vital capacity is known to be <1 L and respiratory rate >20 breaths/min.[25]

NIV in Palliative Care

Palliative care aims to provide enhanced quality of life for patients with serious and incurable illnesses. NIV can be an option in selected cases to reduce dyspnoea, while allowing verbal communication and better comfort during the last hours of life.

NIV may be used in terminally ill patients with different objectives: (1) life support with no limitation of life-sustaining treatment, (2) life support when patients refuse intubation, and (3) as a pure 'palliative measure', for breathing control. As the goals of care might change, patient transition from one category to another is possible. When NIV has only palliative purposes, physician must clearly explain to the patient and relatives that they should only expect relief of symptoms. Therefore, NIV will be considered successful only if it relieves to some extent dyspnoea without generating excessive discomfort. The most appropriate setting for palliative NIV is not, in most cases, the ICU as if it fails, only a rapid intensification of sedative and analgesic drugs is required. Moreover, due to shortage of ICU beds or ICU physicians' reluctance to admit cancer patients with ARF, NIV is often added to routine care in haematology or oncology wards.

Meduri et al. first reported that NIPPV could reduce dyspnoea and improve gas exchange in a case series of 11 terminally ill (mainly COPD) patients with ARF who refused endotracheal intubation.[26] Similar findings have been noted in patients with cancer, where NIPPV not only improves gas exchange and dyspnoea but is also associated with successful hospital discharge in a substantial proportion of patients. However in a randomized trial, assigning 30 hospitalized patients with end-stage cancer complicated by ARF to receive either NIV or COT, Hui and colleagues found the two treatments equally effective in improving dyspnoea and oxygenation.[27] Liu et al. retrospectively reported data from 79 patients with active haematologic malignancy treated with NIV in ICU.[28] Forty-four (56%) patients who failed NIV had higher mortality as opposed to those who succeeded.[28] Nava et al. randomized 200 patients with solid tumours, ARF, and life expectancy <6 months, to receive either NIPPV or COT. Compared to COT, NIPPV was more effective in reducing dyspnoea, especially in hypercapnic patients, and decreased the required doses of morphine, maintaining better cognitive function.[29]

A multicentre prospective cohort study conducted in 54 ICUs in France and Belgium investigated whether the use of palliative NIV in patients with treatment-limitation decisions could improve the health-related quality of life at 90 days. In patients with a 'do not intubate' (DNI) order, NIV was associated with substantial survival, particularly in COPD patients. Furthermore, at 90 days, NIV prolonged life without increasing symptoms of anxiety, depression, or stress among relatives.[30] Similar results have been observed in elderly patients (≥75 years/old) with DNI orders, and in those with DNI orders presenting to emergency departments with acute or acute-on-chronic respiratory failure. Use of NIV in these patients is associated with survival for reasonable periods of time and without significant decline in health-related quality of life.

In the light of the data present in the literature, recent guidelines suggest offering palliative NIV to patients affected by an end-stage disease.[2]

Conclusions

NIV is the first-line treatment in patients with a severe exacerbation of COPD causing hypercapnic ARF. NIV (in particular, CPAP) is strongly recommended for patients with ARF due to ACPO. NIV may be indicated to treat hypoxaemic ARF secondary to surgical procedures, chest trauma, NMDs, or occurring in immunocompromised patients, to prevent further deterioration and need for endotracheal intubation. NIV is also indicated for a palliative intent in patients with end-stage disease. NIV may help to speed up the weaning process in hypercapnic patients, while its use in patients with hypoxaemic ARF (i.e. ARDS) requires further investigation. NIV should be considered after extubation to prevent the development of post-extubation respiratory failure in 'at-risk' patients, while it is presently not advised in established post-extubation respiratory failure. NIV is controversial in de novo hypoxaemic ARF. Given the uncertainty of evidence, there is presently no recommendation on the use of NIV for de novo hypoxaemic ARF and acute asthma.

REFERENCES

1. Collaborative Research Group of Noninvasive Mechanical Ventilation for Chronic Obstructive Pulmonary Disease. Early use of non-invasive positive pressure ventilation for acute exacerbations of chronic obstructive pulmonary disease: A multicentre randomized controlled trial. *Chin Med J (Engl)*. 2005;**118**:2034–2040.
2. Rochwerg B, Brochard L, Elliott MW, et al. Official ERS/ATS clinical practice guidelines: Noninvasive ventilation for acute respiratory failure. *Eur Respir J*. 2017;**50**(2):160242.
3. Ram FS, Picot J, Lightowler J, et al. Non-invasive positive pressure ventilation for treatment of respiratory failure due to exacerbations of chronic obstructive pulmonary disease. *Cochrane Database Syst Rev*. 2004;**3**:CD004104.
4. Bersten AD, Holt AW, Vedig AE, et al. Treatment of severe cardiogenic pulmonary edema with continuous positive airway pressure delivered by face mask. *N Engl J Med*. 1991;**325**:1825–1830.
5. Cabrini L, Landoni G, Oriani A, et al. Noninvasive ventilation and survival in acute care settings: A comprehensive systematic review and meta analysis of randomized controlled trials. *Crit Care Med*. 2015;**43**:880–888.
6. Frat JP, Thille AW, Mercat A, et al. High-flow oxygen through nasal cannula in acute hypoxemic respiratory failure. *N Engl J Med*. 2015;**372**:2185–2196.
7. Gristina GR, Antonelli M, Conti G, et al. Noninvasive versus invasive ventilation for acute respiratory failure in patients with hematologic malignancies: A 5-year multicenter observational survey. *Crit Care Med*. 2011;**39**:2232–2239.
8. Lemiale V, Mokart D, Resche-Rigon M, et al. Effect of noninvasive ventilation vs oxygen therapy on mortality among immunocompromised patients with acute respiratory failure: A randomized clinical trial. *JAMA*. 2015; **314**:1711–1719.
9. Ireland CJ, Chapman TM, Mathew SF, et al. Continuous positive airway pressure (CPAP) during the postoperative period for prevention of postoperative morbidity and mortality following major abdominal surgery. *Cochrane Database Syst Rev*. 2014;**8**:CD008930.
10. Torres MFS, Porfírio GJM, Carvalho APV, et al. Non-invasive positive pressure ventilation for prevention of complications after pulmonary resection in lung cancer patients. *Cochrane Database Syst Rev*. 2019;**3**: CD010355.
11. Stephan F, Barrucand B, Petit P, et al. High-flow nasal oxygen vs noninvasive positive airway pressure in hypoxemic patients after cardiothoracic surgery: A randomized clinical trial. *JAMA*.2015;**313**:2331–2339.
12. Jaber S, Lescot T, Futier E, et al. Effect of noninvasive ventilation on tracheal reintubation among patients with hypoxemic respiratory failure following abdominal surgery: A randomized clinical trial. *JAMA*. 2016;**315**;1345–1353.
13. Nava S, Ambrosino N, Clini E, et al. Noninvasive mechanical ventilation in the weaning of patients with respiratory failure due to chronic obstructive pulmonary disease. A randomized, controlled trial. *Ann Intern Med*. 1998;**128**:721–728.
14. Girault C, Bubenheim M, Abroug F, et al. Noninvasive ventilation and weaning in patients with chronic hypercapnic respiratory failure: A randomized multicenter trial. *Am J Respir Crit Care Med*. 2011;**184**:672–679.
15. Vaschetto R, Turucz E, Dellapiazza F, et al. Noninvasive ventilation after early extubation in patients recovering from hypoxemic acute respiratory failure: A single-centre feasibility study. *Intensive Care Med*. 2012;**38**:1599–1606.
16. Burns KE, Meade MO, Premji A, et al. Noninvasive positive-pressure ventilation as a weaning strategy for intubated adults with respiratory failure. *Cochrane Database Syst Rev*. 2013; **12**:CD004127.
17. Hilbert G, Gruson D, Portel L, et al. Noninvasive pressure support ventilation in COPD patients with postextubation hypercapnic respiratory insufficiency. *Eur Respir J*. 1998; **11**:1349–1353.
18. Esteban A, Frutos-Vivar F, Ferguson ND, et al. Noninvasive positive-pressure ventilation for respiratory failure after extubation. *N Engl J Med*. 2004;**350**:2452–2460.
19. Nava S, Gregoretti C, Fanfulla F, et al. Noninvasive ventilation to prevent respiratory failure after extubation in high-risk patients. *Crit Care Med*. 2005;**33**:2465–2470.
20. Stefan MS, Nathanson BH, Lagu T, et al. Outcomes of non-invasive and invasive ventilation in patients hospitalized with asthma exacerbation. *Ann Am Thorac Soc*. 2016;**13**:1096–1104.
21. Seneviratne J, Mandrekar J, Wijdicks EF, et al. Noninvasive ventilation in myasthenic crisis. *Arch Neurol*. 2008;**65**:54–58.
22. Wu JY, Kuo PH, Fan PC, et al. The role of non-invasive ventilation and factors predicting extubation outcome in myasthenic crisis. *Neurocrit Care*. 2009;**10**:35–42.
23. Vianello A, Bevilacqua M, Arcaro G, et al. Non-invasive ventilatory approach to treatment of acute respiratory failure in neuromuscular disorders. A comparison with endotracheal intubation. *Intensive Care Med*. 2000;**26**:384–390.
24. Servera E, Sancho J, Zafra MJ, et al. Alternatives to endotracheal intubation for patients with neuromuscular diseases. *Am J Phys Med Rehabil*. 2005;**84**:851–857.
25. Davidson C, Banham S, Elliott M, et al. British Thoracic Society/Intensive Care Society Guideline for the ventilatory management of acute hypercapnic respiratory failure in adults. *BMJ Open Respir Res*. 2016;**3**:e000133.
26. Meduri GU, Fox RC, Abou-Shala N, et al. Noninvasive mechanical ventilation via face mask in patients with acute respiratory failure who refused endotracheal intubation. *Crit Care Med*. 1994;**22**:1584–1590.
27. Hui D, Morgado M, Chisholm G, et al. High-flow oxygen and bilevel positive airway pressure for persistent dyspnea in patients with advanced cancer: A phase II randomized trial. *J Pain Symptom Manage*. 2013;**46**:463–473.
28. Liu J, Bell C, Campbell V, et al. Noninvasive Ventilation in Patients With Hematologic Malignancy: A Retrospective Study. *J Intensive Care Med*. 2019;**34**(3):197-203.
29. Nava S, Ferrer M, Esquinas A, et al. Palliative use of non-invasive ventilation in end-of-life patients with solid tumours: A randomised feasibility trial. *Lancet Oncol*. 2013;**14**:219–227.
30. Azoulay E, Kouatchet A, Jaber S, et al. Noninvasive mechanical ventilation in patients having declined tracheal intubation. *Intensive Care Med*. 2013;**39**:292–301.

10

Medical Gases and Humidification

Lorenzo Ball, Francesco Tasso, Veronica Vercesi, Marco Tixi, Iacopo Firpo, and Paolo Pelosi

KEY MESSAGES

- Oxygen has specific indications and toxicity; hypoxia and hyperoxia should both be avoided.
- Inhaled nitric oxide can improve ventilation perfusion matching and oxygenation in hypoxaemic respiratory failure.
- Heating and humidification of inhaled gases is mandatory in invasively ventilated patients and should be performed using active or passive devices.
- Heating and humidification are also indicated in specific types of non-invasive respiratory support.

CONTROVERSIES

- Do medical gases such as inhaled nitric oxide and helium/oxygen mixtures have any role in respiratory failure?
- Does modification of gas conditioning during mechanical ventilation influence the trajectory of respiratory failure?

FURTHER RESEARCH

- Large-scale studies are ongoing to determine safe and optimal limits of oxygen delivery and oxygen targets in specific populations of acute respiratory distress syndrome (ARDS), critical illness, and respiratory disease.
- Studies are warranted to define clear indications for active humidification during non-invasive respiratory support.

Introduction

Respiratory support can be seen as the administration of medical gases at appropriate concentration, temperature, humidity, and pressure. Humidification and heating of medical gases is referred to as conditioning, and it is a crucial part of non-invasive and invasive respiratory support. This chapter illustrates the role of medical gases and gas conditioning in the treatment of patients requiring different types of respiratory support.

Medical Gases

The most commonly used medical gas is oxygen, typically delivered as a mixture with room air. Other gases are sometimes required, and the knowledge of their indications and limitations is of paramount importance.[1] This section discusses the use of the three most commonly used medical gases: oxygen, nitric oxide, and helium.

Oxygen

The term 'oxygen' was used for the first time at the end of the 18th century, and in the following decades experiments were carried out to clarify its role in biochemical processes. While the use of oxygen is common among hospitalized patients, like any drug, it may be harmful if used inappropriately.[2]

The only evidence-based indication for oxygen administration is correction of hypoxaemia.[3] However, unnecessary use is common especially in non-hypoxaemic dyspnoeic patients or in patients perceived at risk of developing hypoxaemia and in the post-operative setting.[4] Inappropriate prescription is common and has been correlated to increased risk of unnecessary admission to high dependency units, increased length of hospital stay, and possibly higher mortality in patients with chronic obstructive pulmonary disease (COPD).[5] Among patients with acute respiratory distress syndrome (ARDS), targets of PaO_2 from 55 to 80 mmHg are frequently considered the standard of care, based on the trials performed by the ARDS Network.[6,7] However, observational trials report that, also in patients with hypoxaemic respiratory failure and ARDS, clinicians tend to target higher PaO_2 levels, especially in mild-to-moderate ARDS.[8] Among patients with COPD, lower targets of PaO_2 might be acceptable, and the use of indiscriminately high oxygen flow increases mortality.

The common use of oxygenation targets beyond what is strictly necessary to maintain oxygenation raises concerns about potential toxicity. Patients receiving oxygen should also be monitored for the potential occurrence of hyperoxia,[9] which might have specific toxicity mediated by reactive species of oxygen. Extremely elevated PaO_2 values can induce hyperoxic acute lung injury in healthy lungs.[10] However, within the ranges realistically observed in the clinical practice, the actual impact of hyperoxia on clinical outcome is unclear. In a recent randomized trial in ARDS patients, two groups maintaining PaO_2 around 70 and 90 mmHg were compared, without observing differences in mortality.[11] However, the fraction of inspiratory oxygen (FiO_2) should be titrated to maintain oxygenation within the recommended targets, and there is a strong pathophysiological rationale to avoid exposure to extreme values of PaO_2, which were not investigated in randomized trials. It must be stressed that, while strictly correlated, FiO_2 and PaO_2 are two distinct parameters, the first being the inhaled fraction of oxygen and the latter the actual partial pressure of oxygen achieved at the arterial level. How FiO_2 translates into a certain PaO_2 in a specific patient depends on the type of respiratory support used, the application of positive airway pressure, and the degree of impairment of the respiratory function. For these reasons, early studies investigating the effect of pure oxygen administration in healthy lungs, which often results in PaO_2 above 500 mmHg, should not be translated to patients with injured lungs, where high FiO_2 does not necessarily result in supra-physiological PaO_2. In fact, in all ARDS trials investigating the effects of different levels of positive end expiratory pressure (PEEP), the use of lower PEEP was associated with a significant increase in FiO_2 and often lower PaO_2, but this did not result in increased or decreased mortality.[12] Specific patient populations might be particularly sensitive to hyperoxia and might warrant further caution when titrating the FiO_2 and choosing PaO_2 targets. This is the case, in particular, of critically ill patients with brain lesions[13]: in a recent study in post-cardiac arrest patients, early exposure to hyperoxia after resuscitation was associated with worse neurological outcome.[14] Two recent trials[15,16] tested conservative versus liberal oxygen strategies in critically ill patients requiring mechanical ventilation and did not observe differences in ventilator-free days or mortality. However, in both studies there was a small difference in PaO_2 between the intervention and control group, therefore these should not be interpreted as a call to tolerate hyperoxia. Other larger studies are ongoing and will provide further insight on this topic.

Other Medical Gases

Inhaled Nitric Oxide

The role of nitric oxide (NO) in determining pulmonary vasodilation was first identified in the late 1980s.[17] Thereafter, inhaled nitric oxide (iNO) has been proposed to improve oxygenation in patients with ARDS.[18] In these patients, vasodilation induced by NO at the pulmonary level diverts pulmonary blood flow towards ventilated regions, with a relative reduction of perfusion in non-aerated areas. As a consequence, the global ventilation perfusion matching and pulmonary hypertension improve, and venous admixture and shunt are reduced resulting in improved oxygenation. Not all patients with ARDS respond to iNO, and a test dose is often administered. While many patients might show oxygenation improvement during iNO administration, randomized controlled trials failed to show a clear benefit on mortality and raised concerns regarding a potential renal toxicity.[19] Other indications for iNO include persistent pulmonary hypertension of the newborn, bronchopulmonary dysplasia in premature infants and in the post-operative care of congenital heart disease surgery.[1]

Inhaled NO is delivered in doses typically ranging from 1 to 20 parts per million (ppm) and requires dedicated equipment to be administered. The use of iNO is typically restricted to intubated patients; however, there are reports of its use during non-invasive respiratory support in selected patients. Modern machines delivering iNO have a flow sensor to synchronize gas emission with the inspiratory flow, reducing the consumption of iNO tanks, which are expensive. Most sophisticated devices allow real-time monitoring of the actual NO concentration delivered in the inspiratory gases and also measure the levels of nitrogen dioxide (NO_2), an unwanted toxic compound that is generated when NO and oxygen are mixed in the respiratory circuit. Occasionally, a rebound of hypoxaemia and pulmonary hypertension have been observed when discontinuing iNO. Strategies to avoid this phenomenon include titrating the iNO dose to the lowest effective value, which is often around 5 ppm, and slow weaning from iNO, maintaining a concentration of 1 ppm for 1 h before interruption. In has been suggested that co-administration of sildenafil could decrease the likelihood of rebound phenomena.[1] At concentrations above 40 ppm, NO might bind haemoglobin resulting in methemoglobinemia: if this adverse effect is observed, other causes such as drugs co-administrations should be ruled out and the iNO dose reduced. Inhaled NO has been extensively used during the COVID-19 pandemics, also for early studies suggesting a potential direct anti-viral effect at higher doses. However, the clinical relevance of this effect has not been confirmed by trials, and the advantages in terms of oxygenation were reportedly transient.[20] For all these reasons, iNO should only be considered as a rescue therapy for patients with hypoxaemic respiratory failure refractory to conventional mechanical ventilation with high FiO_2.

Helium

The first reports of the use of helium and oxygen mixtures in patients with increased resistance of the respiratory system dates back to 1934.[21] The rationale behind their use is based on the better fluid dynamic properties of helium compared to nitrogen, the main component of air. In fact, the likelihood of a gas to develop a turbulent flow is related to the Reynolds number, which is proportional to gas density, flow, and size of the airway while inversely proportional to gas dynamic viscosity. Helium is 86% less dense than nitrogen but has a similar viscosity: replacing helium to air in oxygen mixtures allows modifying the type of flow observed in smaller airways, converting areas of turbulent flow into more efficient laminar flow.[1] Among patients with increased airway resistance, this translates in less effort to move gases in the respiratory system, reducing the work of breathing in spontaneously breathing patients and allowing ventilation with lower peak pressures in controlled ventilation modes,[22] possibly reducing the risk for barotrauma.[23] For these reasons, it has been proposed as method to treat patients with increased resistances, including asthma, status asthmaticus, respiratory distress of the newborn, upper airway obstruction, and ARDS. Despite the interesting mechanism of action, the evidence from randomized trial concerning the use of oxygen–helium mixtures is very limited. Currently, helium for medical use is distributed in tanks in fixed combination with oxygen (minimum 20% oxygen), to avoid accidental delivery of hypoxic mixtures. Moreover, it must be stressed that heliox has no role in treating the underlying condition but might only offer a temporary advantage increasing tidal volume and airway flow limiting peak pressure (see the section named 'Inhaled Therapies: Therapeutic Aerosol Drug Delivery' in Chapter 22).

Basics of Gas Conditioning

Ventilators invariably deliver cold and dry gases. Humidity affects the functioning of respiratory epithelium, therefore warming and humidification of inspired gases must be considered in all invasively ventilated patients.[3] The act of warming and humidifying respiratory gases is referred to as conditioning. In spontaneous breathing, the upper airways provide, in physiological conditions and in a variety of climates, a flow of warm, humid, and filtered gas mixture to the lower airways, ensuring gas exchange while protecting the respiratory system (Figure 10.1). When the airways are bypassed by an artificial airway such as an endotracheal tube or a tracheostomy cannula, this role is only played by the lower respiratory tract, which is insufficient for this scope.[24] Humidity can be measured as absolute humidity (AH) and relative humidity (RH). AH is the total content of water vapour in a certain volume of gas and is measured in mg H_2O/L. RH is the ratio between the actual water vapour contained in the gas mixture and the whole capacity of it at that temperature and is expressed as a percentage.

The total capacity of a gas mixture to retain water vapour is a function of its pressure and temperature. In the clinical setting, the leading role is played by temperature, which affects importantly the AH of the respiratory gases. The air inside the alveoli at 37 °C is fully saturated (100% RH) and has an AH of 44 mg H_2O/L; when exhaled, it has an average temperature of 33 °C, for an AH of 37 mg H_2O/L. This has practical repercussions in the assessment of humidity delivered to the patient via the humidification devices and in the patient fluid balance. The upper respiratory tract is responsible for 75% of conditioning of inspiratory gases. When air enters the nose, air is exposed to the highly vascularized mucosa covering the convoluted surface of the turbinates, having sufficient interface to deliver heat and moisture to the inspired air. After the upper respiratory tract, the trachea is responsible for the last 25% of gas conditioning, providing warm and fully saturated airflow to the lower respiratory tract. In physiological conditions, this process is achieved few centimetres below the carina, at the isothermal saturation boundary, where air is delivered at core temperature (37 °C) and 100% RH (44 mg H_2O/L AH). During expiration, about 25% of heat and moisture is transferred from the airflow to the mucosae. In this process, the air temperature falls from 37 to 33 °C, its RH remains 100%, and its AH falls from 44 to 37 mg H_2O/L, mainly condensing. If the gradient of temperature between core temperature and expired air is too wide, it exceeds the mucosae capability of retaining condensed vapour. The water lost at every breath is about 27 mg H_2O/L with inspired air carrying 10 mg H_2O/L versus 37 mg H_2O/L in the expired air. This loss is greater as the gradient of temperature and humidity widens or the minute ventilation rises.

Indications During Invasive Mechanical Ventilation

Underhydration and overhydration cause structural and functional damage to the airways (Figure 10.1), resulting in clinical repercussions: mucous thickening, increased resistance and work of breathing, cough, reduced lung compliance, inflammation, atelectasis, and consequently more susceptibility to infections.[25] These factors may lead to worse outcome, longer in-hospital length of stay, and increased healthcare-associated costs. Moreover, secretion retention may result in endotracheal tube occlusion, which can be an abrupt and potentially deadly event, in most cases without predictable signs. Underhydration occurs when a conditioning device is not used during mechanical ventilation, and when the

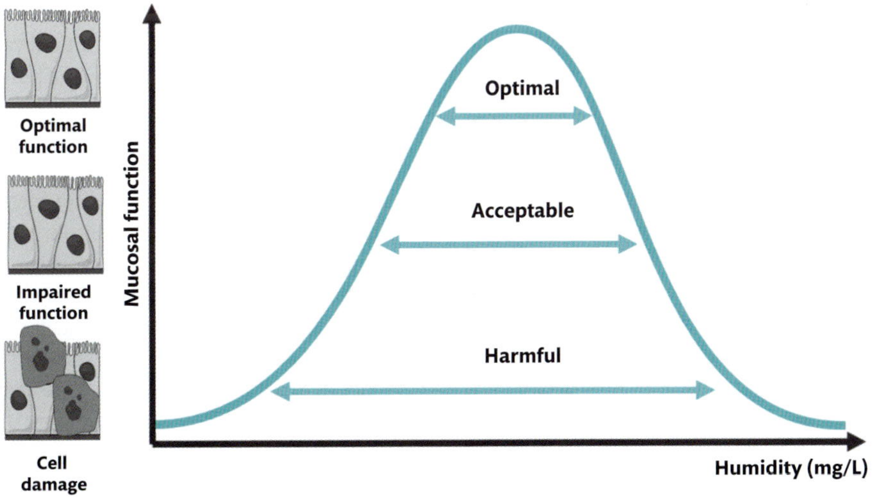

Figure 10.1 Mucociliary function versus humidity. Within optimal ranges, the mucociliary function is preserved. At higher or lower values, progressive impairment of mucosal function is observed.

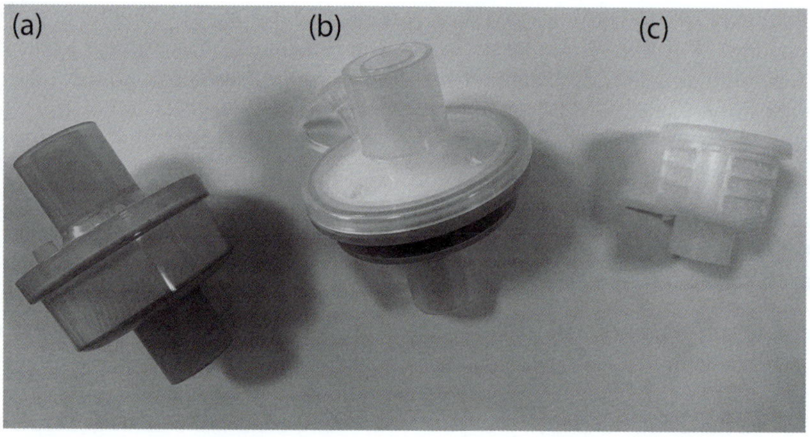

Figure 10.2 Three heat and moisture exchangers intended for use during invasive or non-invasive ventilation (A, B) and with a tracheostomy cannula (C).

humidifying devices are not enough performing, not properly set, or not suited for the patient condition. Overhydration usually occurs only in active humidification, with heated and aerosol humidifiers.[26] Unconditioned cold inspired gases can also lead to heat loss, inversely proportional to the RH of the gas.[27] Overheating is a consequence of inappropriate active humidification, as overhydration, due to incorrect setting or maintenance of the device.

Devices

Available conditioning devices can be classified in passive and active humidifiers. Their goal is to provide at least 33 mg H_2O/L AH and 100% RH to the lower respiratory tract, similarly to physiological conditions.[28] The exposure to humidity levels below 25 mg H_2O/L AH for 1 h or 30 mg H_2O/L AH for 24 h leads to airway mucosal dysfunction, and the conditioning must be started as soon as possible in every patient receiving invasive ventilation.[29]

Passive Devices

Passive humidifiers available are heat and moisture exchangers (HMEs; Figure 10.2) and are widely used because of their limited costs, low maintenance needs, and satisfactory performance in a broad range of patients and clinical settings. These devices act retaining heat and moisture during exhalation and delivering it back to the patient during the following inspiration. They are formed by a condensing element, which can be hydrophobic, hygroscopic, or a combination of the two.[30] HMEs are placed between the patient and the Y-piece, with an increase in dead space and airflow resistances, varying according to the different devices and the operating conditions. They can also act as filters for pathogens, and most of the currently available HMEs include this function. Some HMEs are provided with an active booster and are called active HMEs.[31] These devices showed an improvement in performances compared to normal HMEs, providing supplemental heat and moisture. In patients with acute respiratory failure, HMEs result in increased requirements of minute ventilation, ventilator drive, and work of breathing, and increase the dead space (varying from 30 to 100 mL according to different devices) and $PaCO_2$.[32] HME performance can be affected by several factors. The patient's temperature directly affects that (and the AH) of the gas delivered to her: the lower the temperature, the worst the conditioning. Minute ventilation has not an absolute influence on HME performance. However, higher tidal volume and reductions in respiratory rate can negatively affect humidification capabilities of the devices. Checking for the presence of condensate in the HME and patient respiratory circuit is an adequate system for checking if it is delivering the minimum required amount of heat and moisture. It is highly recommended to keep the HME in vertical position above the endotracheal tube (ETT) in order to prevent obstruction due to condensate accumulation, with consequent increase in circuit resistances. HMEs should be routinely checked for the presence of secretions, blood, or signs of evident contamination to prevent occlusions, contamination, and augmentation of resistance and work of breathing. If these signs are not reported, studies shows that it can be safely used up to a week.[33] However, most manufacturers recommend replacing the HMEs every 24 or 48 h for contamination concerns. Variations in thickness and quantity of secretions should be monitored to choose if a higher level of humidification is needed. During aerosol delivery, the HME should be bypassed to avoid condensate accumulation and consequent increase in airway resistance. In the presence of refractory hypercapnia, use of low tidal volumes, presence of thick secretions, and bronchospasm, active humidifiers should be preferred over HMEs (Box 10.1).

Active Humidifiers

Heated humidifiers (HHs) are more efficient than passive humidifiers, reaching the highest levels of AH and allow delivering of appropriate levels of heat and moisture in all the situations where HMEs are not indicated. Patients with thick and copious or bloody secretions, patients receiving protective ventilation with small tidal volumes, and patients with respiratory acidosis, hypercapnia, and that can benefit a reduction of the dead space are commonly selected for using an HH (Box 10.1). There are different types of HH: bubble humidifiers, passover humidifiers, counter flow humidifiers, and inline vaporizers. Most of the HH currently used in clinical practice are passover humidifiers: they are composed by a heated chamber, typically placed under the ventilator, filled of sterile water; the electric plate inside the chamber heats the water and fills the chamber

Box 10.1 Relative contraindications for the use of heat and moisture exchangers (HMEs)

Patients with thick, bloody, or copious secretions due to risk of occlusion of the ETT.
Patients with major expiratory leaks (as bronchopleural fistulas, ETT cuff leaks, uncuffed ETT).
Low tidal volume ventilation because of the increase in dead space with the HME. In patients with hypercapnia, the reduction of dead space is particularly relevant.
Hypothermia, <32 °C.
High minute volume ventilation, especially in assisted spontaneous breathing (>10 L/min).
During aerosol treatments, the HME should be temporarily removed or placed between the nebulizer and the Y-piece.
Simultaneously with heated humidifiers due to risk of occlusion of the ETT.
When used during non-invasive positive pressure, an increase in pressure support to overcome the additional dead space.

ETT, endotracheal tube.

with water vapour (Figure 10.3). The gas mixture coming from the ventilator passes through the chamber and over the water, raising its temperature and water vapour content. It is delivered to the patient through the inspiratory limb of the circuit. Probes monitor the temperature inside the chamber and at the Y-piece: this is the temperature manually selected, which is about 2 °C higher than that actually

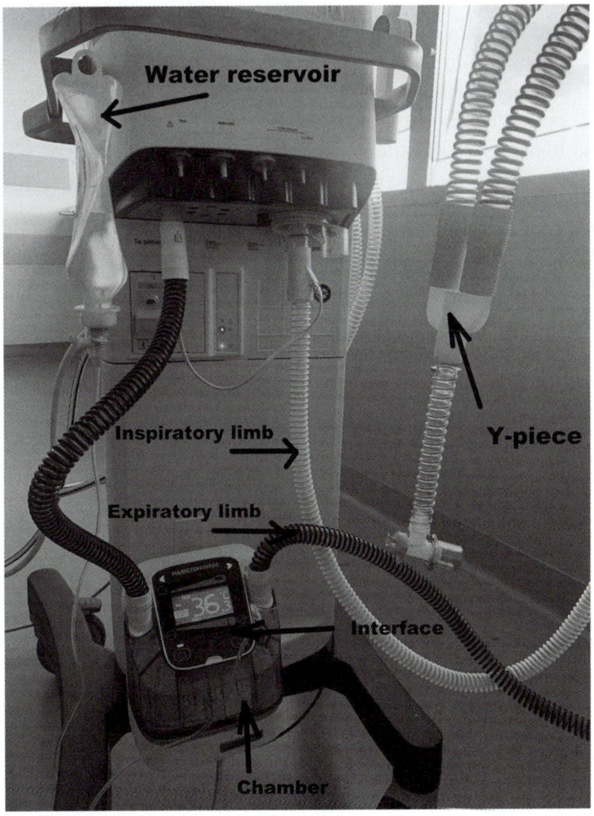

Figure 10.3 Typical set-up of a passover heated humidifier. The gas flow is forced in the heating chamber where it is in contact with the surface of heated water and then delivered towards the Y-piece through the inspiratory limb. In this specific model, both the inspiratory and expiratory limbs are heated with a wire enclosed in the tubing.

delivered to the lower respiratory tract. Guidelines recommend delivering a temperature of at least 34 °C and not above 41 °C.[25] Common settings are 39 °C at the Y-piece, allowing delivering of inspired gases at the temperature of 37 °C with a 100% RH. Gas temperature decreases in the inspiratory and expiratory limbs because of lower surrounding temperature, causing water accumulation in the circuits that can act as a contamination source, increase airflow resistance, and cause ventilator malfunction. In order to prevent the formation of condensate, there are different systems available: reservoirs (water traps) and heated circuits. Reservoirs in the inspiratory and expiratory limbs collect condensate; the drawbacks are the need of close monitoring and the possible cross-contamination to the personnel during emptying. Heated wire circuits increase the temperature from the chamber to the Y-piece; these can be used in both the inspiratory and expiratory limbs of the circuits or inspiratory alone. Usually, a gradient of temperature (2 °C in most cases) is manually selected to raise the temperature from the chamber to the Y-piece; if condensate is still present, this gradient must be further increased.

The correct temperature between 34 and <41 °C, at 100% RH, to the patient will avoid thermal airway damage. Adequate water levels in the chamber must be routinely checked to avoid the dangerous delivery of overheated and dry gases. HHs must be placed under the ventilator to prevent accumulation of water condensate in the ventilator. In HH, the monitoring and feedback system is based on temperature probes. Checking for condensate in the catheter mount is an important way to assess that the minimum conditioning targets have been met. If the expiratory limb is too wet, the heated circuit functioning must be checked, chamber temperature can be lowered, or the difference between the humidifier and the circuit can be increased. If there are no signs of condensate, the level of water in the chamber must be checked, chamber temperature can be increased, or the difference between the humidifier and the circuit can be lowered. Increase of minute ventilation and FiO_2 negatively affect HH performance, lowering the AH delivered to the patient, and must be taken in account. Careful attention must be paid not to use an HME and an HH simultaneously because of the high risk of sudden ETT occlusion. In conclusion, when indicated, HHs are better performing and effective than HMEs. That said, a recent meta-analysis has not shown superiority of HHs over HMEs in critically ill patients in terms of clinical outcomes.[34] For this reason, HMEs should be considered the standard of care for their availability and low cost, while HHs should be used based on specific clinical needs in selected patients.

Conditioning in the Tracheostomized Patient

During mechanical ventilation, patients ventilated through a tracheostomy cannula require the same conditioning parameters as others ventilated patients. The upper respiratory tract is bypassed by the tracheal cannula, but the amount of humidity required in the lower respiratory tract is unchanged. In spontaneously breathing tracheostomized patients, inspired gases may need a smaller amount of conditioning depending on oxygen supplementation and ambient temperature, but heating and humidifying inspiratory gases is necessary for preventing the formation of condensate and so for successful mobilization and removal of secretions. During spontaneous breathing at low flows of supplemental oxygen, in most cases adequate humidification is reached with passive HMEs (some of them provided with a speaking valve) as illustrated in Figure 10.2C, mostly depending on the patient's hydration status and on secretion viscosity and quantity. If enhanced gas conditioning is needed, an HH can be used. In patients receiving mechanical ventilation, HMEs and HHs can be used with the same settings as in patients ventilated through an endotracheal tube.

Gas Conditioning During Non-invasive Respiratory Support

During non-invasive ventilation (NIV), the upper airways are not bypassed, but the high flows received through the upper respiratory tract overwhelm its conditioning capabilities, leading to mucosal dryness, heat loss, higher work of breathing, and eventually to higher nasal airway resistance and discomfort to the patient. Increased resistance translates in a lower pressure transmitted to the distal airways; this may easily lead to failure of effective NIV, with specific risks of increased difficulty in intubation due to copious and dense secretions. During NIV, mouth or mask leaks can impact HME performance, reducing expiration flow through the device and reducing in this way the amount of heat and moisture given or delivered back the following inspiration. In the case of leaks of the system, an HH must be considered; in this case, HHs must be set according to patient's comfort and clinical effectiveness. Usually, home ventilators are provided with an HH.[21]

Conditioning During High-flow Oxygen Therapy

High-flow oxygen therapy is able to deliver high flow to the airways, ensuring a stable FiO_2 throughout the respiratory cycle in patients using it.[35] High-flow nasal cannulas (HFNCs) have been widely used to deliver flows around 30–60 L/m to patients with respiratory failure[36] (see Chapter 7). Delivering this high flow without appropriate heating and humidification would result in rapid damage to the respiratory system. Typical settings include temperature from 34 to 37 °C and RH of 100%. Stand-alone devices capable of generating the flow while heating and humidifying are widely available intermediate care settings, while in the ICU HFNCs are often connected to a ventilator set in the oxygen therapy mode used in conjunction with an HH. Other interfaces used to deliver high-flow oxygen therapy include T-tubes or specific devices intended for use in tracheostomized patients and non-sealed facemasks. Regardless of the device used to generate flow and the interface used, active humidification is mandatory in all patients to prevent severe injury to the airways.

REFERENCES

1. Gentile MA. Inhaled medical gases: More to breathe than oxygen. *Respir Care*. 2011;**56**:1341–1357; discussion 1357–1359.
2. Blakeman TC. Evidence for oxygen use in the hospitalized patient: Is more really the enemy of good? *Respir Care*. 2013;**58**:1679–1693.
3. Tobin MJ. *Principles and Practice of Mechanical Ventilation*. New York: McGraw-Hill Medical; 2013.
4. McDonald V, Cousins J, Wark P. Acute oxygen therapy: A review of prescribing and delivery practices. *Int J Chron Obstruct Pulmon Dis*. 2016;**11**:1067–1075.
5. Wijesinghe M, Perrin K, Healy B, et al. Pre-hospital oxygen therapy in acute exacerbations of chronic obstructive pulmonary disease. *Intern Med J*. 2011;**41**:618–622.
6. Acute Respiratory Distress Syndrome Network, Brower RG, Matthay MA, et al. The ARDS Clinical Trials Network; National Heart, Lung, and Blood Institute; National Institutes of Health. Ventilation with lower tidal volumes as compared with traditional tidal volumes for acute lung injury and the acute respiratory distress syndrome. *N Engl J Med*. 2000;**342**:1301–1308.
7. Brower RG, Lanken PN, MacIntyre N, et al. Higher versus lower positive end-expiratory pressures in patients with the acute respiratory distress syndrome. *N Engl J Med*. 2004;**351**:327–336.
8. Bellani G, Laffey JG, Pham T, et al. Epidemiology, patterns of care, and mortality for patients with acute respiratory distress syndrome in intensive care units in 50 countries. *JAMA*. 2016;**315**:788–800.
9. Ball L, Sutherasan Y, Pelosi P. Monitoring respiration: What the clinician needs to know. *Best Pract Res Clin Anaesthesiol*. 2013;**27**:209–223.
10. Kallet RH, Matthay MA. Hyperoxic acute lung injury. *Respir Care*. 2013;**58**:123–141.
11. Schjørring OL, Klitgaard TL, Perner A, et al. Lower or higher oxygenation targets for acute hypoxemic respiratory failure. *N Engl J Med*. 2021;**384**:1301–1311.
12. Ball L, Serpa Neto A, Trifiletti V, et al. Effects of higher PEEP and recruitment manoeuvres on mortality in patients with ARDS: A systematic review, meta-analysis, meta-regression and trial sequential analysis of randomized controlled trials. *Intensive Care Med Exp*. 2020;**8**:39.
13. Robba C, Ball L, Pelosi P. Between hypoxia or hyperoxia: Not perfect but more physiologic. *J Thorac Dis*. 2018;**10**:S2052–2054.
14. Roberts BW, Kilgannon JH, Hunter BR, et al. Association between early hyperoxia exposure after resuscitation from cardiac arrest and neurological disability: Prospective multicenter protocol-directed cohort study. *Circulation*. 2018;**137**:2114–2124.
15. Barrot L, Asfar P, Mauny F, et al. Liberal or conservative oxygen therapy for acute respiratory distress syndrome. *N Engl J Med*. 2020;**382**:999–1008.
16. The ICU-ROX Investigators and the Australian and New Zealand Intensive Care Society Clinical Trials Group. Conservative oxygen therapy during mechanical ventilation in the ICU. *N Engl J Med*. 2020;**382**:989–998.
17. Palmer RM, Ferrige AG, Moncada S. Nitric oxide release accounts for the biological activity of endothelium-derived relaxing factor. *Nature*. 1987;**327**:524–526.
18. Brett SJ, Hansell DM, Evans TW. Clinical correlates in acute lung injury: Response to inhaled nitric oxide. *Chest*. 1998;**114**:1397–1404.
19. Karam O, Gebistorf F, Wetterslev J, et al. The effect of inhaled nitric oxide in acute respiratory distress syndrome in children and adults: A Cochrane Systematic Review with trial sequential analysis. *Anaesthesia*. 2017;**72**:106–117.
20. Lotz C, Muellenbach RM, Meybohm P, et al. Effects of inhaled nitric oxide in COVID-19-induced ARDS—Is it worthwhile? *Acta Anaesthesiol Scand*. 2021;**65**:629–632.
21. Barach AL. The use of helium in the treatment of asthma and obstructive lesions in the larynx and trachea. *Ann Intern Med*. 1935;**9**:739.

22. d'Angelo E, Pecchiari M, Bellemare F, et al. Heliox administration in anesthetized rabbits with spontaneous inspiratory flow limitation. *J Appl Physiol Bethesda Md.* 1985. 2021;**130**:1496–1509.
23. Gluck EH, Onorato DJ, Castriotta R. Helium–oxygen mixtures in intubated patients with status asthmaticus and respiratory acidosis. *Chest.* 1990;**98**:693–698.
24. Chiumello D, Pelosi P, Gattinoni L. Conditioning of inspired gases in mechanically ventilated patients. In Vincent JL, Eds. *Intensive Care Med.* Springer, New York, NY; 2002:275–286. https://doi.org10.1007/978-3-642-56011-8_25
25. American Association for Respiratory Care, Restrepo RD, Walsh BK. Humidification during invasive and noninvasive mechanical ventilation: 2012. *Respir Care.* 2012;**57**:782–788.
26. Branson RD. Conditioning inspired gases: The search for relevant physiologic end points. *Respir Care.* 2009;**54**:450–452.
27. Severgnini P, D'Onofrio D, Frigerio A, et al. [A rationale basis for airways conditioning: Too wet or not too wet?]. *Minerva Anestesiol.* 2003;**69**:297–301.
28. Wilkes AR. Humidification in intensive care: Are we there yet? *Respir Care.* 2014;**59**:790–793.
29. Bein T, Grasso S, Moerer O, et al. The standard of care of patients with ARDS: Ventilatory settings and rescue therapies for refractory hypoxemia. *Intensive Care Med.* **2016**;42:699–711.
30. Brusasco C, Corradi F, Vargas M, et al. In vitro evaluation of heat and moisture exchangers designed for spontaneously breathing tracheostomized patients. *Respir Care.* 2013;**58**:1878–1885.
31. Chiumello D, Pelosi P, Park G, et al. In vitro and in vivo evaluation of a new active heat moisture exchanger. *Crit Care Lond Engl.* 2004;**8**:R281–288.
32. Pelosi P, Solca M, Ravagnan I, et al. Effects of heat and moisture exchangers on minute ventilation, ventilatory drive, and work of breathing during pressure-support ventilation in acute respiratory failure. *Crit Care Med.* 1996;**24**:1184–1188.
33. Lemmens HJM, Brock-Utne JG. Heat and moisture exchange devices: Are they doing what they are supposed to do? *Anesth Analg.* 2004;**98**:382–385. https://doi.org/10.1213/01.ANE.0000096560.96727.37
34. Vargas M, Chiumello D, Sutherasan Y, et al. Heat and moisture exchangers (HMEs) and heated humidifiers (HHs) in adult critically ill patients: A systematic review, meta-analysis and meta-regression of randomized controlled trials. *Crit Care Lond Engl.* 2017;**21**:123.
35. Nishimura M. High-flow nasal cannula oxygen therapy in adults: Physiological benefits, indication, clinical benefits, and adverse effects. *Respir Care.* 2016;**61**:529–541.
36. Rochwerg B, Einav S, Chaudhuri D, et al. The role for high flow nasal cannula as a respiratory support strategy in adults: A clinical practice guideline. *Intensive Care Med.* 2020;**46**:2226–2237.

PART 4

Basic Concepts in Positive-pressure Ventilation

11

Mechanical Ventilation: How to Set Up the Ventilator

Christoph Boesing, Thomas Luecke, and Joerg Krebs

KEY MESSAGES

- Mechanical ventilation is a common intervention in critically ill patients, but may contribute harmful consequences such as ventilator-induced lung injury and haemodynamic alterations.
- Understanding the physiology of the respiratory system is key to operating a ventilator.
- Ventilator modes are classified based on the control variable, breath sequence, and targeting scheme.
- The optimal ventilator settings for parameters including tidal volume and positive end-expiratory pressure (PEEP) may vary substantially between critically ill patients and need to be assessed individually.

CONTROVERSIES

- What is the optimal ventilatory strategy in distinct groups of critically ill patients regarding key components including tidal volume and PEEP?
- What are the relevant parameters in estimating the risk of ventilator-induced lung injury?

FURTHER RESEARCH

- Personalizing the ventilatory strategy for individual patients.
- Correct indications for advanced treatment options (e.g. extracorporeal carbon dioxide elimination).

How to Select Patients for Invasive Mechanical Ventilation

Invasive mechanical ventilation (MV) is indicated in patients with the need for airway protection, ventilatory support, oxygenation support, or any combination thereof. Box 11.1 gives an overview of typical pathologies that may necessitate MV.

The beneficial effects of MV are mediated through the modulation of end-expiratory and end-inspiratory lung volume through the application of positive end-expiratory pressure (PEEP) and tidal volume (V_T). These improve oxygenation and the elimination of carbon dioxide, reduce respiratory work by unloading the respiratory musculature, and support both the right and left ventricles in decompensated heart failure. However, despite all these beneficial effects, MV is potentially harmful, especially in inflamed lung parenchyma and can produce ventilator-induced lung injury (VILI), alter haemodynamics, and result in atrophy of the respiratory musculature and the diaphragm.

Aims of Mechanical Ventilation

Oxygenation of the blood is critical to the delivery of oxygen to the tissue in order to maintain homeostasis. Targeting a partial pressure of oxygen (PaO_2) in the range of 60–70 mmHg (8–9 kPa) corresponding to an arterial oxygen saturation (SaO_2) of approximately 92% is usually sufficient for adequate oxygen delivery (DO_2). Higher PaO_2 values do not result in major improvements of DO_2 and oxygen consumption (VO_2) in most cases, given the sigmoidal shape of the oxygen–haemoglobin dissociation curve. Furthermore, hyperoxia exacerbates inflammation and may increase mortality and should therefore be avoided.[1] That said, the debate as to the lowest acceptable SaO_2 levels to prevent adverse outcomes in critically ill patients remains, with concerns for targeted SaO_2 below 94% in ARDS, or other situations other than chronic obstructive pulmonary disease (COPD).

Elimination of carbon dioxide is achieved through alveolar ventilation aiming at a physiological partial pressures of carbon dioxide ($PaCO_2$) (35–45 mmHg, 4.5–6.0 kPa) and a balanced pH (7.35–7.45). In contrast to oxygenation, where hypoxia as well as hyperoxia should be avoided, the $PaCO_2$ target may vary substantially depending on the clinical situation and the underlying disease necessitating MV. Permissive hypercapnia with a higher $PaCO_2$ is routinely used in patients with acute respiratory distress syndrome (ARDS) to allow for lung protective ventilation and minimize VILI, at a normal pH or acceptably maintained mild respiratory acidosis. Likewise, in patients with chronic pulmonary diseases (e.g.

Box 11.1 Indications for invasive mechanical ventilation

Airway protection	**Loss of reflexes** • Decreased level of consciousness (pharmacological and neurological) **Airway obstruction** • Infection (e.g. peritonsillar abscess and epiglottitis) • Neoplasms (e.g. glottic and supraglottic tumours) • Immunological (e.g. angioedema and anaphylaxis) • Iatrogenic sequelae (e.g. bilateral vocal cord paralysis) • Traumatic complications (e.g. facial trauma, haematoma, and inhalation injury)
Ventilatory failure	**Impairment of central or peripheral nervous system** • Impairment of the respiratory centre due to central nervous injury • Peripheral nerve conduction disorder (e.g. myasthenia gravis) **Dysfunction of respiratory musculature** • Muscle fatigue as a result of high work of breathing • Myopathies **Chest wall abnormalities** • Pneumothorax • Flail chest
Oxygenation failure	**Ventilation–perfusion mismatch** • Pneumonia and acute respiratory distress syndrome (ARDS) **Shunt** • Congenital heart disease **Increased dead space ventilation** • Exacerbation of chronic obstructive pulmonary disease (COPD) **Impaired diffusion** • Pulmonary fibrosis

bronchial asthma and COPD), metabolic (renal) compensation of respiratory acidosis maintains pH at often substantial $PaCO_2$ levels.

MV can reduce the work of breathing (WOB) by unloading the respiratory musculature and the diaphragm. This might be beneficial in spontaneously breathing patients with acute respiratory failure and impending exhaustion of the respiratory musculature. High WOB increases VO_2, which might be harmful if DO_2 is insufficient (e.g. distributive or cardiogenic shock). Furthermore, effort-dependent lung injury might occur in patients with pulmonary dysfunction through large swings in transpulmonary pressure resulting in patient self-inflicted lung injury (P-SILI). On the other hand, the temporary use of MV to unload the respiratory musculature and the diaphragm should be as short as necessary to prevent muscle atrophy and ventilator-induced diaphragmatic dysfunction.

Respiratory Mechanics

The mechanical properties of the respiratory system (RS) can be characterized by the pressure–volume curve. Like all elastic biological systems, the RS (i.e. lungs and chest wall) show a marked hysteresis, indicating that the pressure needed to retain a given volume of gas in the RS is less than the pressure needed to inflate the RS with that volume. So, on a pressure–volume curve the expiratory part is shifted to the left compared to the pressure–volume relationship of the inspiratory limb (Figure 11.1).

The elastic hysteresis is especially pronounced in injured and inhomogeneous pulmonary parenchyma. As a result, the opening pressure of the atelectatic lung is higher than the pressure stabilizing the alveoli at end-expiration.

Equation of Motion

The interaction between flow (*F*), resistance (*R*), volume (*V*), elastance (*E*), and pressure (*P*) is based on the equation of motion for the passive RS:

$$P_{\text{airway}} = F \bullet R + V \bullet E$$

According to the equation, if either volume, pressure, or flow is set (constant), the other two variables are dependent. Given that volume and flow are inverse functions, flow is derived as a function of volume and time. Resistance and elastance are distinct properties of the patient's RS and can be calculated if volume, pressure, and flow are known.

In ventilator modes with a set V_T and hence a constant inspiratory gas flow, the increase in airway pressure during inspiration is caused

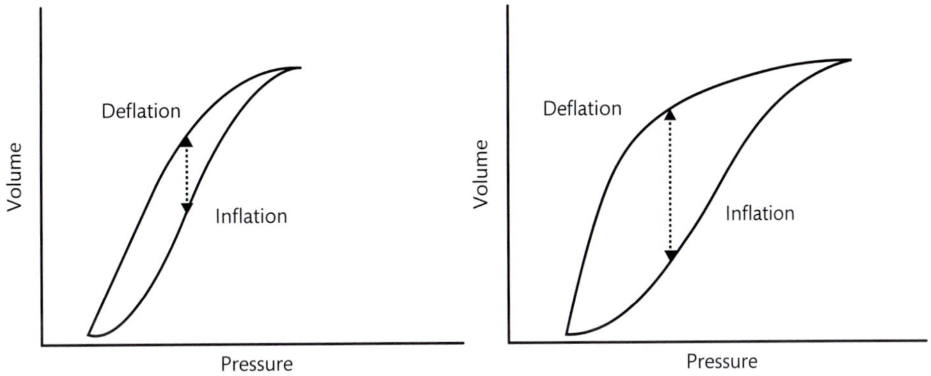

Figure 11.1 Pressure–volume curves of the respiratory system, normal lung (left), and injured lung with inhomogeneous parenchyma (right) showing the respective hysteresis.

by the cumulative pressure to overcome resistance and elastance of the RS according to the equation of motion (Figure 11.2).

The peak inspiratory pressure (P_{peak}) is reached when the set V_T has been applied and the flow is about to terminate (Figure 11.2):

$$P_{peak} = R + (V_T \bullet E)$$

In the absence of inspiratory flow, inspiratory plateau pressure (P_{plat}) can be measured. Compared to P_{peak}, P_{plat} depends solely on the elastance of the RS as the pressure increment caused by the resistance of the RS can be eliminated from the equation of motion:

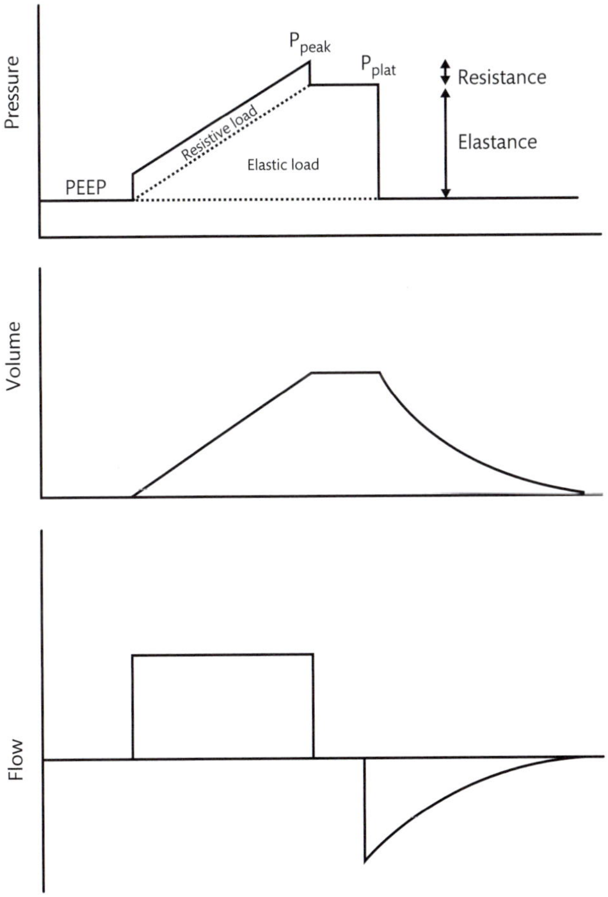

Figure 11.2 Increasing airway pressure during the application of a set V_T.

$$P_{plat} = V_T \bullet E$$

A subtle decrease in the pressure waveform from the end of inspiratory flow to P_{plat} might be visible because of the redistribution of gas in inhomogeneous lungs (Pendelluft) due to inflammation and oedema.

The difference between PEEP and P_{plat} is called driving pressure (P_{driv}) and reflects the increase in airway pressure that is induced by the application of V_T. As the change in airway pressure depends on the elastic properties following the sigmoid shape of the patient's individual pressure–volume curve, the static elastance or compliance of the RS at a distinct level of PEEP can be calculated as follows:

$$\text{Elastance}_{\text{respiratory system}} = P_{plat} - \text{PEEP} \,/\, V_T$$
$$\text{Compliance}_{\text{respiratory system}} = 1 \,/\, \text{Elastance}_{\text{respiratory system}}$$

As P_{plat} solely depends on the elastic properties of the RS, the resistance of the RS can be calculated as the difference between P_{peak} and P_{plat} under the assumption that inspiratory flow (F) is constant:

$$\text{Resistance}_{\text{respiratory system}} = P_{peak} - P_{plat} \,/\, F$$

By assessing the pressure and flow waveform or measuring P_{peak} as well as P_{plat}, the clinician can distinguish between different conditions that cause high airway pressures.

A rise in P_{plat} with a constant difference between P_{peak} and P_{plat} might be caused by an increased elastic load due to oedema formation, inflammation, or infiltration of the lung parenchyma (Figure 11.3). As a result of the dependency between P_{driv} and the RS elastance, P_{driv} will rise. Conversely, a change in P_{peak} with a constant P_{plat} and therefore a constant P_{driv} is indicative of an increase in airway resistance causing higher resistive load. Common causes are bronchoconstriction or mucus plugging.

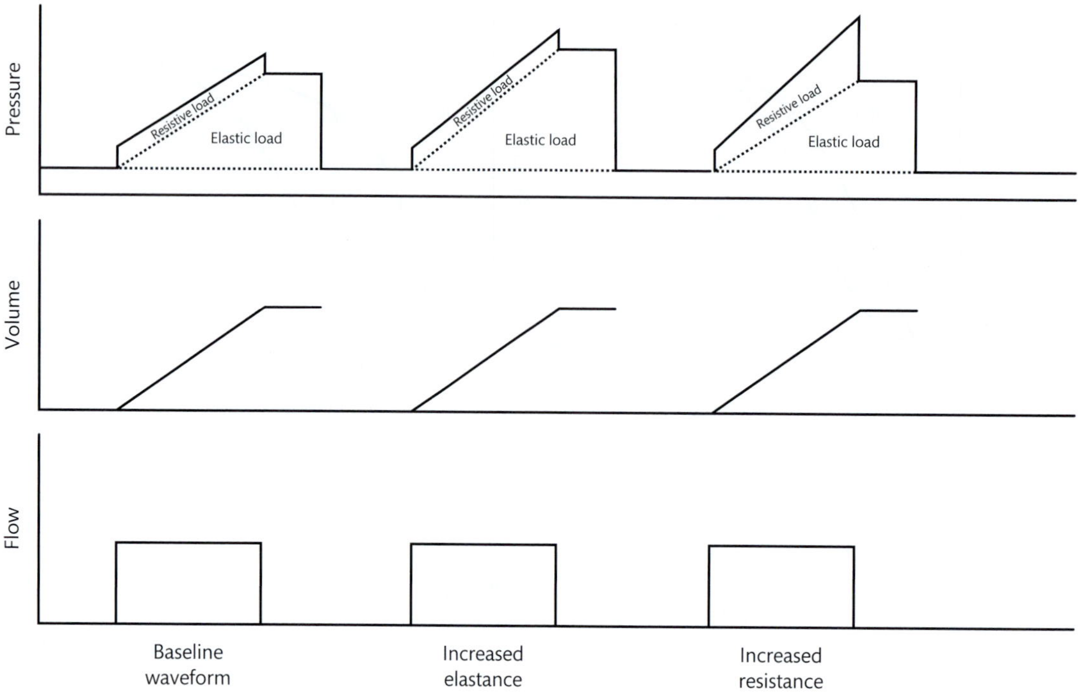

Figure 11.3 Differentiation between increased elastic and resistive loads.

Elastance and resistance of the RS can be estimated in a similar way in ventilator modes with set inspiratory pressure. Due to the fact that V_T and flow are dependent upon the properties of the RS, the flow waveform can provide valuable information regarding elastance and resistance. As the set airway pressure will be reached earlier with increased resistive load, the flow waveform will be flattened and show a decreased peak flow. In conditions with increased elastic load, the peak flow will be lower, and the time of flow will be reduced as the set airway pressure is reached earlier due to the higher elastance (Figure 11.4).

Modes of Mechanical Ventilation

Understanding the differences between mandatory and spontaneous breathing and the criteria that initiate and terminate inspiration and expiration is key to successfully setting up a ventilator.

Mandatory breathing is characterized by initiation and cycling (termination) of the inspiration by the ventilator as opposed to spontaneous or assisted breathing, where the patient triggers and cycles the inspiration. The combined duration of inspiration and expiration is called the 'total cycle time' and can be calculated as 60 s/respiratory rate/minute.

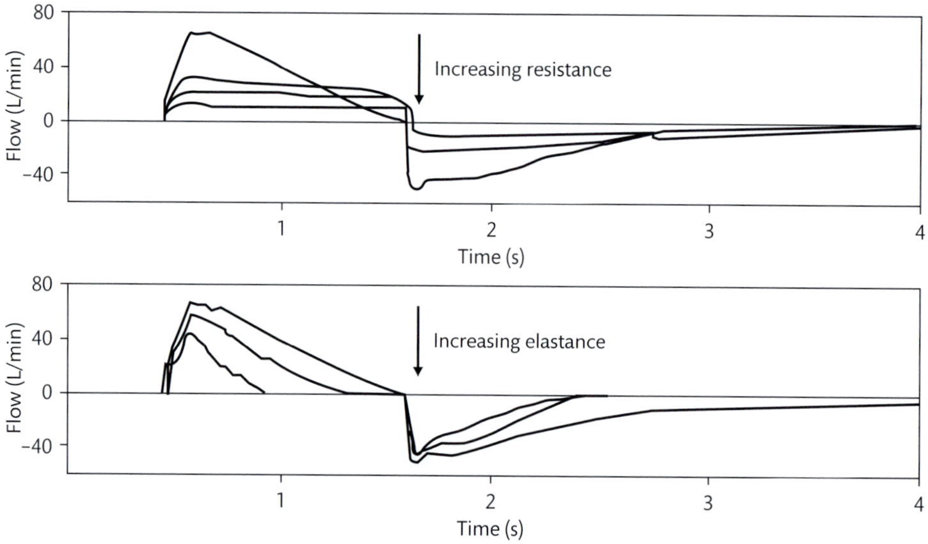

Figure 11.4 Changes in flow with increased resistive and elastic loads in ventilator modes with constant inspiratory pressure.
Adapted from Hess, D.R., Respiratory mechanics in mechanically ventilated patients. *Respir Care*, 2014. 59(11): p. 1773–94.

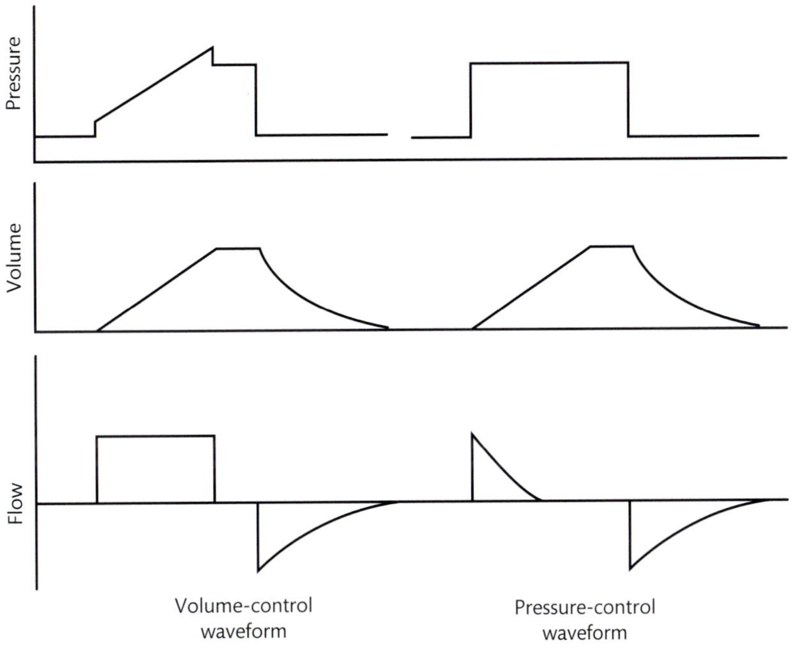

Figure 11.5 Pressure and flow waveforms of volume- and pressure-controlled ventilation modes.

Ventilator modes can be classified based on a three-level scheme consisting of the control variable, the breath sequence, and the targeting scheme.

Control Variable

The ventilator mode is classified according to the control variable that determines the delivered tidal breath. V_T and inspiratory pressure (P_{insp}) are commonly used as control variables; hence, the corresponding ventilator modes are named volume- or pressure-controlled.

As V_T and the total cycle time (due to the respiratory rate) are set in volume-controlled ventilation (VCV), the flow provided by the ventilator is constant during inspiration, resulting in a rectangular shaped flow curve and a P_{peak} based on the mechanical properties of the RS. Conversely, pressure-controlled ventilatory (PCV) modes deliver a predetermined airway pressure (P_{insp}) for a predetermined time. As P_{insp} is constant during the respiratory cycle, the V_T and flow provided by the ventilator vary according to the resistance and elastance of the RS. Therefore, flow decelerates as a result of the airway resistance and the increasing elastance when the lung is progressively inflated (Figure 11.5).

Breathing Sequence

Continuous mandatory ventilation (CMV) is the simplest mode of MV as the operator controls the total cycle time. The delivery and termination of inspiratory flow is based on the set respiratory rate (RR). The patient cannot modify the preset cycle time by inspiratory or expiratory efforts between mandatory breathing. The inspiration will be terminated by the ventilator based on the set cycle time, and a continuing inspiratory effort or premature initiation of expiration by the patient will lead to patient–ventilator asynchrony.

Given these characteristics, CMV is almost exclusively applied in patients who are deeply sedated with/without neuromuscular blockade; the intention being full control of the delivery of MV.

Intermittent mandatory ventilation (IMV) is a form of MV with partial ventilatory support as the patient is allowed to breathe spontaneously between mandatory breaths without a mandatory breath being triggered.

Continuous spontaneous ventilation (CSV, otherwise termed assisted spontaneous breathing, ASB or pressure support ventilation, PSV) describes ventilatory modes where the patient can initiate and terminate inspiratory flow based on their own breathing pattern. A level of pressure support during inspiration can be applied to support inspiratory efforts and reduce WOB. If no inspiratory pressure support is needed, the patient can breathe based on their own needs at a set level of PEEP.

Based on the control variable and the breathing sequence, five basic modes of MV can be derived. The delivery of ventilation in CMV modes and the mandatory breath in IMV can either be volume-controlled (VC-CMV or VC-IMV) or pressure-controlled (PC-CMV or PC-IMV). In CSV modes, only pressure is available as a control variable as volume control would require control of the cycle time.

Targeting Scheme

The five basic modes of MV can be further specified based on the targeting scheme that describes the type of feedback for the control variable and breathing sequence (Table 11.1).

Table 11.1 Targeting scheme

Targeting scheme	Method
Set value	Delivery of MV is controlled by setting V_T, P_{insp}, or the respiratory rate
Dual targeting	Different control variables during the delivery of a tidal breath allowing different targets for mandatory and spontaneous breaths
Servo targeting	Delivery of MV proportional to inspiratory effort of the patient
Adaptive targeting	Target value adjusted with each breath to match another target value (e.g. inspiratory pressure adjusted to guarantee a set V_T)
Optimal targeting	Ventilator adjusts target values automatically in an attempt to constantly optimize the delivery of MV based on a high priority variable (e.g. work of breathing)
Intelligent targeting	Ventilator adjusts target values based on an algorithm to reach a goal set by the operator (e.g. adjustment of pressure support to achieve a set V_T or minute ventilation)

Almost all modes of MV can be set up on a range between CMV and CSV with varying ventilatory support as shown in Figure 11.6. If the ventilatory mode targets CMV and is hence operator controlled, it is characterized as a controlled mode. The operator is able to fully adjust the delivery of MV in controlled modes to match the patient's needs (Table 11.2). Assisted breathing describes a patient-initiated breath with additional inspiratory support (pressure or volume) provided by the ventilator to reach a set target. In contrast, in unassisted (spontaneous) breathing the ventilator only provides flow without additional inspiratory pressure support in order to match the inspiratory effort of the patient.

Time as triggering variable to initiate the inspiration is typically used in CMV to allow full control of the cycle time. Pressure or flow is frequently chosen as the trigger variable in assisted breathing. The patient has to decrease the pressure or increase flow in the ventilator circuit to a level chosen by the operator. Flow triggering is preferential as it tends to reduce WOB compared to pressure triggering especially in pressure support ventilation.

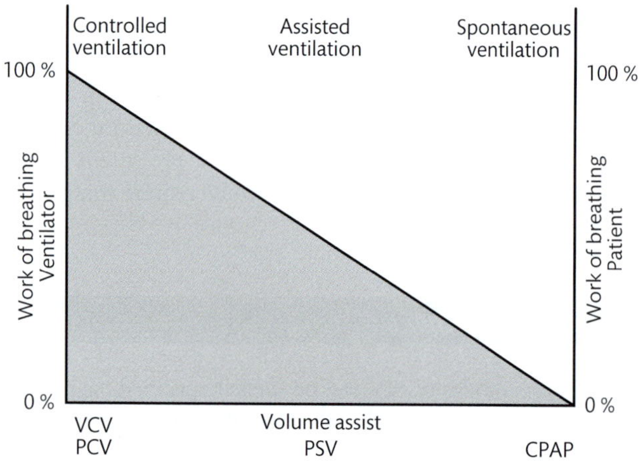

Figure 11.6 Work of breathing in selected ventilatory modes.

In addition to the triggering variable to initiate inspiration, a variable to terminate the delivery of positive pressure, called the cycling-off variable, has to be chosen. If time is chosen for cycling off, the duration of inspiration is dependent on the set RR and the inspiration-to-expiration ratio. After the inspiratory time, the exhalation valve opens and allows expiration. Pressure can be used as a cycling variable to terminate inspiration when the patient increases airway pressure above a set threshold through activation of the expiratory musculature. Similar to pressure, flow can be used to initiate opening of the exhalation valve if the inspiratory flow decreases below a set threshold. For the flow threshold, a fixed value or a percentage of the inspiratory flow can be used.

If the clinical target is assisted breathing and an appropriate ventilation mode is used, the inspiratory time of the ventilator has to be matched with the inspiratory time of the patient in order to allow patient–ventilator synchrony. Ideally, in treatment with improving lung function, the patient is transferred from a controlled mode to an assisted mode with weaning of the inspiratory pressure support to achieve spontaneous breathing.

Based on this three-level classification scheme, all ventilatory modes can be classified according to the control variable, breathing sequence, and targeting scheme (Tables 11.2 and 11.3).

Patient–Ventilator Asynchronies

Patient–ventilator asynchronies occur as result of mismatch between the respiratory efforts of the patient and the assistance delivered by the ventilator and are associated with increased mortality.[3]

They can be detected by assessing the patient's breathing pattern and the airway pressure, flow, and volume waveforms. Subsequently, patient–ventilator asynchronies can be classified according to their appearance in the respiratory cycle: trigger phase, inspiratory phase, and cycling off to the expiratory phase. Another useful tool for differentiating patient–ventilator asynchronies is the measurement of oesophageal pressure (P_{eso}) as a surrogate for pleural pressure or using electromyography of the diaphragm (EAdi) to relate inspiratory efforts of the patient with ventilator waveforms.

Patient–ventilator asynchronies can be distinguished by the respiratory drive of the patient and the assistance provided by the ventilator.

A high respiratory drive of the patient is usually caused by high metabolic demand, gas exchange abnormalities, stimulation of mechanoreceptors in the lung, pain, and anxiety. Patient–ventilator asynchronies in patients with high respiratory drive are commonly associated with insufficient assistance provided by the ventilator.

Flow starvation occurs when the inspiratory airflow provided by the ventilator is too low to match the patient's inspiratory effort. As a consequence, the pressure waveform shows a typical concavity (Figure 11.7) that increases simultaneous to the inspiratory effort of the patient (shown by the P_{eso} tracing). Flow starvation is mostly seen in the assist-volume control mode with a low peak inspiratory flow.

The term 'short cycling' describes the situation when the inspiratory time of the patient is longer than the inspiratory time of the ventilator and thus continues during the expiration phase of the ventilator (Figure 11.8).

Table 11.2 Basic ventilatory modes and variables

Variables/ventilatory mode	V_T	P_{insp}	Minute ventilation	Trigger	Cycling off	RR	Inspiratory time
Volume control	Set	Derived	Set	Time	Time	Set	Set
Pressure control	Derived	Set	Derived	Time	Time	Set	Set
Volume assist	Set	Derived	Derived	Flow or pressure	Volume	Patient	Patient
Pressure support	Derived	Set	Derived	Flow or pressure	Flow	Patient	Patient
PAV	Derived	Derived	Derived	Flow or pressure	Flow	Patient	Patient
NAVA	Derived	Derived	Derived	EaDi	EaDi	Patient	Patient

Table 11.3 Dual ventilatory modes

	Control mode				Assist mode				Total	
Variables/ ventilatory mode	V_T	P_{insp}	Trigger/cycling off	RR	V_T	P_{insp}	Trigger/cycling off	RR	RR	Minute ventilation
Assist-VC	Set	Derived	Time	Set	Set	Derived	Flow or pressure	Patient	Derived	Derived
Assist-PC	Derived	Set	Time	Set	Derived	Set	Flow or pressure	Patient	Derived	Derived
Bi-level (APRV)	Derived	Set	Time	Set	Derived	Set	Flow or pressure	Patient	Derived	Derived
SIMV	Set	Derived	Time	Set	Derived	Set	Flow or pressure	Patient	Derived	Derived
MMV	Set	Derived	Time	Derived	Derived	Set	Flow or pressure	Patient	Derived	Set

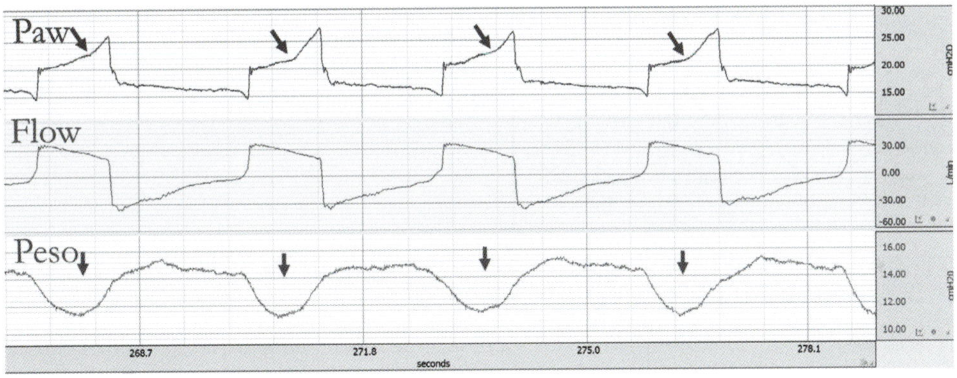

Figure 11.7 Patient-ventilator asynchrony because of flow starvation.
Reprinted from *Critical Care Clinics*, 33, 3, Pham T, et al., Asynchrony Consequences and Management. p. 325–341, Copyright 2018, with permission from Elsevier.

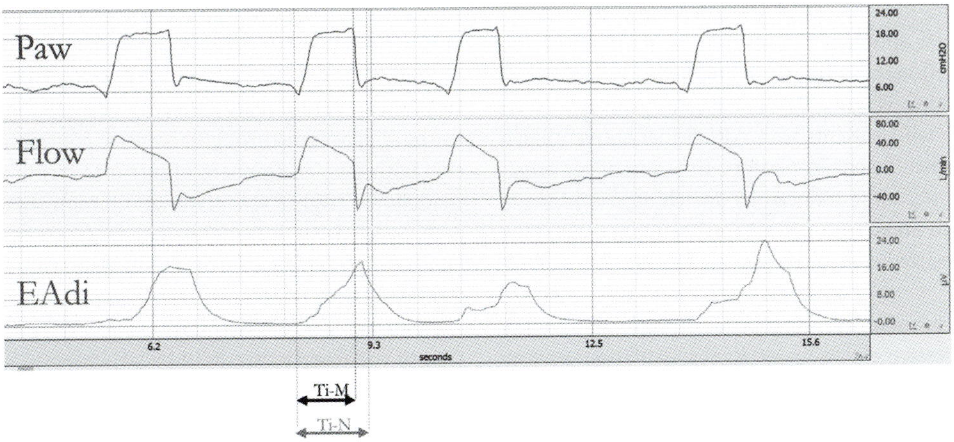

Figure 11.8 Patient-ventilator asynchrony because of short cycling detected by electromyography of the diaphragm. Inspiration time of the patient (Ti-N), derived through measurement of the EAdi, exceeds the inspiration time of the ventilator (Ti-M).
Reprinted from *Critical Care Clinics*, 33, 3, Pham T, et al., Asynchrony Consequences and Management. p. 325–341, Copyright 2018, with permission from Elsevier.

Asynchrony	Graphic representation	Description	Causes
Ineffective efforts	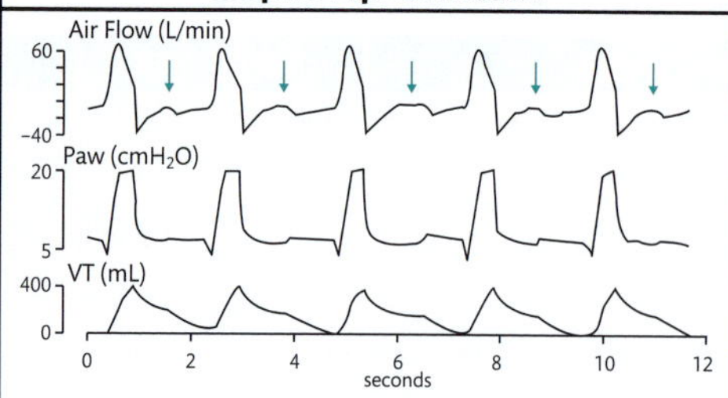	Inspiratory muscle efforts not followed by a ventilator breath (solid arrows)	Inadequate trigger sensitivity Excessive assistance Overdistension/air trapping Low respiratory drive Low level of $PaCO_2$ Oversedation
Double triggering	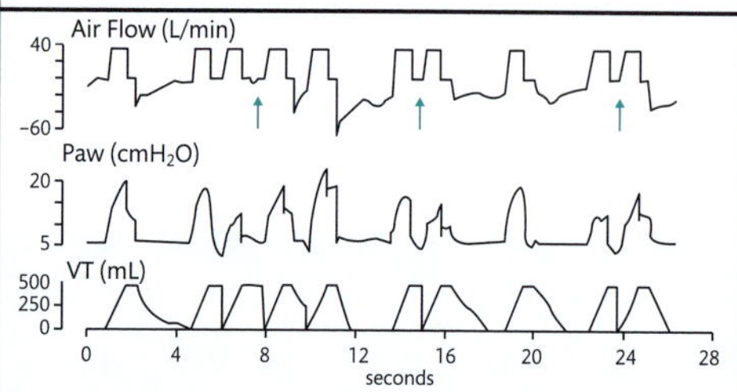	Inspiratory effort that continues beyond the ventilator inspiratory time producing a second or a third ventilator breath (solid arrows) without expiration. Consequently, the volume of the first breath is added to the second or third breath.	Inadequate setting of ventilator inspiratory time Inadequate trigger sensitivity (too sensible) Inadequate circuit pressurization Patient effort too strong Reverse triggering
Reverse triggering	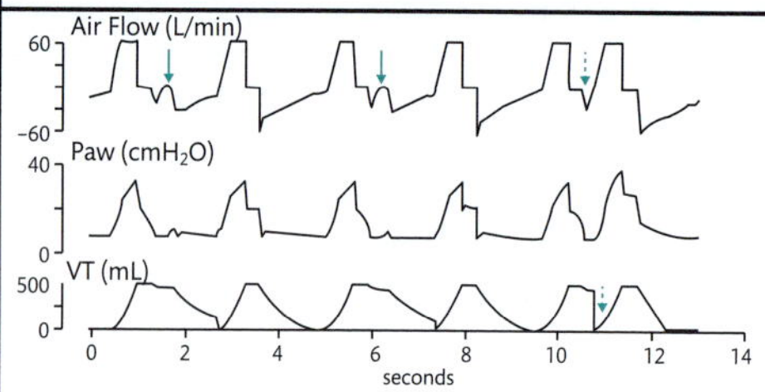	Ventilator insufflations that trigger diaphragmatic muscle contractions (solid arrows) in response to passive insufflation of the lungs. When the diaphragmatic muscle contraction occurs at the end of inspiration, a double triggered breath can occur (dotted arrow).	Oversedation Overdistension/air trapping
Inspiratory airflow dyssynchrony	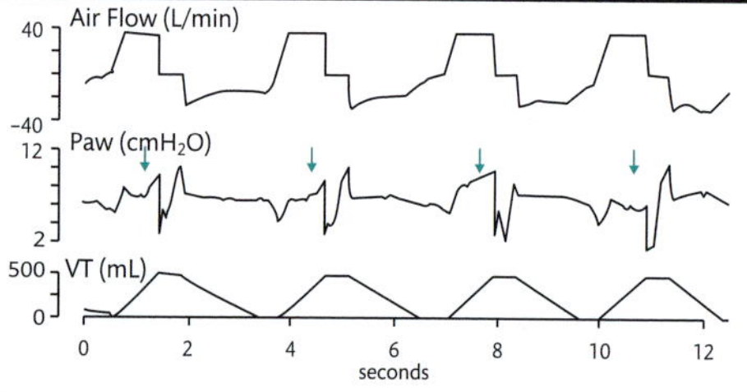	Strong patient inspiratory effort (concavity in pressure tracing) due to insufficient inspiratory airflow in a patient ventilated in assist-volume controlled mode.	Inadequate gas flow Dyspnea Delirium/pain

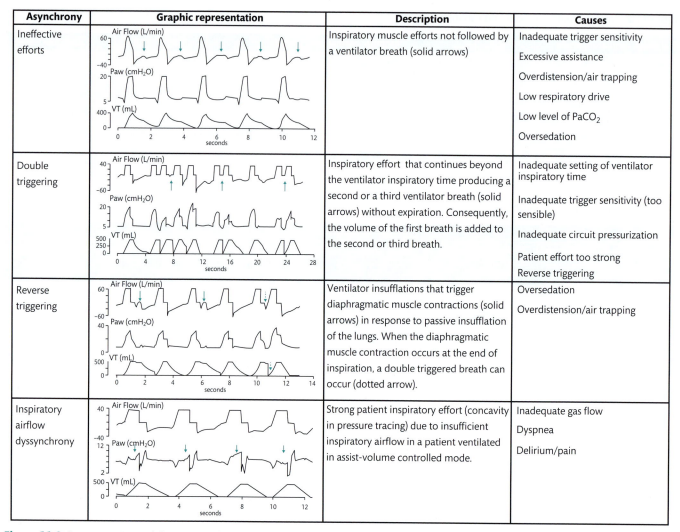

Figure 11.9 Representation and description of the most common asynchronies. Ineffective efforts, double triggering, reverse triggering, and inspiratory airflow dyssynchrony are graphically represented and described together with their causes. Solid arrows indicate where the asynchrony described is present.

Fierce inspiratory efforts of the patient might lead to 'double triggering'. It describes the delivery of a second mandatory breath triggered by sustained spontaneous inspiratory efforts with no or incomplete expiration, resulting in a markedly increased V_T through breath stacking (Figure 11.9). Potential causes include high inspiratory efforts in patients with ARDS that are ventilated with low V_T and an insufficient inspiratory time or trigger sensitivity. 'Breath stacking' can be reduced by switching from the assisted control mode to pressure support ventilation, increasing the inspiratory time in assisted control modes or adapting the sedation regime.

Patient–ventilator asynchronies with low inspiratory drive are typically due to excessive sedation, or hyperventilation leading to hypocapnia. The inspiratory effort is not sufficient to trigger the ventilator, resulting in wasted muscle effort and asynchrony. Inspiratory efforts are visible as a positive flow in the flow waveform with a simultaneous decrease in airway pressure that do not result in triggered inspiration (solid arrows in Figure 11.10). Ineffective inspiratory efforts before the end of expiration can lead to injury to the diaphragm through eccentric contractions and hyperinflation with the development of intrinsic PEEP. Typical causes are an inadequate trigger sensitivity and circumstances that lead to low respiratory drive. In patients with high airway resistance, the presence of high intrinsic PEEP might also prevent patients from triggering the ventilator.

A simple way to avoid ineffective inspiratory efforts is a reduction of the trigger threshold or switching to a flow trigger. When reducing the trigger threshold, 'autotriggering' (triggering of the

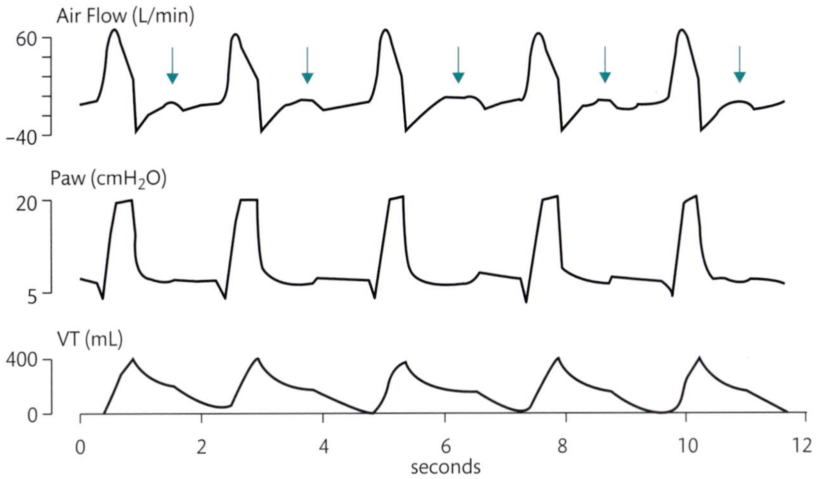

Figure 11.10 Patient–ventilator asynchrony because of insufficient triggering of the ventilator. Solid arrows indicate insufficient inspiratory muscle efforts.

ventilator in the absence of patient's inspiratory efforts) must be avoided.

Reducing the pressure support from the ventilator to avoid overassistance might be another way to reduce ineffective efforts.

In patients with low respiratory drive, delivery of a mandatory breath might trigger inspiratory muscular effort, most likely through activation of the respiratory centre as a response to passive insufflation of the lung.[4,7] This asynchrony is called 'reverse triggering', and the consequences are similar to 'double triggering' as they both might lead to increased V_T through breath stacking. 'Reverse triggering' might even propagate lung injury despite a constant V_T due to an injurious inflation pattern caused by asymmetric stretch of the lung. The main difference between these asynchronies is the initiation of the first breath that leads to the patient–ventilator asynchrony. In 'double triggering', the first breath is initiated by the patient, whereas in 'reverse triggering', the first breath is a mandatory breath delivered by the ventilator. 'Reverse triggering' is easily detectable by assessing the ventilator waveforms, where the inspiratory effort through the induced diaphragmatic contraction triggers an inspiration from the ventilator and breath stacking occurs (dotted arrows in Figure 11.11).

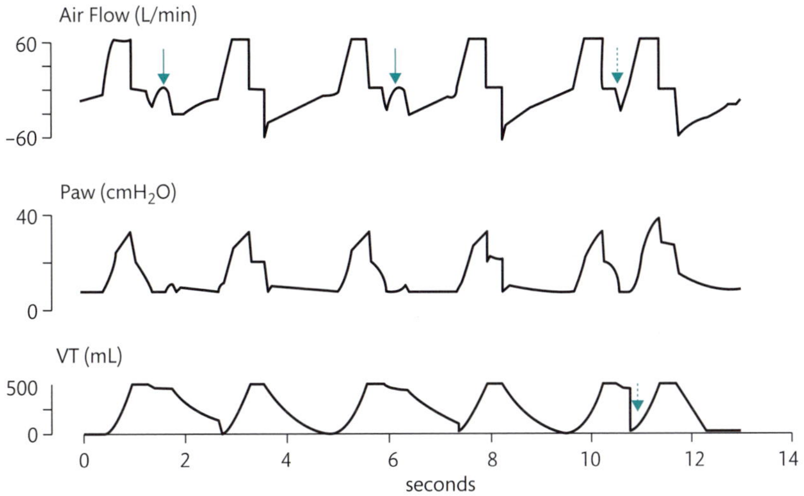

Figure 11.11 'Reverse triggering' without and with breath stacking. Solid arrows indicate diaphragmatic muscle contractions as a response to passive inflation of the lung. Dotted arrows indicate breath stacking due to 'reverse triggering'.

This might not be true for 'reverse triggering' without breath stacking (solid arrows in Figure 11.11) leading to an underestimated incidence of this patient–ventilator asynchrony. Monitoring P_{eso} swings or EAdi may be a route to early recognition.

Analogous to 'short cycling', 'delayed cycling' describes the situation when the set inspiration time of the ventilator is longer than the inspiration time of the patient. Thus, mechanical insufflation continues in the absence of inspiratory efforts or even during expiration of the patient. The inspiratory time of the patient might be reduced through high inspiratory flow rates associated with high pressure support. Consequences of 'delayed cycling' can be overinflation of the lung and a reduced respiratory drive as a result of iatrogenic hyperventilation.

Setting Up the Ventilator

Oxygenation

Oxygenation of the patient is mainly determined by the level of PEEP and the fraction of inspiratory oxygen (FiO_2). FiO_2 is set to achieve sufficient oxygenation, which is usually a PaO_2 in the range of 60–70 mmHg (8–9 kPa) corresponding to an SaO_2 of approximately 92–96% according to the oxygen–haemoglobin dissociation curve (note: the safe range of SaO_2 in critically ill patients remains debated).

To prevent end-expiratory collapse of previously reopened alveoli and alveolar cycling, the application and careful titration of PEEP is recommended.[8] Inadequate, low PEEP leads to atelectasis formation due to negative end-expiratory transpulmonary pressure and increases shunt volume.

Conversely, inappropriately high PEEP causes overinflation and increases lung stress and strain. Furthermore, it can induce right ventricular failure caused by reducing preload and increasing afterload and thus decreasing left ventricular stroke volume. Hypotension, tachycardia, increased fluid balance, and demand of inotropes are known side effects of high PEEP and ventilatory strategies using high mean airway pressures.

An important denominator for the successful application of PEEP is the amount of recruitable lung tissue, which quantifies the amount of atelectatic parenchyma that can be reopened. Patients with low recruitability will most likely not benefit from a 'high PEEP strategy'. RS mechanics (pressure-volume curves, transpulmonary pressure, and recruitment-to-inflation ratio) or imaging modalities such as computed tomography or lung ultrasound are valuable tools to determine recruitability (Figure 11.12).

A minimum PEEP of 5 cmH_2O is usually applied in MV for critically ill patients without airflow restriction caused by high airway resistance. After assessment of lung recruitability, beneficial effects and potential risks of PEEP should be considered individually, taking into account the patient's cardio-respiratory system performance and interaction.

Several ways to titrate PEEP have been proposed.[8,11] First, the Acute Respiratory Distress Network presented a table that empirically paired the demand of the fraction of inspired oxygen to keep the arterial oxygen saturation (SaO_2) above 88% with a given level of PEEP (Table 11.4).

In a study comparing different methods of PEEP titration, the PEEP/FiO_2 tables consistently provided an adequate PEEP according to the corresponding recruitability of the patients.[12] However, PEEP titration according to PEEP/FiO_2 tables lacks any individualization and fails to account for heterogeneity in RS mechanics and haemodynamics in mechanically ventilated patients. Furthermore, the PEEP/FiO_2 tables have been exclusively validated for patients with ARDS and may not suit patients with uninjured lungs.

Another approach for PEEP selection is titration of PEEP according to the mechanics of the RS. Collapsed as well as overinflated lung units have a higher elastance as they need more pressure to be inflated with a given volume of gas. By applying a PEEP that results in the lowest elastance, the amount of atelectasis and overinflation in an inhomogeneous lung should theoretically be minimized. Importantly, PEEP titration according to elastance should always be performed with a decremental PEEP trial following a recruitment manoeuvre (Figure 11.13) because of the hysteresis of the pulmonary system (Figure 11.1).

A strategy for PEEP titration which aimed to prevent alveolar collapse by ensuring a positive end-expiratory transpulmonary pressure was proposed by Talmor et al.[13] The difference between airway and pleural pressure at end-expiration and end-inspiration describes end-expiratory and end-inspiratory transpulmonary pressure, respectively. As direct pleural pressure measurement is not clinically feasible, P_{eso} is used as a surrogate as it closely reflects the pleural pressure in dependent to middle parts in healthy and injured lungs.[14] Measurement of transpulmonary pressure may be indicated to estimate the PEEP required to limit alveolar collapse in situations with altered chest wall properties, as described below.

The titration of PEEP using on pressure–volume curves aims to set the PEEP above the lower inflection point (Figure 11.14). The lower inflection point denotes the airway pressure above which the slope of the pressure–volume curve steepens, indicating low elastance of the RS, through the successful recruitment of atelectatic lung parenchyma. A PEEP above the lower inflection point should theoretically limit alveolar cycling. This method has several limitations in clinical practice. First, the inspiratory pressure–volume curve differs from the expiratory pressure–volume curve because of the hysteresis of the RS, and tidal inflation appears to be in between the two curves. Second, lung recruitment is not exclusively achieved just above the lower inflection point but also at additional segments of the pressure–volume curve. Lastly, neuromuscular blockade or at least heavy sedation is necessary to avoid interference with inspiratory efforts.

The stress index quantifies the slope of the pressure–time curve during tidal inflation, which reflects changes in the elastance of the RS during inspiration (Figure 11.15). A slope of the pressure–time curve that increases during tidal inflation (stress index > 1) denotes increasing RS elastance, indicating potential overdistension of the lung. On the other hand, a decreasing slope of the pressure–time curve during inspiration (stress index < 1) implies a decrease in RS elastance which could be indicative of tidal recruitment of

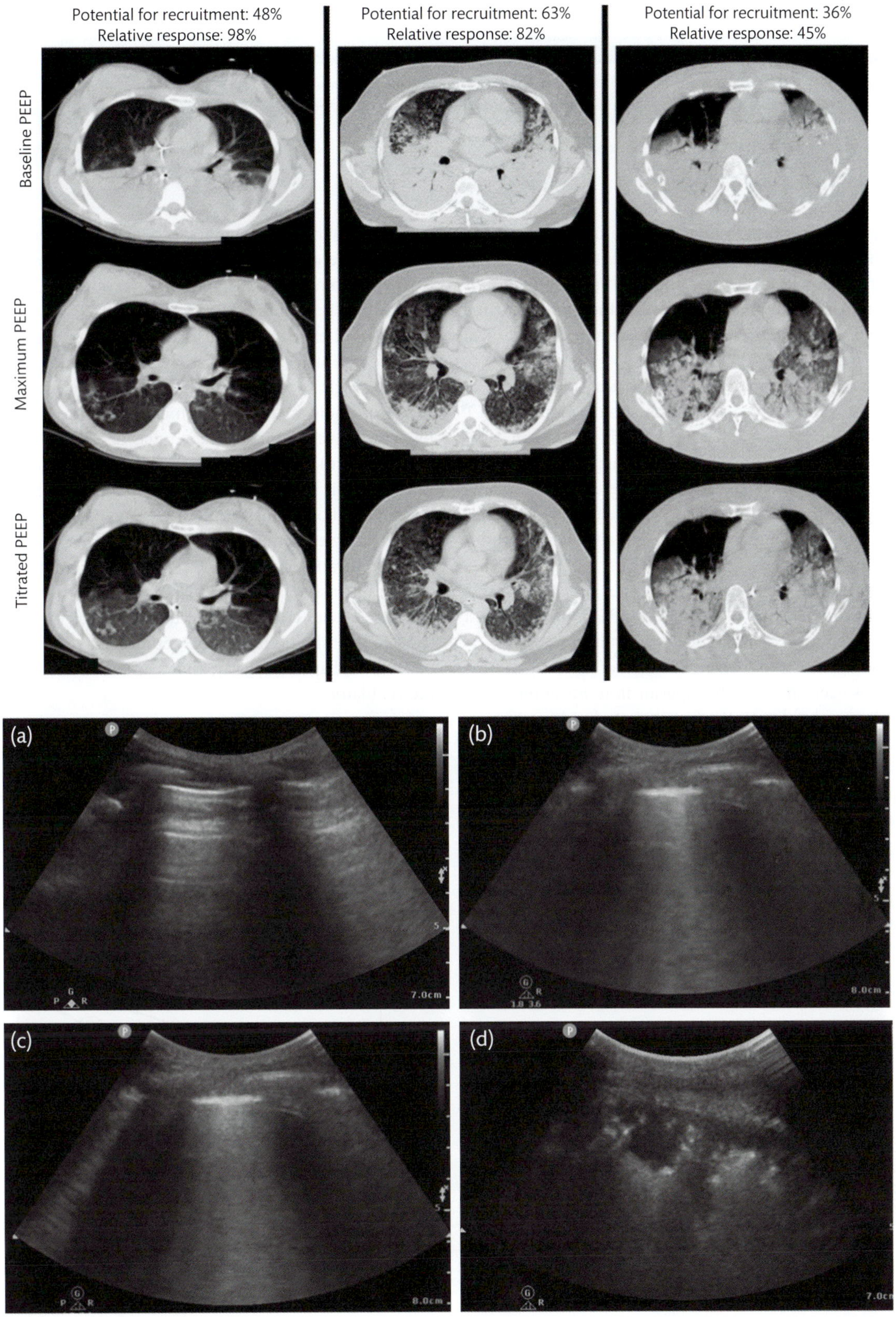

Figure 11.12 Assessing recruitability by computed tomography scan or lung ultrasound. (a) A-lines indicating normal lung aeration; (b) and (c) B-lines indicating interstitial lung oedema; (d) atelectatic or consolidated lung tissue.

Table 11.4 PEEP titration according to the FiO_2 demand using a PEEP/FiO_2 table.

FiO_2	0.3	0.4	0.5	0.6	0.7	0.8	0.9	1.0
PEEP [cmH_2O]	5–10	10–18	18–20	20	20	20–22	22	22–24

Source: Data from Chiumello D, Cressoni M, Carlesso E, et al. Bedside selection of positive end-expiratory pressure in mild, moderate, and severe acute respiratory distress syndrome. *Crit Care Med.* 2014;42(2):252–264.

atelectatic lung areas. Titrating PEEP with the aim of a stress index that equals 1 during tidal inflation may be a potential option balancing lung recruitment with overdistension. The approach requires dedicated monitoring equipment to assess the pressure–time curve; thus, the practical applicability is limited in routine clinical practice.

CT imaging can potentially assess the aeration of the lung at different levels of PEEP. Given the cumbersome nature of CT scans in critically ill patients, the approach is limited in clinical practice.[15] Lung ultrasound, as an easy applicable imaging method at the bedside, has been shown to detect lung recruitment following PEEP titration based on a scoring system.[16] Unfortunately, lung ultrasound cannot detect alveolar overinflation when titrating PEEP.

Electrical impedance tomography can be used to assess ventilation–perfusion matching while titrating PEEP but is limited by its availability in critical care practice at the moment.

At present, no approach to titrate PEEP in the critically ill ventilated patient has been shown to be superior in terms of mortality reduction.[8] This may be due to the fact that studies have not assessed lung recruitability and that possible beneficial effects of high PEEP in patients with high recruitability in preventing VILI and improving lung mechanics might have been masked by detrimental effects in patients with low recruitability. A suggested approach is to primarily choose the PEEP based on PEEP/FiO_2 tables (see above) and then further individualize PEEP based on lung elastance or transpulmonary pressure in selected patients.

In patients with elevated pleural pressure (e.g. obesity, intraabdominal hypertension, or pleural effusions) or reduced chest wall compliance (e.g. burns and scoliosis), the altered RS mechanics frequently result in a reduction of aerated lung area due to negative end-expiratory transpulmonary pressure.[17] In these patients, special care is required when titrating PEEP in order to achieve a positive end-expiratory transpulmonary pressure and prevent derecruitment, atelectasis formation, and alveolar cycling.[18]

If the static expiratory airway pressure determined by an end-expiratory hold manoeuvre is higher than the extrinsic PEEP applied by the ventilator, the patient has developed an intrinsic PEEP (Figure 11.16). Persistent expiratory gas flow at the beginning of the next breath is highly indicative of dynamic hyperinflation and the development of intrinsic PEEP. This is typically observed in patients with airflow restriction due to high airway resistance.

When titrating extrinsic PEEP, it is important to assess the presence of intrinsic PEEP in these patients. When ventilating a patient with airflow restriction in assisted ventilator modes, matched extrinsic PEEP should be used to counterbalance intrinsic PEEP, stabilize the collapsible airway, and decrease WOB required to trigger the ventilator.

Settings for Ventilation

Minute ventilation can be divided into two components, the alveolar ventilation and dead space ventilation. The alveolar ventilation equals the amount of inspired gas that participates in gas exchange and is the main determinator of carbon dioxide elimination.

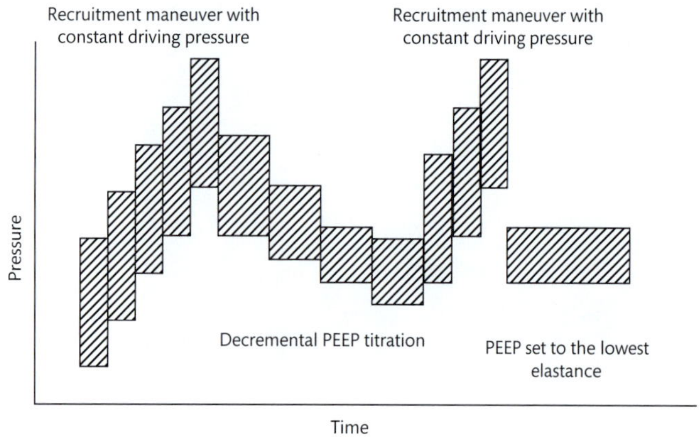

Figure 11.13 Dynamic recruitment manoeuvre and decremental PEEP trial.

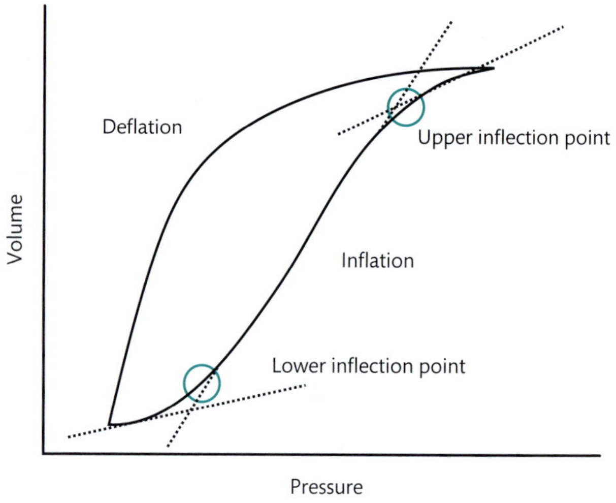

Figure 11.14 Determination of the lower inflection point on a volume–pressure curve.

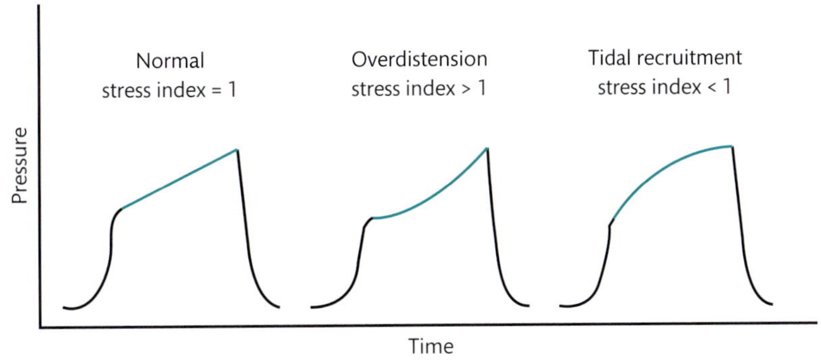

Figure 11.15 Determination of the stress index using intra-tidal pressure curve analysis.

Several studies comparing a ventilatory strategy using a V_T of 6 mL/kg PBW with an historic 'conventional' ventilatory strategy using a V_T of 12 mL/kg PBW have shown significantly reduced 28-day mortality, reduced incidence of barotrauma, and a higher rate of weaning from MV when using a low V_T.[19] These findings were in line with a wealth of experimental data showing an increase in pro-inflammatory mediators in lung parenchyma and systemic circulation associated with end-inspiratory alveolar overdistension with subsequent injury to the alveolar cytoskeleton. Furthermore, there is an increasing amount of data showing a reduction of postoperative respiratory complications by limiting V_T even in patients with healthy lungs.[20] Therefore, a ventilation strategy with low V_T of 4–8 mL/kg PBW aiming for a P_{plat} of less than 30 cmH_2O is recommended in current guidelines for critically ill patients with or without ARDS.

In severe ARDS, however, the recommended V_T might not sufficiently prevent cyclic alveolar overdistension.[21–23] Targeting a P_{driv} of <15 cmH_2O has been proposed and a further reduction in V_T may be favourable if this limit is exceeded. P_{driv} normalizes the applied V_T to the aerated lung volume and can easily be calculated at the bedside as described above. A further reduction of the applied V_T (i.e. 3 mL/kg PBW) as part of an ultra-protective ventilator strategy, whilst feasible by utilizing extracorporeal carbon dioxide elimination ($ECCO_2$-R) devices, has not shown patient benefit.[24,25]

To prevent hypercapnia and respiratory acidosis, RR has to be increased when using low V_T. The RR is inevitably linked to the inspiratory-to-expiratory ratio and has to be adjusted considering RS mechanics. The physiological inspiratory-to-expiratory ratio ranges between 1:1.5 and 1:2. RR is mainly limited by the time needed for passive expiration. If the expiration time is insufficient to allow for full expiration, air trapping with the development of intrinsic PEEP occurs (Figure 11.16). Subsequently, dynamic hyperinflation leads to an increased lung volume with a substantial risk for VILI.[26]

Elastance and resistance of the RS determine the duration of passive expiration. High elastance and low resistance result in a short time needed for full passive expiration. A low inspiratory-to-expiratory ratio may be necessary in patients with high airway resistance with the consequence of a short inspiratory time. This will allow for a full passive expiration and prevent dynamic hyperinflation, but due to the short inspiratory time, higher airway pressures in VCV or restricted V_T in PCV will occur.

As expiration is always passive in mechanically ventilated patients and solely depends on the mechanical properties of the RS, dynamic hyperinflation represents the main limitation in increasing the RR, the minute ventilation, and carbon dioxide elimination of the patient.

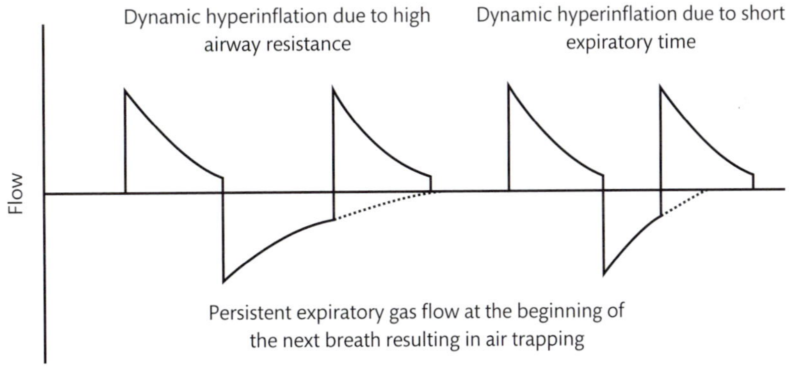

Figure 11.16 Dynamic hyperinflation with development of intrinsic PEEP.

REFERENCES

1. Helmerhorst HJ, Roos-Blom MJ, van Westerloo DJ, et al. Association between arterial hyperoxia and outcome in subsets of critical illness: A systematic review, meta-analysis, and meta-regression of cohort studies. *Crit Care Med.* 2015 Jul;**43**(7):1508–1519. doi:10.1097/CCM.0000000000000998. PMID: 25855899.
2. Hess DR. Respiratory mechanics in mechanically ventilated patients. *Respir Care.* 2014 Nov;**59**(11):1773–1794. doi:10.4187/respcare.03410. Epub 2014 Oct 21. PMID: 25336536.
3. Blanch L, Villagra A, Sales B, et al. Asynchronies during mechanical ventilation are associated with mortality. *Intensive Care Med.* 2015 Apr;**41**(4):633–641. doi:10.1007/s00134-015-3692-6. Epub 2015 Feb 19. PMID: 25693449.
4. Pham T, Telias I, Piraino T, et al. Asynchrony consequences and management. *Crit Care Clin.* 2018 Jul;**34**(3):325–341. doi:10.1016/j.ccc.2018.03.008. PMID: 29907268.
5. Yoshida T, Fujino Y, Amato MB, et al. Fifty years of research in ARDS. Spontaneous breathing during mechanical ventilation. risks, mechanisms, and management. *Am J Respir Crit Care Med.* 2017 Apr 15;**195**(8):985–992. doi:10.1164/rccm.201604-0748CP. PMID: 27786562.
6. de Haro C, Ochagavia A, López-Aguilar J, et al. Asynchronies in the Intensive Care Unit (ASYNICU) Group. Patient-ventilator asynchronies during mechanical ventilation: Current knowledge and research priorities. *Intensive Care Med Exp.* 2019 Jul 25;7(Suppl 1):**43**. doi:10.1186/s40635-019-0234-5. PMID: 31346799; PMCID: PMC6658621.
7. Murias G, de Haro C, Blanch L. Does this ventilated patient have asynchronies? Recognizing reverse triggering and entrainment at the bedside. *Intensive Care Med.* 2016;**42**(6):1058–1061.
8. Sahetya SK, Goligher EC, Brower RG. Fifty years of research in ARDS. Setting positive end-expiratory pressure in acute respiratory distress syndrome. *Am J Respir Crit Care Med.* 2017;**195**(11):1429–1438.
9. de Matos GF, Stanzani F, Passos RH, et al. How large is the lung recruitability in early acute respiratory distress syndrome: A prospective case series of patients monitored by computed tomography. *Crit Care.* 2012 Jan 8;**16**(1):R4. doi:10.1186/cc10602. PMID: 22226331; PMCID: PMC3396229.
10. Yin W, Zou T, Qin Y, et al; Chinese Critical Ultrasound Study Group (CCUSG). Poor lung ultrasound score in shock patients admitted to the ICU is associated with worse outcome. *BMC Pulm Med.* 2019 Jan 3;**19**(1):1. doi:10.1186/s12890-018-0755-9. PMID: 30606165; PMCID: PMC6318853.
11. Caramez MP, Kacmarek RM, Helmy M, et al. A comparison of methods to identify open-lung PEEP. *Intensive Care Med.* 2009 Apr;35(4):740–747. doi:10.1007/s00134-009-1412-9. Epub 2009 Jan 31. PMID: 19183951; PMCID: PMC3956709.
12. Chiumello D, Cressoni M, Carlesso E, et al. Bedside selection of positive end-expiratory pressure in mild, moderate, and severe acute respiratory distress syndrome. *Crit Care Med.* 2014 Feb;**42**(2):252–264. doi:10.1097/CCM.0b013e3182a6384f. PMID: 24196193.
13. Talmor D, Sarge T, Malhotra A, et al. Mechanical ventilation guided by esophageal pressure in acute lung injury. *N Engl J Med.* 2008 Nov 13;**359**(20):2095–2104. doi:10.1056/NEJMoa0708638. Epub 2008 Nov 11. PMID: 19001507; PMCID: PMC3969885.
14. Yoshida T, Amato MBP, Grieco DL, et al. Esophageal manometry and regional transpulmonary pressure in lung injury. *Am J Respir Crit Care Med.* 2018 Apr 15;**197**(8):1018–1026. doi:10.1164/rccm.201709-1806OC. PMID: 29323931.
15. Cressoni M, Chiumello D, Carlesso E, et al. Compressive forces and computed tomography-derived positive end-expiratory pressure in acute respiratory distress syndrome. *Anesthesiology.* 2014 Sep;**121**(3):572–581. doi:10.1097/ALN.0000000000000373. PMID: 25050573.
16. Bouhemad B, Brisson H, Le-Guen M, et al. Bedside ultrasound assessment of positive end-expiratory pressure-induced lung recruitment. *Am J Respir Crit Care Med.* 2011 Feb 1;**183**(3):341–347. doi:10.1164/rccm.201003-0369OC. Epub 2010 Sep 17. PMID: 20851923.
17. Krebs J, et al. Positive end-expiratory pressure titrated according to respiratory system mechanics or to ARDSNetwork table did not guarantee positive end-expiratory transpulmonary pressure in acute respiratory distress syndrome. *J Crit Care.* 2018;**48**:433–442.
18. Boesing C, Graf PT, Schmitt F. et al. Effects of different positive end-expiratory pressure titration strategies during prone positioning in patients with acute respiratory distress syndrome: a prospective interventional study. *Crit Care.* 2022;**26**:82. https://doi.org/10.1186/s13054-022-03956-8
19. Umbrello M, Marino A, Chiumello D. Tidal volume in acute respiratory distress syndrome: How best to select it. *Ann Transl Med.* 2017;5(14):287.
20. Yang D, Grant MC, Stone A, Wu CL, Wick EC. A meta-analysis of intraoperative ventilation strategies to prevent pulmonary complications: Is low tidal volume alone sufficient to protect healthy lungs? *Ann Surg.* 2016 May;**263**(5):881–887. doi:10.1097/SLA.0000000000001443. PMID: 26720429.
21. Sahetya, S.K., J. Mancebo, and R.G. Brower, Fifty Years of Research in ARDS. Vt Selection in Acute Respiratory Distress Syndrome. *Am J Respir Crit Care Med.* 2017;**196**(12):1519–1525.
22. Terragni PP, Rosboch G, Tealdi A, et al. Tidal hyperinflation during low tidal volume ventilation in acute respiratory distress syndrome. *Am J Respir Crit Care Med.* 2007 Jan 15;**175**(2):160–166. doi:10.1164/rccm.200607-915OC. Epub 2006 Oct 12. PMID: 17038660.
23. Terragni PP, Del Sorbo L, Mascia L, et al. Tidal volume lower than 6 ml/kg enhances lung protection: role of extracorporeal carbon dioxide removal. *Anesthesiology.* 2009 Oct;**111**(4):826–835. doi:10.1097/ALN.0b013e3181b764d2. PMID: 19741487.
24. Combes A, Fanelli V, Pham T, et al; European Society of Intensive Care Medicine Trials Group and the "Strategy of Ultra-Protective lung ventilation with Extracorporeal CO2 Removal for New-Onset moderate to severe ARDS" (SUPERNOVA) investigators. Feasibility and safety of extracorporeal CO_2 removal to enhance protective ventilation in acute respiratory distress syndrome: the SUPERNOVA study. *Intensive Care Med.* 2019 May;**45**(5):592–600. doi:10.1007/s00134-019-05567-4. Epub 2019 Feb 21. PMID: 30790030.
25. McNamee JJ, et al. Effect of lower tidal volume ventilation facilitated by extracorporeal carbon dioxide removal vs standard care ventilation on 90-day mortality in patients with acute hypoxemic respiratory failure: The REST Randomized Clinical Trial. *JAMA.* 2021;**326**(11):1013–1023. doi:10.1001/jama.2021.13374
26. Slutsky AS, Ranieri VM. Ventilator-induced lung injury. *N Engl J Med.* 2013;**369**(22):2126–2136.

12

Pulmonary Effects of Positive-pressure Ventilation

Pedro Leme Silva, Gary Nieman, Paolo Pelosi, and Patricia RM Rocco

KEY MESSAGES

- Mechanical ventilation is a life-saving system to ensure blood gas exchange and to reduce work of breathing during the acute phase of lung disease or following surgery.
- Mechanical ventilation can cause a secondary iatrogenic lung injury known as ventilator-induced lung injury (VILI).
- Several mechanisms have been hypothesized for VILI: (1) inspiratory stress (i.e. the respiratory system plateau pressure), (2) dynamic strain (i.e. the ratio between tidal volume and the end-expiratory lung volume), (3) static strain (i.e. the end-expiratory lung volume determined by PEEP), (4) driving pressure (i.e. the difference between plateau pressure and PEEP), (5) energy (i.e. the changes in airway pressure as a function of tidal volume with addition of PEEP), and (6) and power (the amount of energy as a function of time (i.e. respiratory rate).

CONTROVERSIES

- Not only controlled mechanical ventilation but also assisted mechanical ventilation may promote lung injury.
- Uncertainty of the specific contribution of each ventilatory parameter on VILI.
- Personalized individual patient setting of PEEP and ventilatory parameters to improve outcomes in acute respiratory distress syndrome (ARDS).
- The role of energy and mechanical power as compared to driving pressure and respiratory rate alone to induce VILI in ARDS.
- The role of protective mechanical ventilation during surgery to influence outcomes.

FURTHER RESEARCH

- Identification of different phenotypes to individualize mechanical ventilation settings in ARDS and in patients undergoing high-risk surgery.
- Identification of biomarkers of VILI.
- Large RCTs exploring the effectiveness of precision medicine applied to mechanical ventilation in critically ill patients and patients undergoing high-risk surgery (predictive and prognostic enrichment trials).

Introduction

Positive-pressure mechanical ventilation represents a life-support system essential for blood gas exchange and resting respiratory muscles during the acute phase of lung disease or following surgery. Positive-pressure mechanical ventilation considerably differs from the physiologic negative-pressure breathing exhibited by humans. In normal ventilation, humans are able to vary the breathing pattern within specific amplitude and time domains,[1] and increase/decrease the ventilation rate as a consequence of metabolic fluctuations. On the other hand, mechanical ventilators pressurize the respiratory system using a tidal volume (V_T), positive end-expiratory pressure (PEEP), respiratory rate (RR), and inspiratory airway flow (V'), which are adjusted by the operator. Application of these mechanical breath variables can cause injury to pulmonary tissue, which is not clinically apparent and associated with a negative prognosis. Importantly, respiratory system plateau pressure (P_{plat}), driving pressure (ΔP), and, more recently, energy and power have been shown to correlate with ventilator-induced lung injury (VILI). These mechanical breath parameters, if improperly adjusted, have been shown to exacerbate the main mechanisms associated with VILI: (1) volutrauma, inappropriate tidal volumes leading to alveolar overdistension, or (2) atelectrauma, cyclic closing and opening of small airways and alveoli due to low PEEP levels. These two mechanical injuries to lung tissue can trigger biotrauma, which is characterized by the decompartmentalization of the inflammatory markers formerly located in the alveolar space and then translocated to adjacent bloodstream, which can result in distal organ injury.

The following mechanical breath parameters and their impact on VILI is discussed in this chapter: (1) inspiratory stress (transpulmonary pressure), (2) dynamic strain (ratio between V_T and the end-expiratory lung volume), (3) static strain (the end-expiratory lung volume alone determined by PEEP), (4) ΔP (difference between P_{plat} and PEEP), (5) energy (the changes in airway pressure as a function of V_T), and (6) power (the amount of energy as a function of RR). The impact of these mechanical breath parameters on alveolar Type I and II epithelial cells, extracellular matrix, and endothelial cells will be presented. The role of volutrauma, atelectrauma, and biotrauma as well as the strategies to mitigate these mechanisms with protective mechanical ventilation will be analyzed by reviewing the current literature.

Variables to Be Adjusted

Tidal Volume

During general anaesthesia, neuromuscular blocking agents are frequently administered in order to paralyze respiratory muscles, with mechanical ventilation required to ensure appropriate delivery of oxygen and elimination of carbon dioxide (CO_2). The lungs are inflated with a certain volume of gas and specific number of times per minute in order to address patient's oxygenation and ventilation needs. V_T is approximately 5–6 mL/kg of body weight in healthy non-anaesthetized patients.[2] Anaesthesia and shallow breathing during surgery may induce physiological changes, including alveolar collapse, also known as atelectasis, which mostly occurs in the dependent lung zones. During positive-pressure ventilation, the insufflated gas preferentially goes to the uppermost parts of the lung (non-dependent parts of the lung), while blood flow (due to gravity and the branching structure of the vessels) will preferentially go to the lower lung (dependent parts of the lung). Thus, the initiation of mechanical ventilation in an anaesthetized individual increases the mismatch between the ventilation (non-dependent parts of the lungs) and perfusion (dependent parts of the lungs).

One of the initial decisions is the correct setting of V_T when the patient with acute respiratory distress syndrome (ARDS) is placed on mechanical ventilation. It has been shown that ARDS patients ventilated with 6 mL/kg had a lower mortality compared to those ventilated with 12 mL/kg (p value = 0.007). Recently, a meta-analysis pooled data from large randomized studies comparing different V_Ts, which showed that low V_T (defined as <10 mL/kg) should be preferentially used during surgery before the development of acute lung injury (ALI).[3] Pre-emptive application of low V_T decreased the need for post-operative ventilatory support (invasive and non-invasive). One study in this meta-analysis[4] showed that volumes of 6–8 mL/kg of ideal body weight versus tidal volumes of 10–12 mL/kg resulted in fewer pulmonary and extrapulmonary complications. However, patients ventilated with low V_T also had PEEP levels ranging from 6 to 8 cmH_2O with periodic recruitment manoeuvres (RMs), while the group of patients ventilated with high V_T had no PEEP. Therefore, the optimal ventilator strategy remains uncertain since it is unknown if the main contributor of lung protection is low V_T or the addition of RM and PEEP or all three.

Positive End-expiratory Pressure

To evaluate whether the absence of PEEP worsens prognosis when combined with high V_T, a study was performed separating these two mechanical ventilation parameters. The PROVIHLO trial[5] was designed to test the hypothesis that a ventilation strategy with a high PEEP level (12 cmH_2O) plus RMs compared to low PEEP level (2 cmH_2O) combined with the same V_T (7.1 mL/kg of PBW) during general anaesthesia for open abdominal surgery protected against post-operative pulmonary complications. Since V_T was comparable in the two arms of the study, the positive effect, if any, could only be attributed to the PEEP applied during surgery. They showed that the incidence of post-operative pulmonary complications in the first 5 days after surgery was comparable between the two groups. Although the hypothesis in the PROVHILO trial was not supported, the authors did answer several relevant questions: (1) dynamic respiratory system compliance improved with 12 cmH_2O PEEP, which suggests effective lung recruitment without relevant overdistension; (2) in non-obese patients under open abdominal surgery, low V_T combined with 2 cmH_2O PEEP was not associated with poorer clinical outcome; and (3) less haemodynamic impairment was observed in the low PEEP compared to high PEEP arm plus RMs. The ventilator strategy may lead to different outcomes depending on the patient's underlying condition. For instance, in morbidly obese patients, functional residual capacity was reduced associated with airway closure and ventilation/perfusion mismatching during normal tidal ventilation.

Unlike during surgery, PEEP settings in critically ill patients, mainly in ARDS patients, remain unclear. Three large, randomized, controlled trials studied higher versus lower PEEP in ARDS patients.[6–8] Although the methods used to adjust PEEP level differed between studies and some imbalances were observed between the compared arms, no beneficial improvement was observed in survival. Nevertheless, patients allocated to higher PEEP strategies required less rescue therapies,[7,8] presented more ventilator-free and organ failure–free days, and improved respiratory system compliance.[8] Pooling all these data, and analyzing the most severe ARDS patients ($PaO_2/FiO_2 \leq 200$), randomization to higher PEEP strategies was associated with lower mortality (34.1% vs 39.1%) with an adjusted relative risk of 0.90 (95% CI, 0.81–1.00; $p = 0.049$). On the other hand, in those with mild ARDS when assigned to higher PEEP strategies (PaO_2/FiO_2 between 201 and 300), there was a trend towards higher mortality with an adjusted relative risk of 1.37 (95% CI, 0.98–1.92; $p = 0.07$). Although there has been no consensus, these analyses suggest that the use of higher PEEP strategy in severe ARDS patients is beneficial.

The impact of PEEP on lung recruitment in ARDS patients can vary greatly. In 19 patients with severe ARDS ($PaO_2/FiO_2 \leq 150$), 9 exhibited significant alveolar recruitment, while in the remaining 10 the alveolar volume recruited was reduced without improvement in oxygenation. Similar behaviour has been observed in computed tomography studies, where the degree of alveolar recruitment varied among ARDS patients. This variable effect on lung recruitment may explain the negative results found in these three large trials comparing lower and higher PEEP strategies in ARDS patients.

Respiratory Rate

Respiratory rate is adjusted in addition to tidal volume and PEEP in order to maintain an appropriate minute ventilation to meet the patients' metabolic demand. In the landmark study demonstrating that low tidal volume reduced mortality in acute respiratory failure,[9] the authors did not discuss the RR, which was approximately 30 breaths/min, in order to facilitate CO_2 clearance. With the RR of 30 breaths/min, the respiratory cycle lasts 2 s. If the inspiratory:expiratory ratio (I:E) is adjusted to 1:1, this gives 1 s in both inspiration and expiration. If I:E is adjusted to 1:2, this gives 0.66 and 1.33 s in inspiration and expiration, respectively. Therefore, either the expiration time is shortened, which may induce intrinsic PEEP, or the inspiration time is reduced, which may compromise ventilation. To test if high RR can improve CO_2 clearance without a cardiovascular impairment, Vieillard-Baron et al.[10] compared conventional low-rate RR (15 breaths/min) with high RR strategy (30 breaths/min). Interestingly, the authors made efforts to control the inspiratory flow (at 50 L/min) in both groups. They showed that the increase in RR, up to a range commonly used in an intensive care unit, was inefficient in improving CO_2 elimination and produced intrinsic PEEP (PEEPi). Furthermore, the increased RR was associated with significant haemodynamic consequences, including venous return impairment and abdominal vena cava enlargement.

High-frequency oscillatory ventilation (HFOV) is a ventilation strategy using a very fast RR and is used as a rescue mode for ARDS patients. HFOV delivers small tidal volumes (1–3 mL/kg) in addition to the high RRs (180–900 breaths/min). Usually, during HFOV, high mean airway pressures (mean P_{aw}) is applied to limit cyclic alveolar collapse as well as very small tidal volumes in order to restrain overdistention. An early randomized, controlled trial of 148 adults with moderate ARDS showed that HFOV decreased mortality compared to conventional ventilation at 30 days (37% vs 52%).[11] The benefits of HFOV may be secondary to maximizing the ventilator frequency, while minimizing tidal volume delivery. Thereafter, two large multicentre trials 'Oscillation for ARDS Treated Early Trial' (OSCILLATE) and the 'High Frequency OSCillation in ARDS trial' (OSCAR) aimed to compare HFOV with conventional lung protective ventilation.[12,13] In the OSCILLATE trial, patients with early moderate ARDS were randomly assigned to conventional lung protective ventilation versus HFOV. After 548 enrolled patients from 1200 planned, an interim analysis showed higher mortality in the HFOV compared to conventional groups (47% vs 35%; $p = 0.005$). In the OSCAR trial, 795 patients with moderate ARDS were randomly assigned to HFOV or conventional lung protective strategy. Both trials have limitations, such as (1) high mean airway pressure with frequent RMs, which may be harmful to non-recruitable ARDS patients with areas of consolidation; (2) excessive sedatives and neuromuscular blockers in the HFOV group, which may increase the need for haemodynamic support; and (3) relative low oscillator frequency on days 1 and 3 (5.5 and 6.8 Hz, respectively) since many patients can tolerate higher frequencies.[14] In short, HFOV should be limited to patients that have not responded to other rescue interventions, such as neuromuscular blockade and prone positioning.

Inspiratory and Expiratory Airway Flows

The flow scalar takes on either a predictable, repeatable shape or a variable shape depending on the ventilation mode employed. In volume control modes of ventilation, the flow waveform would typically be square or descending ramp in conformation.[15] Many ventilators allow the operator to choose the flow profile in this setting. Independent of the flow pattern, flow itself is an important determinant of stress in the lung since it enhances the transmission of kinetic energy. This energy is tightly associated with the shear stress applied to the cells within respiratory bronchi. There are some reports relating inspiratory flow profiles to gas exchange, work of breathing, and cardiovascular functions. Among these studies, from a macroenvironment point of view, an accelerating flow waveform has been associated with haemodynamic compromise and higher chance of barotrauma.[16] On the other hand, decelerating flow waveform has been associated with better lung mechanics and gas exchange in positive-pressure ventilation.[17]

Not only the inspiratory airway flow associated with major physiologic consequences but also expiratory flow is an important indicator of changes in lung mechanics as ALI progresses. Expiration is a passive process that uses elastic energy stored during inflation to drive expiratory airflow. If the potential energy stored after inspiration is low, and not sufficient to return the system to a relaxed equilibrium before the next inspiration begins, flow continues throughout expiration and alveolar pressure remains positive at end expiration, exceeding the clinician-selected PEEP value. This is the so-called auto-PEEP or intrinsic PEEP (PEEPi), which can lead to hyperinflation, after several respiratory cycles. This hyperinflation may lead to two major consequences: (1) shifting the lung to a high work point on the low compliance portion of the pressure–volume curve and (2) alteration in the ventilation/perfusion ratio (V/Q) creating areas of high perfusion (i.e. West Lung Zone 3) and low perfusion (i.e. West Lung Zone 1), which increase both pulmonary shunt and dead space ventilation.

Ventilatory Parameters: The Consequence

Plateau Pressure

Plateau pressure is measured by extending the time at inspiration in order for lung pressure to equilibrate at that volume. The magnitude of P_{plat} depends on respiratory system, lung, and chest wall compliance, as well as tidal volume, and represents the elastic recoil pressure of the lung. Although, a high P_{plat} can suggest a risk of alveolar overdistension, the threshold used to guide mechanical ventilation adjustments is still a matter of discussion. In the ARDSNet study, in addition to low tidal volume ventilation, P_{plat} was controlled. In the low V_T arm, the authors used P_{plat} lower or equal to 30 cmH_2O.[9] However, depending on the patients' respiratory system mechanics, keeping P_{plat} below 30 cmH_2O may not be protective of all patients with ARDS. It has been shown that some patients can develop tidal hyperinflation even with low tidal volume (6 mL/kg) and P_{plat} lower than 30 cmH_2O. Therefore, authors suggested that the P_{plat} should be reduced to 28 cmH_2O.[18] Moreover, P_{plat} >25 cmH_2O at 24 h after admission was an independent risk factor for mortality. Recently, Villar et al. used a screening tool for identifying individual patients at greater risk of death by using age, oxygenation index, and plateau pressure.[19] They divided the P_{plat} into three ranges (P_{plat}, <27 cmH_2O; P_{plat}, 27–30 cmH_2O; P_{plat}, >30 cmH_2O). Mortality increased as P_{plat} increased,[19] supporting the previous study.

Driving Pressure

After major surgery with prominent atelectasis or in patients with ARDS, there is reduced available area for ventilation. This is reflected, at the bedside, in low respiratory system compliance. Usually, the tidal volume is normalized to predicted body weight in order to scale the lung size. However, not all lung tissue is available for ventilation. Thus, driving pressure represents the tidal volume normalized by the respiratory system compliance. This index may indicate the functional size of the lung and may be a better predictor of outcome in patients with and without lung injury. Recent studies reported that driving pressure is an excellent marker of ventilator settings that may cause VILI and can unify the forces that cause tissue damage in the ARDS-affected lung. In a retrospective study analyzing the data from the low V_T ARDSnet study, it was found that driving pressure >15 cmH_2O was associated with higher mortality rate in patients with ARDS.[20] Tidal volume, P_{plat}, and PEEP were not independently correlated with increased mortality. Increasing PEEP will have different effects in driving pressure, depending on the degree of lung pathology. If increasing PEEP results in lung tissue recruitment, a decrease in the driving pressure is expected. On the other hand, if increasing PEEP does not recruit lung tissue, the lung may become overstretched, and the driving pressure will remain unchanged or increase. Driving pressure seems to be an important parameter for the optimization of mechanical ventilation in non-injured and injured lungs, as well as for intraoperative ventilation. In a meta-analysis of individual patient data, including 2250 patients in 17 randomized controlled trials, Neto et al. showed that changes in the PEEP level resulting in increased driving pressure were associated with post-operative pulmonary complications. As stated above, increased PEEP levels may yield different effects on the driving pressure. Increased PEEP levels associated with no changes or reduced driving pressure lead to less post-operative pulmonary complications. Interestingly, no major changes were observed in P_{plat} after changing the PEEP level. Since P_{plat} is not associated with outcome, it is not a good parameter to use when adjusting ventilator settings.

The Concept of Energy

Tidal volume and plateau pressure have been associated as surrogate measures of strain and stress, respectively. Strain is defined as the change in size or elongation of the lung tissue as compared with the resting size and shape. Thus, an appropriate surrogate for lung strain might be the ratio between the tidal volume and end-expiratory lung volume (EELV). Stress is the distending force of the lung and equal to transpulmonary pressure. In addition to strain and stress, factors such as RR and inspiratory flow are all components of the energy load and may contribute to ventilator-induced lung injury. All these factors together generate the energy applied to the respiratory system during one breath cycle. In Figure 12.1, the energy applied to the respiratory system was computed based on the airway pressure–volume curve, considering that it is linear up to the total lung capacity region. In order to compute the actual energy being injected into the lungs, the following energies must be subtracted: (1) the energy necessary to move the chest wall, (2) the energy necessary to overcome tracheal tube and tracheobronchial tree during inspiration, and 3) the energy necessary recovered at mouth.

Mechanical Power

The energy applied into the lungs at each frequency is called mechanical power, which is effectively energy expressed per minute. Different parameters may contribute differently to the mechanical power, such as V_T/driving pressure, flow, PEEP, and RR. In a recent study,[21] the authors varied the mechanical power applied to the respiratory system by changing the RR while keeping the tidal volume and transpulmonary pressure constant, in order to identify a power threshold for VILI. They showed that in healthy piglets widespread oedema developed only when the delivered transpulmonary mechanical power exceeded 12.1 J/min. Once injured lungs need a high mechanical power in order to be ventilated at the same tidal volume, lung collapse results in a reduction of lung area that can be ventilated, which requires more pressure and flow. This in turn increases

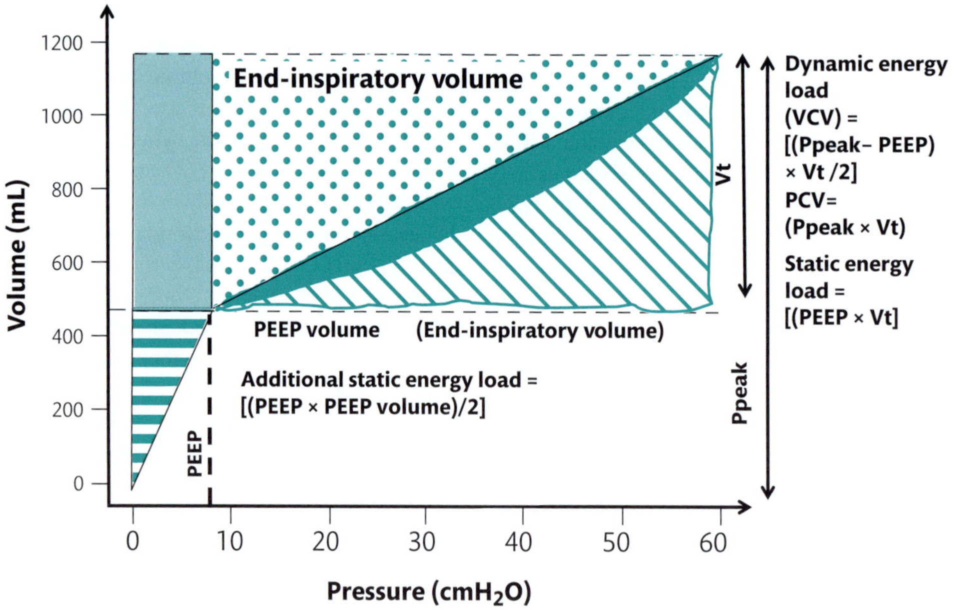

Figure 12.1 Representative scheme of static and dynamic energy calculation. P_{peak}, peak pressure; V_t, tidal volume; PEEP, positive end-expiratory pressure. The static energy load is the area of green triangle: PEEP value × PEEP volume divided by 2. Dynamic energy (area of the trapezoid) is the sum of the area of the rectangle (PEEP × V_t) plus the area of the dotted triangle (P_{peak} – PEEP) × V_t/2.

Adapted from Giosa L, et al., Mechanical power at a glance: a simple surrogate for volume-controlled ventilation. *Intensive Care Medicine Experimental*, 7(1):61. doi: 10.1186/s40635-019-0276-8.

the delivered mechanical power, without a change in tidal volume. This vicious cycle might explain the increase in lung damage as the impact of mechanical power is amplified. In short, VILI originates from the interaction between the mechanical power transferred to the lung and its histopathological changes. Better understanding of mechanical power and related factors, such as temperature, flow, and RR, will help in the understanding of injury induced by the mechanical ventilator.

Ventilator-induced Lung Injury

Ventilator-induced lung injury (VILI) is commonly attributed to the application of excessive V_T (volutrauma) or airway pressure (barotrauma). Volutrauma and barotrauma are primarily caused by unphysiologic lung distortion or strain (the ratio between V_T and functional residual capacity) and stress (transpulmonary pressure), acting either globally or locally. In a large animal model, the formation of oedema in healthy lungs was shown to occur only when the global strain ratio of between 1.5 and 2 was reached or exceeded.[22] Global strain adds a new tool in analyzing the impact of the mechanical breath on VILI since neither V_T nor plateau pressure are well-known surrogates of lung distortion.[23]

The development of VILI can be triggered by a complex interplay of potentially injurious factors: (a) regional overdistension of the alveoli caused by application of high volumes and/or alveolar pressures; (b) modifications of local stress, which deforms cells and their supporting matrix into abnormal shapes and dimensions compared to normal spontaneous breathing; (c) abrasion of the epithelial airspace, observed in particular with ventilation at low tidal volumes (V_T) and due to the repeated recruitment and de-recruitment of unstable lung units; (d) conversion of surfactant molecules into inactive surfactant aggregates as a consequence of large alveolar surface area oscillations; and (e) increased stresses between neighbouring cells and between cells and the surrounding tissue caused by the interdependence phenomenon. Two main mechanisms actually cause VILI-induced tissue trauma: (1) direct damage to the alveolar capillary membrane and ECM and (2) mechano-transduction, which is the conversion of a mechanical stimulus into intracellular biochemical and molecular signals. In the microenvironment, several mechanical forces act on Type I and II epithelial cells, and endothelial cells during positive-pressure ventilation.

Type I Epithelial Cells

Alveolar epithelial cells form a relatively impermeable barrier that is dependent on the formation and maintenance of tight junctions. More than 95% of the surface area of the alveolus is covered by Type I epithelial cells. These cells can adapt to cyclic stretch through gene expression, depending not only on the amount of stress (amplitude) but also the time of the applied stress (period). It has been observed that there is an increase in reactive oxygen species (ROS), superoxide, and nitric oxide after stretch of Type I epithelial cell (12%, 25%, and 37% change in surface area [ΔSA]). In addition, increased ROS concentration is associated with cell monolayer permeability via NF-κB activation and ERK phosphorylation. One pathway closely associated with epithelial tight junctions is Wnt signalling. A previous study showed that high-V_T ventilation for 4 h caused upregulation of Wnt5a protein levels and was associated with increased levels of total β-catenin, which can modulate adherens junctions and tight junctions between epithelial cells. In addition, claudin 18 and claudin 4 have been shown to play important roles in regulating the composition and permeability of alveolar epithelial tight junctions.

Type II Epithelial Cells

Although Type I epithelial cells cover 93% of the alveolar surface,[24] due to their spread distribution and elongation at the alveolar capillary membrane, they are less numerous than Type II epithelial cells at the alveolar scale. Typically, Type II cells tend to reside near the corner-like areas of the alveolus. It is reasonable to think that, if repetitive cyclic deformation is allowed to continue, more injury will be imposed to the epithelial cells and that both the amplitude and the period of perturbations are relevant. Although it is difficult to extrapolate what is the proportion of alveoli expansion in terms of monolayers cells stretch, previous studies have demonstrated that mild stretch (4%) can correspond to a low V_T (5–6 mL/kg of ideal body weight). Interestingly, epithelial cell distortion within physiological range is desired since Type II alveolar cells can release dipalmitoylphosphatidylcholine, a surfactant lipid, thus improving lung function. Furthermore, limiting the deformation amplitude resulted in significant reductions in cell death at identical peak deformations. Adding one more piece to puzzle, Roan et al. not only studied Type II cells stretch but also combined it with high oxygen concentration (80%–90%). This is relevant since most of the ARDS patients in mechanical ventilation can have oxygen supplementation for long periods. They demonstrated that cyclic stretch of hyperoxia-treated cells caused increased detachment of the cells, which correlated to significant alterations in F-actin and microtubules in cytoskeleton.[25]

Endothelial Cells

Each alveolus has around it a dense capillary network. Therefore, if excessive mechanical stretch is taking place, there will be higher chance of endothelial dysfunction and increased vascular leak. Excessive cyclic stretch can act on the endothelial cell surface. In this context, a study found that excessive mechanical stretch (18% elongation from baseline condition) stimulated the formation of microparticles shed from the cell surface of injured tissue, which is a sign of endothelial dysfunction. Interestingly, when these microparticles were intratracheally injected in a healthy animal, it induced lung inflammation. In addition to microparticle release, specific inflammatory mediators are produced as a consequence of cyclic stretch. One of these mediators is the high-mobility group box protein 1 (HMGB-1), which is closely associated with triggering of several proinflammatory cytokines, including TNFα, IL-8, and monocyte chemotactic protein 1 (MCP1). In experimental settings, HMGB-1 expression was positively regulated by cyclic excessive mechanical stretch (18%),[26] but not after physiological cyclic mechanical stretch (5%). Similar behaviour was observed in secretory phospholipases A2 (PLA2). Group V phospholipase A2 (gVPLA2) is a 14-kDa proinflammatory enzyme implicated in cell adhesion, transcellular communication, and generation of lipid mediators, and its activity is also modulated positively by excessive cyclic mechanical stretch (18%). High gVPLA2 activity leads to increased production of the lipid lysophosphatidylcholine and its derivatives, which act as intermediates towards downstream inflammatory signalling, as detected by higher expression of intercellular adhesion molecule (ICAM)-1.

Due to their prognostic value,[27] there is great interest in the angiopoietin (Ang)/Tie-2 system in lung injury induced by overstretch. It is well known that both angiopoietin-1 and angiopoietin-2 can bind to the Tie-2 receptor, with different consequences on endothelial cells. To test this issue, Hegeman et al. evaluated whether treatment with Ang-1, a Tie-2 receptor agonist, would protect ventilated mice against important hallmarks of VILI. Ang-1 administration at the start of ventilation diminished granulocyte infiltration, as well as chemokine (keratinocyte chemoattractant, or KC), monocyte chemoattractant protein (MCP)-1 and MIP-2), cytokine (interleukin (IL)-1β, vascular endothelial growth factor (VEGF), and Ang-2 expression in lungs of healthy animals after overinflation. On the other hand, Ang-1 treatment failed to prevent increases in bronchoalveolar lavage fluid (BALF) protein level or pulmonary wet-to-dry ratio, and had no effect on the reduction in the PaO_2/FIO_2 ratio induced by overinflation.

The degree of cyclic stretch per se can lead to higher inflammatory state of endothelium cells. So, which of the pulmonary cells respond most rapidly to injurious ventilation? A recent study suggested that pulmonary endothelial cells initiate inflammatory signalling pathways at least as fast as alveolar epithelial cells, within 15 min, and may be the most sensitive cell type in response to stretch. Furthermore, the authors found that, 15 min of overinflation, increases are observed in phosphorylation of the mitogen-activated protein kinases p38 and ERK1/2, MK2 (the immediate downstream substrate of p38), and transcription factor NF-κB.

Translational to Clinical Practice

One common question about adjusting mechanical ventilation is whether the clinician should apply low PEEP values and ventilate some alveolar units towards opening/closing (i.e. prioritizing atelectrauma) or apply high PEEP values and ventilate some alveolar units towards overdistension (i.e. prioritizing volutrauma). Which of these two mechanisms is more injurious to the lung? Seeking to address these issues, Wakabayashi et al. showed that volutrauma, but not atelectrauma, directly activates monocytes within the pulmonary vasculature, leading to cytokine release into the systemic circulation.[28] However, one could argue that there was no control of tidal volume (low: 7 mL/kg vs high: 30–32 mL/kg), and therefore the injury could be related to the high tidal volume applied. Guldner et al. overcame this issue by applying a different protocol, and the authors were able to match the tidal volume between atelectrauma and volutrauma forms of ventilation, therefore only changing the point the lung was being ventilated on the respiratory system pressure–volume curve (opening/closing or overdistension). The authors showed that volutrauma increased lung inflammation and was associated with more tidal hyperaeration and less tidal recruitment.[29]

This study has important clinical relevance. The results of the PROVIHLO trial showed that the incidence of post-operative pulmonary complications in the first 5 days after surgery was comparable between patients receiving a high level of PEEP and RMs and those receiving a low level of PEEP.[5] In addition, the authors pointed out the higher chance to cause harm during surgery in the high PEEP level group.[30] Which part of pressure–volume curve is better to ventilate, closer to atelectrauma or volutrauma? According to the latest evidence from RCTs, strategies that tend to lean towards volutrauma may cause high haemodynamic compromise, and further lung injury, compared to strategies with low PEEP level leaning more towards atelectrauma, in the operating room with patients with healthy lungs.

Conclusion

Mechanical ventilation is an essential supportive therapy during the peri-operative period, and it can help to reduce mortality among ARDS patients. Several ventilator variables are available for the clinician. Among these, that can be controlled, are tidal volume, level of PEEP, RR, inspiratory, and expiratory airway flow, while others represent the consequence with prognostic value, plateau, and driving pressures. A better understanding of the mechanisms of VILI in healthy lungs is necessary if protective ventilator strategies are to be developed further. The precise mechanism of VILI in the Type I and II epithelial cells and endothelial cells deserves attention. Pooling these data with the in vivo animal studies, and with the results of the last large trials, there is a core avenue being delineated. In healthy lungs, a consensus exists regarding the use of mechanical ventilation with low V_T (6 mL/kg); nevertheless, controversies persist as to the use of higher or lower levels of PEEP and as to whether RMs should be performed during the peri-operative period.

REFERENCES

1. Tobin MJ, Mador MJ, Guenther SM, et al. Variability of resting respiratory drive and timing in healthy subjects. *J Appl Physiol (1985)*. 1988 Jul;**65**(1):309–317.
2. Aliverti A, Kostic P, Lo Mauro A, et al. Effects of propofol anaesthesia on thoraco-abdominal volume variations during spontaneous breathing and mechanical ventilation. *Acta Anaesthesiol Scand*. 2011 May;**55**(5):588–596.
3. Guay J, Ochroch EA. Intraoperative use of low volume ventilation to decrease postoperative mortality, mechanical ventilation, lengths of stay and lung injury in patients without acute lung injury. *Cochrane Database Syst Rev*. 2018 Jul 9;7(7):CD011151. doi:10.1002/14651858.CD011151.pub3. PMID: 29985541.
4. Futier E, Pereira B, Jaber S. Intraoperative low-tidal-volume ventilation. *N Engl J Med*. 2013 Nov 7;**369**(19):1862–1863.
5. Hemmes SN, Gama de Abreu M, et al. High versus low positive end-expiratory pressure during general anaesthesia for open abdominal surgery (PROVHILO trial): A multicentre randomised controlled trial. *Lancet*. 2014 Aug 9;**384**(9942):495–503.
6. Brower RG, Lanken PN, MacIntyre N, et al. Higher versus lower positive end-expiratory pressures in patients with the acute respiratory distress syndrome. *N Engl J Med*. 2004 Jul 22;**351**(4):327–336.
7. Meade MO, Cook DJ, Guyatt GH, et al. Ventilation strategy using low tidal volumes, recruitment maneuvers, and high positive end-expiratory pressure for acute lung injury and acute respiratory distress syndrome: A randomized controlled trial. *JAMA*. 2008 Feb 13;**299**(6):637–645.
8. Mercat A, Richard JC, Vielle B, et al. Positive end-expiratory pressure setting in adults with acute lung injury and acute respiratory distress syndrome: A randomized controlled trial. *JAMA*. 2008 Feb 13;**299**(6):646–655.

9. Acute Respiratory Distress Syndrome Network, Brower RG, Matthay MA, et al. Ventilation with lower tidal volumes as compared with traditional tidal volumes for acute lung injury and the acute respiratory distress syndrome. *N Engl J Med*. 2000 May 4;**342**(18):1301–1308.
10. Vieillard-Baron A, Prin S, Augarde R, et al. Increasing respiratory rate to improve CO2 clearance during mechanical ventilation is not a panacea in acute respiratory failure. *Crit Care Med*. 2002 Jul;**30**(7):1407–1412.
11. Derdak S, Mehta S, Stewart TE, et al. High-frequency oscillatory ventilation for acute respiratory distress syndrome in adults: A randomized, controlled trial. *Am J Respir Crit Care Med*. 2002 Sep 15;**166**(6):801–808.
12. Ferguson ND, Cook DJ, Guyatt GH, et al. High-frequency oscillation in early acute respiratory distress syndrome. *N Engl J Med*. 2013 Feb 28;**368**(9):795–805.
13. Young D, Lamb SE, Shah S, et al. High-frequency oscillation for acute respiratory distress syndrome. *N Engl J Med*. 2013 Feb 28;**368**(9):806–813.
14. Fessler HE, Derdak S, Ferguson ND, et al. A protocol for high-frequency oscillatory ventilation in adults: Results from a roundtable discussion. *Crit Care Med*. 2007 Jul;**35**(7):1649–1654.
15. Koh SO. Mode of mechanical ventilation: Volume controlled mode. *Crit Care Clin*. 2007 Apr;**23**(2):161–167, viii.
16. Smith RA, Venus B. Cardiopulmonary effect of various inspiratory flow profiles during controlled mechanical ventilation in a porcine lung model. *Crit Care Med*. 1988 Aug;**16**(8):769–772.
17. Al-Saady N, Bennett ED. Decelerating inspiratory flow waveform improves lung mechanics and gas exchange in patients on intermittent positive-pressure ventilation. *Intensive Care Med*. 1985;**11**(2):68–75.
18. Terragni PP, Rosboch G, Tealdi A, et al. Tidal hyperinflation during low tidal volume ventilation in acute respiratory distress syndrome. *Am J Respir Crit Care Med*. 2007 Jan 15;**175**(2):160–166.
19. Villar J, Ambros A, Soler JA, et al. Age, PaO2/FIO2, and plateau pressure score: A proposal for a simple outcome score in patients with the acute respiratory distress syndrome. *Crit Care Med*. 2016 Jul;**44**(7):1361–1369. doi:10.1097/CCM.0000000000001653. PMID: 27035239.
20. Amato MB, Meade MO, Slutsky AS, et al. Driving pressure and survival in the acute respiratory distress syndrome. *N Engl J Med*. 2015 Feb 19;**372**(8):747–755.
21. Cressoni M, Gotti M, Chiurazzi C, et al. Mechanical power and development of ventilator-induced lung injury. *Anesthesiology*. 2016 May;**124**(5):1100–1108.
22. Protti A, Cressoni M, Santini A, et al. Lung stress and strain during mechanical ventilation: Any safe threshold? *Am J Respir Crit Care Med*. 2011 May 15;**183**(10):1354–1362.
23. Chiumello D, Carlesso E, Cadringher P, et al. Lung stress and strain during mechanical ventilation for acute respiratory distress syndrome. *Am J Respir Crit Care Med*. 2008 Aug 15;**178**(4):346–355.
24. Crapo JD, Crapo RO, Jensen RL, et al. Evaluation of lung diffusing capacity by physiological and morphometric techniques. *J Appl Physiol (1985)*. 1988 May;**64**(5):2083–2091.
25. Roan E, Wilhelm K, Bada A, et al. Hyperoxia alters the mechanical properties of alveolar epithelial cells. *Am J Physiol Lung Cell Mol Physiol*. 2012 Jun 15;**302**(12):L1235–1241.
26. Ding N, Wang F, Xiao H, et al. Mechanical ventilation enhances HMGB1 expression in an LPS-induced lung injury model. *PLoS One*. 2013;**8**(9):e74633.
27. Zinter MS, Spicer A, Orwoll BO, et al. Plasma angiopoietin-2 outperforms other markers of endothelial injury in prognosticating pediatric ARDS mortality. *Am J Physiol Lung Cell Mol Physiol*. 2016 Feb 1;**310**(3):L224–231.
28. Wakabayashi K, Wilson MR, Tatham KC, et al. Volutrauma, but not atelectrauma, induces systemic cytokine production by lung-marginated monocytes. *Crit Care Med*. 2014 Jan;**42**(1):e49–57.
29. Guldner A, Braune A, Ball L, et al. Comparative effects of volutrauma and atelectrauma on lung inflammation in experimental acute respiratory distress syndrome. *Crit Care Med*. 2016 Sep;**44**(9):e854–865. doi:10.1097/CCM.0000000000001721. PMID: 27035236; PMCID: PMC5105831.
30. Hemmes S, Serpa Neto A, Gama de Abreu M, et al. Intraoperative ventilation: Improving physiology, or preventing harm? *Br J Anaesth*. 2016 Mar;**116**(3):438–439.
31. Giosa L, Busana M, Pasticci I, et al. Mechanical power at a glance: A simple surrogate for volume-controlled ventilation. *Intensive Care Med Exp*. 2019 Nov 27;7(1):61. doi:10.1186/s40635-019-0276-8. PMID: 31773328; PMCID: PMC6879677.

13

Extrapulmonary Effects of Positive-pressure Ventilation

Pedro Leme Silva, Gary Nieman, Paolo Pelosi, and Patricia RM Rocco

KEY MESSAGES

- Positive-pressure ventilation has effects on organs other than the lungs, most notably the heart and cardiovascular system, cerebral circulation, and renal system.
- Indirect damage to other organ systems can occur through inflammatory activation at the alveolar–capillary membrane, leading to distal organ damage, so called 'biotrauma'.
- Interactions between the thoracic and abdominal cavities, and pressure differences between these two spaces can lead to hard to manage ventilation and perfusion in the context of intra-abdominal hypertension (IAH).

CONTROVERSIES

- The optimal mode of mechanical ventilation for minimizing extrapulmonary complications has not been defined.
- Although positive-pressure ventilation can help judge fluid responsiveness, it is unclear how best to optimize fluid balance in early resuscitation and the balance between use of fluids and vasopressors to maintain perfusion in ventilated patient.

FURTHER RESEARCH

- Future research should aim to understand the interactions between positive-pressure ventilation and IAH and identify the optimal approaches to ventilatory, fluid, and abdominal pressure management to improve clinical outcomes.
- Methods for alleviating the 'biotrauma' from mechanical ventilation beyond avoidance of injurious tidal volumes and pressures should be investigated.

Introduction

In addition to its direct effects on the lungs, mechanical ventilation may affect several other organs, including the heart,[1] central nervous system,[2] kidney,[3] and liver.[4] If the cause of respiratory failure is related to one of these organs, inappropriate mechanical ventilation can exacerbate this organ damage. Furthermore, clinical conditions that lead to high intra-abdominal pressure (IAP) deserve special attention during respiratory system monitoring, as the abdominal compartment is an integral part of the chest wall. Finally, another negative extrapulmonary effect of mechanical ventilation is diaphragm muscle injury, widely known as ventilator-induced diaphragm dysfunction.[5]

In this chapter, we discuss the interactions of mechanical ventilation with the cardiovascular system, central nervous system, kidney, liver, and diaphragm. We also analyze how intra-abdominal hypertension (IAH) alters the impact of mechanical ventilation on these organ systems.

Positive-pressure Ventilation and the Cardiovascular System

The heart and lungs are in close proximity within the thorax, and the lungs serve as a conduit between the right and left heart chambers, which dictates the interdependence of these organs. Different mechanical ventilation strategies affect the cardiovascular system differently. Spontaneous and mechanical ventilation induce changes in intrapleural or intrathoracic pressure (ITP) and lung volume, which can independently affect cardiovascular function through changes in atrial filling or preload, impedance to ventricular emptying or afterload, heart rate, and myocardial contractility. Spontaneous inspiration yields a negative pleural pressure and reduction in ITP.

Conversely, positive-pressure ventilation increases ITP and right atrial pressure, regardless of the addition of positive end-expiratory pressure (PEEP). ITP increases at every passive mechanical breath, which, in turn, changes the end-diastolic volume and compliance of the right and left ventricles (RV and LV, respectively).[1,6] During positive-pressure inspiration, vena cava flow and right ventricular dimension reduce with an increased transseptal pressure gradient. As a consequence, the septum shifts rightwards, increasing left ventricular volume and tending to increase stroke volume as well.[1] RV afterload also increases, mainly due to alveolar vessel compression, as lung volume rises.

Impact of Lung and Chest Wall Volume

The impact of positive-pressure ventilation on the cardiovascular system depends on whether the applied pressure opens the lung and chest wall. Pulmonary vascular resistance (PVR) is lowest at functional residual volume (FRC) and increases at either higher or lower lung volumes.[7] Thus, the curve of PVR to lung volume is 'U'-shaped, with high PVR at both low and high lung volumes and is lowest at FRC. Increased PVR at high or low lung volume is caused by decreased distending pressure of small vessels not exposed to intrapleural pressure, decreased distensibility of pulmonary vessels that might have a reduced diameter, or a change in vascular geometry. At low lung volume, PVR can also be decreased due to geometry changes ('gnarliness') with lung collapse.

In a porcine translational acute respiratory distress syndrome (ARDS) model, it was shown that the airway pressure release ventilation mode when compared to low tidal volume (LVt) ventilation resulted in a higher plateau pressure (P_{plat}) without an increase in transpulmonary pressure suggesting that the higher pleural pressure was being transmitted to and recruiting the chest wall (Figure 13.1).[8] In this study, the higher P_{plat} was not associated with lung injury but rather was highly protective by maintaining a normal lung volume, whereas the lung volume with LVt was significantly reduced. Thus, it is not just the size of the V_T and P_{plat} during positive-pressure ventilation, but also the size of the lung that is being mechanically ventilated. This concept was supported recently in a study on obese patients and in an obese porcine ARDS model.[9] It was shown that high PVR was reduced with lung recruitment, while avoiding lung overdistension and maintaining haemodynamic stability.

Assessment of Fluid Responsiveness

Understanding the fundamentals of these cardiopulmonary interactions is critical to assessing fluid responsiveness in critically ill patients. A positive response to fluids is not directly associated with fluid needs. This information should be obtained from laboratory and clinical data. For pulse pressure (PPV) and systolic volume variation (SVV) to be accurate predictors of fluid responsiveness, patients must be sedated and paralyzed under controlled mechanical ventilation with tidal volume ≥8 mL/kg, regular cardiac rhythm, and respiratory system compliance ≥30 mL/cmH_2O. Both PPV and SVV are defined as the ratio of their maximal minus the minimal values to the mean values. Several studies have showed that an SVV greater than 10% or a PPV greater than 13%–15% is predictive of fluid responsiveness, which is superior to static indices such as central venous pressure.

PPV and SVV have independently important predictive values, but some studies have focused on their ratio, known as the dynamic central arterial elastance (Eadyn), to predict arterial pressure response to volume loading in preload-dependent patients.[10] In this study, even though all patients had an increase in cardiac output in response to the fluid challenge, only those patients with normal or increased dynamic central arterial elastance had an increase in blood pressure. No other bedside parameter, such as mean arterial pressure, was able to predict fluid responsiveness. Figure 13.2 depicts how dynamic central arterial elastance is constructed. For the same increase in SVV (18%), if PPV increases from 18.6% to 27%, the Eadyn will increase up to 1.5. Assuming that SVV was not influenced by Khi, a constant quantifying arterial elastance and vascular resistance, percent SVV is related to percent PPV percentage. This makes the PPV/SVV ratio (as shown in Figure 13.2) possible to calculate and similar to Eadyn, as long as they are sampled during the same timeframe. Eadyn can predict arterial pressure response to volume loading and has interesting physiological underpinnings.

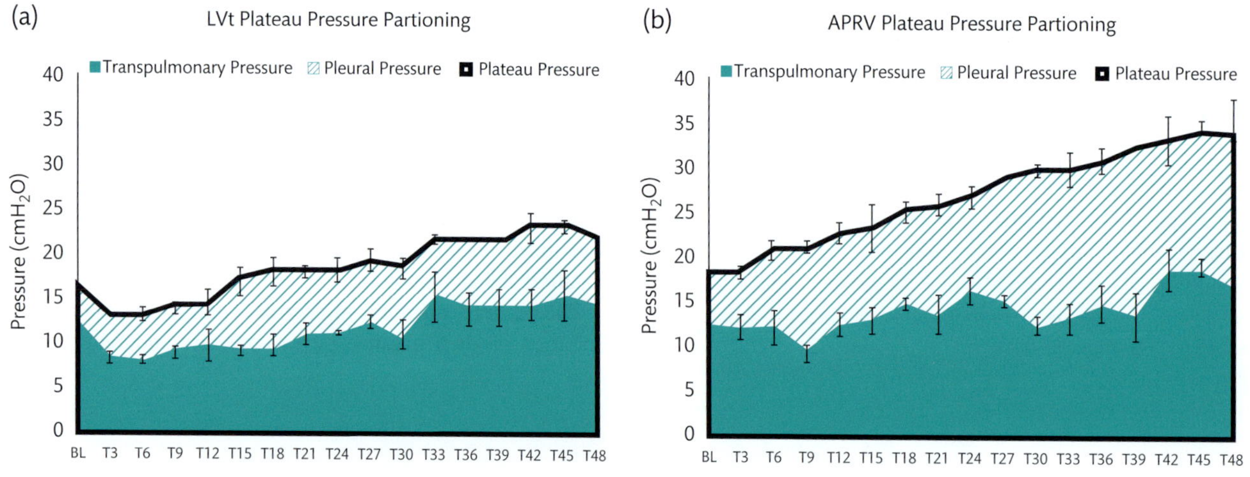

Figure 13.1 The plateau pressure (black line at top of the hatched area curve) in LVt (a) is significantly lower than that of APRV (b) yet the transpulmonary pressures (solid) are statistically similar between groups. This demonstrates that the increase in plateau pressure in APRV reflects an increase in pleural pressure (hatched).

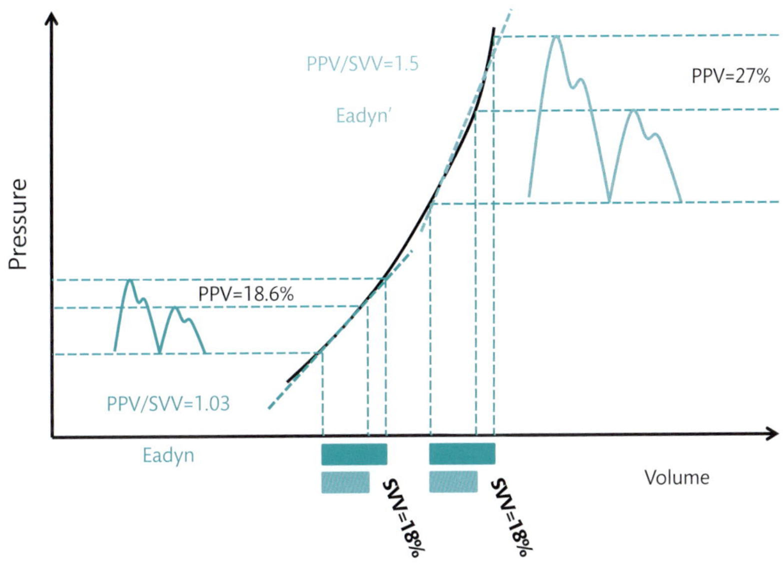

Figure 13.2 Model of two different arterial elastance values (Ea and Ea′) on the pulse pressure variation (PVV) relationship curve with the same stroke volume variation (SVV). The PPV/SVV ratio mirrors dynamic central arterial elastance (Eadyn).

Positive-pressure Ventilation and the Central Nervous System

Cerebral Blood Flow

The adequacy of the respiratory rate and tidal volume during controlled mechanical ventilation maintains systemic CO_2 levels within normal ranges. If the CO_2 level changes, vascular reactivity is expected throughout the body. One important area subject to the effects of this reactivity is the central nervous system vasculature. Cerebral blood flow (CBF) depends on a pressure differential between the arterial and venous sides of the cerebral circulation and is inversely proportional to cerebral vascular resistance. Since pressure on the venous side is difficult to measure, intracranial pressure (ICP) is used to estimate cerebral perfusion pressure (CPP). CPP is equal to the difference of mean arterial pressure and ICP. Normal ICP values in adults are <10 mmHg, and a CPP of 60 mmHg is commonly accepted as the minimum threshold for adequate cerebral perfusion. As CBF is closely related to regional cerebral metabolism, it is highly dependent on CO_2 levels and changes in $PaCO_2$. It has been observed that increasing CO_2 tension relaxes cerebral arteries in vitro. In vivo, localized perivascular changes in $PaCO_2$ or pH can change vascular diameter, indicating that elements of the vessel wall are responsible for effecting changes in vessel diameter. Both endothelial/smooth-muscle cells and extravascular cells (perivascular nerve cells, neurons, and glia) may be involved. For each mmHg change in $PaCO_2$, the CBF changes by 3% over the range of 20–60 mmHg. Therefore, hypoventilation resulting in hypercapnia causes vasodilatation and higher CBF, while hyperventilation leads to vasoconstriction and lower CBF.

Hyperventilation has been used in the management of severe traumatic brain injury (TBI) for over 40 years. A 0.5-mL change in blood volume is enough to change ICP by 1 mmHg. However, the vasoconstrictive effect is blunted after 24 h as the pH of the perivascular spaces normalizes. Despite routine use of hyperventilation in acute TBI, there are a very few randomized clinical trials to support a clear recommendation. In fact, better outcomes have been observed in patients who are not hyperventilated.[11] In addition, the effects of hyperventilation and mannitol have been evaluated comparatively.[12] The authors showed that moderate hyperventilation (an increase in minute volume ventilation to reduce end-tidal CO_2 by 5 mmHg) was sufficient to decrease CBF. On the other hand, the administration of mannitol resulted in a significant albeit moderate improvement in cerebral perfusion. Current guidelines state that prophylactic hyperventilation ($PaCO_2$ < 35 mmHg) should be avoided within the first 24 h after severe acute TBI due to CBF impairment.

Intracranial Inflammatory Response

The systemic inflammatory response seems to be important in the development of pulmonary failure after acute brain injury. An intracranial inflammatory response occurs after brain injury, and pro-inflammatory cytokines—interleukin (IL)-1, IL-6, IL-8, and tumour necrosis factor—are produced locally in injured cerebral tissue. This scenario, compounded by a massive sympathetic response, creates an inflammatory environment that increases lung susceptibility to further injurious events. All components of protective ventilation (low tidal volume, moderate to high PEEP, and recruitment manoeuvres with permissive hypercapnia) may interact with the underlying course of acute brain injury. One multicentre, prospective, observational study showed that neurologic, compared with non-neurologic, patients are ventilated with similar tidal volumes (~9 ± 5 mL/kg) but lower respiratory rates and PEEP levels. In addition, a higher mortality rate has been observed in patients with stroke, especially haemorrhagic stroke, which is probably related to neurologic dysfunction.[2]

High tidal volume (30 mL/kg) causes increased cortical and thalamic c-fos expression when compared to ventilation with low tidal volumes (8 mL/kg) for the same PEEP level.[13] Expression of c-fos can be induced by several factors, including metabolic stress, ischaemia, and inflammation. Thus, the specific nature of brain–lung crosstalk has not been fully elucidated. González-López et al.[14] showed that positive-pressure ventilation selectively triggers hippocampal neuronal cell apoptosis, mainly through the stimulation of afferent vagus signalling. After as little as 15 min of high tidal volume (12 mL/kg) followed by protective ventilation (7 mL/kg), signs of injury in the thalamus can be detected by magnetic resonance spectroscopy.[15] The clinical consequences of this phenomenon have been observed in critically ill patients. One study showed that, after severe brain injury, high V_T (11 mL/kg) was associated with increased risk of lung injury. Thus, high tidal volumes should not be used in brain-injured patients. This caveat notwithstanding, the optimal level of PEEP for brain-injured patients remains unclear. One study[16] evaluated the effect of two levels of PEEP, low (0 cmH_2O) and moderate (8 cmH_2O), on brain-injured patients ventilated with similar tidal volume (8 mL/kg), by analyzing exhaled breath condensate (EBC) to detect pulmonary inflammation during mechanical ventilation. The authors found that the moderate PEEP level did not induce changes in most EBC mediators but attenuated the systemic inflammatory response.

Positive-pressure Ventilation and the Kidney

Patients with acute kidney injury (AKI) have twofold higher odds of developing respiratory failure requiring mechanical ventilation compared to those without AKI. Indeed, needing mechanical ventilation is an independent predictor of mortality in these patients; in one study, a need for mechanical ventilation was the main factor associated with 89% mortality in patients with AKI.[17]

As previously exposed, positive-pressure ventilation increases ITP, which reduces renal blood flow, glomerular filtration rate, sodium excretion, and urinary output. Increases in ITP are expected to have a congestive effect on the RV and right atrium, which may lead to renal congestion in backwards fashion. This, in turn, can lead to increasing intracapsular pressure via the formation of renal interstitial oedema.[3] Renal haemodynamics can be further impaired by IAP. High levels of IAP can be caused by the magnitude of positive-pressure ventilation, respiratory system elastance, and pre-existing abdominal pressure due to high-volume fluid infusion. Elevated IAP can compromise microvascular blood flow, leading to kidney oedema as a consequence of reduced venous drainage. Therefore, besides positive ITP, high levels of IAP can be an additional etiogenic factor in kidney oedema.

Inflammatory alterations can be a consequence of systemic effects of inflammatory mediators released in response to different ventilatory strategies acting on the lungs. In a mouse model of experimental intra-tracheal hydrochloric acid instillation, high tidal volume (17 mL/kg), compared to a protective tidal volume (6 mL/kg), increased IL-6 and VEGFR2 levels in the lungs and kidney.[18] Other authors have observed increases not only in inflammation but also in lung and kidney apoptosis after injurious ventilation. Several mediators can exert potential effects that contribute to kidney injury. Among these, two deserve a particularly closer look: sFasL, a mediator of apoptosis, and IL1-β, a pro-inflammatory cytokine. The FasL–Fas system can induce glomerular apoptosis associated with proteinuria and loss of mesangial cells. In addition, IL1-β may facilitate the apoptosis process by acting towards platelet-activating factor and triggering an inflammatory reaction.

Among clinical studies, one meta-analysis evaluated the contribution of V_T and PEEP to the development of AKI in critically ill adult patients.[19] One systematic review and meta-analysis showed that invasive mechanical ventilation increases the odds of AKI. Neither V_T nor PEEP had any effect on the risk of developing AKI. However, this meta-analysis failed to include two important clinical trials.[20,21] The ARDS Network trial[20] demonstrated that patients ventilated with low V_T (6 mL/kg) had more renal failure-free days as opposed to those in the high-V_T group (12 mL/kg; 20 ± 11 vs 18 ± 11 days, $p = 0.005$). The EXPRESS study[21] showed no difference between patients ventilated with low or high PEEP in relation to renal failure-free days. In short, the relationship between lung injury and AKI remains poorly understood and deserves attention.

Positive-pressure Ventilation and the Liver

Impairment in gas exchange due to pulmonary dysfunction is a common complication in acute liver failure. For instance, refractory hypoxaemia and increasing ventilatory support needs represent absolute contraindication for transplantation. Deterioration in gas exchange in acute liver failure can be caused by hydrothorax, atelectasis, ARDS, and reduced respiratory system compliance due to raised IAP. In addition, intrapulmonary shunting and the hepatopulmonary syndrome have also been reported.

One large study[22] evaluated patients admitted to a specialized liver intensive care unit (ICU) over a 6-year period and found an association between mechanical ventilation in ICU for patients with cirrhosis and high ICU mortality within 1 year (89%). Furthermore, the authors observed that a duration of mechanical ventilation >9 days during ICU stay represents a risk factor for death in the year after ICU discharge. A similar scenario can be observed in cirrhotic patients.

Experimental studies have sought to understand the impact of specific ventilatory strategies on liver function. Kredel et al.[4] examined the hepatic consequences of pressure-controlled ventilation with a V_T of 6 mL/kg and PEEP adjusted to 3 cmH_2O above the lower inflection point of the pressure–volume curve or as high-frequency oscillatory ventilation (≥12 Hz) with a mean airway pressure 3 cmH_2O above the lower inflection point combined with arteriovenous extracorporeal lung assist. Aspartate aminotransferase increased approximately threefold in the pressure-controlled ventilation group and fivefold in patients who received high-frequency oscillatory ventilation with arteriovenous extracorporeal lung assist. Correspondingly, creatine kinase increased about twofold and fourfold, respectively. Lactate dehydrogenase levels were higher in patients who received high-frequency oscillatory ventilation with arteriovenous extracorporeal lung assist than in those who received pressure-controlled ventilation.

Positive-pressure Ventilation and Intra-abdominal Hypertension

In critically ill patients, the IAP is approximately 5–7 mmHg. IAH is defined by a sustained or repeated pathological elevation in IAP ≥12 mmHg, while abdominal compartment syndrome is defined as a sustained IAP >20 mmHg (with or without a difference between mean arterial pressure and IAP, i.e. abdominal perfusion pressure of 60 mmHg or greater) that is associated with new organ dysfunction or failure. IAH can be further graded as follows: grade I, IAP 12–15 mmHg; grade II, IAP 16–20 mmHg; grade III, IAP 21–25 mmHg; and grade IV, IAP > 25 mmHg. There are well-recognized risk factors for IAH and abdominal compartment syndrome, such as abdominal surgery, major trauma, gastroparesis, gastric distention, ileus, acute pancreatitis, damage control laparotomy, massive fluid resuscitation or positive fluid balance, and mechanical ventilation. Once developed, IAH can promote a cephalic shift of the diaphragm, with a reduction in lung volumes and increase in pleural pressure, causing atelectasis and impaired lung function.

One way to counteract these forces is to apply PEEP (Figure 13.3). It has been shown that PEEP levels up to 15 cmH_2O (11 mmHg) cannot prevent the functional residual capacity decline caused by IAH (18 mmHg) and are actually associated with reduced oxygen delivery as a consequence of reduced cardiac output. In a subsequent study, the PEEP level was adjusted to match the IAP in a porcine model of IAH with healthy lungs. End-expiratory lung volume was maintained, but no improvements in arterial oxygen tension were observed, and, in fact, cardiac output decreased. However, with acute lung injury, IAP-matching PEEP reduced shunt and dead space fraction as well as respiratory system elastance due to a reduction in chest wall elastance. Furthermore, high IAP-matching PEEP caused a reduction in CO. By comparing different lung injury aetiologies in IAH models, it has been shown that higher PEEP levels (10 cmH_2O) in direct lung injury increased lung elastance, while intermediate PEEP levels (7 cmH_2O) in indirect lung injury increased inflammatory markers expression. This evidence suggests that, in healthy lung conditions, IAP-matching PEEP may not be tolerated. In a condition of lung injury, the IAP-matching PEEP approach can be effective, but close cardiac output monitoring is needed.

During mechanical ventilation, it is important to dichotomize the information that comes from the respiratory system from that originating in the lungs. Changes in the respiratory system can be monitored by the measurement of airway driving pressure, which represents the tidal volume divided by respiratory system compliance. However, this index can be affected in conditions of altered chest wall compliance and should not be generalized to the lungs. Transpulmonary driving pressure would represent a better option as it eliminates the chest wall compartment. Stiffening the chest wall by elevating IAP can increase the calculated airway driving pressure of a fixed tidal volume and PEEP combination more than did transpulmonary driving pressure. This is important as there are recommended safety values for airway driving pressure in critically ill patients[23] and surgical patients[24]; however, increases in this level can

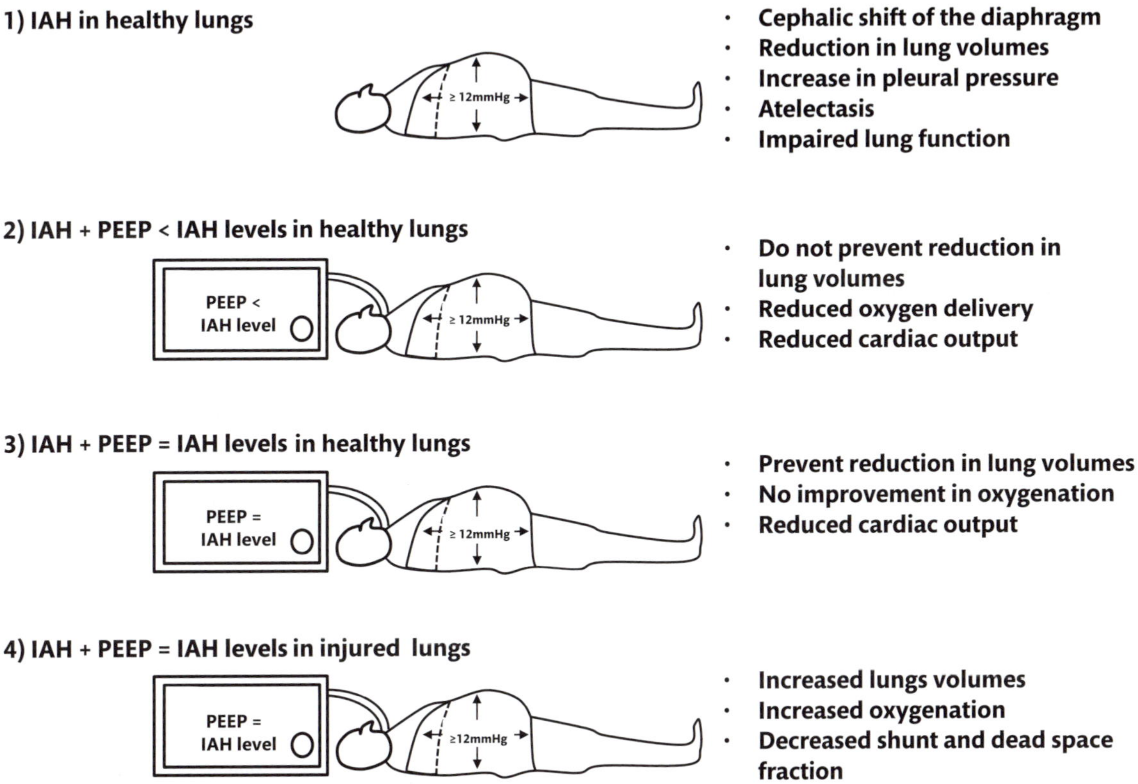

Figure 13.3 Schema showing the effects of intra-abdominal hypertension (IAH), and its association with PEEP levels below and similar to IAH level, associated or not with lung injury. In the first schema, IAH is developed when intra-abdominal pressure is higher than 12 mmHg. This condition is associated with cephalic shift of the diaphragm, reduced lung volumes, and increased pleural pressure, leading to atelectasis and impaired lung function. In the second schema, if PEEP level is lower than the intra-abdominal pressure in healthy lungs, oxygen delivery and cardiac output may reduce, and lung volumes are not affected. In the third schema, if PEEP level is similar to intra-abdominal pressure in healthy lungs, oxygenation and cardiac function are not affected, but this PEEP level prevents lung volume reduction. In the fourth schema, if PEEP level is similar to intra-abdominal pressure in injured lungs, oxygenation improved, lung volumes increased, and shunt reduced.

be driven not only by lung abnormalities but also by the presence of IAH, for instance.

Positive-pressure Ventilation and Ventilator-induced Diaphragm Dysfunction

Mechanical ventilation can result in the rapid development of diaphragmatic weakness due to both atrophy and contractile dysfunction (see Chapter 51). This causative relationship was first observed in a 1994 experimental study in which animals were ventilated in controlled mode for 48 h and a significant loss of diaphragm mass was observed, as well as a large reduction in maximal diaphragmatic specific force production.[25] This phenomenon remained unconfirmed in humans for 14 years until Levine et al. revealed that prolonged mechanical ventilation resulted in rapid diaphragmatic atrophy.[5] But how rapid?

Previous studies have indicated that diaphragmatic fibre atrophy develops within ≥24 h during controlled ventilation (full ventilator support) and correlates significantly with the duration of mechanical ventilation. During controlled ventilation, one way to rule out this effect is to promptly institute partial ventilator support by allowing the patient's effort to participate in the total diaphragm workload. One recent study added a valuable piece to this complex puzzle. Goligher et al.[26] corroborated that diaphragm dysfunction occurs early in the course of ventilation and seems to be modulated by the intensity of respiratory muscle work done by the patient, even under partially assisted modes of ventilation. Furthermore, diaphragm thickness increased in some patients, and both decreased (mainly during controlled ventilation) and increased diaphragm thicknesses (mainly during active breathing) were associated with significant diaphragm dysfunction, possibly secondary to oedema or inflammatory infiltration. The maintenance of adequate (but not excessive) levels of inspiratory effort by titrating ventilator support might prevent changes in diaphragm configuration during mechanical ventilation (Figure 13.4). There are exciting pathways to be understood regarding the underlying mechanism of diaphragm dysfunction.

Skeletal muscle fibre size is maintained by the balance of protein degradation and synthesis. Although not confirmed in humans, animal models have shown that myosin heavy chain protein synthesis rapidly declines within the first 6 h of controlled mechanical ventilation and remains depressed during the next 12 h of mechanical ventilation. Controlled mechanical ventilation has also been shown to activate at least four major proteolytic systems in the diaphragm:

(1) Full mechanical ventilation increases expression of key autophagy proteins (e.g. ATG5, ATG7, and beclin 1) and the number of autophagosomes in the human diaphragm. However, one recent study called into question the notion that autophagosome activation is always detrimental. Azuelos et al. proposed that autophagy might instead be a beneficial adaptive response that can potentially be exploited for therapy of VIDD.[27] The authors made this claim after observing that treatment with the autophagy-inducing agent rapamycin prevented the diaphragmatic force loss associated with mechanical ventilation.

(2) Calpains are responsible for the release of myofilament proteins that are then degraded by the ubiquitin–proteasome system. In this line, it is well established that prolonged mechanical ventilation activates calpain in the human diaphragm.[28]

(3) Caspase-3 plays an important role in apoptosis and may contribute to muscle protein degradation during several conditions. There is ample evidence showing that controlled mechanical ventilation activates caspase-3 in the human diaphragm.[28]

(4) The ubiquitin–proteasome system is dependent on binding of ubiquitin to protein substrates by specialized ubiquitin ligases (E3s). Controlled mechanical ventilation has been shown to increase expression of muscle-specific E3 ligases as well as increase ubiquitinated proteins in the human diaphragm.[29]

Activation of the reactive oxygen species (ROS) system has been recognized as one of the most important pathways

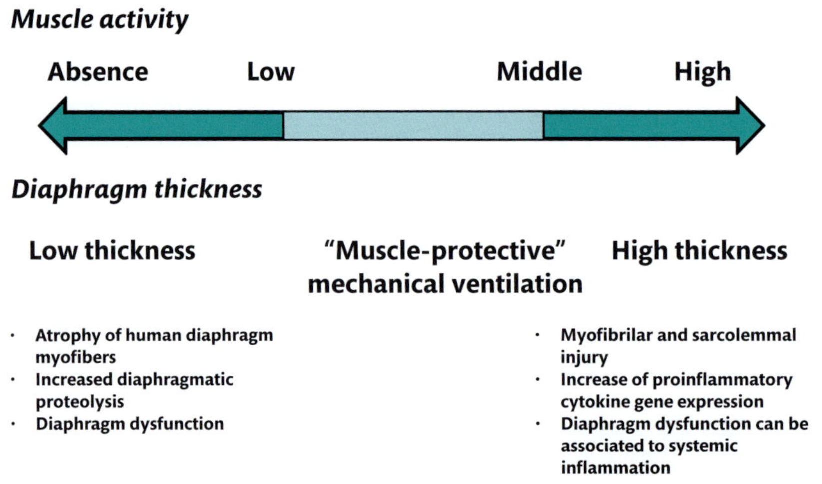

Figure 13.4 Diaphragm activity and thickness scale. Low thickness is associated with the absence of muscle activity, which can lead to atrophy of human diaphragm myofibers, proteolysis, and dysfunction. On the other hand, higher thickness is associated with increased muscle activity, which can be associated with myofibrillar and sarcolemmal injury, elevation of proinflammatory cytokine expression, and if systemic inflammation is present, the diaphragm injury can be even worse. Diaphragm thickness can be evaluated at bedside using ultrasonography.

regulating diaphragm function as it can modulate, in different ways, all four proteolytic systems described above. Oxidant production can occur via NADPH oxidase, xanthine oxidase, or mitochondria. Of these, the dominant site of production in the diaphragm during prolonged mechanical ventilation is the mitochondrion. In rats, increases in ROS production from diaphragm mitochondria to levels able to cause lipid peroxidation and protein oxidation have been observed after 12 h of controlled mechanical ventilation. In addition, two independent studies have confirmed that prolonged (15–176 h) mechanical ventilation also results in mitochondrial damage in the human diaphragm.[30] Once an increase in oxidative stress has been detected, several key proteins involved in both autophagy and the ubiquitin–proteasome system are expressed, which can occur via redox-sensitive transcriptional activating factors (NFkB and FoxO3a). The link between ROS production and calpain activation may be mediated by increases in cytosolic-free calcium. Oxidative stress can activate caspase-3 in the diaphragm, mainly via the caspase-9-dependent intrinsic apoptosis pathway, as observed after prolonged mechanical ventilation.[28]

Conclusion

Evidence suggests that positive-pressure ventilation can exert negative effects not only on the lungs but also in distal organs. These effects may be intermediated by haemodynamic fluctuations or by inflammatory infiltration through different mechanisms. Other compartments that bound the lungs and chest wall can be affected by their mechanical properties. In addition, recent observational studies have shown a causative effect of mechanical ventilation on diaphragm dysfunction, although the underlying mechanism is still unclear. Further research in this area may help minimize the long-term negative consequences of mechanical ventilation in critically ill patients.

REFERENCES

1. Mitchell JR, Whitelaw WA, Sas R, et al. RV filling modulates LV function by direct ventricular interaction during mechanical ventilation. *Am J Physiol Heart Circ Physiol.* 2005 Aug;**289**(2):H549–557.
2. Pelosi P, Ferguson ND, Frutos-Vivar F, et al. Management and outcome of mechanically ventilated neurologic patients. *Crit Care Med.* 2011;**39**:1482–1492.
3. Husain-Syed F, Slutsky AS, Ronco C. Lung-kidney cross-talk in the critically ill patient. *Am J Respir Crit Care Med.* 2016 Aug 15;**194**:402–414.
4. Kredel M, Muellenbach RM, Johannes A, et al. Hepatic effects of lung-protective pressure-controlled ventilation and a combination of high-frequency oscillatory ventilation and extracorporeal lung assist in experimental lung injury. *Med Sci Monit.* 2011;**17**:BR275–281.
5. Levine S, Nguyen T, Taylor N, et al. Rapid disuse atrophy of diaphragm fibers in mechanically ventilated humans. *N Engl J Med.* 2008;**358**:1327–1335.
6. Brower R, Wise RA, Hassapoyannes C, et al. Effect of lung inflation on lung blood volume and pulmonary venous flow. *J Appl Physiol.* 1985;**58**:954–963.
7. Simmons D, Linde L, Miller J, et al. Relation between lung volume and pulmonary vascular resistance. *Circ Res.* 1961;**9**:465–471.
8. Kollisch-Singule M, Emr B, Jain SV, et al. The effects of airway pressure release ventilation on respiratory mechanics in extrapulmonary lung injury. *Intensive Care Med Exp.* 2015;**3**:35.
9. De Santis Santiago R, Teggia Droghi M, Fumagalli J, et al. High pleural pressure prevents alveolar overdistension and hemodynamic collapse in ARDS with Class III obesity. *Am J Respir Crit Care Med.* 2021 Mar 1;**203**(5):575–584. doi:10.1164/rccm.201909-1687OC. PMID: 32876469; PMCID: PMC7924574.
10. Monge Garcia MI, Gil Cano A, Gracia Romero M. Dynamic arterial elastance to predict arterial pressure response to volume loading in preload-dependent patients. *Crit Care.* 2011;**15**:R15.
11. Muizelaar JP, Marmarou A, Ward JD, et al. Adverse effects of prolonged hyperventilation in patients with severe head injury: A randomized clinical trial. *J Neurosurg.* 1991;**75**:731–739.
12. Soustiel JF, Mahamid E, Chistyakov A, et al. Comparison of moderate hyperventilation and mannitol for control of intracranial pressure control in patients with severe traumatic brain injury—a study of cerebral blood flow and metabolism. *Acta Neurochir (Wien).* 2006;**148**:845–851
13. Quilez ME, Fuster G, Villar J, et al. Injurious mechanical ventilation affects neuronal activation in ventilated rats. *Crit Care.* 2011;**15**:R124.
14. Gonzalez-Lopez A, Lopez-Alonso I, Aguirre A, et al. Mechanical ventilation triggers hippocampal apoptosis by vagal and dopaminergic pathways. *Am J Respir Crit Care Med.* 2013;**188**:693–702.
15. Skiold B, Wu Q, Hooper SB, et al. Early detection of ventilation-induced brain injury using magnetic resonance spectroscopy and diffusion tensor imaging: An in vivo study in preterm lambs. *PLoS One.* 2014;**9**:e95804.
16. Korovesi I, Papadomichelakis E, Orfanos SE, et al. Exhaled breath condensate in mechanically ventilated brain-injured patients with no lung injury or sepsis. *Anesthesiology.* 2011;**114**:1118–1129.
17. Walcher A, Faubel S, Keniston A, et al. In critically ill patients requiring CRRT, AKI is associated with increased respiratory failure and death versus ESRD. *Ren Fail.* 2011;**33**:935–942.
18. Gurkan OU, O'Donnell C, Brower R, et al. Differential effects of mechanical ventilatory strategy on lung injury and systemic organ inflammation in mice. *Am J Physiol Lung Cell Mol Physiol.* 2003;**285**:L710–8.
19. van den Akker JP, Egal M, Groeneveld AB. Invasive mechanical ventilation as a risk factor for acute kidney injury in the critically ill: A systematic review and meta-analysis. *Crit Care.* 2013;**17**:R98.
20. The Acute Respiratory Distress Syndrome Network, Brower RG, Matthay MA, et al. Ventilation with lower tidal volumes as compared with traditional tidal volumes for acute lung injury and the acute respiratory distress syndrome. *N Engl J Med.* 2000;**342**:1301–1308.
21. Mercat A, Richard JC, Vielle B, et al. Positive end-expiratory pressure setting in adults with acute lung injury and acute respiratory distress syndrome: A randomized controlled trial. *JAMA.* 2008;**299**:646–655.
22. Levesque E, Saliba F, Ichai P, et al. Outcome of patients with cirrhosis requiring mechanical ventilation in ICU. *J Hepatol.* 2014;**60**:570–578.
23. Amato MB, Meade MO, Slutsky AS, et al. Driving pressure and survival in the acute respiratory distress syndrome. *N Engl J Med.* 2015;**372**:747–755.
24. Neto AS, Hemmes SN, Barbas CS, et al. Association between driving pressure and development of postoperative pulmonary

complications in patients undergoing mechanical ventilation for general anaesthesia: A meta-analysis of individual patient data. *Lancet Respir Med*. 2016;**4**:272–280.

25. Le Bourdelles G, Viires N, Boczkowski J, et al. Effects of mechanical ventilation on diaphragmatic contractile properties in rats. *Am J Respir Crit Care Med*. 1994;**149**:1539–1544.
26. Goligher EC, Fan E, Herridge MS, et al. Evolution of diaphragm thickness during mechanical ventilation. impact of inspiratory effort. *Am J Respir Crit Care Med*. 2015;**192**:1080–1088.
27. Azuelos I, Jung B, Picard M, et al. Relationship between autophagy and ventilator-induced diaphragmatic dysfunction. *Anesthesiology*. 2015;**122**:1349–1361.
28. Nelson WB, Smuder AJ, Hudson MB, et al. Cross-talk between the calpain and caspase-3 proteolytic systems in the diaphragm during prolonged mechanical ventilation. *Crit Care Med*. 2012 Jun;**40**(6):1857–1863. doi:10.1097/CCM.0b013e318246bb5d. PMID: 22487998; PMCID: PMC3358441.
29. Hussain SN, Mofarrahi M, Sigala I, et al. Mechanical ventilation-induced diaphragm disuse in humans triggers autophagy. *Am J Respir Crit Care Med*. 2010;**182**:1377–1386.
30. Picard M, Jung B, Liang F, et al. Mitochondrial dysfunction and lipid accumulation in the human diaphragm during mechanical ventilation. *Am J Respir Crit Care Med*. 2012;**186**:1140–1149.

PART 5

Monitoring the Mechanically Ventilated Patient

14

Monitoring Airway Inflammation and Infection

Anthony Rostron, Thomas Hellyer, and A John Simpson

KEY MESSAGES

- The respiratory tree is not a sterile environment.
- Distinguishing colonization from infection, particularly in the setting of critical illness, is a challenge.
- Lack of disease resolution, even in infection, does not always warrant administration of antibiotics.

CONTROVERSIES

- Clinical behaviour is often engrained and difficult to modify.
- The invasiveness of the diagnostic approach ought to be proportionate to the clinical scenario, and current evidence may not be sufficiently granular to guide this.
- Relevant outcomes in antimicrobial prescribing are not limited to morbidity and mortality of studied patients.

FURTHER RESEARCH

- Development of simple, automated, high-fidelity, rapid, near-patient testing for infection.
- Host genome and metabolic profiling may facilitate the development of non-antibiotic treatment to improve patient outcome.

Introduction

Lung inflammation is the major cause of respiratory failure, which in turn is the most common reason for admission to the intensive care unit (ICU). Monitoring, which includes clinical assessment, can be undertaken at repeated intervals or continuously, with the intention of detecting deterioration or improvement and triggering an appropriate response. Monitoring is facilitated by accurate diagnosis, an assessment of disease severity and a clear treatment strategy.

Patients with acute respiratory failure and inflammatory lung disease are commonly assumed to have an infective precipitant. Further investigation may only be prompted by treatment failure with antibiotics. Intervention on critical care can further compromise innate immune defence and thus infection can coexist with other disease entities or complicate their critical care stay. Dissecting out infective from non-infective causes of inflammation remains a major clinical challenge, especially in an era of growing antimicrobial resistance.

Respiratory problems present with dyspnoea, chest pain, wheeze, and cough, which may be productive of sputum. Previous medical history (including childhood illness), vaccination, occupational, smoking, travel, and medication histories along with the risk of exposure to environmental triggers should be considered. Examination may help to determine the severity of illness, elicit extrapulmonary manifestations, refine diagnostic hypotheses, and guide investigations, but it is limited in distinguishing infective from non-infective causes of inflammation. An overview of the assessment of the pulmonary and systemic compartments is displayed in Figure 14.1.

Respiratory Sampling and Microbiological Diagnosis

Respiratory and blood cultures have a low yield, and microbiological sensitivities take 48–72 h to turn around, but the identification of a causative organism facilitates rational antimicrobial therapy. In severe community-acquired pneumonia, current American Thoracic Society (ATS) practice guidelines suggest pre-treatment blood cultures, culture and Gram stain of expectorated sputum, and urinary antigen tests for *Streptococcus pneumoniae* and *Legionella pneumophila* should be taken.[1]

Laboratories should exercise quality control over sputum samples. The presence of saliva, mucus, blood, and pus should be assessed macroscopically. Sputum should be screened by microscopic examination for the relative number of polymorphonuclear cells and squamous epithelial cells in a low-power (100× magnification) field. Invalid specimens (>10 squamous epithelial cells and <25 polymorphonuclear cells/field) should not be examined further.

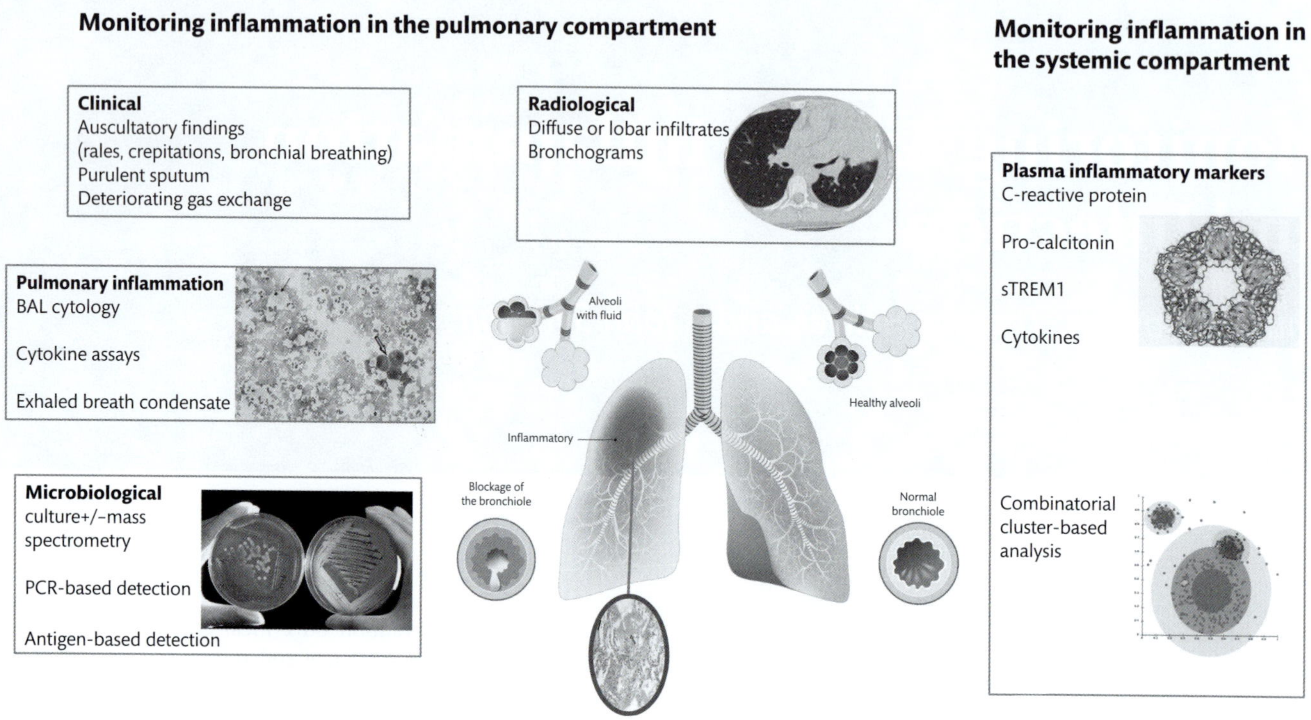

Figure 14.1 Diagrammatic representation of approaches to monitoring inflammation in the pulmonary and systemic compartments. BAL, bronchoalveolar lavage; PCR, polymerase chain reaction; sTREM-1, soluble triggering receptor on myeloid cells-1.

Agar plate: This image was released into the public domain by the National Cancer Institute (https://www.cancer.gov), an agency part of the National Institutes of Health, with the ID 2230.

BAL cells: Reprinted by permission from Springer Nature: *Critical Care*, Bronchoalveolar lavage cytological alveolar damage in patients with severe pneumonia, Bogdan Grigoriu et al., © 2005.

CT scan: Reproduced from Wang B, et al., Computed tomography-based predictive nomogram for differentiating primary progressive pulmonary tuberculosis from community-acquired pneumonia in children. *BMC Med Imaging*, 19, 63 (2019). https://doi.org/10.1186/s12880-019-0355-z Reproduced under the terms of the Creative Commons Attribution 4.0 International License (http://creativecommons.org/licenses/by/4.0/)

CRP image: Reproduced under the Creative Commons Attribution 3.0 Unported license (https://creativecommons.org/licenses/by/3.0/deed.en). Wikimedia Commons / User: Astrojan. Data from: http://www.rcsb.org/pdb/explore/explore.do?structureId=1lj7

Cluster image: Reproduced under the Creative Commons Attribution-Share Alike 3.0 Unported license (https://creativecommons.org/licenses/by-sa/3.0/deed.en). Wikipedia Commons / User: Chire.

Histology: Reproduced from Scendoni, R., et al. Histopathology of COVID-19 pneumonia in two non-oncological, non-hospitalised cases as a reliable diagnostic benchmark. *Diagn Pathol* 15, 73 (2020). https://doi.org/10.1186/s13000-020-00990-4. Reproduced under the terms of the Creative Commons Attribution 4.0 International License (http://creativecommons.org/licenses/by/4.0/).

Image created by A Conway Morris

Deep respiratory samples are more accessible following endotracheal intubation. Endotracheal aspirates (ETAs) are the correlate of sputum and form part of the standard diagnostic approach for pneumonia. ETA samples are often taken for microbiological surveillance. Bacteria identified by surveillance may help identify the causative microorganism if ventilator-associated pneumonia (VAP) develops. Non-quantitative ETA cultures nevertheless lack a validated threshold for positivity, and they may not distinguish colonization by oropharyngeal flora from infection.

A more invasive strategy involves bronchoscopic techniques including bronchoalveolar lavage (BAL) or a protected specimen brush (PSB). Although a standardized approach to BAL has been reported, there is considerable variation in UK practice.[2] Quantitative culture is used to distinguish between colonization and infection. In a landmark study, Chastre et al. compared BAL and PSB specimens to post-mortem histology and microbiological culture of lung tissue from the same bronchopulmonary segment.[3] Operating characteristics were determined for BAL or PSB (cfu/mL) to detect significant tissue microbiology ($>10^4$ cfu/g). For BAL at a threshold of $>10^4$ cfu/mL, sensitivity was 91% and specificity was 78%; for PSB at a threshold of $>10^3$ cfu/mL, sensitivity was 82% and specificity was 77%. Variations in differential cell counts of BAL for different conditions have not yet shown diagnostic value (Figure 14.2).

'Blind' BAL (i.e. not visually directed by bronchoscopy), mini-BAL, and blind PSB have been proposed to be as good, but firm evidence is lacking. Pneumonia, particularly VAP, is usually a patchy process, and the operator is unaware whether a radiologically involved region of the lung is being sampled by a blind technique.

The ATS has previously recommended invasive respiratory sampling as best practice due to higher specificity reducing false positive cultures from proximal airway colonization. More recently, this recommendation has been challenged by a meta-analysis that did not support the use of invasive sampling.[4] As a consequence, updated ATS guides suggest a non-invasive sampling approach whereas European guidelines suggest an invasive, distal sampling approach with a greater emphasis on antibiotic stewardship from a more accurate sample. However, both of these guidelines

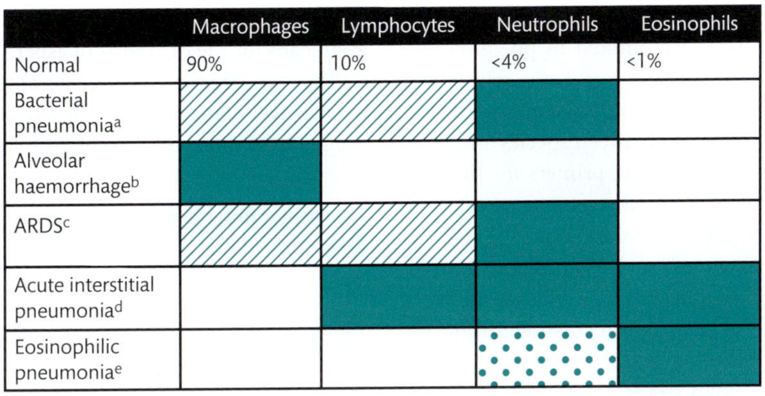

Macrophages
Lymphocytes
Neutrophils
Eosinophils
Normal
90%
10%
<4%
<1%
Bacterial pneumonia[a]
Alveolar haemorrhage[b]
ARDS[c]
Acute interstitial pneumonia[d]
Eosinophilic pneumonia[e]

Figure 14.2 Changes in bronchoalveolar cell composition in varied respiratory conditions associated with acute respiratory failure. Solid cells indicate increased absolute or relative cell counts, hatched cells indicate decreased absolute or relative cell counts, white cells indicate unchanged proportions and absolute counts.

[a] Bacterial pneumonia—neutrophils typically exceed 50% of total cell count.

[b] Alveolar haemorrhage—red blood cells typically predominate, haemosiderin containing macrophages are pathognomic and develop within 48 hours of haemorrhage.

[c] Acute respiratory distress syndrome (ARDS)—neutrophils typically account for around 70% of total cell count.

[d] Cellular make-up in AIP is variable, although classically both neutrophils and eosinophils are elevated in equal proportions, isolated neutrophilia may indicate infection rather than autoimmune disease. Lymphocytic AIP is seen in 10% of cases.

[e] Eosinophils typically make up 20–90% of cell count, although neutrophils may be elevated they are always lower than % of eosinophils.

Data from J Dakin and M Griffiths, The pulmonary physician in critical care 1: Pulmonary investigations for acute respiratory failure. *Thorax* 2002;57:79–85.

grade these recommendations as weak and based on low-quality evidence.

An invasive diagnostic strategy is still supported in patients with interstitial lung disease or in lung transplant recipients, particularly as they may require augmentation of immunosuppressive treatment. Targeted antimicrobial treatment is also less likely to lead to drug toxicity. Bronchoscopy and BAL are also considered the gold standard for the diagnosis of *Pneumocystis jiroveci*. When invasive aspergillosis is suspected, BAL should be sent for microscopy for hyphae and fungal culture; a BAL galactomannan test may further improve the diagnostic yield.

Almost 40% of patients hospitalized with pneumonia have evidence of a pleural effusion. Although empyema (bacterial invasion of the pleura) is relatively uncommon, the specificity of pleural cultures is very high. A pathogen in pleural fluid is likely to be the causative organism of the pneumonia. If a 10–20 mL sample can be aspirated easily and safely under ultrasound guidance, it is sufficient to test pH, protein, lactate dehydrogenase, differential white cell count, Gram stain, and culture.

In patients with severe pneumonia and treatment failure in whom a microbiological diagnosis has not been possible, transthoracic needle aspiration (TNA) offers another, albeit invasive, approach. Ruiz-Gonzalez obtained a microbiological diagnosis in 36 of 55 patients (65%) with pneumonia in whom the aetiology had proven elusive by conventional methods.[5] The risk of complications does mean that TNA should only be undertaken in severely ill patients with a focal, consolidative infiltrate, when the usual approach has failed.

In immunocompromised individuals, BAL is commonly useful, but where diagnostic uncertainty and treatment failure persist, an invasive diagnostic procedure such as transbronchial biopsy (TBB), percutaneous needle biopsy, video-assisted thorascopic biopsy (VATS), or open lung biopsy is sometimes required to obtain a sample of lung tissue for diagnosis.[6] The optimal procedure is determined by the nature (focal/diffuse) and location (central/peripheral) of the lesion, modified by the skills available locally, and risk of pneumothorax. Diffuse lesions may be sampled by TBB, whereas nodules are better located by CT-guided percutaneous needle biopsy, VATS, or open lung biopsy. VATS is also useful for sampling peripheral pulmonary lesions, but surgical biopsies have a higher incidence of complications.

In areas with high prevalence of tuberculosis, TBB should be considered. Isolated BAL is also less often diagnostic in invasive fungal or cytomegalovirus infection than for *Pneumocystis* pneumonia or bacterial infection. Biopsy allows distinction between colonization and invasion of fungal or viral infection.

Some bacterial species are difficult to isolate or grow slowly in culture. Others may not culture because of prior empirical antimicrobial treatment. Culture-negative lower respiratory tract infections present a particular barrier to effective treatment. Molecular diagnostic techniques can assist in diagnosis, with three broad classes in use and development:

(i) Fluorescent in situ hybridization (FISH) using nucleic acid probes.
(ii) Nucleic acid amplification techniques or polymerase chain reaction (PCR), which extend into post-amplification techniques such as sequencing and spectrometry.
(iii) Non-nucleic acid techniques including mass spectrometry and proteomics.

Current methods of FISH allow the detection of pathogens in respiratory samples within 10 h with a sensitivity of 94% and specificity of 88%.[7] However, cost and technical complexity currently limit its introduction into routine clinical practice.

Matrix-assisted laser desorption/ionization time-of-flight mass spectrometry (MALDI/TOF MS) has been used to shorten incubation time for identification of fungi, anaerobic bacteria, and *Mycobacterium* spp., which require long incubation times.

Identification of bacteria directly from specimens has led to variable results, and performance is particularly limited in polymicrobial infections.

The 16S component of bacterial ribosomal DNA contains nucleotide sequences that are highly conserved between species and other sequences that are species-specific. By using primers for the conserved sequences, PCR can be used to amplify genetic material and DNA sequencing can be used to determine the species.

Challenges for molecular techniques are determining antimicrobial susceptibility and automation of technology. The sensitivity of molecular techniques presents a challenge in distinguishing between viable and non-viable infection and colonization, particularly as the respiratory tract is not a sterile site. Over-reliance on molecular techniques may actually lead to the over-diagnosis of infection and compromise antibiotic stewardship.

The major respiratory viral pathogens (Chapter 34) include influenza virus, respiratory syncytial virus (RSV), coronavirus, adenovirus, and rhinovirus. Adenovirus and rhinovirus commonly cause infections with lower mortality but significant morbidity, particularly in patients with chronic respiratory problems. However, as with coronavirus, influenza, and RSV, they can present with severe pneumonia and acute respiratory distress syndrome (ARDS).

Clinical diagnosis of viral pneumonia is notoriously inaccurate. Conventional techniques of virus detection, such as culture and immunofluorescence assays, have a long turnaround time and are of limited use for individual patient management and institution of timely preventative measures. Rapid and accurate diagnosis, with nucleic acid amplification and enzyme-linked immunosorbent assay (ELISA), can help with epidemiological monitoring, infection control, implementing appropriate treatment, and antimicrobial stewardship.

Methods of sampling the respiratory tract for viral infection include a nasal/nasopharyngeal swab placed in viral transport medium, a nasal/nasopharyngeal aspirate or wash, or an ETA or BAL. The aim is to collect fluid containing epithelial cells or mucus containing viral particles. Test positivity can be dependent on the type of sample and the clinical presentation.

The *S. pneumoniae* urinary immunochromatographic membrane test detects the cell wall polysaccharide common to all serotypes. On a single unconcentrated urine specimen, the test performs with a sensitivity of >70% and a specificity >80%. Evidence would suggest reserving *S. pneumoniae* urinary antigen testing for the sickest patients in whom sputum Gram stain results are inconclusive. The test lacks specificity in children as a result of the high carriage rate of pneumococci in the nasopharynx.

Urinary antigen detection is currently the most helpful test for the diagnosis of *Legionella* infection. It is recommended for patients admitted to intensive care and in those for whom the history is suggestive of *L. pneumophila*, but it is only designed to detect an antigen from the most common serotype of *L. pneumophila*. It performs best on concentrated urine specimens. Occasionally, repeated testing is worthwhile.

Specific fungal cell wall components can be detected in serum (e.g. galactomannan in the diagnosis of invasive *Aspergillus* infection), urine (e.g. *Histoplasma* carbohydrate antigen), or BAL (e.g. newer uses of galactomannan assays for *Aspergillus* or *Histoplasma* carbohydrate antigen for histoplasmosis). Additional assays are being designed to detect other components of the cell wall, such as β-glucans for the diagnosis of aspergillosis and candidiasis.

The measurement of specific antibody responses has a limited role in the management of lower respiratory tract infections because of the time lag to develop and detect a response.

Indirect Monitoring of Airway Inflammation

Thoracic imaging is integral to the diagnosis of pulmonary pathology and is covered separately in Chapter 18.

Abnormalities or improvements in gas exchange can be detected by non-invasive (pulse oximetry and transcutaneous carbon dioxide monitors) or invasive (capnography and arterial blood gas analysis) means.

Airflow limitation can occur in asthma, chronic obstructive pulmonary disease, anaphylaxis, bronchiolitis, bronchiectasis, and bronchiolitis obliterans syndrome. Invasive mechanical ventilation can exacerbate dynamic hyperinflation and gas trapping. Monitoring airway pressure and gas flow can help assess severity of disease and response to treatment.

Composite scoring systems offer another approach to the assessment of severity and monitoring patient trajectory. APACHE II has predictive value for mortality in acute exacerbations of chronic obstructive pulmonary disease (COPD), although disease-specific scores, such as Dyspnoea, Eosinopenia, Consolidation, Atrial fibrillation (DECAF),[8] may offer further refinement.

CURB65 and the pneumonia severity index have been developed to predict in-hospital mortality for pneumonia. They have been used to infer which patients need hospital admission. However, they do not perform as well when trying to predict which patients need critical care admission. Other tools such as those developed by the Infectious Diseases Society of America/American Thoracic Society (IDSA/ATS) guideline committee and SMART-COP may perform better in this regard.[9]

Organ failure scores are designed to describe organ dysfunction serially. The most widely used organ failure score is the sequential organ failure assessment score that was initially developed for use in septic patients but has been used to describe non-septic patients.

The clinical pulmonary infection score (CPIS) was developed to make the diagnosis of VAP (Chapter 32) more objective. The score is composed of temperature, white blood cell count, appearance of tracheal secretions, PaO_2/FiO_2 ratio, signs on the CXR, and culture of tracheal aspirate. In the derivation study, a CPIS >6 correctly identified VAP with a sensitivity of 93% and a specificity of 100%.[10] This has not been validated in subsequent studies. The CPIS correlates poorly with quantitative cultures from BAL. Another potential use of CPIS is as an aid to antibiotic de-escalation, but evidence for this is currently limited to the early discontinuation of antibiotics in patients who had an initial CPIS of ≤6 which persisted 3 days after antibiotics had been commenced.[11]

An increase in extravascular lung water (EVLW) is the pathophysiological hallmark of ARDS and an independent risk factor for 28-day mortality. The gold standard method of measurement is the gravimetric method based on measuring wet and dry weights of lung but requires biopsy specimens. The transpulmonary thermodilution technique compares favourably and has been used as a primary end point in clinical trials investigating ARDS[12] with a suggestion that management based on EVLW may reduce ICU length of stay and improve mortality,[13] but RCT evidence is currently lacking.

Direct Monitoring of Airway Inflammation

Early clinical signs of infection, such as fever, tachycardia, and leucocytosis, are non-specific for the diagnosis of lung infection. Kaukonen et al. highlighted the limitations of using systemic inflammatory response syndrome criteria to diagnose sepsis.[14]

Biomarkers of disease can facilitate early diagnosis and provide insight into disease progression, prognosis, and response to therapy. The performance of biomarkers can be described by a confusion matrix and area under the receiver operating characteristic (ROC) curve, with values >90% representing good performance. In emergency medicine and critical care, a rule-out test for infection, prioritizing sensitivity (and negative predictive value) over specificity, would be an appropriate compromise.

Systemic Compartment

C-reactive protein (CRP) levels rise in response to inflammation. It is of hepatic origin and increases following interleukin-6 (IL-6) secretion. CRP is generally regarded to lack the necessary specificity to be an effective biomarker for the diagnosis of infection, but potentially has more promise in predicting bacteraemia. In a small cohort study of patients with a clinical diagnosis of VAP,[15] a decrease in CRP from day 0 to day 4 seemed to have some prognostic value with respect to 28-day mortality. In patients with moderate or severe pneumonia, it is generally recognized that CRP should be falling after 3 days of adequate antibiotic therapy, and, if not, an explanation should be sought. Notably, anti-IL-6 therapies, such as tocilizumab, suppress the normal CRP response to infection, and therefore in patients with a history of recent use of these agents a low CRP should not be taken to indicate the absence or resolution of bacterial infection.

Normal procalcitonin (PCT) levels in the blood are less than 0.05 ng/L. PCT is produced and released in response to inflammatory stimuli, and the magnitude of this response is thought to be greater when the stimulus is bacterial in origin. Viruses also modulate its release through interferon gamma. PCT is detectable within 2–4 h of infection, peaks within 6–24 h, and can be present for up to 7 days.

The area under the curve for summary ROC curves for a single PCT level in distinguishing infective from non-infective causes of inflammation was 0.85 for patients with critical illness (sensitivity of 0.77; specificity of 0.79).[16]

In addition to its potential role in diagnosis, PCT has been used to predict prognosis. Liu et al. undertook a meta-analysis and demonstrated that an elevated PCT was associated with an increased risk of death in critically ill patients with pneumonia. The prognostic performance was similar in VAP and community-acquired pneumonia, although this only showed moderate accuracy.[17]

The value of PCT in tailoring individual antibiotic therapy has been assessed, with a reported reduction in antibiotic exposure and a significant improvement in survival. The PCT thresholds for determining prognosis and guiding treatment are variable. Biomarkers with varying optimal cut points in different populations may lead to confusion. Interestingly, there is poor adherence, even in trials, to recommendations with respect to PCT-guided antibiotic prescription in critical care. While PCT kinetics can be used to de-escalate antibiotic treatment, no mortality benefit has been shown in using PCT to trigger further investigation and escalation of antibiotic treatment.

Triggering receptor expressed on myeloid cells type 1 (TREM-1) is up-regulated in various inflammatory diseases, including bacterial and fungal sepsis. A meta-analysis suggested that the soluble form (sTREM-1) was a useful aid to diagnosis of infection in adults,[18] but there was heterogeneity in sampling, and the studies that analyzed plasma were equivocal.

Recent studies in ARDS have used latent class analysis to identify two distinct endotypes based upon systemic IL-8 and tumour necrosis factor (TNF) receptor measurement, more pronounced shock and metabolic acidosis.[19] Emerging evidence indicates these endotypes respond differently to fluid management, application of positive end-expiratory pressure, and pharmacological treatments such as simvastatin. Surprisingly, the hyperinflammatory phenotype does not appear to be particularly prevalent in COVID-19-associated ARDS.[20]

Pulmonary Compartment

Exhaled breath condensate has three principal components:

(i) non-volatile aerosolized droplets or particles from the airway fluid lining the respiratory tract,
(ii) water, and
iii) exhaled volatiles from airway lining fluid.

It is therefore a matrix of potential biomarkers than can be sampled non-invasively and repeatedly, though determining the site of origin (conducting airways vs alveolar, gas exchanging lung) can be a challenge. There is a risk of oropharyngeal contamination, which is bypassed during invasive mechanical ventilation. Condensing water vapour has the potential to dilute the samples leading to both intra-subject and inter-subject variability. Other limitations include the lack of a gold standard with which to compare assays, variability between collection of samples and assays, and the absence of normal ranges; relative change is therefore a better way to express trends. Samples can be collected in spontaneously breathing patients or those who are mechanically ventilated.

Markers of oxidative stress, for example, hydrogen peroxide (H_2O_2), have been detected in the exhaled breath condensate from patients with inflammatory lung conditions, such as asthma, COPD, cystic fibrosis, bronchiectasis, and ARDS, but they lack the specificity to be diagnostic.

Nitric oxide (NO) has direct and indirect oxidant potential and thus it is cytotoxic and antimicrobial. Fractional exhaled NO (FeNO) is increased in patients with eosinophilic airway inflammation in asthma and COPD, and this correlates with responsiveness to inhaled corticosteroids (ICS). A systematic review showed no statistically significant benefit from FeNO-guided management in terms of severe exacerbations or ICS use, but did show a statistically significant reduction in exacerbations of any severity.[21] A clear place for FeNO in critical care has yet to be established.

Bacteria produce a characteristic signal of volatile organic compounds that can be detected by gas chromatography and mass spectrometry in the exhaled breath of mechanically ventilated patients. Exhaled breath condensate analysis therefore offers real potential for a minimally invasive method of detecting infection. In mechanically ventilated patients following traumatic brain injury, exhaled breath condensate was analyzed by thermal desorption/gas chromatography/time-of-flight mass spectrometry. VAP was confirmed by semi-quantitative culture of blind-BAL samples. A clear separation in signal was observed between patients who were culture positive and those who were not.[22]

In addition to BAL analysis for microbiological purposes, cytology with a differential leucocyte count may occasionally help if a neutrophilia (broadly favouring bacterial infection) is not observed. For example, lymphocytosis may favour a viral diagnosis or forms of interstitial lung disease, while eosinophilia may suggest a corticosteroid-responsive or helminthic aetiology. BAL fibrocyte numbers are elevated in ARDS, and a cell count in excess of 6% was observed in non-survivors.[23] However, detailed cytological or biomarker assessment is largely reserved for research purposes.

Although serum CRP and PCT have been used to guide treatment in infection, they do not appear to have any discriminatory value for the diagnosis of VAP when measured in BAL.

In a study of 148 mechanically ventilated patients in whom pulmonary infection was suspected, sTREM-1 showed promise as an aid to diagnosis of pneumonia.[24] Blind-BAL sTREM-1, TNF-α, and IL-1β were raised in pneumonia in comparison to those without pneumonia. On constructing ROC curves, the AUROC for sTREM-1 was 0.93 (95% confidence interval (CI) 0.92–0.95), and a cut-off of 5 pg/mL had a sensitivity of 98% and a specificity of 90%. In contrast, two studies did not demonstrate any diagnostic value of BAL sTREM-1. In one study, there was no significant difference in sTREM-1 between the VAP and non-VAP groups,[25] and in the other, although there was a significant difference between groups, when an ROC was constructed, the AUROC was poor (0.58, 95% CI 0.50–0.65).[26] In both studies, BAL was more selectively retrieved using a flexible bronchoscope.

A small study of 35 patients with suspected VAP attempted to determine the prognostic value of serial sTREM-1 in BAL.[27] A BAL was performed at enrolment, with two more on day 4/5 and days 7–9. ROC curves were constructed for sTREM-1 at each time point with the aim of distinguishing survivors from non-survivors. sTREM-1 levels fell over time in survivors and continued to rise in non-survivors. At baseline the AUROC was 0.54 (not statistically significant), at days 4–5 the AUROC was 0.77 (95% CI 0.57–0.97), and at 7–9 days the AUROC was 0.89 (95% CI 0.72–1.07). In this study, the rate of VAP, confirmed by positive BAL culture, was unusually high at 70%.

In a prospective, observational cohort study, Conway Morris et al. measured a range of biomarkers of the innate immune response in the lung, sampled by BAL.[28] Patients were recruited if VAP was suspected, but excluded if it was anticipated that bronchoscopy and BAL would be poorly tolerated. Seventy-two patients were included in the analysis. VAP was confirmed by quantitative culture of BAL with a pathogen growth of $>10^4$ cfu/mL. BAL was assayed for TNF-α, IL-1β, IL-6, IL-8, IL-10, granulocyte colony-stimulating factor (G-CSF), MIP-1α, sTREM-1, and monocyte chemo-attractant peptide. Significant differences were found between patients with and without VAP for BAL IL-1β and IL-8. IL-1β and IL-8 had AUROC of 0.81 (95% CI 0.71–0.91) and 0.83 (95% CI 0.74–0.95), respectively, for the diagnosis of VAP. For IL-1β, an optimal cut point determined by the Youden index at 10 pg/mL had a sensitivity of 94% and a specificity of 64%. This corresponds to a negative predictive value of 97% to rule out VAP. A multicentre validation study from a broad ICU population, using a standardized, selective distal airway sampling technique, yielded similar results.[29] A subsequent randomized controlled trial seeking to determine whether BAL IL-1β and IL-8 could reduce unnecessary antibiotic use (by excluding VAP) confirmed the diagnostic usefulness of both biomarkers. However, despite this, clinicians did not reduce antibiotic use based on BAL IL-1β and IL-8, suggesting complex influences on clinicians' antibiotic prescribing behaviour in critically ill patients.[30]

Future Directions and Current Recommendations

Future developments are likely to focus on non-invasive, point of care tests with a rapid turnaround time. The pursuit of isolated, disease-specific biomarkers is likely to remain elusive due to the variation in pathogens and host genetics. It is more realistic that panels of biomarkers, adding novel biomarkers of function and damage to classic biomarkers, will prove to be more effective. Host genome sequencing and metabolic profiling are likely to offer further refinement.

Automated processing in molecular detection techniques such as nucleic acid amplification may facilitate their more widespread introduction into clinical practice, although careful, targeted patient sampling is likely to be required to minimize false positive diagnosis of infection. Assessment of respiratory microbiota through amplification of bacterial RNA and sequencing may improve the value of surveillance cultures, with identification of emerging dominant bacterial species particularly in patients with underlying lung disease or at risk of nosocomial pneumonia. However, repeated sampling will necessitate a standardized approach to ensure that results are representative.

While current iterations of guidelines have steered away from the use of routine invasive sampling, this is likely to be a product of using mortality as an end point in clinical trials. Given the need for improved antimicrobial stewardship, it may be more appropriate to consider antibiotic exposure as an alternative end point with the proviso that mortality is not observed to increase.

REFERENCES

1. Metlay JP, Waterer GW, Long AC, et al. Diagnosis and treatment of adults with community-acquired pneumonia. *Am J Respir Crit Care Med*. 2019;**200**:E45–67.
2. Browne E, Hellyer TP, Baudouin SV, et al. A national survey of the diagnosis and management of suspected ventilator-associated pneumonia. *BMJ Open Respir Res*. 2014;**1**:e000066.
3. Chastre J, Fagon JY, Bornet-Lecso M, et al. Evaluation of bronchoscopic techniques for the diagnosis of nosocomial pneumonia. *Am J Respir Crit Care Med*. 1995;**152**:231–240.

4. Berton DC, Kalil AC, Teixeira PJ. Quantitative versus qualitative cultures of respiratory secretions for clinical outcomes in patients with ventilator-associated pneumonia. *Cochrane Database Syst Rev*. 2014 Oct 30;(10):CD006482. doi:10.1002/14651858.CD006482.pub4. PMID: 25354013.
5. Ruiz-Gonzalez A, Falguera M, Nogues A, et al. Is Streptococcus pneumoniae the leading cause of pneumonia of unknown etiology? A microbiologic study of lung aspirates in consecutive patients with community-acquired pneumonia. *Am J Med*. 1999;**106**:385–390.
6. Janzen DL, Adler BD, Padley SP, et al. Diagnostic success of bronchoscopic biopsy in immunocompromised patients with acute pulmonary disease: Predictive value of disease distribution as shown on CT. *AJR Am J Roentgenol*. 1993;**160**:21–24.
7. Koncan R, Parisato M, Sakarikou C, et al. Direct identification of major Gram-negative pathogens in respiratory specimens by respiFISH(R) HAP Gram (-) Panel, a beacon-based FISH methodology. *Eur J Clin Microbiol Infect Dis*. 2015;**34**:2097–2102.
8. Echevarria C, Steer J, Heslop-Marshall K, et al. Validation of the DECAF score to predict hospital mortality in acute exacerbations of COPD. *Thorax*. 2016;**71**:133–140.
9. Chalmers JD, Mandal P, Singanayagam A, et al. Severity assessment tools to guide ICU admission in community-acquired pneumonia: Systematic review and meta-analysis. *Intensive Care Med*. 2011;**37**:1409–1420.
10. Pugin J, Auckenthaler R, Mili N, et al. Diagnosis of ventilator-associated pneumonia by bacteriologic analysis of bronchoscopic and nonbronchoscopic 'blind' bronchoalveolar lavage fluid. *Am Rev Respir Dis*. 1991;**143**:1121–1129.
11. Singh N, Rogers P, Atwood CW, et al. Short-course empiric antibiotic therapy for patients with pulmonary infiltrates in the intensive care unit. A proposed solution for indiscriminate antibiotic prescription. *Am J Respir Crit Care Med*. 2000;**162**:505–511.
12. Craig TR, Duffy MJ, Shyamsundar M, et al. A randomized clinical trial of hydroxymethylglutaryl-coenzyme a reductase inhibition for acute lung injury (The HARP Study). *Am J Respir Crit Care Med*. 2011;**183**:620–626.
13. Eisenberg PR, Hansbrough JR, Anderson D, et al. A prospective study of lung water measurements during patient management in an intensive care unit. *Am Rev Respir Dis*. 1987;**136**:662–668.
14. Kaukonen K-M, Bailey M, Pilcher D, et al. Systemic inflammatory response syndrome criteria in defining severe sepsis. *N Engl J Med*. 2015;**372**:1629–1638.
15. Seligman R, Meisner M, Lisboa TC, et al. Decreases in procalcitonin and C-reactive protein are strong predictors of survival in ventilator-associated pneumonia. *Crit Care*. 2006;**10**:R125.
16. Wacker C, Prkno A, Brunkhorst FM, et al. Procalcitonin as a diagnostic marker for sepsis: A systematic review and meta-analysis. *Lancet Infect Dis*. 2013;**13**:426–435.
17. Liu D, Su L, Han G, et al. Prognostic value of procalcitonin in adult patients with sepsis: A systematic review and meta-analysis. *PLoS One*. 2015;**10**:e0129450.
18. Jiyong J, Tiancha H, Wei C, et al. Diagnostic value of the soluble triggering receptor expressed on myeloid cells-1 in bacterial infection: A meta-analysis. *Intensive Care Med*. 2009;**35**:587–595.
19. Calfee CS, Delucchi K, Parsons PE, et al. Subphenotypes in acute respiratory distress syndrome: Latent class analysis of data from two randomised controlled trials. *Lancet Respir Med*. 2014;**2**:611–620.
20. Sinha P, Calfee CS, Cherian S, et al. Prevalence of phenotypes of acute respiratory distress syndrome in critically ill patients with COVID-19: A prospective observational study. *Lancet Respir Med*. 2020;**8**:1209–1218.
21. Essat M, Harnan S, Gomersall T, et al. Fractional exhaled nitric oxide for the management of asthma in adults: A systematic review. *Eur Respir J*. 2016;**47**:751–768.
22. Fowler SJ, Basanta-Sanchez M, Xu Y, et al. Surveillance for lower airway pathogens in mechanically ventilated patients by metabolomic analysis of exhaled breath: A case-control study. *Thorax*. 2015;**70**:320–325.
23. Quesnel C, Piednoir P, Gelly J, et al. Alveolar fibrocyte percentage is an independent predictor of poor outcome in patients with acute lung injury. *Crit Care Med*. 2012;**40**:21–28.
24. Gibot S, Cravoisy A, Levy B, et al Soluble triggering receptor expressed on myeloid cells and the diagnosis of pneumonia. *N Engl J Med*. 2004;**35**:451–458.
25. Horonenko G, Hoyt JC, Robbins RA, et al. Soluble triggering receptor expressed on myeloid cell-1 is increased in patients with ventilator-associated pneumonia: A preliminary report. *Chest*. 2007;**132**:58–63.
26. Oudhuis GJ, Beuving J, Bergmans D, et al. Soluble triggering receptor expressed on myeloid cells-1 in bronchoalveolar lavage fluid is not predictive for ventilator-associated pneumonia. *Intensive Care Med*. 2009;**35**:1265–1270.
27. Wu C-L, Lu Y-T, Kung Y-C, et al. Prognostic value of dynamic soluble triggering receptor expressed on myeloid cells in bronchoalveolar lavage fluid of patients with ventilator-associated pneumonia. *Respirology*. 2011;**16**:487–494.
28. Conway Morris A, Kefala K, Wilkinson T, et al. Diagnostic importance of pulmonary interleukin-1beta and interleukin-8 in ventilator-associated pneumonia. *Thorax*. 2010;**65**:201–207.
29. Hellyer TP, Morris AC, McAuley DF, et al. Diagnostic accuracy of pulmonary host inflammatory mediators in the exclusion of ventilator-acquired pneumonia. *Thorax*. 2015;**7**:41–47.
30. Hellyer TP, McAuley DF, Walsh TS, et al. Biomarker-guided antibiotic stewardship in suspected ventilator-associated pneumonia (VAPrapid2): A randomised controlled trial and process evaluation. *Lancet Respir Med*. 2020;**8**:182–191.

15

Monitoring Lung-protective Ventilation

Paolo Formenti and John J Marini

KEY MESSAGES

- Repeated tidal recruitment–derecruitment of unstable alveoli promotes epithelial small airway damage and inflammation. Both these processes may contribute to progressive lung injury in unstable lung units.
- The static inspiratory pressure–volume (*P/V*) curve provides a useful descriptor of respiratory mechanics in patients afflicted by acute respiratory distress syndrome (ARDS). However, measurements based on airway pressure alone have limited ability to provide reliable insights for any given individual.
- Measuring oesophageal pressure (P_{es}) and calculating transpulmonary (P_{tp}) as a part of a rational strategy for setting the parameters of ventilator support must be interpreted with caution.
- The driving pressure (ΔP) reflects lung strain relevant to the end-expiratory volume: in a given individual, the greater the strain, the greater the driving pressure.
- The energy delivered to the lungs over a given interval ('power') is determined by the frequency of breathing as well as the pressures and volumes of the individual tidal cycle.

CONTROVERSIES

- The most effective and safest recruitment strategies using PEEP.
- The accuracy of P_{es} (oesophageal pressures) in representing the heterogeneity of the transpulmonary pressure associated stresses within the injured lung.

FURTHER RESEARCH

- Techniques for integrating the risk of intensity of ventilation, as tracked by energy, power, and driving power, are emerging.
- The role of such techniques in the bedside monitoring of protective/harmful ventilation of the injured lung requires evaluation.

Introduction

Mechanical ventilation (MV) remains the primary first-line support for maintaining acceptable pulmonary gas exchange while treatment is undertaken that addresses the underlying lung disease or disorder. Acute lung injury is associated with a reduced number of functional lung units and therefore with a decline in respiratory-system compliance that often obligates high pressures for delivery of traditional tidal volumes. In such patients, MV may lead to injury due to over-distension, stretch, and shearing forces on the alveolar walls and micro-vessels (Figure 15.1). Ventilator-induced lung injury (VILI) is one among several iatrogenic factors that can exacerbate lung damage; others include fluid overload, transfusion of blood products, and ventilator-associated pneumonia.

Better understanding of the pathophysiology of acute respiratory distress syndrome (ARDS) and VILI have led to the justified conviction that airway pressures and tidal volumes should be restrained when managing the ventilation of patients with ARDS.[1] Increasing the number of functional lung units by sustained recruitment of unstable lung units usually improves the capacity for (if not always the efficiency of) gas exchange. Furthermore, because tidally cyclic inflation–deflation of injured lung units has been proposed to exacerbate lung injury,[6] medium to high levels of positive end-expiratory pressure (PEEP) are usually advised in the early stage of illness to keep unstable but recruitable alveoli open throughout the ventilatory cycle. Used in conjunction with limitation of plateau and driving pressures, this approach has been termed a lung-protective ventilation strategy (Figure 15.1).

Why We Should Consider Lung-protective Mechanical Ventilation?

Alveolar over-distension, apart from overt rupture and air leakage (barotrauma), may inflict parenchymal damage through inflammatory signalling or by repeated application of excessive mechanical forces, especially at points of stress focusing within the mechanically heterogeneous lung. Increased alveolar–capillary permeability results from excessive tissue strain believed to be mediated in large

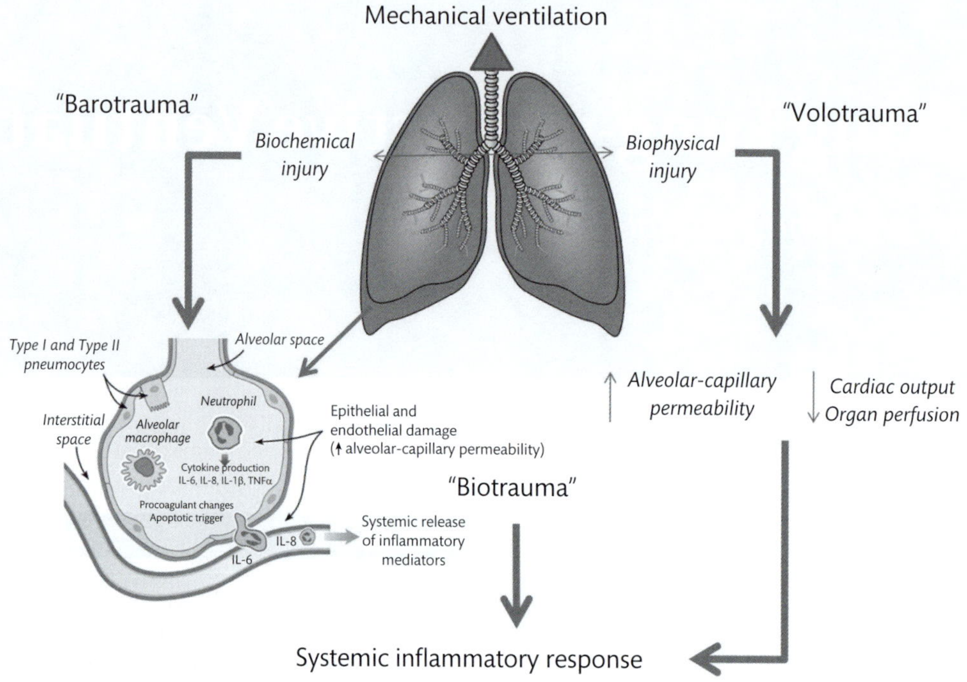

Figure 15.1 Lung injury associated with mechanical ventilation. The postulated mechanisms whereby volutrauma, atelectrauma, and biotrauma caused by mechanical ventilation contribute to multiple organ dysfunction syndrome. Biotrauma not only aggravates ongoing lung injury but also contributes to the development of MODS, possibly through the release of proinflammatory mediators from the lung. IL, interleukin; PEEP, positive end-expiratory pressure; P_{plat}, plateau pressure; TNF, tumour necrosis factor; VT, tidal volume.

part by high tidal alveolar pressures ('driving pressure' = plateau pressure minus PEEP). Repeated tidal recruitment–derecruitment of unstable alveoli promotes epithelial small airway damage and inflammation. Both these processes in unstable lung units may contribute to progressive lung injury. For a given tidal cycle, frequency, minute ventilation, and rate of inspiratory pressure build-up are other potentially influential and measurable parameters that have received less attention. Yet, these mechanical factors affect the overall energy delivery, which can inflict lung injury. Hence, increasing interest towards the roles of the workload and power exposure that the lung must sustain during ventilation. Total machine energy, total power, and the power component related to driving pressure can potentially be measured at the bedside. A lung-protective ventilation strategy using low tidal volume and limited maximal alveolar pressure (plateau, P_{plat}) has been reported to improve survival in patients with ARDS in a highly influential randomized controlled trial conducted by the ARDS Network, whose conclusion has been supported by individualized meta-analysis of multiple other studies.[2] Although evidence for firm causation of VILI due to the ventilation strategy, and higher mortality, reducing ventilator-associated lung injury does appear to be a key intervention to further improve survival in this syndrome.

Animal and Clinical Studies

Almost without exception, pre-clinical studies conducted in small and large animals have shown that using lower tidal volumes and driving pressures (as opposed to higher ones) reduces the injurious effects of ventilation, even when lungs are initially intact. Because it is transpulmonary (transalveolar) pressure that generates lung tissue stress, vigorous patient efforts also contribute to VILI risk. Experimental findings are in line with results from trials in ICU and operative patients without ARDS, which demonstrate the association of lower tidal volumes with less pulmonary complications and trends to improved survival.[3] However, published evidence mostly derives from non-randomized clinical trials, and concern has been expressed regarding non-selective use of lower tidal volumes in all ventilated critically ill patients. While it seems plausible that indiscriminate use of low tidal volumes may reduce oxygenation efficiency and/or increase needs for sedation and/or neuromuscular blockade in some, convincing population-based documentation is lacking. Furthermore, higher levels of PEEP during MV often adversely influence haemodynamics and may amplify the global mechanical stress imposed on healthy lungs as well as contribute to the formation of stress risers within the mechanically heterogeneous injured lung. Yet, although higher-volume ventilation may act as pro-inflammatory stimulus, selective increases of PEEP cause only modest changes in pulmonary cytokine production over the short term in isolated mouse lungs.[4]

Uniform Ventilatory Targets as the 'Holy Grail'

It is broadly accepted that ventilation with tidal volumes <6 mL/kg predicted body weight while targeting a plateau pressure <30 cmH_2O reduces mortality and increases ventilator-free days in patients with severe and moderate ARDS.[5] However, adherence to low tidal volume strategies remains inconsistent. The objective of setting a single numerical guideline for tidal volume to apply to all patients is irrational as the stresses generated by a given tidal

Data relevant for *all* patients

- **Mechanics data**
  - –*Minute ventilation*
  - –Airway and lung pressures
    - Body size, structure, and position
    - Waveforms –secretions, asynchrony, timing
- **Hemodynamic data**
  - –Heart rate, rhythm, blood pressure
  - –Perfusion adequacy
- **Blood gases**
  - –FiO2 & PEEP
- **Cardiopulmonary physical exam**
  - –Effort, sounds, and synchrony

→ Disease progression; VILI risk; Effort & asynchrony

Figure 15.2 Assessment of variables that may contribute to ventilator-induced lung injury in the critically ill patient. Ventilator and respiratory system variables together with hemodynamic status, gas exchange, and cardiopulmonary physical examinations assist clinicians in determining disease progression, in reducing the risk of ventilation-induced lung injury (VILI), and in improving patient–ventilator interaction.

volume relate to the aerated capacity (i.e. functional capacity) of the lungs in question.

In survivors of ARDS, lung function after tissue recovery returns to near normal performance within 5 years. The effect of critical illness on skeletal and diaphragmatic muscle wasting is associated with lingering weakness and reduced physical functioning.[6] Optimal management of acute lung injury might speed up resolution of lung injury and the associated inflammatory response, which in turn could mitigate skeletal muscle loss and better preserve exercise capacity.[21] Excessive or dyssynchronous MV might also increase the risk of ventilator-induced diaphragmatic dysfunction.[7] Assessment of the ventilated patient for the prevention or mitigation of lung injury requires a multi-modal approach beyond simple assessment of ideal body-weight-indexed tidal ventilation and airway pressures (Figure 15.2). The still unproven hypotheses as to the aetiology VILI of might help explain how adherence to a strategy of lung-protective ventilation could provide long-term benefits for physical functioning as well as decrease extra-pulmonary organ dysfunction.

Monitoring the Lung to Enforce Protective Strategies

Classical Airway Pressure and Flow-derived Measures

The static inspiratory pressure–volume (*P*/*V*) curve provides a useful descriptor of respiratory mechanics in patients afflicted by ARDS. However, measurements based on airway pressure alone have limited ability to provide reliable insights for any given individual. Other factors influencing the impact on lung tissues of airway pressures and volumes include altered chest wall compliance, muscular activity, positional changes in absolute lung volume, body mass, mechanical asymmetry of lung disease, pleural effusion, and abdominal distension. Functional residual capacity and calculated transpulmonary pressure are two components of bedside monitoring recently introduced into clinical practice that, could in theory, help to address these shortcomings.

Analysis of the *P*/*V* curve has been used to provide a physiological rationale for recommendations made to avoid settings that incite VILI (Figure 15.3). The static *P*/*V* curve of the respiratory system is characterized by lower (LIP) and upper (UIP) inflection contours that are thought to demarcate zones above which extensive tidal re-opening is less prevalent and below which extensive over-stretching/over-distension do not occur, respectively.[8] Conceptually, tidal inflations that begin below the LIP on the *P*/*V* curve lead to recruitment/derecruitment cycles of unstable alveoli, whereas tidal ventilation that occurs above the UIP amplifies the stresses applied to the unopened tissues and risks over-stretching of those already open. Potentially, both processes promote a spectrum of pulmonary and systemic problems (such as tissue damage, air leaks, alterations in lung fluid balance, and increases of endothelial and epithelial permeability). In truth, the recruitment of lung units and regional over-distension probably occurs simultaneously throughout the course of lung inflation to the total lung capacity. The shape of the volume curve in response to increasing pressure reflects the relative proportions of overall incremental recruitment and over-distention. Although numerous studies have correlated *P*/*V* curves to laboratory manifestations of VILI, a few randomized clinical trials have shown a protective ventilatory strategy individually tailored to the *P*/*V* curve, to reduce pulmonary and systemic inflammation and to decrease mortality in patients with ALI.[9,25] The LIP and UIP zones correlate with quantitative computed tomographic analyses of atelectasis and over-distension, respectively, lending support to using the *P*/*V* curve to estimate alveolar recruitment (and VILI risk) with PEEP.[10]

Constructing the Static Pressure/volume Curve

Deep sedation and paralysis are required to construct the *P*/*V* relationship in stepwise fashion using the traditional 'super syringe' technique. While cumbersome and rarely deployed in the clinical setting, using a syringe allows stepwise deflation to delineate the expiratory limb of the *P*–*V* loop, which holds some logical appeal for the deflation-oriented task of setting PEEP. The constant inspiratory flow technique for the construction of the inflation limb of the loop is based on the assumption that when inspiratory flow is slow and held constant during passive inflation, volume is the direct analogue of the applied pressure so that the airway opening pressure relates

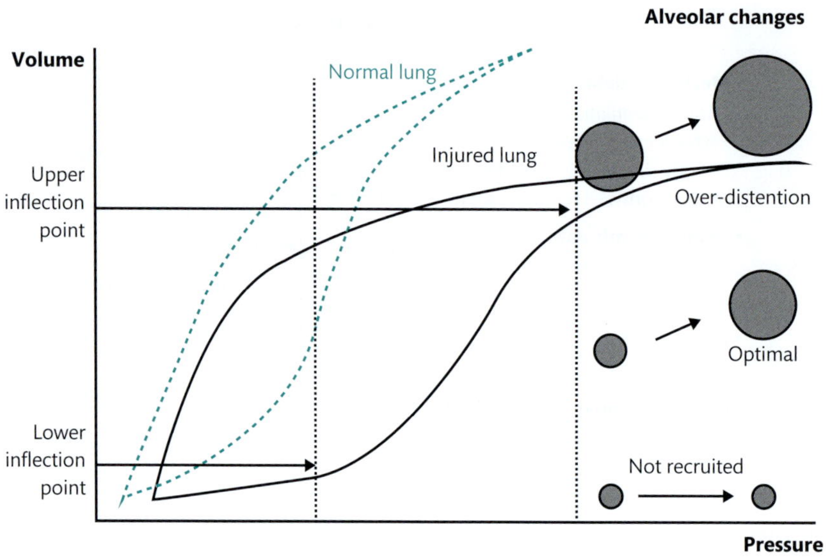

Figure 15.3 Pressure–volume (PV) relationship and its interpretation. The PV relationship is usually traced from the elastic equilibrium lung volume that corresponds either to the functional residual capacity or to the end-expiratory volume of the respiratory system. The classic shape of the PV curve in ARDS patients is more or less sigmoidal (solid line) with an overall compliance that is markedly reduced compared with normal subjects. The inflation PV curve is generally viewed as consisting of three segments separated by two inflection points: the first segment, characterized by low compliance, is separated from a more linear part of the curve by the lower inflection point. The intermediate segment can be considered linear. Beyond the upper inflection point, the PV curve tends to flatten again.

primarily to the elastance of the respiratory system. There is no need to disconnect the patient from the ventilator, special devices are not required, and LIP and UIP zones can usually be identified at the bedside. Yet, this method also requires deep sedation and/or paralysis, and only a few ventilator displays are equipped with such a monitoring tool. A quasi-static *P*/*V* curve can also be constructed with stepwise increments and decrements of PEEP while maintaining a fixed tidal volume (or ideally, fixed driving pressure). Indeed, such methodology may help in selecting the optimal PEEP to be maintained after a recruiting manoeuvre. All curve-generating methods carry an intrinsic risk of adverse effects, including hypoxaemia, haemodynamic sequelae, alveolar rupture, and derecruitment at low lung volumes (Figure 15.3).

Plateau Pressure, Oesophageal Pressure, and Tidal Mechanics

During MV, the total pressure applied to the respiratory system (P_{total}) is the sum of the pressure provided by the ventilator (P_{aw}) and the pressure generated by the patient's inspiratory muscles (P_{mus}):

$$P_{total} = P_{aw} + P_{mus} \quad (1)$$

The total pressure applied to the respiratory system to deliver a tidal breath must overcome the opposing forces produced by the elastic and resistive properties of the series-coupled respiratory system. This relationship is described in the modified equation of motion:

$$P_{total} = P_{aw} + P_{mus} = P_0 + E_{rs} \times V + R_{rs} \times V^{o} \quad (2)$$

where P_0 is the value of P_{aw} at the beginning of the breath (zero or a positive value of end-expiratory pressure), E_{rs} is the respiratory-system elastance, R_{rs} is the respiratory-system resistance, V is the volume difference between the instantaneous and relaxation volumes of the respiratory system, and V^{o} is airflow. At the end of a controlled inflation using constant flow, Equation (2) can be applied using delivered tidal volume for V and set inspiratory (peak) flow for V^{o}. Under these conditions, the values of R_{rs} and E_{rs} are readily estimated during passive MV by using the end-inspiratory (and end-expiratory) occlusion technique.[30] Although dynamic hyperinflation does not usually present a major problem in ARDS, any auto-PEEP generated during ventilation adds to the applied PEEP level to yield the total P_0 of Equation (2). Unaccounted for increases in total alveolar PEEP caused by auto-PEEP raise end-expiratory lung volume but may reduce the risk associated with measured 'driving' pressure (Plateau minus PEEP) that does not consider it (see below).

The pressure that relates most closely to that applied to the lung itself, which is always passive, is the transpulmonary value ($P_{aw} - P_{pl}$). It stands to reason, therefore, that the pleural pressure is conceptually important to consider during active as well as passive breathing. Indeed, in certain settings of vigorous breathing, the inspiratory pressures generated during spontaneous effort hold the potential for mechanical damage to the lung—the so-called 'patient self-inflicted lung injury' (P-SILI) (11.5).

Pleural pressure (P_{pl}) has been estimated both in the laboratory and at the bedside using an oesophageal balloon catheter system. The respiratory changes in oesophageal pressure measured in its lowest third (P_{es}) are representative of changes in P_{pl} applied to the lung surface. The difference between P_{aw} and P_{es} is a valid estimate of transpulmonary pressure (P_{tp}) in the region surrounding the balloon catheter and perhaps surrounding the lung all across the same horizontal plane.[11] Absolute values of P_{es} can be influenced by respiratory mechanics, lung volume, overlying weight of the mediastinum, the abdomen, posture, reactivity of the oesophageal smooth

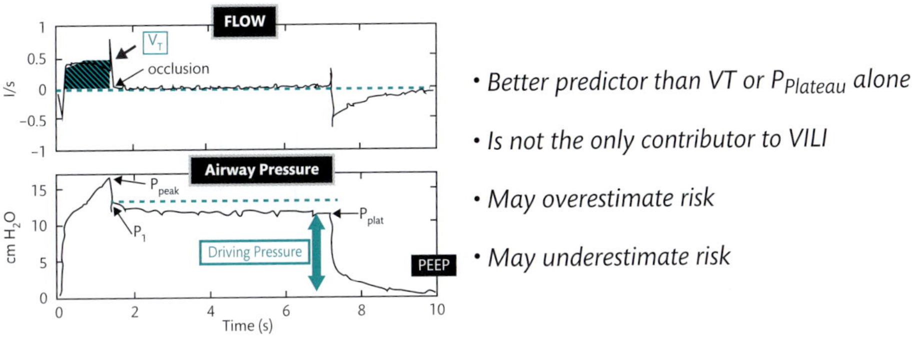

Figure 15.4 The driving pressure analysis and its interpretation, including limits of its use in the clinical setting.

muscle wall, and mechanical properties of the balloon.[12] Our knowledge about the impact of position, asymmetry of lung disease, lung and chest wall distortion, increased abdominal pressure, and large pleural effusion on the observed P_{es} and its respiratory variation is limited for clinical applications. Experimental data in large animals strongly suggests that the transpulmonary pressure calculated using the P_{es} tracks events and capacities in the aerated compartment under each of these challenging conditions. Because of the paucity of clinical data, an active debate continues about whether the absolute values of P_{es} can be interpreted as reliable for specific clinical purposes (Figure 15.4).

The feasibility of using P_{es} in guiding the therapy in ARDS was demonstrated in the initial Esophageal Pressure–Directed Ventilation (EPVent) study.[13] Because of reduced chest wall compliance, oedema, or abdominal distension, P_{es} is often elevated in patients with ARDS, and the calculated (regional) P_{tp} can be negative at end expiration. This negativity may indicate closed airways or flooded or atelectatic lung. In principle, to optimally 'open' the lung, PEEP could be increased until end-expiratory P_{tp} becomes positive, indicating open airways in the region of the P_{es} catheter. In their single-centre, randomized controlled trial, the EPVent investigators compared MV guided by P_{es} measurements with ventilation based on the protocol of the ARDS Network, which is sponsored by the National Institutes of Health (USA). Although this trial showed a trend towards reduced 28-day mortality, it was not sufficiently powered to show significant change using that rather demanding outcome standard, nor of other key outcome variables such as ventilator-free days, length of stay, duration of ventilation, or long-term clinical status. Setting PEEP to ensure a positive value of end-expiratory transpulmonary pressures is likely to require higher mean airway pressures than other PEEP-setting techniques in common use. Nonetheless, focusing on transpulmonary pressure for clinical decision making seems prudent for other reasons; peak end-inspiratory stresses applied to the lung are better indexed by P_{pl} than by airway pressures alone. This is undeniably true during spontaneous breathing efforts. Even if clinically feasible and logical to acquire during both controlled and spontaneous breathing, measuring P_{es} and calculating P_{tp} to help determine a rational strategy for setting the parameters of ventilator support must be adopted with caution.[14] We cannot expect a single local pressure to accurately represent absolute stresses everywhere across the topography of a thorax or deep within the heterogeneous lung itself.

Dynamic Pressure/volume Curve and Pressure/time Profile

Modern ventilators develop well-controlled inspiratory flow or pressure profiles and are equipped with monitoring tools able to display informative tracings. In fact, under passive constant-flow conditions with unchanging resistances, time is a direct analogue of volume so that changes in airway opening pressure reflect respiratory-system elastance as the breath proceeds. When respiratory-system compliance decreases (i.e. elastance rises) during the breath under these constant-flow conditions, the airway pressure profile becomes concave upwards. Conversely, when compliance improves during tidal inflation, the airway pressure contour appears concave downwards with respect to the time axis. During volume-controlled inflation ventilation with constant flow, the changes in the contour of pressure applied across the respiratory system are usually caused primarily by changes in lung compliance and reflect events within a mechanically non-uniform compartment[15] (Figure 15.5). Recently, it has been proposed to replace the use of the static P/V curve by the analysis of the dynamic airway opening pressure–time (P/t) profile during constant-flow inflation, as under those conditions of steady flow, time becomes a linear analogue of volume. The stress index (SI) is a parameter that characterizes the shape of the airway pressure–time profile (P/t) during passive constant-flow MV. The SI is the exponent of a power equation that characterizes the curvilinear slope progression (contour) of the curve. The unique rationale for the clinical use of SI monitoring is its potential for dynamic detection of tidal inflation patterns and settings that promote (or avoid) VILI, accomplished without the need for disconnecting the patient from the ventilator.

Setting aside the potentially important influence of the chest wall on the airway pressure, a convex P/t curve is reflected by an SI < 1, indicating steadily increasing compliance, likely caused by a preponderance of tidal recruitment (TR). On the other hand, an upwardly concave shape in the P/t curve (associated with an SI > 1) indicates decreasing compliance, suggesting preponderant tidal hyperinflation.[15] Careful calculation of the SI value requires the fitting and smoothing of an exponential equation with integrated, dedicated machine software.

The validity of the 'single compartment' SI concept as a reflection of the balance between TR and over-distension of the lung requires several assumptions. SI is clearly of interest when relatively uniform lungs are inflated passively and are surrounded by a normal chest wall. However, these conditions do not always apply in the clinical

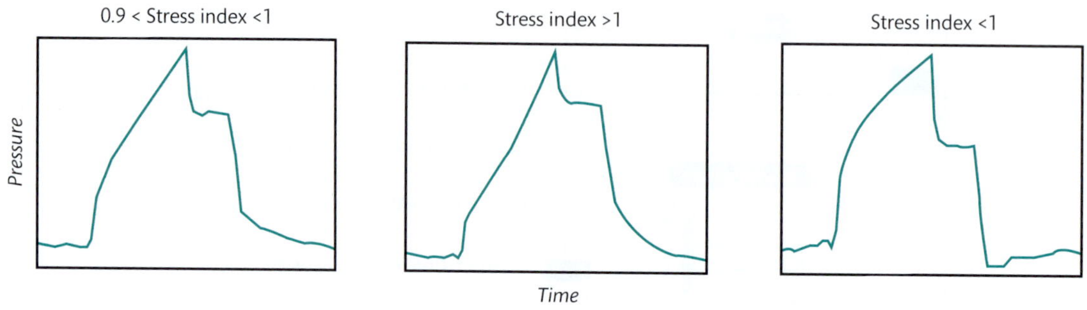

Figure 15.5 The pressure/time curve profile analysis and interpretation. The shape of pressure/time curve can be described by the stress index during constant ('square') inspiratory flow. The stress index between 0.9 and 1 suggests a balance of recruitment and distention; the stress index >1 describes an upward concavity shape that corresponds to prevalent tidal recruitment; the stress index <1 describes a downward concavity shape that corresponds to prevalent tidal overdistension.

setting. Moreover, linearity of the airway pressure profile (SI = 1.0) does not ensure safe ventilation, as regional hyperinflation and TR of similar degrees may offset one another. Of equal concern, the SI characterizes not only the applied airway pressure, but also it reflects the properties of all components of the series-coupled lung, pleural compartment, and chest wall.[16]

The SI has been evaluated in ARDS patients without chest wall abnormalities, and confirmatory experimental work has been confined to small animal lungs. In a recent experimental study, CT scans were compared to the SI values of the inflations that produced them.[17,48] In that work, quantitative analysis demonstrated an inhomogeneous distribution of pulmonary alterations of the lung which were consistent with the SI. However, other studies in which the mechanics of the chest wall and pleural compartments were altered have failed to confirm these observations.[18]

Driving Pressure and PEEP Titration

There is general consensus and good scientific justification that lower tidal volumes and plateau pressures are safer than higher ones in the same individual. However, the translation of group results to individual cases can be challenging. Use of lower tidal volumes, end-inspiratory airway pressures, and higher PEEP during the early phase of treatment have been associated with improved survival rates in ARDS.[13] However, although the tidal volume has generally been based on predicted body weight, patients with ARDS have less functionally available lung for gas exchange, which is the primary reason for their lower respiratory-system compliance. From this 'baby lung' perspective, the burden of gas exchange is left with the remaining aerated portion. The absolute volume of the aerated lung by gas dilution is routinely evaluated in outpatient pulmonary function laboratories but seldom measured at the bedside. Nonetheless, commercial ventilators are now available to estimate the functional residual volume (FRC)—a parameter of potential clinical value in tracking the progression and resolution of lung injury as well as the response to therapeutic interventions. Tidal compliance may provide much of the same information. It has been reported that the aerated 'baby lung' of ARDS is normally expandable (not stiff, but small) so that measured respiratory-system compliance when the chest wall is flexible reflects the size of the chamber able to receive the tidal volume. Higher pressures are generated when the same tidal volume is forced into a lung of smaller size. The ratios of tidal volume (VT) to measured FRC and of VT to respiratory-system compliance hold obvious appeal for judging the risk of any given VT to over-stress the lung available to accept it.

The driving pressure can be described during positive pressure ventilation as the quotient of VT and respiratory-system compliance $(C_{RS}): \Delta P = VT / C_{RS}$.[19] Numerically, ΔP is equivalent to the difference between the two static pressures required to deliver tidal volume under passive conditions: P_{plat} – PEEP. The defining equation of ΔP implies that driving pressure relates VT to the capacity of the lung to receive it, as compliance of the lung reflects more closely the number rather than the pliability of functioning lung units. Therefore, ΔP reflects lung strain relevant to the end-expiratory volume: the greater the strain, the greater the driving pressure. Minimized driving pressure during volume-controlled ventilation serves as the basis for identifying optimal PEEP in the decremental PEEP-setting strategy.[20] It is tempting to speculate that the excess mortality observed in the high tidal volume, higher driving pressure cohorts of trials comparing ventilatory strategies in ARDS, was due, at least in part, to biotrauma resulting from excessive strain, but that assumption remains to be directly confirmed. For several reasons, speculation that driving pressure has a causal role in the mortality outcome—though reasonable and attractive conceptually—can neither be accepted nor refuted without reservation. Firstly, the link between actual strain (the damaging variable) and driving pressure is indirect. Secondly, the value of P_{plat} required to calculate driving pressure is not only a function of lung mechanics but also of chest wall stiffness and muscle tone. Thirdly, no prospective study has prospectively determined the impact of different driving pressures on ARDS outcome. Fourthly, ventilator settings in investigations relevant to driving pressure varied from study to study. This makes it impossible to cleanly dissect the effect of driving pressure from other ventilatory variables on patient outcome. In other words, while it might seem reasonable to aim for a driving pressure below approximately 15 cmH_2O, it is necessary to bear in mind that such a threshold zone is based on conjecture, biological plausibility, and post hoc analysis of studies that were not designed to identify the ideal driving pressure to use in patients with ARDS. Any contention that the risk of driving pressure is not influenced by the range over which it operates must also be questioned, for lack of strong biologic rationale.

In an important and influential recent study, driving pressure has been identified as a key predictor of lung injury caused by MV itself. Using sophisticated statistical methodology, Amato and colleagues[21] retrospectively analyzed individual data from previously reported randomized trials that compared differing ventilation strategies for ARDS. Both a standard risk analysis with multivariate adjustments and multilevel mediation methodology were used to estimate the isolated effects of changes in ΔP and other variables resulting from ventilator setting changes, independent of the extent of the underlying lung injury and of the specific lung-protection protocol. They found that driving pressure was more strongly linked (inversely) to survival than to either P_{plat} or PEEP or other recorded ventilation variables. If this is the case and causal linkage is assumed, limiting ΔP may be a rational and convenient way to scale the delivered breath to the size of the lung that is available to participate in gas exchange, rather than scaling to body size, which may be less relevant to the low-capacity, injured lungs. The ability of ΔP to predict outcome could be attributable to the fact that the P_{plat} that is key to defining it itself tracks with severity of illness and by that connection ΔP may be predictive of survival. As the authors correctly emphasized, the component studies used in their meta-analysis were not designed to assess ΔP as an independent variable, and thus, the reported findings must be considered hypothesis-generating rather than definitive. Their results should form the basis for a robust debate regarding the design of future trials to definitively test the issue.

Whatever its role in VILI generation, ΔP seems a valid and practical means for setting the PEEP value associated with best tidal compliance, the parameter found nearly 40 years ago to indicate the PEEP value associated with optimal oxygen delivery during volume-cycled ventilation.[54] When a PEEP trial is performed using stepwise escalation of PEEP and a fixed tidal volume, the best compliance value corresponds to the minimum ΔP; conversely, if a fixed driving pressure mode of ventilation is used (e.g. pressure control with zero end-inspiratory flow), then the PEEP value associated with the greatest VT defines the optimum tidal compliance. As noted above, PEEP can be selected using a variety of techniques based on the P–V curve or by tracking pulmonary gas exchange. A decremental method performed after a recruiting manoeuvre that employs a fixed low tidal volume or fixed ΔP (e.g. 6 mL/kg PBW or ΔP = 12–15 cmH_2O) and compliance assessment of the respiratory system (or preferably of the lung) is both rational and has a strong supporting experimental and clinical evidence base for optimizing both oxygen delivery and lung protection with minimal haemodynamic impairment. Unfortunately, a recently published randomized trial ('ART') reported findings contrary to those expected, showing higher mortality with the decremental PEEP approach after an aggressive recruiting manoeuvre.[22] Serious concerns regarding design and execution of that trial preclude its acceptance as definitive without confirmation.

Flow, Minute Ventilation, Energy, and Power

Although the characteristics of the individual tidal cycle such as tidal volume, plateau pressure, and PEEP are of unquestioned importance to lung protection, it is intuitively obvious that once stresses and strains of the individual cycle exceed tolerance, the frequency of their application must also have an important impact on their safety or hazard. The abruptness with which the driving pressure is applied—as reflected by the flow profile—may also be influential. Yet, until very recently, these 'intensity' issues have received relatively little attention. Minute ventilation can be considered an intensity variable that determines whether an identical driving pressure for ventilation may cause injury or be well tolerated. The energy delivered to the lungs over a given interval (power) is determined by the frequency of breathing as well as the driving pressure utilized during the individual tidal cycle. Of the pressure components that determine the energy delivered per tidal cycle, the driving pressure may be the one most directly related to VILI risk. It stands to reason that driving power, the product of driving pressure and minute ventilation ('normalized' to the reduced capacity of the baby lung by the ratio of expected to measured compliance), may even more closely determine the true risk for VILI than does the ΔP of the individual tidal cycle or the total energy load. Recent experimental work suggests that dynamic power, a measure that includes PEEP, may be even more influential.

The flow magnitude and profile of each individual breath determines the rate at which alveolar pressure is developed, and both parameters theoretically and experimentally have been shown to be important determinants of VILI. At the bedside, however, the inspiratory to expiratory ratio and inspiratory flow profile are seldom considered in the effort to protect the lung. This neglect is in some sense understandable, in that no randomized clinical trial has yet compared these intensity variables. Extending the duration of inspiration and 'squaring' the inspiratory flow profile have been shown in both small and large animal models to blunt the degree of injury inflicted by the same driving pressure. How fast strain is achieved appears to be especially important when the lung is subjected to high stretching forces. In fact, experimental studies suggest that the driving airway or transpulmonary pressures—both based on static variables of plateau pressure and PEEP—do not closely predict ventilation-inflicted lung damage when the flow rate is altered through a wide range. It can be concluded from such experimental and observational scientific work that these 'intensity' variables deserve to be considered in the effort to protect the lung. The current challenge is that, as yet, no simplified and practical indices have been developed with which to implement their monitoring at the bedside.

Intra-abdominal Pressure and Respiratory Mechanics

It is only recently that the prevalence and impact of increased intra-abdominal pressure (IAP) as well as its implications for lung-protective monitoring have become better understood. Substantially abnormal IAP increases chest wall elastance (decreases respiratory-system compliance) and promotes cranial shifting of the diaphragm, with consequent reduction in lung volume and formation of basilar atelectasis. The linkage between the abdominal and thoracic compartments across the diaphragm often poses a substantial interpretive challenge for monitoring airway pressures during the MV of ARDS. Despite considerable variation among published studies, on average approximately 50% of increments of IAP that occur above 5–7 cmH_2O can be expected to be transmitted to the pleural space of a passively ventilated subject. Patients with primary abdominal compartment syndrome often develop a secondary ARDS, and while general principles of lung protection remain the same, require modestly different ventilatory strategy and pressure guidelines than other patients with ARDS.[23] The major problem lies in the IAP-caused reductions of diaphragmatic excursion and functional residual capacity. Acting together with the alterations caused by secondary ARDS, peri-diaphragmatic compression reduces aerating capacity and predisposes to pulmonary infection. The relative increase of IAP also helps translocate blood from the abdominal cavity to the chest, potentiating oedema formation.

In the morbidly obese, increased IAP is a major determinant of the associated reductions in FRC and impairment of lung and chest wall mechanics. In ARDS patients, the measurement of IAP—and by inference, chest wall mechanics—should be considered for better interpretation of respiratory mechanics and haemodynamics, as well as for appropriate setting of the ventilator. Although raised IAP decreases chest wall and total respiratory-system compliance, lung compliance remains relatively unchanged unless substantial peri-diaphragmatic collapse occurs. To provide lung-protective ventilation, the plateau pressures should be limited to keep transmural plateau pressures across the lung below 20–25 cmH_2O. Recent work using oesophageal balloon catheters has indicated that even morbidly obese patients without ARDS require very high PEEP levels to keep the basilar regions open throughout the tidal cycle.[24]

Regional Lung Mechanics

The lungs of patients with ARDS are not mechanically homogeneous and display heterogenous regional properties. Indeed, such local disparities are responsible in large part for the difficulty of selecting single airway pressure and flow profiles that simultaneously achieve adequate recruitment of unstable alveoli without over-distending units in other zones that were already open. Whereas computed tomography is clearly impractical for continuous bedside monitoring, two recent radiation-free innovations hold promise to bring regional mechanics into better focus for the clinician. These are electrical impedance tomography and thoracic ultrasound (US).[25] Both have obvious limitations regarding quantitative imprecision and restricted ability to interrogate the air spaces. Although each has been demonstrated to have useful qualitative imaging capability, and both offer brief dynamic views throughout the tidal cycle, neither of these complementary techniques appears to be suitable for continuous monitoring at the present time, and their quantitative outputs currently lack standardization. Nonetheless, advances in this area have been rapid. Both hold potential to boost the value of current measures of lung mechanics and therefore to take clinical monitoring of the lung-injured patient to the next higher level of precision regarding lung protection.

Conclusions

Though lifesaving, MV can also exacerbate lung injury or delay healing though the process of VILI. Current knowledge suggests that preventing VILI during MV requires avoidance of cyclical opening and closing of unstable lung units and avoidance of excessive stretching of lung parenchyma during the tidal cycle. Growing experimental evidence suggests that these goals may be closely approximated by careful titration of ventilator support guided by appropriate monitoring of pulmonary mechanics. Calculating P_{tp} based on P_{es} measurements by oesophageal balloon manometry, recording of abdominal pressure, and refocusing on the driving pressure across the lung itself are complementary pieces of the diagnostic/monitoring puzzle to be added to traditional pulmonary mechanics stemming from measuring P_{aw} and tidal air flow in the external circuit. Using P_{es} (and P_{aw}) to determine the pressures applied across the lung during active as well as passive breathing may allow personalization and improve analysis of the mechanics of pulmonary injury. Electrical impedance tomography (EIT) and thoracic ultrasound are at the threshold of widespread deployment. Realization that the intensity of ventilation, as tracked by energy, power, and driving power, is a key integrating indicator of ventilation risk may soon lead to its bedside measurement. It seems clear that these newly available tools, used separately and/or together, have potential to improve delivery of respiratory care by characterizing the response to interventions or in tracking the course of disease. Moreover, recognizable patterns and trends in correlated indexes of FRC and P_{tp}, in addition to traditional monitoring tools and US, could help diagnose and/or provide an early warning to the clinician of impending danger in the settings of chest wall abnormalities and the asymmetrically distributed lung diseases often encountered in critical care. Instead of the first response being crisis intervention or expensive testing, earlier evaluation and prevention could be achieved by using and understanding these newer indicators.

REFERENCES

1. Artigas A, Bernard GR, Carlet J, et al. The American-European Consensus Conference on ARDS, part 2. Ventilatory, pharmacologic, supportive therapy, study design strategies and issues related to recovery and remodeling. *Intensive Care Med.* 1998;24(4):378–398.
2. Petrucci N, De Feo C. Lung protective ventilation strategy for the acute respiratory distress syndrome. *Cochrane Database Syst Rev.* 2013 Feb 28;2013(2):CD003844. doi:10.1002/14651858.CD003844.pub4. PMID: 23450544; PMCID: PMC6517299.
3. Briel M, Meade M, Mercat A, et al. Higher vs lower positive end-expiratory pressure in patients with acute lung injury and acute respiratory distress syndrome: Systematic review and meta-analysis. *JAMA.* 2010;303(9):865–873.
4. Meier T, Lange A, Papenberg H, et al. Pulmonary cytokine responses during mechanical ventilation of noninjured lungs with and without end-expiratory pressure. *Anesth Analg.* 2008;107(4):1265–1275.
5. Villar J, Kacmarek RM, Pérez-Méndez L, et al. A high positive end-expiratory pressure, low tidal volume ventilatory strategy improves outcome in persistent acute respiratory distress syndrome: A randomized, controlled trial. *Crit Care Med.* 2006;34(5):1311–1318.
6. Putensen C, Muders T, Kreyer S, et al. Lung protective ventilation—protective effect of adequate supported spontaneous breathing. *Anasthesiol Intensivmed Notfallmed Schmerzther.* 2008;43(6):456–462; quiz 463.
7. Supinski GS, Morris PE, Dhar S, et al. Diaphragm dysfunction in critical illness. *Chest.* 2018;153(4):1040–1051.
8. Brochard L, Lemaire F. Tidal volume, positive end-expiratory pressure, and mortality in acute respiratory distress syndrome. *Crit Care Med.* 1999;27(8):1661–1663.
9. Wrigge H, Uhlig U, Zinserling J, et al. The effects of different ventilatory settings on pulmonary and systemic inflammatory responses during major surgery. *Anesth Analg.* 2004;98(3):775–781, table of contents.
10. Ranieri VM, Giuliani R, Fiore T, et al. Volume-pressure curve of the respiratory system predicts effects of PEEP in ARDS: 'occlusion' versus 'constant flow' technique. *Am J Respir Crit Care Med.* 1994;149(1):19–27.

11. Chiumello D, Guérin C. Understanding the setting of PEEP from esophageal pressure in patients with ARDS. *Intensive Care Med.* 2015;41(8):1465–1467.
12. Mauri T, Yoshida T, Bellani G, et al. Esophageal and transpulmonary pressure in the clinical setting: Meaning, usefulness and perspectives. *Intensive Care Med.* 2016;42(9):1360–1373.
13. Acute Respiratory Distress Syndrome Network, Brower RG, Matthay MA, et al. Ventilation with lower tidal volumes as compared with traditional tidal volumes for acute lung injury and the acute respiratory distress syndrome. *N Engl J Med.* 2000;342(18):1301–1308.
14. Umbrello M, Formenti P, Bolgiaghi L, Chiumello D. Current Concepts of ARDS: A Narrative Review. *Int J Mol Sci.* 2016 Dec 29;18(1):64. doi:10.3390/ijms18010064. PMID: 28036088; PMCID: PMC5297699.
15. Grasso S, Terragni P, Mascia L, et al. Airway pressure–time curve profile (stress index) detects tidal recruitment/hyperinflation in experimental acute lung injury. *Crit Care Med.* 2004;32(4):1018–1027.
16. Terragni PP, Filippini C, Slutsky AS, et al. Accuracy of plateau pressure and stress index to identify injurious ventilation in patients with acute respiratory distress syndrome. *Anesthesiology.* 2013;119(4):880–889.
17. Formenti P, Graf J, Santos A, et al. Non-pulmonary factors strongly influence the stress index. *Intensive Care Med.* 2011;37(4):594–600.
18. Formenti P, Umbrello M, Graf J, et al. Reliability of transpulmonary pressure–time curve profile to identify tidal recruitment/hyperinflation in experimental unilateral pleural effusion. *J Clin Monit Comput.* 2017;31(4):783–791.
19. Marini JJ. Mechanical ventilation: Past lessons and the near future. *Crit Care.* 2013;17(Suppl 1):S1.
20. Writing Group for the Alveolar Recruitment for Acute Respiratory Distress Syndrome Trial (ART) Investigators, Cavalcanti AB, Suzumura ÉA, et al. Effect of lung recruitment and titrated positive end-expiratory pressure (PEEP) vs low PEEP on mortality in patients with acute respiratory distress syndrome: A randomized clinical trial. *JAMA.* 10 2017;318(14):1335–1345.
21. Amato MBP, Meade MO, Slutsky AS, et al. Driving pressure and survival in the acute respiratory distress syndrome. *N Engl J Med.* 2015;372(8):747–755.
22. Cavalcanti AB, Amato MBP, de Carvalho CRR. Should the ART trial change our practice? *J Thorac Dis.* 2018;10(3):E224–226.
23. Cortes-Puentes GA, Cortes-Puentes LA, Adams AB, et al. Experimental intra-abdominal hypertension influences airway pressure limits for lung protective mechanical ventilation. *J Trauma Acute Care Surg.* 2013;74(6):1468–1473.
24. Fumagalli J, Berra L, Zhang C, et al. Transpulmonary pressure describes lung morphology during decremental positive end-expiratory pressure trials in obesity. *Crit Care Med.* 2017;45(8):1374–1381.
25. Pesenti A, Musch G, Lichtenstein D, et al. Imaging in acute respiratory distress syndrome. *Intensive Care Med.* 2016;42(5):686–698.

16

Monitoring Respiratory Muscle Function

Benjamin Garfield and Sunil Patel

KEY MESSAGES

- Respiratory muscle wasting is an underreported but common complication in critical illness.
- Pressure measurements of the respiratory system and the diaphragm can be made invasively and non-invasively with increasing accuracy.
- Measures of energy expenditure, electromyography, and imaging can be useful in multi-modal assessment.
- Non-invasive ultrasonography is a reliable method of quantifying respiratory and non-respiratory muscle wasting.

CONTROVERSIES

- Current gold standard diagnostic techniques are invasive in nature, and no single test can accurately assess respiratory muscle strength.

FURTHER RESEARCH

- Standardized guidelines and methodology are essential but are currently lacking. However, patient-centred and individualized approaches are possible through evolving artificial intelligence methods.

Introduction

Muscle wasting is a common complication of critical illness. It occurs early, causes significant morbidity, and is associated with a higher mortality in the intensive care unit (ICU). Critically ill patients can lose up to 2%–3% of their total muscle mass per day in the first 10 days of their admission. Furthermore, significant restriction in physical activity after critical illness may persist for as long as 5 years after hospital discharge. Studies have identified as high as 25%–50% of patients admitted to the ICU as having significant ICU acquired weakness (ICUAW). These patients are less likely to return to work and are more likely to utilize healthcare services within 1 year after hospital discharge.

Peripheral skeletal muscle wasting is often identified on clinical assessment at the bedside, whereas weakness in respiratory muscle function may be more difficult to ascertain. Some patients may exhibit recruitment of accessory respiratory muscles such as the sternocleidomastoid or trapezius, and others may have paradoxical abdominal breathing. However, in early critical illness, many patients are often deeply sedated and/or receiving neuromuscular blocking agents such that recognition of accessory muscle use and volitional testing of strength will not be possible. During spontaneous breathing, respiratory muscle dysfunction will manifest as an increased respiratory rate and a fall in the tidal volume, but neither the breathing pattern nor the pressure flow waveforms on the ventilator can accurately distinguish between respiratory muscle dysfunction and increased work of breathing (WOB) due to respiratory loading. In addition, the intensivist may also, from time to time, be confronted by respiratory muscle failure as a manifestation of a primary neuromuscular disorder (e.g. Guillain-Barré syndrome or myasthenia gravis). Many patients may also present with co-morbidities that have primary or secondary muscle weakness as part of a chronic condition (e.g. chronic obstructive pulmonary disease), thereby influencing short- and long-term outcomes[1] (see Chapter 51).

Like skeletal muscle, respiratory muscle dysfunction is a common finding in patients receiving mechanical ventilation (MV) but is thought to occur earlier in critical illness. In clinical studies, patients have been shown to lose up to 30% of their diaphragm strength after 5–6 days on a ventilator. However, histological analysis of diaphragm muscle demonstrates significant atrophic change in diaphragm myofibers and occurs as early as 18–72 h after initiating MV. Overall, significant respiratory muscle weakness contributes to prolonged ICU stay due to failure to wean from MV, leading to increased risk of complications and healthcare costs. It is therefore important to be able to measure and then track respiratory muscle function in these patients to identify those at risk, monitor recovery or deterioration, and provide prompt intervention.[2]

Respiratory muscles mainly consist of the diaphragm (the principal respiratory muscle) and intercostal muscles. Other muscles involved in the respiratory cycle, the accessory muscles, are also illustrated in Figure 16.1 (see also Chapter 2).

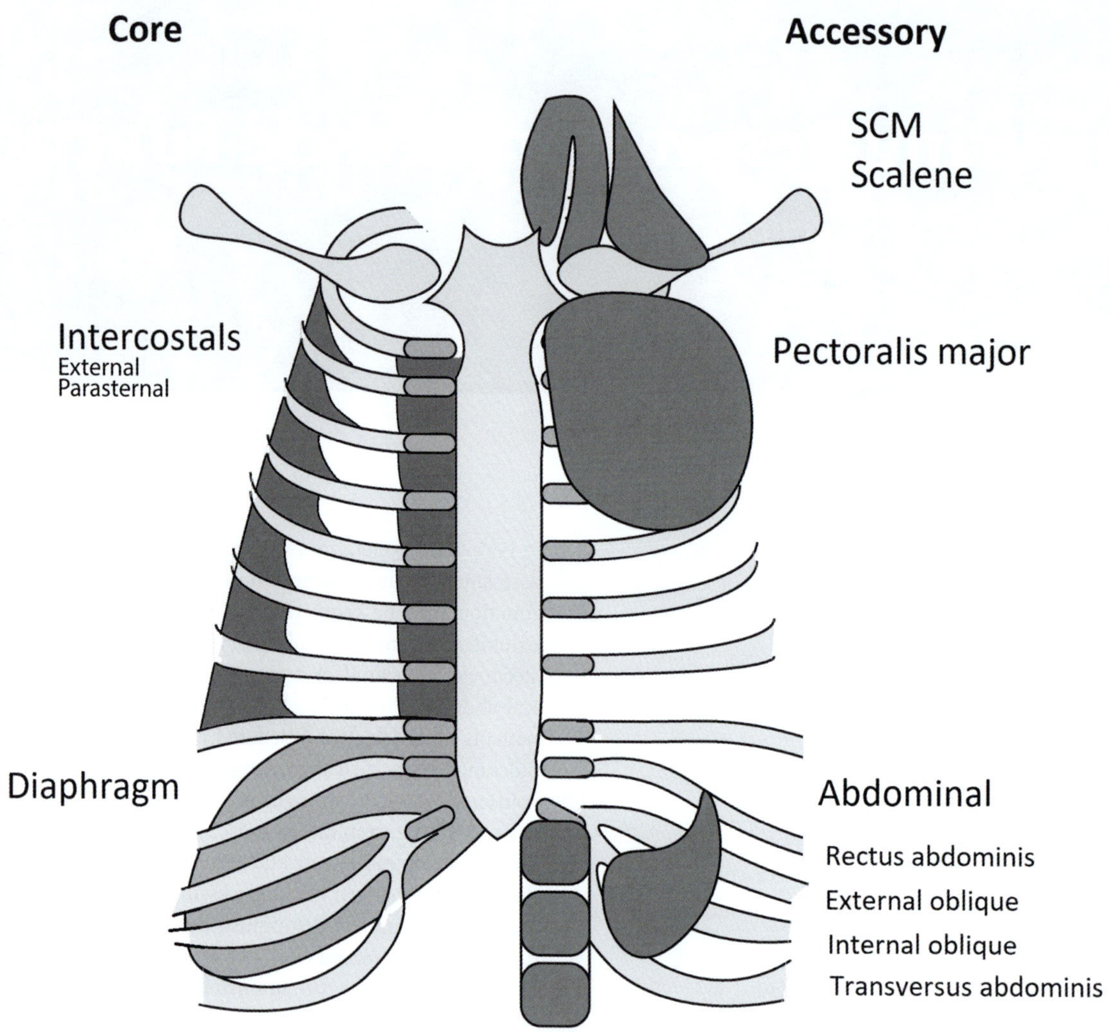

Figure 16.1 The core and accessory muscles of respiration. SCM, sternocleidomastoid.

In critical illness, primary neuromuscular diseases, a lack of neurological stimulation, increased loading, inflammation and hypoxia, protein deficit, and drugs (such as steroids and neuromuscular blockers) lead to muscle weakness. This sets up a vicious cycle: upregulation of pro-atrophic and anti-hypertrophic pathways within the muscle leading to an imbalance in protein synthesis and degradation, and propagating a loss of functional muscle units resulting in further weakness (Figure 16.2).[2]

Monitoring Muscle Function

Monitoring of respiratory muscle function outside of the ICU is well established with a number of methods available. These utilize pressure, volume, flow, electrophysiological outputs, ultrasound, and computed tomography (CT) imaging often concurrently with volitional and non-volitional manoeuvres to generate data about the strength, structure, function endurance, and fatiguability of different parts of the respiratory system. In critically ill patients, especially those on a mechanical ventilator, voluntary effort is likely to be significantly curtailed, so measuring actual intrinsic respiratory muscle function proves more challenging.

The major methods and reference ranges for monitoring respiratory muscle function in the critically ill patients are listed in Table 16.1.

Pressure Monitoring

Global Assessment with Manometers and Ventilators

Most modern mechanical ventilators have the facility to measure pressures throughout the respiratory cycle, which can give important, if crude, information on the overall strength and effectiveness of the respiratory system.

In ventilated patients, maximal inspiratory pressure (MIP) and maximal expiratory pressure (MEP) can be measured by attaching a manometer to the endotracheal tube. MIP can also be measured, potentially more accurately, by doing an expiratory hold at end expiratory volume, for up to 20 s and instructing the patient to breath against the closed system. The MIP can then be calculated by

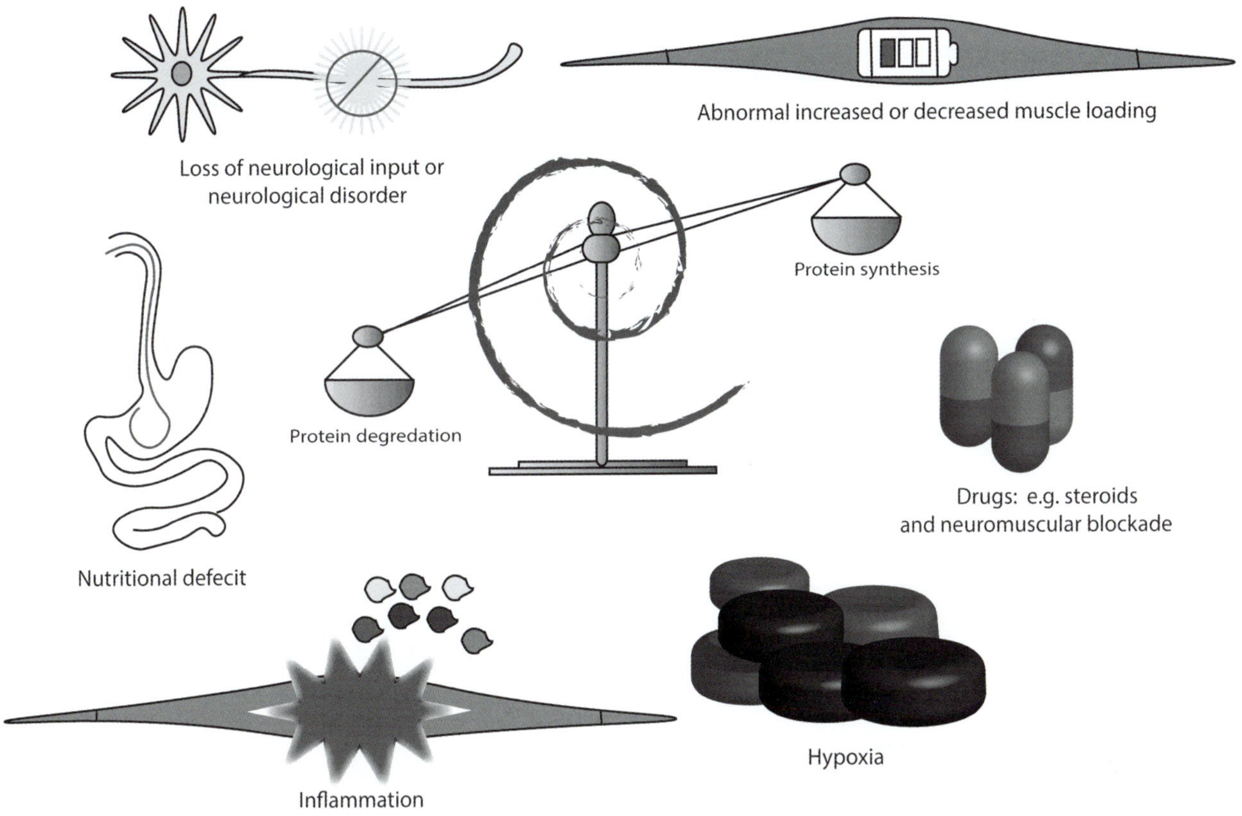

Figure 16.2 Drivers of respiratory muscle dysfunction in critical illness. The diagram shows the vicious cycle of respiratory muscle weakness that is a consequence of critical illness. This leads to an imbalance of protein synthesis and degradation resulting in muscle loss and hence further weakness.

reviewing the pressure–time scalar and the positive end-expiratory pressure (PEEP). The formula for calculating MIP is as follows:

MIP = total PEEP − peak airway pressure drop*

(*peak airway pressure drop is negative)

In general, an MIP of ≤30 cmH_2O has been associated with poor outcomes both in the short and long terms. However, some authors have suggested that MIPs are underestimated when the patient is mechanically ventilated. Whilst MIP is a sensitive, if not specific, measure in identifying patients who may fail to wean from MV, MEPs have traditionally been used to provide a reliable measure of cough efficiency and airway clearance.[2] Despite their simplicity, MIPs and MEPs have a number of drawbacks. Firstly, they require full cooperation of the patient, which may be hampered by sedation, delirium, and pain. Secondly, despite the cut-off value quoted above, there is no standard definition of normal values in ventilated patients. Thirdly, whilst normal values may indicate preserved respiratory muscle function, interpreting low levels may be unreliable.[11]

A low airway occlusion pressure ($P_{0.1}$) is another surrogate marker of respiratory muscle wasting. $P_{0.1}$ is the airway pressure generated in the first 100 ms of inspiration against a closed system and has been used for nearly 50 years as a surrogate for neural drive to breathe in ventilated patients, who have functional respiratory muscles. Whilst high levels, above 3.5–4.0 cmH_2O, are associated with increased respiratory drive and risk of potential self-induced lung injury, levels less than 1.1–1.5 cmH_2O are associated with a reduction in neural drive within the respiratory system. Recent evidence points to a close relationship between ventilator and reference-derived $P_{0.1}$ when the ventilator performs a true occlusion manoeuvre. At constant lung volumes, chest wall elastance, and in the absence of hyperinflation and over-sedation, low $P_{0.1}$ levels may be considered a sign of global respiratory muscle weakness. There are, however, a number of caveats, where expiratory muscle recruitment during positive pressure ventilation can lead to a falsely elevated $P_{0.1}$ in the context of an overall reduction in neural drive to breathe.[3]

Diaphragmatic Pressure Monitoring

The specific problem of ventilator-induced diaphragmatic dysfunction (VIDD) is an increasingly recognized and clinically significant complication of critical illness. The current best standard technique for measuring of diaphragm strength in the ICU is transdiaphragmatic pressure (P_{di}) monitoring. P_{di} measurement involves the insertion of a specialized nasogastric tube with two pressure transducers, which can be used to determine oesophageal (P_{oes}) and gastric (P_{ga}) pressures (Figure 16.3). The P_{di} can then be calculated by using the following formula:

$$P_{di} = P_{ga} - P_{oes}$$

The spontaneously breathing patient can be asked to perform a *maximal voluntary inspiration* against a closed circuit (MaxPdi) or a *forceful sniff* (SnPdi), the latter of which may be more reproducible and therefore more useful. Alternatively, and potentially

Table 16.1 Summary of measurements of respiratory muscle function with published clinical cut-off values

Technique	Measurement/parameter	Comments	Useful values
Airway pressure and flow	MIP MEP	Volitional but reproducible. Indication of global respiratory muscle strength. High values (>30 cmH_2O) exclude weakness, but technique may limit the interpretation of low values. Unlikely to be achievable in early critical illness	Gender and age specific
	$P_{0.1}$	Marker of respiratory drive. Requires several measurements to determine reliability. Caution in patients where intrinsic PEEP (i.e. dynamic hyperinflation) is high as there is a delay in the fall of P_{aw} which underestimates $P_{0.1}$	1.1–1.5 to 3.5–4.0 cmH_2O are often used to wean ventilatory support and indicate adequate drive[3]
	P_{di}	Invasive. Requires specialized nasogastric tube. Utilizes the difference between P_{es} and P_{ga} to calculate P_{di}	P_{di} (max) < 60 cmH_2O may indicate weakness[4]
	P_{es}	Gold standard to assess respiratory effort and work of breathing. P_{es} is often used as a surrogate for P_{pl} and therefore in the calculation of transpulmonary pressure	
Electromyography (EMG)	EA_{di}	Measure of respiratory output from the brain stem. Normal ranges/values not reported. Requires specialized catheter with EMG electrodes. Comparable measurements to P_{di}. Useful for detecting patient–ventilator asynchrony. Parasternal muscles may be an accessible, reproducible alternative site[5]	
	Neurovenitilatory and neuromechanical efficiency	Evolving technique[6]	
Phrenic nerve stimulation	Diaphragm strength (P_{diTw})	Non-volitional quantification of function. Standardized measure independent of patient effort. Invasive and often limited to specialist centres and requires expertise for interpretation. Longitudinal and repeated measurements may not be well tolerated	P_{diTw} < −10 cmH_2O is associated with diaphragm weakness[7]
Imaging Chest X-ray Fluoroscopy Ultrasound Computed tomography	Diaphragm position	Elevation of the hemi-diaphragm may be difficult to detect due to confounders such as consolidation, atelectasis, etc.	N/A
	Diaphragm motion	Requires a brief occlusion manoeuvre. Radiation exposure. Gross interpretation of movement	N/A
	Diaphragm thickness, excursion	Well-described techniques with good reproducibility. Left-sided views difficult. TF_{di} and EXC_{di} limited to spontaneous breathing. Evidence to suggest use as predictive tool in weaning failure and extubation success during SBT. Expiratory thickness and its change may also predict weaning success. Patient body habitus may prevent adequate views	TF_{di} < 20%–36% when measured during an SBT may predict extubation failure. Alternatively 10% increase or decrease in TF_{di}[8]
	Parasternal thickness	Less well described but emerging as a reproducible technique and quantitative assessment of small respiratory muscles	EXC_{di} < 1 cm during an SBT may predict extubation failure[9]
	Intercostal and accessory muscle cross-sectional area[8]	Paucity of literature in critically ill patients. Potential to study longitudinally by utilizing routine imaging	Paucity of data to date. TF_{Psm} of >8% with concurrent diaphragm dysfunction may help predict failure of an SBT[10]

MIP, maximal inspiratory pressure; MEP, maximal expiratory pressure; $P_{0.1}$, inspiratory pressure in first 100 ms; P_{di}, trans-diaphragmatic pressure; P_{es}, oesophageal pressure; P_{Pl}, transpulmonary pressure; P_{aw}, airway pressure; EA_{di}, electrical activity of diaphragm; P_{diTw}, trans-diaphragmatic twitch pressure; TF_{di}, diaphragm thickening fraction; EXC_{di}, diaphragm excursion; TF_{Psm}, thickening fraction of parasternal muscle.

more accurately, the trans-diaphragmatic twitch pressure (P_{diTw}) can be measured. This non-volitional technique uses bilateral supra-maximal magnetic stimulation of the phrenic nerve to cause diaphragmatic contraction, whilst simultaneously occluding the inspiratory limb of the ventilator resulting in a maximal P_{diTw}. P_{diTw} has been shown to be closely correlated with diaphragmatic thickening fraction (TF_{di}) when assessed via ultrasound (see below).[12]

Most often MaxPdi and P_{diTw} have been used as a research tool rather than within regular clinical practice. They may be felt to be unnecessarily invasive. There is, therefore, limited evidence for the use of MaxPdi and P_{diTw} in clinical practice. However, they have been used to set ideal PEEP and to guide ventilation weaning strategies. This has led to interest in the less invasive surrogate measures of diaphragm function. One of these measures is the twitch airway pressure (P_{aTw}) that is closely correlated with the P_{oesTw} and P_{diTw}; these do not require the use of an extragastric or oesophageal manometer. However, P_{di} like MIPs and MEPs have limitations. Firstly, voluntary measurements are influenced by MV and should be ideally taken during a spontaneous breathing trial (SBT). Secondly, magnetic stimulation can be painful, especially if sustained. Thirdly, P_{di}

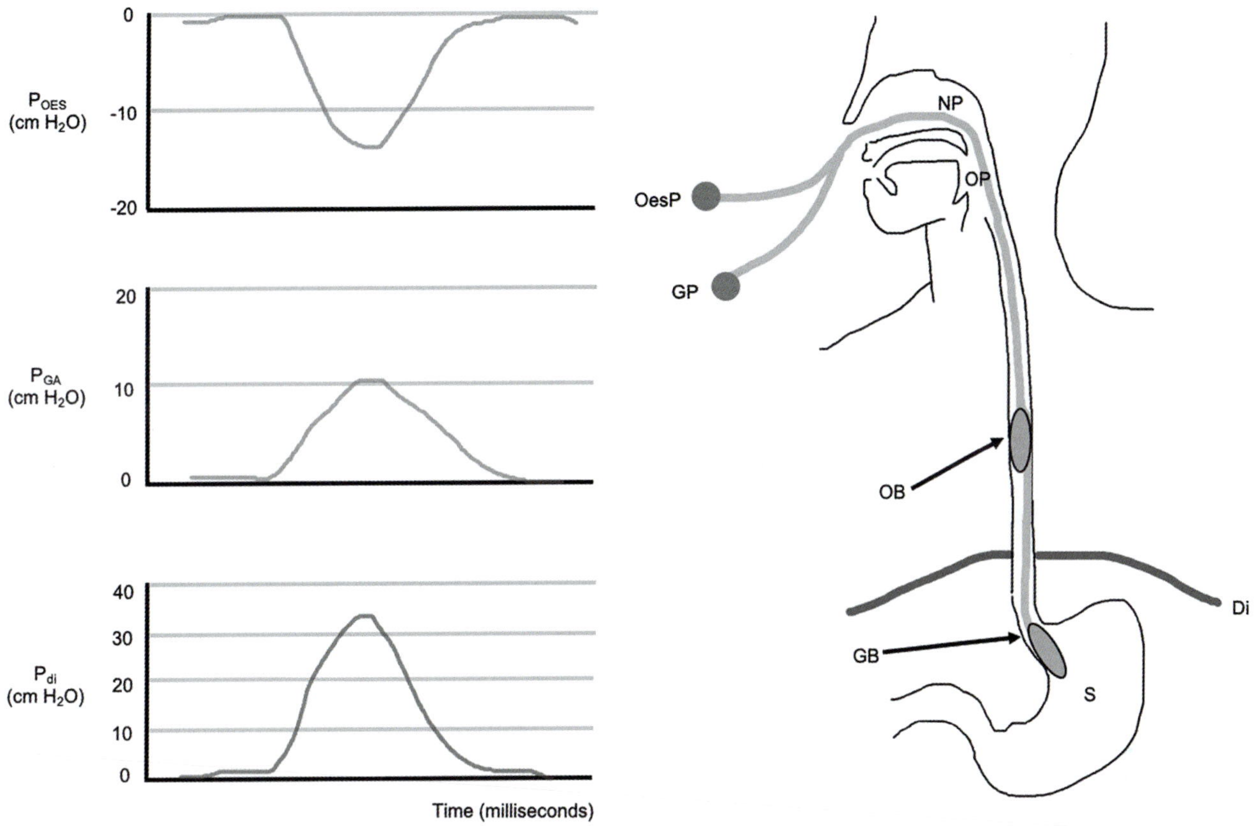

Figure 16.3 Transdiaphragmatic pressure measurement. Transdiaphragmatic pressure (P_{di}) is calculated by subtracting the oesophageal pressure (P_{OES}) from the gastric pressure (P_{ga}) which are reliable surrogate measures for abdominal and pleural pressures, respectively. The more negative Pdi (converted to a positive) reflects a greater transdiaphragmatic pressure generated for inspiration. Oesophageal pressure is considered the gold standard in the assessment of respiratory effort and work of breathing. A dual lumen catheter is inserted via a nasogastric or orogastric route so that the oesophageal balloon (OB) lies in the mid-thorax and the gastric balloon (GB) lies below the diaphragm (Di) and adjacent to the cardia of the stomach (S). The oesophageal port (OesP) and gastric port (GP) are then inflated, and the pressure signal is transduced. Nasopharynx, NP; oropharynx, OP.

has been shown to poorly correlate with respiratory muscle energy expenditure as it fails to take into account respiratory rate, intrinsic PEEP, and chest wall compliance, thus potentially limiting its usefulness as a stand-alone measure.[13]

Measures of Respiratory Muscle Energy Usage

Too much (a reduction in neural stimulation) or too little MV (overloading the respiratory pump) can lead to significant diaphragmatic dysfunction via different mechanisms. Setting the ventilator to offload the respiratory system enough but not too much is one of the goals of MV. The pressure–time scalar gives a simple and rough but practical guide to patient effort.

Although not used routinely in clinical practice, there are also a number of research tools available to quantify the offloading of the respiratory muscles. The pressure–time product (PTP) can be defined as follows:

$$PTP = P_{MUS} \times T_i$$

where P_{MUS} is the average inspiratory muscle pressure and T_i is the inspiratory time. It is normally reported over 1 min, is sensitive to respiratory frequency and duration, which means it closely correlates with energy expenditure of the respiratory muscles. It also requires an accurate measurement of chest wall compliance. The PTP does not take into account volume or flow although this helps minimize the effects of isometric contractions and intrinsic PEEP. It also means that oxygen consumption at similar PTPs can differ widely depending on these variables. This has led some researchers to define the upper and lower PTPs, which they argue may give a more accurate representation of energy expenditure.[14]

The tension time index (TTI) is a ratio that gives an estimate of the respiratory muscle force that has been related to fatigue. It can be measured invasively with a diaphragm pressure monitor (equation (A)) or less invasively using airway pressures (equation (B)):

$$TTI_{di} = (\text{Mean di pressure/MaxPdi}) \times (T_i / T_{tot}) \qquad (A)$$

$$TTI = (\text{Mean airway pressure/MIP}) \times (T_i / T_{tot}) \qquad (B)$$

Studies show that TTI of 0.15–0.18 can be maintained under normal circumstances indefinitely, whilst higher levels will lead to respiratory muscle fatigue. The aforementioned problems with measuring inspiratory pressures both with and without specialized equipment limit the applicability of this measure in clinical practice.

Finally, WOB can be defined as the energy required by the respiratory muscles for inspiration and expiration. The equation for WOB and power can be expressed as follows:

$$\text{Work (Joules)} = \int \text{Pressure} \times \text{Volume}$$
$$\text{Power (Watts)} = \text{Work/Time}$$

This measure takes into account the elastic recoil of the lungs and the chest wall and the resistance to flow in both inspiration and expiration. Work will therefore be significantly influenced by lung and chest wall compliance, intrinsic PEEP, bronchoconstriction and artificial airways. Some drawbacks of this measure include insensitivity to isometric contraction and the duration of the respiratory cycle. Despite this work rate, a function of power and respiratory rate is now felt to be a major determinant in the development of ventilator-associated lung injury and closely correlates with oxygen consumption.[12,13]

Electrophysiology

Electromyography Measurement of Respiratory Muscle Function

Electromyography (EMG) is the recording of the summation of electrical activity coming from the brain to a muscle. In the respiratory system diaphragm, EMG can be measured on the skin or by an electrode on a nasogastric tube, or in some cases a needle inserted intercostally. These impulses can be measured continuously and processed to provide a measure referred to as the amplitude of the electrical activity of the diaphragm (EAdi). Whilst skin electrodes can be used to determine the action potentials of the entire respiratory system, they come with disadvantages. There may be variability in signal caused by fat, oedema, and movement. They also lack standardization both in terms of electrode placement and reference ranges. Needles inserted intercostally into the insertion of the diaphragm has proven safe in the past but needs further study and may be unnecessarily invasive for use in routine clinical practice. Nasogastric electrode monitoring, originally developed as part of neutrally adjusted ventilatory assist, is attractive as it is minimally invasive. EAdi measured by this method has been shown to closely correlate with P_{di} and diaphragm function, whilst also providing information on patient–ventilator dyssynchrony.

The ratio of baseline to maximal EAdi (defined by the EMG amplitude after a 20 s of inspiratory hold) shown below can be used to define failed unloading or over-ventilation:

$$\text{EAdi ratio} = \text{EAdi-base/EAdi-max}$$

Using EAdi as an accurate marker of the neural onset of inspiration and expiration can help diagnosing a number of dysynchronous ventilator patterns, including trigger delays, early and late cycling off, auto-triggering, double triggering, and wasted efforts.

Combining EMG with volume and pressure measurements can provide additional information on the function of the respiratory muscles in intubated patients. Neuroventilatory efficiency (NVE) can be defined as follows:

$$\text{NVE} = \text{Tidal volume/EAdi}$$

with higher levels associated with fewer failed extubations.[6] The neuromechanical efficiency (NME), defined as

$$\text{NME} = P_{di}/\text{EAdi},$$

can be used to monitor the development of diaphragm weakness and recovery over time, which may provide information independent of mechanical load.

Whilst these variables have a number of theoretical advantages, none has found its way into clinical practice and further information and assessment is required. This may be because the ideal and target measures for EMG amplitudes and ratio have not, as yet, been defined. Furthermore, the EMG is influenced by sedatives and analgesics. Their use has not been shown to significantly alter patient outcomes. More work is needed in this expanding area.[13,15]

Imaging

The role of imaging in the detection and quantification of muscle wasting in critical care has gained increasing interest. Muscle quantity and quality can be studied from CT and MRI imaging and has been associated with longer ICU stay and prolonged MV and mortality in some ICU cohorts. The widespread availability of imaging makes this an attractive diagnostic tool in the detection of critical-illness-associated muscle wasting.

Chest X-ray

Whilst a normal chest X-ray is neither sensitive or specific in ruling out significant respiratory muscle weakness, a raised hemi-diaphragm may be a first sign of respiratory muscle dysfunction. Alternative causes of a raised hemi-diaphragm (such as phrenic nerve crush in historical treatment of tuberculosis, phrenic nerve injury during cardiac surgery, or electrophysiological ablation) must always be sought.[16] Fluoroscopy has been used, in the past, as a dynamic test of diaphragmatic function but is impractical for bedside use on the intensive care.

Computerized Tomography Imaging

CT imaging is commonly performed in critically ill patients. The widespread availability of such a modality allows quantitative measurements of muscle to be studied over time. Muscle quantity is often expressed as the cross-sectional area (CSA of a given muscle group (or groups)), and single slice images at the third lumbar vertebra are the most widely reported as they are used in the calculation of the skeletal muscle index (SMI).[17] SMI can be used to determine total body muscle and is calculated by dividing the CSA of the muscle groups at L3 by the height (in metres squared). SMI is then compared against published thresholds to decide whether patients have a low muscle mass. Furthermore, changes in muscle quality can be quantified by the calculation of Hounsfield units in muscle which infers density of the tissue in question. To date, there is a paucity of data describing the application of CT imaging in the quantification of smaller respiratory muscles.

Ultrasound

During MV, ventilatory 'over-assistance' can be as high as 50% of the time on MV and may lead to VIDD.[18] As VIDD is a diagnosis of exclusion, its incidence is probably underestimated. Some studies have shown diaphragm dysfunction to be more prevalent than limb weakness in patients undergoing active weaning from MV, possibly as the diaphragm is continually active compared to peripheral skeletal muscle. It is reported that approximately 40% of the total time spent on MV is during the weaning process, and difficulties in complete separation are encountered in around 25%. Thus, early recognition of diaphragm dysfunction is important as it is associated with prolonged MV and longer periods of weaning.

Ultrasound can be performed quickly at the bedside, is non-invasive, and can be used longitudinally, without significant risk to the patient or the operator. Despite small measurements, the intra- and interobserver reliability of ultrasound-based measures has been shown to be high. The diaphragm is the most widely studied respiratory muscle using ultrasound both in B and M mode ultrasonography, but other respiratory muscles, such as the intercostal muscles, are gaining interest. Diaphragmatic and intercostal thickness can be used to show muscle wasting in a proportion of patients on the ICU, and this represents a widely available and reproducible approach. The studies using this technique have noted a high proportion of patients losing significant muscle size between subsequent scans (and as early as day 3). The size of the muscles and the variation within the respiratory cycle mean that readings can, however, be unreliable outside of expert hands, which highlights the importance of reliability and reproducibility studies before clinical application.[19]

Diaphragmatic thickness and/or excursion (EXC_{di}) in the zone of apposition or the sub-costal or low intercostal position respectively in between the mid-clavicular and mid-axillary lines is widely described. This can easily distinguish between normal diaphragmatic movement and paralysis, and within a short period of time the operator can be trained to measure diaphragmatic thickening. The thickening fraction of the diaphragm (TF_{di}) is the difference between the diaphragmatic thickness at the end of inspiration and expiration divided by the diaphragmatic thickness at the end of expiration (Figure 16.4). Furthermore, TF_{di} has been correlated with other measures of diaphragm function (such as P_{di} and P_{diTw}) in a number of other studies. Normal diaphragm thickness at functional residual capacity ranges from 1.8 to 3 mm, but generally the mean thickness at rest is quoted as 2.2–2.8 mm with a thickness less than 2 mm often used to define atrophy, and a 10% change in TF_{di} is associated with a higher chance of failed extubation, prolonged ICU stay, and higher incidence of tracheostomy. The quoted threshold of TF_{di} and excursion that may predict successful extubation (when assessed during an SBT) is variable but generally quoted to be one greater than 30%–36% (or a 10% change) and 10 mm, respectively. Diaphragmatic measurements have high sensitivity in predicting

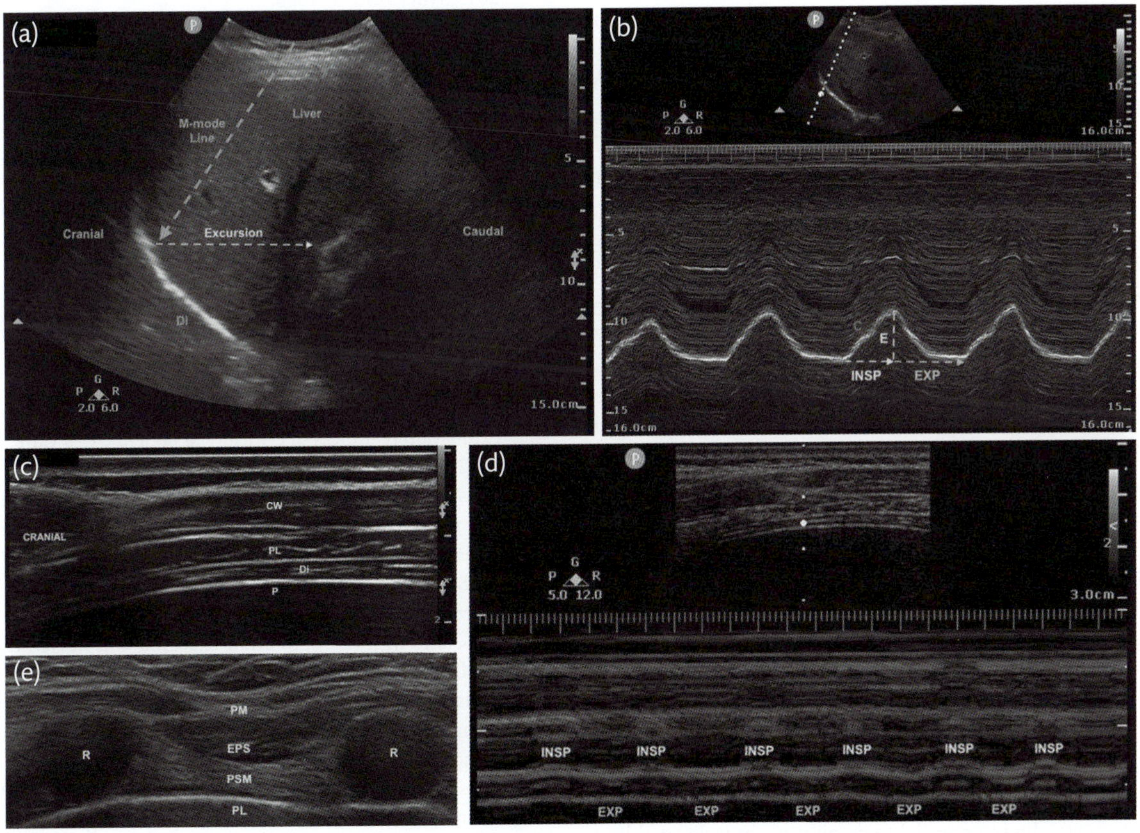

Figure 16.4 Quantitative and qualitative respiratory muscle ultrasound. (A) B-mode ultrasound of diaphragm excursion. (B) M-mode ultrasound to quantify diaphragm excursion. (C) B-mode ultrasound in the zone of apposition to measure diaphragm thickness. (D) M-mode ultrasound in the zone of apposition to quantify inspiratory and expiratory thickness and thus diaphragm thickening fraction. (E) B-mode ultrasound of the parasternal muscle in the right third intercostal space. Di, diaphragm; C, contractility; E, excursion; INSP, inspiration; EXP, expiration; CW, chest wall; PL, pleura; PM, pectoralis major; PSM, parasternal muscle; EPS, external parasternal muscle surface; R, rib.

successful weaning from MV and may be a highly useful clinical tool in tracking atrophy over time. Other emerging ultrasound-based measures of diaphragmatic function include contraction speed and pulse wave tissue Doppler imaging, which may add to the usefulness of ultrasound in a comprehensive assessment of the respiratory system.[20]

Monitoring respiratory muscle function in the critically ill patients is fraught with challenges. The reliance on patient cooperation as well as the requirement for invasive techniques has meant respiratory muscle function monitoring primarily remains a research tool. This is evidenced by the fact that no current guideline on weaning from MV mentions any specific respiratory muscle strength test,[21] with only a passing comment in the European guideline published in 2007.[22] More specific and sensitive non-invasive tests are therefore needed to truly define the wasting seen. The clinical importance of diaphragm dysfunction is likely to be underestimated, and as we refine our techniques for minimizing damage to the lungs during MV, defining the presence and clinical sequelae of respiratory muscle weakness will be ever more important.

Future Areas of Research

Precision, or tailored patient approaches through utilization of computer-based, open-loop decision support tools, is an evolving area of research and has already been shown to advise in the weaning of pressure support and PEEP. Randomized control trials have begun to assess whether a tailored approach leads to reduced length of MV and reduced periods of weaning.

Inspiratory muscle training in various forms has been shown to increase MIP, rapid shallow breathing index, and weaning success. In some studies, it has also been shown to reduce length of ICU stay, hospital stay, and time spent on non-invasive ventilation after weaning. Patients who will benefit from training need to be defined, as does the ideal timing for, the duration of inspiratory muscle training. Those who are most likely to benefit will probably be in the clear weaning phase, with resolution of the underlying requirement for MV.[23] A natural extension of inspiratory muscle training is diaphragmatic pacing. This has been suggested as a potential treatment but also as a preventative measure to stop respiratory muscle atrophy in the first place, and clinical trials are currently underway in a critical care domain.[24]

The widespread availability of ultrasound in ICUs has certainly allowed respiratory muscle research to expand over the last 10–15 years. Formal guidelines and education in respiratory muscle ultrasound are yet to be developed, but techniques and approaches are widely published, and reliability studies have continually shown high levels of agreement and reproducibility. Furthermore, the non-invasive nature, portability, and ease of repeatability confer a significant advantage over other imaging modalities. Indices from invasive techniques such as P_{di} and P_{diTw} have also been shown to closely correlate with TF_{di}, thus making ultrasound an attractive option in future research trials. Ultrasound also allows peripheral skeletal muscle to be studied in parallel to respiratory muscle, enabling longitudinal study with minimal risk to the patient.

Finally, there are a number of experimental drugs in development and in the testing phase, which may affect both the skeletal and respiratory muscles. These include anti-oxidants, inhibitors of proteolytic pathways, theophylline, and calcium channel sensitizers. So far none has reached clinical practice but as we discover more about the extent and molecular pathways involved in respiratory muscle dysfunction, novel treatment pathways and targeted therapies are likely to emerge.[2,11,15,25]

Conclusion

Monitoring of respiratory muscle function has been a somewhat neglected part and inconsistently utilized aspect of the assessment of critically ill patients. As we learn more about the importance of the respiratory muscles not only in weaning but also in the generation of self-induced lung injury, the multi-modal assessment of respiratory muscle function in critical care will become more clinically relevant and important. With better understanding of the impact of respiratory muscle weakness, further study, and ultimately simplification of currently unproven multi-modal tools for measurement, guidelines will be required to establish the place of respiratory muscle function testing in the ICU.

REFERENCES

1. Puthucheary ZA, Rawal J, McPhail M, et al. Acute skeletal muscle wasting in critical illness. *JAMA.* 2013;**310**(15):1591–1600.
2. Doorduin J, van Hees HW, van der Hoeven JG, et al. Monitoring of the respiratory muscles in the critically ill. *Am J Respir Crit Care Med.* 2013;**187**(1):20–27.
3. Sassoon CS, Younes M. Airway occlusion pressure revisited. *Am J Respir Crit Care Med.* 2020;**201**(9):1027–1028.
4. American Thoracic Society/European Respiratory Society. ATS/ERS Statement on respiratory muscle testing. *Am J Respir Crit Care Med.* 2002 Aug 15;**166**(4):518–624. doi:10.1164/rccm.166.4.518. PMID: 12186831.
5. Bellani G, Bronco A, Arrigoni Marocco S, et al. Measurement of diaphragmatic electrical activity by surface electromyography in intubated subjects and its relationship with inspiratory effort. *Respir Care.* 2018;**63**(11):1341–1349.
6. Liu L, Liu H, Yang Y, et al. Neuroventilatory efficiency and extubation readiness in critically ill patients. *Crit Care.* 2012;**16**(4):R143.
7. Dres M, Goligher EC, Dube BP, et al. Diaphragm function and weaning from mechanical ventilation: An ultrasound and phrenic nerve stimulation clinical study. *Ann Intensive Care.* 2018;**8**(1):53.
8. Guerri R, Gayete A, Balcells E, et al. Mass of intercostal muscles associates with risk of multiple exacerbations in COPD. *Respir Med.* 2010;**104**(3):378–388.
9. Boussuges A, Gole Y, Blanc P. Diaphragmatic motion studied by m-mode ultrasonography: Methods, reproducibility, and normal values. *Chest.* 2009;**135**(2): 391–400.
10. Dres M, Dube BP, Goligher E, et al. Usefulness of parasternal intercostal muscle ultrasound during weaning from mechanical ventilation. *Anesthesiology.* 2020;**132**(5): 1114–1125.
11. Bissett B, Gosselink R, van Haren FMP. Respiratory muscle rehabilitation in patients with prolonged mechanical ventilation: A targeted approach. *Crit Care.* 2020;**24**(1):103.

12. Hess DR. Respiratory mechanics in mechanically ventilated patients. *Respir Care.* 2014;**59**(11):1773–1794.
13. de Vries H, Jonkman A, Shi ZH, et al. Assessing breathing effort in mechanical ventilation: Physiology and clinical implications. *Ann Transl Med.* 2018;**6**(19):387.
14. Grinnan DC, Truwit JD. Clinical review: Respiratory mechanics in spontaneous and assisted ventilation. *Crit Care.* 2005;**9**(5):472–484.
15. Jonkman AH, Jansen D, Heunks LM. Novel insights in ICU-acquired respiratory muscle dysfunction: Implications for clinical care. *Crit Care.* 2017;**21**(1):64.
16. Wilcox P, Baile EM, Hards J, et al. Phrenic nerve function and its relationship to atelectasis after coronary artery bypass surgery. *Chest.* 1988;**93**(4):693–698.
17. Schweitzer L, Geisler C, Pourhassan M, et al. What is the best reference site for a single MRI slice to assess whole-body skeletal muscle and adipose tissue volumes in healthy adults? *Am J Clin Nutr.* 2015;**102**(1):58–65.
18. Petrof BJ, Jaber S, Matecki S. Ventilator-induced diaphragmatic dysfunction. *Curr Opin Crit Care.* 2010;**16**(1):19–25.
19. Sarwal A, Parry SM, Berry MJ, et al. Interobserver reliability of quantitative muscle sonographic analysis in the critically ill population. *J Ultrasound Med.* 2015;**34**(7): 1191–200.
20. Schepens T, Verbrugghe W, Dams K, et al. The course of diaphragm atrophy in ventilated patients assessed with ultrasound: A longitudinal cohort study. *Crit Care.* 2015;**19**:422.
21. Ouellette DR, Patel S, Girard TD, et al. Liberation from mechanical ventilation in critically ill adults: An Official American College of Chest Physicians/American Thoracic Society Clinical Practice Guideline: Inspiratory pressure augmentation during spontaneous breathing trials, protocols minimizing sedation, and noninvasive ventilation immediately after extubation. *Chest.* 2017;**151**(1):166–180.
22. Boles JM, Bion J, Connors A, et al. Weaning from mechanical ventilation. *Eur Respir J.* 2007;**29**(5):1033–1056.
23. Elkins M, Dentice R. Inspiratory muscle training facilitates weaning from mechanical ventilation among patients in the intensive care unit: A systematic review. *J Physiother.* 2015;**61**(3):125–134.
24. Evans D, Shure D, Clark L, et al. Temporary transvenous diaphragm pacing vs. standard of care for weaning from mechanical ventilation: Study protocol for a randomized trial. *Trials.* 2019;**20**(1):60.6–13.
25. Schellekens WJ, van Hees HW, Doorduin J, et al. Strategies to optimize respiratory muscle function in ICU patients. *Crit Care.* 2016;**20**(1):103.

17

Monitoring Cardiovascular Function in Critically Ill Patients

Rodney A Gabriel and Michael R Pinsky

KEY MESSAGES

- Haemodynamic monitoring needs to be linked to physiology.
- Disease states reflect various constellations of physiologic changes.
- The options for monitoring by variable and method are extensive, and the clinician needs to understand the strengths and weaknesses of their devices.

CONTROVERSIES

- Does haemodynamic monitoring improve outcome?
- Is there a minimal monitoring data set that all unstable patients should receive?
- What is the cause of decreased oxygen extraction in sepsis?

FURTHER RESEARCH

- Targeting specific organs for resuscitation.
- Personalized resuscitation.

Introduction

Respiratory failure, its causes, and the associated mechanical ventilatory therapies may all affect cardiovascular homeostasis. Thus, in the critically ill patients with respiratory failure, haemodynamic monitoring is an essential aspect of care. Such monitoring allows the clinician to assess the cardiovascular state of the patient and characterize any insufficiencies, their causes, and responses to therapy aimed at restoring and supporting cardiovascular function. Since the adequacy of cardiovascular homeostasis is essential to host survival and end-organ function, this focus usually becomes a diagnostic and treatment priority.

Patients in respiratory failure offer unique challenges to the clinician. Respiratory failure is often associated with hypoxaemia, which by itself may make oxygen (O_2) delivery insufficient to meet metabolic demands of the body independent of primary cardiovascular causes. Furthermore, positive-pressure ventilation increases intrathoracic pressure, so impeding venous return, particularly if right atrial pressure also increases. Hyperinflation, by increasing pulmonary vascular resistance, can impede right ventricular (RV) ejection, which increases right atrial pressure further. A full discussion of heart–lung interactions is beyond the scope of this chapter but underscores the importance of accurate and continuous haemodynamic monitoring in the unstable patient with acute respiratory failure.

The type of haemodynamic monitoring selected for these scenarios must be personalized based on the underlying pathophysiology and treatment options. The focus of this chapter is to discuss such haemodynamic monitoring tools used to assess cardiac output (CO), ventricular function, and vascular pressures in ventilator-dependent patients. The principal haemodynamic monitoring biomarkers discussed include arterial pressure, central venous pressure (CVP), pulmonary artery pressure (PAP), various ways to estimate CO, and ways of determining oxygenation and tissue blood flow.

Although it is not clear that any specific monitoring and management approach is superior to overall excellent bedside titration of care for the critically ill, no care can be effectively given without measuring its effects relative to the current state. In this context, haemodynamic monitoring is essential in defining both the current state and the change in response to cardiovascular treatment.

Haemodynamic Monitoring Biomarkers

Understanding the cardiovascular state of a critically ill patient requires an understanding of the relationships between various haemodynamic measures and tissue perfusion. In order to optimize vital organ perfusion, treatments need to focus on reversing cardiovascular insufficiency and maintaining organ blood flow sufficiency without over-resuscitation. To accomplish these goals, certain specific forms of haemodynamic monitoring will allow manipulation of cardiovascular and respiratory therapy, while monitoring the progression of disease.

Arterial Blood Pressure

Organ blood flow is determined by both organ perfusion pressure and intra-organ arterial resistance. For the body as a whole, the primary driving force for tissue blood flow is arterial blood pressure. However, each organ system has its own unique perfusion pressure, and it varies its own intra-organ resistance to maintain its own blood flow relative to its metabolic requirements. Thus, hypotension, by removing this high arterial input pressure, can impair autoregulation of organ blood flow because local changes in vascular resistance will have minimal effects on organ blood flow if the input pressure is too low.

The left ventricle (LV) ejects its stroke volume into a relatively stiff central arterial capacitor—the aorta, which stores most of the energy of LV ejection so as to drive organ perfusion throughout both ejection (systole) and diastole. Arterial pressure is neither a single value nor it is the same throughout the arterial circuit. The primary components of arterial pressure are systolic pressure (the maximum pressure during the contraction of ventricles), diastolic pressure (lowest pressure between heart beats during ventricular filling), mean arterial pressure (MAP), and the pulse pressure, which is the pressure rise from diastole to the next systole. The MAP can be calculated as the sum of the diastolic arterial pressure plus one-third the pulse pressure.

The pulse pressure is the difference between the systolic and the diastolic pressure, which is largely determined by central arterial capacitance, rate of LV ejection, and LV stroke volume. From one heart beat to the next, the primary cause of changes in pulse pressure is LV stroke volume. Accordingly, pulse pressure variation is often used as a measure of LV stroke volume variation, which is useful in the diagnosis of cardiac tamponade and volume responsiveness.

Non-invasive Estimation of Arterial Pressure

The sphygmomanometer is the commonest non-invasive technique of measuring blood pressure. It has three components: an inflatable cuff, a measuring unit, and a mechanism for inflation. A manual approach for measuring blood pressure with a sphygmomanometer involves auscultation of an artery (i.e. brachial artery) distal to the cuff (if placed in the upper arm). The cuff is inflated until greater than systolic pressure and then the pressure is slowly released. The pressure at the first Korotkoff sound is the systolic blood pressure, while the pressure when the sounds disappear is the diastolic blood pressure. Digital instruments utilize the oscillometric method for measuring blood pressure. When compared to more invasive methods of blood pressure measuring, the non-invasive approach usually gives higher systolic and lower diastolic readings. In unstable patients, the oscillatory sensing algorithm degrades. Thus, if patient is hypotensive or on vasopressor therapy and if measures of blood pressure need to be made accurately, then they should be done manually using auscultation or an indwelling arterial catheter.

Continuous analysis of the arterial pressure waveform is also possible non-invasively by systems using either the volume clamp method (Clearsight (Edwards Lifesciences, USA), CNAP (CNSystems, Austria)) or the radial artery applanation tonometry (T-Line, Tensys, USA). The volume clamp method derives the finger arterial pressure waveform from the cuff pressure that is needed to keep the blood volume (assessed by photo-plethysmography) in the finger arteries constant throughout the cardiac cycle. The continuous radial artery applanation tonometry technique records the arterial pressure waveform using a sensor that is electromechanically driven over the radial artery. As described below, these devices can also be used to estimate CO using proprietary algorithms for pulse contour analysis. Validation studies for the volume clamp method showed good agreement when compared with indwelling arterial catheters, but poorer results in both cardiac surgery and ICU patients, presumably due to alterations in vasomotor tone. The radial applanation tonometry method is novel and at present needs further validation. The main limitations of the volume clamp method are peripheral oedema and severe vasoconstriction; thus, in these settings, if continuous arterial pressure waveform analysis is required, indwelling arterial pressure monitoring is indicated.[1]

Invasive Estimates of Arterial Pressure

Intra-arterial blood pressure monitoring is a more invasive approach to measuring this haemodynamic marker. Figure 17.1 illustrates a typical arterial waveform and the various components. This provides a beat-to-beat assessment of blood pressure, arterial pulse pressure, pulse pressure variation, and, through proprietary algorithms, CO.[2] Furthermore, it allows the clinician to perform repeat blood sampling more easily. Due to the viscoelastic properties of the central arterial circuit and reflected hydraulic pressure waves, systolic arterial pressure tends to increase and diastolic arterial pressure decrease as the measuring site moves more distal to the aortic valves. However, since flow in the central arterial compartment is relatively slow and vascular resistance almost nil, no measurable change in MAP occurs from the central aorta to the radial artery. Thus, one can use a radial arterial site to estimate MAP with accuracy. However, under conditions of profound vasoconstriction or hypothermia, distal arteries constrict, and radial arterial pressure may underestimate MAP. Under these conditions, usually associated with the immediate post-operative state following prolonged cardiac surgery with circulatory arrest, a more central arterial pressure measuring site is recommended, such as the femoral or brachial arterial sites.

Central Venous Pressure

CVP is the vascular pressure at the level of the intrathoracic vena cavae. It is used as a close estimate of right atrial pressure. Previously, CVP had been used as a marker for preload and as a predictor to volume responsiveness when measuring changes in CVP in response to volume resuscitation. However, overwhelming evidence has demonstrated that CVP is a poor predictor of both volume status and volume responsiveness. The use of CVP as an estimate for either volume status or volume responsiveness has as such been abandoned.[3] However, as a measure of right atrial pressure, CVP can be used to assess RV function. Normal CVP values range from 0 to 4 cmH_2O in supine healthy patients and slightly higher in intubated patients on mechanical ventilation due to the associated increase in intrathoracic pressure. CVP values greater than 12 mmHg are pathological and connote right heart dysfunction.

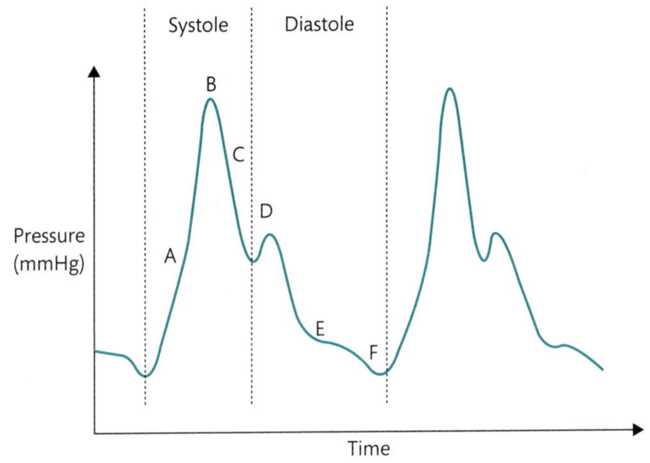

Figure 17.1 Arterial waveform. (A) Systolic upstroke (opening of aortic valve), (B) peak systolic pressure, (C) systolic decline, (D) dichroitic notch (aortic valve closes here), © diastolic runoff, and (F) end-diastolic pressure. Arterial pulse pressure is the difference between the initial diastolic pressure and its subsequent peak systolic pressure. Mean arterial pressure can be calculated as the diastolic pressure plus one-third the pulse pressure.

Non-invasive Measures of CVP

Non-invasive methods of measuring CVP include inspection of jugular venous pulsation. With the patient sitting upright, at least 45° above horizontal, the height of the meniscus of jugular venous distention above the sternal angle in centimetres can be used to estimate CVP. Since CVP varies in the setting of arterio-venous dissociation, cor pulmonale, and with vigorous respiratory efforts, the accuracy of jugular venous distention method to measure CVP is poor. Its primary uses are to note a decrease in the height with spontaneous inspiration, thus suggesting volume responsiveness or an increase with instantaneous inspiration, suggesting acute cor pulmonale.

Invasive Measures of CVP

Invasive methods of measuring CVP require an indwelling central venous catheter, which may be placed either in the femoral, internal jugular, or subclavian vein, and a pressure manometer or transducer. Since such central venous vascular sites are needed for fluid and drug infusion, CVP recordings are commonly available. Since the vena cavae reside within the chest, both spontaneous breathing efforts and mechanically generated breaths will all alter intrathoracic pressure causing parallel changes in CVP. Of note, CVP changes with changes in intrathoracic pressure; therefore, this haemodynamic marker is usually measured at end-expiration to minimize influence of changing pressures in the intrathoracic space. Just like arterial pressure, there is no one value for CVP. It is a dynamic pressure signal altered by RV contraction and intrathoracic pressure. Figure 17.2 illustrates a typical CVP waveform and its various key components as seen during apnoea.

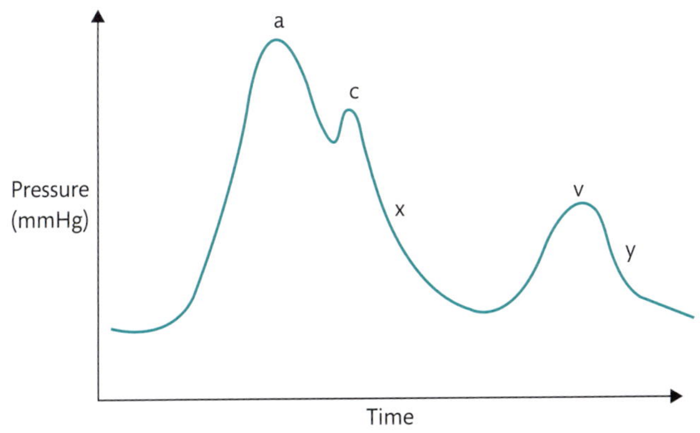

Figure 17.2 Central venous pressure waveform: a wave, atrial contract during end diastole; c wave, tricuspid valve bulging during early systole; x-descent, atrial relaxation; v wave, systolic filling of the atrium during late systole; y-descent, early ventricular filling during early diastole.

Pulmonary Artery Pressure

PAP is the intravascular pressure within the pulmonary arterial circuit. The normal PAP ranges from 9 to 18 mmHg and considered elevated when generally greater than 25 mmHg. Pulmonary hypertension can be due to increases in pulmonary vascular resistance (primary) or increases in the back pressure to pulmonary blood flow seen with elevated left atrial pressure. Pulmonary hypertension is not a uniform disease but can be due to many processes. Typically, it is classified into four groups: primary pulmonary hypertension, including chronic haemolytic anaemia (i.e. sickle cell disease), pulmonary hypertension due to left heart disease, pulmonary hypertension due to lung diseases (i.e. chronic obstructive lung disease and acute respiratory distress syndrome), and chronic pulmonary thromboembolic disease.

Measuring PAP in patients with pulmonary hypertension and respiratory failure may help titrate appropriate interventions. Since the RV myocardium is primarily perfused during systole, elevated PAP relative to MAP may lead to RV ischaemia and RV failure, leading to decreased CO and potentially death. The clinician should also monitor other biomarkers known to increase PAP, including hypoxia, hypercarbia, hypervolemia, and metabolic acidosis. To the extent they are minimized, pulmonary vasomotor tone usually remains low.

Non-invasive Estimates of PAP

PAP can be estimated indirectly from the degree of tricuspid regurgitation present at end-expiration using echocardiographic measuring techniques. However, the accuracy of these estimates is poor. Presently, there are no accurate non-invasive measuring tools for PAP.

Invasive Measures of PAP

PAP is usually measured invasively with balloon floatation pulmonary artery catheterization (PAC), which involves the insertion of a catheter into the pulmonary artery from a central venous site. The catheter must pass through the right atrium and right ventricle before resting in one of the pulmonary arteries. The purpose of a PAC is diagnostic and allows the clinician to assess various haemodynamic markers in the patient with respiratory failure, including CVP, RV pressure, PAP, filling pressures of the left atrium (pulmonary artery occlusion pressure), mixed venous O_2 saturation (SvO_2), and CO. CO is estimated by the thermodilution technique, while SvO_2 is estimated by reflective spectroscopy.[4] Complications of PAC placement include arrhythmias during the passing of the catheter tip through the right heart, rupture of the pulmonary artery if the balloon is inflated while the PAC tip is already wedged in a small pulmonary artery, thrombosis, infection, pneumothorax, and pericardial effusion leading to cardiac tamponade.

Cardiac Output

The primary function of the ventricles of the heart is to maintain circulation of blood to the organs of the body. The LV receives oxygenated blood from the pulmonary circulation and further distributes it throughout the systemic arterial tree. The systolic function of the ventricles involves ventricular ejection, whereas diastole involves ventricular filling. The resultant LV stroke volume is a function of diastolic filling and LV ejection. LV ejection is a function of intrinsic LV contractility, contraction synchrony, and the arterial pressure load (afterload).

CO is equal to the stroke volume times the heart rate. Thus, CO is determined by ventricular filling, systolic ejection, and heart rate. Under normal conditions, systolic function and heart rate play a minor role in regulating CO, therefore filling due to venous return primarily determines CO. In heart failure state, however, both systolic function and heart rate play a greater role. Since CO values vary greatly with body size, owing to proportional metabolic demands, CO is often normalized to body surface area. The ratio of CO to body surface area is called cardiac index (CI). Normal values of CI in a healthy subject at rest are 2.5–4.2 L/min/m^2.

Preload

The preload is determined by end-diastolic wall stress, which itself is roughly proportional to LV end-diastolic volume. LV end-diastolic volume is itself dependent on LV diastolic compliance, mitral and aortic valvular function, and LV filling pressure. Pulmonary artery occlusion pressure may be used as a surrogate for LV filling pressure. However, it poorly approximates LV end-diastolic volume because the relationship between LV distending pressure and volume is curvilinear at best and may rapidly change with RV volume changes, pericardial volume restraint, and hyperinflation. Rapid changes in LV end-diastolic volume result in proportional changes in LV ejection force. This concept is referred to the Frank–Starling mechanism (i.e. Starling's law of the heart). Specifically, the force of LV contraction dynamically varies with changes in LV wall stretch such that stroke volume increases in response to an increase in the end-diastolic volume given that all other factors are constant (Figure 17.3). However, this process only works dynamically and not in the steady state. Its goal is to match the constantly varying RV and LV outputs to each other over a few beats.

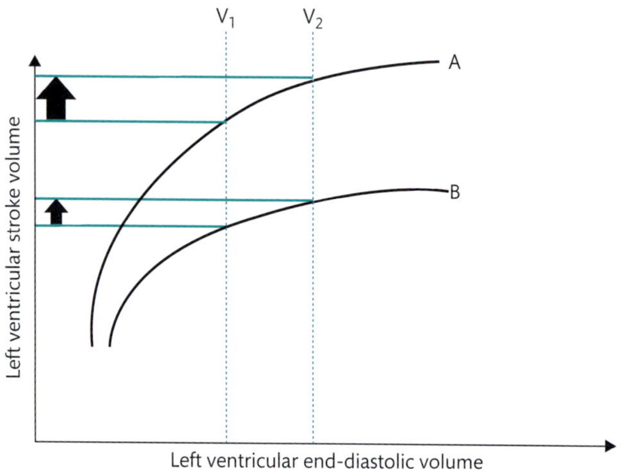

Figure 17.3 Frank–Starling curves for two different cardiac states showing the relationship between left ventricular (LV) end-diastolic volume and LV stroke volume. Part (A) refers to normal cardiac function, while (B) illustrates a patient with heart failure. At lower levels of LV end-diastolic volume changes, stroke volume variation will be greater than the flatter portions of the curve. The same increase in volume will increase stroke volume to a greater extent than if volume is increased at a flatter portion of the curve. As illustrated by the two curves, at the same end-diastolic volume, stroke volume is not increased as much in the heart failure patient than the normal patient.

The Starling mechanism is limited by the absolute volume limitation of the pericardial sac. Once end-diastolic volume increases passed a certain threshold, increases in CO no longer occur though CVP and pulmonary artery occlusion pressure continues to increase. For example, when the heart rate and arterial tone are constant, the CO is directly proportional to the combined effects of preload and contractility. However, if arterial pressure were to increase, as may occur with the response to pain or the use of exogenous vasopressor therapy (e.g. phenylephrine), then CO will decrease. Persistent increases in LV filling or afterload increase intrinsic LV contractility causing stroke volume to remain elevated despite a decrease in LV end-diastolic volume. This concept is referred to as the Anrep effect.[5]

Afterload

Afterload refers to the maximal LV wall stress during ejection. By the law of LaPlace, wall stress is a function of the maximal product of transmural pressure gradient (e.g. arterial pressure) and LV radius of curvature, approximated as LV volume, which usually equates to the product of LV end-diastolic volume and arterial diastolic pressure since once LV systolic pressure exceeds arterial diastolic pressure ejection ensues and LV volume rapidly decreases. So, in essence, the LV unloads itself during ejection. This is why diastolic hypertension is considered so dangerous to the normal heart's ejection.

With sustained arterial hypertension, LV hypertrophy develops, which minimizes local wall stress because the stress is distributed over a greater volume of muscle. Thus, we can express LV afterload or ventricular wall stress as the ratio of the product of maximal pressure and volume to wall thickness, where LV pressure is equal to ventricular transmural pressure and LV volume is ventricular radius. Thus, increases in LV afterload can independently occur if aortic pressure increases, aortic valve stenosis impedes ejection, or the LV dilates. Accordingly, for the same pressure and wall thickness, if LV volumes increase, then LV afterload also increases. Furthermore, in dilated cardiomyopathies, LV ejection does not decrease LV radius very much because LV end-diastolic volume remains high. Thus, in these patients, maximal wall stress usually occurs at end systole when the transmural pressures–LV radius product is greatest. This is why afterload reduction therapy is effective in improving LV systolic function in patients with dilated cardiomyopathies but not those with LV hypertrophy. For the same CO, if arterial tone increases, then arterial pressure also increases. In the clinical setting, one way to measure arterial tone is to calculate resistance as the ratio of CO to pressure, either total peripheral resistance (CO/MAP) or systemic vascular resistance (SVR) (CO/[MAP – CVP]).

Contractility

Cardiac contractility, otherwise known as inotropy, is the intrinsic ability of the myocardium to contract. It is directly related to intracellular calcium trafficking and basal energy state of the cardiac myocytes. Myocardial contractility is compromised in states of anoxia, acidosis, and cardiac ischaemia/infarction. Regional wall motion abnormalities are the physical manifestation of regional ischaemia, occurring as a consequence of localized cardiac ischaemia/infarction, and may alter the overall contractility of the heart.

Tissue Oxygenation

Decreased CO levels relative to metabolic demand leads to inadequate O_2 delivery to perfused tissues. This leads to an increased O_2 extraction, usually manifested by a decrease in SvO_2 <70%. Low SvO_2 levels normally occur in the setting of exercise, anaemia, and arterial hypoxaemia. Outside of these settings, a low SvO_2 usually connotes increased circulatory stress. If associated with other measures of tissue hypoperfusion, such as elevate blood lactate levels (i.e. >2 mmol/L), increased venous to arterial PCO_2 gradients (i.e. >5 mmHg), metabolic acidosis, and impaired end-organ function (e.g. oliguria, altered sensorium, and ileus), then the presumptive diagnosis of circulatory shock can be made.

Importantly, arterial pressure need not be decreased early on as normal sympathetic reflexes will increase arterial tone to sustain an adequate cerebral perfusion pressure despite decreasing CO values. Furthermore, not all hypotension is due to low CO values. In the fluid-resuscitated septic shock patient, CO is often excessively high with associated high SvO_2 values (e.g. >80%) despite a low arterial pressure. Thus, measuring MAP, CO, or SvO_2 alone may give misleading information as to the presence of circulatory insufficiency and if present its aetiology.

Cardiovascular Insufficiency

It is crucial that the clinician is aware of the dynamic interactions between CO, MAP, metabolic demands, and circulating blood volume as various forms of circulatory shock affect these determinants of cardiovascular health differently.[6] The basic aetiologies of circulatory shock can be grouped into four broad categories: distributive, cardiogenic, hypovolemic, and obstructive. These groupings are not mutually exclusive, and critically ill patients may have more than one type of shock occurring at the same time or sequentially. Circulatory shock is a state of decreased tissue perfusion leading to cellular hypoxia and end-organ dysfunction. Adequate tissue perfusion is largely due to adequate CO and vasomotor tone. CO is determined by preload, myocardial contractility, and afterload. Vasomotor tone and blood flow distribution are also a function of vessel length, blood viscosity, and sympathetic tone. Any change in these variables can contribute to the pathophysiology of shock. Importantly, each shock subtype affects these variables differently. Thus, to be effective in the diagnosis and management of the critically ill patient, the clinician needs to be knowledgeable in these processes. Table 17.1 outlines how each category of shock affects key haemodynamic variables. In all four conditions, systemic hypotension usually occurs, if not early, then as a late-stage event. Whereas cardiogenic, hypovolemia, and obstructive shock all share a low CO, distributive shock has a high CO. In general, if CO is decreased, SvO_2 is also decreased (e.g. <65%), and if CO is increased, SvO_2 is increased (e.g. >80%).

Distributive Shock

This type of shock involves loss of vascular smooth muscle tone inducing an associated peripheral vasodilation and hypotension, with the hallmark being a low diastolic arterial pressure. Many unrelated processes can cause distributive shock. These include the following: sepsis causing mediator activation and generalized loss of vascular reactivity and energetic failure (septic shock); loss of neurologic output preventing normal reflex vasoconstriction to support basal vascular tone (neurogenic shock); overwhelming mast cell degranulation in response to a hypersensitive immune reaction (anaphylactic shock); loss of intrinsic hormonal endocrine-related metabolic support from corticosteroids (endocrine shock); and finally, drug and toxin-induced cytotoxic shock.

With distributive shock, circulating blood volume is often unchanged early on and loss of vascular barrier integrity may decrease later on. Thus, assessing effective circulating blood volume as well as MAP and CO in these patients is difficult to do at the bedside. With the initial fluid resuscitation, patients in distributive shock usually manifest an increase in CO, with its associated increase in SvO_2. Measures of vascular tone, such as SVR, decrease as the MAP

Table 17.1 Categories of shock and the effects each has on haemodynamic variables

Type	Examples	Preload	Cardiac output	Tissue perfusion	Systemic vascular resistance
Distributive	Sepsis, anaphylaxis, neurogenic shock, adrenal insufficiency	Unchanged	Increases	Increases or decreases	Decreases
Cardiogenic	Infarction, cardiomyopathy, valvulopathy, arrhythmias	Increases	Decreases	Decreases	Increases
Hypovolemic	Haemorrhage, vomiting, diarrhoea, diabetes insipidus	Decreases	Initially unchanged but eventually decreases	Decreases	Increases
Obstructive	Pulmonary embolism, tamponade, tension pneumothorax	Increases	Decreases	Decreases	Increases

remain low while CO increases to high levels. As evidence of impaired cellular function, lactic acidosis and end-organ dysfunction are commonly present. However, at the present time, increased CO is going through functional peripheral arterio-venous shunts such that areas of hypoperfusion reside next to areas of excess perfusion or if the cells themselves are unable to utilize the oxygen delivered owing to primary mitochondrial dysfunction. In both cases, lactic acidosis and end-organ dysfunction would occur. This is an area of speculation and ongoing study.

Cardiogenic Shock

Cardiogenic shock is secondary to cardiac pump failure due to an intracardiac pathology, resulting in reduced CO and systemic hypotension. Causes of cardiogenic shock can be further divided into mechanical (i.e. severe valvular disorders), arrhythmic (i.e. complete heart block or unstable ventricular rhythms), and cardiomyopathic (i.e. acute decompensation from congestive heart failure or myocardial infarction) aetiologies. With cardiogenic shock, systemic hypotension is a defining characteristic, whereas vasomotor tone is usually increased owing to increase sympathetic tone. The primarily impaired ventricular pump function results in both a decreased CO and increased ventricular filling pressures. SvO_2 is usually <65%.

Hypovolemic Shock

This category of shock is secondary to inadequate intravascular volume, which involves a decreased pressure gradient for systemic venous return leading to decreased ventricular preload and consequently decreased CO. The two large categories of hypovolemic shock are haemorrhagic and non-haemorrhagic (i.e. gastrointestinal losses, skin losses from severe burns, and polyuria). With hypovolemic shock, both preload and CO remain unchanged early on but decrease in late stages of hypovolemic shock. Tachycardia is common as an early marker of increased sympathetic tone, and once CO begins to decrease, calculated SVR increases. Importantly, in an otherwise healthy subject, hypotension in hypovolemic shock occurs late and represents loss of compensatory mechanisms. Thus, waiting for hypotension to occur before treating hypovolemic shock is an error because end-organ hypoperfusion must have already occurred.

Obstructive Shock

Obstructive shock, unlike cardiogenic shock, is due to extracardiac causes of cardiac pump failure, and includes pulmonary vascular and mechanical causes. Examples of pulmonary vascular aetiologies include pulmonary embolism or severe pulmonary hypertension. Mechanical causes include restrictive cardiomyopathies, pericardial tamponade, or tension pneumothorax. From a peripheral vascular perspective, obstructive shock resembles cardiogenic shock. In the diagnostic separation of the two aetiologies, echocardiographic analysis is often definitive. Although not described in the chapter, point-of-care echocardiography is a powerful tool in the assessment of cardiogenic and obstructive shock aetiologies.

Measuring Cardiac Output

CO is stroke volume multiplied by the heart rate and is the volume of blood ejected by the heart every minute. It is a critical measure of cardiovascular health. There are multiple methodologies for measuring CO that are presently being used and which the clinician needs to be aware. Adolf Eugen Fick was the first to estimate CO in 1870 using the principle of conservation of mass. His logic, known today as the 'Fick principle', states that the amount of oxygen, which is added or removed from the organ, is equal to the difference between the amount brought into the organ and the amount carried away from the organ. Oxygen consumption (VO_2) may also be calculated to measure CO with the following equation:

$$VO_2 = CO \times Ca - CO \times Cv.$$

$$CO = VO_2 / (Ca - Cv)$$

where Ca is the amount of O_2 from the arterial blood and Cv is the amount of O_2 in the mixed systemic venous blood. Thus, by measuring the arterial and mixed venous O_2 contents and measuring VO_2 at the mouth, Fick could calculate CO. Since that time, the Fick approach has been largely abandoned in favour of simpler and more rapid techniques, which is described below.

Echocardiography

Echocardiography can be performed both using a probe placed on the chest wall and abdomen, called transthoracic echocardiography (TTE), or from a probe inserted into the oesophagus, called transoesophageal echocardiography (TOE). TTE is a safe procedure but is limited by not always allowing proper imaging of the intrathoracic structures. TOE is an invasive medical procedure used as a diagnostic tool for assessing cardiac function and abnormalities in intubated patients.[7] TOE gives very clear echo images of cardiac structures and can measure pulmonary and aortic flows using the Doppler technique. TOE has rare but potentially life-threatening complications. It can be used to quickly identify cardiac causes of hypotension in the critically ill patient.

Among the multiple haemodynamic markers echocardiography can estimate, CO is an important one. With TOE, stroke volume may be estimated by the Doppler-derived pulmonary artery, aortic, and mitral flow signals. The principle is based on the fact that the velocity–time integral (VTI) of blood flow times the cross-sectional area of the conduit estimates stroke volume (Figure 17.4). A VTI is measured as the integral of all of the velocities during a specified time across a conduit as defined as the region of interest window. During this flow period, the Doppler will measure all velocities along its scan line or at the location of the sample volume. The integral of all these velocities yields the VTI. If the cross-sectional area of the conduit in question is known, then the stroke volume through that conduit may be calculated. VTI can also be estimated using a simple handheld echo-Doppler device (USCOM, Sydney, Australia). This device is limited in only making flow measures, but its portability and ease of use make it an attractive spot method to estimate CO.

The most important limiting factor in calculating the stroke volume using the VTI signal is the estimation of vessel cross-sectional area. Since area is calculated as radius squared, and CO is heart rate times stroke volume, small errors in the estimation of diameter result in large errors of stroke volume and CO estimations.

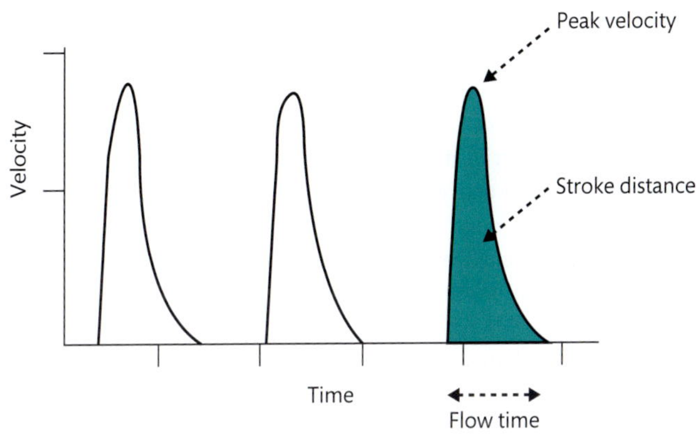

Figure 17.4 Graphic illustration of waveforms developed from Doppler echocardiography. In order to estimate stroke volume from Doppler, the volume time integral (VTI) is multiplied by the cross-sectional area of the conduit. The VTI is calculated by the area under the velocity–time curve of a waveform (as highlighted by the shaded area on a waveform in the illustration).

CO calculation is only accurate in non-regurgitant valves as a diseased valve can falsely elevate CO calculation. Furthermore, in conditions where the heart rate is variable, such as that of atrial fibrillation, one estimation of stroke volume may not accurately depict CO. In these cases, it is important to use an average stroke volume calculation multiplied by an average heart rate to produce a more reliable CO.

Pulsed Oesophageal Doppler

Oesophageal Doppler monitoring measures the descending aortic flow using an indwelling specialized oesophageal Doppler probe. It is a quick and simple method for estimating CO that requires a relatively short period of training and takes minutes to insert and perform.[8] Based on the size and shape of the produced waveforms, clinicians may infer relative contractility, preload and afterload states allowing them to guide therapy, especially when ventilator settings are changed.[9] In 1971, Side and Gosling used a 1 cm diameter oesophageal probe emitting continuous wave Doppler and recorded velocity waveforms of blood flow in the aortic arch. The oesophageal Doppler devices display a velocity–time waveform in real time when inserted in the oesophagus at the mid-thoracic level parallel to the descending thoracic aorta. The area under the waveform (the VTI or 'stroke distance') is proportional to blood flow travelling down the descending thoracic aorta. If the assumption is made that the aortic diameter changes little during systole, then the waveform area is proportional to LV stroke volume.

Other components of the waveform may be measured to assess other haemodynamic biomarkers. For example, peak velocity and acceleration may provide information on left ventricular contractility. A positive inotrope would increase both peak velocity and acceleration, while myocardial depression resulting from cardiodepressant drugs or ischaemia would reduce both variables. The flow time, defined as the base of the waveform, is affected by the heart rate. The corrected flow time is inversely related to SVR. Figure 17.5 illustrates the oesophageal Doppler waveform and its various components.

The oesophageal Doppler device has limitations. This technique assumes that (1) the angle of ultrasound beam to the blood flow direction is the same as that of the transducer and probe, (2) there is a defined amount of blood travelling caudally and not in the cephalad direction, and (3) it is assumed that aortic diameter minimally changes (as changes in diameter is associated with stroke volume changes).[10] Furthermore, this procedure is operator dependent and continuous monitoring is difficult for long-term placement. It is even more difficult in the awake and non-intubated patient. Adverse events and morbid complications are otherwise rare.

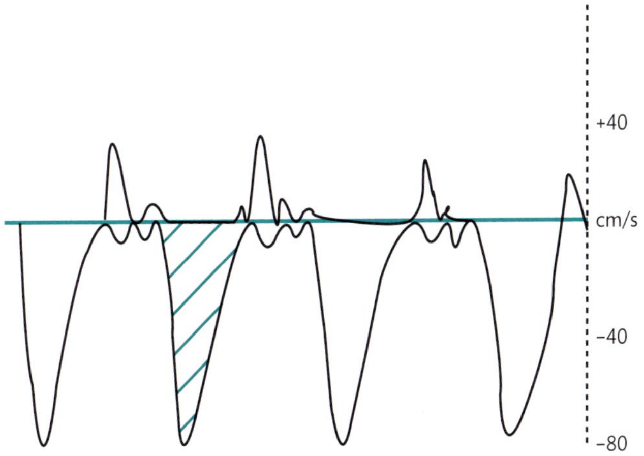

Figure 17.5 Graphic illustration of waveforms derived from oesophageal Doppler. The device displays a velocity–time waveform in real time when it is inserted in the oesophagus at the mid-thoracic level parallel to the descending thoracic aorta. The stroke distance (or velocity–time integral) is the area under the waveform and is proportional to blood flow travelling down the aorta. This area is proportional to left ventricular stroke volume if the assumption is made that aortic diameter minimally changes. The peak velocity provides information regarding contractility and the flow time is inversely related to systemic vascular resistance.

Arterial Pulse Pressure Waveform Analysis

Given the complications associated with PAC placement, other less invasive means have been developed to measure CO. The arterial waveform is commonly measured in critically ill patients and, as described above, can be done either non-invasively or using arterial catheterization.[11] Waveform analysis allows for the calculation of various haemodynamic parameters, including pulse pressure variation, LV stroke volume, stroke volume variation, CO, and arterial resistance.[1,12] This technique has gained a large interest in the evaluation and management of critically ill patients at risk for haemodynamic collapse.

The pulse contour method for estimating CO is based on the principle that arterial pressure and its pulse pressure are a function of LV stroke volume and heart rate. These interactions were understood since 1904 but finally quantified by Remington et al. in 1944. In 2001, the first commercial pulse contour analysis algorithm for CO calculation was developed. This study compared measured CO from pulse contour analysis to that of thermodilution and concluded that the former can estimate CO accurately. The premise of pulse contour analysis is that pulse pressure depends upon the amount of blood ejected into the aorta. The relationship, however, between pulse pressure and stroke volume is complex as the magnitude of pulse pressure given a stroke volume depends on aortic compliance, which in itself varies in a non-linear way, and arterial elastance, which is the non-linear viscoelastic property of the large arterial walls. Finally, pulse wave reflection can markedly alter the observed arterial pulse pressure. For all these reasons, external calibration of the arterial pressure contour analysis always results in more accurate estimates of CO.

Importantly, changes in pulse pressure proportionately reflect changes in LV stroke volume when the resistance and compliance of the arterial tree and blood components remain constant. This condition is present on a beat-to-beat basis such that pulse pressure variation tracks stroke volume variation. The major advantage of pulse contour analysis over PAC-based monitoring is that it is less invasive and carries fewer complications. Disadvantages include its sensitivity to changes in vascular compliance, over- and under-dampening of the arterial pressure waveforms will decrease precision, and some pathologies such as aortic regurgitation may further decrease accuracy.

Several companies have now introduced their own pulse contour analysis algorithms that estimate CO to a similar degree. They include, in order of appearance, PiCCO (Getinge, Sweden), LiDCOplus (Masimo Medical, Irvine, CA), FloTrac (Edwards Lifesciences, Irvine, CA), and MostCare (Vytech, Padua, Italy). These commercially available devices use proprietary algorithms that analyse pulse contour of the arterial pressure waveform to estimate CO. Each device differs in its requirements for calibration. These devices need to be calibrated based on patient's blood pressure, age, sex, and height. Although they use slightly different approaches, their common estimates of CO appear to display the same level of accuracy and variance, making the choice of which to use based on issues of ease of use and availability.[13]

PiCCO

The PiCCO device utilizes an algorithm that analyses the pulse contour and integrates the area under the systolic portion of the curve and divides this by the aortic compliance. PiCCO uses transpulmonary thermodilution for calibration. To accomplish this, 20 mL of cold saline is injected via a central vein and the thermal profile is reported in a large artery (may not use the radial artery, but the femoral, axillary, and brachial arteries may be used). This needs to be calibrated every 8 h. The device allows measurement of the CO, stroke volume variation, and the pulse pressure variation. The limitations to this device include multiple recalibration requirements and diminished accuracy in the hypothermic patient.

LiDCOplus

The LiDCOplus uses pulse power analysis to provide continuous CO data. It converts the arterial waveform into a volume–time waveform and uses autocorrection to determine the stroke volume. Calibration of this device requires a lithium transpulmonary dilution technique. Because lithium is used, calibration is not affected by coadministration of room temperature or cold fluids. Furthermore, the radial artery may be utilized for measurement. This device also allows measurements of CO, stroke volume variation, and pulse pressure variation.

FloTrac

The FloTrac, also known as the 'Vigileo', is another device that utilized pulse contour analysis to assess various haemodynamic variables. The FloTrac probe requires a separate device to do this called the 'Vigileo monitor', and therefore, their names are often times used synonymously—even though they are not the same thing. Unlike the previous devices discussed, this device does not require calibration to correct CO and therefore can easily be and quickly attached to an arterial line and ready to measure CO. Vigileo uses pressure recording analytical method (PRAM) systems, which involve an algorithm developed for arterial waveform analysis without external calibration. The reliability of uncalibrated devices, in general, is debated in literature more than that of calibrated devices.[12] The reliability of FloTrac/Vigileo diminishes if there are extensive vasomotor tone changes. In any case, it has been shown that surgical complications are reduced when utilizing measured stroke volume variation (SVV) and pulse pressure variation (PPV) from Vigileo.[14] Other devices that do not require calibration include LiDCOrapid, ProAQT/Pulsioflex, and MostCare.

MostCare

The MostCare PRAM monitors in real-time CO using a proprietary algorithm that takes into account the area under the systolic part of the arterial pressure curve and the MAP based on PRAM systems. It requires an extremely high data sampling rate (~600 Hz), but has as its advantage in that it does not require external calibration.

In summary, the calibrated devices tend to give more accurate data but often are more invasive. Because non-calibrated devices may be less accurate in patients with extensive vasomotor tone changes, they are likely more useful in healthier subjects. In addition, they are more quickly able to set up and less expensive.[15]

Pulmonary Artery Catheter (Thermodilution)

CO measured by thermodilution from a PAC is considered by regulatory agencies as the gold standard for measuring CO, and it is the most common tool for measuring cardiac output intraoperatively.[4] It has a declining utilization in the intensive care unit due to evidence demonstrating risk outweighing the benefits.[16] Still, there is no single monitoring device with such an array of potential physiologic parameters that it can provide to the clinician (Table 17.2).

In order to measure CO, the PAC uses a thermodilution technique. Fegler first described the use of thermodilution for estimating CO. The technique was further refined by Ganz et al.[17] The PAC has a thermistor located 4 cm from the tip and a proximal port 30 cm from the tip. An injection bolus is delivered, and the thermal profile or semi-random intermittent thermal pulses from the upstream thermistor detects changes and allows continuous CO measurement. The bolus consists of a cold saline sample of known amount and temperature. Some limitations of this technique include the following cases: blood flow variations will affect CO measurement as this technique measures pulmonary blood flow over a short-defined period of time; ventilator cycle-specific patterns has an effect on the measurement; and measurements may be inaccurate in the setting of tricuspid regurgitation (which can be identified by observing the respiratory-cycle-specific prominent v-wave in the right atrial pressure tracing). In the setting of tricuspid regurgitation, measurements of CO via thermodilution may be overestimated. If measured randomly, measurements of pulmonary blood flow may be accurate. Furthermore, CO can be estimated continuously by providing a continuous cold infusion upstream from the sensing thermistor.

Another continuous technique involves a thermal filament or thermal coil that warms blood in the superior vena cava (SVC) and

Table 17.2 Possible haemodynamic measurements derived from a pulmonary artery catheter*

Haemodynamic biomarker	Method of measurement
Cardiac output	Bolus or continuous thermodilution
Central venous pressure	Pressure waveform measured at most proximal port
Pulmonary arterial pressure	Pressure waveform measured at most distal port
Pulmonary artery occlusion pressure	Balloon occlusion stop flow pulmonary artery pressure
Right ventricular pressures	Pressure in the right ventricle during insertion or withdrawal
Mixed venous oxyhaemoglobin saturation	O_2 measurement from the most distal port without occlusion
Systemic vascular resistance	SVR = 80 × (MAP – CVP)/CO
Pulmonary vascular resistance	PVR = 80 × (mean PAP – Ppao)/CO
Left ventricular stroke work index	LVSWI = [MAP – Ppao] × SVI × 0.136
Right ventricular stroke work index	RVSWI = [mean PAP – CVP] × SVI × 0.136
Cardiac index	CI = CO/body surface area
Stroke volume	SV = CO/HR
Stroke volume index	SVI = CI/HR
Right ventricular ejection fraction	RVef = 1 – residual indicator during bolus thermal injection
Right ventricular end-diastolic volume	RV EDV = SV/RVef
Oxygen delivery	DO_2 = CO × Hbg ×S aO_2 × 1.39
Oxygen consumption	VO_2 = CO × Hbg × (SaO_2 – SvO_2) × 1.39

*Arterial oxygen saturation (SaO_2) and haemoglobin (Hbg) levels can be estimated non-invasively using a pulse oximeter. All other variables can be measured directly from the pulmonary artery catheter.

Abbreviations: SVR, systemic vascular resistance; MAP, mean arterial pressure; RA, right atrium; PA-C, pulmonary artery catheter; CVP, central venous pressure; CO, cardiac output; LVSWI, left ventricular stroke work index; PVR, pulmonary vascular resistance; Ppao, pulmonary artery occlusion pressure; SV, stroke volume; SVI, stroke volume index; PAP, pulmonary artery pressure; RVSWI, right ventricular stroke work index; CO, cardiac output; CI, cardiac index; RVef, right ventricular ejection fraction; RV EDV, right ventricular end-diastolic volume; DO_2, oxygen delivery; Hbg, haemoglobin; SaO_2, arterial O_2 saturation; VO_2, oxygen consumption; SvO_2, mixed venous oxygen saturation.

measures changes in the blood temperature at the PAC tip using the thermistor. Average values are taken over the previous 10 min. Continuous CO monitoring technique has largely replaced the intermittent bolus technique. In addition, PAC can estimate RV end-diastolic volume and ejection fraction, LV stroke work, pulmonary vascular resistance, PAP, CVP, pulmonary artery occlusion pressure, and SvO_2.

Measurement of Extravascular Lung Water

Extravascular lung water (EVLW) values include all fluid within the lung that is outside of the pulmonary vasculature, which includes fluid residing in the interstitial and alveolar spaces. The pathophysiology of pulmonary oedema formation includes that of increased lung endothelial and epithelial permeability or increased hydrostatic pressure in the pulmonary capillaries, or a combination of both. Measurements of EVLW coupled to measures of filling pressures would identify the presence or absence of oedema and then its presumed aetiology. For example, if EVLW were elevated in the setting of low filling pressures, it would suggest primary pulmonary oedema (i.e. capillary leak), whereas high filling pressure would suggest secondary pulmonary oedema (i.e. hydrostatic). ARDS and septic shock patients often have high EVLW values and low filling pressures.

Chest radiograph is a common diagnostic tool in determining presence of lung water; however, it is extremely insensitive to determining the quantity of water and there is considerable inter-observer variability. The gold standard for measuring EVLW is an ex vivo method termed gravimetry.[18] This involves measuring the difference in the lung weight before and after drying out. Other methodologies include estimation of water via computed tomography or magnetic resonance imaging. Of course, this would be an expensive and cost-ineffective method if repeated measurements are required.

Transpulmonary Thermodilution

To perform this technique, the patient requires central venous access with the catheter tip in the SVC and a thermistor-tipped arterial catheter usually placed in the femoral artery. A cold indicator and a colorimetric indicator are injected simultaneously. The thermal marker equilibrates with fluid volumes in both the intravascular and extravascular spaces while the dye remains intravascular, measuring total thoracic blood volume. The difference between the two values is EVLW.[18] The downside of this technique is its high cost of using two indicators and two separate sensing devices.

To address this concern, a simplified approach was developed. This also requires central venous access with the tip in the SVC and a thermistor-tipped arterial catheter (which can be placed in the femoral, axillary, brachial, or radial arteries). A cold injectate is delivered via the central line, and subsequently the thermistor-tipped arterial catheter detects the change in blood temperature and creates a thermodilution curve. The EVLW is estimated from the thermodilution curve based on the Stewart-Hamilton and Newman principles. This technique has been demonstrated to be correlated with values determined by the thermo-dye dilution technique and gravimetry after autopsy.[19] The two transpulmonary thermodilution devices that are currently commercially available include $PICCO_2$ (Getinge, Sweden) and VolumeView/EV 1000 (Edwards Lifesciences, Irvine, CA, USA). There are some limitations with the transpulmonary thermodilution technique. The accuracy of EVLW measurement depends on the volume of distribution of the cold indicator, which essentially means that well perfused areas would get preferential distribution than other regions. EVLW may be overestimated in patients with lung resections.

Indirect Estimations of Volume Overload

The utilization of biomarkers, such as brain natriuretic peptide (BNP), has also been used to clinically assess patients in decompensated heart failure to assess functional volume status. Additionally, BNP levels have correlated with lung water in these patients.[20] This peptide is a 32-amino acid polypeptide that is secreted by the ventricles of the heart in response to excessive stretching of the cardiomyocytes. The main clinical utility of measuring BNP is that normal serum levels essentially rule out acute decompensation of heart failure. However, BNP has low specificity as the sole determinant of diagnosing decompensated heart failure. A BNP <100 pg/mL indicates a low likelihood of acute heart failure, whereas values >400 pg/mL suggests it as a likely diagnosis, and there is a linear correlation between BNP levels and mortality. When determining cause of pulmonary oedema in patients in respiratory failure, higher BNP levels were associated with a cardiogenic or hydrostatic oedema cause than that of acute lung injury.[21] When determining cause of pleural effusions, BNP levels in the pleural fluid are higher in those with heart failure as the cause. Furthermore, the combined use of BNP and impedance cardiography during the first assessment of a patient in heart failure identified those with a worse prognosis. The downside of measuring BNP for assessing heart failure progression is that it is not a continuous monitor but rather data that must be routinely collected with a delay of up to 60 min for results.

Functional Haemodynamic Monitoring

Since the goal in haemodynamic monitoring is not just to identify a problematic haemodynamic process, but also to predict how patients would respond to a therapeutic action. Knowing if a patient is volume-responsive is very useful information. During positive-pressure breathing, cyclic changes on venous return occur owing to the associated dynamic inspiration-induced increases in intrathoracic pressure.

The best way to predict how the body will adapt to an intervention is not from a static view of haemodynamics, but to see how it responds to a defined extrinsic stress.[22] Functional haemodynamic monitoring involves the repeated measurement of cardiovascular variables in response to a defined and quantifiable physiological perturbation. Examples of perturbations shown to identify volume responsiveness include a fluid challenge, a passive leg raising manoeuvre, positive-pressure ventilation-induced changes in arterial pulse pressure and LV stroke volume, changes in CVP in response to changes in intrathoracic pressure during respiration, and a vascular occlusion test.

The Fluid Challenge

The traditional approach to assess volume responsiveness is to infuse a small fluid bolus rapidly and see if the cardiovascular response is positive. If there were a positive response, one would expect an increase in arterial pressure, CO or SvO_2, or a decrease in the heart rate. The main goal in the fluid challenge is to see if blood flow improves with volume loading. If there is an improvement, then the patient must be resuscitated with fluids.

There are a few disadvantages in using fluid challenges to identify fluid responsiveness. First, only half of all haemodynamically unstable patients will be volume responders.[23] If a volume challenge is given to a non-volume responder, intravascular volume overload may occur. For all these reasons, it would be preferable to have a simple and rapid way of assessing volume responsiveness without giving a fluid challenge.

Passive Leg Raising Manoeuvre

The passive leg raise (PLR) causes stored venous blood in the lower extremities to be transferred into the central compartment. If the subject is volume-responsive, then CO will increase, otherwise it will not.[24] The trial starts with the subject supine, and then having the legs passively raised to 30° above the chest and held there for 1–2 min. This approximates a 300 mL fluid bolus in a 70 kg man. If the PLR manoeuvre is sustained, the increased preload lasts for about 2–3 min, after which time blood volume is redistributed back to the venous circuit. PLR is both easy to perform and reversible, thus it imposes no harm from excess fluids, and it can be repeated as many times as necessary to determine the appropriate time to cease volume resuscitation. Because PLR improves venous return by recruiting blood from the splanchnic and lower extremity circulation, it can be falsely negative in the setting of intra-abdominal hypertension.

Arterial Pulse Pressure and LV Stroke Volume Variation

Ventilated patients experience normal variations in CO during the respiratory cycle, which can be exaggerated under hypovolemic conditions. The extent of this variation predicts volume responsiveness. During positive-pressure inspiration, intrathoracic pressure increases CVP, which usually decreases the pressure gradient for venous return. This causes a transient inspiration-associated decrease in venous return to the right heart. This transiently decreases RV stroke volume which, after a few heart beats, decreases LV stroke volume. The magnitudes of the variation in either LV stroke volume or arterial pulse pressure are excellent predictors of volume.

Since the cause of the cyclic changes in LV output is the dynamic change in the pressure gradient of venous return, tidal volume is a primary determinant of this variation. A PPV >13%, or a SVV >10%, in patients receiving tidal volumes of 8 mL/kg accurately predicts preload responsiveness.[25] Both PPV and SVV can be assessed non-invasively using the above-mentioned finger cuff methods. PPV and SVV, unlike PLR changes, in CO can be confounded by a number of factors, including tidal volume, arrhythmias, and vasopressor use. A prudent clinician should become knowledgeable of the uses and limitations of these powerful monitoring techniques and apply them to define fluid responsiveness only in the correct settings.

Inferior Vena Cava and Superior Vena Cava Diameter

The dynamic changes in inferior vena cava (IVC) and SVC diameter have been shown to be highly predictive of volume responsiveness in various clinical scenarios.[22] Ultrasonographic measure of IVC diameter is an alternative method in measuring pulse pressure or LV stroke volume. This is a useful tool in measuring both preload and predicting volume responsiveness in ventilated patients (by measuring respiratory variations).[26] Positive-pressure ventilation increases the intrathoracic pressure, which results in reduced venous return to the right atrium and decreases IVC diameter. In contrast, expiration causes a decrease in intrathoracic pressure which increases venous return and thus increases IVC diameter. Based on this principle, the dynamic change in IVC diameter is greater in patients who are more volume-responsive. This was demonstrated in studies that identified volume-responsive versus non-volume-responsive septic patients.[27] Similarly, dynamic changes in SVC diameter may be used; however, adequate ultrasonographic imaging of this vascular structure is usually only possible with TOE. The threshold SVC collapsibility of 36%, which is calculated as (maximum diameter on expiration – minimum diameter of inspiration)/maximum diameter one expiration, allowed appropriate discrimination of responders and non-responders to volume in septic patients.[28]

Summary

When assessing the cardiovascular function in critically ill patients in respiratory failure, there are a myriad of tools that a clinician may use to determine haemodynamic biomarkers, such as CO, to tailor therapy. Each method has its advantages as well as disadvantages—mainly related to invasiveness of procedure, accuracy, and expense. In any case, it is essential for diagnostic and therapeutic steps. However, none substitute for a thorough knowledge of their technical limitations and the physiologic basic for normal cardiovascular homeostasis and how disease and treatment alter it.

REFERENCES

1. Teboul JL, Saugel B, Cecconi M, De Backer D, Hofer CK, Monnet X, Perel A, Pinsky MR, Reuter DA, Rhodes A, Squara P, Vincent JL, Scheeren TW. Less invasive hemodynamic monitoring in critically ill patients. *Intensive Care Med.* 2016 Sep;**42**(9):1350–1359. doi:10.1007/s00134-016-4375-7. Epub 2016 May 7. PMID: 27155605.
2. Suess EM, Pinsky MR. Hemodynamic monitoring for the evaluation and treatment of shock: What is the current state of the art? *Semin Respir Crit Care Med.* 2015;**36**:890–898.
3. Marik PE, Baram M, Vahid B. Does central venous pressure predict fluid responsiveness? A systematic review of the literature and the tale of seven mares. *Chest.* 2008;**134**:172–178.
4. Hadian M, Pinsky MR. Evidence-based review of the use of the pulmonary artery catheter: Impact data and complications. *Crit Care.* 2006;**10**(Suppl 3):S11–18.
5. Monroe RG, Gamble WJ, LaFarge CG, et al. The Anrep effect reconsidered. *J Clin Invest.* 1972;**51**:2573–2583.
6. Cecconi M, De Backer D, Antonelli M, et al. Consensus on circulatory shock and hemodynamic monitoring. Task force of the European Society of Intensive Care Medicine. *Intensive Care Med.* 2014;**40**:1795–1815.
7. Vignon P. Hemodynamic assessment of critically ill patients using echocardiography Doppler. *Curr Opin Crit Care.* 2005;**11**:227–234.
8. Marquez J, McCurry K, Severyn DA, et al. Ability of pulse power, esophageal Doppler, and arterial pulse pressure to estimate rapid changes in stroke volume in humans. *Crit Care Med.* 2008;**36**:3001–3007.
9. Monnet X, Rienzo M, Osman D, et al. Esophageal Doppler monitoring predicts fluid responsiveness in critically ill ventilated patients. *Intensive Care Med.* 2005;**31**:1195–1201.
10. Monnet X, Chemla D, Osman D, et al. Measuring aortic diameter improves accuracy of esophageal Doppler in assessing fluid responsiveness. *Crit Care Med.* 2007; **35**:477–482.
11. Wesseling KH, Jansen JR, Settels JJ, et al. Computation of aortic flow from pressure in humans using a nonlinear, three-element model. *J Appl Physiol.* 1993;**74**:2566–2573.
12. Esper SA, Pinsky MR. Arterial waveform analysis. *Best Pract Res Clin Anaesthesiol.* 2014;**28**:363–380.
13. Hadian M, Kim H, Severyn DA, et al. Cross-comparison of cardiac output trending accuracy of LiDCO, PiCCO FloTrac and pulmonary artery catheters *Crit Care.* 2010;**14**:R212.
14. Romano SM, Pistolesi M. Assessment of cardiac output from systemic arterial pressure in humans. *Crit Care Med.* 2002;**30**:1834–1841.
15. Benes J, Chytra I, Altmann P, et al. Intraoperative fluid optimization using stroke volume variation in high risk surgical patients: Results of prospective randomized study. *Crit Care.* 2010;**14**:R118.
16. Shah MR, Hasselblad V, Stevenson LW, et al. Impact of the pulmonary artery catheter in critically ill patients: Meta-analysis of randomized clinical trials. *JAMA.* 2005;**294**:1664–1670.
17. Ganz W, Donoso R, Marcus HS, et al. A new technique for measurement of cardiac output by thermodilution in man. *Am J Cardiol.* 1971;**27**:392–396.
18. Lange NR, Schuster DP. The measurement of lung water. *Crit Care.* 1999;**3**:R19–R24.
19. Tagami T, Kushimoto S, Yamamoto Y, Atsumi T, Tosa R, Matsuda K, Oyama R, Kawaguchi T, Masuno T, Hirama H, Yokota H. Validation of extravascular lung water measurement by single transpulmonary thermodilution: human autopsy study. *Crit Care.* 2010;**14**(5):R162. doi:10.1186/cc9250. Epub 2010 Sep 6. PMID: 20819213; PMCID: PMC3219254.
20. Dres M, Teboul JL, Anguel N, et al. Extravascular lung water, B-type natriuretic peptide, and blood volume contraction enable diagnosis of weaning-induced pulmonary edema. *Crit Care Med.* 2014;**42**:1882–1889.
21. Rana R, Vlahakis NE, Daniels CE, et al. B-type natriuretic peptide in the assessment of acute lung injury and cardiogenic pulmonary edema. *Crit Care Med.* 2006;**34**:1941–1946.
22. Pinsky MR. Functional hemodynamic monitoring. *Crit Care Clin.* 2015;**31**:89–111.
23. Michard F, Teboul JL. Predicting fluid responsiveness in ICU patients: A critical analysis of the evidence. *Chest.* 2002;**121**:2000–2008.
24. Monnet X, Rienzo M, Osman D, et al. Passive leg raising predicts fluid responsiveness in the critically ill. *Crit Care Med.* 2006;**34**:1402–1407.

25. Michard F, Boussat S, Chemla D, et al. Relation between respiratory changes in arterial pulse pressure and fluid responsiveness in septic patients with acute circulatory failure. *Am J Respir Crit Care Med.* 2000; **162**:134–138.
26. Pinsky MR. The hemodynamic consequences of mechanical ventilation: An evolving story. *Intensive Care Med.* 1997; **23**:493–503.
27. Barbier C, Loubieres Y, Schmit C, et al. Respiratory changes in inferior vena cava diameter are helpful in predicting fluid responsiveness in ventilated septic patients. *Intensive Care Med.* 2004;**30**:1740–1746.
28. Vieillard-Baron A, Chergui K, Rabiller A, et al. Superior vena caval collapsibility as a gauge of volume status in ventilated septic patients. *Intensive Care Med.* 2004;**30**:1734–1739.

18

Imaging Critically Ill Patients

Arjun Nair

KEY MESSAGES

- Despite its technical limitations, portable chest radiography remains the most vital and convenient form of serial thoracic imaging on the critical care unit.
- CT protocols can be tailored to specific scenarios to (a) guide ventilator strategy, (b) assess underlying causative pathology, (c) assess complications, and (d) aid prognostication.
- Paired low- and high-ventilatory-pressure computed tomographic (CT) imaging is an important component of assessing alveolar recruitment to guide ventilator strategies.
- Ultrasound has gained an invaluable role in the bedside assessment of both pleural and pulmonary pathology in critically ill patients.

CONTROVERSIES

- Newer techniques such as electrical impedance tomography and dual-energy CT, as well as well-developed but less utilized techniques of positron emission tomography and magnetic resonance imaging, provide valuable pathophysiologic insights but are currently mainly confined to research applications.

FURTHER RESEARCH

- Future research should focus on the optimal use of newer imaging techniques in clinical decision making, especially the role of electrical impedance tomography, positron emission tomography, and magnetic resonance imaging of lungs. The ability of data from these techniques to complement and enhance that available from currently standard techniques (plain X-ray, cross-sectional and sonographic imaging) requires evaluation.
- The impact of ultrasound imaging on patient outcomes should be studied in the context of well-conducted trials, to extend data beyond case series and retrospective reports.

Technical Considerations

The principles and techniques of thoracic imaging as a whole are beyond the scope of this chapter and are more comprehensively covered elsewhere.[1] Here, technical aspects of imaging relevant to the critically ill patient are discussed.

Portable Chest Radiography

Portable chest radiography (CXR) is the mainstay of the critical care setting since it is easy to both perform and interpret the examination. Computed radiography (CR) systems, which use a re-usable photostimulable phosphor image receptor plate that functions as a large-area detector within a cassette, are the most widely used portable radiography system. Once processed, the CXR image is transmitted in a Digital Imaging and Communications in Medicine (DICOM) format to a Picture Archiving and Communications System (PACS). However, portable direct radiography (DR) systems, although still quite expensive, are becoming more popular. Such DR systems allow direct transmission of an image to PACS, circumventing the need to process any image receptor plate. They have become increasingly portable by either using DR detectors that are compatible with existing CR cassettes or with wireless flat panel detectors that can transmit images immediately to PACS.

However, there are multiple limitations of the portable CXR. Positioning of bed-bound patients is challenging, leading to inadequate coverage, marked rotation, or poor penetration. The reduced focus–film distance can falsely magnify anatomical structures. High-kilovoltage techniques are not possible since portable machines are unable to deliver such a tube potential. The portable X-ray tube can sustain only a limited current, and so longer exposure times that can potentially increase motion blur artefact are required.

Principles of Thoracic Computed Tomography (CT)

An exhaustive discussion of thoracic CT is beyond the scope of this chapter, but we discuss here the principles and techniques that are relevant to the use of CT in critical care imaging.

CT relies on the concept that the attenuation of X-rays by a given material depends on its density; the higher the density, the greater the attenuation, and vice versa. The CT scanner is fundamentally composed of a rotating gantry with a fan beam X-ray source at one end and a detector bank (or array) at the opposite end; modern CT scanners with dual X-ray sources have recently also been developed to markedly reduce acquisition time. The patient is translated through the ring of the gantry such that X-rays penetrate the patient and are incident on the detectors. The relative energies of the photons incident on the detectors are converted into an image that is a 'map' of different densities, representing the degree of attenuation of the X-rays by the various materials within the scanned volume. These densities are displayed using multiple three-dimensional volumetric pixels, or *voxels*, in the transverse (also termed *axial*) plane and can be reconstructed in any plane on modern CT scanners (see section titled High-resolution, Interspaced, and Volumetric CT).

The density of a material on CT is expressed as its relative difference from the attenuation of water (arbitrarily assigned a value of 0), on a logarithmic scale, called a *CT number* (or Hounsfield number), and expressed in Hounsfield units (HUs). The different densities are displayed on a greyscale, and the available greyscale is adjusted according to the desired structures to be viewed. A particular greyscale setting is termed a *window*. Wider window settings (spreading the greyscale over a wider range of densities) are required for the lung parenchyma, as opposed to narrower windows for the mediastinum.

CT Image Reconstruction and Post-processing

CT raw data is reconstructed by applying appropriate algorithms, sometimes also called 'kernels' or 'filters' by different manufacturers, to the image. Low-spatial-resolution algorithms (so-called 'smooth' or 'soft tissue' algorithms) reduce image noise and improve contrast, at the expense of spatial resolution, while high-spatial-resolution reconstruction algorithms (so-called 'lung' or 'sharp' algorithms) enhance fine structural detail at the expense of increased image noise. Slices of varying thickness can be reconstructed, with thicker slices produced for speedier review and thinner slices reserved for better spatial resolution and multiplanar reconstructions (MPRs) in any plane. As a general rule, the thicker the slice, the higher the contrast resolution, the lower the image noise, and the poorer the spatial resolution.

By and large, transverse datasets are used for CT interpretation, but MPRs and volume-rendered images can be useful for problem-solving, particularly in non-orthogonal planes for identifying line malposition, elucidating the nature of puzzling appearances on transverse CT, understanding the cephalocaudal extents of complex pleural or pulmonary collections, and visualizing skeletal injury (Figure 18.1). Most modern PACS systems can now perform quick MPRs from axial CT datasets.

High-resolution, Interspaced, and Volumetric CT

'High-resolution' CT (HRCT), a technique inextricably associated with thoracic CT, optimizes all three components of resolution—spatial, temporal, and contrast—to provide detailed evaluation of the lung parenchyma. Since the lung is innately a high-contrast structure, contrast resolution can be sacrificed (to a certain extent) for superior spatial resolution; high spatial resolution requires thin sections and a sharp reconstruction algorithm (decreasing the contrast-to-noise ratio for improved spatial resolution). However, optimal temporal resolution requires motion-free imaging, which can only be achieved in suspended respiration. Historically, CT using conventional (one slice at a time) or helical single-slice scanners did not have the ability to obtain thin-section imaging of the entire thorax in one breath-hold. As such, the HRCT technique usually involved an *interspaced acquisition*, where thin sections (0.6–1.2 mm) were performed with a 10 or 20 mm gap in between slices so that respiration/ventilation can be suspended every two to three sections. Such an interspaced technique thus 'samples' 5%–10% of the lung.

Imaging of the critical care patient with single-slice or spiral CT involved performing thick-section (5–10 mm) acquisitions of the whole thorax, termed *volumetric acquisition*, with less spatial resolution. Thin-section HRCT acquisitions through any focal area of abnormality could then be re-acquired. Interspaced HRCT would be performed sparingly since it did not image at least 90% of the lung.

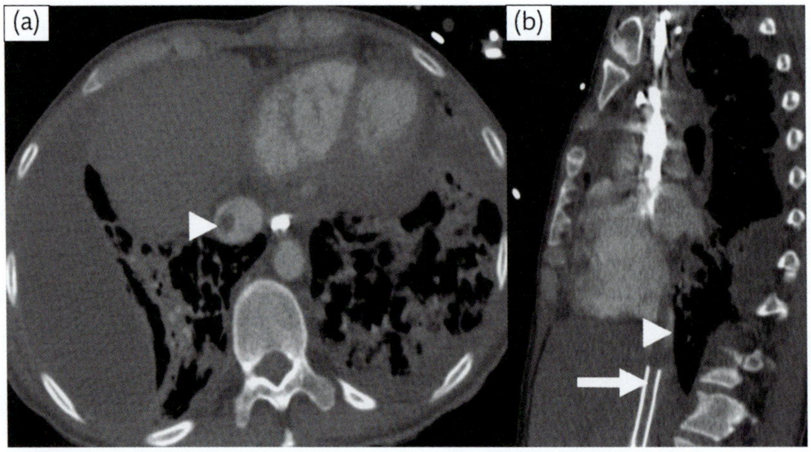

Figure 18.1 (a) Axial contrast-enhanced CT slice demonstrating possible filling defect (arrowhead) that could be misinterpreted as thrombus in the suprahepatic inferior vena cava (IVC). A sagittal reconstruction (b) however reveals that this is a beam-hardening artefact associated with the high density of the extracorporeal membranous oxygenation (ECMO) cannula (white arrow) within the intrahepatic IVC.

However, modern CT scanners—especially those servicing critical care units—will almost certainly be multidetector (MDCT, also called multislice) systems. Such systems, even those with older four-slice detector banks, can acquire volumetric thin-section images through the whole thorax in a single breath-hold or suspended ventilation. These datasets can then be reconstructed as thin-section CTs on both soft and sharp algorithms. In this way, every volumetric acquisition on an MDCT scanner is potentially an 'HRCT' (as long as the appropriate reconstructions are performed), obviating the need to specifically request HRCT when scanning the thorax.

The Role of Intravenous Contrast

HRCT is usually performed without intravenous (IV) iodinated contrast since the lung parenchyma is inherently already high in contrast. However, IV contrast is necessary for the evaluation of vascular structures and is of course mandatory for CT pulmonary angiography or CT aortography. However, IV contrast can spuriously increase lung parenchymal density (Figure 18.2). As increased density may imply worsening inflammation or oedema in acute respiratory distress syndrome (ARDS) or diffuse lung disease, IV contrast can thus confuse interpretation of such areas in the critical care patient. Furthermore, IV contrast may be relatively contraindicated due to renal impairment or a history of allergic reaction.

Suggested CT Protocols in the Critical Care Patient

The initial thoracic CT in critical care settings is usually performed as a volumetric acquisition about 20 s post-IV contrast optimized for evaluation of the pulmonary vasculature, with soft and sharp algorithm reconstructions to evaluate the mediastinum and lung parenchyma, respectively. Subsequent follow-up scans often do not require IV contrast unless vascular complications (e.g. pulmonary embolus) need to be excluded. Certain modifications to technique can be performed:

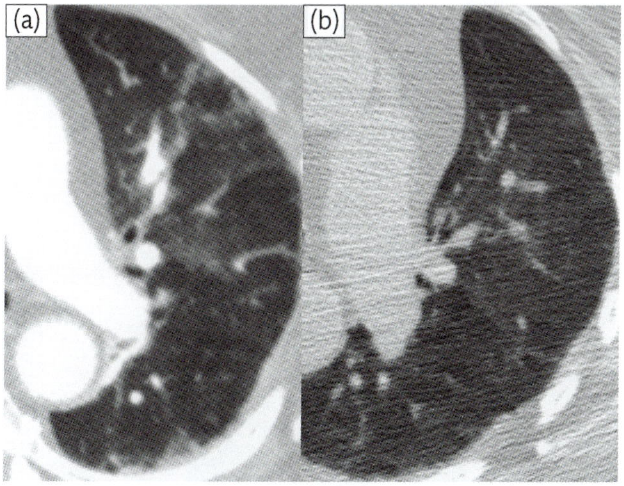

Figure 18.2 Contrast-enhanced CT (a) demonstrating apparently increased and heterogeneous left lung density, which is much less conspicuous on a repeat non-contrast CT (b) performed 5 days later. Whether or not the change in lung density is due to a reduction in pathological ground-glass opacity or simply due to the absence of iodinated contrast is uncertain.

Low- and High-ventilatory-pressure Imaging

Thoracic CT can be performed to assess alveolar recruitment. This involves performing an initial volumetric CT at a high inspiratory plateau pressure (the recruitment manoeuvre), typically 45 cmH_2O, during an end-inspiratory pause, followed by a second acquisition at a positive end-expiratory pressure (PEEP) value of 5 cmH_2O during an end-expiratory pause. Both scans are usually performed without IV contrast.

Imaging Patients on Extracorporeal Membranous Oxygenation (ECMO)

In patients placed on ECMO, baseline CT evaluation is more extensive. Unenhanced CT brain is performed as a baseline since these patients are at risk of intracerebral haemorrhage from the heparin used as an anticoagulant in the ECMO circuit. In addition to post-IV contrast CT thorax, portal venous phase (50–60 s post-contrast) imaging of the abdomen and pelvis is also performed, to assess for any unsuspected intra-abdominal pathology and also to demonstrate the positions of ECMO cannula and femoral lines (Figure 18.1). Paired low- and high-ventilatory-pressure imaging may be performed if safe to do so and is better performed before IV contrast has been administered.

Cardiac Gating

Gating of the CT acquisition to the cardiac cycle, using ECG-gating, to minimize cardiac or vascular motion artefact is not usually performed. However, spurious appearances of aortic dissection due to pulsation artefact on post-contrast CT may necessitate cardiac gating as a problem-solving tool. If CT coronary angiography is required to exclude coronary artery disease in critical care patients that are too unwell for invasive coronary angiography, cardiac gating is of course mandatory.

Radiation Considerations

Radiation dose is measured in a number of ways. To estimate cancer and hereditary detrimental effects, *effective dose* is used. Effective dose is calculated by multiplying the average organ equivalent dose by a tissue weighting factor, summing the doses across the whole body, and averaging for age and sex. It is expressed in sieverts.

A standard CXR has an effective dose of around 0.02–0.1 milisieverts (mSv), equivalent to 3–10 days background radiation. In contrast, a standard volumetric chest CT can have an average dose of 7 mSv, or 2-year background radiation, while an interspaced HRCT has a dose of about 1–2 mSv. These doses reflect averaged values, but actual doses vary depending on patient size and shape and acquisition parameters.

In practice, modern MDCT scanners are equipped with a variety of dose reduction strategies that significantly reduce radiation dose on volumetric CT; effective doses of 1–3 mSv on standard volumetric chest CT are thus now achievable. Nevertheless, when deciding whether to subject a critical care patient to ionizing radiation, particularly for follow-up CT, the 'As Low as Reasonably Achievable' (ALARA) principle of ionizing radiation should be adhered to; that is, all reasonable steps should be taken to administer the lowest possible radiation dose required to obtain a diagnostic examination.

Imaging and Diagnosis in the Mechanically Ventilated Patient

CXR and CT are by far and away the most frequently used imaging modalities to diagnose lung injury and identify its potential causes, whether intra- or extrapulmonary, in the mechanically ventilated patient. Indeed, the diagnosis of ARDS mandates the presence of bilateral opacities, on either CXR or CT, that cannot be entirely attributed to effusions, lobar or whole lung collapse, or nodules.[2] The distribution of such opacities is not specified in the ARDS definition, and it is worth recognizing that different distributions and patterns may signify different underlying aetiology.

Identifying ARDS and Elucidating Its Causes

Irrespective of its underlying cause, ARDS follows the established common pathologic cascade of lung injury, which comprises the familiar sequence of exudative, fibroproliferative, and resolving/organizing phases. CXR and CT both reflect this cascade but to different degrees; given the comprehensively well-established correlations between CT (particularly thin-section CT) and histopathologic patterns, CT appearances unsurprisingly parallel these histopathologic phases more sensitively and contemporaneously than CXR, although all imaging changes can variably lag behind their clinical, functional, and serological counterparts.

CXR

As the exudative phase of ARDS develops (typically over the first 24 h), the CXR may be striking by virtue of its normality unless other causes of direct lung insult, such as pneumonia or massive pulmonary haemorrhage, are responsible (in which case corresponding radiographic opacities may already be immediately present). Over the next 48–72 h, as the proliferative phase leads to a vicious downwards spiral of progressive interstitial and alveolar oedema and inflammation, the CXR progresses from hazy density obscuring lung markings (the radiographic definition of ground-glass opacification) to frank consolidation. Depending on underlying severity, the development of complications, and the success of therapy, the tertiary organizing phase is often accompanied by radiographic improvement, although some abnormalities may persist for days or even weeks. The persistence of some abnormalities such as reticular opacities and cysts may signify the effects of barotrauma or fibrosis, while the sudden development of new areas of consolidation where serial CXRs were hitherto showing progressive improvement should alert one to the possibility of nosocomial pneumonia or aspiration. Regardless, with successful treatment the CXR can return to total normality over the longer term. A 'typical' radiographic sequence is illustrated in Figure 18.3.

CT

To understand the appearances of ARDS on CT, it is imperative to first appreciate what the relevant CT patterns represent at a lobular level. The parenchymal abnormalities seen in the exudative and proliferative phases of lung injury reflect two related phenomena: (1) the loss of aerated lung and (2) an excessive increase in lung tissue, the latter a combination of inflammatory exudate with or without oedema. Consequently, the CT parenchymal patterns that correlate

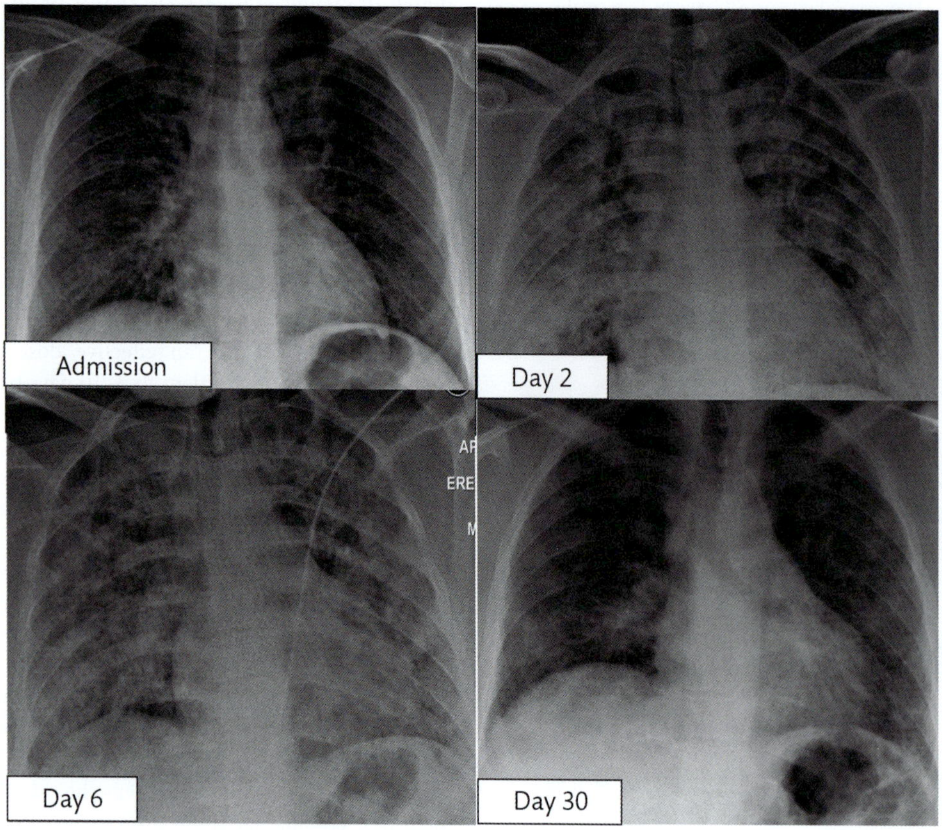

Figure 18.3 Serial chest radiographic progression of ARDS over 6 days with subsequent almost complete resolution by day 30.

with these phenomena are ground-glass opacity (GGO), consolidation, and collapse.

- *GGO* represents, quite simply, partial displacement of air from the pulmonary lobule. It stands to reason that non-pathological GGO could thus be caused by an under-ventilated lobule, for instance, in expiration. Pathologically, GGO could be caused by air being displaced by any other cell within the alveolus (e.g. an intra-alveolar exudate), but it could also be due to the ventilated portion of the lobule becoming proportionally smaller as a result of a thickened interstitium (again due to inflammation and oedema). The CT appearance of GGO is defined by the presence of hazy increased lung attenuation within which the bronchial and vascular margins are still preserved.[3]
- *Consolidation*, on the other hand, represents the total replacement of air from the pulmonary lobule such that it becomes solid and is characterized on CT by increased attenuation which is dense enough to obscure the margins of the bronchial and vascular structures, with or without the presence of an air bronchogram.
- *Collapse* (or atelectasis) represents the total displacement (rather than replacement) of air from the lobule. It is also characterized by an increase in lung attenuation, but will usually be accompanied by the displacement of structures such as the fissures, diaphragm, or airways.

As such, these CT patterns may be seen to different extents within a given patient, depending on the cause and level of severity of ARDS, and of course can vary with ventilation. As with the CXR, overall lung density and the extent of these CT patterns both increase as lung injury progresses from its exudative to its proliferative phases. The morphological changes seen on both CXR and CT may or may not be accompanied by the presence of septal lines (indicating interlobular septal thickening from interstitial oedema) and can be indistinguishable from concurrent pulmonary oedema due to raised pulmonary venous pressure resulting from left-sided cardiac failure.

As CT is usually performed by the time a patient is already in established ARDS, the distribution of these abnormalities is often extensive. However, early studies with CT have played a vital role in demonstrating that the distribution of abnormalities is far from homogeneous in every patient. The 'typical' distribution of ARDS on CT is now well recognized: increasing density in the dependent lung, that is, the dorsal and caudal regions, with often total opacification (a combination of both consolidation and collapse) in the lower lobes and relatively preserved aeration in the upper lobes (Figure 18.4). However, this pattern may only be seen in one-third of patients, with others having a more diffuse or patchy, non-lobar distribution of abnormalities interspersed with normally aerated lung (Figure 18.5). It is important to recognize that in some patients the increased caudal opacification may not be the result of excess (i.e. inflammatory) tissue but purely due to compression (i.e. mechanical) from upward excursion of the diaphragm, increased abdominal pressure (especially in extrapulmonary ARDS), and overall increases in lung and mediastinal (especially cardiac) weight.[4] These differences have implications for ventilation strategies.

It has also been suggested that the extent and distribution of intense parenchymal opacities (in other words, consolidation) may help differentiate pulmonary from extrapulmonary causes of ARDS. An earlier study suggested that consolidation is more extensive in patients with pulmonary causes, while GGO is more extensive in patients with extrapulmonary ARDS, in a head-to-head comparison between the two groups.[5] However, subsequently Desai and colleagues showed that, while non-dependent foci of consolidation were more extensive in patients with pulmonary ARDS, this difference did not persist when adjusted for the duration of disease prior to CT scanning. Nevertheless, it is noteworthy that, in that study, radiologists' impression of whether or not ARDS had a typical pattern had a sensitivity of 72% and a specificity of 69% for diagnosing extrapulmonary ARDS.[6] Such a general impression may thus confer some value in searching for an underlying aetiology and directing therapy when the cause of ARDS is not apparent on initial investigations. Of course, certain ancillary signs may also be highly useful in elucidating the cause of pulmonary ARDS, as shown in Figure 18.6.

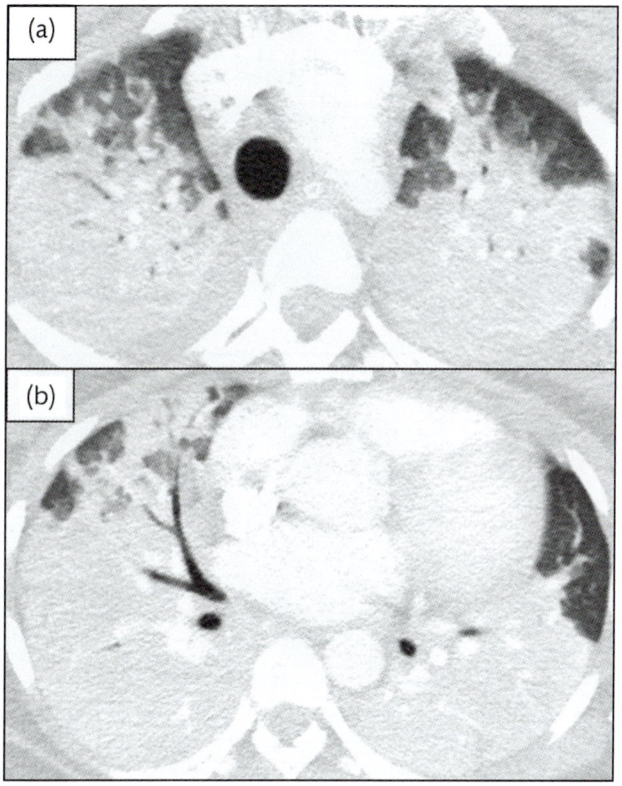

Figure 18.4 'Typical' appearances of ARDS demonstrating increased density in the dorsal (a) and caudal (b) lung compared to the ventral and cranial lungs, respectively.

Given the superior sensitivity of CT to changes in lung injury, it is tempting to conclude that CT should replace the CXR in evaluation of ARDS patients. However, the ease of its acquisition and interpretation, its lower radiation dose, and its ability to demonstrate serial improvement on a day-to-day basis mean that the CXR still retains its place as the first-choice imaging investigation to monitor all patients with ARDS during the acute stage, with CT reserved for problem-solving.

Imaging in Some Specific Critical Care Scenarios

Pulmonary Infection

The type and aetiology of pulmonary infection can determine the patterns and extent of abnormality seen on thoracic CT, which in

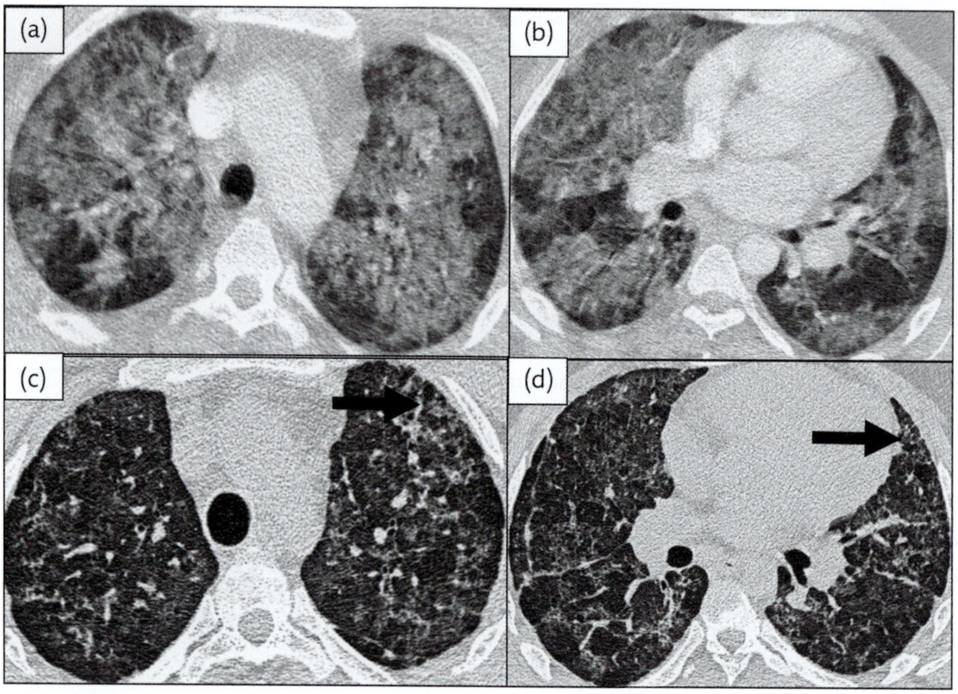

Figure 18.5 Diffuse alveolar damage due to influenza A; 4 days after presentation, extensive patchy ground-glass opacity and consolidation, with no gradient, is seen in the upper (a) and lower (b) lungs; 30 days later, the ground-glass opacity has receded, but there are now areas of coarse reticulation (arrows) suspicious for developing fibrosis (c and d).

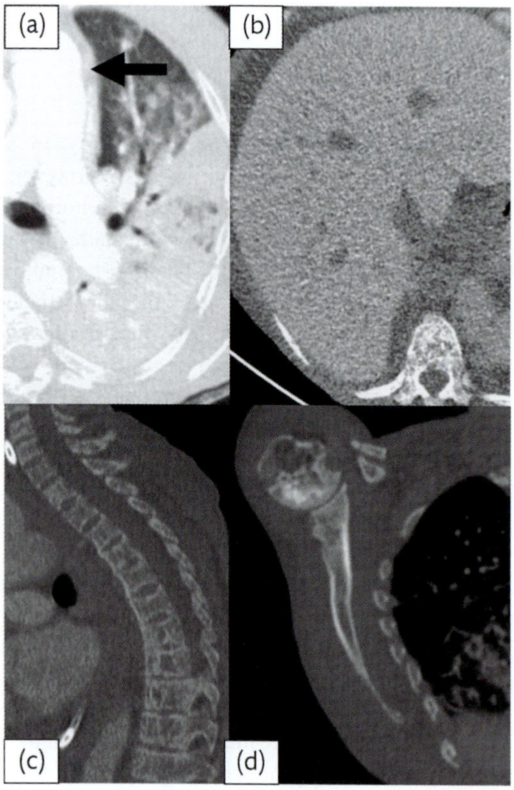

Figure 18.6 Patchy diffuse alveolar damage in a 35-year-old man of African origin. In addition to the diffuse ground-glass opacity and left-sided consolidation (a), note the enlarged pulmonary artery (arrow) implying pulmonary hypertension, very dense liver implying secondary haemochromatosis due to successive blood transfusions in this context (b), vertebral end-plate depression (c), and sclerosis of the right humeral head due to previous avascular necrosis (d), all hallmarks of sickle cell disease; a chest crisis has caused diffuse alveolar damage in this case.

turn lead to non-typical patchy or lobar distributions of parenchymal changes in lung injury. Bacterial or fungal infection may lead to lobar or multifocal consolidation as the predominant feature and, although these foci may be embedded within dependent lung that is already densely opacified (from lung injury itself), they are not infrequently seen in non-dependent lung as well.

It is worth noting that while viral respiratory infections tend to cause centrilobular ground-glass nodularity, influenza A (H1N1) infection is associated with predominantly GGO, either alone or in combination with consolidation.[7] This GGO may be virtually indistinguishable from that caused by lung injury itself, although it can appear more heterogeneous in density (Figure 18.5). Similarly, *Pneumocystis jiroveci* pneumonia can present as diffuse, often perihilar, GGO in the immunocompromised patient with lung injury.

Interstitial Lung Disease (ILD)

All ILDs are susceptible to acute exacerbations that manifest as acute lung injury in combination with their established CT findings. For instance, acute exacerbations of usual interstitial pneumonia (UIP) should be suspected on CT when new patchy GGO is seen, particularly in non-dependent regions, superimposed over the established UIP findings of subpleural, basal-predominant honeycombing, reticulation, and traction bronchiectasis; the basal fibrosis may of course be obscured by the dense parenchymal opacification of lung injury by the time CT is performed. Such acute exacerbation is a diagnosis of exclusion and should only be considered once other causes of GGO such as pulmonary oedema, infection, and pulmonary haemorrhage—all difficult to distinguish from lung injury—have been excluded. Spurious causes of increased lung density, such as imaging being performed post-bronchoalveolar lavage and intravenous contrast, should also have been eliminated.

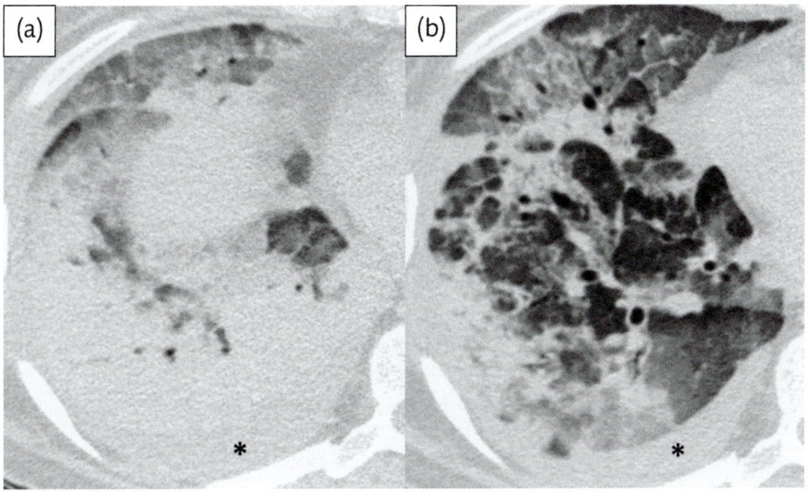

Figure 18.7 Acute interstitial pneumonitis at low (5 cmH_2O) (a) and high (45 cmH_2O) ventilation pressures, demonstrating extensive parenchymal opacification with a patchy but overall increasing ventral to dorsal density gradient. Note the pleural effusion (asterisk).

Acute interstitial pneumonitis (AIP), the idiopathic form of lung injury, is considered an acute ILD and pathologically indistinguishable from the diffuse alveolar damage (DAD) seen in ARDS (Figure 18.7). Acute lung injury may also be the first presentation of an autoimmune disease; such patients, even if not meeting criteria for a defined connective tissue disease, may still be classified as having interstitial pneumonitis with autoimmune features (IPAFs).[8] In this regard, the identification of CT features of organizing pneumonia (OP), such as the perilobular pattern,[9] may reinforce the need to look for an autoimmune aetiology that could potentially be immunomodulated. Such patterns may also become only more prominent on high-pressure ventilation imaging (Figure 18.8). It should be stressed that evidence for this approach is thus far anecdotal, and the ability of CT to distinguish between OP associated with an autoimmune signal and OP associated with lung injury/DAD itself is probably, at best, extremely limited.

Trauma

Penetrating thoracic trauma manifests as various combinations of skeletal injury, pneumothorax, pneumomediastinum, and disruption of mediastinal, particularly vascular, structures. A flail segment—that is, fractures of at least three contiguous ribs in at least two locations, leading to paradoxical chest wall motion on ventilation—should carefully be sought on CT, especially multiplanar reconstructions (MPR), as they can influence mechanical ventilation strategies.

Blunt trauma to the chest, particularly acceleration–deceleration injury, can also be associated with vascular injuries, particularly aortic disruption at the aortic isthmus. However, it is often associated with pulmonary contusions and lacerations, and such trauma is a risk factor for ARDS. Pulmonary contusions occur when traumatic injury to alveoli causes alveolar haemorrhage but leaves the wall intact and may be coup (at the site of impact) or contrecoup (opposite to the site of impact). Contusions manifest as ill-defined non-segmental areas of consolidation or GGO and are thus difficult to distinguish from the early phases of ARDS.

Lacerations, on the other hand, involve tearing of the lung parenchyma; normal pulmonary elastic recoil causes lung tissue

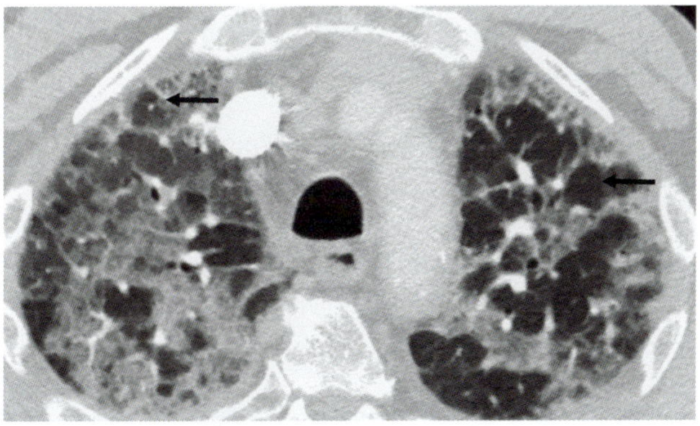

Figure 18.8 Diffuse alveolar damage in a previously well patient with no stigmata of connective tissue disease but positive anti-Jo1 antibodies, suggesting an interstitial pneumonitis with autoimmune features (IPAF) phenotype. Note the extensive perilobular pattern (exemplified by arrows) that are associated with organising pneumonia.

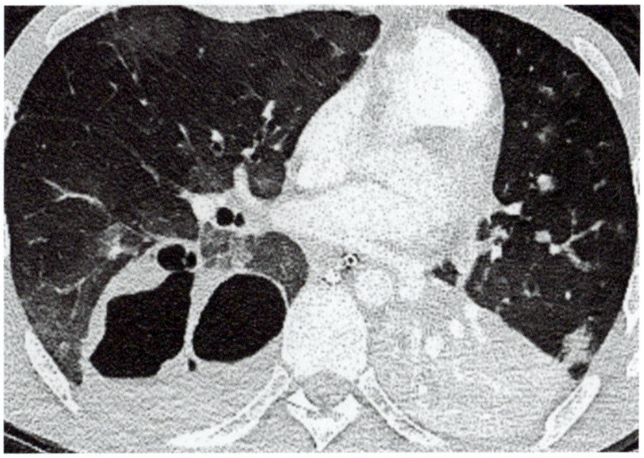

Figure 18.9 Multiloculated thick-walled cysts in the right lower lobe containing dependent high-density fluid, consistent with lacerations, as well as patchy ground-glass opacity due to aspirated blood from haemoptysis, following a fall from a moped.

Table 18.1 Complications assessed on CXR and CT

Complication	Remarks
Pneumothorax	Can be extremely difficult to detect on supine portable CXR, suggested only by increased translucency of hemithorax (Figure 18.10). CT can demonstrate complex pneumothorax and possibly identify alveolo-pleural or bronchopleural fistulae
Pneumomediastinum/pneumopericardium	Can be suspected on semi-recumbent CXR by the presence of a continuous diaphragm sign (Figure 18.11)
Pulmonary embolism	CT pulmonary angiography required but may also be incidentally detected on standard post-contrast CT
Line malposition	CXR usually sufficient to detect line position; CT reserved for exploring line position in more detail, for example, whether intercostal drain tip is abutting mediastinum or diaphragm
Lung necrosis and abscess	Difficult to distinguish from consolidation on CXR unless cavitating; on CT, can still be difficult to ascertain if a thoracic collection represents a pulmonary abscess or empyema, as localizing the collection to the parenchymal or pleural space can be challenging (Figure 18.12)
Occult haemorrhage	May occur due to heparinization used for anticoagulation in extracorporeal membranous oxygenation (ECMO); commonly occurs at catheter insertion and intracranial or gastrointestinal sites. Non-contrast followed by arterial (20 s post-contrast) and delayed (60–100 s post-contrast) phase CT may be required to demonstrate bleeding source

to retract from the tear, resulting in a cavity that may fill with blood or fluid.[10] These cavities are thin-walled and as such can be difficult to distinguish from barotrauma cysts on imaging alone. However, barotrauma cysts would usually not be present on an initial CT, unless the patient had already been on mechanical ventilation for some time prior to CT, while lacerations are readily visible on admission CT (Figure 18.9). Lacerations are often surrounded by contusions and can be associated with haemoptysis; in such cases, the CT appearances may be complicated by airspace opacification from re-aspirated blood products.

Visualizing Complications

Both CXR and CT are integral to visualizing various iatrogenic and disease-related complications, many of which can be clinically insidious. Some of these complications are summarized in Table 18.1. (Figures 18.10, 18.11 and 18.12 illustrate the radiographic appearance of these complications.)

Imaging in Therapeutics and Prognostication

In addition to diagnosing ARDS, determining underlying aetiology, and visualizing complications, numerous radiologic-functional and radiologic-pathologic insights (primarily from CT) have been gleaned over the past three decades. While an exhaustive discussion of these insights is beyond the scope of this chapter, the interested reader is directed to comprehensive reviews on this subject.[11–13] Collectively, these insights have augmented the role of imaging in helping to potentially (1) decide the best ventilation strategy, (2) assess longitudinal progression of lung injury, and (3) provide prognostic information, in mechanically ventilated patients.

Determining Ventilation Strategies

CT is very useful in assessing whether or not recruitment manoeuvres with PEEP are likely to succeed. On paired CTs performed at low and high PEEP, alveolar recruitment can be defined either (1) as a reduction in non-aerated lung during increased PEEP or (2) more widely as an increase in gas volume in both poorly aerated and non-aerated lungs (Figure 18.13). Although quantification

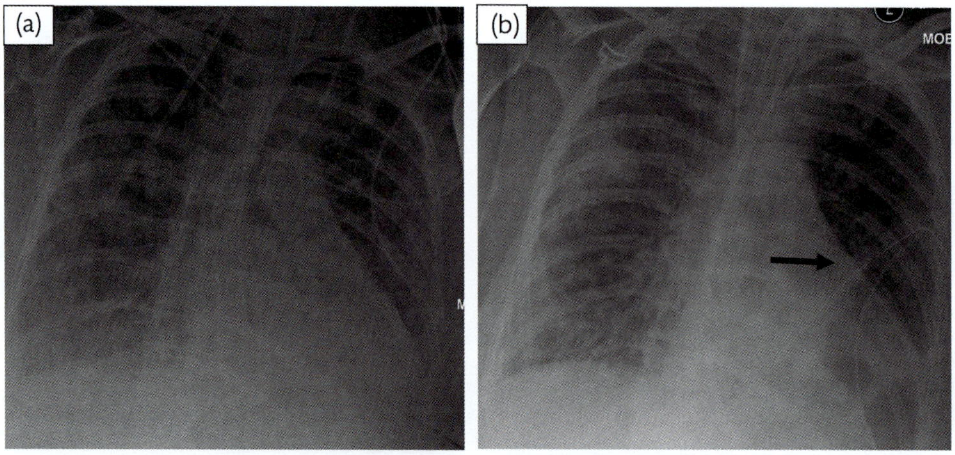

Figure 18.10 Diagnosing a pneumothorax on a supine CXR is difficult. (A) Supine CXR demonstrates only subtly increased translucency in the left hemithorax, in addition to left basal retrocardiac airspace opacity. Such an appearance raises the suspicion of a pneumothorax as the intrapleural air rises anteriorly. However, rotation may also cause such a spurious appearance. (B) Subsequent supine CXR demonstrates increased translucency in the left lung, following confirmation of a pneumothorax with ultrasound. A left intercostal drain (arrow) has now been inserted.

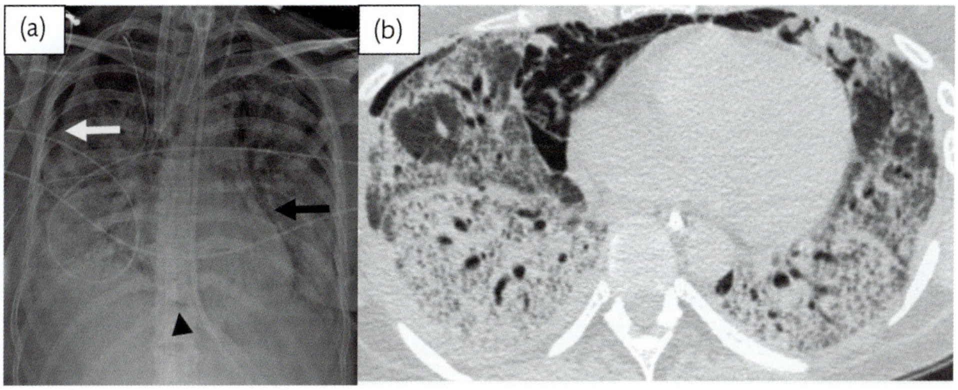

Figure 18.11 (a) Portable erect CXR demonstrates a right pneumothorax (white arrow) in addition to a pneumomediastinum, characterized by increased lucency along the left cardiomediastinal contour (black arrow) and air between the pericardium and the diaphragm, giving rise to the 'continuous diaphragm' sign (arrowhead). (b) Ct confirms the pneumothorax and pneumomediastinum, in addition to a 'crazy paving' pattern of diffuse alveolar damage in this case.

of these abnormalities is software-, time-, and labour-intensive, simple qualitative visual assessment can be just as powerful, reproducible, and easy to perform.[14] The parenchymal abnormality in a recruitable region of lung decreases in density: dense parenchymal opacification (either consolidation or collapse) changes to GGO, and GGO becomes less intense and may even revert to normal lung density. However, increased PEEP can also cause undesirable overdistension of normal lung, a potential risk factor for barotrauma and thus ventilator-induced lung injury (VILI). Detrimental effects of high PEEP on cardiac preload and right ventricular (RV) function should also be considered.

The regional distribution of abnormalities on CT can indicate whether or not the lung is likely to respond to recruitment manoeuvres using PEEP and prone positioning. CT scans that show diffuse attenuation demonstrate the greatest alveolar recruitment without alveolar overdistension, while those with lobar attenuation demonstrate the least recruitment with a propensity towards overdistension of normal lung exclusively in the upper lobes; patients with patchy attenuation have relatively intermediate volumes of recruitment and overdistension.[15,16] By implication, patients with diffuse increased attenuation are more likely to respond to PEEP recruitment manoeuvres without the danger of overdistension, while PEEP is unlikely to confer benefit in patients with lobar or focal abnormality, especially if the increased abnormality is due to compression atelectasis rather than an inflammatory exudate. In the latter group of patients, prone positioning may hypothetically be more beneficial, although as yet the benefit of CT-derived morphological classification to predict response to prone positioning in ARDS, let alone the benefit of prone positioning at all,[17] has not been convincingly proven.

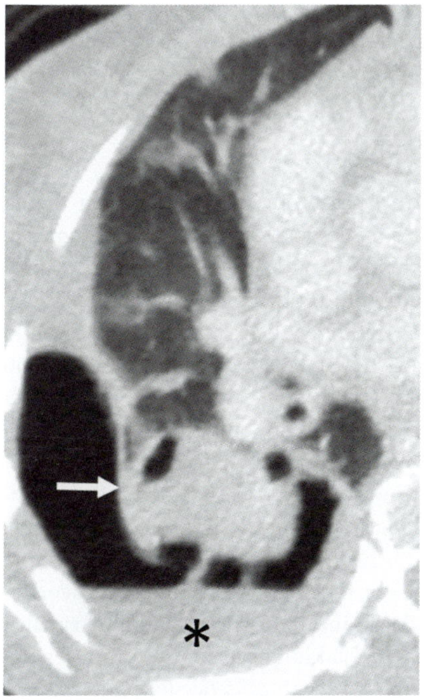

Figure 18.12 Right pulmonary abscess (arrow) that has ruptured into the right pleural space, causing a pyopneumothorax (asterisk).

Imaging Predictors of Potential Fibrosis and Mortality

Within several days to a few weeks, the fibroproliferative phase of ARDS may either progress to pulmonary fibrosis (and barotrauma), or resolution, depending on whether a maladaptive or adaptive tissue host defence response predominates, respectively. As fibrosis heralds an adverse prognosis, its early identification may help in prognostication, and potentially justify immunomodulatory strategies (although the latter is still a subject of debate). Increased density—either GGO or consolidation—associated with traction bronchiectasis, and honeycombing are CT biomarkers of fibroproliferation and are more extensively seen in non-survivors of ARDS compared to survivors.[18] Tellingly, the extent of these CT surrogates of fibroproliferation is also independently predictive of mortality, number of ventilator-free days, and risk of barotrauma in both prospective and retrospective analyses.[18–20]

It is important, however, to recognize that airway dilatation per se may occur on CT within areas of parenchymal abnormality when sufficiently high PEEPs are applied, as is elegantly illustrated when comparing low- and high-pressure imaging. This airway dilatation is simply a pressure-related phenomenon, rather than 'traction' bronchiectasis, and may even be reversible (Figure 18.14). Thus, one should be careful to not over-interpret airway dilatation as a definite sign of fibrosis, unless it can be said for certain that zero or

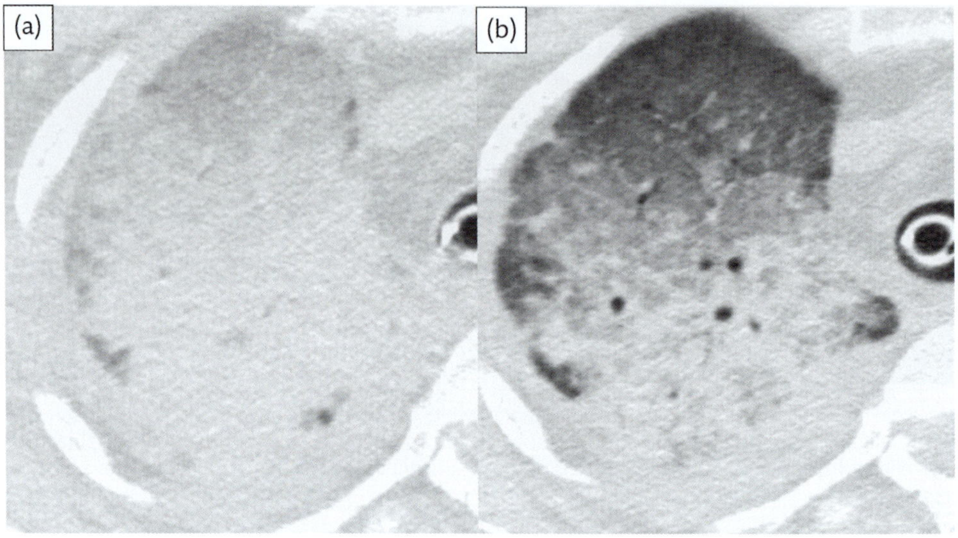

Figure 18.13 CT images at a PEEP of 5 cmH_2O (a) and inspiratory plateau pressure of 45 cmH_2O (b), showing a marked decrease in non-aerated and poorly aerated lung at high pressure, suggesting highly recruitable lung.

very low ventilatory pressures were applied during CT acquisition, or the peripheral airways appear distorted and non-tapering along their entire length.

There is some evidence to support the notion that patients with an OP pattern in association with DAD at surgical biopsy in ARDS may have a survival advantage over patients with DAD alone.[19,21] Selection bias towards patients who are suitable for lung biopsy, and who therefore probably have less severe illness, is of course a limitation in such investigations. Whether or not CT can distinguish DAD from DAD combined with OP has not been exhaustively studied; one study suggests that it cannot,[19] but did not specifically look for signs of organizing pneumonia, including the perilobular pattern. Regardless of any survival advantage, the identification of such a pattern may also invigorate the effort to look exhaustively for an autoimmune aetiology to the lung injury that could be arrested with immunomodulation, thus potentially influencing outcome. It should be stressed that evidence for this approach is thus far anecdotal.

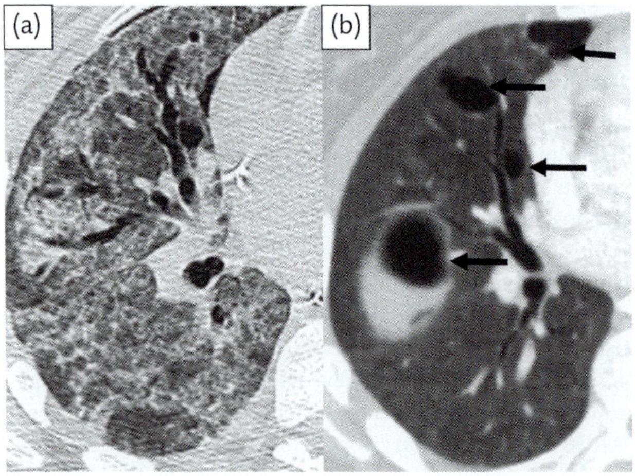

Figure 18.14 CT of ARDS at day 2 (a) demonstrating extensive ground-glass opacity with some interlobular septal thickening and associated extensive varicose dilatation of the airways that may be construed as concerning for developing fibrosis. Note that although the airways are dilated, they still taper towards the periphery. CT at day 10 (b) demonstrates both marked reduction of the parenchymal opacification and normalisation of airway calibre, suggesting that the airway dilatation was simply a pressure-related phenomenon; note the development of barotrauma-related pneumatoceles (arrows) due to high-pressure ventilation.

It has also been suggested that RV strain, defined by the ratio of the maximal short axis diameter of the RV to the left ventricle of greater than 1 and a transverse pulmonary artery diameter of greater than 3 cm, may be associated with poorer survival, although these differences do not achieve statistical significance.[19] Contrast-enhanced CT is ideally placed to assess RV strain, especially if poor acoustic windows, for example due to pneumothorax or pneumomediastinum, impede echocardiographic assessment.

Imaging in Survivors of Lung Injury

More extensive disease on CT performed in the acute phase of ARDS is not only associated with increased mortality, but may also independently herald decreased quality of life in survivors, even when adjusted for other risk factors such as age and severity of disease.[22] Intriguingly, the reticulation observed in survivors of ARDS has been shown to have a striking anterior distribution, that is, the non-dependent lung, with the extent of reticulation being independently related to not only the total duration of mechanical ventilation, but the duration of pressure-controlled inverse-ratio ventilation[23] (Figure 18.15). As such, the reticulation may indicate VILI to the lung that remains 'unprotected' (i.e. relatively better aerated).

Whether or not reticulation on CT of survivors at 6 months is associated with significant restrictive pulmonary function derangements (decreased total lung capacity, gas transfer, and forced vital capacity) is uncertain, with evidence for[22] and against.[23]

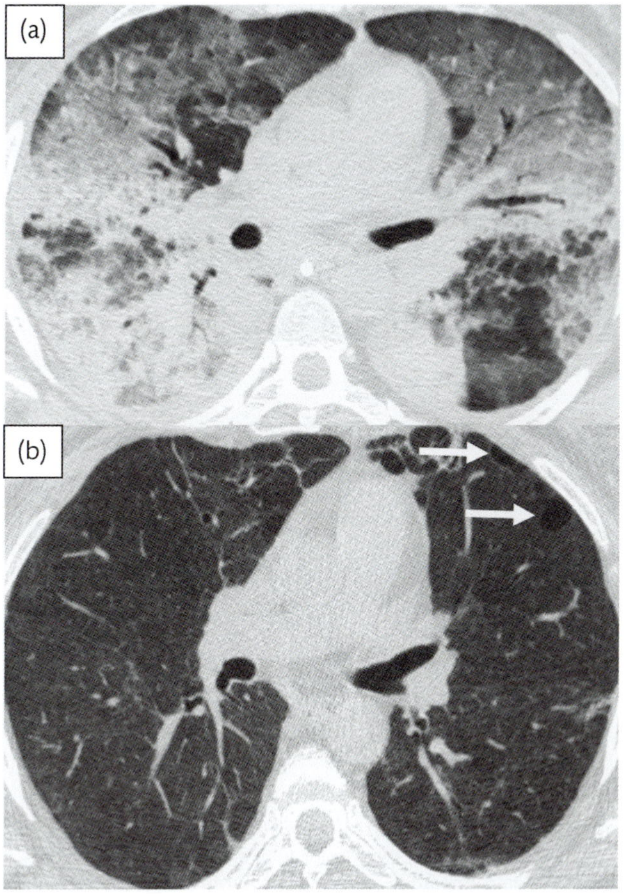

Figure 18.15 Extensive ARDS (a) with patchy but generally increasing density from the ventral non-dependent lung to the dorsal dependent lung. CT 18 months later (b) demonstrates subpleural reticulation in the ventral non-dependent lung. Barotrauma-associated thin-walled cysts have persisted (arrows).

Although thin-walled cysts—essentially pneumatoceles—are a cardinal feature of barotrauma, they often regress over time, although some may persist after well over a year from the critical care episode (Figure 18.14b).

Ultrasound

Technique

Thoracic ultrasound is invaluable in the critical care setting because it requires minimal, if any, repositioning of patients and can be performed at the bedside. In the critical care setting, it is desirable to visualize both pleural and parenchymal pathology. This is usually carried out with a convex (or microconvex) transducer at a frequency anywhere between 4 and 15 MHz (and usually at 5–9 MHz). The probe is aligned parallel with the intercostal space in order to obtain a view of the lungs and pleura unobstructed by ribs. A systematic examination covering six regions on either hemithorax (upper and lower anterior and lateral and posterior chest walls) as delineated by the anterior and posterior axillary lines is suggested. Two-dimensional B-mode ultrasonography is usually used, but additional tools, such as M-mode and colour or power Doppler, can be helpful, for example in distinguishing consolidation from echogenic pleural effusions with colour Doppler.

Box 18.1 Recognized signs in sonographic assessment

B-mode

- *Pleural line*: Horizontal echogenic line usually about 5 mm deep to rib cortex
- *Lung sliding*: 'Twinkling' movement of visceral pleura against parietal pleura, synchronized with respiration
- *Lung pulse*: Perception of cardiac motion at the pleural line (NB: usually more prominent when lung sliding is absent due to atelectasis)
- *Horizontal reverberation artefacts (A-lines)*: Acoustic reverberation from the pleural line
- *Vertical comet-tail artefacts (B-lines)*: Arise from the pleural surface (only normal if <4 lines), move with respiration

M-mode

- *'Seashore' sign*: The grainy pattern of the sliding lung (the 'sand' of the 'shore') is seen deep to the normal layered pattern of the motionless chest wall (the 'waves' of the 'sea')

Sonographic Appearances of the Normal and Pathologic Lung

The characteristic normal signs on lung ultrasound are described in Box 18.1, while pathologic conditions and their related sonographic signs are shown in Box 18.2. Ultrasound is extremely useful in the evaluation of pneumothorax (Figure 18.16), pleural effusion (including guiding intercostal aspiration or drain insertion), consolidation (Figure 18.17), and the presence of increasing interstitial exudate, termed the *interstitial syndrome* (Figure 18.18).

Ultrasound to Assess Recruitment

Given the not insignificant difficulties in transporting critical care patients to the CT scanner, the radiation-free, bedside assessment of lung recruitment using ultrasound is an attractive

Box 18.2 Main pathologic patterns and their sonographic signs

Pneumothorax

- Figure 18.16
- Loss of lung sliding (in the absence of previous pleurodesis)
- Exaggerated reverberation artefact (A-lines)
- Loss of comet-tail artefacts (B-lines)
- Presence of the lung point: Intermittent, often fleeting, visualization of mobile partially collapsed lung sliding into view, against the pleura
- Stratosphere sign: Total replacement of the seashore sign with a 'grainy' appearance

Consolidation

- Increased tissue echogenicity (isoechoic to tissue such as liver or spleen) accompanied by dynamic air bronchograms, manifest as hyperechoic tubular structures (Figure 18.17)

Interstitial syndrome

- Interstitial syndrome: Caused by pulmonary oedema (cardiogenic or non-cardiogenic) or diffuse parenchymal lung disease (e.g. pulmonary fibrosis or interstitial pneumonitis)
- Sonographic findings: Multiple B-lines (4 or more lines); may be coalescent (Figure 18.18)

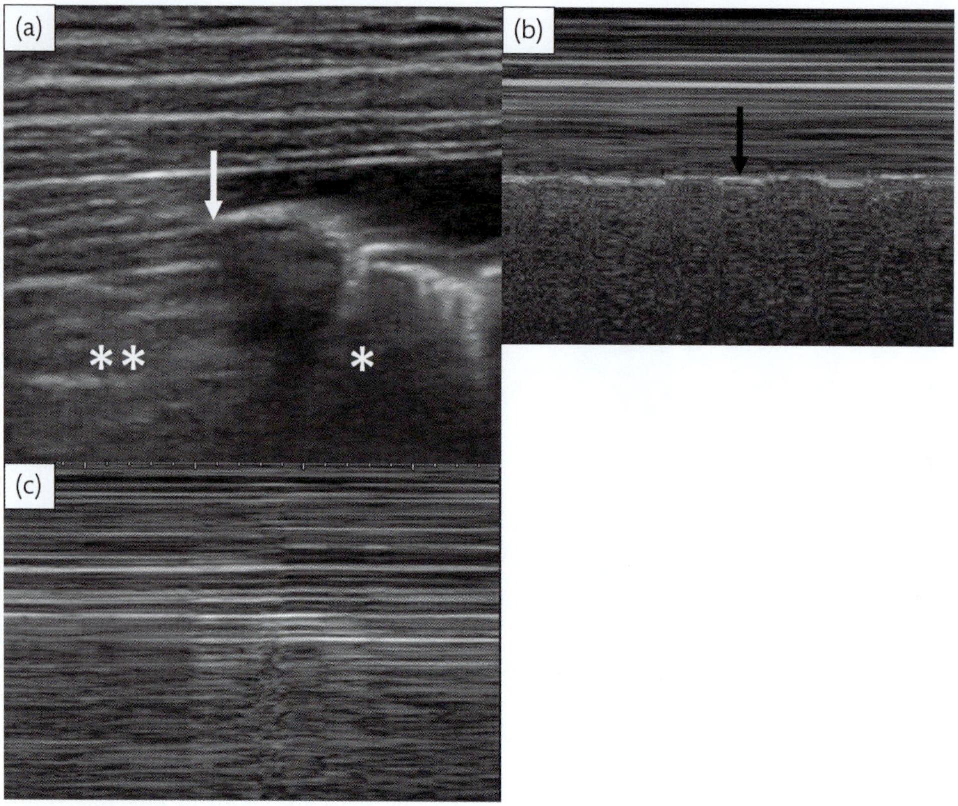

Figure 18.16 Sonographic appearances of pneumothorax. (a) B-mode sonography demonstrates the normal mobile lung (asterisk) sliding in and out of view, with a clearly visible pleural line (arrowhead). There is a clear point of demarcation, the lung 'point' (white arrow), separating the normal lung from the non-mobile air within the pleural space (double-asterisk). (b) M-mode sonography of normal lung from a different patient for reference. The 'seashore' appearance of normal lung is characterized by a clear demarcation of the stratified pattern of the motionless chest wall (the 'waves' of the 'sea'), from the grainy pattern of the mobile lung (the 'sand' of the 'shore'), by the visceral pleural line (black arrow). (c) In pneumothorax, the 'seashore' appearance is totally replaced by multiple narrowly spaced horizontal lines resembling a 'bar code' on M-mode ultrasonography—the so-called stratosphere sign. Images are courtesy of Dr Liju Ahmed, Consultant Respiratory Physician, Guy's & St Thomas Hospitals, London, UK and used with permission.

Images are courtesy of Dr Liju Ahmed, Consultant Respiratory Physician, Guy's & St Thomas Hospitals, London, UK and used with permission.

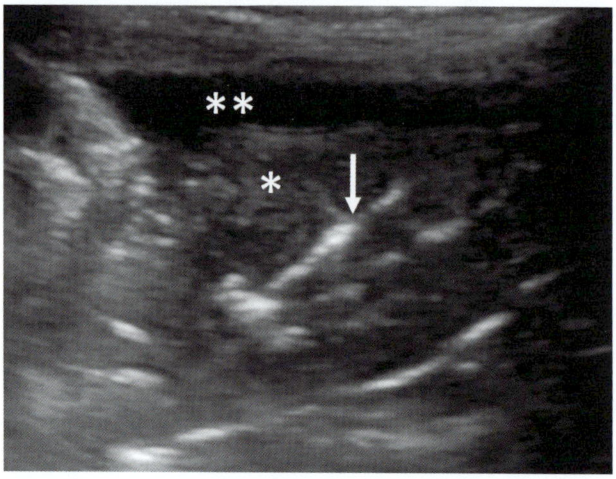

Figure 18.17 Sonographic appearance of pulmonary consolidation. The consolidated lung (asterisk) is similar in echoreflectivity to liver. A branching echogenic structure passing through the consolidation (arrow) is consistent with an air bronchogram. Note the incidental anechoic pleural effusion (double-asterisk) and the tip of atelectatic, echogenic lung (arrowhead).

Images are courtesy of Dr Liju Ahmed, Consultant Respiratory Physician, Guy's & St Thomas Hospitals, London, UK and used with permission.

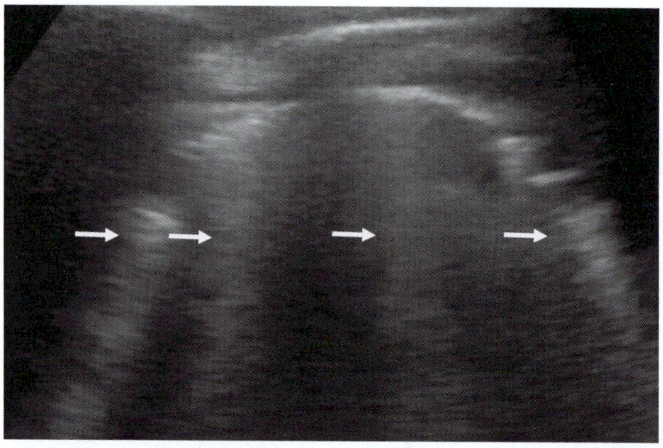

Figure 18.18 Interstitial syndrome on ultrasound. At least four B-lines (arrows)—resembling comet tails—extend from the visceral pleural line (arrowhead). Some of these lines appear thicker due to the coalescence of a few lines. The lines imply increased acoustic impedance due to air and water as a result of oedematous interlobular septa surrounded by alveolar air.

Image is courtesy of Dr Liju Ahmed, Consultant Respiratory Physician, Guy's & St Thomas Hospitals, London, UK and used with permission.

premise to guide mechanical ventilation. An ultrasound-derived lung reaeration score has been proposed and validated, with high correlation with CT-quantified reaeration and pressure–volume curves.[24] This score involves, firstly, recognizing four entities, namely (1) consolidation; (2) multiple, irregularly spaced B-lines; (3) multiple coalescent B-lines; and (4) normal aeration. The thorax is scanned at 12 different regions of interest, including upper and lower posterior regions, and scores at each level are assigned based on changes observed on recruitment manoeuvres, such as from consolidation to normal or from consolidation to multiple B-lines (Figure 18.19).

Ultrasound Assessment of Diaphragmatic Function

Ultrasound may help identify reduced diaphragmatic excursion, which in turn could be causing compressive atelectasis of dependent lung. Before commencing such assessment, ventilator pressure should be minimized to their safest lowest levels, to avoid misinterpreting ventilator-induced diaphragmatic motion as normal motion. A paralyzed diaphragm is suspected when there is absent or even paradoxical movement, or when a diaphragm of reduced thickness (<2 mm) is seen and does not thicken with inspiration.

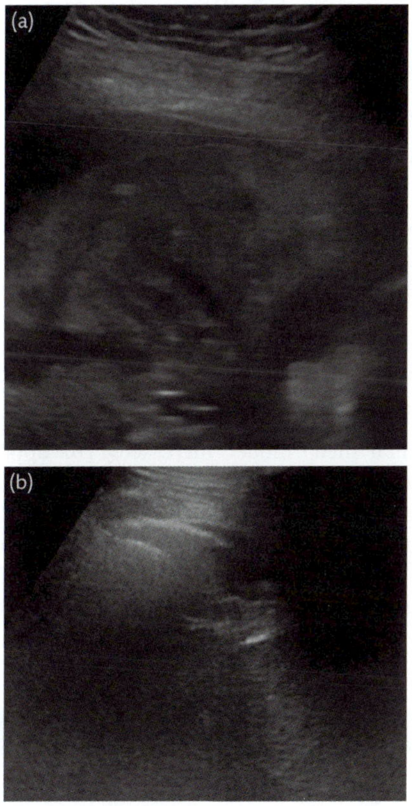

Figure 18.19 Sonographic assessment of recruitment. (a) Dense lung consolidation and a small effusion are noted. (b) After PEEP 15 cm H2O, the same lung region is characterized by multiple coalescent B lines emanating from the pleural line due to penetration of gas throughout the lung.

Courtesy of Dr Carole Ridge, Royal Brompton and Harefield Hospitals.

Electrical Impedance Tomography (EIT)

EIT is a radiation-free, non-invasive technique for monitoring the ventilated patient. Although it was invented 30 years ago, and is primarily used as a research tool, it is gaining clinical acceptance in certain centres.

Technique

EIT relies on the simple principle that the electrical conductivity of a given tissue alters proportionally with the composition of that tissue. Thus, for a given volume of lung, an increase in intrapulmonary gas volume decreases electrical conductivity, while an increase in blood or fluid volume (i.e. excess lung tissue) increases conductivity. Such periodic changes in lung composition can be captured by applying small alternating currents through adjacent pairs of electrodes, with voltage measured on the remaining electrodes. Each current application can result in one EIT image or frame. Multiple frames can be acquired through successive current application, resulting in a dynamic acquisition. Image reconstruction algorithms can then produce an anatomical representation of conductivity, with corresponding tomographic maps of ventilation and perfusion. The EIT technique is summarized in Figure 18.20.[25]

Potential Applications

In the critical care setting, EIT can most practically be used to monitor mechanical ventilation. EIT is able to illustrate both the temporal and spatial heterogeneity of lung ventilation: by illustrating how regional areas of collapse and overdistension continuously change over successive PEEP levels during recruitment manoeuvres, EIT can be used to titrate PEEP for optimal ventilation (Figure 18.21). Although lung perfusion imaging using EIT has been studied, and therefore could potentially be used to assess ventilation–perfusion mismatch, clinical data on such an application is currently in development.

Other Imaging Techniques

Magnetic Resonance Imaging (MRI)

MRI of the thorax is of limited use in the critical care patient due to the practical limitations of moving a ventilated patient into the MRI scanner, the incompatibility of a large number of critical care paraphernalia with MRI, the longer duration of MRI acquisitions, and the relatively poorer availability of MRI scanners (as opposed to CT) in many institutions. As the healthy lung is inherently an organ containing high tissue contrast and low proton density, the use of MRI in the evaluation of lung parenchyma is also of limited value. That said, MRI offers a radiation-free alternative for the evaluation of morphological abnormalities in the diseased state, when the lung may contain increased proton density due to inflammation and fluid. It can also simultaneously be used to assess cardiac and pulmonary haemodynamics. The use of hyperpolarized noble gases, such as xenon-129, on MRI to study ventilation–perfusion mismatch, pulmonary end-capillary diffusion of oxygen, and lung microstructure is currently confined to research applications.

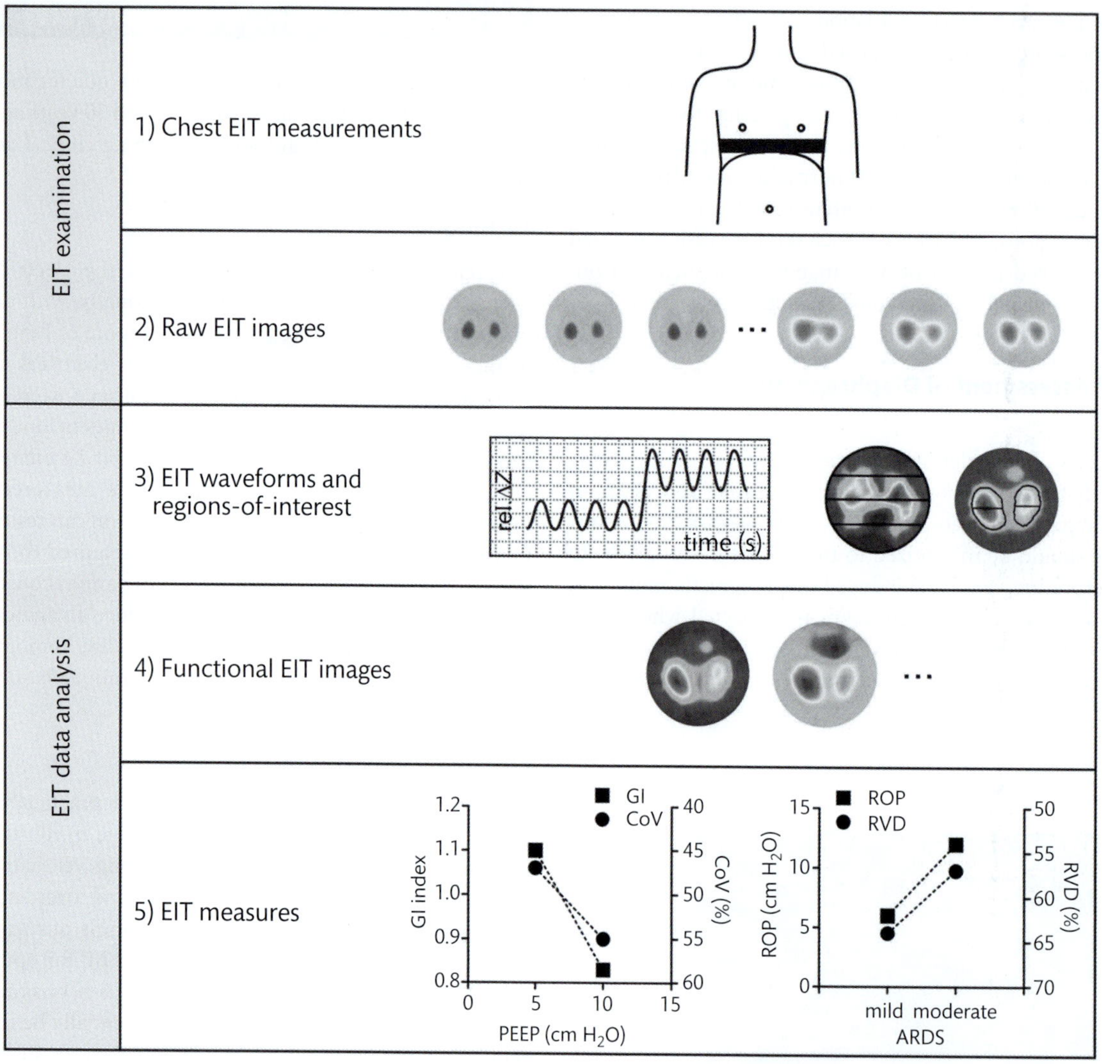

Figure 18.20 Schematic presentation of the chest EIT examination and data analysis. ARDS, acute respiratory distress syndrome; EIT, electrical impedance tomography; rel. ΔZ, relative impedance change; GI, global inhomogeneity index; CoV, centre of ventilation; PEEP, positive end-expiratory pressure; ROP, regional opening pressure; RVD, regional ventilation delay. See plate section.

Reproduced from *Thorax*, Frerichs I, et al., Chest electrical impedance tomography examination, data analysis, terminology, clinical use and recommendations: consensus statement of the TRanslational EIT developmeNt stuDy group. 72(1):83–93, copyright 2017, with permission from BMJ Publishing Group Ltd.

Positron Emission Tomography (PET) and PET-CT

2-[18F]-Fluoro2-deoxy-D-glucose (FDG) PET identifies areas of increased metabolic activity by identifying foci of increased glucose uptake and utilization. PET is now routinely integrated with PET-CT to provide anatomic correlates of metabolic activity.

As with MRI, PET and PET-CT are not useful in the routine clinical evaluation of critical care patients, but may have some value in identifying a source of occult sepsis and also in assessing response to immunomodulatory therapy. PET has also been used to demonstrate that (1) inflammation (as evidenced by increased FDG uptake) in ARDS is not confined to the regions of parenchymal abnormality, but is also seen in normally aerated lung,[26] and (2) oedema in ARDS is evenly distributed, with no overt ventrodorsal gradient of pulmonary vascular permeability present (in contrast to a ventilatory gradient).[27] Interestingly, in an experimental sheep model, increased FDG uptake was seen and associated with increased neutrophil infiltration when lung overdistension was caused by excessive mechanical ventilation after only 90 min despite normal regional gas exchange and respiratory compliance. This observation suggests that the altered FDG signal may precede regional impairment and support a future role for FDG PET-CT in the early detection of ventilator-induced lung injury (VILI).[28]

Future Directions

Dual-energy CT

Dual-energy CT (DECT) is a technique where simultaneous low- and high-kilovoltage CT datasets can be obtained in a single acquisition. This technique has a few potential applications in the thorax,

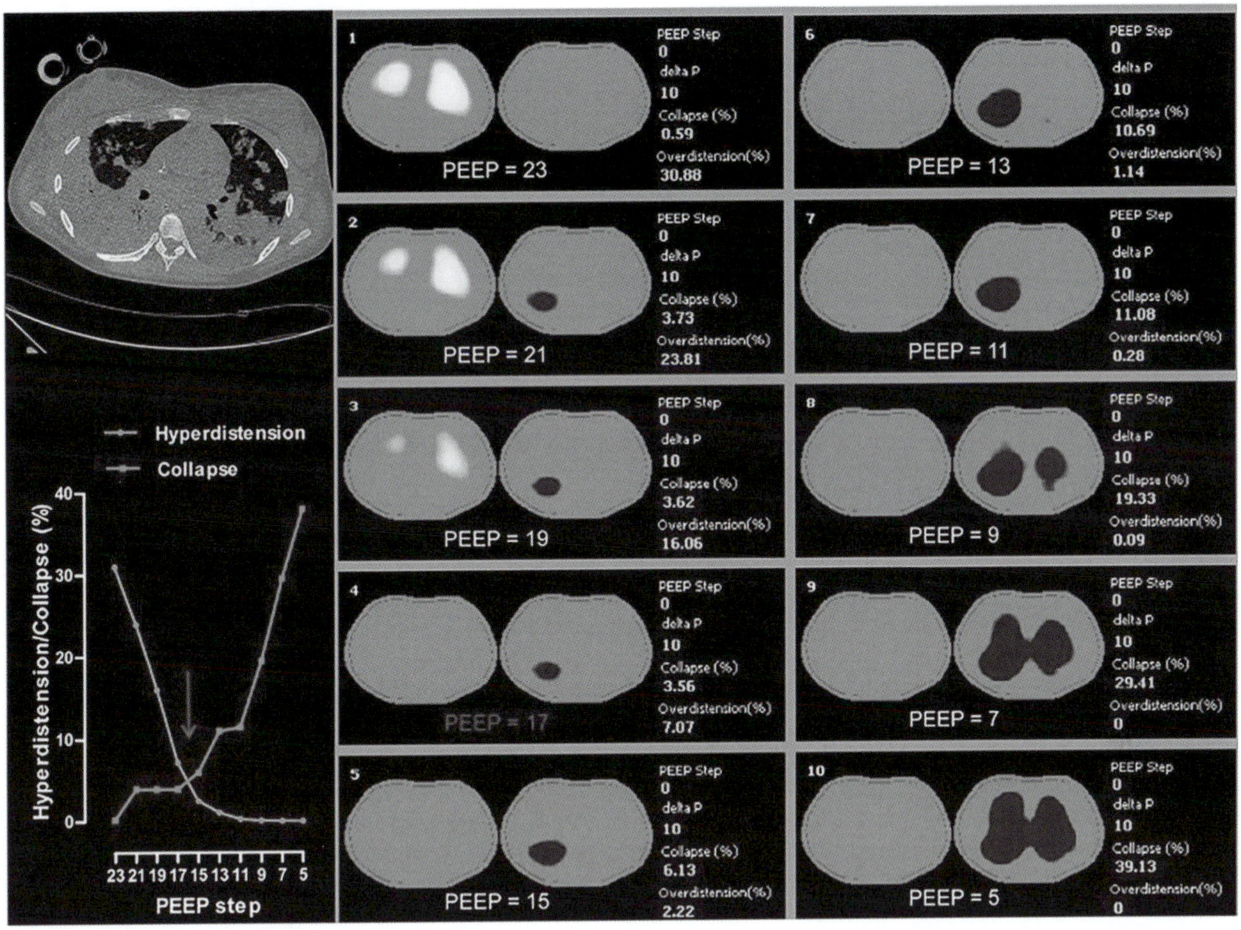

Figure 18.21 Using electrical impedance tomography (EIT) (Enlight, Timpel, Sao Paulo, Brazil) to assess the effect of decremental PEEP in a patient with severe ARDS (CT image, top left). Panels 1–10 show regional lung hyperdistention and collapse at each PEEP step in white and blue colours, respectively, obtained with the EIT electrode belt at the same level as the CT. The percentages of collapse and overdistension are provided at the right side of each panel and in the diagram (bottom left). With decreasing PEEP, hyperdistention fell (blue curve) and collapse rose (green curve). The crossover point between the curves is highlighted by the arrow. The corresponding PEEP step preceding the crossover shows the value of 17 cmH_2O in red in panel 4. See plate section.

although as yet the use of this technique in the critical care setting is limited.

- With DECT, high-attenuation materials can be specifically differentiated.[29] As such, the amount of iodine within the lung (from iodinated contrast) can be quantified in a DECT-pulmonary angiogram (DECTPA), and used as a surrogate for pulmonary perfusion, indicating perfusion defects from pulmonary emboli, the heterogeneous distribution of pulmonary blood volume overall, or areas of relative enhancement versus under-enhancement in the ARDS patient (Figure 18.22).
- DECT also enables reconstruction of image datasets at multiple kilovoltage levels (so-called 'monoenergetic' datasets). Iodine attenuation is higher at lower kilovoltage levels, meaning that suboptimal enhancement on conventional CT can be optimized to a certain degree at lower kilovoltage reconstructions. More importantly for the critical care patient, however, lower iodinated contrast volumes may be used to achieve the same level of enhancement on lower monoenergetic datasets; such smaller volumes of contrast may be more desirable when patients are in established, or at risk of, renal impairment.

Portable CT Systems

Portable CT systems would allow CT scanning at the bedside on the critical care unit, eliminating the dangers and difficulties of transporting the ventilated patient to the CT scanner. Such scanners are however currently limited in availability and expensive.

Imaging the Critically Ill COVID-19 Patient

Here, we consider the imaging aspects most relevant to patients with COVID-19 who are critically ill. The CXR and CT appearances of COVID-19 infection are summarized in Table 18.2 for reference.[30,31]

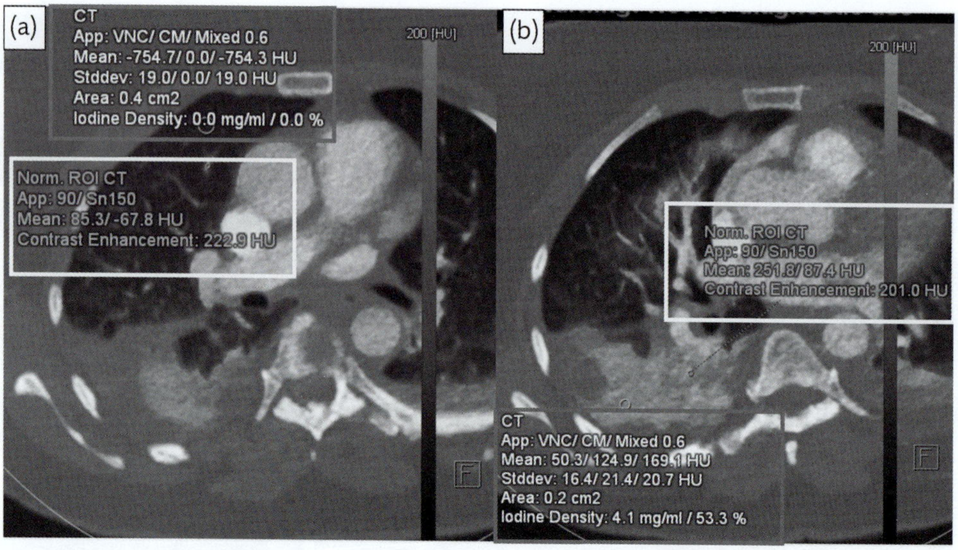

Figure 18.22 Dual-energy CT pulmonary angiography in a patient with ARDS. The images represent the combination of CT and iodine distribution images using dedicated, commercially available software (Liver VNC, Syngovia, Siemens, Forcheim, Germany). Dual-energy CT allows the calculation of specific materials within tissue, such as iodinated contrast within vessels and parenchyma, as a surrogate for perfusion. By first placing a region of interest (ROI) in a nearby artery to measure contrast enhancement (white rectangles), iodine density within a specific region can be measured in both mg/mL and as a relative percentage of the total volume of iodine within the lung (red rectangles). The iodine density of 0 in the ventral, well-aerated lung (red rectangle in (a)) as compared to the iodine density of 4.1 mg/mL, representing 53% of the iodine in the lung, within the dorsal, non-aerated lung (red rectangle in (b)) suggests that blood is being shunted through the non-aerated lung. See plate section.

Although patterns associated with OP are frequently seen in COVID-19 infection (see section titled organizing pneumonia), there is no data to suggest that the patterns of ARDS in COVID-19 are any different to that of ARDS from other pulmonary causes. However, anecdotal reports of an increased predisposition to interstitial emphysema and pneumothorax have been reported.

It is now well established that the extent of involvement on both CXR and CT is useful in understanding prognosis.[32–34] Indeed, the extent of opacification on CXR alone at presentation can predict which patients are likely to require intubation, using a simple six-zone severity score[35] (Figure 18.23). Furthermore, the binary presence/absence of airspace opacification on CXR (but not the degree of severity) was 1 of only 10 variables independently predicting a composite critical end point of admission to the intensive care unit (ICU), invasive ventilation, or death in one study.[35]

With regard to imaging in therapeutic monitoring, some general considerations should be acknowledged. Imaging critically ill patients, already a difficult undertaking (as described earlier in this chapter), is made all the more complex in COVID-19 by infection control imperatives, that is, limiting nosocomial transmission by minimizing patient and staff (especially radiographer/technologist) traffic between the imaging department and ICU, and minimizing contact with shared equipment (portable CXR and ultrasound devices). Thus, the decision to perform sequential imaging in these patients is not taken lightly, and only in circumstances where the additional information from a CXR, CT, or ultrasound scan, over and above clinical and laboratory monitoring, is very likely to contribute to management.

The indications for portable CXR and CT in assessing COVID-19-associated ARDS are broadly the same as for ARDS from any other cause. However, given the increased propensity to immunothrombosis in COVID-19,[36] an additional role for CT pulmonary angiography (CTPA) in identifying the subset of critically ill patients with pulmonary vascular involvement has been proposed. Intriguingly, there

Table 18.2 Chest radiograph (CXR) and computed tomography (CT) findings in COVID-19

CXR findings	CT findings		
	Typical	Less frequent	Rare
Initially subtle ground-glass opacity, progressing to more dense airspace opacity as infection becomes more severe	Ground-glass opacification and/or consolidation; multifocal, lower zone, peripheral, bilateral; may be segmental or subsegmental; +/− inter- and intralobular septal thickening ('crazy-paving')	Patterns of organizing pneumonia: reverse halo/atoll signs, perilobular pattern	Pleural effusion
Usually bilateral, may be asymmetrical or unilateral		Air bronchogram; 'air bubble'; reticulation	Lymphadenopathy
Usually predominantly lower zone and peripheral		Peripheral arteriolar enlargement; reticulation; halo sign	Cavitation

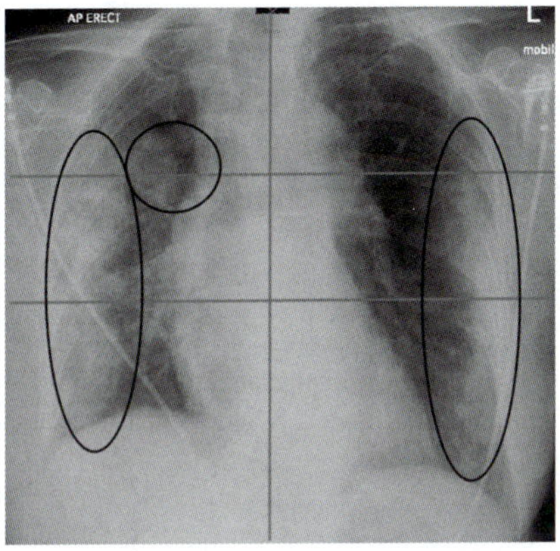

Figure 18.23 Chest radiograph of a patient severely ill with COVID-19 infection, demonstrating the typical pattern of peripheral and mid-lower zone predominant bilateral airspace opacity. Using the method proposed by Toussie et al.[32], each lung is divided into three zones. Opacities are noted in all six zones (circles), giving a total score of 6. A score greater than 3 predicted the need for intubation in admitted patients aged 21–50 years in their cohort.

is a high frequency of branching vascular dilatation—the vascular 'tree-in-bud' pattern—in these patients[37,38] even when macrovascular pulmonary arterial filling defects are not visible, potentially indicating peripheral vascular immunothrombosis. This observation, coupled with potentially decreased lung perfusion (as measured using DECTPA or subtraction CTPA),[38–40] could provide a potent imaging biomarker for anticipating a vascular dysfunction phenotype in these patients (Figure 18.24).

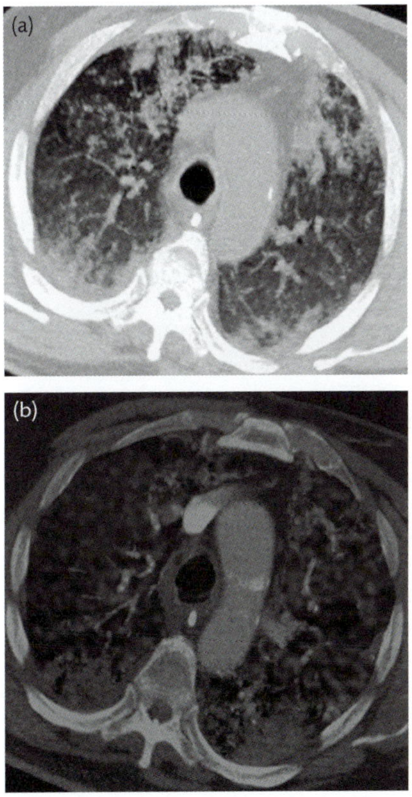

Figure 18.24 Dual-energy CT (DECT) pulmonary angiography in a Covid-19 patient with severe respiratory failure. (a) Maximal-intensity-projection CT images showing vascular tree-in-bud pattern in the upper lobes anterolaterally and (b) corresponding DECT blood volume colour map showing nodular decreased perfusion. See plate section.
Courtesy of Dr Carole Ridge, Royal Brompton and Harefield Hospitals.

Given the above, it is thus tempting to surmise that imaging phenotypes can guide therapy in COVID-19 associated ARDS. Indeed, models identifying clinical and biochemical markers to phenotype COVID-19-associated ARDS—with mortality implications—have been proposed[41,42] but are yet to include rigorous imaging biomarker assessment at the time of writing.

Importantly (and as with any ventilated patient with ARDS), transient dilatation and distortion of airways should not be overenthusiastically interpreted as an indicator of evolving fibrosis, given that early follow-up data already suggests that clear reversal can be seen in survivors.

For all of the reasons mentioned earlier (see section titled Ultrasound), many units have turned to point-of-care ultrasound for serial monitoring of COVID-19 patients in critical care settings. Indeed, some prognostic implications of ultrasound appearances at diagnosis have been suggested,[43,44] and there is emerging evidence that ultrasound scores positively correlate with increased PEEP requirements in patients who clinically deteriorate.[43]

REFERENCES

1. Nair A, Aziz ZA, Hansell DM. Techniques in thoracic imaging. In: Adam A, Dixon AK, Gillard JH, Schaefer-Prokop CM, eds. *Grainger & Allison's Diagnostic Radiology*. 6th ed. London: Churchill Livingstone; 2014:149–161.
2. Ranieri VM, Rubenfeld GD, Thompson BT, et al. Acute respiratory distress syndrome: The Berlin Definition. *JAMA*. 2012;**307**:2526–2533.
3. Hansell DM, Bankier AA, MacMahon H, et al. Fleischner Society: Glossary of terms for thoracic imaging. *Radiology*. 2008;**246**:697–722.
4. Puybasset L, Cluzel P, Gusman P, et al. Regional distribution of gas and tissue in acute respiratory distress syndrome. I. Consequences for lung morphology. CT Scan ARDS Study Group. *Intensive Care Med*. 2000;**26**:857–869.
5. Goodman LR, Fumagalli R, Tagliabue P, et al. Adult respiratory distress syndrome due to pulmonary and extrapulmonary causes: CT, cli-nical, and functional correlations. *Radiology*. 1999;**213**:545–552.
6. Desai SR, Wells AU, Suntharalingam G, et al. Acute respiratory distress syndrome caused by pulmonary and extrapulmonary injury: A comparative CT study. *Radiology*. 2001;**218**:689–693.
7. Marchiori E, Zanetti G, Hochhegger B, et al. High-resolution computed tomography findings from adult patients with Influenza A (H1N1) virus-associated pneumonia. *Eur J Radiol*. 2010;**74**:93–98.
8. Fischer A, Antoniou KM, Brown KK, et al. An official European Respiratory Society/American Thoracic Society research statement: Interstitial pneumonia with autoimmune features. *Eur Respir J*. 2015;**46**:976–987.
9. Ujita M, Renzoni EA, Veeraghavan S, et al. Organizing pneumonia: Perilobular pattern at thin-section CT. *Radiology*. 2004;**232**:757–761.
10. Kaewlai R, Avery LL, Asrani AV, et al. Multidetector CT of blunt thoracic trauma. *RadioGraphics*. 2008;**28**:1555–1570.

11. Caironi P, Langer T, Gattinoni L. Acute lung injury/acute respiratory distress syndrome pathophysiology: What we have learned from computed tomography scanning. *Curr Opin Crit Care*. 2008;**14**:64–69.
12. Gattinoni L, Caironi P, Pelosi P, et al. What has computed tomography taught us about the acute respiratory distress syndrome? *Am J Respir Crit Care Med*. 2001;**164**:1701–1711.
13. Chiumello D, Froio S, Bouhemad B, et al. Clinical review: Lung imaging in acute respiratory distress syndrome patients—an update. *Crit Care*. 2013;**17**:243.
14. Chiumello D, Marino A, Brioni M, et al. Visual anatomical lung CT scan assessment of lung recruitability. *Intensive Care Med*. 2013;**39**:66–73.
15. Puybasset L, Gusman P, Muller JC, et al. Regional distribution of gas and tissue in acute respiratory distress syndrome. III. Consequences for the effects of positive end-expiratory pressure. CT Scan ARDS Study Group. Adult Respiratory Distress Syndrome. *Intensive Care Med*. 2000;**26**:1215–1227.
16. Constantin JM, Grasso S, Chanques G, et al. Lung morphology predicts response to recruitment maneuver in patients with acute respiratory distress syndrome. *Crit Care Med*. 2010;**38**:1108–1117.
17. Bloomfield R, Noble DW, Sudlow A. Prone position for acute respiratory failure in adults. *Cochrane Database Syst Rev*. 2015 Nov 13;**2015**(11):CD008095. doi:10.1002/14651858.CD008095.pub2. PMID: 26561745; PMCID: PMC6464920.
18. Ichikado K, Suga M, Muranaka H, et al. Prediction of prognosis for acute respiratory distress syndrome with thin-section CT: Validation in 44 cases. *Radiology*. 2006;**238**:321–329.
19. Chung JH, Kradin RL, Greene RE, et al. CT predictors of mortality in pathology confirmed ARDS. *Eur Radiol*. 2011;**21**:730–737.
20. Ichikado K, Muranaka H, Gushima Y, et al. Fibroproliferative changes on high-resolution CT in the acute respiratory distress syndrome predict mortality and ventilator dependency: A prospective observational cohort study. *BMJ Open*. 2012;**2**:e000545.
21. Mandal RV, Mark EJ, Kradin RL. Organizing pneumonia and pulmonary lymphatic architecture in diffuse alveolar damage. *Hum Pathol*. 2008;**39**:1234–1238.
22. Burnham EL, Hyzy RC, Paine R, III, et al. Chest CT features are associated with poorer quality of life in acute lung injury survivors. *Crit Care Med*. 2013;**41**:445–456.
23. Desai SR, Wells AU, Rubens MB, et al. Acute respiratory distress syndrome: CT abnormalities at long-term follow-up. *Radiology*. 1999;**210**:29–35.
24. Bouhemad B, Brisson H, Le-Guen M, et al. Bedside ultrasound assessment of positive end-expiratory pressure-induced lung recruitment. *Am J Respir Crit Care Med*. 2011; **183**:341–347.
25. Frerichs I, Amato MB, van Kaam AH, et al. Chest electrical impedance tomography examination, data analysis, terminology, clinical use and recommendations: Consensus statement of the TRanslational EIT developmeNt stuDy group. *Thorax*. 2017;**72**:83–93.
26. Bellani G, Messa C, Guerra L, et al. Lungs of patients with acute respiratory distress syndrome show diffuse inflammation in normally aerated regions: A [18F]-fluoro-2-deoxy-D-glucose PET/CT study. *Crit Care Med*. 2009;**37**:2216–2222.
27. Sandiford P, Province MA, Schuster DP. Distribution of regional density and vascular permeability in the adult respiratory distress syndrome. *Am J Respir Crit Care Med*. 1995;**151**:737–742
28. Musch G, Venegas JG, Bellani G, et al. Regional gas exchange and cellular metabolic activity in ventilator-induced lung injury. *Anesthesiology*. 2007;**106**:723–735.
29. Godoy MC, Naidich DP, Marchiori E, et al. Basic principles and postprocessing techniques of dual-energy CT: Illustrated by selected congenital abnormalities of the thorax. *J Thorac Imaging*. 2009;**24**:152–159.
30. Salehi S, Abedi A, Balakrishnan S, et al. Coronavirus disease 2019 (COVID-19): A systematic review of imaging findings in 919 patients. *AJR Am J Roentgenol*. 2020;**215**:87–93.
31. Yang W, Sirajuddin A, Zhang X, et al. The role of imaging in 2019 novel coronavirus pneumonia (COVID-19). *Eur Radiol*. 2020;**30**:4874–4882.
32. Liu F, Zhang Q, Huang C, et al. CT quantification of pneumonia lesions in early days predicts progression to severe illness in a cohort of COVID-19 patients. *Theranostics*. 2020;**10**:5613–5622
33. Toussie D, Voutsinas N, Finkelstein M, et al. Clinical and chest radiography features determine patient outcomes in young and middle-aged adults with COVID-19. *Radiology*. 2020;**297**:E197–E206.
34. Balbi M, Caroli A, Corsi A, et al. Chest X-ray for predicting mortality and the need for ventilatory support in COVID-19 patients presenting to the emergency department. *Eur Radiol*. 2021;**31**:1999–2012
35. Liang W, Liang H, Ou L, et al. Development and validation of a clinical risk score to predict the occurrence of critical illness in hospitalized patients with COVID-19. *JAMA Intern Med*. 2020;**180**:1081–1089.
36. Loo J, Spittle DA, Newnham M. COVID-19, immunothrombosis and venous thromboembolism: Biological mechanisms. Thorax. 2021. DOI: thoraxjnl-2020-216243 [pii];10.1136/thoraxjnl-2020-216243 [doi]
37. Patel BV, Arachchillage DJ, Ridge CA, et al. Pulmonary angiopathy in severe COVID-19: Physiologic, imaging, and hematologic observations. *Am J Respir Crit Care Med*. 2020;**202**:690–699.
38. Ridge CA, Desai SR, Jeyin N, et al. Dual-energy CT pulmonary angiography (DECTPA) quantifies vasculopathy in severe COVID-19 pneumonia. *Radiol Cardiothorac Imaging*. 2020;**2**:e200428.
39. Lang M, Som A, Carey D, et al. Pulmonary vascular manifestations of COVID-19 pneumonia. *Radiol Cardiothorac Imaging*. 2020;**2**:e200277.
40. Arru CD, Digumarthy SR, Hansen JV, et al. Qualitative and quantitative DECT pulmonary angiography in COVID-19 pneumonia and pulmonary embolism. *Clin Radiol*. 2021;**76**:392.
41. Sinha P, Calfee CS, Cherian S, et al. Prevalence of phenotypes of acute respiratory distress syndrome in critically ill patients with COVID-19: A prospective observational study. *Lancet Respir Med*. 2020;**8**:1209–1218.
42. Ranjeva S, Pinciroli R, Hodell E, et al. Identifying clinical and biochemical phenotypes in acute respiratory distress syndrome secondary to coronavirus disease-2019. *EClinicalMedicine*. 2021;**34**:100829.
43. Lichter Y, Topilsky Y, Taieb P, et al. Lung ultrasound predicts clinical course and outcomes in COVID-19 patients. *Intensive Care Med*. 2020;**46**:1873–1883.
44. Yasukawa K, Minami T, Boulware DR, et al. Point-of-care lung ultrasound for COVID-19: Findings and prognostic implications from 105 consecutive patients. *J Intensive Care Med*. 2021;**36**:334–342.

19

Bronchoscopy in Critical Care

Suveer Singh

KEY MESSAGES

- Flexible bronchoscopy (FB) is a well-established and safe technique for diagnosis and therapy in critically ill patients.
- Bronchoscopy is recommended as part of a strategy for upper airway intubation if standard means are unsuccessful or if pre-planned.
- Bronchoscopic sampling for diagnosis of ventilator-associated pneumonia has not demonstrated significant differences in patient outcomes versus non-invasive sampling and qualitative analysis despite recommendation as best practice.
- Preparation by understanding risks, adverse effects, how to manage them, periprocedural checklists, and timeouts are recommended.
- Training in a simulated setting with skills attainment and contextual knowledge are part of a satisfactory training programme.
- Disposable FBs are single use only and should be discarded after use to prevent the known risk of contamination and infection.

CONTROVERSIES

- The role of rapid diagnostic sampling for ventilator-associated pneumonia, both biomarker and molecular platform based, in antibiotic stewardship.
- Does regular therapeutic bronchial lavage have added value to physiotherapy and mucolytic treatments in mechanically ventilated patients?
- Safe practice of therapeutic bronchoscopy in the acutely deteriorating non-intubated patient.

FURTHER RESEARCH

- The safety and role of diagnostic cryobiopsy in an ICU setting.
- Do perfluorocarbons offer advantages over saline in the safety and effectiveness of diagnostic sampling?

History of Bronchoscopy in Intensive Care

Tracheoscopy and foreign body removal was first performed with a rigid oesophagoscope in 1895 by Gustav Killian, and Shigeto Ikeda developed the first commercial FB in 1968. Integration of a charge-coupled device (CCD) permitted video monitoring of the airway without a proximal eyepiece.[1] Sackner and colleagues described the use of FB on ICU in 1971.[2] FB became a tool for assessing airway integrity in post-thoracic surgical patients without need for rigid bronchoscopy. Transnasal insertion of the FB, facilitation of airway intubation, aspiration of mucus plugs, visualization of local tumours, clearing lung collapse, managing airway stenoses, localization of haemoptysis, and selective sampling of the lower airways ensued.

Advances in the miniaturization of improved video-optics and computer processing have resulted in so-called 'hybrid' bronchoscopes that combine the flexibility and small size of the FB with high-definition images of the videoscopes.

Equipment

Bronchoscopes are rigid or flexible. Rigid bronchoscopes are a straight metal tube with a bevelled distal tip inserted into the trachea through the oropharyngolaryngeal pathway. In the critical care unit, it is less used than FB; usually for massive haemoptysis, foreign body or airway thrombus removal, dilatation, or stent procedures are not possible by FB. The FB provides visualization to segmental and subsegmental bronchi.

Newer single-use disposable bronchoscope systems have certain particular advantages such as ease of access, portability, absence of cross-contamination, and a small footprint. The optics and image quality are currently inferior to, but are approaching those of the reusable videobronchoscope systems. They are increasingly used for urgent therapeutic bronchoscopy and during percutaneous tracheostomy.

In disposable systems, the distal CCD is illuminated by an LED (light emitting diode) rather than fibreoptic cables of the hybrid reusable FBs. Image transmission via cable to the monitor enables quality of image (still inferior to reusable FBs) with low manufacturing costs. Comparative economic studies of disposable and reusable bronchoscopes take into account factors such as volume of use, availability, and infection risks and consequences. The unit costs of disposable devices are assessed against capital and service maintenance costs for videobronchoscope systems.

Disposable bronchoscopes should be discarded and *not* reused due to a significantly increased infection risk by reuse.[3]

Indications

In the ICU, indications fall into diagnostic or therapeutic categories (see Table 19.1). The main indications of FB are for the following cases:

1. Sampling respiratory secretions for diagnostic purposes (e.g. infection, malignancy).
2. Airway inspection, restoration, and maintenance of the patency.
3. Managing advanced and complex airways.
4. Haemoptysis.
5. More advanced procedures (i.e. endobronchial ultrasound [EBUS], cryoextraction, airway stenting, and endobronchial valves[4]).

Infection—Pneumonia

Diagnostic sampling for suspected respiratory infection is the most common reason for bronchoscopy in this setting. Sampling modalities include endotracheal aspirate (ETA), non-directed bronchial lavage (NBL), bronchial washings, mini bronchoalveolar lavage (miniBAL), and, less commonly, protected brush catheter specimens (PSB).

Ventilator-associated Pneumonia (VAP)

VAP develops in ~5%–35% of critically ill patients receiving mechanical ventilation for over 48 h, with attributable mortality of 2%–27%. Less than two-thirds of suspected cases are confirmed by semi-quantitative microbiology due to mimics such as non-infective and non-pulmonary causes or tracheobronchitis without alveolar pathology. The premise for distal airway sampling is for more accurate microbiological diagnosis of pneumonia. Clinical diagnosis of VAP and HAP (hospital acquired pneumonia) is discussed in accompanying chapters. MiniBAL (bronchoalveolar lavage) has not demonstrated diagnostic superiority over less invasive sampling techniques, such as bronchial washings, NBL, or blind catheter brushings. When compared against post-mortem histology, BAL has sensitivities of 50% and positive predictive values of 70%.[5] Single site sampling, compared with multiple lobe sampling, may only provide 61% positive predictive microbiological value although single site sampling does not appear to affect the antibiotic prescribing or outcomes, and so remains acceptable.[6]

Table 19.1 Indications for bronchoscopy in intensive care

	Diagnostic	Therapeutic	Airway
Infection	✔ Bronchial wash/miniBAL		
Malignancy ILD Undiagnosed lung disease Unilateral wheeze	✔ BAL for cytology Biopsies/TBNA		
Atelectasis/ Segmental lobar collapse	✔	✔ Therapeutic lavage	
Difficult airway assessment			✔
Double lumen tube/balloon blocker		✔ Part of haemorrhage control	✔
Percutaneous tracheostomy			✔
Upper airway obstruction Expiratory dynamic airway collapse	✔		✔
Haemoptysis Airway haemorrhage	✔	✔	
Foreign body	✔	✔	
Inhalation injury	✔	✔ Therapeutic lavage	
Persistent pneumothorax/air leak	✔ Balloon isolation of alveolopleural fistula segment	✔ Expiratory-only endobronchial valves	
Tracheobronchial injury	✔		
Airway stent insertion		✔	✔
Lung transplant surveillance	✔		
Problem-solving: Non-resolving respiratory failure Non-resolving infection Cavitatory disease Suspected trachea-oesophageal fistula EDAC	✔	✔	

Bronchoscopy is more invasive and requires proficiency to obtain high yielding samples, but may reduce the overdiagnosis of infection, based upon the presence of organisms in an NBL or bronchial wash. MiniBAL usually involves serial insertion of 20–40 mL aliquots up to 120 mL of warm saline into the relevant bronchial segment (depending on tolerance and oxygenation), through the bronchoscope, ideally wedged in the segment. An assessment of collapsibility of the segmental walls on suction will allow anticipation of the likely yield based upon the degree of suction applied. Hand suction allows adjustable suction titrated to the degree of airway collapse and fluid aspiration, and is non-inferior to conventional automatic suction in the daycase setting. There is no mortality difference in VAP, when comparing qualitative (i.e. presence or absence of pathogens in the culture) with quantitative analysis (i.e. a threshold count of the bacterial growth to differentiate between infection and colonization of the lower airways), obtained by bronchoscopic versus non-bronchoscopic techniques.[7] Nevertheless, the possibility of reducing unnecessary antibiotic prescriptions favours directed bronchoscopic sampling if semi-quantitative measures are utilized. Although miniBAL and semi-quantitative cultures have become a research standard, it is not a widely used clinical standard.[8–10] Thus, while bronchoscopic sampling may improve diagnostic accuracy in VAP, it has not proven superior to less invasive sampling in either mortality or antibiotic prescribing.[11] The current recommendations are for ETA as first-line sampling technique, with BAL reserved for more complex cases, that is, ETA is inconclusive, or if the initial treatment fails.[12] Our practice suggests that directed miniBAL can and should be used where practicable in the context of safety and theoretical advantages.

Immunocompromised Host

In patients immunosuppressed by treatments for haematological and other malignancies, bone marrow and/or solid organ transplants, vasculitic or other rheumatological conditions, and clinical suspicion of respiratory infection, particularly if critical illness supervenes, should warrant early consideration of diagnostic bronchoscopic sampling. With new or worsening pulmonary infiltrates, early bronchoscopic sampling obtains positive microbiological yields of 21%–85%. This can change antibiotic prescribing in >50% of cases, in non-intubated critically ill patients.[13] Early sampling (<4 days), particularly in haematological malignancy, can improve yields and survival, while lobar rather than interstitial or diffuse radiological abnormalities predicts better diagnostic yields.

The early diagnosis of viral pneumonia through airway sampling is possible by real-time PCR platforms, which can contain wide array panels for common respiratory viruses including SARS-COV2, influenza, respiratory syncytial virus, and CMV,[14] and bacterial PCR is also increasingly available. BAL PCR for *Pneumocystis jirovecii* pneumonia (PJP) has a similarly high performance.[15]

Invasive respiratory fungal infection is difficult to diagnose with a high mortality (>80%) if un(der)treated. Diagnostic criteria are determined by the revised European guidelines.[12] The sensitivity of cultures is low. Current diagnostic methods are optical density assays to identify fungal cell wall elements (β-D-glucan for any fungi and galactomannan (GM) for invasive pulmonary aspergillosis (IPA)) or PCR. In likely or probable disease, using optical density cut-offs of 1.0 or 1.5, BAL GM is 70%–92% sensitive and up to 98% specific. BAL specificity is better than serum BDG, GM, or PCR. Combining BAL GM and PCR provides the current best diagnostic accuracy.[15]

Airway Assessment and Management

Flexible bronchoscopy should be considered diagnostically for assessment of the airways, mucosa, and/or upper airway, particularly if the clinical scenario suggests a possible endobronchial explanation. Airway secretions, mucoid (e.g. chronic obstructive pulmonary disease, COPD), purulent, or slough causing atelectasis are the commonest reasons for FB. If the work of breathing (WOB) is unexplainedly high, FB may identify inspissated secretions, extensive tracheal tube/mucosa lined secretions, that if cleared may improve the WOB by reducing airway resistance. Further, expiratory dynamic airway collapse (EDAC) is a cause of the increased WOB and is more likely due to distal secretion load than tracheobronchial malacia, the main other differential.

Post-extubation breathlessness or stridor may be due to tracheal stenosis or vocal cord dysfunction following critical illness. Further, acute airway obstruction after decannulation of tracheostomy tubes may be due to a tracheal flap or membrane, which together with cross-sectional imaging can be diagnosed by planned FB and visualization through the vocal cords as the tracheal tube is withdrawn.

Lobar Collapse

While therapeutic bronchial lavage, the so-called 'pulmonary toiletting', is important, the available evidence has not shown it to be superior to chest physiotherapy in the absence of lobar collapse. Lobar collapse by radiography is better resolved when FB is added to routine physiotherapy.[16] Indeed, in situations of acute hypoxaemia due to suspected secretion load/obstruction, therapeutic FB may be essential rather than being contraindicated. Directed suction is usually combined with forced saline flushing. Repeated episodes may be necessary with intermittent periods of re-recruitment following temporary removal of the bronchoscope from the airway (or into the catheter mount only without full removal, to prevent aerosolization in high-risk circumstances such as COVID-19). Sufficient time should be allowed for distally agitated secretions to move proximally and suction, before completion. Concurrent use of mucoactives (e.g. nebulized *N*-acetylcysteine) or hypertonic saline (3%) can be used to treat airway plugging when non-purulent mucus is tenacious (e.g. in COPD). NAC is considered not to be useful when there are purulent secretions or if FIO_2 > 40%, at which its activity is reduced.

The use of endobronchial DNase has been reported to improve the success of bronchoscopic lobar re-expansion in resistant cases of collapse. It is safe and shown to improve chest radiography appearance compared with hypertonic or normal saline, but with no difference in other outcomes.[17] There have been no completed RCTs of DNAse in the critical care setting at the time of writing.

Foreign Body Removal

The removal of foreign body bronchoscopically in the ICU setting is uncommon. The nature of the foreign body, its location, potential impact, available bronchoscopic tools, and expertise should be considered. A range of retrieval devices including grasping forceps, wires, baskets, and endobronchial balloons may be needed. Most commonly in this setting, blood clots or retained tenacious mucoid impaction are dealt with by en-bloc suctioning or forceps extraction. If available, cryoadhesion and extraction may be an effective alternative. This entails a through-the-bronchoscope probe, whose tip freezes on the foreign body by delivering high-pressure CO_2 or nitrous oxide. It is safe and effective in reported cases and in the author's experience[18] (Figure 19.1).

Burn Inhalation Injury (BII)

FB should ideally be performed within the first 24 h as a gold standard to confirm the diagnosis and assess the severity of injury and prognosticate in BII. Standard bronchoscopic grading using the Abbreviated Injury Score (AIS) scale (0–4) correlates with increased attributable mortality for moderate/severe grades 2–4.[19] This has been more recently confirmed using similar classification into mild, moderate, or severe grades. A combination of nebulized heparin 5–10,000 units and *N*-acetylcysteine 20% is common but not universal practice and is discussed in Chapter 61. The use of therapeutic lavage has been shown to reduce extubation failure rates.[20]

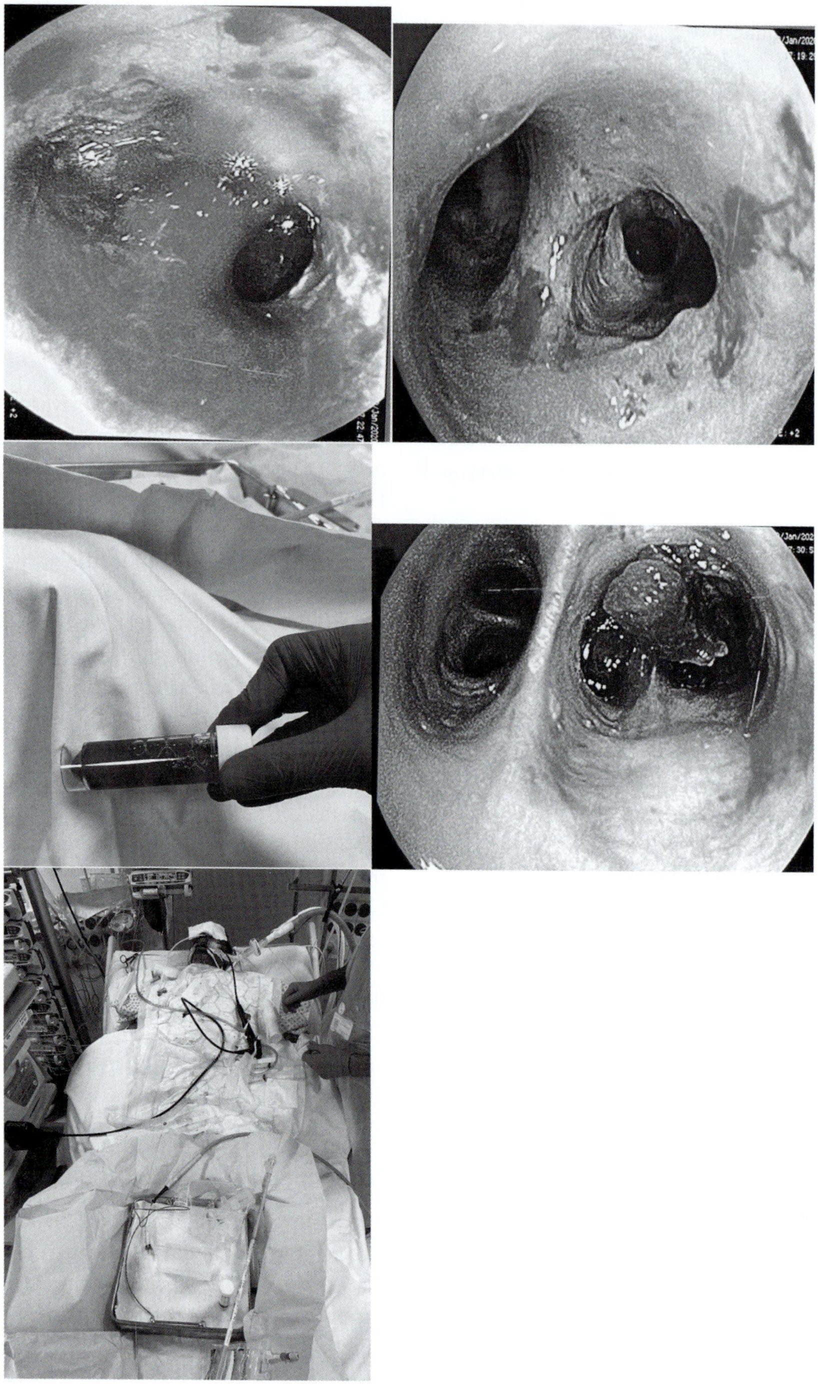

Figure 19.1 Cryoextraction. See plate section.

Tracheobronchial Injury/Trauma

FB is an important diagnostic tool in identifying tracheobronchial injury following trauma. An index of suspicion is necessary. High-impact deceleration chest injuries, difficult or repeated intubation attempts, unexplained pneumothorax, and extensive subcutaneous or persistent endotracheal tube cuff leaks may all warrant diagnostic FB, with regular therapeutic lavage being part of a multidisciplinary strategy in non-surgical cases.[21]

Transbronchial Diagnostic Sampling

Transbronchial biopsies or cryobiopsies are possible in selected mechanically ventilated patients, both having an acceptable histological yield and risk profile in lung transplant recipients and, more generally, influencing change of management in concordance with open lung biopsies.

Artificial Airway Assistance

Difficult Airway

FB can be used to facilitate endotracheal intubation and correct placement of double lumen tubes in the airway.

FBs are part of difficult airway protocols. Awake fibreoptic intubation is a recognized standard for the anticipated difficult airway. Failed intubation in the operating room is reported at <1%, whereas up to 25% of airway complications reported in hospitals in the UK were in the ICU or emergency department. Here, a combination of unpreparedness, lack of a backup plan, and/or lack of appropriate airway skills, including bronchoscopy, is implicated.[22]

The pre-placement of an ETT (endotracheal tube) over the bronchoscope allows it to be advanced into the trachea under direct vision. In experienced hands, the use of multimodality tools can improve the chances of success. For instance, the flexible tip of the bronchoscope may not be easily manoeuvred through the vocal cords due to distortion or excess soft tissue/debris. Here, the use of a laryngoscope (direct or indirect viewing) or a supraglottic airway device to allow better and quicker controlled direction of the bronchoscope to its target can be helpful. Airway adjuncts to assist the insertion of the FB in the non-intubated patient even through an NIV (non invasive ventilator) mask can be very effective (Figures 19.2 and 19.3). However, use must be governed by the level of expertise and familiarity of the user, adopting published guidance and protocols (e.g. the Difficult Airway Society, www.das.uk.com; or the Airway Management Academy, www.airwaymanagementacademy.com).

Percutaneous Tracheostomy

Direct visualization of the endotracheal airway during tracheostomy has several inherent advantages over 'blind' insertion. These include accurate percutaneous needle insertion, observation of cartilaginous ring integrity, prevention of posterior membranous tracheal wall damage, confirmation of accurate final placement, and post-procedure bronchial segmental therapeutic lavage. While randomized studies have not shown an outcome difference between ultrasound guidance and bronchoscopic guidance, the TRACHUS randomized non-inferiority controlled trial demonstrated reduced complications with bronchoscopic guidance.[23]

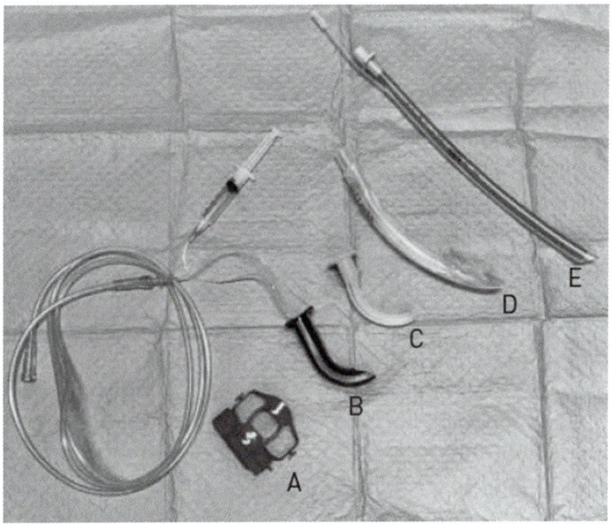

Figure 19.2 Airway adjuncts for bronchoscopy in the non-intubated patient.

A few practical points should be highlighted. (1) The procedure may require a third operator, apart from the tracheostomist and assistant holding the ETT. (2) The bronchoscope tip should be within the distal end of the ETT at the time of needle insertion, to prevent FB damage. The use of disposable bronchoscopes is useful here. (3) Awareness of the partially occluded airway during withdrawal of the ETT and intra-procedurally should necessitate ongoing assessment of the airway pressure/volume and oxygen/carbon dioxide (CO_2) profiles.

Airway Haemorrhage

In the critical care setting, airway haemorrhage must be acted upon quickly from a diagnostic and therapeutic perspective. Major haemorrhage is fortunately rare but may quickly become catastrophic. The clinical situation (e.g. medical or surgical patient, potential aetiology, iatrogenicity, risk factors for coagulopathy, and likely source of bleeding) needs to be considered when planning the strategy for haemorrhage control and patient management.

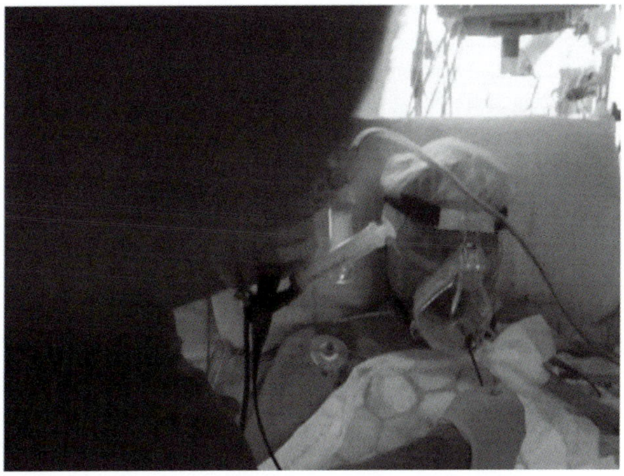

Figure 19.3 Bronchoscopy through NIV.

Likely causes of haemorrhage may be local mucosal, tumour related, from cavitatory lung disease, anomalous vessels, diffuse alveolar haemorrhage, or traumatic. The risk of hypoxaemia and asphyxiation must be managed alongside haemodynamic control. Systematic approaches for control are published, but there is no formal training in these strategies beyond various training workshops.[24] More practically useful than haemorrhage volume is a change in the rate of bleeding and the time from intervention to control. Alternating suction and ice-cold saline instillation are the main initial interventions (Box 19.1).

Once bleeding is settling, it is important to survey the other airway segments and clear spillover blood before it clots. The aims of FB are to identify the source of bleeding, isolate the remaining lung, and create a tamponade effect until there is haemorrhage control.

Management involves suction above the point of bleeding, administration of ice-cold saline, tranexamic acid 0.5–1 mg iv or bronchial, diluted adrenaline (serial 2 mL 1:100K to 1:200K up to 1:10K cognizant of arrythmias), and tamponade of the source segment with the FB. If necessary, tamponade with an inflatable balloon blocker through-the-bronchoscope (expect loss of ability to suction) or paraxial is created. Surgical gauze packing has been proposed as a further measure for controlling the bleeding. Other techniques, such as turning onto the side of the bleeding, DLTs, and non-contact strategies, that is, argon plasma coagulation, are reported outside the critical care setting. In the specific situation of diffuse alveolar haemorrhage, due to vasculitides, post-haemopoietic stem cell transplant, and drugs or toxins, untreated mortality is >50%. Success by serial endobronchial recombinant factor VII with systemic glucocorticoids and aminocaproic acid is reported. Some form of tamponade is the most effective way of controlling immediate local endobronchial bleeding (Figure 19.4).

The patient's cardiorespiratory status, source, and rate of control of bleeding will determine the need for sequential actions. Rapid recourse to alternatives, such as rigid bronchoscopy, interventional radiology (bronchial artery embolization), or surgery, may be needed if initial bronchoscopic strategies fail. Surgical resection must also be available if necessary and feasible, with good reported success rates of bleeding control related to mycetoma.

Box 19.1 Airway Haemorrhage Protocol

General principles

Assess patient, staff, and equipment
LocSIPP, WHO checklist, and timeout pre-procedure
Risk assessment—optimize conditions and have your PLAN B
Once bleeding control obtained, clean the other airway of clot
Endobronchial blockers:
If high-risk procedure—pre-positioned endobronchial blocker
If unexpected—option of 'through the working channel' balloon but no suction
Once deployed, if paraxial (i.e. outside the bronchoscope), clean the 'good' side
Check control by partial deflation after 2–3 min

When clinically significant haemorrhage occurs:

Stay calm and call for help
Be prepared
The drill
Do not remove the bronchoscope
Suction, cold saline, and suction
Assess rate of bleeding control
Suction, cold saline, and suction
Assess rate of bleeding control
Tranexamic acid 0.5–1 mg iv or bronchial, adrenaline 1–2 mL 1; 100K bronchial
Assess rate of bleeding

Other techniques

Endobronchial blocker (through the working channel) or paraxial (e.g. Fogarty 6F or Cook Arndt/Cohen)
Surgical airway packing
Isolate bleeding side by single lumen intubation (advancing ETT)
Turn patient onto side of bleeding source once known
Rigid bronchoscopy
Interventional radiology

Prophylactic measures

Endotracheal tube and balloon blockers

Other Indications

Pneumothorax, Air Leak, and Resolution

Persisting pneumothorax is discussed in detail elsewhere in Chapter 56. The air leak is either due to a bronchopleural fistula, usually following surgery, or a common air leak known as an alveolopleural fistula. Endobronchial (expiratory-only) valves can be placed if usual treatments have not worked or if unsuitable for thoracic surgical repair. In the critical care setting, they have reported success rates up to ~50%.[25] Identification of the bronchial segment(s) involves placing a through-the-bronchoscope balloon blocker to occlude the suspected segment(s) airflow until reduction/cessation of flow at the external pleural flow drain. The valves are then deployed to those segments via the FB and monitored for effect and position/clearance of mucus.

Stents and Tracheo-oesophageal Fistulae

More complex procedures are possible in patients on the ICU. There is evidence in selected cases of malignancy that endobronchial stent insertion can lead to liberation from mechanical ventilation.[4]

Physiological Effects and Complications of Bronchoscopy

Physiological Effects of Bronchoscopy

The physiological effects of bronchoscopy are categorized as (1) increased airway resistance, (2) reduced lung compliance, (3) hypoxaemia and hypercapnia, and (4) cardiovascular effects.

A standard 5.7 mm outer diameter bronchoscope will occlude ~15% of the trachea. This increases serially to ~40% and ~66% in size 9 and 7 ETTs, respectively.

The airway resistance will increase accordingly and flow will reduce notably (Poiseuille's law), as well as due to a longer ETT and non-laminar flow.

A rise in peak airway pressures theoretically increases the risk of pneumothorax. Distal airway collapse and de-recruitment caused by repeated suction and the effect of saline lavage on denuding any remaining alveolar surfactant layer may contribute to changes in lung compliance. Consider post-procedure recruitment manoeuvres, if deemed safe.

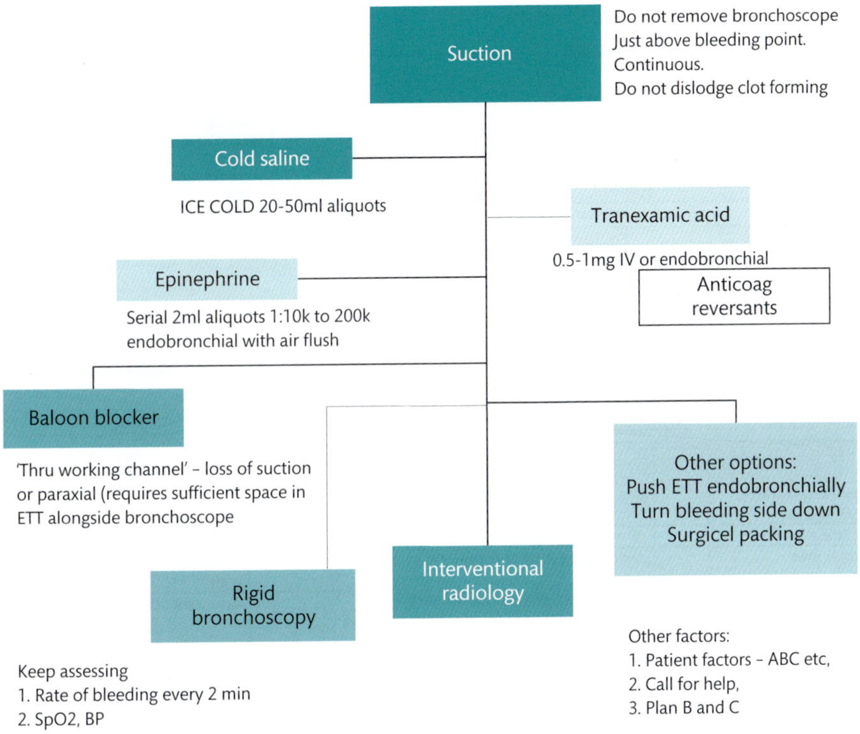

Figure 19.4 An algorithm for the management of endobronchial airway haemorrhage.

Hypoxaemia is expected by reduced alveolar oxygen, due to multiple factors of reduced inspiratory flow and volume, and flooding of alveoli during BAL. Hypercapnia is a result of hypoventilation primarily caused by airway obstruction. The end-tidal CO_2 will rise quickly and may necessitate adjustment of the set minute ventilation or temporary removal of the bronchoscope if haemodynamic consequences ensue, although this is clinically infrequent.

Cardiovascular alterations in heart rate and blood pressure are the result of the balance between sympathetic stimulation and sedation-related vascular effects.

Complications

Bronchoscopy is safe (mortality rate 0.01%; major complication rate 0.08%–2%),[26] whereas complication rates of 4%–10% occur with its use in intensive care.[27] Thus, severe respiratory failure, hypercapnic acidosis, poorly controlled bronchospasm, ETT <8 mm, pneumothorax, haemodynamic instability, arrhythmogenic potential, and raised intracranial pressure should all be recognized, managed, and accounted for with regard to the timing and duration of FB. The most common complications are bronchospasm, hypoxaemia, hypotension, bleeding, cardiac arrhythmias, pneumothorax, and myocardial ischaemia/pulmonary oedema.

Bronchospasm is rare but may be relevant in known obstructive airway disease.

Hypoxaemia (<90%) occurs in 4.5%–6% of those with acute respiratory distress syndrome (ARDS). Hypotension requiring vasoactive support has been noted in 22% in the ICU. Untreated raised intracranial pressure is a contraindication. Appropriate sedation, neuromuscular blockade, and blood pressure control are crucial. Major bleeding is rare (1:500–1000 cases). Interventions will cause reported bleeding in 3%–5% of all bronchoscopies, which is a likely underestimate for the ICU. Preparedness for bleeding control is essential. Pneumothorax after transbronchial biopsies occur in ~0.4% of daycase bronchoscopies but up to 14% in mechanically ventilated patients. This may be delayed. Topical Tranexamic acid (TXA) is similar to 1:10k epinephrine after cold saline failure for controlling most iatrogenic bleeding in daycase bronchoscopy. TXA can also be given i.v serially.[32] A judgement regarding the timing of chest radiograph or lung ultrasound should be considered. Other complications, such as fever and transient bacteraemia, may occur.

Preparation, Safety, and Procedure

Patient safety and crisis risk management dictate the need for appropriate planning and preparation. Consistent with perioperative guidance, bronchoscopy in the ICU should adopt a World Health Organization (WHO)–like checklist with 'timeouts' and reporting, as part of Local safety standards for invasive procedures (LocSIPP). A suggested, bronchoscopy checklist is provided in Figure 19.5. Preparation should include patient, staff, and equipment assessments in advance. A risk evaluation, mitigating strategies, as well as a plan for anticipated complications should be undertaken.

Ventilatory settings in a control mode can be adjusted according to the anticipated length of the procedure, and periprocedural oxygenation at FiO_2 1.0, adequate sedation, and usually short acting neuromuscular blockade are important. Ensuring all equipment, sampling containers, and emergency paraphernalia are available in advance will reduce unnecessary delays.

Practical aspects of FB involve centring it within the lumen and withdrawing to a recognized point of anatomical reference. Basic knowledge of endobronchial anatomy, with 10 right-sided segments

Adult Intensive Care Unit COVID-19 Bronchoscopy Checklist

Patient name			**Indication**	Diagnostic Y/N Therapeutic Y/N
DOB			HAVE YOU ADOPTED COVID PPE PRECAUTIONS? HAVE YOU GOT ENOUGH STAFF – [OPERATOR/ASSISTANT/RUNNER AVAILABLE OUTSIDE] HAVE YOU GOT BRONCHOSAMPLER/SERIAL COLLECTIONS SPECIMEN POTS AND BAGS?	
Hospital Number				
Date				

Please complete for all patients having a Bronchoscopy performed on the ICU

Equipment (tick, initial after checking need)		
Bronchoscopy specific equipment Bronchoscope + video monitor Bronchoscopy catheter mount Sputum collection pots x3 (Bronchosampler or serial connecion) Suction tubing Lubricant Swabs 1L sterile saline & Jug 20ml non luer lock syringes x 5 (50ml non luer lock syringes)	**Airway kit** Difficult Airway trolley Ventilator settings FiO2 1.0, Sedation, Paralysis	
	Haemorrhage kit – fridge ONLY IF BLEEDING ANTCIPATED Ice cold saline Balloon blocker Tranexamic acid (500mg x 3-4) Epinephrine 1:100k(1mg in 100ml 0.9% N/S x 2mLs aliquots)	**Emergency drugs** - ICU crash trolley OUTSIDE **Pneumothorax kit** - ICU (chest drain box)

Before the procedure	✓	Preprocedure	✓	After the procedure (Confirmed by procedure team lead)	✓
Sufficient staff for the procedure to take place; roles identified USUALLY 2 PEOPLE ONLY				Patient review. Consider recruitment manouevre/Ventilatory change / CXR?	
Team member Introductions/ Role allocation		All essential imaging reviewed		Samples labelled, processed and bagged	
Indication for bronchoscopy confirmed		Anticipated critical or unexpected events		On-going management plan communicated to staff	
Patient identity and consent /assent confirmed		Bronchoscopy protocol (please circle): Diagnostic, VAP, Collapse, Tracheostomy, Hemorrhage Other		Bronchoscopy report completed	
Monitoring equipment and medication checks		**Nurse in charge**		Any problems with equipment that has been identified that need to be addressed	
Does the patient have a known allergy? Yes / No		Disposable bronchoscope only +monitor+ samplers			
Anticoagulation and/or anti-platelet agent Yes / No		PLAN: Preprepare Bronchoscope – place tip in bronch catheter mount. Connect serial sample containers, suction and monitor. INSPIR HOLD/TUBE CLAMP CATH MOUNT EXCHANGE. Procedure and samples. DO NOT REMOVE 'SCOPE. Withdraw into tip of catheter mount. INSPIR HOLD or VENTILATOR PAUSE. Circuit change.		Comments:	

	Procedure Team Lead	Bronchoscopist	Nurse in charge	Runner	Other staff
Name /sign					

Figure 19.5 Bronchoscopy checklist.

and 9 or 10 left-sided segments, is very important (often missing a medial left basal segment) (Figure 19.6). Learned handling, dexterity, and situational awareness of ergonomic positioning can ensure optimal visualization. A helpful rule of thumb for remembering the segmental anatomy is to consider the endobronchial tree as two descending corkscrews. When approached from the back of the patient, with the posterior wall of the trachea at the 6 pm position on an imaginary clockface, the right endobronchial corkscrew descends rotating clockwise (the caveat being middle lobe lateral, RB4, and then medial, RB5) and the left endobronchial corkscrew descends anticlockwise.

Infection Control

Cross-infection, particularly with multi-resistant organisms, is an important risk if standard procedures for cleaning and decontamination are not followed correctly.

Thus, pre- and post-procedure decontamination and disinfection will minimize cross-infection.

Single-use-only accessories should be used where possible to prevent cross-contamination. Disposable FBs eliminate the need for disinfection between procedures. However, they must be discarded shortly after single use as there is very high risk of persisting organisms if left, and hence of re- or cross-infection.[3]

Bronchoscopy in Special Circumstances

The Non-intubated Patient (NIV and High Flow)

Bronchoscopy can be performed in the emergency setting without a definitive airway. The indication is usually for airway clearance of tenacious secretions causing acute airway obstruction/collapse or for diagnostic sampling. The aim is generally to prevent intubation/re-intubation. One study reported respiratory status deterioration in ~50% after FB in non-intubated patients with acute respiratory failure, and one-third needed ventilatory support.[28]

Adjunctive oxygenation by HFNO (high flow humidified nasal oxygen), up to 70 L/min, has superseded the use of the cut-out mask of the non-rebreather bag at 15 L/min. Assisted ventilation is caused via NIV masks, which can be modified to accommodate a bronchoscope using a swivel adaptor and mouth guard (Figure 19.2).

Regarding safety, one-third of non-intubated patients with acute respiratory failure (PaO_2/FiO_2 ratio ≤ 300), who underwent 169 FBs and BAL, required escalation of the therapy (i.e. increased oxygen need or NIV) within 24 h, usually <4 h, and 15% required intubation. The presence of COPD (odds ratio (OR) 5.2) and immunosuppression (OR 5.4), but not the duration of FB or the volume of BAL, independently predicted intubation.[29]

In patients with infective exacerbations of COPD and difficult-to-clear secretions, NIV with early therapeutic FB can prevent intubation and need for tracheostomy in a proportion, although the duration of ventilation, hospital mortality, and stay may not change.

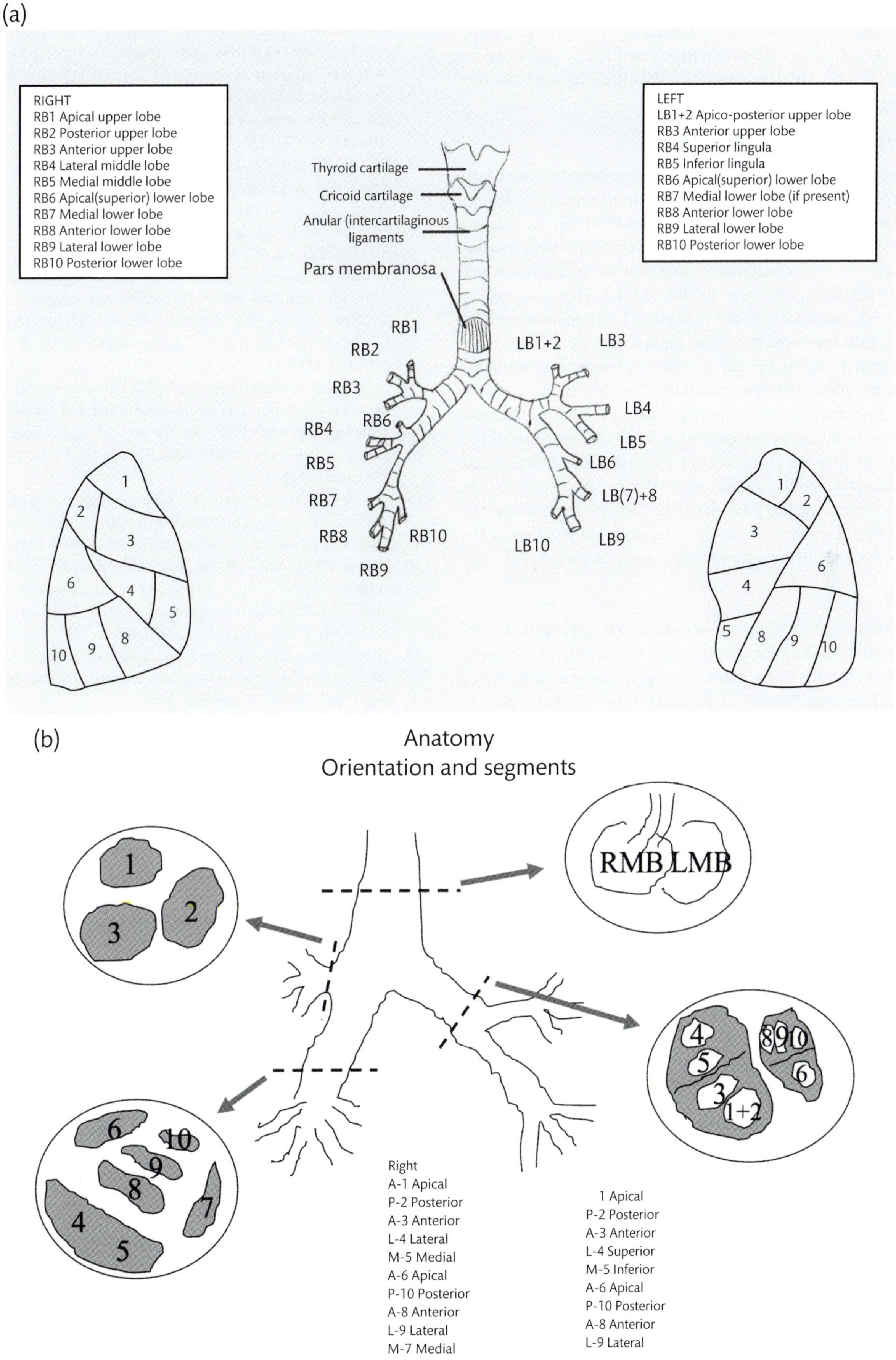
(a)
RIGHT
RB1 Apical upper lobe
RB2 Posterior upper lobe
RB3 Anterior upper lobe
RB4 Lateral middle lobe
RB5 Medial middle lobe
RB6 Apical(superior) lower lobe
RB7 Medial lower lobe
RB8 Anterior lower lobe
RB9 Lateral lower lobe
RB10 Posterior lower lobe
Thyroid cartilage
Cricoid cartilage
Anular (intercartilaginous ligaments
Pars membranosa
LEFT
LB1+2 Apico-posterior upper lobe
RB3 Anterior upper lobe
RB4 Superior lingula
RB5 Inferior lingula
RB6 Apical(superior) lower lobe
RB7 Medial lower lobe (if present)
RB8 Anterior lower lobe
RB9 Lateral lower lobe
RB10 Posterior lower lobe
RB1
RB2
RB3
RB4
RB6
RB5
RB7
RB8
RB10
RB9
LB1+2
LB3
LB4
LB5
LB6
LB(7)+8
LB10
LB9
(b)
Anatomy
Orientation and segments
RMB LMB
Right
A-1 Apical
P-2 Posterior
A-3 Anterior
L-4 Lateral
M-5 Medial
A-6 Apical
P-10 Posterior
A-8 Anterior
L-9 Lateral
M-7 Medial
1 Apical
P-2 Posterior
A-3 Anterior
L-4 Superior
M-5 Inferior
A-6 Apical
P-10 Posterior
A-8 Anterior
L-9 Lateral

Figure 19.6 Practical bronchial anatomy.

Up to one-third of patients on NIV with mild ARDS were intubated within 24 h of FB, making HFNO more practical. Clearly, a plan of escalation to a definitive airway or limit of care must be established beforehand. Having an ETT sheathed over the bronchoscope may facilitate this.

Bronchoscopy During COVID-19

Bronchoscopy is designated as an aerosol-generating procedure by the World Health Organization. As such, its use in mechanically ventilated patients with COVID-19 has been advised against or recommended only following a careful risk–benefit assessment. Expert recommendations for safe practice of bronchoscopy during the pandemic have been published.[30] Key elements include a benefit–risk assessment of the indication for bronchoscopy, the use of full PPE (personal protective equipment) for all personnel involved, and, if feasible, the use of negative pressure environments in which to undertake the procedure. Further, single-use-only bronchoscopes may have an important role. In the ICU, additional safe practice to minimize aerosolization involves preloading of the bronchoscope into the bronchoscopy adaptor of the endotracheal tube, pausing the ventilator and wall suction for the circuit change prior to commencing the procedure. Similarly on completion, the bronchoscope and adaptor are only withdrawn and replaced by the standard circuit again during a ventilator pause manoeuvre.

Training

Many international training schemes specify FB as a required competency skill, including for percutaneous tracheostomy. However, the processes for acquiring and assessing procedural competency vary. The European Society of Intensive Care Medicine has recommended formal training competencies through its link with CoBaTrICE (www.cobatrice.org), the international competency training programme. The value of computer-based virtual bronchoscopy modules, bronchoscopy simulators, dexterity tools, and high-fidelity simulation scenarios is recognized as a valuable part of skills acquisition, compared with no training. However, the evidence base for outcomes in which bronchoscopy simulation may be beneficial beyond conventional clinical instruction is lacking. It is suggested that such simulation-based training be complemented by programmes such as the Bronchoscopy Skills and Tasks Assessment Tool and the Mastery of Learning model, whereby progression to the next level requires the demonstration of proficiency. There is further needed to increase accessibility to all trainees, utilizing cheaper low-fidelity simulation tools and contextual structured scenarios. The pursuit of competencies in training is essential to fulfil the safe effectiveness of the invaluable tool of FB in the ICU.

REFERENCES

1. Becker HD. Bronchoscopy: The past, the present, and the future. *Clin Chest Med.* 2010 Mar;**31**(1):1–18, Table of Contents. doi:10.1016/j.ccm.2009.11.001. PMID: 20172428.
2. Amikam B, Landa J, West J, et al. Bronchofiberscopic observations of the tracheobronchial tree during intubation. *Am Rev Respir Dis.* 1972;**105**:747–755.
3. McGrath BA, Ruane S, McKenna J, et al. Contamination of single-use bronchoscopes in critically ill patients. *Anaesthesia.* 2017;72(1):36–41.
4. Du Rand IA, Barber PV, Goldring J, et al. BTS Interventional Bronchoscopy Guideline Group. Summary of the British Thoracic Society guidelines for advanced diagnostic and therapeutic flexible bronchoscopy in adults. *Thorax.* 2011;**66**(11):1014–1015.
5. Klompas M, Kalil AC. The 'last breath' of the ventilator-associated pneumonia surveillance definition. *Crit Care Med.* 2014; **42**(3):722–723.
6. Bello G, Pennisi MA, Di Muzio F, et al. Clinical impact of pulmonary sampling site in the diagnosis of ventilator-associated pneumonia: A prospective study using bronchoscopic bronchoalveolar lavage. *J Crit Care.* 2016;**33**:151–157.
7. Berton DC, Kalil AC, Teixeira PJ. Quantitative versus qualitative cultures of respiratory secretions for clinical outcomes in patients with ventilator-associated pneumonia. *Cochrane Database Syst Rev.* 2012 Jan 18;**1**:CD006482. doi:10.1002/14651858.CD006482.pub3. Update in: *Cochrane Database Syst Rev.* 2014;10:CD006482. PMID: 22258968.
8. Grover V, Pantelidis P, Soni N, et al. A biomarker panel (Bioscore) incorporating monocytic surface and soluble TREM-1 has high discriminative value for ventilator-associated pneumonia: A prospective observational study. *PLoS One.* 2014 7;**9**(10):e109686.
9. Conway Morris A, Gadsby N, McKenna JP, et al. 16S pan-bacterial PCR can accurately identify patients with ventilator-associated pneumonia. *Thorax.* 2017;**72**(11):1046–1048.
10. Hellyer TP, McAuley DF, Walsh TS, et al. Biomarker-guided antibiotic stewardship in suspected ventilator-associated pneumonia (VAPrapid2): A randomised controlled trial and process evaluation. *Lancet Respir Med.* 2020; **8**:182–191
11. The Canadian Critical Care Trials Group. A randomized trial of diagnostic techniques for ventilator associated pneumonia. *N Eng J Med.* 2006;**355**(25):2619–2630.
12. Torres A, Niederman MS, Chastre J, et al. International ERS/ESICM/ESCMID/ALAT guidelines for the management of hospital-acquired pneumonia and ventilator associated pneumonia. *Eur Respir J.* 2017;**50**(3):pii:1700582.
13. Cracco C, Fartoukh M, Prodanovic H, et al. Safety of performing fiberoptic bronchoscopy in critically ill hypoxemic patients with acute respiratory failure. *Intensive Care Med.* 2013;**39**(1):45–52.
14. Singh S, Shah PL. Viral pneumonia in severe respiratory failure. *Respiration.* 2014;**87**(4):267–269.
15. Fan LC, Lu HW, Cheng KB, et al. Evaluation of PCR in bronchoalveolar lavage fluid for diagnosis of *Pneumocystis jirovecii* pneumonia: A bivariate meta-analysis and systematic review. *PLoS One.* 2013 Sep 4;**8**(9):e73099.
16. Marini J, Pierson DJ, Hudson LD. Acute lobar atelectasis: A prospective comparison of fiberoptic bronchoscopy and respiratory therapy. *Am Rev Respir Dis.* 1979;**119**(6):971–978.
17. Prodhan P, Greenberg B, Bhutta AT, et al. Recombinant human deoxyribonuclease improves atelectasis in mechanically ventilated children with cardiac disease. *Congenit Heart Dis.* 2009;4(3):166–173.
18. Schmidt LH, Schulze AB, Goerlich D, et al. Blood clot removal by cryoextraction in critically ill patients with pulmonary hemorrhage. *J Thorac Dis.* 2019 Oct;**11**(10):4319–4327.
19. Endorf FW, Gamelli RL. Inhalation injury, pulmonary perturbations, and fluid resuscitation. *J Burn Care Res.* 2007;**28**(1):80–83.
20. Carr J, Phillips BD, Bowling WM. The utility of bronchoscopy after inhalational injury complicated by pneumonia in burn patients: Results from the National Burn Repository. *J Burn Care Res.* 2009;**30**:967–974.

21. Singh S, Gurney S. Management of post-intubation tracheal membrane ruptures: A practical approach. *Indian J Crit Care Med.* 2013;**17**(2):99–103. doi:10.4103/0972–5229.114826
22. Cook TM, Woodall N, Harper J, et al. Major complications of airway management in the UK: Results of the Fourth National Audit Project of the Royal College of Anaesthetists and the Difficult Airway Society. Part 2: Intensive care and emergency departments. *Br J Anaes.* 2011;**106**:632–642.
23. Gobatto AL, Besen BA, Tierno PF, et al. Ultrasound-guided percutaneous dilational tracheostomy versus bronchoscopy-guided percutaneous dilational tracheostomy in critically ill patients (TRACHUS): A randomized noninferiority controlled trial. *Intensive Care Med.* 2016;**42**:342–351.
24. Singh S, Hetzel J, Shah PL. Controlled pressure: The solution for a high-pressure situation—aetiology and techniques for control of airway haemorrhage. *Respiration.* 2017;**93**:398–400.
25. https://www.nice.org.uk/guidance/ipg448. Published: 27 Mar 2013.
26. Focciolongo N, Patelli M, Gasparini S, et al. Incidence of complications in bronchoscopy. Multicentre prospective study of 20,986 bronchoscopies. *Monaldi Arch Chest Dis.* 2009;**71**(1):8–14.
27. Schnabel RM, van der Velden K, Osinski A, et al. Clinical course and complications following diagnostic bronchoalveolar lavage in critically ill mechanically ventilated patients. *BMC Pulm Med.* 2015;**15**:107.
28. Azoulay E, Mokart D, Rabbat A, et al. Diagnostic bronchoscopy in hematology and oncology patients with acute respiratory failure: Prospective multicenter data. *Crit Care Med.* 2008;**36**(1):100–107.
29. Cracco C, Fartoukh M, Prodanovic H, et al. Safety of performing fiberoptic bronchoscopy in critically ill hypoxemic patients with acute respiratory failure. *Intensive Care Med.* 2013;**39**:45–52.
30. Luo F, Darwiche K, Singh S, et al. Performing bronchoscopy in times of the COVID-19 pandemic: Practice statement from an international expert panel. *Respiration.* 2020;**99**(5):417–422.
31. Frerichs I, Amato MBP, van Kaam AH, et al. Chest electrical impedance tomography examination, data analysis, terminology, clinical use and recommendations: Consensus statement of the TRanslational EIT developmeNt stuDy group. *Thorax.* 2017;**72**(1):83–93.
32. Badovinac S, Glodić G, Sabol I, et al. Tranexamic Acid vs Adrenaline for Controlling Iatrogenic Bleeding During Flexible Bronchoscopy: A Double-Blind Randomized Controlled Trial. *Chest.* 2023 Apr;**163**(4):985–993. doi: 10.1016/j.chest.2022.10.013.

[illegible]

PART 6
Advanced Mechanical Ventilation

20

Airway Management in the Intensive Care Unit

Johannes M Huitink and Lorenz G Theiler

KEY MESSAGES

- Airway management in intensive care patients should be classified as an advanced procedure because of the many complexity factors.
- In recent years, newer techniques for oxygenation during airway management and emergency procedures have become available.
- Videolaryngoscopes have an important place in airway management in intensive care unit (ICU) patients.
- Percutaneous tracheostomy is a safe procedure in carefully selected patients.
- It is important to learn airway rescue techniques, and all doctors working in the ICU should be trained in an emergency front-of-neck access technique.
- Advanced airway management skills may be needed to intubate ICU patients.
- Standardized peri-procedural checklists and protocols should be implemented and practised.

CONTROVERSIES

- What is the definitive role of non-invasive ventilation (NIV) or high-flow oxygenation in the peri-intubation management of critically ill patients compared with conventional pre-oxygenation techniques?

FUTURE RESEARCH

- Future research should focus on developing techniques to minimize peri-intubation complications such as cardiovascular collapse, marked hypoxaemia, and failure to intubate.
- The use of modified rapid-sequence induction, including routine use of cricoid pressure, avoidance of manual ventilation during the apnoeic phase, and optimal induction drugs, should be subjected to rigorous clinical trial-based investigation.

Introduction

Airway management can be challenging in critically ill patients, both establishing the airway and maintaining it safely over days or even months. In the intensive care unit (ICU), airway management is often performed in very sick patients under difficult circumstances or emergency settings. A number of factors make airway management challenging relative to elective intubation in the operating theatre. These include location away from the operating theatre, time pressure precluding through airway examination, the proficiency and/or experience of airway management skills in ICU staff, and the physiological condition of the patient. Appropriate training and regular renewal of skills will reduce complications. In the ICU, airway incidents are among the most common problems reported in ICUs, with human error playing an important role.[1]

The unstable physiology of critically ill patients presents specific problems for airway management. The patient may have laboured breathing, reduced oxygen saturations, have copious secretions, be haemodynamically unstable, and have a compromised airway. Even low doses of sedation can have a profound effect, causing upper airway and respiratory muscle depression, hypotension, and rapid oxygen desaturation. Induction of anaesthesia is complex, requiring modification of normal drug choices and doses.

Moreover, airway management in the ICU is often performed under time pressure, when the patient is often near a cardiac-respiratory (peri)arrest situation. Oral awake intubation can be considered first, although in reality this is not commonly done in this setting due to patient instability and agitation as well as lack of operator familiarity with the techniques.

Even when airway management is successful, the initiation of positive pressure ventilation may also be poorly tolerated.

In the British national anaesthesia audit project number four (NAP4) concerning airway management,[2] nearly 20% of all reported major airway incidents occurred in the ICU, with a disproportionate burden of neurological damage or death (61% compared with only 14% during anaesthesia and 31% in the emergency department).[2] Main reasons for devastating airway outcomes were unrecognized oesophageal intubations without the use of capnography, failed surgical airway as a rescue manoeuvre, and accidental extubation especially during patient transfer. The authors of NAP4 have made several suggestions how to improve airway management in the ICU, which is highlighted in this chapter.

In contrast to the enormous literature on anaesthetic airway management, focusing on airway management in ICU is rather modest. The NAP4 study[2] is important as it identified major risk factors for complications. Compared with the operating theatre setting, ICU was notable for failure to identify high-risk patients, higher rates of night-time events, management by unskilled junior trainees without supervision, failure to adhere to a structured guideline plan, and for lack of equipment. The quality of airway management was judged to be poor during more events on ICU than in anaesthesia.

Recent years have seen many changes in guidance because of rapid developments in airway management devices. These include videolaryngoscopes, supraglottic airway devices, and ultrasound (US). New tracheostomy and oxygenation devices have come to market. This has changed the way we work. In this chapter, we provide an overview of the latest insights in adult airway management and recent developments in the field. We recognize that technological advances such as viewing tipped endotracheal tubes continue to emerge. Their place in standard care will require robust evaluation prior to recommendation.

Upper Airway Evaluation and Assessment

Paul L Marino once stated his famous rule no. 1—the indication for intubation and mechanical ventilation is thinking of it.[3] If invasive mechanical ventilation is warranted, a secure airway is usually necessary, which by definition requires a cuffed tube in the trachea. Before securing the airway, the upper airways must be assessed.

Failure to recognize a difficult airway may lead to significant injury or death. One of the recommendations of NAP4 is to clearly identify patients at risk for difficult airway management.[2]

Rosenblatt formulated five questions to ask before performing any airway management manoeuvres in the ICU: (1) Is airway management necessary? (2) Will direct laryngoscopy and tracheal intubation be straightforward? (3) Can supralaryngeal ventilation be used? (4) Is there an aspiration risk? (5) In the event of airway failure, will the patient tolerate an apnoeic period?[4]

The classic tests for the prediction of difficulties during airway management in ICU patients often fail or are impossible. It is important to acknowledge the fact that predictive tests for difficult intubation are often not so. Such scoring systems include Naguib's score, Arne Risk Sum, or the MACOCHA score.[5,6] To assess the pharyngeal space, a thin flexible fibreoptic endoscope can be introduced through the nose. Most often, local anaesthesia is not even necessary for this task. Tumour, oedema, and stenosis are then easily assessed before starting any airway management procedure. In ICU, mouth opening is often limited, patient confusion can add to the difficulty, while the risk of aspiration is high. Unstable vital parameters may make urgent care necessary. Rapid-sequence intubation is often advocated. When patients are at high risk for aspiration and desaturation, maintenance of oxygen levels is paramount. Thus, critically ill patients often have advanced airways with many complexity factors such as unstable physiology, and time pressure, that can complicate the airway management procedure.[6,7]

Considering the issues discussed above, the LEMON[8] mnemonic may be helpful:

L.
(L)ook externally to identify easily recognizable conditions that would predict a difficult airway. These may be obesity, facial or neck trauma, short neck, neck deviation secondary to malignancy; protruding tongue or teeth, missing teeth, overbite, small mandible; presence of a beard; and old age with abundant loose facial and neck tissue, and being edentulous.

E.
(E)valuate the 3–3–2 rule. This practical rule does not exclude an advanced airway but may help predict potential difficulty. Although there are variations with age, gender, and build, the average patient should have at least:

- 3 fingerbreadth wide mouth opening (inter-incisor distance) with good mandibular motion;
- 3 fingerbreadth distance from the mentum to the hyoid bone; and
- 2 fingerbreadth distance from the floor of the mouth to the thyroid cartilage.

M.
(M)allampati class:

- Class 1: Able to visualize the soft palate, uvula, fauces, anterior, and posterior tonsillar pillars.
- Class 2: Able to visualize the soft palate, fauces, and uvula. The anterior and posterior tonsillar pillars are hidden by the tongue.
- Class 3: Only the soft palate and base of uvula are visible.
- Class 4: Only the hard palate can be seen (no parts of uvula seen).

O.
(O)bstruction: Consider possible airway obstruction when the patient has epiglottitis, midneck haematoma (e.g. gun or knife wound trauma and bleeding tendency) or malignancy and oedema of the airway (angioedema especially in patients taking angiotensin-converting enzyme inhibitors, in allergic patients, and in burn patients).

N.
(N)eck mobility, extension. The patient with trauma to the area or with rheumatoid arthritis and cervical spine involvement requires special care.

If difficult airway management is predicated or known, additional precautions must be taken, including adaptation of the chosen technique to secure the airway and the help of adequately trained personnel.

Direct laryngoscopy may be possible in many patients; however, many ICU units start with a videolaryngoscope as their first airway device. This has the advantage that a clear view can be obtained during intubation, but tracheal intubation may still be difficult without proper training. In a general population, >99% of the patients can be intubated with a direct laryngoscopy technique by a trained doctor. This is different for ICU patients. Techniques other than direct laryngoscopy may be needed to secure the airway.

Two particular aspects of airway management in the ICU are unplanned extubation and blocked tracheal tubes. In a study of unplanned extubation events in an ICU, it was found that 85% were self-extubation and 15% were accidental.[9] Accidental extubation occurred during day shift in less alert patients and were associated with transport procedures and the use of rotary beds. Of all these patients, almost half had to be re-intubated within the first hour. Re-intubation is often difficult due to oedema of the larynx or saliva and blood secretions in the upper airway. Unplanned extubation is an adverse event that should be preventable by adequately sedating patients during transport and using pre-transfer checklists.

Prolonged use of heat and moisture exchanger (HME) filters has been associated with an increased incidence of blocked endotracheal tubes.

General Airway Management Considerations

Team Factors

ICU airway management is a challenging procedure in a challenging environment. A good knowledge of anatomy and physiology is the starting point for airway management. The team approach is also important. The leader of the team should be established, and team coordination under their guidance should be expected. Often a multidisciplinary team is necessary to treat the ICU patient, which can make team work more challenging because all team members may have a different approach to airway management.

Before attempting laryngoscopy, it is crucial to have several contingency action plans (plan A, plan B, or even plan C), thus creating an airway management strategy (Figure 20.1). These plans should always

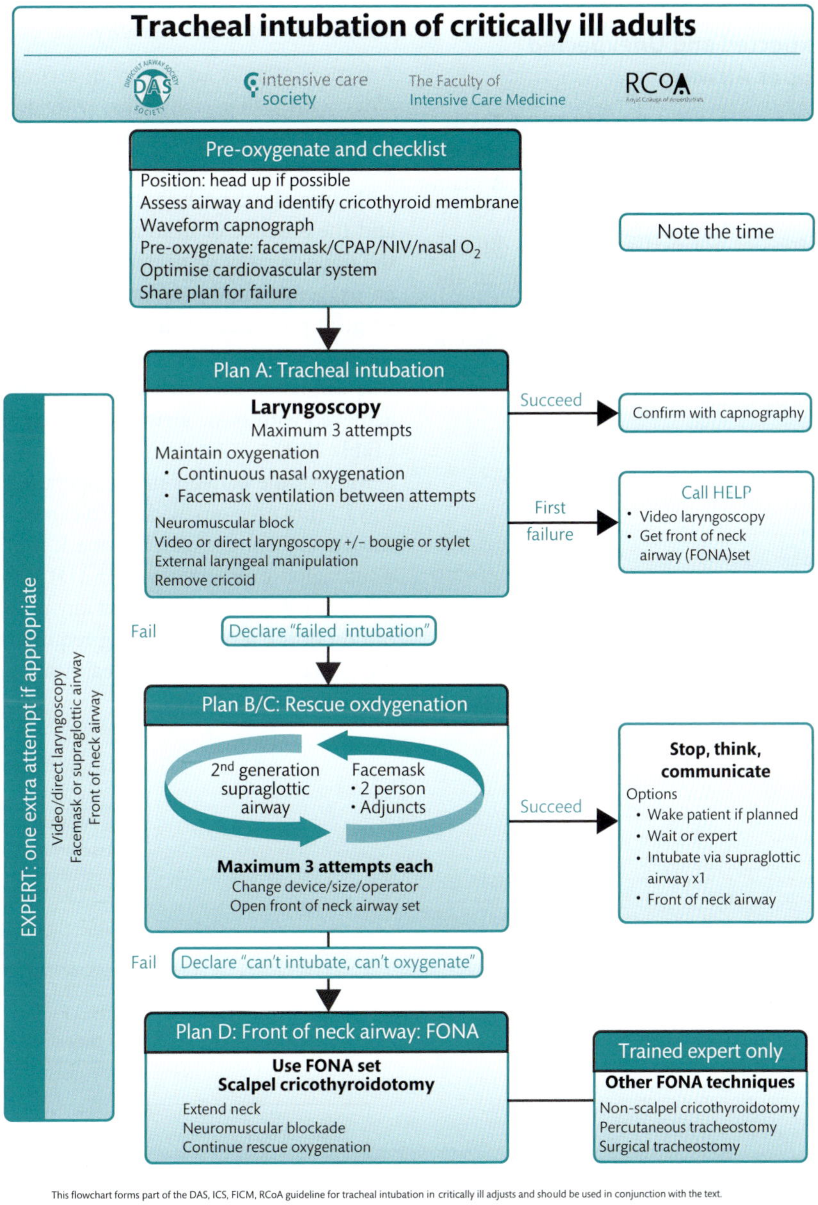

Figure 20.1 Algorithm for tracheal intubation of the critically ill adult.

Reprinted from *British Journal of Anaesthesia*, 120, 2, Higgs A, et al., Guidelines for the management of tracheal intubation in critically ill adults, pp. 323–352, Copyright 2018, with permission from the Board of Management and Trustees of the British Journal of Anaesthesia.

be discussed with the team. The team should think of possible failed intubation and be prepared in advance. It can be necessary to change the initial plan after first inspection of the airway. This is called *prevention of plan continuation error*. For example, a videolaryngoscope may be a great device to help intubate a patient. However, when bleeding occurs, a change of equipment may become necessary.

During the attempts at tracheal intubation, the person intubating should describe his actions and findings. It is very important for the other members of the team to be alerted if the airway is difficult. Videolaryngoscopy may have a role here because the larynx can be seen by everyone on a monitor screen. This is a big advantage, as everyone around the patient becomes actively involved in securing the airway and senior clinicians may take over sooner when the airway appears difficult to intubate. For teaching purposes, it is great to capture the intubation procedure on video images or photographs. This may also become important as evidence of good practice done during the intubation procedure.

Guidelines to Manage Expected and Unexpected Difficult Access to the Upper Airway

The most well-known airway management guidelines are the revised difficult airway guidelines of the American Anesthesiology association (ASA) and Difficult airway society UK (DAS).[6] A main algorithm may be used when the patient, who needs to be intubated, is not in severe distress or nor peri-arrest and a difficult airway is not anticipated. This may be the patient to whom the intensivist will explain the procedure and the reason for which it will be performed. It may be useful to use a checklist and differentiate between basic and advanced airway (Tables 20.1 and 20.2 and Figure 20.2).[7]

Table 20.1 Requirements for a classification of a basic airway, according to the PHASE criteria

Patient	ASA physical status 1–2 Age >12 years Cooperative BMI < 25 kg/m^2 Height > 130 cm, <200 cm Weight >30 kg, <100 kg Airway management in a hospital environment
History	No prior history of airway management complications or problems, no prior reconstructive surgery and/or radiation therapy to upper airway or neck, and no medical syndrome that is associated with airway management problems
Airway	Mallampati 1–2 with mouth opening >3 cm No loose teeth or buck teeth Good neck flexion/extension >S cm from tip of chin to sternal notch No large beard that affects good face oxygenation No short neck-thyromental distance >4 cm No tumours or lumps in the upper airway or neck region No active bleeding in the upper airway No inspiratory stridor
Surgical Procedure	Outside upper airway or neck region
Evaluation of vital signs	Oxygen saturations >95% off oxygen at the start of the procedure and stable vital signs—systolic blood pressure >95 mmHg, heart rate 40–140/mm, Respiratory rate 14–20/mm

Pregnant patients will most likely have a BMI >25 kg/m^2 and are often classified as an advanced airway.

Source: Reproduced from Huitink JM, Bouwman RA. The myth of the difficult airway: Airway management revisited. *Anaesthesia*. 2015;70:244–249, with permission from Wiley.

Table 20.2 Complexity factors that are a threat to patient safety during airway management: the HELP-ET checklist

Factor	Example(s)
Human factors	Language barrier, fatigue, stress, etc.
Experience	Lack of skills (e.g. flexible awake intubation is needed but the team has never done this procedure)
Location	Remote part of the hospital, new environment, and expert help not available
Patient factors	Prior radiation therapy to the neck and airway obstruction
Equipment	Technical problems
Time pressure	Rapid desaturation and unstable vital signs

Source: Reproduced from Huitink JM, Bouwman RA. The myth of the difficult airway: Airway management revisited. *Anaesthesia*. 2015;70:244-249, with permission from Wiley.

Definition of Basic Airway

A basic airway is an airway in a cooperative patient, 12 years or older with stable vital signs, with normal body mass index and no extremes in weight or length, ASA I or II, Mallampati I or II without a large beard that makes face mask ventilation difficult, without a short neck, but with good neck flexion and extension and the absence of head and neck tumours or active bleeding in the upper airway or neck region in an hospital environment with an oxygen saturation of >95% without supplemental oxygen. If a surgical procedure in these patients is done, it should be outside the upper airways or neck region. Without complexity factors, it is estimated that airway management in these patients can be achieved with basic airway management skills in almost all cases (Table 20.1).

Most of the patients in the operating theatre will have basic airways. From previous evidence it can be deduced that a trained medical person can perform bag-mask ventilation (BMV), insertion of a supraglottic airway device (SAD), or tracheal intubation in these patients within 1 min, without any problem. We will not give a definition of the level of training required, but it seems reasonable to argue that this should be a healthcare professional trained in acute care medicine.

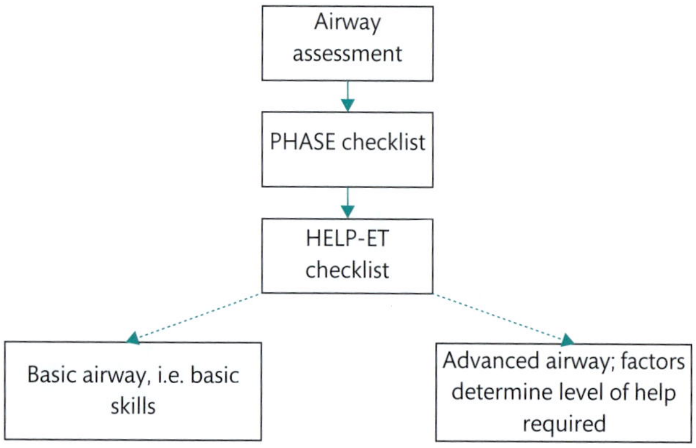

Figure 20.2 A framework for determining the airway type based upon PHASE and HELP-ET checklists.

Reproduced from Huitink JM and Bouwman RA. The myth of the difficult airway: airway management revisited. *Anaesthesia* 2015; 70: 244–9, with permission from the Association of Anaesthetists and Wiley.

For the basic airway, basic airway management skills can be used: BMV, SAD insertion, tracheal intubation with a Macintosh 3 or 4 blade, and sometimes a bougie for difficulty in introducing the tracheal tube. And even in a basic airway case with unexpected difficulties, it should be possible to call for help early or to wake up the patient and start again and do it differently. Postoperatively, these airways will almost never be a challenge or a problem because the airway anatomy is normal and the surgical procedure has been performed away from the respiratory tract.

All other airways can be classified as advanced airways. In patients with advanced airways, it must be anticipated that airway management can be challenging because of the presence of one or more airway management complexity factors (Table 20.1).

With this classification, it can be clearly seen that ICU patients will almost always be classified as advanced airways. In this situation, it is very important to assess airway management complexity factors, which may be a threat to patient safety during airway management. Checklists may be helpful in assessing the presence of an advanced airway from a basic one such as PHASE (Table 20.1). Further factors that can contribute to the complexity of the task are defined by the HELP-ET criteria (Table 20.2). These may be helpful in determining the pathway for airway management (Figure 20.2).

Airway Management Complexity Factors

1. *Patient factors*: for example, prior radiation therapy to the neck and airway obstruction;
2. *Experience*: for example, experience of the team and their skills, such as flexible awake intubation;
3. *Time pressure*: for example, because of unstable vital signs or rapid desaturation, anatomical considerations, or uncooperative patients;
4. *Equipment*: for example, technical problems and missing equipment;
5. *Location*: for example, remote hospital, no resources and no expert help available;
6. *Human factors*: for example, language barriers, fatigue, and stress.

In these cases, special measurements or advanced skills may be needed to guarantee safe airway management during or after a procedure. This could be the immediate availability of a dedicated airway management trolley with extra equipment and in cases with many complexity factors, the help of an airway management expert, and or a head and neck surgeon.

Each ICU unit should have their own unexpected difficult airway algorithm, which is adapted to local conditions. Think globally but act locally.

In every ICU, a trolley or box should be immediately available with emergency equipment for the anticipated and unanticipated difficulties with the airway. Second-generation supraglottic airway devices, which are 'SADs that have been designed for safety and which have design features to reduce the risk of aspiration' are preferable. A videolaryngoscope, a flexible bronchoscope, and equipment to perform surgical access to the airway should be available, as well as a device for emergency ventilation, for example, Ventrain (Ventinova©) or Manujet (VBM©). All staff should be trained regularly.

Airway team members, monitors, and equipment should be appropriately positioned to maximize visual cues and not hinder access to the patient. Alarm limits should be predetermined as appropriate for patient age and anticipated difficulties. It should be acknowledged that noise can be substantial and that acoustic alarms are easily missed. Standard monitoring (oximetry, waveform of end-tidal carbon dioxide, blood pressure, and ECG) should be applied and rapid-sequence induction (RSI) optimized according to the abnormalities wherever possible. If time permits, this may include commencement of vasopressor infusions. A timer should be used both for pre-oxygenation and to facilitate rapid progression through agreed airway plans.

Avoidance of hypoxia and hypotension is essential in the critically ill patient. Pre-oxygenation strategies are discussed below. With regard to hypotension, many clinicians will consider the impact of induction and paralysis on both cardiac contractility and venous tone, along with effects of positive pressure ventilation, as mandating an intravenous fluid bolus to improve preload prior to induction, unless contraindicated. Measurements of blood pressure should be made regularly, with either non-invasive blood pressure set to cycle at 1 min intervals or placement of an arterial line if time allows.

Airway Management Techniques

Pre-oxygenation

The purpose of pre-oxygenation is to remove nitrogen from the lungs and to create a reservoir of oxygen, so allowing a margin of safety before critical desaturation during attempts to secure the airway. Key steps include mandatory use of pre-oxygenation to extend safe apnoea time during RSI, along with appropriate positioning, and may involve the use of positive end-expiratory pressure (PEEP). There is growing evidence for the use of ventilation, via bag-valve mask (BVM) or non-invasively, and the use of passive apnoeic oxygen diffusion by nasal cannulae in reducing peri-intubation hypoxia.[10]

The period of pre-oxygenation should adequately remove nitrogen from the lungs. An empiric approach applying high-flow oxygen for 3 min or eight vital capacity breaths is common anaesthetic practice. However, critically ill patients may require a longer period for this and are often unable to perform eight vital capacity breaths. If available, the measurement of expired end-tidal oxygen should be used as a guide to adequate pre-oxygenation, aiming for a value of at least 90% ($FetO_2$ of 0.9).

Pre-oxygenation technique may be governed by available equipment, personnel, and patient requirements. Valid techniques include the following:

- The use of a Mapleson B or C anaesthetic circuits. These lack the separate inspiratory or expiratory ports of traditional BVM devices, with exhaled gas flushed out of the circuit by high fresh gas flow via the pressure-release valve, ensuring maximal oxygen delivery.
- The use of standard BVM devices commonly used in the emergency department, ICU, or by emergency medical services. Caution is needed as such devices may entrain room air during spontaneous ventilation. Addition of a PEEP valve to the expiratory port of BVM assembly obviates this.

- The use of standard reservoir face masks on maximal oxygen flow and supplemented with nasal cannula on maximal flow, which remains during the intubation effort. This may be a preferred in the prehospital environment, where limitations of personnel preclude alternatives.
- The use of existing non-invasive ventilation (NIV) modes. For many critically ill patients, RSI may represent the end result of a failure of NIV. NIV masks may be left in situ and used to pre-oxygenate. CPAP/NIV may be very useful in pre-oxygenation of the morbidly obese patient.

An important concept in the ICU is high-flow nasal cannula therapy (HFNC). Patients with high-flow nasal oxygen (HFNO) are less likely to be intubated, and 90-day mortality could be decreased (see Chapter 7). HFNO proved to increase saturation levels during intubation in ICU patients. In apnoeic patients, even ventilatory effects have been discovered when using HFNC for prolonged duration up to 1 h: transnasal humidified rapid-insufflation ventilatory exchange (THRIVE) to provide HFNO has thus revolutionized airway management with the ability to dramatically increase apnoea time during the intubation efforts, providing the airways are open. That said, recent randomized studies and meta-analyses have not demonstrated a reduction in the frequency of desaturations through the use of HFNC and/or NIV and so firm recommendations have not been made.[10]

On occasions, the uncooperative patient (e.g. intoxicated, head-injured, and hypoxic) will thwart best attempts at both positioning and pre-oxygenation. Pre-treatment with small, titrated aliquots of a sedative agent can be effective (so-called 'delayed sequence intubation'), with ketamine the preferred agent to facilitate assessment, monitoring, positioning, and pre-oxygenation. The technique is not without risks, though, and high experience levels are necessary to walk the line between giving enough sedation for pre-oxygenation tolerance and too much that diminishes ventilatory drive.

Pre-treatment with appropriate drugs like lidocaine can be used for blunting airway reflexes, and the intracranial pressure response to laryngoscopy in head injury patients, opioids, atropine, and vasopressors can be used in the case of haemodynamic instability.

Positioning and protection of the airway (occiput elevation and the sniffing position) should be used, if feasible.

Oral intubation under direct laryngoscopy should be attempted as this is the most common approach and most intensivists are familiar with the technique. The intubation is considered successful if the tracheal tube is seen passing through the vocal cords. After that point, post-intubation management should commence immediately.

Rapid-sequence Induction

RSI involves the rapid administration of an induction agent to induce unconsciousness and a neuromuscular blocker to provide fast muscle relaxation. It is also named 'Crash induction', first described by Woodbridge.[11] This combination is intended to eliminate the chance of active vomiting. For the same reason, BMV is also avoided. Interestingly, the concept of RSI has never been validated and it remains unclear whether the risk of haemodynamic or other complications is justified by shortening the time until intubation. Patients in the ICU are often at high risk for aspiration and desaturation because they may have been enterally fed and may have gastroparesis, ileus or bowel obstruction. Cricoid pressure during the attempt may help prevent passive regurgitation and assists visualization. Cricoid pressure has become controversial, and much debate is still going on if it is helpful to prevent aspiration.

The first attempt at intubation should be the best, so muscle paralysis is often necessary to create optimal intubation conditions.

It is important to appreciate that repeated attempts at laryngoscopy may increase risk of aspiration and it may cause swelling or bleeding. Thus, maximizing the potential for first-pass success is essential in RSI of the critically ill patient. Direct laryngoscopy using an appropriate blade and light source (modern-day LED optics offer excellent illumination and contrast) remains the cornerstone of intubation. Careful and sequential visualization of landmarks and avoidance of repeated attempts causing airway trauma are key skills. Adjuncts such as a bougie or malleable stylet are commonly used in cases of difficult intubation. For intubation of the critically ill patient, such adjuncts should be used routinely. Understanding appropriate use is vital as infrequent users may not appreciate the nuances of these devices, which are designed to facilitate navigation to the laryngeal inlet in difficult cases. Stylets, if used, should be shaped 'straight-to-cuff', that is, the stylet should remain straight as far as the proximal part of the endotracheal tube cuff where it should be angled to no more than 35° (angles >35° increase difficulty). Traditional teaching has been to avoid pre-loading endotracheal tubes onto bougies, as the weight of the tube may impair control of the bougie tip; however, hang-up of the bougie on the endotracheal tube connector may impede smooth railroading of the endotracheal tube, causing delay in tube passage and risking a loss of situational awareness in the operator. A refinement is to preload an endotracheal tube onto a bougie and hold them in such a grip that control of the bougie is maintained during navigation to the laryngeal inlet. It is not uncommon for the leading edge of bevel-shaped endotracheal tubes to hang up on the right arytenoid cartilage; gentle slight withdrawal and a anticlockwise rotation of the endotracheal tube/bougie complex allow the free edge to enter the glottic opening and advance.

There is evidence for variation in how individuals, institutions, and even nations practise RSI. The technique of RSI is centred on reduction of risk; that of regurgitation/aspiration; and that associated with the procedure itself, including failure to rapidly secure the airway, hypoxia, airway trauma, and hypotension from induction agents. Analysis of airway complications reveals a higher incidence of difficulty in ICU and emergency department intubations than in the operating theatre: the incidence of death or brain damage is 38-fold higher in the ED and 58-fold higher in the ICU compared with operating theatre.[12]

Variations in RSI are inevitable given the heterogeneous mix of patient pre-morbid physiology, teams, environment, and available options. Indeed, it is appropriate that RSI is modified to the circumstances, particularly in the critically ill patient.[13] Unfortunately, the existence of such appropriate heterogeneity in practice can lead to debate, whether between clinical experts, between health institutions, between medical specialties, or medico-legally.

Documented modifications to RSI technique include patient position, pre-oxygenation strategies, pre-RSI decompression of gastric contents with a nasogastric tube, choice and method of administration of induction agent, application of cricoid pressure, choice of paralysing agent, use of manual ventilation, and options for failed RSI.

The following mnemonic (the '4P') may be used as a checklist:

1. *Preparation*: All required equipment should be ready and functioning. Suction, medications, bougie or stylet and a functioning laryngoscope should be available with different size blades. A direct and preferably also an indirect laryngoscope should be available, or a combined device.
2. *Pre-oxygenation*: The patient should be preoxygenated with 100% oxygen by a non-rebreather mask or 15 L/min oxygen by nasal prongs. More recently, transnasal humidified respiratory inspiratory ventilation exchange THRIVE was recently proposed to increase apnoea time.[10] Pre-oxygenation with HFNO (up to 60 L/min) and removal of nitrogen may prolong the time to critical desaturation. This remains to be confirmed consistently.
3. *Prevention* of hypoxia and hypotension during the induction and intubation sequence.
4. *Passage* of a cuffed endotracheal tube with confirmation of placement.

Regardless of the individual expertise of the person intubating, team factors will impact on performance of the RSI process. Team members should be adequately trained prior to involvement in airway management, preferably involving simulation training under increasing degrees of cognitive load to reinforce the importance of human factors in performance.

Use of a standardized approach to RSI may be appropriate within an institution or service and an RSI checklist is recommended,[6,7] but any such checklist should be short, clear, and contain a check only of essential items (Figure 20.3). Checklists should be designed to be read aloud to verify 'essential items completed' rather than being presented as a 'recipe in a cookbook'.

Airway teams should regularly engage in simulation training, using their own equipment and personnel, and simulating both common and uncommon scenarios. This may include common critical care presentations, but will also incorporate changes in team members, equipment failure, and other measures to encourage understanding of human factors in team performance.

Cricoid Pressure

Cricoid pressure has become an area of contention in airway management. Sellick's original description was of a 'firm' amount of pressure applied to the cricoid cartilage of a cadaver while in a steep head-down position to occlude the oesophagus and prevent regurgitation of fluid into the oropharynx.[14] Sellick's procedure was repeated during induction of 26 patients deemed at high risk of aspiration. None of the patients experienced regurgitation with application of cricoid force; three experienced immediate reflux upon release of cricoid force after tracheal intubation. Cricoid force was incorporated into Stept and Safar's description of RSI and has since been considered an essential component.[15] Refinements describe a force of 10 N applied at the commencement of induction, which increased to 30 N with loss of consciousness.

However, the application of cricoid force is not considered routine practice in some countries or organizations. There are concerns that cricoid force does not effectively occlude the oesophagus and thus prevent aspiration, is variably applied by assistants (often incorrect timing, incorrect position, or force), and that cricoid force can impede view at laryngoscopy thus delaying first-pass success. Also, cricoid pressure may make intubation more difficult as the cricoid is pushed downwards, contrary to the BURP manoeuvre: i.e., *b*ackwards, *u*pwards, *r*ightwards *p*ressure, which eases intubation because the larynx is moved upwards.

Some suggest that cricoid force is a low-risk procedure that works in a proportion of patients but is confounded by poor technique and relative infrequency of regurgitation. Thus, it is proposed that cricoid force should be removed early if it impedes laryngoscopy, if there is active vomiting, or if there is impediment of rescue ventilation via laryngeal mask airway or BVM. It can be argued that in certain arenas, particularly prehospital or with limited/untrained personnel (e.g. rural and small ICU), the application of cricoid pressure is more likely to hinder laryngoscopy and that the policy of 'apply, then release' adds additional cognitive load to an already high-stake tightly coupled procedure. On the basis of this, some airway experts may opt to omit cricoid force in such circumstances, based on limited evidence of efficacy and risk–benefit balance in regard to optimizing first-pass intubation success.

Patient Positioning and Optimization

Most clinicians perform RSI in the supine position. In the bariatric patient, 'ramping' of the upper body to around 45° may be required to improve functional residual capacity via displacing the weight of the anterior chest wall off the thoracic cavity and the weight of the intra-abdominal contents off the diaphragm. This ramped position is often referred to as the 'ear-to-sternum position' as it results in the external auditory meatus being at the same horizontal level as the sternum. Head-up positioning may be preferable for the non-hypotensive head-injured patient, to improve venous outflow from the brain, thus helping to reduce intracranial pressure.

The head-up position has been suggested as an alternative, or in addition to, to the application of cricoid pressure in reducing passive regurgitation. However, if the patient vomits, it theoretically increases the chances of aspiration from the effects of gravity rather than particulate matter draining from the mouth.

Patient positioning continues to be debatable. Even head-down position has been proposed to avoid tracheal aspiration although regurgitation may be increased.

Pregnant patients should be positioned head-up or in left lateral tilt to avoid aortocaval compression. Regardless of whether positioned supine, head-up to limit regurgitation, head-down to limit aspiration, or in a left lateral position if pregnant, working suction should always be available. Specific guidelines for difficult airway management in pregnancy have been produced.[16]

Manual Bag-mask Ventilation

Manual ventilation has traditionally been avoided in classical RSI due to concerns of gastric insufflation and aspiration. However, gentle ventilation has been advocated in both obstetric and paediatric RSI due to concerns of rapid desaturation in these populations. A decision on whether to gently ventilate will be guided by aspiration risk—the patient with ileus, with gastroparesis, or with upper gastrointestinal bleeding is clearly at higher risk than the fasted patient. For the critically ill patient, risks of hypoxia and hypercapnia may require gentle manual ventilation. Critically ill patients commonly have an existing metabolic acidosis with respiratory compensation, and periods of apnoea can result in significant reductions in pH, which amplify haemodynamic risk. A recent randomized trial intensive care society — care when it matters

Intubation Checklist: critically ill adults - to be done with whole team present.

The Faculty of Intensive Care Medicine — RCoA Royal College of Anaesthetists

Prepare the patient

- ❑ **Reliable IV /IO access**
- ❑ **Optimise position**
  - ❑ Sit-up?
  - ❑ Mattress hard
- ❑ **Airway assessment**
  - ❑ Identify cricothyroid membrane
  - ❑ Awake intubation option?
- ❑ **Optimal preoxygenation**
  - ❑ 3 mins or ETO_2 >85%
  - ❑ Consider CPAP/NIV
  - ❑ Nasal O_2
- ❑ **Optimise patient state**
  - ❑ Fluid/pressor/inotrope
  - ❑ Aspirate NG tube
  - ❑ Delayed sequence induction
- ❑ **Allergies?**
  - ❑ ↑ Potassium risk? -avoid suxamethonium

Prepare the equipment

- ❑ **Apply monitors**
  - ❑ SpO_2/waveform $ETCO_2$/ ECG/BP
- ❑ **Check equipment**
  - ❑ Tracheal tubes x 2 -cuffs checked
  - ❑ Direct laryngoscopes x 2
  - ❑ Videolaryngoscope
  - ❑ Bougie/stylet
  - ❑ Working suction
  - ❑ Supraglottic airways
  - ❑ Guedel/nasal airways
  - ❑ Flexible scope/Aintree
  - ❑ FONA set
- ❑ **Check drugs**
  - ❑ Consider ketamine
  - ❑ Relaxant
  - ❑ Pressor/inotrope
  - ❑ Maintenance sedation

Prepare the team

- ❑ **Allocate roles**
  One person may have more than one role.
  - ❑ Team Leader
  - ❑ 1st Intubator
  - ❑ 2nd Intubator
  - ❑ Cricoid force
  - ❑ Intubator's assistant
  - ❑ Drugs
  - ❑ Monitoring patient
  - ❑ Runner
  - ❑ MILS (if indicated)
  - ❑ Who will perform FONA?
- ❑ **Who do we call for help?**
- ❑ **Who is noting the time?**

Prepare for difficulty

- ❑ **Can we wake the patient if intubation fails?**
- ❑ **Verbalise** "Airway Plan is:"
  - ❑ **Plan A:** Drugs & laryngoscopy
  - ❑ **Plan B/C:** Supraglottic airway; Face-mask; Fibreoptic intubation via supraglottic airway
  - ❑ **Plan D:** FONA; Scalpel-bougie-tube
- ❑ **Does anyone have questions or concerns?**

Figure 20.3 Intubation checklist for the critically ill adult.

Reprinted from *British Journal of Anaesthesia*, 120, 2, Higgs A, et al., Guidelines for the management of tracheal intubation in critically ill adults, pp. 323–352, Copyright 2018, with permission from the Board of Management and Trustees of the British Journal of Anaesthesia.

including 400 patients demonstrated manual ventilation during induction-reduced hypoxaemia and severe hypoxaemia with no associated increase in aspiration.[17]

Airway Devices in the ICU

Supraglottic Airway Devices

Supraglottic airway devices (SADs) are rarely used in the ICU. Because the secure airway is defined as a cuffed tube in the trachea, SADs do not fulfil the criteria of a secured airway. However, it can be used as an airway rescue device. There is evidence, however, that SAD may lead an important role in the ICU and perhaps they should be used more often. In 2009, Russo et al.[18] prospectively studied 40 randomized patients who were weaned either with a tracheal tube or ProSeal Laryngeal Mask Airway. Use of the SAD was associated with less cardiovascular change compared to the endotracheal tube, while ventilation was possible without reported adverse events despite the prolonged use in the ICU. In fact, the ProSeal has been used up to 40 h postoperatively without negative effects. Tracheal tubes can safely be exchanged for an SAD for smoother extubation in elective settings. The ProSeal laryngeal mask airway (LMA) has been used successfully to aid in percutaneous tracheostomy in the ICU either as an intermediate ventilation mean after tracheal intubation or as a backup in the case of failed intubation. SAD is the major backup device used in the case of failed intubation, regardless of the environment.[6] In the ICU and in any other environment as well, second-generation devices are to be preferred. Second-generation devices are defined by featuring specific aspects to avoid gastric regurgitation and aspiration, such as a gastric access tube. There are no third-generation devices available as there is no definition of a third-generation device. Regardless of the specific device, SAD may be used as backup ventilation devices in the case of failed intubation. They can also be used to intubate either blindly or fibre-optically, which may be the preferred technique. The learning curve is steep, and failure rates are low, although no data exists for the elective use of SAD in this context in the ICU. While SAD may not be the first-line device to secure an airway device in the ICU, an SAD should be readily available and its use should be without hesitation in the case of failed intubation.[6] As outlined above, the SAD may be used electively in selected cases for smooth extubation and facilitated weaning and perhaps for percutaneous tracheostomy procedures in trained hands.

Videolaryngoscopy

Videolaryngoscopy has virtually revolutionized airway management in anaesthesia over the last decade. Arulkumaran et al. conducted a systematic review and meta-analysis in 2018, covering over 15,000 intubations.[19] They found that videolaryngoscopy was of particular value in the intensive care setting, with a significantly enhanced chance of successful intubation. Although this analysis found a significant reduction in peri-procedural complications, this was predominantly due to a reduction in oesophageal intubations (1.4% vs 4.7%). Rates of airway and dental trauma, hypoxaemia, and aspiration did not differ between video and direct laryngoscopy, although arterial hypotension was more common in the videolaryngoscopy group.[19] The 32 studies included a range of videolaryngoscopes, with the glidescope and C-MAC being the dominant devices examined and the C-MAC demonstrating clearer evidence of superiority over direct laryngoscopy. Although Arulkumaran's analysis demonstrated that first-past intubation was commoner in less experienced operators using videolaryngoscopy, they found no effect for experienced operators. Sakles and colleagues demonstrated that the learning curve for videolaryngoscopy may be increased compared with direct laryngoscopy in the emergency department where the experience with intubations is less than in anaesthesia, but similar to the ICU.[20] It is uncertain whether a typical fellowship on an ICU results in enough training in direct laryngoscopy to reach an expert skill level as should be expected for optimal care. The use of video laryngoscopes could ease intubation and therefore improve patient safety by addressing the potential problem of inadequate training in the use of direct laryngoscopy. While the evidence for superiority of videolaryngoscopes in anaesthesia is abundant, there are no prospective randomized controlled trials available for the ICU. A major obstacle for success is the inability to advance the tracheal tube into the trachea despite a good or even excellent view on the glottic opening. This phenomenon of difficult intubation despite good visibility has been dubbed 'you see that you fail'.[20] Clinicians used to direct laryngoscopy might then be tempted to procrastinate with prolonged and repeated fruitless attempts at intubation. 'You see that you fail' occurs more often with angulated blades, which enhance the view on the glottis in the case of difficult intubation. At the same time, these blades obtain a view on the glottic opening from below, unlike direct laryngoscopy, where the oro-pharyngeal curve and the pharyngo-glotto-tracheal curve need to be aligned to allow a glottic view. In indirect laryngoscopy with videolaryngoscopes, these curves are not necessarily aligned and stylets to mimic the curve of the blade are mandatory for intubation with angulated blades. Examples for such angulated blades are the C-MAC D-Blade (Karl Storz, Tuttlingen, Germany)™ or the Glidescope™ (Verathon Inc., Bothell, WA, USA). Attempts have been made to overcome these obstacles by attaching guiding channels for the tracheal tube at the blade of the videolaryngoscope. However, at least one recent large prospective study in 720 patients with simulated difficult airway showed no higher intubation success rate of videolaryngoscopes with guiding channels.[21] Regardless of the device, supervised practice with videolaryngoscopes is essential to acquire the necessary skills, and videolaryngoscopes featuring blades that resemble a Macintosh blade are easiest for beginners. Using Macintosh blades such as the C-MAC™ or the McGrath™ MAC (Aircraft Medical Ltd., Edinburgh, UK) also enables the physician to fall back to direct laryngoscopy in the case of failure of the videolaryngoscope due to excessive blood or other fluids in the hypopharyngeal space. When using angulated blades, several manoeuvres have been proposed to facilitate tracheal intubation such as bending the tracheal tube's stylet the same way as the videolaryngoscope's blade to reach the glottic opening, using BURP and rotation of the tracheal tube to advance the tube into the trachea. Further possibilities are reversed loading the tracheal tube on the stylet, which will lead to a downwards movement of the tip of the tube when retracting the stylet, inflating the pilot balloon of the tracheal tube and passive flexion of the head and neck. Regardless of the method, videolaryngoscopes should be used often to ensure adequate practice and they therefore should be used as first-line intubation tools, not as backup devices in the ICU setting.

Flexible Optical Bronchoscopy

A flexible bronchoscope (see also Chapter 19) can be used for diagnostic purposes before intubation or when neck extension should be avoided, but also for the treatment of aspirations or awake or asleep flexible optical intubation. A combination of techniques such as videolaryngoscopy-assisted fibreoptic intubation may be very helpful for airway management in ICU patients. The tip of the flexible scope is advanced in the airway with guidance of the monitor of the videolaryngoscope. A two-camera technique has the advantage that a view is always obtained. And with the videolaryngoscope, it is possible to manipulate the base of tongue. In complicated patients, it should always be considered to plan airway management in the ICU environment or rather in theatre where more and specialized equipment is available. The bronchoscope can be directed orally or nasally. When using nasal access, the probe assumes a straighter course, and this may facilitate the procedure. One important adjunct may be the administration of an anti-sialogue, usually glycopyrrolate.

Induction and Sedative Medication

When sedation or induction agents are required in the ICU, the ideal medication should be safe, have a rapid and predictable onset and recovery, a dose-dependent effect, a short half-life, and minimal cardiovascular, respiratory, and central nervous system stimulatory effects. Insufficient analgesia may lead to the development of vomiting or agitation after sedative administration.

A special concern in ICU patients is the usually transient post-induction hypotension caused by sedatives during RSI as outlined above.

There are no data to compare the potential aspiration risks of a longer induction time via dose titration versus the risks of either awareness or haemodynamic instability with a predetermined bolus technique.

Clinicians will determine the optimal choice of induction agent for the situation, often guided by personal expertise, institutional guidelines, available agents, and appropriate patient selection. Regardless of induction agent used, delay between administration, loss of consciousness, and administration of paralysing agent may prolong the period of aspiration risk and increase the risk of desaturation.

New agents continue to evolve. Dexmedetomidine (Dexdor™) is a highly selective centrally acting alpha$_2$-adrenergic agonist and enantiomer of medetomidine. Related to clonidine, it induces a state of cooperative sedation. Dexmedetomidine has been approved as a short-term sedative. It provides sedation during which the patients are easily aroused, and it does not depress the respiratory system. Hypotension with bradycardia is a reported side effect, especially in combination with opioids.

Etomidate is a particularly attractive agent for haemodynamically unstable patients because it does not have much cardiovascular depressant effect. In the past, etomidate has been associated with adverse outcomes, which were thought to be related with adrenal suppression. In a recent meta-analysis, no increased mortality could be shown that was related with a single induction bolus of etomidate for intubation. So, it can probably be deducted that the effect of a single induction bolus of etomidate has no clinically important effects of patient outcome in the ICU. A Cochrane review concluded there might be effects on adrenal gland function after application of etomidate, but no effect on mortality.[22]

Other commonly used induction agents include thiopentone, propofol, benzodiazepines such as midazolam (relatively slow onset compared to other agents), and ketamine. Ketamine is gaining favour within emergency and critical care circles due to relative cardiovascular stability. It should be noted that all induction agents (including midazolam and ketamine) have potential for cardiovascular depression and hypotension if a too high dose is used. In addition, combinations of agents may be synergistic with amplification of effect. Previous concerns of deleterious effects of ketamine on intracranial pressure in head injury have been challenged and as such use of ketamine has much to commend it for RSI in the critically ill patient.

Adjunct Opioid Agents

Adjunct agents are not described in the traditional teaching of RSI, yet many practitioners incorporate rapid acting opioids to attenuate the reflex sympathetic responses to laryngoscopy and intubation. This may be especially useful in critically ill patients with head injuries. The very short-acting opioid remifentanil provides adequate analgesia without the risk for prolonged side effects after its use. Arguments against use of opioids include historical concerns due to slow onset and longer duration with older opioids, as well as concerns of decreased respiratory drive if intubation fails. This is less of a concern in the critically ill patient as options to awaken the patient are generally not appropriate.

It should be noted that the use of opioids such as alfentanil and fentanyl may produce synergistic effects in combination with induction agents, and cautious dosing should be used in haemodynamically unstable patients to minimize hypotension.

Paralysis

Use of succinylcholine (a depolarizing neuromuscular blocking agent) as the preferred agent to facilitate vocal cord relaxation and endotracheal tube passage has been the accepted norm for RSI with traditional teaching being that the short duration of action will allow return of spontaneous ventilation in the case of a failed RSI. While awakening may be an option for some patients in the operating theatre, it is rarely the case for the unfasted, haemodynamically compromised patient for whom RSI represents a commitment to securing the airway.

It should be noted that there are concerns regarding the use of neuromuscular blocking agents in the ICU, as there is a high risk for apnoea if the patient cannot be intubated and ventilated after their administration. For succinylcholine in particular, some authors advocate totally abandoning the drug in the ICU, calling it obsolete.[23] Succinylcholine has been shown to cause hyperkalaemia and cardiac arrest in ICU patients, the degree of hyperkalaemia correlating with the length of ICU stay and immobilization. The drug should be avoided in renal failure, burns, and in patients with neuromuscular disease. On the other hand, the rapid onset and short duration of action of succinylcholine may be irreplaceable in an unexpectedly difficult intubation in situations where a reversal agent to alternative neuromuscular blocking drugs is not available. It appears that it should be probably avoided in the ICU and used only for strict indications and in the hands of an experienced physician.[23]

Rocuronium at a dose of 0.9–1.2 mg/kg gives the same onset of muscle relaxation as succinylcholine and is suggested as the preferred choice of non-depolarizing neuromuscular blocking agents for RSI in the critically ill. A commitment to full paralysis and rapid progression to a surgical airway in the case of failed intubation and ventilation in the critically ill patient is congruent with pre-agreed airway plans between team members, appropriate for the patient whose pathology requires a cuffed tube in the trachea by whatever means and avoids the possibility of attempting a surgical airway in a combative, coughing patient.

High-dose rocuronium can be acutely reversed with sugammadex, but appropriate measures should be taken for its safe use. When high-dose rocuronium is antagonized with sugammadex, it may still not be possible to have an open airway.

Difficult Airway Management

An important aspect when dealing with a difficult airway (difficult intubation and difficult BMV) is to be able to predict it. Several morphometric criteria and techniques have been developed and evaluated mostly for the patient in the OR. It is important to distinguish between predicted difficult mask ventilation, difficult direct laryngoscopy, difficult intubation with a videolaryngoscope, difficult use of supraglottic airway device, and difficult surgical airway, although they may be an overlap of risk factors (Tables 20.1 and 20.2).

Successful BMV is particularly important when there is a difficult airway. When BMV fails, the first response should be better BMV. This can often be accomplished by simple measures including repositioning the patient's head, inserting a nasal or oral airway, or holding the mask with two hands.

Failed RSI and Failed Airway Algorithm

A difficult airway plan should be discussed, and a checklist should be completed prior to RSI such that a shared mental model of actions to be undertaken exists between team members, both for routine and in the case of difficulty.[2] Many such difficult airway plans exist. Another cognitive aid showing promise is 'The Vortex approach' (Figure 20.4).[24] The Vortex approach (www.vortexapproach.org) is designed to optimize rescue techniques either by intubating the patient, placement of a supraglottic airway device, rescue BMV, or emergency front-of-neck access (FONA). Time-limited plans should be agreed on prior to RSI and then completed sequentially. In a 'cannot intubate, cannot oxygenate' situation, the practitioner is prompted towards the establishment of a surgical airway.

Standards exist for equipment to manage the difficult airway, and such equipment should be available wherever airways are managed. Such rehearsal may facilitate swift transition through airway plans and crisis algorithms, with early use of appropriate equipment and decisions. There is no substitute for experience. In particular, rescue surgical airway techniques must be regularly practised as they are infrequently used and as such remain a common area of unease. This is a true emergency, as the patient is in respiratory arrest. The first step is calling for help. Special expertise is necessary to manage a failed airway, and a calmer and more experienced colleague is often what is required. If both intubation and ventilation with a mask and

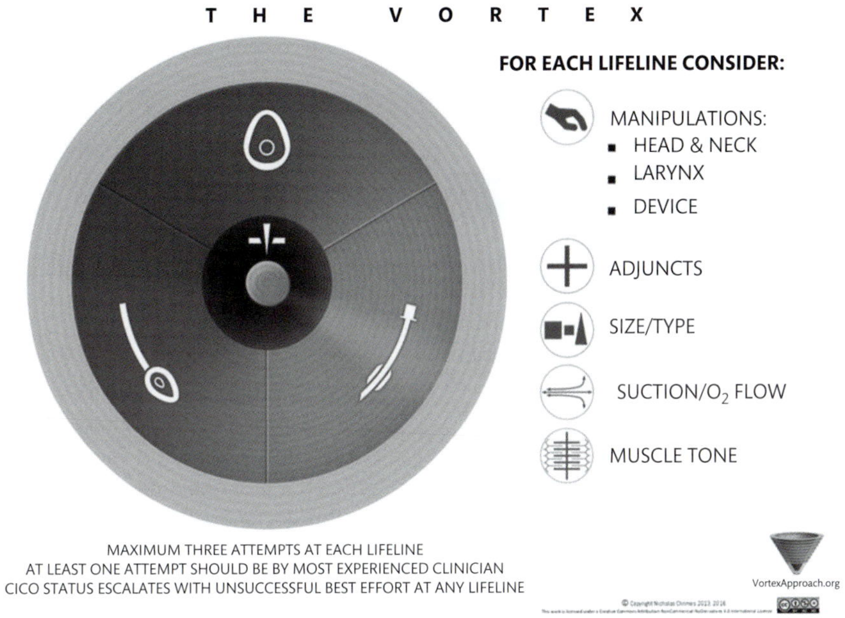

Figure 20.4 The vortex cognitive aid.

Reprinted from *British Journal of Anaesthesia*, 117, Suppl 1, Chrimes N, The Vortex: a universal 'high-acuity implementation tool' for emergency airway management, pp. i20–i27, Copyright 2016, with permission from the Board of Management and Trustees of the British Journal of Anaesthesia.

oral airway become impossible, providers should have an alternative means of oxygenation. This may include a supraglottic airway device, a laryngeal tube, the tracheal-oesophageal Combitube, transtracheal oxygenation, retrograde intubation, the lighted stylet, and others.

Fibreoptic bronchoscopy in this setting may be very difficult because of the presence of secretions, inadequate local anaesthesia, and an increased risk for hypoxemia in a potentially apnoeic patient.

Cricothyroidotomy

Cricothyroidotomy is the procedure of choice when an emergency surgical airway is needed. The main reasons to use the cricothyroid membrane as the target for emergency FONA are the easily identifiable anatomy and the relatively simple skills required. A meta-analysis that included 24 studies found no difference between emergency cricothyroidotomy techniques in terms of time to securing airway or success.[25] However, the authors noted that small study sizes and the use of non-clinical models (animals or human cadavers) limited their ability to draw firm conclusions. Recent prominent airway expert statements seem to favour the surgical approach to FONA.[26] In the NAP4 study, there was a higher failure rate of percutaneous techniques compared to surgical emergency FONA.[2] Therefore, the surgical approach has been adopted as the main final emergency pathway in the recent Difficult Airway Guidelines by the Difficult Airway Society.[6] There is univocally agreement that regardless of the technique, the important skill of emergency FONA needs to be rehearsed and practised by everyone confronted with airway management. Percutaneous wire-over-needle techniques may have an advantage in that there may be less hesitancy among anaesthesia-trained personnel using a needle technique instead of a scalpel technique. A combined technique, where a scalpel is used to cut skin and soft tissue, thereby facilitating detection of the cricoid membrane, and a percutaneous technique is used afterwards, may be the ideal technique, but this has not been studied prospectively yet.

Alternatively, percutaneous transtracheal jet ventilation is used, although barotrauma may then occur. Preparation, experience, and the existence of the special kit are the most important factors for predicting a successful outcome when any of these techniques are used.

Confirmation of Correct ETT Placement

Auscultating breath sounds bilaterally may be difficult or misleading. The sensitivity and specificity of the technique improves when it is combined with epigastric auscultation. Disposable colorimetric CO_2 detectors may be helpful, but they are unreliable in cardiac arrest patients. End-tidal capnography to confirm tracheal intubation is mandatory as was shown by the NAP4 investigators.[2] The safest way of confirming correct placement is visualization of the ETT passing through the vocal cords during direct laryngoscopy and subsequent fibreoptic visualization through the ETT of the tracheal rings and the carina. The postplacement chest radiograph will also assist in confirmation, but it takes time and it may miss oesophageal misplacement. Ultrasound may be used for quick detection of correct ventilation after tracheal intubation.

Proper fixation and securing of the airway is of paramount importance: the airway should be secured in place preferably using a special securing device. Mechanical ventilation and appropriate sedation should follow.

Accidental Extubation and Difficult Extubation Guidelines

Patients who are weaned from the ventilator are at increased risk for accidental extubation because sedative medication is stopped. In the case of accidental extubation, re-intubation is often necessary, and precautions should be taken to avoid these events, including staff surveillance, restraining methods, and sedation.[27]

Many patients with difficult airways undergo elective delayed extubation in the ICU. Proper planning for re-intubation must be instituted before extubation attempts. Guidelines have been published to differentiate easy extubation from expected difficult extubation.[28]

Ultrasound for Airway Management

Ultrasound has emerged as an easily accessible valuable tool in airway management. It may be used in all levels of airway management, from evaluating the airway to facilitating airway management, and verifying proper tracheal intubation and lung ventilation.

Oral and nasal cavities, pharynx, larynx, and trachea are nearly completely filled with air. However, various other structures can be visualized in relation to their anatomic location.

Ultrasonography has emerged as a reliable tool for assessing the narrowest diameter of the cricoid lumen (transverse diameter). Lakhal et al. compared the transverse diameter of the cricoid lumen assessed by ultrasonography and magnetic resonance imaging in healthy young adults and found it a reliable tool to assess the diameter of the subglottic upper airway.[29] Accurate identification of anterior neck structures during percutaneous dilatational tracheostomy can eliminate potential dreaded complications like haemorrhage, tracheal stenosis, erosion into high mediastinal vessels, and injury to the thyroid isthmus. With advanced US technology, it will be possible in the future to have real-time guidance in the placement of dilators and tracheostomy tubes.

Most frequently used methods of confirmation of tracheal intubation are auscultation of chest and end-tidal carbon dioxide detection. US imaging can visualize the motion of the diaphragm and pleura indicating lung expansion, are indirect but dynamic anatomic evidence of the correct physiologic function of the tracheal tube in paralyzed or apnoeic patients. Bilateral equal motion of the diaphragm towards the abdomen can be seen by US if the tracheal tube is inside the trachea. Further, with intercostal ultrasonographic view at the lung–chest wall interface, 'to-and-fro' movement of the pleura synchronized with ventilation (lung-sliding) can be visualized.

Tracheostomy

Indications for Tracheotomy

Indications for placing tracheostomy tubes can be grouped into four general categories: ventilation, airway obstruction, airway protection, and secretions. The first category applies to patients who require long-term mechanical ventilation because of chronic respiratory failure (see Chapters 51 and 65), who cannot maintain respiratory function unassisted, or who cannot be weaned from ventilatory support (see Chapter 64). Numerous studies have been done to determine the optimal interval from orotracheal intubation to placement of a tracheostomy tube, but no definitive recommendations have been made because of varied results in different populations of patients and in patients with different comorbid conditions, although there is some consensus to wait for at least 2 weeks before attempting tracheostomy. Benefits of establishing a tracheostomy rather than using an endotracheal tube include decreasing direct laryngeal injury, improving comfort and thereby allowing sedation to be weaned, and improving activities of daily living, such as mobility, speech, and eating.

Patients who have tumours within the airway, paralyzed vocal cords, swelling, stricture, or unusual airway anatomy are another category for tracheostomy because of airway obstruction that compromises normal respiration. A third category includes patients who cannot protect their airway and patients with an inefficient swallow and/or cough mechanism, and common situations in patients who have a high spinal cord injury, cerebrovascular accident, or traumatic brain injury. Last, patients who cannot mobilize or manage their secretions may also require a tracheostomy.

A tracheostomy tube may be placed surgically or percutaneously[30]. A recent Cochrane review found lower rates of wound infection when percutaneous techniques were used, but otherwise no difference in serious adverse events or mortality could be found due to insufficient data.[31] Surgical placement is performed in the operating room or at the bedside, generally with the use of general anaesthesia. A stoma is created by using an open surgical technique. Landmarks are identified, and a skin incision is made below the cricoid cartilage. The isthmus of the thyroid gland is exposed, cross-clamped, and ligated. The trachea can then be visualized. A common technique is to create a 'trap door' (Bjork flap) in which a small part of the tracheal cartilage is pulled down and sutured to the skin. This flap is thought to facilitate reinsertion of the tracheostomy tube if accidental decannulation occurs, especially in patients with difficult anatomy or obesity.

Percutaneous (dilatational) tracheostomy is generally performed solely on intubated patients and, unlike surgical tracheotomy, can be performed without direct visualization of the trachea. There is no evidence whether a tracheal tube or a supraglottic airway device is superior for aiding the tracheostomy procedure.[32] Bronchoscopy or ultrasound may be used to guide and confirm the placement of the tracheostomy tube within the trachea. Contraindications to percutaneous tracheostomy include uncorrected coagulopathy, infection at the incision site, high ratio of PEEP to fraction of inspired oxygen, elevated intracranial pressure, tracheal obstruction, unusual neck anatomy, and the need for emergency airway management.

Immediate postoperative priorities of care for a patient with a new tracheostomy include ensuring that the tracheostomy tube is securely in place and is patent. Routine care, as well as prompt management of postoperative complications, can be facilitated by ensuring that proper equipment and supplies are quickly available.

Scheduled Changes of Tracheostomy Tubes

Currently, no empirical evidence indicates a standardized time for changing a tracheostomy tube, and changes are typically done according to the preference of the healthcare provider. Indications for changing a tracheostomy tube include the need for a different size tube, tube malfunction, need for a different type of tube, and routine changes for ongoing airway management and prevention of infection. Many would change tracheostomy tubes 7–14 days after initial insertion, but there is no evidence supporting that recommendation. It often depends astleast on the anticipated time likely on mechanical ventilation with a desire to waken the patient (without intolerance of the endotracheal tube), so offering differential respiratory and neurological weaning. A tracheostomy tube that is inserted percutaneously fits more tightly within the stoma than does a tube that was inserted through a surgical incision. If a tracheostomy tube is changed prematurely, the tissue of the dilated stoma tract is more likely to recoil than it would if the change were done later. Most manufacturers recommend changing the tubes every 1–2 months; however, Yaremchuk found that routine tube changes every 2 weeks decreased the formation of granulation tissue.[33]

Changing tracheostomy tubes can correct problems that cause ventilator asynchrony, improve comfort by reducing tube size, and correct a cuff leak due to tracheomalacia or malposition or fracture of the tracheostomy tube or flange.

Cleaning and Replacing the Inner Cannula

The primary purpose of the inner cannula is to prevent tube obstruction by allowing regular cleaning or replacement. Many episodes of tube obstruction can be prevented with simple inspection and cleaning or changing of the inner cannula. For these reasons, it is important to check manufacturers' instructions for cleaning tracheostomy tubes.

With certain tubes, such as the disposable inner cannula (DCT), low-pressure cuffed (LPC), extended length (XLT) by Shiley (Covidien), or the TRACOE Twist (TRACOE Medical GmbH), patients cannot receive ventilatory support via a manual resuscitation bag or a mechanical ventilator when the inner cannula is not in place. In these tubes, the 15 mm connector, the standard connector for all respiratory equipment, is part of the inner cannula. A temporary inner cannula can be used while the standard inner cannula is being cleaned.

Problems with Tracheostomy Tubes

There are many different tracheostomy tubes available. The depth of the stoma should be assessed in all cases either by ultrasound or manual palpation before the incision is made. The stomal section of most tubes is short and only suitable for thin necks. A tube that is too short will increase the risk at accidental decannulation, which is a medical emergency. Longer adjustable flange tubes should be considered for patients with thick necks or in cases anatomy is abnormal due to radiation therapy or prior surgery. For each patient, a description of the used tube and technique should be immediately available. This can be done with a leaflet attached to the bed, which also indicates if the patient can still be intubated orally or he has undergone complete laryngectomy. These checklists may be used in the case of airway emergencies encountered with tracheostomy tubes, especially in those recently placed.[32]

Tracheostomy and endotracheal tubes have subglottic suction ports, which are used for intermittent or continuous supra-cuff clearance of secretions, so reducing the contamination of the tracheobronchial tree from the upper airway.

Airway Obstruction in the Intubated Patient with Respiratory Support

This is a common finding in ICU patients and may have different causes. Biting, kinking, dislodgement, a blood clot, or thick mucus may obstruct the tube. Careful tube care avoids most problems, and it is important to recognize these problems immediately. Warning signs are falling tidal volumes, loss of capnography, inability to inflate the chest manually, or desaturation. If ventilation is impossible, and the tube is totally obstructed, remove the tracheal tube and manually ventilate the patient and call for help. Re-intubation may be a challenge. The mnemonic 'DOPE' (Dislocation, Obstruction, Pneumothorax, Equipment failure) has been used to quickly find reason behind an acute airway problem in patients already intubated.

Conclusions

Securing and maintaining a definitive airway in the critically ill patient is necessary, complex, and risky. Indeed, there is evidence of frequent peri-intubation complications with at least one event in at least 45% of cases globally.[34]

Understanding the risks and utilizing effective guidelines with adequate training and tested protocols are an increasingly recognized necessity in the peri-intubation care of the critically ill patient. A comprehensive updated guideline that includes a pre-procedure checklist (Figure 20.2) and algorithm (Figure 20.3), as well as CICO and assessment protocols, endorsed by the Faculty of Intensive Care Medicine, The Intensive Care Society, The Royal College of Anaesthetists, and the Difficult Airway Society all in the United Kingdom, is available as open access.[6]

REFERENCES

1. Cook TM, MacDougall-Davis SR. Complications and failure of airway management. *Br J Anaesth.* 2012;**109**(Suppl 1): i68–i85.
2. Cook TM, Woodall N, Harper J, et al. Fourth National Audit P. Major complications of airway management in the UK: Results of the Fourth National Audit Project of the Royal College of Anaesthetists and the Difficult Airway Society. Part 2: Intensive care and emergency departments. *Br J Anaesth.* 2011;**106**:632–642.
3. Marino PL. *The ICU Book.* Philadelphia: Lippincott Williams & Wilkins; 2013.
4. Rosenblatt WH. Preoperative planning of airway management in critical care patients. *Crit Care Med.* 2004;**32**:S186–92
5. Detsky ME, Jivraj N, Adhikari NK, et al. Will this patient be difficult to intubate? The rational clinical examination systematic review. *JAMA.* 2019;**321**:493–503.
6. Higgs A, McGrath BA, Goddard C, et al. Difficult Airway Society; Intensive Care Society; Faculty of Intensive Care Medicine; Royal College of Anaesthetists. Guidelines for the management of tracheal intubation in critically ill adults. *Br J Anaesth.* 2018;**120**:323–352.
7. Huitink JM, Bouwman RA. The myth of the difficult airway: Airway management revisited. *Anaesthesia.* 2015;**70**:244–249.
8. Reed MJ, Rennie LM, Dunn MJ, et al. Is the 'LEMON' method an easily applied emergency airway assessment tool? *Eur J Emerg Med.* 2004;**11**:154–157.
9. de Groot RI, Dekkers OM, Herold IH, et al. Risk factors and outcomes after unplanned extubations on the ICU: A case-control study. *Crit Care.* 2011;**15**:R19.
10. Rochwerg B, Einav S, Chaudhuri D, et al. The role for high flow nasal cannula as a respiratory support strategy in adults: A clinical practice guideline. *Intensive Care Med.* 2020;**46**:2226–2237.

11. Woodbridge PD. 'Crash induction' for tracheal intubation. *JAMA.* 1967;**202**:845
12. Cheney FW, Posner KL, Caplan RA. Adverse respiratory events infrequently leading to malpractice suits. A closed claims analysis. *Anesthesiology.* 1991;**75**:932–939.
13. Apfelbaum JL, Hagberg CA, Caplan RA, et al. Practice guidelines for management of the difficult airway: An updated report by the American Society of Anesthesiologists Task Force on Management of the Difficult Airway. *Anesthesiology.* 2013;**118**:251–270.
14. Sellick BA. Cricoid pressure to control regurgitation of stomach contents during induction of anaesthesia. *Lancet.* 1961;**2**:404–406.
15. Stept WJ, Safar P. Rapid induction-intubation for prevention of gastric-content aspiration. *Anesth Analg.* 1970;**49**:633–636.
16. Mushambi MC, Kinsella SM. Obstetric Anaesthetists' Association/Difficult Airway Society difficult and failed tracheal intubation guidelines—the way forward for the obstetric airway. *Br J Anaesth.* 2015;**115**:815–818.
17. Casey JD, Janz DR, Russell DW, et al. Bag-mask ventilation during tracheal intubation of critically ill adults. *N Engl J Med.* 2019 Feb 28;**380(9)**:811–821.
18. Russo SG, Goetze B, Troche S, et al. LMA-ProSeal for elective postoperative care on the intensive care unit: A prospective, randomized trial. *Anesthesiology.* 2009;**111**:116–121.
19. Arulkumaran N, Lowe J, Ions R, et al. Videolaryngoscopy versus direct laryngoscopy for emergency orotracheal intubation outside the operating room: A systematic review and meta-analysis. *Br J Anaesth.* 2018;**120**:712–724.
20. Sakles JC, Mosier J, Patanwala AE, et al. Learning curves for direct laryngoscopy and GlideScope(R) video laryngoscopy in an emergency medicine residency. *West J Emerg Med.* 2014;**15**:930–937.
21. Kleine-Brueggeney M, Greif R, Schoettker P, et al. Evaluation of six videolaryngoscopes in 720 patients with a simulated difficult airway: A multicentre randomized controlled trial. *Br J Anaesth.* 2016;**116**:670–679.
22. Bruder EA, Ball IM, Ridi S, et al. Single induction dose of etomidate versus other induction agents for endotracheal intubation in critically ill patients. *Cochrane Database Syst Rev.* 2015;**1**:CD010225.
23. Hung O, McKeen D, Huitink J. Our love-hate relationship with succinylcholine: Is sugammadex any better? *Can J Anaesth.* 2016;**63**:905–910.
24. Chrimes N. The Vortex: A universal 'high-acuity implementation tool' for emergency airway management. *Br J Anaesth.* 2016;**117**(Suppl 1):i20–i7.
25. Langvad S, Hyldmo PK, Nakstad AR, et al. Emergency cricothyrotomy—a systematic review. *Scand J Trauma Resusc Emerg Med.* 2013;**21**:43.
26. Baker PA, O'Sullivan EP, Kristensen MS, et al. The great airway debate: Is the scalpel mightier than the cannula? *Br J Anaesth.* 2016;**117**(Suppl 1):i17–i9.
27. da Silva PS, Fonseca MC. Unplanned endotracheal extubations in the intensive care unit: Systematic review, critical appraisal, and evidence-based recommendations. *Anesth Analg.* 2012;**114**:1003–1014.
28. Difficult Airway Society Extubation Guidelines G, Popat M, Mitchell V, et al. Difficult Airway Society Guidelines for the management of tracheal extubation. *Anaesthesia.* 2012;**67**:318–340.
29. Lakhal K, Delplace X, Cottier JP, et al. The feasibility of ultrasound to assess subglottic diameter. *Anesth Analg.* 2007;**104**:611–614.
30. Brass P, Hellmich M, Ladra A, et al. Percutaneous techniques versus surgical techniques for tracheostomy. *Cochrane Database Syst Rev.* 2016;**7**:CD008045.
31. Strametz R, Pachler C, Kramer JF, et al. Laryngeal mask airway versus endotracheal tube for percutaneous dilatational tracheostomy in critically ill adult patients. *Cochrane Database Syst Rev.* 2014(6) Jun 30:CD009901.
32. McGrath BA, Bates L, Atkinson D, et al, National Tracheostomy Safety P. Multidisciplinary guidelines for the management of tracheostomy and laryngectomy airway emergencies. *Anaesthesia.* 2012;**67**:1025–1041.
33. Yaremchuk K. Regular tracheostomy tube changes to prevent formation of granulation tissue. *Laryngoscope.* 2003;**113**:1–10.
34. Russotto V, Myatra SN, Laffey JG, et al. INTUBE study investigators. Intubation practices and adverse peri-intubation events in critically ill patients from 29 countries. *JAMA.* 2021;**325**:1164–1172.

21

Acute Respiratory Distress Syndrome

Michele Umbrello, Paolo Formenti, and Davide Chiumello

KEY MESSAGES

- Acute respiratory distress syndrome (ARDS) is characterized by non-cardiogenic pulmonary oedema with bilateral chest X-ray opacities, reduction in respiratory system compliance, and hypoxaemia refractory to oxygen therapy.
- Mechanical ventilation (both non-invasive and invasive), in association with adjuvant therapies, remains the main standard supportive treatment.
- Therapeutic approaches to ARDS include lung-protective ventilation, prone positioning, inhaled vasodilators, neuromuscular blockade, steroids, and recruitment manoeuvres.
- Estimation of lung recruitability at bedside should be considered, avoiding excessive lung stress and strain, by monitoring airway driving pressure and/or transpulmonary pressure.
- In the most severe cases, neuromuscular blockade, prone positioning, and extracorporeal membrane oxygenation (ECMO) (alone or in combination) should be considered.

CONTROVERSIES

- Definition of ARDS according to individual pathologies, lung imaging, extravascular lung water (pulmonary oedema), and recruitability.
- The role of assisted ventilation in the early phases of ARDS.
- The role of ECMO, including onset time and indications.

FURTHER RESEARCH

- Personalized mechanical ventilation in ARDS according to different clinical and genetic phenotypes.
- The individualization of positive end-expiratory pressure (PEEP) according to recruitability response, respiratory mechanics, transpulmonary pressure, or lung imaging.
- Haemodynamic monitoring and targeted fluid strategies in early ARDS.
- Mechanical ventilation in late ARDS.
- Large randomized controlled trials evaluating adjuvant new supportive therapies as well as commonly used mechanical ventilation strategies.

Pathophysiology

Cellular and Molecular Pathophysiology

Increased capillary permeability is the hallmark of acute respiratory distress syndrome (ARDS). Damage to the capillary and alveolar epithelia in conjunction with impaired alveolar fluid removal results in accumulation of protein-rich fluid. This leads to diffuse alveolar damage with release of pro-inflammatory cytokines. Neutrophils are thought to play a key role in the pathogenesis of ARDS, as suggested by studies of bronchoalveolar lavage and lung biopsy specimens in early phases.[1]

Transcription of genes for pro-inflammatory mediators are detectable in the lungs of ARDS patients, alongside other factors that increase vascular permeability and destroy micro-vascular architecture, enhancing inflammation and lung damage. Cytokines (including tumour necrosis factor, leukotrienes, and macrophage inhibitory factor), along with platelet sequestration and activation, are also important. Over-activation of both pro- and anti-inflammatory mechanisms occurs after a precipitating insult that may be localized to the lungs themselves or distant from them. The primary site of injury may be at the vascular endothelium or the alveolar epithelium, depending on whether the precipitant is pulmonary or extra-pulmonary.

Alveolar epithelial cells are found in two forms, and damage to these cells produces distinct patterns of injury. Damage to type I cells allows both increased entry of fluid into the alveoli and decreased clearance of fluid from the alveolar space. Type II alveolar epithelial cells are relatively more resistant to injury, but when damaged the decreased production of surfactant leads to decreased compliance and alveolar collapse. Interference with the normal repair processes in the lung may ultimately lead to the development of fibrosis (Figure 21.1).

Time Course

Lung injury is a dynamic condition and the pathological features of ARDS pass through three overlapping phases—an inflammatory or exudative, a proliferative, and, lastly, a fibrotic phase. These phases may be complicated by additional insults—for example, episodes of nosocomial pneumonia and the deleterious effects of ventilator-induced lung injury (VILI). Heterogeneity in the pathological picture arises from both the variable precipitating insult and the distribution

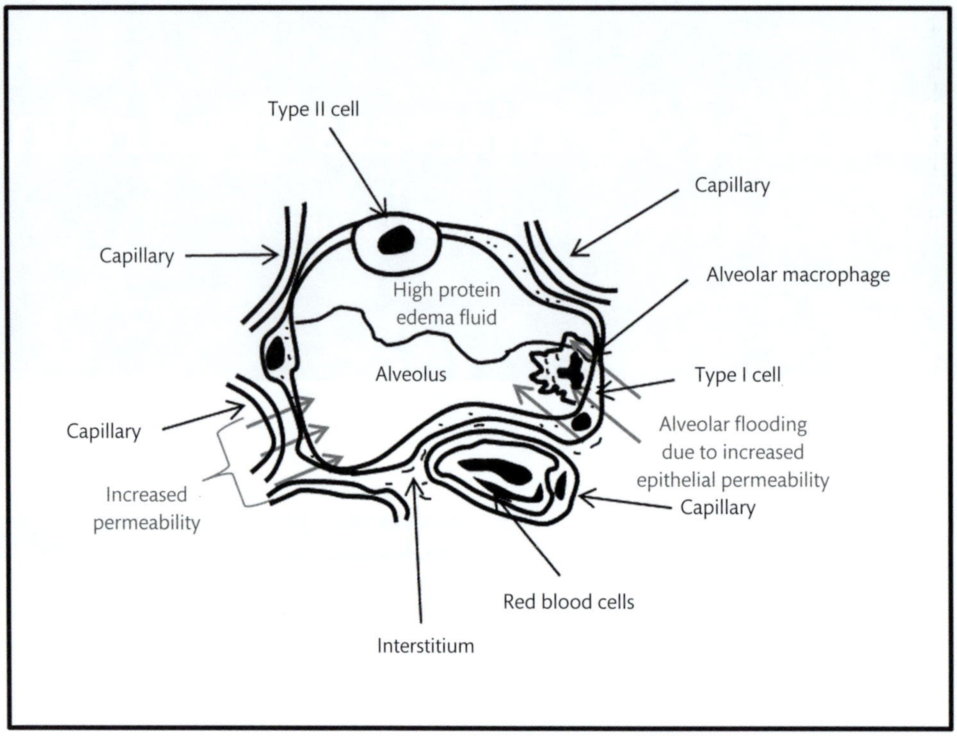

Figure 21.1 Pathophysiology of ARDS development. The cartoon depicts an ideal alveolus developing ARDS. The site of injury is on either the vascular endothelium or the alveolar epithelium. Two types of alveolar epithelial cells exist. Damage to type I cells allows both increased entry of fluid into the alveoli and decreased clearance of fluid from the alveolar space. Type II alveolar epithelial cells are relatively more resistant to injury. However, damage to type II cells results in decreased production of surfactant with resultant decreased compliance and alveolar collapse.

of alveolar injury. Ventilatory strain is applied in an inhomogeneous manner. For instance, relatively normal alveoli may become overdistended by the delivered tidal volume, resulting in barotrauma, while alveoli already damaged by ARDS may experience further injury from the shear forces exerting cyclical atelectasis and reopening.

The initial phase of fluid accumulation is followed by a proliferative phase characterized by resolution of pulmonary oedema, proliferation of type II alveolar cells, fibroblasts and myofibroblasts, and new matrix deposition. This phase starts early (within 72 h) and lasts for >7 days. Factors influencing the progression to fibroproliferation versus resolution and reconstitution of normal pulmonary parenchymal architecture are poorly understood, but patients who develop pulmonary fibrosis exhibit deterioration of pulmonary compliance, progressive hypoxia and ventilator dependence, and increased mortality.[2] Multiple organ failure (MOF) is the leading cause of death in ARDS, but the pathophysiologic link between the two is not well defined: it is likely that in some patients ARDS is a manifestation of MOF, whereas in others MOF arises as a result of ARDS.

Survival from ARDS commonly leads to complete resolution of pathological features. Less commonly, residual pulmonary fibrosis occurs, in which the alveolar spaces are filled with mesenchymal cells and new blood vessels leading to longer-term impairment of pulmonary function.

Pathophysiology Related to Pathology

It is well recognized that mechanical ventilation can, itself, exacerbate the damage which occurs in ARDS. VILI has variously been attributed to excessive tidal volumes, stress, driving pressures, respiratory rates, and gas flows.[3] A recent unifying theory is that VILI results from excessive mechanical power applied to the 'baby lung'. The 'baby lung' concept was first introduced to describe the small portion of aerated lung with near-normal compliance, which is open during the end-expiration phase.[4] This underlying concept is that in ARDS lungs are not stiff, but small, introducing the concept of relativity in VILI based on lung size.

Alveolar overdistension can generate a pro-inflammatory response that is exacerbated by repetitive opening and closing of alveoli as occurs through the use of inappropriately low levels of positive end-expiratory pressure (PEEP).[5] Both overdistension and alveolar opening/closing can induce structural damage to the lung. The effect of high inspired concentrations of oxygen on the disease process is uncertain, particularly in humans. However, prolonged exposure to 100% oxygen is fatal in most animal models, producing neutrophil influx and alveolar oedema that can be blocked, at least in rodents, by using anti-inflammatory strategies.

The key to understanding the pathophysiology of VILI lies in understanding the nature of the stress distribution in the lung and the cellular and molecular biological responses of the blood-gas barrier to tensile stress; the stress distribution displays considerable heterogeneity that is not immediately appreciable to the clinician. The interaction of the relatively rigid chest wall and abdomen with the lungs is more influential in the topographic deformational stress and strain than the lung weight. Examination of confocal images of oedematous, injured lungs, indicates the presence of both collapsed and overdistended alveoli with a range of air pockets of differential radius surrounded by fluid and foam. The presence of non-uniform gas pressures and/or surface tension may require high pressures to drive the foam out of the alveoli. Fluid-filled alveoli create areas with high surface tension. Understanding the pathophysiology of these flooded, unstable lung units and the airways that are repetitively opening and closing is central to the concepts of ventilator management and the prevention of VILI.

For decades, pressure-based respiratory mechanics have assisted the judgement of clinicians when monitoring mechanical ventilation and making decisions in respiratory care. However, measurements based on airway pressure alone provide limited insights into patient populations with varying pathologic conditions. While the passive lungs are the primary target of attention, airway-pressure-based interpretations may be influenced by differences in breathing pattern, alterations in chest wall activity (including diaphragm function), changes in lung volume, heterogeneity of lung disease, and abdominal distension. All of these factors may complicate the interpretation of respiratory mechanics and make fixed criteria for safe ventilation difficult to apply. The transpulmonary pressure (alveolar–oesophageal pressure (P_{es})) is a conceptual step closer to monitoring the object of interest, that is, the lung itself. Transpulmonary pressure monitoring has been proposed as a promising approach to guide ventilation strategy in ARDS, as airway-pressure-based plateau and PEEP values are insufficiently representative of pulmonary strain. Despite studies supporting P_{es} as a reliable surrogate for pleural pressure, oesophageal balloon estimation of pleural pressure may be influenced by regional characteristics of the sampled horizontal plane when supine, as well as by pulmonary and/or extra-pulmonary conditions, such as elevated intra-abdominal pressure, obesity, and heterogeneity of lung disease.

Refractory hypoxaemia may be multifactorial, but intrapulmonary shunting with ventilation–perfusion mismatching is believed to be the primary cause. Studies on patients with ARDS have shown that the degree of intrapulmonary shunting is sufficient to account for the entire alveolar-arterial oxygen gradient, suggesting that a decrease in transfer factor may be of secondary importance. Microscopic studies have shown that the alveolar airspaces are filled with oedema, debris, and hyaline membranes, creating a huge physiological dead space. The effects on gas exchange are maximized by loss of hypoxic pulmonary vasoconstriction and by the widespread patchy vascular defects.

Histopathologic Findings

Lung morphology in ARDS reflects the rapid evolution from interstitial and alveolar oedema to end-stage fibrosis. The histologic correlate of ARDS is termed diffuse alveolar injury (DAD), a pattern of injury in which there is widespread and severe damage to the whole alveolo-capillary unit. Pulmonary lesions correlate with the phase of alveolar damage rather than its specific cause; moreover, the pathologic features are consistent with the effects of a host of injurious stimuli and the complex interaction of inflammatory mediators on alveolar epithelial and capillary endothelial cells.

DAD is characterized by an orderly sequence of pathologic changes that occur following lung injury, divided into two or three overlapping phases: an early or exudative, an organizing/proliferative, and a fibrotic phase. These phases are not necessarily progressive as the process can stop and recovery may occur at any time; moreover, acute and organizing aspects may coexist. Involvement of the pulmonary vasculature is an important aspect of ARDS, from the initial phase of oedema to the terminal stage of intractable pulmonary hypertension. Vascular lesions include thrombotic, fibro-proliferative, and obliterative changes that, like the parenchymal lesions, correlate with the temporal phase of DAD. Box 21.1 summarizes the typical microscopic findings of the different stages of DAD.

The acute, exudative phase occurs in the first week post-injury. The main histologic findings are capillary congestion with interstitial and intra-alveolar oedema associated with fibrin and thickened alveolar septa. Sparse interstitial inflammatory cell infiltrate consisting of lymphocytes, plasma cells, and macrophages is present. The lungs, on gross examination, appear heavy, airless, and diffusely dark red-blue, and the main histologic feature is the formation of hyaline membranes (the histologic hallmark of the acute phase), eosinophilic structures that form along the alveolar ducts and walls and are composed of cellular debris, plasma proteins, and surfactant.

The late, proliferative/organizing stage generally occurs 1–2 weeks after injury. On gross examination, the lungs are densely consolidated with patchy red-brown or yellow-grey discoloration. The histologic picture is characterized by development of a reparative process with the formation of organized granulation tissue (fibroblast and myofibroblasts admixed with scattered mononuclear cells) involving predominantly the alveolar septa. Hyaline membranes are generally less prominent, while vascular macroscopic and microscopic thrombo-emboli are common.

The fibrotic stage develops after 3–4 weeks. The lung is completely remodelled by granulation tissue. On gross examination, the pleural surface has a cobblestone appearance. The parenchyma is pale and replaced by alternating areas of microcysts and irregular zones of diffuse scarring. On microscopic examination, the lung is characterized by enlarged airspaces surrounded by thickened alveolar septa due to collagen deposition and few fibroblasts. Characteristically, the fibrosis is uniform and associated with areas of honeycomb. On autopsy, intra-alveolar and interstitial fibrosis may be very difficult to differentiate due to the extensive fibrotic remodelling. Vascular lesions are frequent and include fibro-cellular intimal and mural fibrous thickening involving small muscular arteries, veins, and lymphatics, and complete, irreversible, muscularization of

Box 21.1 Summary of microscopic findings of diffuse alveolar damage

Acute stage

- Hyaline membranes along alveolar ducts and septa
- Interstitial and intra-alveolar oedema

Organizing stage

- Diffuse proliferation of fibroblasts and myofibroblasts (granulation tissue), predominantly in the interstitium and focally involving airspaces
- Hyperplasia and reactive atypia of type II pneumocytes
- Squamous metaplasia
- Macro- and microthrombus, associated with lung infarcts with atypical shapes

Fibrotic stage

- Dense uniform fibrosis
- Thickening of the intima and the muscularis propria of the arterioles
- Honeycomb changes

the smaller arteries, which in turn are responsible for pulmonary hypertension.[6]

Epidemiology of ARDS

Patients with ARDS represent approximately 5% of hospitalized, mechanically ventilated patients. Mild forms represent only 25% of patients, with approximately 75% of patients having moderate or severe ARDS. However, approximately one-third of patients with initially mild ARDS will later progress to moderate/severe disease.

The incidence of ARDS has declined steadily over the past decades. This decline is primarily due to a decrease in nosocomial ARDS. In contrast, the incidence of community-acquired ARDS, defined as diagnosis within 6 h of hospital admission, has not changed. However, a decrease in the use of routine chest radiographs and arterial blood-gas analyses may lead to underdiagnosis of nosocomial ARDS, partially accounting for this trend. Moreover, adoption of restrictive fluid management strategies may have reduced the incidence of hydrostatic pulmonary oedema misdiagnosed as ARDS. However, several major advances in critical care practice are likely to have contributed to this finding, such as timely resuscitation and antimicrobial administration, restrictive transfusion strategies, ventilator care bundles, and the widespread use of lung-protective ventilation.

Recent data suggests an incidence of ARDS in the United States, ranging from 15.3 to 58.7 cases per 100,000 person-years.[7] Attributable mortality also varies, with reported ranges of 41%–58%. Indeed, data from patients enrolled in the ARDS Network documents a significant trend towards improved 60-day mortality during the period 1996–2005.[8] Interestingly, a comprehensive systematic review of observational studies noted similar improvements in survival from 1984 to 1993, but no further changes between 1994 and 2006. Moreover, mortality was found to be lower in RCTs than observational studies: RCTs may underestimate "real-world" mortality because they are often performed in specialized centres, and the selection criteria, designed to improve safety and maximize potential treatment effects, may generate a group of patients who are less sick relative to the overall ARDS population. Mortality due to ARDS remained static at 44.0% for observational studies and 36.2% for RCTs since the standard AECC definition was introduced in 1994 (see the next section).

The recent LUNG SAFE (Large Observational Study to Understand the Global Impact of Severe Acute Respiratory Failure) was a large multinational prospective cohort study, including 29,144 patients from 459 ICUs across 50 countries.[9] The study confirmed that ARDS is common, accounting for 10.4% of all ICU admissions and 23.4% of mechanically ventilated patients. However, despite the relatively high prevalence, only 60% of ARDS cases were identified at any point during their clinical course, and only 34% were identified at the initial time that ARDS criteria were met, suggesting that the diagnosis of ARDS was frequently delayed and often was not made.

Mortality varies according to severity of oxygenation deficit. In the Berlin definition clinical study cohort (see below), mortality was on average 27% in mild, 32% in moderate, and 45% in severe ARDS. Although worsening oxygenation is a risk factor for mortality, patients generally die from MOF or progressive underlying illness; only a minority (13%–19%) die from refractory hypoxaemia.

ARDS Definition

Since its first description, ARDS has been redefined several times in order to improve the accuracy of the clinical diagnosis.[10–12] However, independent of the different definitions, the hallmark of ARDS is arterial hypoxaemia refractory to oxygen therapy due to pulmonary shunt.

ARDS is a syndrome of acute onset, bilateral, inflammatory pulmonary infiltrates, and impaired oxygenation. The first known description dates back to the invention of the stethoscope itself: indeed, Laennec described fatal 'idiopathic pulmonary oedema' and anasarca of the lungs in his Treatise on Diseases of the Chest back in 1821. The wars of the 20th century provided ample evidence that severe traumatic insults could result in oedematous lung injury, and terms such as 'shock lung' were developed. In 1967, the first widely accepted description of ARDS was published describing a case-series of 12 patients that developed a common pattern of respiratory failure stemming from a variety of insults. 'Respiratory distress syndrome' was clinically characterized by the acute onset of severe dyspnoea, tachypnoea, oxygen-refractory cyanosis, loss of lung compliance, and infiltration on chest radiographs; this was associated with a high short-term mortality in adults.[10] The term ARDS eventually achieved a shared definition during the American–European Consensus Conference (AECC) (Table 21.1) in 1994.[11] The AECC definition facilitated the completion of seminal epidemiological and clinical studies, significantly increasing our understanding of this condition. The AECC defined ARDS by the four criteria set out in Table 21.1, and ARDS was considered the more severe form of an overarching entity called acute lung injury (ALI) defined by a less severe hypoxaemia.

Although the AECC definitions allowed for a concerted research effort, the validity of the definition was criticized. Widely recognized limitations included the vague nature of the term 'acute', wide inter-observer variation in ascertaining 'bilateral radiographic infiltrates', the frequent misclassification of left atrial hypertension, and sensitivity of the PaO_2/FiO_2 ratio criteria to small changes in FiO_2 and PEEP.

Because of these and other concerns, the European Society of Intensive Care Medicine convened an international expert panel in 2011 in Berlin, which led to the drafting of the Berlin definition of ARDS[12] (Table 21.1, comparing the two definitions). The Berlin criteria addressed the criticisms of the AECC definition and were unique in that they were iteratively drafted and then empirically evaluated in order to provide a definition that would be feasible, reliable, and prognostic. Major changes included were as follows: (1) elimination of the term 'acute lung injury' and replacing it with three levels of severity based on PaO_2/FiO_2 measured with at least 5 cmH_2O of applied PEEP, (2) defining 'acute' as ≤7 days from the predisposing clinical insult, and (3) eliminating pulmonary wedge pressure cut-off values that discriminate ARDS from cardiogenic oedema. The Berlin criteria provide a modest although significant improvement in predictive ability for mortality when compared to the AECC.

Table 21.1 American-European Consensus Conference (AECC) definition of acute lung injury and the Berlin definition of acute respiratory distress syndrome (ARDS)

Characteristic	The AECC definition 1994	The Berlin definition 2012
Onset	Acute	≤7 days from the predisposing clinical insult
Radiographic abnormality	Bilateral infiltrate on frontal chest radiograph	Bilateral opacities on radiograph or computed tomography scan not fully explained by effusion, atelectasis, or nodules
Non-cardiogenic source of pulmonary oedema	No clinical evidence of elevated left atrial pressure or a pulmonary capillary wedge pressure <18 mmHg	Respiratory failure not fully explained by cardiogenic pulmonary oedema or volume overload
Oxygenation	PaO_2/FiO_2 ratio Acute lung injury: ≤300 Acute respiratory distress syndrome (ARDS): ≤200	PaO_2/FiO_2 ratio with ≥5 cmH_2O PEEP Mild ARDS: 201–300 Moderate ARDS: 101–200 Severe ARDS: ≤100
Predisposing condition	Not specified	If none identified, then need to rule out cardiogenic oedema with additional data (e.g. echocardiography)

Source: Data from Bernard GR, Artigas A, Brigham KL, et al. The American-European Consensus Conference on ARDS. Definitions, mechanisms, relevant outcomes, and clinical trial coordination. *Am J Resp Crit Care Med* 1994;*149*(3 Pt 1):818–824; and Ranieri VM, Rubenfeld GD, Thompson BT, et al. Acute respiratory distress syndrome: The Berlin Definition. *JAMA* 2012;*307*(23):2526–2533.

Despite the improvements brought by the new ARDS definition, some problems still remain. Most evident is the lack of a biomarker to confirm the diagnosis. Even combinations of clinically available measures with the latest research-generated biomarkers, though promising, have not been compelling enough to be moved into clinical practice. Moreover, clinicians still cannot readily measure permeability that is often considered the hallmark of ARDS. The role of hydrostatic pressure remains a major confounder and is not readily clarified by the use of echocardiograms or CT scans. Perhaps tools that hold potential for diagnosing increased lung water and/or permeability may take hold clinically in the near future.

Therapeutic Approaches to ARDS

In the following section, a holistic framework of respiratory support is presented, including both pharmacologic and non-pharmacologic interventions aiming to ensure adequate gas exchange while minimizing the risk of VILI, by promoting lung recruitment and setting protective mechanical ventilation (Table 21.2).

Non-Invasive Support

The possible use of non-invasive ventilation (NIV) in patients with ARDS, although potentially reducing intrapulmonary shunt and decreasing the work of breathing, remains controversial due its high risk of failure and risks associated with a delay in starting invasive mechanical ventilation. Larger controlled studies are required to determine the potential benefit of adding NIV to standard medical treatment in the avoidance of endotracheal intubation. A recent meta-analysis, which included 13 studies with a total of 540 patients mainly treated with NIV rather than CPAP, found that the intubation rate ranged between 30% and 86% and mortality rate from 15% to 71%. Unfortunately, the majority of these studies were not randomized, were heterogenous, and none compared NIV to invasive ventilation; consequently, it is currently not possible to draw firm conclusions. The LUNG SAFE study found that 15% of all patients with ARDS received NIV as a form of respiratory support. Treatment failure occurred in about 20% (mild) and 45% (moderate–severe) of ARDS cases, and failure was associated with more than two-fold increase in hospital mortality. Due to the high risk of failure, NIV should be reserved to patients without non-pulmonary organ failures, and should be provided in an ICU environment, where a strict monitoring and prompt intubation is available. Failure to improve gas exchange and work of breathing within a few hours should prompt a shift from NIV to invasive mechanical ventilation.

Table 21.2 Pharmacologic and non-pharmacologic intervention for ARDS

Non-pharmacologic interventions	Pharmacologic interventions
Non-invasive/invasive mechanical ventilation	Neuromuscular blocking agents
PEEP and tidal volume selection	Inhaled vasodilators
Prone positioning	Corticosteroids
ECMO	

A possible alternative is the high-flow nasal cannula (HFNC) system, which can deliver a high, heated and humidified oxygen flow through the nose. HFNCs increase the end-expiratory lung volume, reduce the work of breathing, and improve CO_2 clearance and oxygenation. In addition, and in contrast to NIV, HFNCs do not require any mask interface. This significantly improves long-term tolerance and use. The HFNCs, originally developed for neonatal and paediatric settings, have recently been evaluated in adult patients. In an observational study in ARDS patients (33% severe and 29% moderate), HFNCs failed in 40% of cases, leading to subsequent intubation mainly because of worsening hypoxaemia and haemodynamic or neurologic failure. This rate of intubation was similar to the values previously found for NIV. Presently, only one randomized study compared HFNCs (gas flow rate 50 L/min) to NIV (pressure support to ensure a tidal volume of 7–10 mL/kg and PEEP 2–10 cmH_2O) and oxygen therapy.[13] Intubation rate was not different between the three groups (38%–50%), but intensive care mortality was significantly lower in the HFNC group.

The indications and the standards of monitoring for the HFNCs in ARDS patients are similar to those of NIV.

Mechanical Ventilation

Mechanical ventilation does not cure ARDS: it buys time by maintaining sufficient gas exchange for survival. This benefit is achieved, in part, by taking over the function of the respiratory muscles. In patients with ARDS, the respiratory muscles are unable, for several reasons, to provide sufficient power to move gas in and out of the lungs. The effects of mechanical ventilation on oxygenation are two-fold: they allow the precise titration of FiO_2 in the delivered gas, while providing sufficient inspiratory pressure to open some of the collapsed pulmonary units, thus oxygenating the perfusing blood. However, these units will collapse again during the expiratory phase if PEEP is insufficient. Consequently, the effects of tidal ventilation alone on oxygenation are limited, unless it is applied together with an appropriate PEEP level. Ventilation, on the other hand, is essential for CO_2 elimination. In ARDS, the increased respiratory drive and pulmonary dead space increase the necessary minute ventilation to a level that far exceeds normal.

Unfortunately, a completely 'safe' lung-protective ventilation does not exist, and ventilatory support should be individualized to achieve the most optimal balance between respiratory mechanics, recruitability, gas exchange, and haemodynamics. Experimental evidence has accumulated over the past 30 years that mechanical ventilation at high volumes and pressures can injure the lung. The consequences of high-volume ventilation include increased permeability pulmonary oedema in the uninjured lung and enhanced oedema formation in the injured lung. Initial attempts to explain these deleterious effects focused on alveolar overdistension, with injury attributed predominantly to capillary stress failure with resultant endothelial and epithelial injury. However, more recent evidence points to high tidal volume ventilation and repeated collapse and reopening of alveoli causing lung injury by initiating a pro-inflammatory cascade. These responses bear a marked resemblance to the primary mechanisms underlying lung injury in ARDS. In a landmark trial, ventilation with a tidal volume of 6 versus 12 mL/kg predicted body weight reduced mortality.[14] This is supported by recent findings that protective ventilatory strategies are associated with lower pulmonary and systemic cytokine levels.

The application of PEEP is an essential component of mechanical ventilation for patients with ARDS. High PEEP levels may open collapsed alveoli and decrease intrapulmonary shunt. Additionally, ventilation-induced alveolar injury is reduced by decreasing alveolar over-distention, as the volume of each subsequent tidal breath is shared by more open alveoli. PEEP may decrease repetitive alveolar opening and closing during the respiratory cycle, thereby limiting lung injury. RCTs have compared modest versus high levels of PEEP in patients with ARDS; while they demonstrated reduced use of rescue therapies for hypoxaemia, such as prone positioning and inhaled nitric oxide, there was no survival benefit. The heterogeneity of ARDS may underpin the apparent absence of benefit from high PEEP levels: it is plausible that any beneficial effects of high PEEP in some ARDS patients might be offset by detrimental effects in others.

PEEP and Lung Recruitment

Although PEEP and lung recruitment are frequently considered separately, they are strictly related. According to a physical model, in order to recruit the lung (i.e. to inflate the collapsed lung regions) and to maintain these regions open, it is necessary to overcome the superimposed pressure generated by the lung and chest wall (Figure 21.2). Several types of recruitment manoeuvres (RMs) have been proposed: the sigh, in which higher tidal volumes are intermittently delivered during ventilation; the sustained inflation, induced by a static increase in airway pressure applied for 20–40 s; and the extended sigh, in which a stepwise increase of PEEP or of both PEEP and plateau pressure is applied (Figure 21.3). Independent of the specific type of RM applied, the main goal is to reinflate the 'closed' pulmonary units by applying a high transpulmonary pressure for an adequate period of time. In the majority of patients, an RM is able to improve oxygenation for a certain period of time without major side effects; however, RMs alone were not associated with a reduction in the mortality.[15]

Few issues in critical care medicine have been more troublesome to the physician attempting to regulate the ventilator than selecting the appropriate level of PEEP: insufficient PEEP allows unnecessary collapse of recruitable tissue, whereas excessive PEEP promotes tissue stretch and dead space generation while elevating the mean airway pressure and right-ventricular (RV) afterload (Figure 21.4). Unless the tidal volume is simultaneously reduced, increasing PEEP also elevates the plateau pressure. When the overstretching of open lung tissue outweighs the benefit from recruitment, PEEP redirects pulmonary blood flow and accentuates mechanical heterogeneity within the acutely injured lung.

During the decades, the 'philosophy' of PEEP has significantly changed. From a tool used to simply increase oxygenation, in the last years PEEP gained a primary role in the framework of lung-protective strategy, avoiding the intra-tidal opening and closing and decreasing the lung inhomogeneities that increase with ARDS severity.

In the injured and inhomogeneous lung, such as that seen in ARDS, the stress and strain are unevenly distributed with possible localized increases.[16] The regional inhomogeneities may act as 'stress raisers': while a given value of transpulmonary pressure may be safe in a homogeneous lung, it may locally reach harmful levels if it is multiplied by regional stress raisers. A CT scan study found that lung inhomogeneities increased with ARDS severity, were positively associated with dead space fraction and poorly aerated tissue, decreased when PEEP was increased, and were independently associated with outcome. Moreover, although the intensity of the lung inhomogeneities was similar in mild, moderate, and severe ARDS, what changed was their extent. The potential benefit of PEEP in the framework of lung-protective strategy is to maintain open, at end-expiration, lung parenchyma that has been recruited during inspiration, thus decreasing inhomogeneity and VILI. Within such framework, the combination of low tidal volume and higher PEEP may exert a lung-protective effect by decreasing both stress and strain.

Due to the different amount of lung oedema, the total lung recruitability (estimated by lung CT scan) was found to range from 0% up to 70% of the total lung weight[17] (Figure 21.5). Although lung CT scan requires the transport of patients outside the ICU

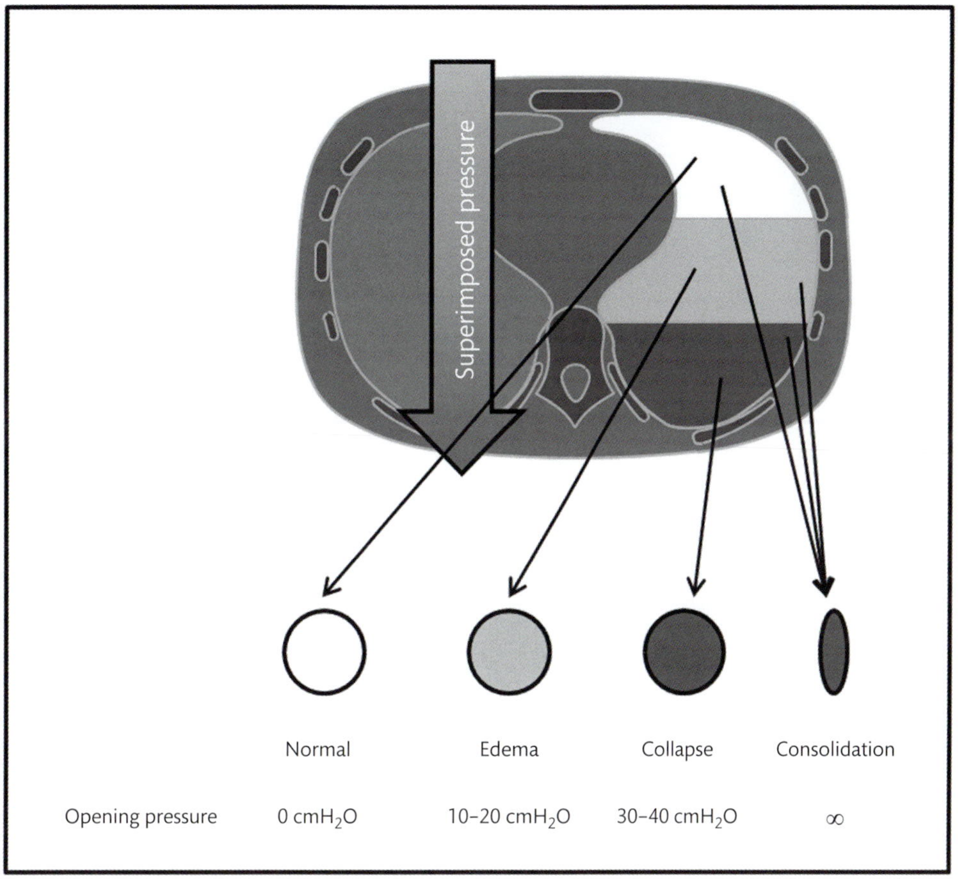

Figure 21.2 Ideal model depicting the effects of increased permeability in terms of increased superimposed pressure, with the inhomogeneous coexistence of areas of hyperinflation, normal inflation, and collapse and areas of consolidation along with the necessary pressure that needs to be applied to the lung in order to overcome the superimposed pressure generated by the lung mass and by the chest wall and recruit the alveolar units (i.e. to inflate the collapsed lung regions) and to maintain these regions open.

and the use of X-rays, it remains the gold standard to compute lung recruitability. The use of a visual scale to estimate recruitment and the application of a low-dose protocol for CT scan acquisition have shown promising results. In addition, recent studies showed that CT scan, independently from estimation of lung recruitment, contributed to diagnosis in 53% of the patients and induced a therapeutic change in 54% of the cases. As an alternative, lung ultrasound showed a reliable accuracy in estimating lung recruitability, but further studies are necessary to confirm its use.

Although several experimental and observational studies found a beneficial effect of the use of higher PEEP in ARDS, the three most recent randomized trials (ALVEOLI, ExPress, and LOV) did not show any outcome difference between a low and high PEEP strategy.[18–20] However, when combining this data and considering only the subgroup of the most severe patients, the use of higher PEEP level significantly decreased mortality.[21] This suggests that the greater the severity (and higher the amount of lung oedema), the higher is the beneficial effect of PEEP in reducing VILI. However, the relationship between lung oedema/mass and recruitability has been questioned by the finding that PEEP levels necessary to keep the lung open are independent from total lung recruitability, suggesting that recruitability also depends on the nature of oedema, time of onset, and distribution of the disease within the lung parenchyma.

In order to tailor PEEP on the individual patient, several approaches have been proposed (Table 21.3). The most common is the use of an oxygenation/saturation target based on a PEEP/FiO_2 table. An alternative method, based on respiratory mechanics, is to increase PEEP by maintaining a constant tidal volume, while not overcoming a safe limit of airway pressure (26–28 cmH_2O), or, after a recruitment manoeuvre, to decrease PEEP until a reduction of compliance appears. Despite the possible uncertainties regarding the end-expiratory absolute oesophageal pressure as a reliable estimation of the pleural pressure, a better oxygenation and compliance were found when PEEP was set according to an end-expiratory transpulmonary pressure between 0 and 10 cmH_2O in a single-centre investigation. Notably, a recent multicentre trial on 200 patients with ARDS randomized to a similar strategy versus standard care resulted in no significant difference in death and days free from mechanical ventilation.[22] Recently, our group compared the previously published methods for selecting PEEP (based on gas exchange, respiratory mechanics, and transpulmonary pressure) to lung recruitability and severity of the disease.[23] The method based on gas exchange (i.e. PEEP/FiO_2 table) was the only one which provided PEEP levels according to the severity of the disease; the other methods suggested similar levels of PEEP, which were not related to severity or lung recruitability.

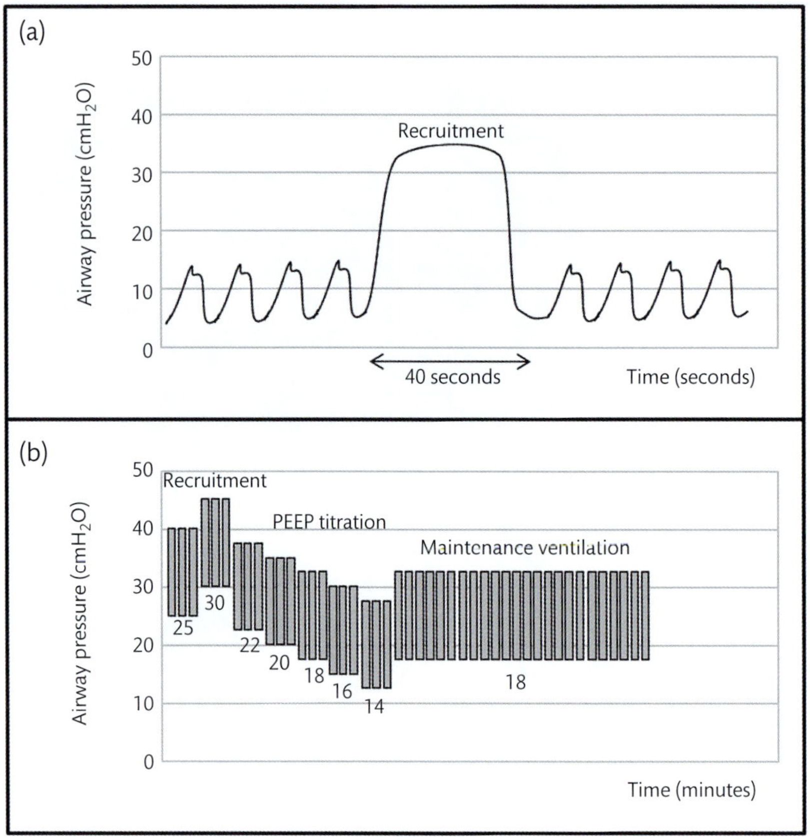

Figure 21.3 Pressure–time curve showing different recruitment manoeuvres. (A) Sustained inflation sigh using continuous positive airway pressure (CPAP) of 35 cmH_2O for 40 s. (B) Stepwise recruitment manoeuvre using both plateau pressure and PEEP increase, keeping a fixed driving pressure of 15 cmH_2O; after recruitment, a decremental PEEP titration is performed until an optimal level is identified (e.g. one associated with the best compliance or best oxygenation).

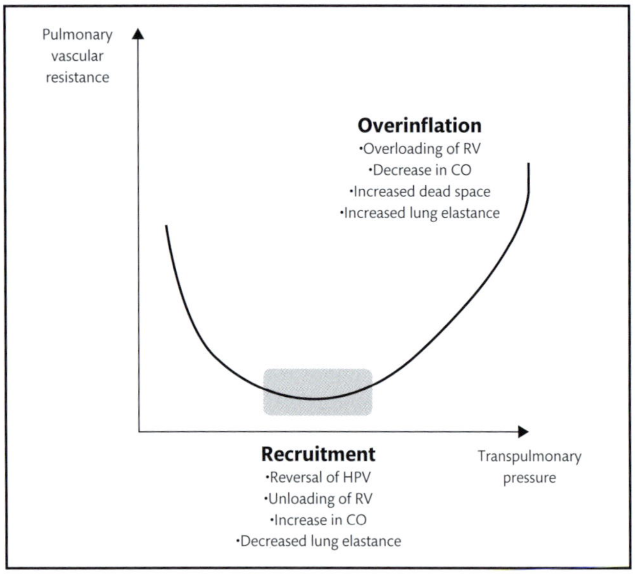

Figure 21.4 Relationship between pulmonary vascular resistance and transpulmonary pressure (TPP). Insufficient PEEP allows unnecessary collapse of recruitable tissue, whereas excessive PEEP promotes tissue stretch and dead space generation while elevating the mean airway pressure and right ventricular afterload. The grey area represents the target stress volume operating area in which the impact of transpulmonary pressure on the right ventricle is minimal. CO, cardiac output; RV, right ventricle; HPV, hypoxic pulmonary vasoconstriction.

A recent multicentre RCT tested the value of an 'open lung' approach: RMs, small tidal volumes, and decremental PEEP adjustment based on optimized tidal compliance were compared to standard care using low levels of PEEP for the management of established moderate/severe ARDS.[24] The study was stopped earlier due to difficulties in enrolment. The open lung approach improved oxygenation and driving pressure, without detrimental effects on mortality, ventilator-free days, or barotrauma, giving evidence to support the need for a larger trial using RMs and a decremental PEEP trial in established ARDS.

Based on the available data, it is apparent that 'perfect PEEP', which can simultaneously provide the best oxygenation, compliance, and reduction of VILI, does not exist. Therefore, a suggested approach in the acute phase is to perform a stratification of patients according to the severity of ARDS before any PEEP selection. This can easily be done by ventilating patients with pure oxygen at PEEP 5 cmH_2O. In the case of severe (or moderate-to-severe) ARDS, lung recruitability should be computed by lung CT scan or ultrasound, and high PEEP levels (i.e. >15 cmH_2O), following the PEEP/FiO_2 table, should be applied. It should always be remembered that the improvement in oxygenation can simply be due to a haemodynamic effect (that is, the reduction of cardiac output and right-to-left shunt) without any effect on lung recruitment. Thus, before any PEEP trial, patients should present haemodynamic stability, and any change in haemodynamics during the trial should be evaluated.

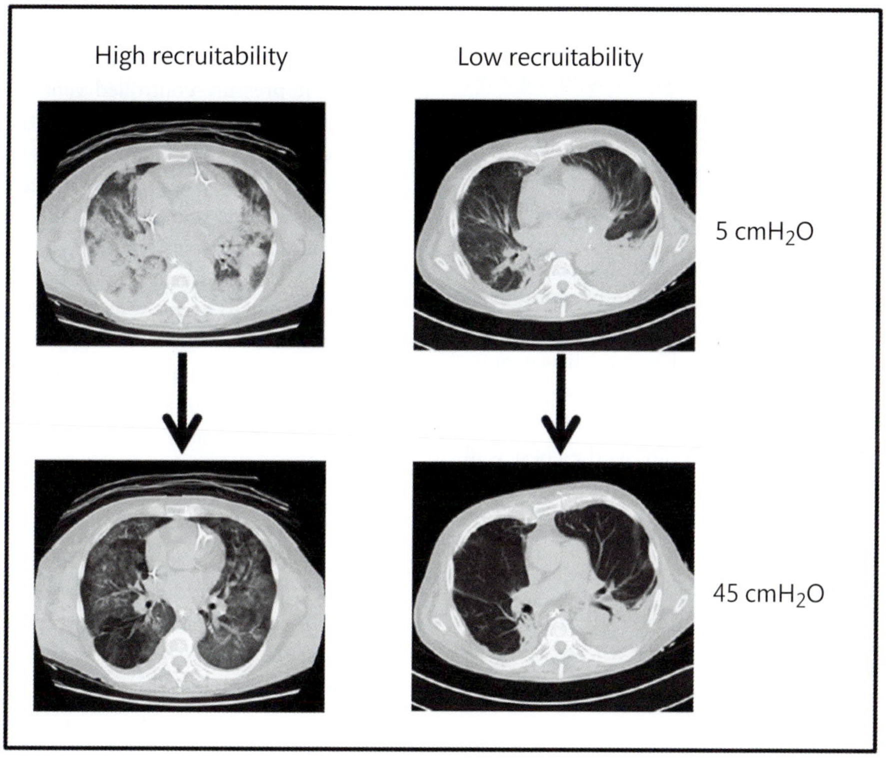

Figure 21.5 Example of lung CT scan of patients with high (upper panel) or low (lower panel) potential of lung recruitment.

In addition, to avoid lung overstress, the transpulmonary pressure should be measured while simultaneously titrating PEEP and tidal volume.

Tidal Volume

One of the main determinants of VILI is the generation of an unphysiologic stress (tension) and strain (deformation), which depend both on the size of delivered tidal volume and the amount of resting lung volume. The lower the tidal volume and/or the higher the resting volume, the lower the generated stress/strain will be. Based on these findings, a seminal study (the ARMA trial) showed a 22% mortality reduction by using a tidal volume of 6 versus 12 mL/kg predicted body weight.[14] A recent meta-analysis of trials comparing ventilation using either a lower tidal volume or lower airway pressure versus a higher tidal volume demonstrated significant 28-day mortality benefit in the lung-protective groups.[25] Ventilation with lower tidal volumes was shown to be clinically safe without any need to increase the dosage of sedatives or neuromuscular blockers, and it should then be a routine strategy of treatment of ARDS, while further trials may be unethical. However, despite two decades since the publication of the ARMA trial, low tidal volume ventilation is still not routinely used.

To better individualize the tidal volume without relying on the ideal body weight, which is poorly related to the resting volume (a similar tidal volume can generate different lung stress/strain), the use of airway driving pressure has been proposed.[26] The latter, defined as the ratio between tidal volume and respiratory system compliance, should better reflect lung stress/strain, as respiratory system compliance is related to available lung gas volume and thus the severity and extent of lung injury. Despite different combinations of tidal volume and levels of PEEP, driving pressure was the factor most strongly associated with outcome in a pooled sample of >3500 patients involved in nine RCTs. Higher plateau pressures were observed in patients with higher driving pressure or higher PEEP but with different consequences: higher mortality was noted only when higher plateau pressures were observed in patients with higher driving pressures. Similarly, the protective effects of higher PEEP were noted only when there were associated decreases in driving pressures. A cut-off for increased mortality

Table 21.3 Different strategies to select PEEP levels at the bedside

Method	Characteristics	Reference
LOV	PEEP/FiO_2 table as in the lung open ventilation arm of the LOV trial	Meade 2008
ExPress	Maintain an inspiratory plateau pressure between 28 and 30 cmH_2O according to the increased recruitment strategy of the ExPress trial	Mercat 2008
Stress index	Obtain a stress index coefficient of about 1	Grasso 2004
Oesophageal pressure	Target an absolute end-expiratory transpulmonary pressure of 0–10 cmH_2O	Talmor 2008

was found at a driving pressure of 15 cmH_2O. Thus, the airway driving pressure could be a useful tool to identify patients at risk of VILI. Nonetheless, driving pressure also has some limitations, namely its uncertain safety in patients with abnormally elevated respiratory system compliance (COPD or emphysema), in whom an extensive cycling alveolar deformation might not be associated with increased driving pressure. Other factors are also crucial in the interaction of mechanical ventilation with lung parenchyma, such as the resulting mean airway pressure applied, peak inspiratory flow, lung recruitability, and haemodynamics. Moreover, transpulmonary pressure, and not airway pressure, is the relevant distending pressure for the lung: uncritical reliance on airway pressures without considering the effect of the chest wall may lead to an erroneous interpretation of the real forces determining lung expansion and stress. This is especially relevant as the chest wall has frequent but unpredictably low compliance in ARDS, while high intrathoracic pressures and low chest wall compliance can be caused by abdominal distension.

In summary, normal (low) VT ventilation is safe and effective in maintaining gas exchange in patients without ARDS. In mechanically ventilated patients at risk of ARDS, exposure to high VT may increase the frequency of ARDS. The recent PReVENT study randomly assigned 961 patients without ARDS and expected to not be extubated within 24 h to a ventilation with 6 versus 10 mL/kg tidal volume.[27] The low tidal volume strategy did not result in a greater number of ventilator-free days than an intermediate tidal volume strategy; however, the study was criticized for its low power and the inadequate overall separation between the low versus intermediate ventilation strategies after day 1. On the other hand, in patients with established ARDS, exposure to high VT clearly increases mortality rates. Height and sex are better predictors of lung size than actual body weight; thus, the predicted body weight should be used to calculate the appropriate VT in mechanically ventilated patients. New strategies based on direct measurement of the size of the baby lung (functional residual capacity) may further optimize VT in individual patients.

Modality of Mechanical Ventilation

Presently, the two most common used modes of mechanical ventilation are the pressure-controlled ventilation (PCV) and volume-controlled ventilation (VCV). With PCV the delivered volume changes according to the characteristics of the respiratory system, and the inspiratory flow presents a decelerating shape; in VCV the delivered volume remains constant, while the airway pressure is variable and the inspiratory flow has a constant shape (Figure 21.6). It has been hypothesized that PCV could present benefits in reducing VILI due to decelerating inspiratory flow and the changes in delivered tidal volume according to the patient disease. On the other hand, volume-controlled mechanical ventilation could be more protective in the presence of changing respiratory compliance as it guarantees that transpulmonary pressure and tidal volume remain at a fixed level. A systematic review and meta-analysis did not demonstrate any difference in mortality or risk of barotrauma between the two modes.[28] Moreover, despite the different working principles of the two modes of ventilation, a recent meta-analysis was unable to find any difference in other physiologic responses, such as patient work of breathing, cardiac output, arterial blood pressure, oxygenation, or $PaCO_2$ levels.[29] Several ventilator manufacturers have developed 'hybrid' modes that deliver guaranteed tidal volumes by using a constant pressure wave form, examples include pressure-regulated volume control (Getinge) and autoflow/volume guarantee (Draeger).

Oxygenation and Carbon Dioxide Target

The commonly recommended oxygenation target ranges between 88% and 95%. However, in clinical practice, a more liberal approach to maintain an arterial saturation >96% is often used due to physician perception of a higher patient safety. A randomized study assigned patients to maintain an arterial saturation >96% and between 88% and 92%. The liberal strategy influenced neither the number of organ failures nor the outcome.

The application of a low tidal volume ventilation strategy can result in hypercapnia, which however does not present major side

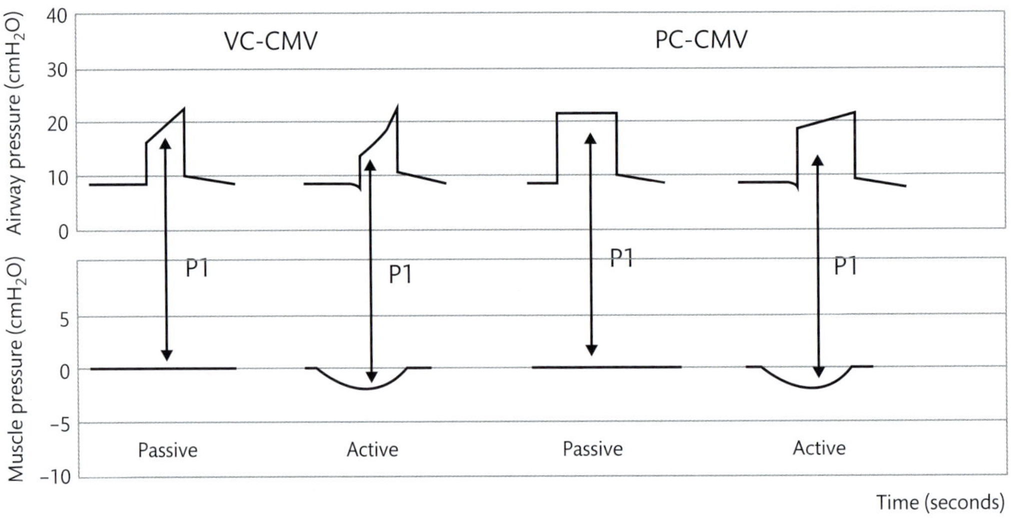

Figure 21.6 Different waveforms and effect of passive and active breathing in volume—VC-CMV and pressure-controlled (PC-CMV) mechanical ventilation. In VC-CMV, airway pressure drops when muscle pressure increases so that transpulmonary pressure (Pl) and tidal volume are maintained. With PC-CMV, changing from passive to active breathing leads to an increase in Pl and consequently tidal volume, while airway pressure is constant.

effects and is well tolerated. Although the optimal carbon dioxide level is still unclear, in the absence of right heart failure and raised intracranial pressure, up to 70 mmHg of arterial carbon dioxide with a pH of 7.20 has been found to be safe. Hypercapnic acidosis potentially increases arterial and tissue oxygenation in a number of ways: (1) improved ventilation/perfusion matching from the combination of the potentiation of hypoxic pulmonary vasoconstriction and increased local alveolar ventilation from inhibition of airway tone; (2) increased oxygen delivery from an increase in cardiac output; (3) increased tissue unloading due to a rightwards shift in the oxygen–haemoglobin dissociation curve and micro-vascular vasodilation; and (4) anti-inflammatory effects. Indeed, it is difficult to determine whether the potential benefits associated with permissive hypercapnia are due to the low minute ventilation or the resulting hypercapnic acidosis as they generally occur together. However, in vitro cell studies and in vivo animal models suggest that hypercapnic acidosis itself may have a beneficial impact independent of the effect of low minute ventilation.

Neuromuscular Blocking Agents

Neuromuscular blocking agents (NMBAs) are frequently used to abolish the inspiratory and expiratory patient efforts in order to improve patient–ventilator synchrony and to minimize muscle oxygen consumption. In addition, NMBAs can reduce the generation of stress/strain by reducing the negative increase in pleural pressure during spontaneous efforts. However, NMBAs increase the risk of ICU-acquired weakness and diaphragmatic dysfunction, prolonging the duration of mechanical ventilation. In the last multicentre RCT of ARDS, NMBAs were given in up to a half of the enrolled patients. Although NMBAs were applied without a predefined protocol, they were more frequently used in patients with a higher APACHE III score and hypoxaemia. To clarify the role of NMBAs in ARDS, several trials have been published in the last years. A 48-h NMBAs infusion added to deep sedation resulted in a higher oxygenation without any difference in the airway plateau pressure, PEEP levels, and amount of drugs used for sedation, as well as a significantly lower local (pulmonary) and systemic (blood) inflammatory response and better oxygenation. In a multicentre trial (ACURASYS), 340 severe ARDS patients were randomized to a 48-h continuous infusion of NMBAs or placebo.[30] The NMBAs group showed a significant 90-day mortality reduction with a higher number of ventilator-free days and lower incidence of pneumothorax. The incidence of ICU-acquired weakness at ICU discharge did not differ. A subsequent meta-analysis found that patients treated with NMBAs presented a 30% lower mortality, and fewer days of mechanical ventilation, with a higher number of ventilator-free days at day 28 and lower episodes of barotrauma. Since a logic drawback of NMBA use is the need for a deeper level of sedation, a strategy of early neuromuscular blockade with heavy sedation, as opposed to current usual care with lighter sedation targets, was compared in the recently published ROSE study.[31] The inclusion criteria and management of muscle relaxant drugs were similar to the previous ACURASYS study; the main difference being that the control group had a light sedation target (RASS 0/-1). No significant difference in 90-day mortality was found between the two groups. While reducing the enthusiasm in favour of early neuromuscular blockade, the results need to be considered in the light of its main limitation: almost half of patients in ACURASYS were placed in prone position, while only 16% of patients in ROSE were proned. Whether early continuous neuromuscular blockade is more effective with prone positioning is unknown, but this is a possible explanation for the divergent results of the two studies.

Based on the available data, NMBAs should be reserved to the most severe ARDS patients, mainly in the acute phase and in the first hours of mechanical ventilation, to ensure adequate patient–ventilator synchrony, avoiding the generation of a harmful transpulmonary pressure. However, the adjustment of ventilator setting and the need of paralysis should, at least, be evaluated every day.

Spontaneous Breathing

It is commonly accepted that trans-alveolar pressure should be minimized during ventilation. Indeed, the same transpulmonary pressure can be achieved, whether it is generated by a positive pressure, by a negative pressure (and therefore the respiratory muscles), or by a combination of the two, so that even spontaneous ventilation has high potential to be damaging early in the disease course. It must be remembered that when patients have high demands, vigorous breathing violates the objectives of lung protection. The work of breathing moderately increases cardiac output and pulmonary vascular flow. More importantly, transpulmonary inspiratory stresses are not only high, but during exhalation the muscular effort often also compresses the thorax below the PEEP-appropriate functional residual capacity. This not only encourages de-recruitment but also increases effective inspiratory transpulmonary forces that drive inspiration. Moreover, during spontaneous breathing, negative pleural pressure swings will have differing vascular effects than those seen during controlled mechanical ventilation, resulting in higher cardiac and pulmonary filling pressures. This vascular congestion may increase the risk of VILI. Indeed, sustained hyperventilation induced by severe acidosis may lead per se to ALI in animals with previously healthy lungs. However, some benefits of spontaneous breathing over muscle paralysis have emerged from various animal and clinical studies. A small randomized study demonstrated that spontaneous breathing improved oxygenation and shortened durations of ventilatory support and ICU stays compared with a muscle paralysis group. However, patients who were randomized mainly had a mild form of ARDS.

In experimental models, allowing spontaneous breathing seems to have different consequences depending on the severity of lung injury.[32] In the case of severe injury, spontaneous breathing appears to worsen damage, while the converse is seen with mild injury. These differences may reflect increases in transpulmonary pressure and tidal volume during spontaneous ventilation, associated with high regional distending pressures and increases of trans-vascular pressure. In summary, the current body of evidence suggests that spontaneous breathing activity is beneficial in mild to moderate and harmful in severe ARDS. It has been hypothesized that it is not the severity of lung injury itself but rather the ability of spontaneous breathing to generate sufficient transpulmonary pressure to open collapsed lung units, and the settings of PEEP and/or expiratory time to maintain them open at end-expiration, that determine whether spontaneous breathing is protective or harmful in ARDS.

Prone Positioning

More than 30 years ago, observational studies reported that prone positioning was able to increase the arterial oxygenation in the majority of patients with acute respiratory failure. This manoeuvre was reserved as a rescue treatment in the case of life-threatening hypoxaemia. The main consequences of prone positioning, which can be all or in part present, include a redistribution of the lung densities with a recruitment of the dorsal regions, an increase in chest wall elastance, a reduction in the alveolar shunt and a better ventilation/perfusion ratio with improvement in oxygenation and CO_2 clearance, a more homogeneous distribution of ventilation with a reduction of VILI, and a reverse of the right heart failure (Box 21.2). Based on these favourable effects, several trials were conducted to test the prone positioning in ARDS patients. The first studies, enrolling patients with moderate-to-severe ARDS without applying a protective mechanical ventilation, did not show any beneficial effect of the short-term use (<8 h/day) of prone position. Similar results were found by subsequent trials, which enrolled more severely hypoxemic patients with longer periods of prone position (20 h/day); however, a meta-analysis suggested a significant survival benefit for patients with a PaO_2/FiO_2 <140 mmHg on admission. On this background, the PROSEVA multicentre randomized trial investigated the use of long-term prone positioning (at least 16 h/day) in severe ARDS. PEEP was selected on the PEEP/FiO_2 table of the low PEEP arm of the ALVEOLI study and tidal volume was strictly controlled to 6 mL/kg of ideal body weight; 28-day mortality was halved in the prone positioning group (16% vs 32%), the rate of successful extubation was higher, and the mean duration of prone positioning was 17 ± 3 h.[33]

Similar to PEEP, the role of prone positioning in ARDS also changed over time as it is now clear that, besides its value in improving gas exchange, prone positioning helps protect against VILI by distributing stress and strain more homogeneously through the lung parenchyma (Figure 21.7). Indeed, it was shown that patients whose $PaCO_2$ was reduced following proning had a reduced 28-day mortality, whereas no association was found with the PaO_2/FIO_2 response to pronation. Due to the reduction of the harmful effects of mechanical ventilation both by prone positioning and NMBAs when separately evaluated, adding NMBAs in prone positioning could have a synergistic effect in improving oxygenation, decreasing the duration of mechanical ventilation, and improving the final outcome.

According to the recent Berlin definition, prone position should be reserved to severe ARDS patients, especially in the acute phase in which the amount of oedema, atelectasis, and lung recruitability is higher, and for longer periods of time. Although improvements in oxygenation are the most readily assessable benefit of proning, even amongst the minority which do not improve this parameter, there are beneficial effects in reducing VILI. Although prone positioning presents some technical challenges, when it is performed by a skilled and experienced team the adverse effects are relatively low and they are significantly outweighed by the beneficial effects. However, before any change in the position of critically ill patients, the presence of any absolute contraindication (e.g. pregnancy, unstable fractures, open abdominal wounds, and extreme haemodynamic instability) has to be considered.

Box 21.2 Physiologic consequences of prone positioning

- Recruitment of the dorsal lung regions
- Increase in chest wall elastance
- Reduction in the alveolar shunt
- Better ventilation/perfusion ratio
- More homogeneous distribution of ventilation
- Reverse of the right heart failure

Inhaled Vasodilators

Inhaled vasodilators exert a localized effect leading to selective pulmonary vasodilation. As they only dilate the pulmonary vasculature in well-ventilated areas of the lung, this reduces pulmonary arterial pressure and pulmonary vascular resistance, thus improving ventilation–perfusion matching and oxygenation. Their short half-life minimizes the systemic effects, compared to other routes such as oral/intravenous administration. Indeed, both inhaled nitric oxide (NO) and either inhaled or intravenous prostacyclin have similar effects on pulmonary arterial pressure, pulmonary vascular resistance, cardiac output, and RV ejection fraction. However, in contrast to inhaled NO and prostacyclin, intravenous prostacyclin caused systemic vasodilation, which lowered mean systemic arterial pressure and worsened arterial oxygenation, likely due to reversal of hypoxic pulmonary vasoconstriction, which increases perfusion to non-ventilated alveoli.

Inhaled NO, the first selective pulmonary vasodilator used in humans, acts by preferentially diffusing to capillary beds of less inflamed alveoli leading to a reduction in ventilation/perfusion mismatch and pulmonary vascular pressures. However, its use in ARDS is highly controversial: it was shown to improve oxygenation and reduce pulmonary hypertension without affecting systemic blood pressure; the decrease in pulmonary arterial pressure is key to reduce pulmonary oedema formation and RV afterload. However, no clear outcome benefits have been demonstrated after its use, and it was associated with significant costs and safety concerns. Recent meta-analysis failed to demonstrate any mortality benefit regardless of severity; moreover, its use was associated with an increase in the incidence of renal failure. Nevertheless, its use was reported to be still as high as 13% of all severe ARDS patients in the recent LUNG SAFE investigation.

The vasodilator effects of inhaled prostacyclins, epoprostenol (prostaglandin I-2), and alprostadil (PGE1) are nearly identical to inhaled NO; despite limited differences in physiologic response, potency, and anti-thrombotic properties, no evidence is available as to whether this translates into better efficacy with epoprostenol than alprostadil. In summary, despite some improvements in haemodynamic parameters and oxygenation, due to the limited number of studies and the lack of trials investigating mortality, the use of inhaled prostacyclins cannot be recommended as standard of care in ARDS, and its use should only be regarded as a rescue therapy for those refractory to traditional treatment.

Corticosteroids

The rationale for the use of corticosteroids in ARDS lies in the clear understanding that inflammation is a key factor in the pathophysiology of the syndrome irrespective of aetiology. This inflammatory injury to the lungs evolves through various stages that include an early exudative phase followed by a late fibro-proliferative phase. Corticosteroids, with their potent anti-inflammatory activity, seem be a logical therapeutic option. Following the above concept, several

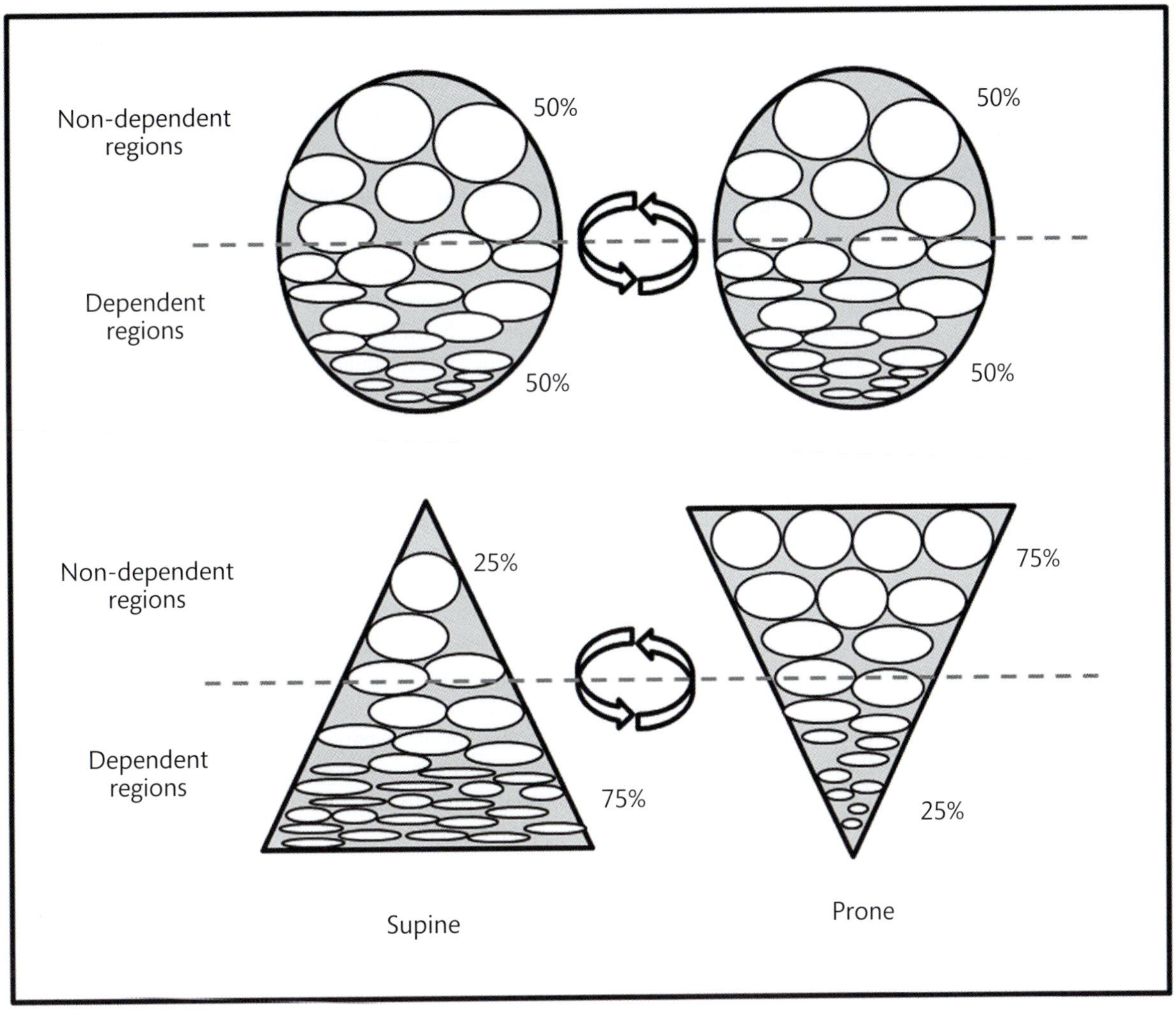

Figure 21.7 Simplified model that shows the influence of lung shape on the distribution of aeration in the parenchyma during supine and prone position. If an elliptical-shaped lung is considered, the portion of well-aerated tissue in non-dependent regions is similar between supine and prone positions. As the amount of open and closed parenchyma will be the same in both positions, the aeration distribution will remain the same. If a triangle-shaped lung is considered instead, the portion of well-aerated tissue in non-dependent regions increases during the turning process as the result of recruitment in dorsal zones is higher than the de-recruitment in ventral zones. As a consequence, parenchyma aeration will increase, and lung compliance will improve.

trials investigated these at various stages of ARDS, with heterogeneous results.

The early, short-course, high-dose administration of corticosteroids to combat the strong pro-inflammatory response of the early stage of the syndrome (methylprednisolone 30 mg/kg every 6 h for 1 day) was not associated with any beneficial effect on mortality or chance of reversal of ARDS as compared with placebo. A trial by ARDS clinical trial network,[34] in 180 patients with both early (73%) and late (27%) ARDS, showed that a prolonged course of methylprednisolone at a lower dose (2 mg/kg bolus, followed by 0.5 mg/kg every 6 h for 14 days, 0.5 mg/kg every 12 h for 7 days, and then tapering over 4 days) had no survival benefits. A more prolonged corticosteroid use (a loading dose of 1 mg/kg, followed by an infusion of 1 mg/kg/day from day 1 to 14, 0.5 mg/kg/day from day 15 to 21, 0.25 mg/kg/day from day 22 to 25, and 0.125 mg/kg/day from day 26 to 28) in early ARDS was associated with a nearly halved ICU mortality.[35] However, the study was poorly matched in terms of severity of patients and a significant percentage of control patients crossed over to receive open-label corticosteroids.

The DEXA-ARDS study randomized 277 patients with moderate-to-severe ARDS to a 10-day course of dexamethasone (20 mg/day for the first 5 days, then 5 mg/day) versus standard care; patients in the treatment group showed a significantly higher amount of ventilator-free days and a 15% lower 60-day all-cause mortality.[36] Notably, similar findings were consistently replicated in recent trials of steroids in patients with septic shock (an accelerated weaning from ventilation and reduced ICU length of stay were found in the ADRENAL and APROCCHSS studies, with the latter also showing a mortality benefit) and with community-acquired pneumonia. Patients assigned to steroids had a similar rate of gastrointestinal bleeding, ICU-acquired muscle weakness, and nosocomial infections than the control group.

A positive effect of corticosteroids in ARDS was also found during the recent COVID-19 pandemic: the landmark RECOVERY trial demonstrated that administration of 6 mg/day dexamethasone in hospitalized patients with COVID-19 significantly reduced 28-day mortality, with the greatest effect observed in patients receiving invasive mechanical ventilation.[37] A further, prospective meta-analysis of seven RCTs further confirmed the benefit of corticosteroid therapy in reducing mortality in critically ill patients with COVID-19.[38] The mortality reduction was similar for studies that used dexamethasone or hydrocortisone, suggesting a class effect.

A different issue is that of persistent ARDS at later stages, which are characterized by more of fibrosis than cellular inflammation, as corticosteroid effect is expected to be different. A significant association was found between late initiation corticosteroids and failure to improve. In conclusion, short-duration, high-dose glucocorticoid therapy is not effective in preventing ARDS and may be harmful, whereas a 10-day course of dexamethasone was associated with significantly improved outcomes in patients with moderate–severe ARDS. Lower doses for persistent ARDS may improve lung function and shorten the duration of mechanical ventilation, but the impact on long-term mortality is unclear.

ECMO

The standard extracorporeal membrane oxygenation (ECMO) support is commonly performed by a veno-venous access in which the blood is drained by the superior or inferior vena cava and reinfused in the right atrium. The artificial lung is able to provide an adequate blood CO_2 removal and oxygenation, allowing to reduce mechanical ventilation and to minimize the VILI. The first applications of ECMO in patients with acute respiratory failure did not show any benefit; later studies (starting from 1985) found a decreased mortality, ranging between 21% and 50%. However, few randomized trials comparing ECMO to standard care have been performed. In the CESAR trial, patients with ARDS were referred to a single centre and managed with ECMO or treated with conventional mechanical ventilation.[39] Mechanical ventilation during ECMO provided lung rest with a peak inspiratory pressure of 20–25 cmH_2O and PEEP 10–15 cmH_2O. At 6 months, the ECMO group presented a higher survival rate compared to control group, while the quality of life and spirometric parameters were not different. Despite these positive results, the trial has been criticized because ventilator treatment in control group was not standardized, 30% of the patients were not ventilated with a lung-protective strategy, and all patients requiring ECMO were allocated only in one skilled centre, making it impossible to draw firm consequences. Indeed, despite the limited evidence and mainly based on the theoretical benefit of lung rest and on several case-series, the use of ECMO has continued to increase worldwide.

It is worthy to remember that VILI is not completely abolished during ECMO treatment: consequently, prone positioning, similarly to conventional mechanical ventilation, should be used. At the present time there is a paucity of data regarding the use of prone position during ECMO; for example, the ELSO registry, the worldwide biggest registry on extracorporeal treatments (http://elsonet.org), did not collect this information.

Recently, the EOLIA trial randomized critically ill patients with the most severe forms of ARDS to the best available supportive care or to an early trial of veno-venous ECMO.[40] The authors could only find a non-significant indication of potential benefit (mortality rate 35% vs 46%, $p = 0.09$); however, a high percentage of patients (28%) crossed over from the control group to ECMO because of refractory respiratory failure or deteriorating haemodynamics, and the trial may have been underpowered since it was stopped earlier. Indeed, a reanalysis of the results conducted using Bayesian methods found that it is highly probable that this form of support lowers mortality in patients with ARDS.[41]

ARDS in the Obese Patient

The prevalence of obesity is steadily increasing worldwide; in the Unites States, it is estimated that about two-thirds of citizens are either overweight or obese (i.e. a body mass index >25 kg/m^2). A potential link between ARDS and obesity was found during the 2009 pandemic H1N1 influenza and later confirmed during the COVID-19 pandemic, leading to the recognition that when critical illness is coincident with obesity, there are additional considerations for disease mechanism, management, and prognosis.[42] While the first, mainly retrospective studies found a significant association between obesity and increased mortality from ARDS, and more recent prospective investigations found that obese patients may even counterintuitively show a better outcome. The protective effect of obesity (which has been defined as the 'obesity paradox') is not a new finding as it has also been reported in obese patients with medical conditions such as acute heart failure and chronic kidney disease; in critically ill patients, a similar reduced mortality has been described for obese patients with septic shock. To solve the 'obesity paradox' debate, several meta-analyses have been performed, which showed either no effect or a protective role of obesity on ICU and hospital mortality.

Indeed, obese patients with ARDS are often challenging to manage due to issues related to their chronic state and some peculiarities of acute care management (Table 21.4). The most significant change in pulmonary mechanics of obese subjects is a decrease in respiratory system compliance, which has been attributed to several factors: fatty infiltration of the chest wall, increased pulmonary blood volume, and extrinsic compression of the thoracic cage by weight from excess soft tissue. As a result, obese subjects exhibit an increased work of breathing. With the increased pleural pressure experienced in obesity, transpulmonary pressure becomes less positive (or more negative), that is, lung parenchyma experiences less distending (and more collapsing) pressure. Patients who are obese, therefore, have considerable atelectasis, which in turn results in impaired gas exchange and decreased lung compliance. As far as pulmonary function tests are concerned, static lung volumes are most affected with reductions in expiratory reserve volume and functional residual capacity. Moreover, obesity has many important effects on non-pulmonary physiology (Table 21.4). In addition to the changes in respiratory mechanics, obese patients experience chronic alterations in circulating inflammatory mediators derived from adipose tissue (collectively known as adipokines) as well as increased circulating levels of pro-inflammatory cytokines. While current data is incomplete, obesity and ARDS appear to share alterations in inflammation, endothelial dysfunction, and oxidative stress. This raises the possibility that obese patients may be at higher risk of developing ARDS and have poorer outcomes, although this currently remains under active investigation.

When obesity and ARDS coexist in the same patient, there are specific issues for mechanical ventilation and management: the heterogeneity normally seen in patients who are obese is amplified in ARDS, in which increased pleural pressure is combined

Table 21.4 Effects and complications of obesity

Type	Chronic effect	Acute management issues
Neurologic	Increased ICP, cerebrovascular disease, disordered breathing, anxiety, and depression	Sedation and abnormal respiratory control
Cardiovascular	Ischaemic heart disease hypertension	Haemodynamic instability, monitoring problems, and elevated filling pressures when measured relative to atmosphere
Pulmonary	OSA, obesity hypoventilation, and atelectasis	Aspiration risk, complicated intubations, and impaired ventilation and gas exchange
Body habitus	Chest wall restriction and limited mobility	Transport and positioning and procedural difficulties (vascular access and imaging)
GI/renal	Cholelithiasis, non-alcoholic steatosis, pancreatitis, and glomerulosclerosis	Altered pharmacokinetics, malnutrition, and abdominal compartment syndrome
Endocrine	Diabetes mellitus and hyperlipidaemia	Glucose disturbances

with increased surface tension due to surfactant dysfunction and alveolar–endothelial damage so that obese patients with ARDS can experience considerable atelectasis and alveolar flooding with resultant gas exchange abnormalities. This also predisposes these patients to significant risk of VILI, which results in part from the shear stresses that occur at the intersection of open and closed alveoli. Failure to account for increased pleural pressure, which is rarely measured, can result in an under-titration of PEEP and increased shear stress and lung injury so that oesophageal pressure measurement becomes of great help in the management of such patients.

A recent paper investigated the effect of a combination of RMs and PEEP titration in a mixed population of medical/surgical, morbidly obese (average BMI 51 kg/m^2) critically ill patients compared to zero PEEP and the baseline PEEP level as set by the attending physician.[43] The authors found that RMs followed by titrated PEEP were effective at increasing end-expiratory lung volumes and oxygenation, while decreasing end-inspiratory transpulmonary pressure, suggesting an improved distribution of lung aeration and reduction of overdistension. PEEP levels set by the clinicians were significantly lower (on average 21 vs 11 cmH$_2$O) and were associated with lower lung volumes, worse elastic properties of the lung, and lower oxygenation, outlining the deleterious pathophysiologic effects of commonly adopted PEEP levels in critically ill morbidly obese patients.

Very few studies specifically investigated the pathophysiologic effect of obesity in ARDS. Indeed, a recent paper specifically analyzed the effect of BMI in a group of ARDS patients on chest wall elastance, lung recruitability, and transpulmonary pressure. Lung and chest wall elastance were not affected by body weight, obese patients had significantly higher total superimposed pressure and lower lung gas volume, and the end-inspiratory transpulmonary pressure (i.e. total stress applied to the lung), lung recruitability, and gas exchange were similar amongst the different BMI groups.[44] If the role of PEEP is to keep the lung open and limit intra-tidal collapse and de-collapse, then the routine use of higher PEEP levels may not be recommended in obese ARDS patients.

Long-term Outcomes after ARDS

Thanks to the therapeutic strategies here reviewed, and improvements in ICU supportive care, several studies have reported a decrease in the short-term mortality rate of ARDS. However, patients who survive ARDS remain at risk for mortality and may have persistent morbidity. When short- and long-term mortality in subjects with ARDS are compared, hospital mortality is generally significantly lower than that at 1 year after hospital discharge (24% vs 41%) regardless of the aetiology of ARDS. To investigate the influence of rescue therapies on mortality at 1 year, ARDS subjects ventilated in prone or supine position were compared, without finding any difference, although an overall high mortality rate (60%) was reported.[45] However, the authors could not establish whether this high rate was mainly due to respiratory function impairment or extra-pulmonary complications. In summary, long-term mortality in patients with ARDS may be significantly higher than expected and mainly depends on non-modifiable factors, including previous co-morbidities and age, rather than on severity of acute illness, which, conversely, is a strong predictor of hospital mortality. In other words, the treatment of ARDS does not resolve the underlying co-morbidities, and the survivors mainly die from these.

Besides crude mortality, the long-term health-related quality of life of ARDS survivors has gained recent attention; however, this is hard to estimate precisely due to the small samples of subjects enrolled in the studies, large losses during follow-up, and the different scales used to quantify it. Indeed, results of a meta-analysis show how significant decrements of long-term health-related quality are found when compared with the general population, especially with higher decrements in the physical domains compared with the mental domains 6 months after ICU discharge.

Development of neuro-psychological disability is significant after ARDS. Its aetiology is incompletely understood but is likely to be contributed to by pathophysiological alterations related to critical illness (hypoxaemia, activation of the hypothalamic–pituitary axis, elevated cytokines, and organ dysfunction) and medications (e.g. catecholamines and sedatives). Disturbances includes neurocognitive impairment and psychiatric dysfunction such as posttraumatic stress disorder (anxiety, pain, and nightmares) and depression. Reports indicate that up to 50% of survivors after ARDS are depressed at 1 year, whereas posttraumatic stress disorder was diagnosed in about 30% of patients.

Little is also known about the pathophysiology of the neurocognitive impairment after ARDS. However, up to 55% of ARDS survivors can show long-term cognitive dysfunction in terms of attention, memory, mental processing speed, and executive function. It is likely that different mechanisms contribute to its development, such as hypoxia, delirium, glucose dysregulation, the effects of sedatives, and pre-existing cognitive impairment. Further research to understand the mechanisms and causes of long-term ARDS consequences could provide new preventive and therapeutic strategies.

Conclusions

Patients suffering from ARDS should receive a holistic framework of medical support ensuring adequate gas exchange while minimizing VILI. This can be achieved by either a volume- or a pressure-controlled form of mechanical ventilation, by setting an adequate PEEP level and considering lung recruitability. Lung overstress should be avoided by regulation of tidal volume and possibly monitoring transpulmonary pressure (or airway driving pressure). In the most severe cases, adjuncts such as NMBAs, prone positioning, and ECMO (alone or in combination) may be considered. The need for NMBAs and prone positioning should be evaluated daily to avoid delaying the waking of the patient and the onset of early mobilization. Inhaled vasodilators should not be routinely used, while a short course of low-dose corticosteroids should be considered.

REFERENCES

1. Huppert LA, Matthey MA, Ware LB. Pathogenesis of acute respiratory distress syndrome. *Semin Respir Crit Care Med.* 2019;**40**(1):31–39.
2. Rocco PR, Dos Santos C, Pelosi P. Lung parenchyma remodeling in acute respiratory distress syndrome. *Minerva Anestesiol.* 2009;**75**(12):730–740.
3. Marini JJ, Rocco PRM, Gattinoni L. Static and dynamic contributors to ventilator-induced lung injury in clinical practice. pressure, energy, and power. *Am J Resp Crit Care Med.* 2020;**201**(7):767–774.
4. Gattinoni L, Pesenti A. The concept of 'baby lung'. *Intensive Care Med.* 2005;**31**(6):776–784.
5. Ranieri VM, Suter PM, Tortorella C, et al. Effect of mechanical ventilation on inflammatory mediators in patients with acute respiratory distress syndrome: A randomized controlled trial. *JAMA.* 1999;**282**(1):54–61.
6. Tomashefski JF, Jr., Davies P, Boggis C, et al. The pulmonary vascular lesions of the adult respiratory distress syndrome. *Am J Path.* 1983;**112**(1):112–126.
7. Rubenfeld GD, Caldwell E, Peabody E, et al. Incidence and outcomes of acute lung injury. *N Eng J Med.* 2005;**353**(16):1685–1693.
8. Erickson SE, Martin GS, Davis JL, et al. Recent trends in acute lung injury mortality: 1996–2005. *Crit Care Med.* 2009;**37**(5):1574–1579.
9. Bellani G, Laffey JG, Pham T, et al. Epidemiology, patterns of care, and mortality for patients with acute respiratory distress syndrome in intensive care units in 50 countries. *JAMA.* 2016;**315**(8):788–800.
10. Ashbaugh DG, Bigelow DB, Petty TL, et al. Acute respiratory distress in adults. *Lancet.* 1967;**2**(7511):319–323.
11. Bernard GR, Artigas A, Brigham KL, et al. The American–European consensus conference on ARDS. Definitions, mechanisms, relevant outcomes, and clinical trial coordination. *Am J Resp Crit Care Med.* 1994;**149**(3 Pt 1):818–824.
12. Ranieri VM, Rubenfeld GD, Thompson BT, et al. Acute respiratory distress syndrome: The Berlin Definition. *JAMA.* 2012;**307**(23):2526–2533.
13. Frat JP, Thille AW, Mercat A, et al. High-flow oxygen through nasal cannula in acute hypoxemic respiratory failure. *N Eng J Med.* 2015;**372**(23):2185–2196.
14. Acute Respiratory Distress Syndrome Network, Brower RG, Matthay MA, et al. Ventilation with lower tidal volumes as compared with traditional tidal volumes for acute lung injury and the acute respiratory distress syndrome. *N Eng J Med.* 2000;**342**(18):1301–1308.
15. Suzumura EA, Figueiro M, Normilio-Silva K, et al. Effects of alveolar recruitment maneuvers on clinical outcomes in patients with acute respiratory distress syndrome: A systematic review and meta-analysis. *Intensive Care Med.* 2014;**40**(9):1227–1240.
16. Mead J, Takishima T, Leith D. Stress distribution in lungs: A model of pulmonary elasticity. *J App Physiol.* 1970;**28**(5):596–608.
17. Gattinoni L, Caironi P, Cressoni M, et al. Lung recruitment in patients with the acute respiratory distress syndrome. *N Eng J Med.* 2006;**354**(17):1775–1786.
18. Brower RG, Lanken PN, MacIntyre N, et al. Higher versus lower positive end-expiratory pressures in patients with the acute respiratory distress syndrome. *N Eng J Med.* 2004;**351**(4):327–336.
19. Mercat A, Richard JC, Vielle B, et al. Positive end-expiratory pressure setting in adults with acute lung injury and acute respiratory distress syndrome: A randomized controlled trial. *JAMA.* 2008;**299**(6):646–655.
20. Meade MO, Cook DJ, Guyatt GH, et al. Ventilation strategy using low tidal volumes, recruitment maneuvers, and high positive end-expiratory pressure for acute lung injury and acute respiratory distress syndrome: A randomized controlled trial. *JAMA.* 2008;**299**(6):637–645.
21. Briel M, Meade M, Mercat A, et al. Higher vs lower positive end-expiratory pressure in patients with acute lung injury and acute respiratory distress syndrome: Systematic review and meta-analysis. *JAMA.* 2010;**303**(9):865–873.
22. Beitler JR, Sarge T, Banner-Goodspeed VM, et al. Effect of titrating positive end-expiratory pressure (PEEP) with an esophageal pressure-guided strategy vs an empirical high PEEP-Fio2 strategy on death and days free from mechanical ventilation among patients with acute respiratory distress syndrome: A randomized clinical trial. *JAMA.* 2019;**321**(9):846–857.
23. Chiumello D, Cressoni M, Carlesso E, et al. Bedside selection of positive end-expiratory pressure in mild, moderate, and severe acute respiratory distress syndrome. *Crit Care Med.* 2014;**42**(2):252–264.
24. Kacmarek RM, Villar J, Sulemanji D, et al. Open lung approach for the acute respiratory distress syndrome: A pilot, randomized controlled trial. *Crit Care Med.* 2016;**44**(1):32–42.
25. Petrucci N, De Feo C. Lung protective ventilation strategy for the acute respiratory distress syndrome. *Cochrane Database Syst Rev.* 2013(2):CD003844.
26. Amato MB, Meade MO, Slutsky AS, et al. Driving pressure and survival in the acute respiratory distress syndrome. *N Eng J Med.* 2015;**372**(8):747–755.
27. Writing Group for the PReVENT Investigators, Simonis FD, Serpa Neto A, et al. Effect of a low vs intermediate tidal volume strategy on ventilator-free days in intensive care unit

patients without ARDS: A randomized clinical trial. *JAMA.* 2018;**320**(18):1872–1880.

28. Chacko B, Peter JV, Tharyan P, et al. Pressure-controlled versus volume-controlled ventilation for acute respiratory failure due to acute lung injury (ALI) or acute respiratory distress syndrome (ARDS). *Cochrane Database Syst Rev.* 2015;**1**:CD008807.
29. Rittayamai N, Katsios CM, Beloncle F, et al. Pressure-controlled vs volume-controlled ventilation in acute respiratory failure: A physiology-based narrative and systematic review. *Chest.* 2015;**148**(2):340–355.
30. Papazian L, Forel JM, Gacouin A, et al. Neuromuscular blockers in early acute respiratory distress syndrome. *N Eng J Med.* 2010;**363**(12):1107–1116.
31. National Heart Lung Blood Institute Petal Clinical Trials Network, Moss M, Huang DT, et al. Early neuromuscular blockade in the acute respiratory distress syndrome. *N Eng J Med.* 2019;**380**(21):1997–2008.
32. Yoshida T, Uchiyama A, Matsuura N, et al. Spontaneous breathing during lung-protective ventilation in an experimental acute lung injury model: High transpulmonary pressure associated with strong spontaneous breathing effort may worsen lung injury. *Crit Care Med.* 2012;**40**(5):1578–1585.
33. Guerin C, Reignier J, Richard JC, et al. Prone positioning in severe acute respiratory distress syndrome. *N Eng J Med.* 2013;**368**(23):2159–2168.
34. Steinberg KP, Hudson LD, Goodman RB, et al. Efficacy and safety of corticosteroids for persistent acute respiratory distress syndrome. *N Eng J Med.* 2006;**354**(16):1671–1684.
35. Meduri GU, Headley AS, Golden E, et al. Effect of prolonged methylprednisolone therapy in unresolving acute respiratory distress syndrome: A randomized controlled trial. *JAMA.* 1998;**280**(2):159–165.
36. Villar J, Ferrando C, Martinez D, et al. Dexamethasone treatment for the acute respiratory distress syndrome: A multicentre, randomised controlled trial. *Lancet Respir Med.* 2020;**8**(3):267–276.
37. Recovery Collaborative Group, Horby P, Lim WS, et al. Dexamethasone in hospitalized patients with Covid-19—preliminary report. *N Engl J Med.* 2021 Feb 25;**384**(8):693–704.
38. WHO. Rapid Evidence Appraisal for COVID-19 Therapies Working Group, Sterne JAC, Murthy S, Diaz JV, et al. Association between administration of systemic corticosteroids and mortality among critically ill patients with COVID-19: A meta-analysis. *JAMA.* 2020;**324**(13):1330–1341.
39. Peek GJ, Mugford M, Tiruvoipati R, et al. Efficacy and economic assessment of conventional ventilatory support versus extracorporeal membrane oxygenation for severe adult respiratory failure (CESAR): A multicentre randomised controlled trial. *Lancet.* 2009;**374**(9698):1351–1363.
40. Combes A, Hajage D, Capellier G, et al. Extracorporeal membrane oxygenation for severe acute respiratory distress syndrome. *N Engl J Med.* 2018;**378**(21):1965–1975.
41. Goligher EC, Tomlinson G, Hajage D, et al. Extracorporeal membrane oxygenation for severe acute respiratory distress syndrome and posterior probability of mortality benefit in a Post Hoc Bayesian analysis of a randomized clinical trial. *JAMA.* 2018;**320**(21):2251–2259.
42. Umbrello M, Fumagalli J, Pesenti A, et al. Pathophysiology and management of acute respiratory distress syndrome in obese patients. *Semin Respir Crit Care Med.* 2019;**40**(1): 40–56.
43. Pirrone M, Fisher D, Chipman D, et al. Recruitment maneuvers and positive end-expiratory pressure titration in morbidly obese ICU patients. *Crit Care Med.* 2016;**44**(2):300–307.
44. Chiumello D, Colombo A, Algieri I, et al. Effect of body mass index in acute respiratory distress syndrome. *Br J Anaes.* 2016;**116**(1):113–121.
45. Chiumello D, Taccone P, Berto V, et al. Long-term outcomes in survivors of acute respiratory distress syndrome ventilated in supine or prone position. *Intensive Care Med.* 2012;**38**(2):221–229.

22

Advanced Respiratory Therapies: Inhaled Therapies, Heliox, ECMO and $ECCO_2$-R, and Non-conventional Ventilatory Modes

Stephan Ehrmann, Nicole P Juffermans, Marcus J Schultz, Nicolò Patroniti, Alex Molin, Martin Scharffenberg, Sabine Nabecker, and Marcelo Gama de Abreu

22.1 Inhaled Therapies: Therapeutic Aerosol Drug Delivery

Stephan Ehrmann

KEY MESSAGES

- Aerosol therapy is common in the critical care setting.
- The driving gas of jet nebulizers interferes with the ventilator which represents an important drawback compared to vibrating mesh nebulizers.
- Placement of a filter on the expiratory limb of the ventilator is mandatory to avoid any dysfunction.
- The benefit of inhaled antibiotics is not established in the critical care setting and should only be considered in selected patients for specific indications.
- Standard operating procedures and checklists should be used to implement inhaled therapy in optimal safety conditions for critically ill patients.

CONTROVERSIES

- Despite several small positive trials and daily implementation in ICUs, a recent large RCT showed no benefit of inhaled antibiotics to treat ventilator-associated pneumonia (VAP).
- The theoretical benefit of interrupting heated humidification during aerosol delivery remains debated as the benefit in drug delivery may be offset by under-humidification associated with side effects.
- The frequent use of mucolytic agents is not backed by strong clinical evidence.

FURTHER RESEARCH

- Development of new devices: dry powder inhalers for mechanical ventilation.
- Nanoparticle and liposomal particle engineering for aerosol therapy.
- Innovative inhaled biotherapies such as inhaled monoclonal antibodies and phage therapy.

Introduction

Delivery of drugs to the lungs using the systemic route such as oral or intravenous administration is hindered by the limited diffusion of many drugs from the blood to the lung. Systemic administration may therefore require high doses, potentially associated with side effects. Delivering drugs directly to the respiratory tract through inhalation is an appealing alternative potentially increasing drug concentrations at the pulmonary site of action while reducing systemic concentrations and associated side effects. While delivering medical gases such as oxygen, nitric oxide or helium (covered in Chapters 10, 21, and 22.2, respectively) by inhalation may seem obvious, such inhaled delivery of solid or liquid medication poses specific challenges. The present chapter covers the pulmonary delivery of drugs through inhalation of drug aerosols.

An aerosol is a cloud of liquid or solid particles of sufficiently small size to be transported by inhaled gases. Physically, this means particles need to be small enough (in the range of a few micrometres) that gravitational forces are negligible compared to the drag forces resulting from the interaction between the aerosol particles and the surrounding gas molecules. Drugs commonly delivered as aerosols include bronchodilators, anti-inflammatory, and anti-infectious medications targeted to treat obstructive, inflammatory, and infectious diseases of the lung. Aerosols may be generated using nebulizer, metered dose inhalers, and dry powder inhalers, all of which have advantages and drawbacks.[1] In the specific setting of critical care, the severity of disease, and the interaction of aerosol therapy with oxygen therapy, invasive or non-invasive ventilation (NIV) poses specific constraints. This chapter discusses the current accepted practice for aerosol therapy in critically ill patients, the evidence base of those recommendations, technical aspects, physiology, and pharmacology of aerosol delivery in particular among ventilated patients. It also covers controversies and future directions to be anticipated for this appealing therapeutic modality. It is divided according to drug classes as each class raises distinct issues in terms of constraints, evidence, and benefit to patients. It covers the most frequently used aerosols in critical care, namely bronchodilators, corticosteroids, and antibiotics. Given the important constraints related to mechanical ventilation and its specificity to critical care, aerosol therapy will be considered separately in ventilated and spontaneously breathing patients.

Current Accepted Practice

Aerosol therapy is very frequent in intensive care units, being used in approximately 25% of all patients and 20% of ventilated patients. Several surveys and observational studies demonstrate that clinical practice is frequently suboptimal and sometimes dangerous.[2] Good practice recommendations are summarized in Tables 22.1 and 22.2 and Box 22.1.

Spontaneously Breathing Patients

Spontaneously breathing patients in critical care frequently experience a degree of respiratory failure that may cause difficulty in using certain inhaled drug delivery devices. Specifically, the use of metered dose inhalers requires good breath–hand coordination while dry powder inhalers require forceful inspiration to generate sufficient inspiratory flows. Their use should be avoided among acutely ill patients, and the use of a nebulizer should be preferred (see below).[3] Acute asthma and exacerbation of chronic obstructive pulmonary disease (COPD) represent the main currently accepted indication for inhaled bronchodilators (Table 22.1). Inhaled corticosteroids may be given in this setting. Inhaled short acting beta-2-agonist (SABA) may also be used as an emergency therapy to lower serum potassium. Inhaled antibiotics among spontaneously breathing patients mainly comprise long-term therapy among patients with cystic fibrosis and/or bronchiectasis with chronic *Pseudomonas aeruginosa* infection. Practical dosage recommendations for those

Table 22.1 Spontaneously breathing patients: current accepted practice for inhaled therapy.

Drugs	Indication	Implementation
Short acting beta-2-adrenergic agonists	Acute asthma	Nebulizer: consider initial continuous nebulization, decrease to 2.5–5 mg albuterol every 2–6 h according to patients' response
		pMDI with spacer: 400 µg albuterol every 30 min, decrease to every 2–6 h according to patients' response
	Chronic obstructive pulmonary disease exacerbation	pMDI with spacer: 100 µg albuterol every hour, decrease to every 2–6 h according to patients' response
		Nebulizer: 2.5–5 mg albuterol every 2–6 h according to patients' response
	Hyperkalaemia in the absence of intravenous access	Nebulizer: 10–20 mg albuterol continuous nebulization
		pMDI with spacer: 1200 µg albuterol over 15–30 min
Anticholinergic drugs	Acute asthma and chronic obstructive pulmonary disease exacerbation	pMDI with spacer: 40 µg every 4 h
		Nebulizer: 0.5 mg every 4 h
Corticosteroids	Acute asthma	pMDI with spacer: high-dose delivery—2–3 mg budesonide, 5–7 mg beclomethasone, and 1–10 mg fluticasone within first 1–6 h in ED
	Chronic obstructive pulmonary disease exacerbation	Nebulizer: budesonide 4–8 mg per day
Antibiotics	*Pseudomonas aeruginosa* colonization in cystic fibrosis or bronchiectasis	Nebulizer: - Tobramycin 300 mg twice daily for 28 days' periods alternating with 28 days off therapy - Aztreonam 75 mg three times a day for 28 days' periods alternating with 28 days off therapy Dry powder inhaler: - Colistimethate sodium 125 mg (1.6625 million units) twice daily for 28 days' periods alternating with 28 days off therapy

Sources: Global Initiative for Asthma. Global Strategy for Asthma Management and Prevention, 2017. Available from www.ginasthma.org; Global Strategy for the Diagnosis, Management and Prevention of COPD, Global Initiative for Chronic Obstructive Lung Disease (GOLD) 2016. Available from: http://goldcopd.org; Mogayzel PJ, Naureckas ET, Robinson KA, et al. Cystic fibrosis pulmonary guidelines: Chronic medication for maintenance of lung health. *Am J Respir Crit Care Med*. 2013;187:680–689; Flume PA, Mogayzel PJ, Robinson KA, et al. Cystic fibrosis pulmonary guidelines: Treatment of pulmonary exacerbation. *Am J Respir Crit Care Med*. 2009;180:802–808; Mahoney BA, Smith WA, Lo DS, et al. Emergency interventions for hyperkalaemia. *Cochrane Database Syst Rev*. 2005;18:CD003235.

Table 22.2 Mechanically ventilated patients: current accepted practice for inhaled therapy

Short acting beta-2-adrenergic agonists	Acute asthma and chronic obstructive pulmonary disease exacerbation	pMDI: 400 μg albuterol ever 3–4 h
		Nebulizer: 2.5–5 mg albuterol every 3–4 h
Anticholinergic drugs	Acute asthma and chronic obstructive pulmonary disease exacerbation	pMDI with spacer: 40 μg every 4 h
		Nebulizer: 0.5 mg every 4 h
Corticosteroids	Chronic obstructive pulmonary disease	pMDI: 1 mg budesonide twice daily
Antibiotics	Ventilator-associated pneumonia and tracheobronchitis: to be discussed on a case-by-case basis among patients with multidrug resistant infection or therapy failure	Nebulizer: - Colistimethate sodium: 2–5 MU three times a day - Amikacin: 400 mg twice or three times a day or 25 mg/kg once a day - Gentamicin: 80 mg three times a day

currently accepted indications, based on international guidelines, are provided in Table 22.1.[4–8]

Mechanical Ventilation

Key practical recommendations for the delivery of inhaled drugs during mechanical ventilation are presented in Box 22.1. While inhaled delivery of bronchodilators represents current accepted practice in ventilated patients with obstructive lung disease, inhaled corticosteroids may be considered in certain patients. With increasing frequencies of multidrug resistant bacteria causing difficult-to-treat nosocomial lung infections, inhaled antibiotic therapy may be considered on a case-by-case basis in ventilator-associated pneumonia (VAP) or tracheobronchitis.[9,10] Dose recommendations are provided in Box 22.1.

Evidence Base

Bronchodilators and Corticosteroids

Spontaneously Breathing Patients

For severe exacerbations of acute asthma or chronic obstructive pulmonary disease (COPD), nebulized SABA therapy may be easier to implement; however, pressurized metered dose inhalers used with an inhalation chamber are effective in most patients. Continuous nebulization has shown inconsistent benefits compared to intermittent delivery in acute asthma. The wide therapeutic range of beta-2-adrenergic agonists enables safe initial, frequently repeated, or continuous delivery tailored to patient's demands and response (Table 22.1). Inhaled epinephrine and inhaled magnesium show no benefit in this setting. Among patients suffering exacerbations of COPD, continuous inhaled bronchodilator delivery is probably of no benefit but has not been rigorously evaluated, and higher initial doses may be considered for significantly worsened wheezing and documented reversibility. Inhaled short acting anticholinergic muscarinic drugs (SAMA, e.g. ipratropium bromide) should be added to a SABA (e.g. salbutamol) for additive effect.

The benefit of inhaled corticosteroids as compared to systemic administration in patients suffering acute asthma or exacerbation of COPD remains debated. Systemic steroids tend to be given in the emergency room for exacerbations of asthma and COPD. Any additive effect of inhaled corticosteroids in patients already receiving systemic corticosteroids is unclear. That said, for COPD exacerbations, inhaled budesonide seems equivalent to systemic therapy with less metabolic side effects.

Mechanical Ventilation

Bronchodilators are delivered to ventilated patients during exacerbations of asthma and COPD. There is efficacy and combined synergy of inhaled SABA and SAMA whether patients undergo invasive ventilation or NIV.[11] In NIV, this is commonly delivered as nebulized therapy while having a break from the ventilator.

In spontaneously breathing patients with acute asthma, inhaled bronchodilators have equivalent efficacy to intravenous but with a better side-effect profile, and this is accepted practice in mechanically ventilated patients as well (Box 22.1). Notably, however, high-dose inhaled beta-2-adrenergic agonist therapy can lead to significant systemic drug concentrations through alveolo-capillary diffusion with consequent tachycardia and raised serum lactate concentrations. Additional delivery of intravenous beta-2-adrenergic agonists simply increases the risk of side effects without improved bronchodilation.

Significant bronchodilation occurs after inhalation of bronchodilators during severe exacerbations of COPD requiring invasive or non-invasive ventilator support.[11] However, their effect on patient-centred outcomes such as duration of ventilation, length of stay, or mortality has not been evaluated in RCTs. There remain questions about routine use of bronchodilators in these exacerbations, given the frequently limited reversibility of bronchial obstruction and potential for side effects.

The evidence for inhaled corticosteroids is even weaker in the setting of mechanical ventilation. Benefits have been demonstrated in terms of improved lung mechanics among patients with COPD ventilated through a tracheostomy. Furthermore, while the benefits associated with systemic corticosteroids remain undisputed in less severe exacerbations, a recent study failed to show benefit of oral corticosteroids exacerbations requiring non-invasive ventilation in critical care.[12] The value of inhaled corticosteroids has not been evaluated among patients undergoing NIV.

Antibiotics

Cystic Fibrosis and Bronchiectasis

Inhaled antibiotics are well established for treating patients suffering from cystic fibrosis (CF) and other bronchiectasis with chronic *P. aeruginosa* bronchial colonization. However, in the case of acute exacerbation or overt pneumonia prompting intensive care unit admission, antibiotics are usually administered

Box 22.1 Patients undergoing mechanical ventilation: practical recommendations to deliver inhaled drug aerosols

Safety

- Use standard operating procedures and a checklist
- Ensure adequate staff training
- Monitor patients closely during aerosol therapy: airway pressure, oxygen saturation, and arterial pressure
- Place a filter between the expiratory limb and the ventilator; change it at least daily
- Do not use gas external to the ventilator to drive a jet nebulizer
- Check for resumption of active or passive humidification if interrupted during aerosol therapy
- Consider therapeutic drug monitoring to avoid systemic toxicity

Implementation

- Remove heat and moisture exchanger if placed between aerosol-generating device and patient
- Suction tracheal tube for bronchial secretions before starting therapy

pMDI (bronchodilators and corticosteroids):

- Use a valve holding chamber placed between the inspiratory limb and the Y-piece or temporarily placed between the Y-piece and the patient (collapsible chambers may be used to avoid dead space increase between administrations without removing the chamber)
- The operator needs to heat the canister in his hands, shack the canister, engage the valve, and prompt the device in the chamber, and each puff is then delivered activating the device at the beginning of inspiration; 30-s to 1-min intervals need to be observed between each puff

Nebulizer (any drug):

- Place continuous nebulizer in the inspiratory limb or between the Y-piece and the patient, and breath synchronized nebulizers need to be placed close to the patient
- Favour drug solutions designed for inhalation use
- Respect sterility standards when filling the nebulizer

Optimization to increase drug delivery (indicated to improve amount of antibiotics delivered to the lungs)

- Use vibrating mesh nebulizer or ultrasonic nebulizer with reduced residual volume
- Place nebulizer upstream in the inspiratory limb, 15–40 cm from the Y-piece
- Use volume-controlled constant flow ventilation; use low respiratory rate, low inspiratory flow, long inspiratory time, and an end inspiratory pause
- Consider temporary patient sedation to optimize patient-ventilator synchrony
- Consider switching of heated humidification or use of a dry circuit dedicated for aerosol therapy

Non-invasive ventilation

The use of a single-limb circuit with an exhalation port requires positioning nebulizer between the exhalation port and the non-invasive interface. For other aspects of aerosol therapy and when using two-limb ventilator circuits on critical care ventilators, similar principles may be implemented during non-invasive ventilation as in intubated patients

intravenously, with or without concomitant inhaled therapy (Table 22.1). In patients with CF and pseudomonal colonization, several trials demonstrated benefit with inhaled tobramycin on outcomes including lung function, exacerbation frequency, and quality of life. Inhaled colistin showed non-inferiority and aztreonam potential benefits when compared to inhaled tobramycin in this setting. These inhaled medications may be continued during exacerbation and critical illness. For non-CF bronchiectasis, evidence is less favourable regarding inhaled antibiotics.

Ventilator-associated Pneumonia

Several studies documented high antibiotic concentrations in bronchial secretions and epithelial lining fluid of ventilated patients suffering ventilator-associated pneumonia (VAP) or tracheobronchitis[13] (see Chapter 32). Similar cure rates for VAP have been demonstrated by inhaled antibiotics versus intravenous therapy.[14] However, those patients frequently receive concomitant intravenous antibiotics to treat pneumonia. Several studies evaluated the benefit of inhaled amikacin and inhaled colistin as adjunctive therapies in patients receiving intravenous antibiotics (beta-lactams, amikacin, or colistin). These studies show conflicting results, although potential benefits observed included faster sterilization of bronchial secretions and clinical resolution, faster improvement in oxygenation, reduced use of systemic antibiotics, faster weaning from mechanical ventilation, and reduced systemic toxicity. Several studies observed a reduced emergence of antibiotic resistant bacteria in the lung when antibiotic therapy was given as an inhaled aerosol compared to the intravenous route. However, these studies comprised small numbers of patients limiting the quality of evidence. Several meta-analyses have shown conflicting results, and divergent recommendations are made by scientific societies.[10,15–17] A recent large-scale RCT did not show any benefit of inhaled antibiotic therapy adjunctive to intravenous therapy to treat VAP, and current evidence does not support widespread implementation of inhaled antibiotics among ventilated patients. However, given the increasing incidence of multidrug resistant bacterial pneumonia in intensive care units, this therapeutic modality may be considered in carefully selected patients. Patients most likely to benefit are those at high risk of failure of intravenous therapy, that is, those with high severity of disease, infected with multidrug resistant bacteria, or who have already experienced failure of conventional therapy. Good practice and implementation of safety recommendations is of paramount importance in this setting (Box 22.1).

Aerosolization Technology

Aerosol therapy is a complex process that starts with different aerosol-generating devices followed by the transport of the aerosol through various interfaces and within conducting airways until deposition in the respiratory system at the site of pharmacological action.

Different types of devices may be used with differing advantages and drawbacks depending on the patient situation (as summarized in Table 22.3).[1,10]

Pressurized Metered Dose Inhalers

They are mainly used in the outpatient setting. Bronchodilators and corticosteroids are available in this form. Here, the main limitation is coordination of device activation with inspiration. Coordination may frequently be suboptimal in critically ill patients.[3] In ventilated patients, the use of pressurized metered dose inhalers requires a valve holding access port to the ventilator circuit. As the nurse

Table 22.3 Advantages and drawback of available aerosolization devices

	Advantages	Drawbacks
Pressurized metered dose inhalers	Handheld Breath synchronized	Require good coordination and correct breathing procedure during inhalation
Dry powder inhalers	Handheld Breath synchronized	Require forceful inspiration
Jet nebulizer	Disposable Low cost	Driving gas interferes with ventilator and oxygen delivery High residual volume
Ultrasonic nebulizer	No gas interference with ventilator and oxygen delivery	Large size Heating of drug solution Need for decontamination
Vibrating mesh nebulizer	No gas interference with ventilator and oxygen delivery Disposable	Membrane alteration over time

activates the device, coordination is less of an issue (see Box 22.1 for practical use).[10]

Dry Powder Inhalers (DPIs)

The drug powder is contained in a cap; after activation of the inhaler rupturing the cap, the powder is aerosolized by the own inspiratory flow generated by the patient. Bronchodilators, corticosteroids, and antibiotics are available for dry powder inhaler use. The main advantage of these devices is that they do not require inspiration–activation coordination. However, for bronchodilators and corticosteroids, patients need sufficiently forceful inspiration (30–60 L/min inspiratory flow) to aerosolize the drug. Antibiotic powders do not require such high flow due to different formulations. DPI systems for use in mechanically ventilated patients are under development.

Jet Nebulizer

These represent the most frequently used aerosolization device type in ICU.[2] They require a source of compressed gas to function; this driving gas interferes with the delivered tidal volume and the fraction of inspired oxygen. Some ventilators enable breath actuated nebulization, which allows good control of the delivered tidal volume but synchronization with inspiration is generally poor. During oxygen therapy in spontaneously breathing patients, driving the nebulizer with air or oxygen influences the fraction of inspired oxygen. The residual volume of jet nebulizers is high; thus, a large amount of drug (30%–60%) placed in the nebulizer remains at the end of nebulization and is lost. This has significant economic consequences with expensive drugs.

Ultrasonic Nebulizer

These systems do not generate extra gas and are therefore well suited for use during mechanical ventilation. Heating of the drug solution during nebulization may alter drugs, although for most drugs this is inconsequential. The exceptions are frail peptides such as recombinant DNase, a mucolytic agent mostly used in patients with CF.

Vibrating Mesh Nebulizer

Vibrating mesh devices are also well suited for use during mechanical ventilation as no driving gas is required. Residual volumes are very low, and disposable devices are now available for use during both spontaneous breathing and mechanical ventilation. Breath synchronized devices are under development.[13]

Specific Constraints Related to Mechanical Ventilation

Safety

Very severe complications have been reported in relation to aerosol therapy in ventilated patients.[9,14] Given the paucity of evidence regarding patient-centred benefits, avoidance of side effects is important (Box 22.1). Aerosol particles generated during expiration, as well as exhaled particles, are cleared through the expiratory limb of the ventilator. To prevent dysfunction of the ventilator's expiratory block, it is mandatory to place a filter between the expiratory limb and the ventilator; this must be changed regularly. Simple antibacterial filters or heat and moisture exchanging filters can be used. Jet nebulizer should not be supplied with gas external to the ventilator as this can result in uncontrolled tidal volumes. Lastly, due to interruptions in humidification during nebulization, therapy should not last longer than an hour. Limiting therapy duration and ensuring humidification is resumed help limit the risk of tracheal tube obstruction.

Delivery Optimization

An important proportion of aerosolized drug may be lost to the patient through deposition in the ventilator circuit. This has little consequences for bronchodilator drugs given their wide therapeutic range (see the section titled 'Pharmacodynamics') but may impair the efficacy of inhaled antibiotic therapy.[10] Indeed, most studies showing benefits of inhaled antibiotic therapy in ventilated patients implement some form of optimization technique (see Box 22.1).

Aerosol particles generated during expiration are cleared by the bias flow through the expiratory limb of the ventilator, and placing a nebulizer upstream in the inspiratory limb (15–40 cm depending on bias flow and circuit section) limits drug loss.

Aerosol deposition in the circuit mostly occurs through inertial impaction mechanisms, thus reducing gas velocity through specific ventilator settings and avoiding patient–ventilator dyssynchrony improve aerosol delivery.

Lastly, as inhaled gas humidification induces an increase in aerosol particle size which in turn favours deposition in the circuit (see the section titled 'Pharmacokinetics'), dry circuit conditions improve aerosol therapy efficacy. While removing heat and moisture exchanger is mandatory if placed between the aerosol-generating device and the patients (as the filter would retain all particles), the value of interrupting a heated humidifier is limited given the time needed for the plate to cool down and humidity to drop. Studies that showed benefit of dry circuit conditions on aerosol delivery use dry circuits specifically put in place and dedicated to aerosol therapy.

Non-invasive Ventilation

A high proportion of patients undergoing NIV receive aerosol therapy, mainly bronchodilators and corticosteroids.[2] Efficacy on lung mechanics has been proven in several studies, and thus interruption of NIV to deliver inhaled bronchodilators seems unnecessary. Conversely, the efficacy of inhaled therapy during ventilation compared to spontaneous breathing depends on circuit configuration (see Chapter 8). While two-limb ventilator circuits show no difference, in single-limb non-invasive ventilator circuits the nebulizer should be positioned between the expiratory leak port and patient for optimal efficiency.

Technical and Device-related Issues

Powder Inhalation during Mechanical Ventilation

Dry powder delivery into mechanical ventilation circuits is not yet commercially available, but some prototype devices are in development. Such systems may enable delivery of high amounts of inhaled drugs in a short period of time. This may be interesting for delivery of antibiotics, where the amount of drug reaching the respiratory system is key. Strategies aiming at delivering high doses of inhaled antibiotics to ventilated patients are currently limited by the very long nebulization durations, which become problematic when lasting more than 60–90 min.

High-flow Nasal Therapy

High-flow nasal therapy is increasingly used in the critical care setting (Chapter 7). It is generally used continuously in patients, and interruption for aerosol delivery may be deleterious. Nasal high-flow therapy combines all factors hindering aerosol delivery, that is, high gas velocity favouring impaction, high gas humidity, and delivery through the natural nasal filter retaining aerosol particles. However, several bench and animal studies demonstrate that aerosol delivery within a nasal high-flow therapy circuit of beta-2-adrenergic agonist drugs is feasible. Optimal nebulizer placement is close to the humidification chamber, and gas flow should be limited to 30 L/min in adults and 4 L/min in infants.[18,19] Some preliminary work shows promising results in terms of bronchodilation observed in patients with those settings.

Particle Engineering/Gas Conditioning

Specific aerosol particles are being designed to improve the efficacy and safety profile of inhaled drugs, most notably using nanotechnologies.[20] Delivery of nanoparticles (diameter below 1 μm) dramatically reduces deposition through impaction and sedimentation, so theoretically targeting distal airway deposition at very slow gas velocities through Brownian diffusion. Matching aerosol particle diffusion to the site of action is another aim. Mucus inert nanoparticles have been designed to improve particle diffusion through the mucus layer thus improving diffusion to the epithelium and reducing muco-ciliary clearance of the drug. Nebulization of liposomes is another field of great interest with the potential of specific intra-cellular targeting of the inhaled drug and increasing the residence time within the lung.

In parallel to altering aerosol particles, it is the modification of the composition and properties of the carrying gas. Helium is better than nitrogen for delivery of aerosol to the distal lung, although clinical benefit is not yet proven. Early work with the use of dry gas conditions to improve delivery of aerosols has not translated into benefit using clinical simulation models with concerns regarding the interruption of gas humidification.

Pharmacology of Inhaled Drugs

Pharmacokinetics

When administering an aerosol to a patient, the first step is the transport of the aerosol from the generating device to the patient through an interface; in this regard, the ventilator circuit may be considered the interface. The aerosol is then further transported through the conducting airways until deposition in the respiratory tract. Aerosol therapy efficacy improves when deposition in the circuit and upper airways is reduced, maximizing pulmonary deposition. Aerosol deposition occurs through three main physical mechanisms: (1) inertial impaction that increases with increasing particle mass and velocity and thus with particle size and gas flow rate. This mechanism is predominant in interfaces and large airways. (2) Sedimentation due to gravitational forces. Again linked to particle size. (3) Diffusion mainly occurs for small particles with low velocity. Thus, particle size plays an important role in regard to particle deposition. Large particles (5 μm and above) mainly deposit in interfaces, ventilator circuit, and upper airways of spontaneously breathing patients; particles 3–5 μm deposit predominantly in large airways; particles 1–3 μm are considered optimal for alveolar deposition; and particles smaller than 1 μm are largely exhaled. Once deposited in the respiratory system, inhaled drugs are cleared through two mechanisms: (1) muco-ciliary clearance that clears the drug to the digestive track where secondary absorption may occur. (2) Alveolo-capillary diffusion to the systemic circulation followed by conventional renal, hepatic, and/or metabolic clearance. Bronchial and upper airway mucosal absorption is quantitatively less important. Several pharmacokinetic approaches enable quantification of pulmonary deposition of inhaled drugs. Lung drug concentrations may be measured in bronchial secretions and broncho-alveolar lavage fluid easily recovered in ventilated patients, by estimating epithelial lining fluid concentration. High drug concentrations after inhalation are documented in bronchial secretions and epithelial lining fluid. In particular, for antibiotic nebulization, concentrations far above minimum inhibitory concentrations are present.[9] Scintigraphic lung imaging after inhalation of a radiolabelled aerosol demonstrates significant pulmonary delivery of inhaled medication in spontaneously breathing and mechanically ventilated patients. However, large airway deposition predominates.[21] Systemic pharmacokinetic studies have been performed (serum and urine concentration measurements) as inhaled drugs pass into the systemic circulation through alveolo-capillary diffusion and eventually through digestive absorption after mucociliary clearance. Such studies enable an assessment of the safety of aerosol therapy as serum drug concentrations remain far lower than after systemic administration.[22] For example, when nebulizing antibiotics to treat lung infection, efficient therapy of a concomitant bacteraemia cannot be achieved without adding systemic antibiotics. However, drug diffusion into the systemic circulation is not negligible, especially in the injured lung. In such settings, nebulized administration of aminoglycosides requires therapeutic drug monitoring to ensure toxic levels are not exceeded. Inhaled antibiotic therapy is better for drugs with low diffusion through biological membranes (e.g. aminoglycosides and colistin), increasing local concentration and reducing systemic loss. The converse holds for systemic delivery.

Pharmacodynamics

Bronchodilators

Bronchodilators have a very wide therapeutic range. Only 40 μg of albuterol reaching the respiratory system induces significant bronchodilation as assessed by combined scintigraphy to quantify deposition and pulmonary function tests for clinical effect.[23] Conversely, tachycardia represents a useful sign for dose limitation to avoid arrhythmias and lactic acidosis.

Antibiotics

High drug concentrations of inhaled antibiotic therapy in the lung may be particularly beneficial for concentration-dependent antibiotics such as aminoglycosides or colistin; high peak concentrations correlate with efficacy and the post-antibiotic effect. Conversely, for time-dependent antibiotics such as beta-lactams, very frequent nebulization would be needed (every 3–4 h) to maintain lung concentrations consistently above minimum inhibitory concentrations, which is impractical.

Drugs

Bronchodilators and Corticosteroids

No large-scale clinical trials have investigated benefits of inhaled bronchodilators or corticosteroids on patient-centred outcomes among critically ill or acute care patients. Their benefit is inferred from ambulatory COPD settings. Side effects and lack of benefit should be considered in treatment decisions and further registry or large-scale data are required.[12]

Antibiotics: Curative and Preventive/Spectrum of the Disease

Inhaled antibiotic therapy as a standard to treat lung infection cannot be recommended due to conflicting evidence and advice from different scientific societies.[9,10,17] It seems reasonable to reserve inhaled antibiotics as an adjunct, for patients with nosocomial lung infection with a high probability of failure of systemic antibiotic therapy, that is, patients infected with multidrug resistant bacteria, with high disease severity, and poor lung penetration of the particular antibiotic.

Their role as prophylactic therapy in patients at risk of developing nosocomial lung infection, patients undergoing mechanical ventilation and/or suffering tracheobronchitis, may deserve evaluation.

Prostaglandins

Vasomotor tone of the pulmonary vessels is greatly influenced by prostaglandins and may be modulated by drugs such as iloprost or treprostinil. Efficacy of inhaled prostaglandins has been shown from a pharmacological point of view. Further work is required on the role of selective and newer pulmonary vasodilators in critically ill patients: acute therapy of patients suffering pulmonary hypertension and right ventricular dysfunction, as well as for improving ventilation–perfusion matching in patients suffering acute respiratory failure.

Mucolytic Drugs

Optimal mechanical properties of the mucus layer are of utmost importance for proper airway physiology. The role and efficacy of different mucoactive agents such as hypertonic saline, N acetylcysteine, and DNase are yet to be determined in the ICU.

Biotherapies

Biotherapies for lung disease is a field of growing research interest. Inhaled delivery of monoclonal antibodies and phages is of interest because their large size limits diffusion from the blood to the lung after systemic delivery. This reduced diffusion may also enable prolonged lung residence times and extend interval administration once inhaled.[24] Reduced systemic degradation of the drug and systemic side effects also favour inhaled biotherapies. Very small therapeutic peptides such as small interfering RNA are also being evaluated for inhaled use in various lung diseases.[25] The role such inhaled biotherapies may play in the future of intensive care medicine remains under investigation, but several pre-clinical works suggest feasibility of aerosolized delivery of such therapeutic agents.

22.2 Heliox for Acute Respiratory Failure

Nicole P Juffermans and Marcus J Schultz

KEY MESSAGES

- Heliox can relieve respiratory distress, improve gas exchange, and avoid or reduce the intensity of mechanical ventilation.
- Its indications are increased upper airway resistance, for exacerbations of asthma and COPD.

CONTROVERSIES

- Evidence-based patient outcomes are limited.
- Helium is a natural resource so potentially limiting its availability for application.

Further Research

- The effect of heliox on patients with exacerbations of severe asthma or COPD, unresponsive to therapy, or unable to wean from mechanical ventilation.

Introduction

Heliox, a mixture of helium and oxygen, has better laminar flow than oxygen or air. It is theoretically beneficial in situations where increased resistance impairs gaseous delivery, such as the upper and larger airways. However, the proportion of oxygen will limit the amount of helium and so may not help in notably hypoxic patients. In general, studies have shown improved ventilation and gas exchange with heliox ventilation. It can relieve respiratory distress, improve gas exchange, avoid intubation, and reduce intensity of mechanical ventilation immediately following application. Despite these promising effects on short-term outcomes, there is a lack of studies on the impact of the use of heliox on relevant clinical outcomes. Given the technical challenges, data from large trials is unlikely.

Helium is an inert gas with a lower density than air. The physical properties of a mixture of helium and oxygen (heliox) depend on the concentration of helium in the mixture, but due to a smaller molecular size, its density will always be lower compared to an oxygen–nitrogen mixture. For any gas mixture, whether flow in the airways is laminar or turbulent can be quantified by the Reynolds number, the ratio of inertial (turbulent) to viscous (laminar) forces.

Heliox has a low Reynolds number and thereby a tendency to laminar flow that has less resistance than turbulent flow.[26] Thus, the driving pressure needed to generate flow is lower with heliox. As flow is laminar in the larger bronchi, heliox decreases resistance in the larger airways. Therefore, it is best applied in conditions characterized by a high resistance in the upper airways. Because of the high resistance of the neonatal pulmonary system compared to adults, most of the applications of heliox and consequent gathering of scientific data of the efficacy has been done in children. Another useful property of heliox is an increased diffusion capacity of CO_2 when compared to oxygen. This feature may further result in improved gas exchange and correction of respiratory acidosis. This section summarizes the efficacy of heliox in various clinical settings.

Clinical Applications of Heliox

Small clinical trials with heliox have been performed. In these trials, outcome measures were most often physiological, studying effects of heliox on gas exchange and mechanical ventilation settings, but rarely clinical outcomes. Nonetheless, a lot can be learned on efficacy of heliox from these studies.

Heliox in Neonatal Respiratory Distress Syndrome

In premature newborn infants with neonatal RDS in need of mechanical ventilation, high doses of heliox (80%) were shown to improve oxygenation when compared to gas mixtures using equal amounts of nitrogen or air.[27] Further, heliox reduced the number of infants that developed bronchopulmonary dysplasia. In pre-term RDS infants ventilated with nasal continuous positive airway pressure (CPAP), heliox reduced peak inspiratory pressures, work of breathing, improved gas exchange, and reduced risk of intubation.[28] In paediatric patients with bronchopulmonary dysplasia, heliox increased tidal volume, dynamic compliance, and peak expiratory flow rate. PaO_2/FiO_2 ratio improved, as did the alveolar–arterial oxygen tension and oxygenation index.[29] All these beneficial effects reversed after switching back to a normal gas mixture. Despite these promising properties of heliox on physiological end points, the effect of heliox on clinically relevant outcomes in neonatal RDS to date is unclear.

Heliox in Paediatric Bronchiolitis

During non-invasive CPAP ventilation, 70% heliox improved saturation, respiratory rate, and $PaCO_2$ levels when compared to use of oxygen.[30] However, a multicentre RCT investigating the effect of 78% heliox versus air–oxygen mix (78% nitrogen; 22% oxygen) through a non-invasive, inflatable head hood did not confirm these results.[31] Compared to air–oxygen, heliox did not generate any significant differences in mechanical ventilation settings or gas exchange. A more physiologically oriented study in infants with RSV ventilated in a pressure-controlled mode showed that during ventilation with heliox the respiratory system resistance reduced.[32] However, there was no improvement of CO_2 elimination, nor decrease in peak inspiratory pressures or end-expiratory air-trapping. Taken together, effects of heliox in RSV-induced bronchiolitis are not unequivocally beneficial.

Heliox in High-frequency Oscillatory Ventilation (HFOV)

Heliox may also be useful as a driving gas during HFOV or high jet ventilation because of the respiratory acidosis that can occur during this ventilation mode. In an animal model of acute lung injury, HFOV with heliox improved gas exchange, which was related to the larger tidal volume delivery by the oscillator with heliox.[33] In paediatric patients with hypoxaemic respiratory failure ventilated with HFOV, heliox as a driving gas resulted in a substantial drop in $PaCO_2$ levels compared to nitrogen–oxygen ventilation.[34]

Heliox in Asthma

In asthma, there is constriction of the bronchioli causing increased inspiratory effort. Some patients with status asthmaticus may benefit from breathing heliox until therapy with bronchodilators and steroids is effective as heliox can reduce airway resistance and subsequent respiratory burden. Use of heliox was found to reduce peak airway pressure and resistance in small studies in adult and paediatric patients mechanically ventilated for status asthmaticus. Also, heliox relieved subjective dyspnoea and respiratory acidosis in non-ventilated patients with asthmatic crises. Thereby, in studies with physiological end points, heliox seems to have a beneficial effect. Results of various studies with more clinically relevant outcomes have been summarized in two meta-analyses.[35,36] These studies concluded that there is insufficient evidence that heliox improves respiratory function and that currently administration of heliox to patients presenting with moderate-to-severe acute asthma in the emergency department cannot be recommended. However, these conclusions are based on between group comparisons and small studies, with considerable heterogeneity, and should be interpreted with caution.

Heliox for Aerosol Delivery

Inhaled beta-agonists are the mainstay of treatment for asthma exacerbations (see Section 22.1). Effective aerosol therapy requires the medication to be deposited in the lower airways. The physical properties of helium suggest that lower driving pressures are necessary to distribute oxygen to the distal alveoli to improve oxygenation.[26] In a trial in which paediatric asthma patients were randomized to nebulized, radiolabelled aerosol with oxygen or heliox as the vehicle of nebulization, ventilatory scintigraphy showed increased deposition of the aerosol with helium as the driving gas in patients with severe airway obstruction but not in mild airway obstruction.[37] An RCT evaluating the efficacy of heliox in driving continuous albuterol nebulization in children with exacerbations of asthma showed that heliox improved short-term respiratory status when compared to oxygen.[38]

Taken together, heliox can be used as a driving gas for aerosol delivery in patients with severe status asthmaticus who do not respond to standard inhalation therapy.

Heliox in COPD

Non-invasive positive-pressure support with heliox reduces the work of breathing, decreases $PaCO_2$ level, and relieves subjective dyspnoea during an exacerbation of COPD.[39] These results were confirmed in a randomized trial in COPD patients, showing that NIV with heliox considerably decreased length of hospital stay.[40]

Another group confirmed, in a retrospective study of 81 COPD patients, that use of heliox lowered the intubation rate as well as mortality.[41] These results support the rationale for using heliox as a driving gas in NIV in COPD.

In COPD patients who are on mechanical ventilation, management is also challenging (see Chapter 41). Due to collapsing airways, expiratory time can be insufficient for complete exhalation of the inspired tidal volume, resulting in increased lung volume, termed dynamic hyperinflation or air-trapping and measured by increased intrinsic positive end-expiratory pressure (PEEP). An approach to decrease the volume of trapped gas may be by lowering resistance to flow in airways with heliox. Due to increased diffusion capacity of CO_2 when compared to oxygen, helium may also be beneficial in patients with respiratory acidosis. In exacerbated COPD patients on controlled mechanical ventilation, 70% heliox decreased the amount of trapped lung volume and intrinsic PEEP, with a concomitant decrease in mean airway pressures compared to baseline.[42] Work of breathing was similarly reduced.[43] Post extubation, heliox reduced the transdiaphragmatic pressure–time index and improved respiratory comfort. Together, heliox could be useful adjunct therapy in COPD patients who are in the weaning process or post extubation. However, there is an absence of trials with a relevant patient outcome. The limited use of heliox in COPD reflects both this paucity of evidence and safety issues.

Safety of Heliox Ventilation

The lower density of helium causes inaccurately high readings from flow meters calibrated for air and/or oxygen.[26] Consequently, the flow transducer within the ventilator needs adjustment to correctly measure the flow in order to prevent discrepancy in measured tidal volumes and misinterpreted minute ventilation. Complications of the use of heliox in asthma or COPD have not been reported. However, safety of heliox in various modes of ventilation has not been studied systematically. Inadvertent delivery of large tidal volumes with subsequent lung injury is a realistic threat from the use of heliox.

The percentage of oxygen within the heliox mixture is a concern when ventilating severely hypoxic patients. The efficacy of heliox is proportional to the percentage used, which may not allow for sufficient FiO_2 in hypoxic patients. Of note, however, adverse outcomes in respiratory failure may be influenced by factors other than hypoxaemia, including multiple organ failure and right ventricular failure. Another aspect of the use of heliox are costs.

Heliox is more costly than oxygen mixtures. A reduction in duration of mechanical ventilation with use of heliox compared as compared oxygen was shown before[40] and may compensate for total hospital costs. However, a more prolonged use of heliox than reported in that particular study would incur additional costs. In addition, a very relevant issue is that helium is a natural gas and thus a limited resource. For these reasons, the use of heliox will probably be limited to exceptional cases of severe upper airway resistance that does not respond to standard therapy.

Conclusion

In general, studies have shown improved ventilation and gas exchange with heliox ventilation. Heliox can relieve respiratory distress, improve gas exchange, avoid intubation, and reduce intensity of mechanical ventilation immediately following application. Despite these promising effects on short-term outcomes, there is a lack of studies on the impact of the use of heliox on relevant clinical outcomes. Small patient numbers, differences in design of the studies, the lack of original data, and differences in quality of the papers limit the interpretation of the existing evidence. Given the technical challenges, chances are small that data from large trials will become available. At this point, we conclude that the summarized evidence suggests that heliox reduces work of breathing and improves gas exchange and may be useful in conditions with high airway resistance in the upper airways that fail to respond to conventional therapy.

22.3 Extracorporeal Membrane Oxygenation (ECMO) and CO_2 Removal ($ECCO_2$-R)

Nicolò Patroniti and Alex Molin

KEY MESSAGES

- Primary indications for VV-ECMO are refractory hypoxaemic respiratory failure and high risk for ventilator-induced lung injury (VILI).
- ECMO treatment should be established in those with reversibility and reserve.
- During VV-ECMO the native lung is 'rested' to prevent VILI. Respiratory rate, tidal volume, plateau airway pressure, and FiO_2 are decreased as much as allowed by CO_2 removal and peripheral O_2 delivery.

CONTROVERSIES

- Ventilatory management of the native lung on VV-ECMO: Should the native lung be allowed to collapse for total lung rest or be maintained open with some level of PEEP and airway pressure?
- Eligibility criteria: Should ECMO be reserved for selected populations of patients?
- Hospital resources: Should ECMO treatment provision be centralized or generalized?

FURTHER RESEARCH

- Compare different ventilatory strategies during ECMO.
- Prone positioning in patients on ECMO.
- The assessment of recruitable lung on CT and its implication for the ventilatory strategy and outcomes.

Introduction

Extracorporeal membrane oxygenation (ECMO) is used to improve oxygenation, ventilation, and haemodynamic support using an extracorporeal circuit comprised of an oxygenator, decarboxylator, and a centrifugal pump. Over the years, advancements in the technology have resulted in reduced complexity and increased safety. The ECMO circuit may be attached to the patient's own peripheral vascular system as a venous access and arterial return (i.e. veno-arterial, VA-ECMO) or venous access and return (i.e. veno-venous, VV-ECMO). VA-ECMO may be considered peripheral cardiopulmonary bypass, where support is for cardio-respiratory support, usually due to acute cardiogenic shock. That is not discussed in this chapter. Veno-venous ECMO is indicated for acute respiratory support. Recent evidence suggests favourable outcomes associated with the use of ECMO for selected patients with severe, refractory acute respiratory failure (SARF), including due to COVID-19.

History of ECMO

ECMO is a technique that has its origins since the 1940s but which has only entered widespread clinical practice since the 1970s.

The main purpose of ECMO is to temporarily support systemic perfusion and gas exchange so reducing the intrinsic work of heart and lungs. ECMO should not, therefore, be considered a cure for the underlying disease but a method designed to 'buy time'[44] and act as a bridge to the recovery of native organ or destination therapy such as transplantation if appropriate.

The first successful application of ECMO in a patient with acute respiratory distress syndrome (ARDS) dates back to 1971.[45] In spite of the encouraging early results, an early randomized clinical trial of 90 patients in 1977 using VA-ECMO did not demonstrate any difference in the high mortality (>85%) in the use of ECMO over conventional mechanical ventilation in adults.[46]

In the 1980s, Kolobow and Gattinoni observed that the transfer of CO_2 is more efficient than that of oxygen: while oxygenation requires high blood flows (3–5 L/min), lower blood flows (0.5–3 L/min) are sufficient for CO_2 removal. The concept of extracorporeal CO_2 removal ($ECCO_2$-R) was introduced, not to support oxygenation, but to remove CO_2 in order to deliver more gentle ventilation to the lung.[47]

In 2009, a multicentre randomized controlled study (CESAR trial) showed an improvement in the survival of patients with ARDS being transferred to a specialist centre, in which VV-ECMO was offered, compared to patients treated with conventional mechanical ventilation strategies.[48] However, these beneficial results were not solely due to the ECMO but included management in the specialist centre. Not all patients transferred for ECMO required it due to improvements at the specialist centre with conventional treatments. In the same year, following the outbreak of H1N1 flu epidemic, the use of VV-ECMO expanded worldwide and led to the creation of five nationally commissioned severe acute respiratory failure/ECMO centres in the United Kingdom.[49–51] In 2018, the multicentre EOLIA Trial conducted in patients with very severe ARDS, who had received prior optimal management, showed a positive trend to benefit of early ECMO, as compared with a strategy of conventional mechanical ventilation, with crossover to ECMO permitted (crossover occurred in 28% of the patients in the control group). At 60 days, 44 of 124 patients (35%) in the ECMO group and 57 of 125 patients (46%) in the control group had died (relative risk, 0.76; 95% confidence interval (CI), 0.55–1.04; $P = 0.09$). There has been extensive debate as to whether the early cessation of the study due to triggering of a priori set statistical futility rules prevented the detection of statistical significance alongside an apparently clinically significant result. Irrespective of the statistical uncertainties of EOLIA, VV-ECMO is now an established treatment for most severe ARDS patients. Most recently, an international cohort study of the Extracorporeal Life Support Organisation (ELSO) Registry during SARS COV-2 pandemic found that a 90-day mortality in ECMO patients with COVID-19 in 213 hospitals worldwide was 40%.[52] In a meta-analysis including 1896 patients with COVID-19 receiving ECMO, pooled in-hospital mortality was 37.1% (95% CI, 32.3%–42.0%). Mortality by included studies ranged from 15.4% to 65%.[52]

Indications for ECMO as Respiratory Support

Following the simplification of machines and the spread of ECMO capability, the respiratory indications for ECMO support have expanded. The main indications are refractory hypoxia and/or injurious ventilation in patients with high risk of death despite optimization of medical treatment. In the recent years, ECMO has been increasingly used for non-ARDS indications such as severe trauma, pulmonary embolism, severe asthma, and as a bridge to lung transplant.

Veno-venous ECMO (VV-ECMO) is the configuration of choice for hypoxaemic respiratory failure. However, in patients with concomitant shock, VA or a hybrid veno–veno-arterial ECMO may be the modality of choice.

According to the ELSO Guidelines,[53] there are no absolute contraindications to ECMO as each patient is considered individually with respect to risks and benefits. There are conditions, however, that are associated with a poor outcome despite ECMO and can be considered relative contraindications such as mechanical ventilation at injurious settings for 7 days or more, intense immunosuppression, recent or expanding central nervous system haemorrhage, non-recoverable comorbidity, and advanced age. The nature (absolute or relative) of these contraindications may vary from centre to centre. Generally, the principles of potential reversibility and prior underlying physiological reserve underpin the decisions to introduce VV-ECMO for SARF, which includes ARDS. Several prognostic scores have been published to help select patients for VV-ECMO.[54–58] Unfortunately, prognostic accuracy for all these scores is too modest to recommend their use for treatment decisions. The RESP score was validated in the largest cohort of patients and remained the score most frequently used and reported. In a recently published retrospective multicentre study, both the RESP and PRESERVE scores demonstrated poor accuracy in predicting mortality in severe COVID-19 patients requiring VV-ECMO.[59]

Technical Aspects

During VV-ECMO, part of the venous blood flow is withdrawn from the patient by a centrifugal pump, flowed across a membrane oxygenator and decarboxylator to exchange oxygen and carbon dioxide, and then returned to the body venously (Figure 22.1). The main components of ECMO circuit are the cannulas for vascular access, the pump to propel the blood, and the artificial membrane to provide gas exchange.[60]

Percutaneous cannulation allows a greater bedside applicability and reduces bleeding complications. Double-lumen cannulas allow for single vessel access for both drainage and reinfusion. Sometimes,

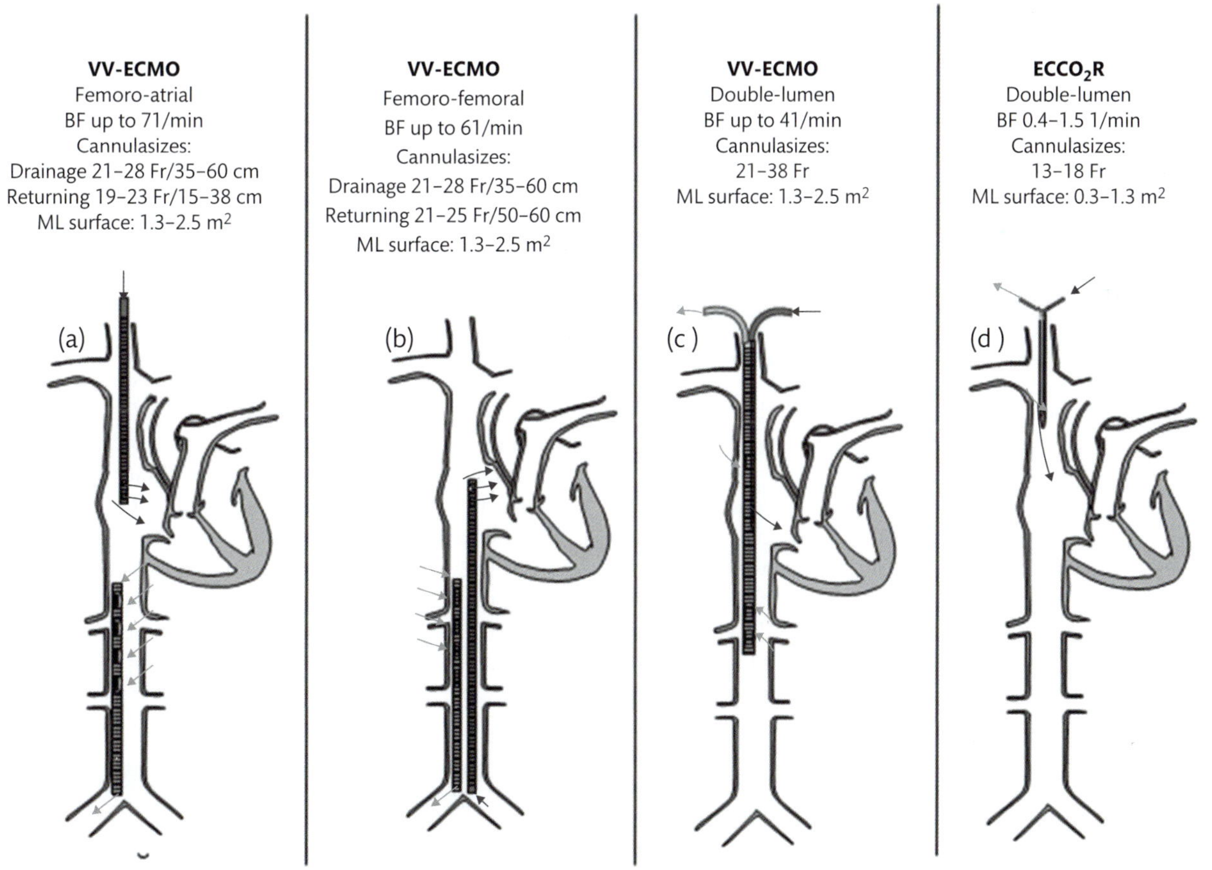

Figure 22.1 Basic cannula configuration for full VV-ECMO (A, B, C) and low-flow ECCO2R (D). Size and length of drainage and returning cannula for each configuration are reported. Independently from the returning cannula, tip of the drainage cannula should be positioned above renal veins, possibly in the intrahepatic portion of inferior vena cava (panel A and B). Range of blood flow (BF) and surface area of artificial membrane lung (ML) are also reported. Arrows indicate direction of blood flow (light grey arrows for drainage, dark grey arrows for returning).

the need for a third cannula for a VVV configuration becomes necessary to increase ECMO blood flow for acceptable oxygenation. This is usually when the protective mechanical ventilation is insufficient for gas exchange in the native lung, and maximal safe suppression of intrinsic cardiac output is still not able to maintain acceptable oxygenation.

Continuous anticoagulation is provided throughout the ECMO treatment. Anticoagulation is commonly achieved by continuous intravenous heparin infusion, targeting a partial thromboplastin time (aPTT) of 45–60 s and/or an activated clotting time (ACT) of 1.5–2 times normal, and anti-Xa levels of 0.2–0.3 or 0.3–0.7 where there is known deep vein thrombosis or pulmonary embolism. That said, VV-ECMO can be performed without anticoagulation if contraindicated once started. Clearly, this increases the risk of circuit failure and the need for more frequent circuit changes during the ECMO run.

Rationale of ECMO Strategy

The aim of the ECMO strategy is to ensure adequate gas exchange, when conventional means cannot, while minimizing the potential harmful effect of mechanical ventilation.

Ventilation is needed in most cases of severe ARDS. However, mechanical ventilation with high volume and/or airway pressure is known to worsen pre-existing lung injury (ventilator-induced lung injury, VILI). The use of lung-'protective' ventilation consisting of low tidal volumes, low plateau pressures, and low driving pressures is the cornerstone of current recommendations regarding mechanical ventilation in patients with ARDS (see Chapter 21 on ARDS).

ECMO provides sufficient stability of gas exchange to allow less minute ventilation (lower tidal volume with or without lower respiratory rate) and lower inflating pressure (plateau and driving airway pressure), facilitating prevention of VILI.

Physiology of VV-ECMO and Patient/ Machine Interaction

During VV-ECMO, the membrane lung (ML) and the native lung (NL) are in series. The total amount of delivered oxygen depends on the contribution of both the ML and the NL.

As the oxygen is mainly transported by the haemoglobin (Hb), the amount of oxygen delivered is limited by Hb saturation. Determinants of oxygen uptake via the ML are the ECMO blood flow (BF) (higher BF means more oxygen delivery), oxygen saturation of venous blood (higher venous saturation implies less oxygen is being delivered, often due to recirculation of returned oxygenated blood back into the access cannula towards the ML and away from the native circulation), the Hb concentration (higher Hb concentration means more oxygen delivery), and the fraction of oxygen of the ECMO gas flow (GF). Once the haemoglobin is fully saturated, increasing GF has no effect in delivered oxygen. During VV-ECMO, BF is the main determinant of oxygen delivery and so of arterial oxygenation.

Carbon dioxide is dissolved in blood, and its removal by the oxygenator is characterized by a linear and steep dissociation curve. The high solubility of carbon dioxide in blood allows for very efficient CO_2 removal by the oxygenator.

In contrast to oxygen, the amount of CO_2 in the blood is not limited by Hb saturation (1 L of blood may contain 2–4 times the body's total CO_2 production per minute) and a high quantity of CO_2 may be effectively removed from relatively low BF (less than 1 L/min, provided that CO_2 partial pressure in the gas compartment is maintained low by means of GF). The major factors determining blood CO_2 removal are the ECMO GF (higher GF means more CO_2 is removed), surface area of the oxygenator, and the ECMO BF (higher BF means more CO_2 removal).

Starting ECMO and Ventilatory Management

ECMO treatment allows a reduction in all parameters of the so-called mechanical power (PEEP, VT, RR, and airway pressure).[61] Management of the NL and the ideal settings of ventilator during ECMO remain a matter of debate. There is general agreement of decreasing driving pressures to below 14 cmH_2O,[62] a plateau pressure (below 24–30 cmH_2O), and maintaining tidal volume (below 4–6 mL/kg). Setting of the respiratory rate may vary greatly, from 4 up to 20 bpm. More debated is the setting of PEEP with some centres decreasing PEEP down to below 10 cmH_2O after starting ECMO (allowing the NL to collapse) while others maintain a higher level of PEEP to avoid lung collapse and theoretically preserve NL function. A strategy aiming to maximize lung rest (low PEEP, low tidal volume, and low FiO_2) will require higher BF and GF but also potentially to accept lower oxygen saturation levels. In certain centres, for example, adopted by some of the UK ECMO centres, a default 'rest' protocol initially is '10,10,10' (PEEP, driving pressure, and respiratory rate) with individual patient adjustments, based upon gas exchange, haemodynamics, ECMO capabilities, and the risks to the NL (e.g. pneumothoraces or pneumomediastinum, bullae, etc.).

Before starting ECMO, patients are generally sedated, paralyzed, and are being ventilated with relatively high respiratory rate and plateau airway pressures, with an FiO_2 close to 1.0. PaO_2 levels are low and $PaCO_2$ commonly high.

The first step after starting ECMO is to decrease tidal volume targeted to a desired level of plateau and driving pressure. The second step is to set ECMO GF according to the desired respiratory rate and $PaCO_2$ level (lower respiratory rate and/or $PaCO_2$ and higher GF). If oxygenation is not a major problem, decreasing of tidal volume and respiratory rate may be obtained with relatively lower BF by adjusting the GF alone. This is the physiological basis of $ECCO_2$-R. However, when also aiming to improve oxygenation, the ECMO BF becomes the most relevant ECMO parameter as the amount of oxygen delivery is mainly dependent on BF. Setting higher BF levels (3–5 L/min) will allow reductions in FiO_2 on the ventilator (commonly below 0.6) followed by adjustment of PEEP level according to the lung rest strategy. Figure 22.2 shows a flow chart of main ventilator settings after starting ECMO.

Weaning from VV-ECMO

Following clinico-radio-physiological evidence of the commencement of healing of the NL, the ECMO contribution to oxygenation and CO_2 removal is progressively reduced. The timing of this weaning strategy is not clearly defined as yet and subject to variations in practice between centres. There is a spectrum of strategies

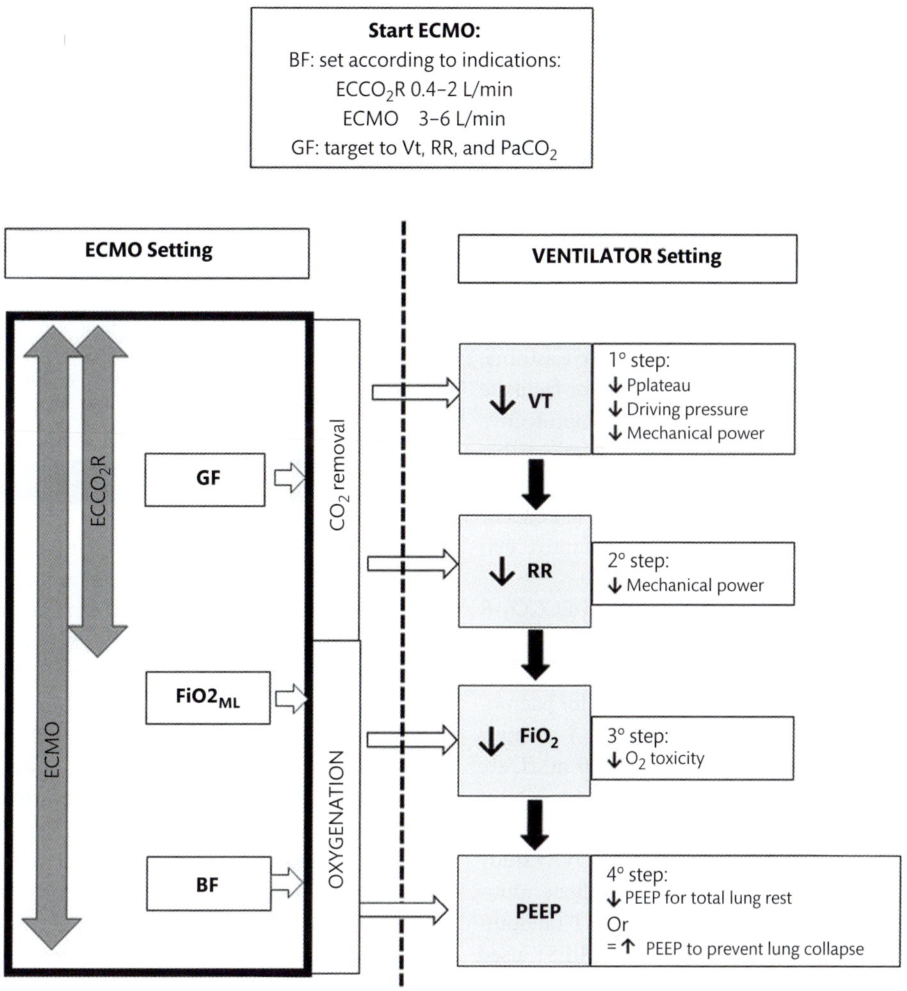

Figure 22.2 Flow chart of ventilator setting after ECMO starting. Tidal volume (VT), respiratory rate (RR), ECMO gas flow (GF), ECMO blood flow (BF), Oxygen fraction of GF (FiO_{ML}).

between early and longer durations on ECMO, based upon the interpretation of the benefits/risks to the patient's further recovery, with or without the extracorporeal circuit. The decision to disconnect a patient from ECMO is based on several factors. During VV-ECMO, patient readiness for weaning is assessed by gradually turning off the sweep GF and reducing the contribution of the ML to both oxygenation and CO_2 removal. Most commonly the patient is awake and receiving assisted spontaneous ventilation. After stopping GF, the patient has to increase respiratory effort and minute ventilation, and ventilator support may be adjusted accordingly. This process may require a few attempts, particularly when intercurrent deterioration occurs (e.g. infection, arrythmia, fluid requirements, etc.). When the patient is considered ready (which may require a period up to 24 h or longer off GF without deterioration or inability for NL gas exchange and satisfactory patient–ventilator interaction), extracorporeal support can be discontinued, and cannulae removed.

ECMO Complications

Bleeding complications remain the most frequent and serious complication in ECMO patients.[63] Localized bleeding, especially from cannula insertion sites or from surgical sites, occurs in approximately 15%–20% of patients. The most serious complication is intracranial bleeding reported in 4% of patients. However, this was not increased compared with the conventional ventilation group during the EOLIA study.[51] Other serious bleeding sites are pulmonary and gastrointestinal occurring in approximately 8% and 5% of patients, respectively.

In the presence of generalized and persistent bleeding, heparin should be reduced or discontinued, and transfusion of fresh frozen plasma and platelets should be considered. Close liaison with haematology is often helpful. Sometimes, uncontrolled bleeding requires anticipated disconnection of ECMO. Careful daily trend measurements of the circuit integrity, coagulation parameters (i.e. APTT, ACT, anti-Xa, D dimer, fibrinogen, platelet function, and Hb), ML pressures (absolute and trends), post oxygenator PaO_2, and visual appearances of clot formation on the visible aspects of the oxygenator and externalized cannulae allow monitoring and anticipation of diminishing ECMO circuit health. These enable controlled changes of the external circuit and oxygenator, without an emergency change being needed. Emergency change is to be avoided where possible in those fully dependent on ECMO for oxygenation. Safety checks and training for emergencies such as a circuit, or oxygenator failure, and air entrainment underpin any credible ECMO service.

Low-flow Extracorporeal CO_2 Removal

Low-flow ECCO$_2$-R techniques take advantage of high efficiency in removing CO_2 at relatively lower ECMO blood flows, smaller cannulas, and less side effects (Figure 22.1). Any clinical situation in which a reduction of minute ventilation may be beneficial is a potential indication for ECCO$_2$-R. These include (1) decrease of ventilatory needs in patients with exacerbations of COPD, severe asthma, and immunocompromised patients, to avoid intubation or facilitate weaning from mechanical ventilation; (2) potentially 'ultraprotective ventilation' in ARDS patients.[64] It is important to underline that while the direct effect of ECCO$_2$-R is the decreasing of $PaCO_2$, the treatment of hypercapnia per se is not the main objective of ECCO$_2$-R applications. Further, it is important to note that definitive evidence of its clinical benefit in all these settings is awaited.

Absolute thresholds to guide initiation and setting of ECCO$_2$-R have not yet been established.[65]

Different devices are available to employ ECCO$_2$-R. Most techniques consist of small roller pumps, similar to that used for haemodialysis applications, a relatively small oxygenator, and a single venous dual-lumen catheter. Blood flows up to 400–500 mL/L are commonly used. Alternatively, standard ECMO systems running at lower BF through smaller cannulas may be used.

Although an international feasibility study (SUPERNOVA) study demonstrated the feasibility of using ECCO$_2$-R to facilitate ultra-lung-protective ventilation,[65] the recently published REST randomized study did not show benefit with this approach.[66] REST used ECCO$_2$-R to aim for tidal ventilation of 3 mL/kg, although the mean achieved was 4.2 mL/kg compared to 6.5 mL/kg in the control arm. The trial was stopped early, having recruited just over one-third of its planned 1120 target, for futility with a non-significant trend to increased mortality in the intervention arm (41.5% vs 39.5%, 2% absolute difference, 95% CI, 7.6%–11.5%). Patients in the ECCO$_2$-R arm experienced fewer ventilator-free days and more serious adverse events than those in the control arm. The role of ECCO$_2$-R in the management of severe acute respiratory failure remains uncertain.

22.4 Non-conventional Modes of Ventilation

Martin Scharffenberg, Sabine Nabecker, and Marcelo Gama de Abreu

KEY MESSAGES

- Despite promising technical features and physiological rationales, non-conventional ventilation modes have been successfully applied in certain cases but without improved patient-centred outcomes in broader patient cohorts.

CONTROVERSIES

- Are methodological limitations hiding potential benefit in certain situations?
- Can study enrichment improve chances of clinically meaningful answers?

FURTHER RESEARCH

- The use of machine learning algorithms and artificial intelligence-based systems to determine effective individual strategies for safe and effective use of other ventilatory modes.

Introduction

Conventional mechanical ventilation modes, namely volume-, pressure- or dual-controlled ventilation, are most frequently used and best understood (see Chapter 11), but sometimes do not fully match the patient's needs.[67] They may be characterized by monotonous respiratory patterns or lack of ideal triggering. Non-conventional ventilator modes, including airway pressure release ventilation (APRV), variable ventilation, high-frequency oscillatory ventilation (HFOV), neurally adjusted ventilatory assist (NAVA), proportional assist ventilation (PAV), and flow-controlled ventilation (FCV), are commercially available in modern ventilators and may further improve respiratory care even if they have not yet been shown improved clinical outcomes. This chapter provides insight into these non-conventional ventilation techniques, including technical aspects, physiological rationale, and clinical effects.

Airway Pressure Release Ventilation

Airway pressure release ventilation (APRV) was first described in 1987 as the application of CPAP with intermittent release of airway pressure and the patient's ability to breathe spontaneously.[68] It therefore can be described as a time-cycled pressure-controlled ventilation mode with a unique pressure–time profile comprising two different levels of airway pressure with superposed unassisted, but unrestricted spontaneous breathing. Therewith, two types of respiratory cycles exist. Mandatory cycles occur at pressure steps (time-triggered, time-cycled), while spontaneous cycles (patient-triggered, patient-cycled) are allowed at any time.[69] Theoretically, a third type of respiratory cycle may be present, namely mixed cycles whenever the inspiratory phase coincides with the triggering from low to high airway pressure. Nowadays, many different definitions and variations of APRV exist since the original definition did not define the exact settings, for example, duration of inspiration and expiration or their ratio, respectively. This uncertainty becomes clear when considering APRV as a mode of partial ventilatory support in the presence of spontaneous breathing on the one hand, or as a pressure-controlled ventilation in the absence of inspiratory efforts and/or a more balanced I:E ratio on the other hand.

In the classical understanding of APRV, the high-pressure level (i.e. inspiratory pressure, P_{high}) is set to create a desired plateau airway pressure and is kept for approximately 90% of the whole respiratory cycle (duration of high pressure, T_{high}). This is followed by the low-pressure level (i.e. expiratory pressure, P_{low}). The very short duration of expiratory phase (T_{low}) prevents equilibration of airway pressure with ambient pressure and thereby creates an intrinsic PEEP. Depending on the respiratory system compliance, inspiratory effort, and the difference between P_{high} and P_{low}, the tidal volume (V_T) is generated. While the ratio of inspiration to expiration duration (I:E) cannot be directly set in APRV, this mode is sometimes imprecisely referred to as *inverse ratio ventilation* (IRV) by some investigators and clinicians.

Airway pressure release ventilation can be found in different ventilators under different names, for example *APRV* (Dräger Evita, Savina and V series, Hamilton G5), *Bi-Vent* (Maquet Servo-i), *BiLevel* (Engström Carestation, Puritan Bennett 840 and 980), *Duo positive Airway Pressure* or *DuoPAP* (Hamilton G5), and *APRV/Biphasic* (Viasys Avea). Notably, some ventilators diverge from classical APRV by adding a patient-triggered pressure support, tube compensation, and/or synchronization algorithms.[70] Although the terms *APRV*, *biphasic*, and *bilevel* are sometimes used interchangeably, it is important to distinguish APRV from BIPAP, another two-pressure-level ventilation technique. BIPAP typically has a shorter duration of high-pressure level, and the I:E ratio rarely exceeds 1:1. Furthermore, PEEP is directly set as the low-pressure level.

In APRV, adjustable ventilator parameters are P_{high}, T_{high}, P_{low}, T_{low}, F_IO_2, and ramp. Regarding exact recommendations for setting parameters, literature is ambiguous. When initializing APRV, P_{high} can be titrated according to a desired airway plateau pressure or the upper inflection point (UIP) on the volume–pressure curve, while P_{low} can be adjusted to or below the lower inflection point (LIP). Usually, P_{high} ranges from 20 to 35 cmH_2O in adults, 20–30 cmH_2O for paediatric, and 10–25 cmH_2O for neonatal patients. In cases with severely decreased respiratory system compliance, P_{high} values up to or above 35 cmH_2O may be necessary,[71] but current guidelines should be followed. In classical APRV, the duration of P_{high} (T_{high}) can initially be set to 90% of total cycle time, for example, 4–6 s for adults, 3–5 s for paediatric, and 1.5–2 s for neonatal patients,[5l], while T_{low} lasts approximately 10% of cycle time or less. However, T_{low} can be alternatively set according to the patient's respiratory mechanics using the slope of the expiratory flow curve and the ratio of end-expiratory flow (EEF) to peak expiratory flow (PEF), respectively. An EEF/PEF ratio of 75% has been shown to sufficiently open and stabilize the alveoli, resulting in a very short T_{low} of 0.3–0.6 s. Because clinicians sometimes are faced with technical problems when recording a clear curve, initial settings of T_{low} can be 0.35–0.6 s for adults, 0.2–0.5 s for children, and 0.2–0.3 s for neonates. However, T_{low} can then be adjusted to achieve a desired end-expiratory pCO_2 (etCO_2). Because expiratory resistance is increased by artificial airway and expiratory time is very brief, the lung retains a fraction of P_{high} pressure, creating a PEEP-like effect (auto-PEEP). Hence, P_{low} can be set to 0 cmH_2O, allowing rapid expiratory GF and effective CO_2 removal, while and preventing end-expiratory alveolar collapse.[71] Therefore, to some authors, proper setting of T_{low} is more important for end-expiratory alveolar stabilization than the level of P_{low}. The inspired fraction of oxygen (F_IO_2) should be adjusted according to clinical standard or patient's requirements. To wean a patient from APRV, some authors promote stepwise reduction of P_{high} and increase of T_{high} until the settings equal CPAP.[72]

Classic APRV relies on the *open lung* concept, recruiting, and stabilizing collapsed alveoli through the application of a prolonged high-pressure phase, which increases the mean airway pressure compared to conventional modes. The short pressure releases allow for tidal ventilation with washout of CO_2. As T_{high} occupies around 90% of the cycle time, most spontaneous breathing takes place at favourable lung volumes with probably optimal respiratory system compliance. As lung volume is maintained above functional residual capacity (FRC), the elastic work of breathing may also be decreased. Increasing duration of P_{high} (T_{high}) increases time for lung recruitment and alveolar stability. Especially in the heterogeneously injured ARDS lung, a long T_{high} may allow recruitment of lung regions with long time constants and may increase the diffusive phase of APRV, promoting alveolar gas exchange. Unassisted spontaneous breaths in APRV distribute ventilation to the more dorsal/dependent lung regions, alter perfusion distribution, and may prevent the so-called ventilator-induced diaphragmatic dysfunction (VIDD), that is, disuse muscle atrophy (see Chapter 16).

APRV has been studied in experimental and clinical trials, but prospective randomized controlled trials are rare and a lack of clear definitions or standardized protocols means results must be interpreted with caution.[69] The most common findings with APRV were improvements in gas exchange, mainly in oxygenation, while reducing peak airway pressure when compared to conventional modes. In experimental studies, APRV has been shown to have beneficial effects on specific pathophysiologic mechanisms of ARDS, altering the ARDS cascade and even mitigating the development of ARDS when applied early. Although the literature is contradictory, in some small clinical studies APRV decreased both the incidence and mortality of ARDS. Furthermore, better patient comfort with reduced sedation requirements, improved haemodynamics, as well as improved perfusion of the kidneys, gut, brain, and spine were found with APRV. In one retrospective single centre study including 50 patients with severe hypoxaemic respiratory failure, initiation of APRV significantly increased oxygenation with a relatively low rate of complications.[73] However, firm data comparing APRV to conventional modes regarding ARDS incidence and outcome, for example, mortality or effects on VILI, is not yet available.[69] Criticisms of APRV include difficulties controlling tidal volume and PEEP, with the risks of volumes exceeding the safety limits of lung-protective ventilation. In common with other pressure-controlled modes, small changes in respiratory mechanics may produce large changes in volumes delivered. The prolonged periods at higher intra-thoracic pressures may worsen hypotension in hypovolaemic patients, while its use in patients with obstructive airways disease such as COPD and acute asthma may promote severe air-trapping and injurious intrinsic PEEP. In the absence of strong evidence, and until optimal settings and use are defined in randomized controlled trials, classic APRV cannot be recommended as a primary ventilation mode in ARDS, especially while the *open lung* concept is controversially discussed and challenged in favour of reduced airway pressures.

Variable-assisted Mechanical Ventilation

Assisted mechanical ventilation, for example, partial respiratory support, unloads the respiratory muscles while the patient's respiratory drive and spontaneous breathing are preserved. In contrast to most of the conventional mechanical ventilation modes, spontaneous breathing patterns are usually highly variable regarding tidal volumes and respiratory rate. The aim of variable artificial ventilation is to resemble some aspects of spontaneous breathing, whose pattern is usually highly variable.[74] Variable ventilation has been shown to have beneficial effects on lung function, and these are mainly explained by lung recruitment and improved ventilation–perfusion matching. Different ways of achieving enhanced variability during assisted spontaneous breathing are discussed.

Neurally Adjusted Ventilatory Assist

In assisted mechanical ventilation modes, effective triggering is important to avoid asynchrony and discomfort. The optimal trigger would be a signal derived from the central nervous system. While this is not feasible with current technology, the electric activity of the diaphragm (EADi) offers a surrogate parameter of inspiratory effort with least delay.[75] This technique is implemented in NAVA, where timing and degree of assistance are primarily patient-controlled. To assess EADi signal, a special gastric tube with electrodes at the distal end is introduced through the nose into the oesophagus until electrodes are placed in the diaphragmatic level (Figure 22.3). The extent of respiratory support provided by NAVA is proportional to the acquired EADi signal and can be adjusted by setting up an amplification factor (NAVA gain). The inspiratory pressure is a function of EADi signal multiplied by the NAVA gain:

Inspiratory Pressure (cmH_2O) = NAVA gain ($cmH_2O/\mu V$) × EADi signal (μV).

Using the neural trigger results in intrinsic variable ventilation as it is dependent on the intrinsic respiratory drive. The inspiration terminates and airway pressure decreases to PEEP, when the EADi signal falls below 70% of its peak value or if pressure limits are reached. If pneumatic triggering occurs prior to electrical signal, no EADi signal is detected or the signal is deemed to be inadequate, and conventional pressure support ventilation (PSV) is activated automatically as a backup to ensure sufficient minute ventilation.

NAVA is implemented in the *Servo-i* ventilator (Maquet Critical Care, Sweden). The EADi catheter is introduced like a common oronasal gastric tube. Different sizes are available, which can be chosen according to the individual distance between *xyphoid process-earlobe-nose tip*. Catheter placement is guided by monitoring the cardiac and EADi electrical potentials via a dedicated ventilator screen. Optimum catheter position is indicated by high-amplitude cardiac signals in the upper and low amplitude in the lower leads, the presence of stable EADi signal highlighted in central leads, and/or the absence of p-waves in the distal lead.

In NAVA, adjustable parameters are NAVA gain, PEEP, F_IO_2, and apnoea time for backup ventilation. The NAVA gain can be increased from initially low values until a desired level of ventilatory support is achieved. Notably, NAVA gain must not be set exclusively according to tidal volume. While PEEP and F_IO_2 can be chosen according to patient's requirements, respiratory rate, inspiratory time, and I:E ratio are primarily patient-controlled and the cycle-off criterion is preset. NAVA can be performed as both invasive and non-invasive respiratory support via nasal probe, face mask, and helmet in both adults and neonates or infants. Patients undergoing NAVA should be closely monitored, as loss of EADi signal or dysregulation of respiratory drive can occur. Furthermore, the detection of both insufficient and excessive ventilatory support is crucial to prevent harm. Optimal catheter position should be verified after changing respiratory settings or patient movement.

NAVA has been studied in both experimental and clinical trials including infants and adults. The most common finding was improved patient–ventilator interaction, that is, less asynchrony, in different clinical circumstances.[76] Compared to conventional pressure support, tidal volume variability is increased, resembling natural breathing patterns. Through preserved spontaneous breathing, NAVA promotes redistribution of ventilation to dorsal lung regions and improved ventilation–perfusion matching. As tidal volume varies as a function of EADi, there is a risk of injurious volumes; however, in practice, the generated volumes tend to be below the limits for lung-protective ventilation, for example, <6 mL/kg predicted body weight (PBW).[75,76] Because NAVA was predominantly used in children, including pre-term neonates, there are many studies in this specific patient cohort. Regardless of the age of the children and invasiveness, NAVA improved patient–ventilator interaction, reduced peak inspiratory pressures (PIP) and tidal volumes, and provided reliable monitoring of the central respiratory drive. Furthermore, non-invasive NAVA seems to prevent intubation while invasive NAVA may facilitate early extubation.

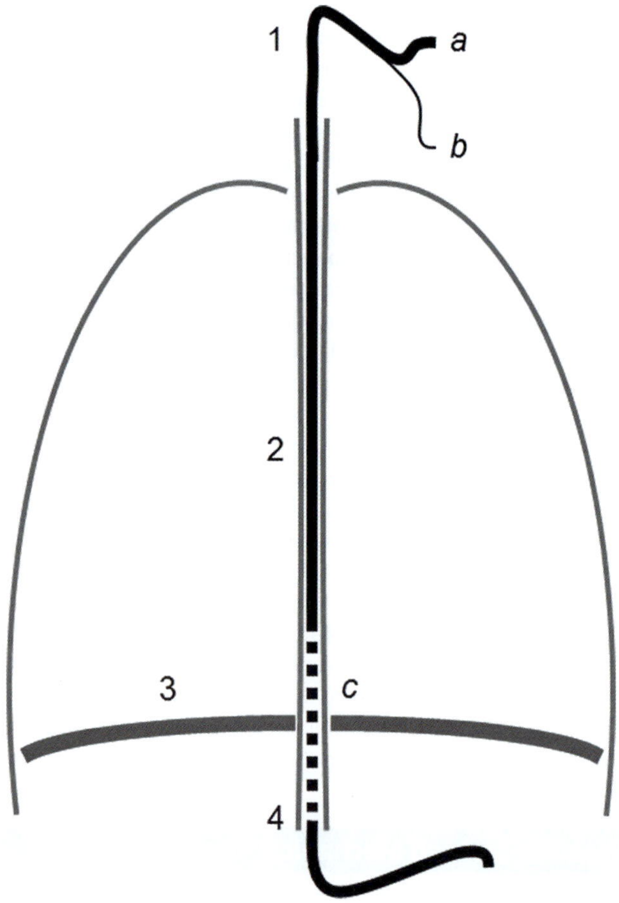

Figure 22.3 EADi catheter position: (1) EADi catheter with (a) gastric lumen, (b) connection to the ventilator, and (c) array of 8–10 electrodes; (2) oesophagus; (3) diaphragm; (4) gastroesophageal junction.

In theory at least, NAVA represents a self-regulating highly synchronized proportional respiratory support system as it majorly relies on the patient's respiratory drive. Thus, the patient can control the amount and frequency of pressure support and the respiratory assistance provided is deemed relatively constant throughout a wide range of NAVA gains. In studies, increasing NAVA gain only leads to limited increases in V_T.[71,72] With this, respiratory over-assistance can be inferred when EADi signal, that is, respiratory drive, significantly declines at a given NAVA gain and vice versa. However, very low and very high gain levels may disturb the self-regulating respiratory system. When breaths are successfully EADi-triggered, NAVA does not depend on the measurement of airway pressure or flow, which allows reliable functioning even in the presence of large air and pressure leaks.[73] Preservation of spontaneous breathing in NAVA prevents diaphragm disuse atrophy.

Due to the obligatory EADi catheter, NAVA is not feasible in patients with contraindications for oesophageal tubes. Dislocation of the EADi catheter or impairment of respiratory drive, for example, due to neurological diseases or deep sedation, may lead to deteriorating respiratory pattern variability and tidal volumes.[76] Conversely, very high levels of NAVA gain may result in unstable periodic breathing patterns, for example, high tidal volumes and apnoea periods, leading to significant patient discomfort. To date, NAVA is available in one ICU ventilator and not for perioperative or home mechanical ventilation. Questions to be answered in future research concern optimal NAVA gain values, timing of NAVA onset in the weaning process,[77,78] and its importance in ARDS therapy. Although some specific advantages were shown for NAVA, clinical outcomes still have to be evaluated in prospective randomized clinical trials.

Proportional Assist Ventilation

Proportional assist ventilation (PAV) was introduced in 1992.[79] In PAV, pneumatically triggered inspiratory pressure is created in proportion to the patient's respiratory demand, resulting in intrinsically variable breathing patterns. PAV and NAVA are the only modes of respiratory support that provide assistance proportionally. Technically, the inspiratory effort moves a free-moving piston in the ventilator while precisely measuring flow and volume. As inspiratory effort is detected, the ventilator immediately rises inspiratory pressure and flow, with breath cycled off as flow drops. As in NAVA, gain control defines the relation between measured signals and applied respiratory support. Contrastingly, levels of flow and volume assist are user- not patient-controlled. Therefore, respiratory system compliance and elastance need to be assessed for proper settings. An updated version of PAV is available, termed proportional assist ventilation with load-adjustable gain factors (PAV+). In this mode, respiratory mechanics are measured non-invasively and semi-continuously, providing automatically adjusted assist level. This development may facilitate more widespread clinical use of PAV+.

PAV+ is implemented in the *Puritan Bennett 840* ventilator and a similar mode, termed Proportional Pressure Support® (PPS®), is available in *Dräger Evita Infinity V500*, *V300* and *Babylog VN500* ventilators (not available in the United States). In PAV, percentages of flow and volume assistance and in PAV+ one general level of assistance can be selected, respectively, and F_IO_2 and PEEP can be set. Other ventilatory parameters are patient-controlled, that is, flow, V_T, and airway pressures are not targeted. For proper automatic estimation of lung mechanics, patient's ideal body weight (IBW), endotracheal tube size, and humidifier volume have to be entered. Recommended initial settings comprise an expiratory sensitivity of 3 (default), flow trigger of 3 L/min, limited protective V_T, airway pressure limit of 40 cmH_2O (default), PEEP of 2–5 cmH_2O, and initial assist level of 60%. The latter may be increased or decreased in steps of 10%–20% if necessary and has to be tailored to the patient's requirements, for example, by blood gas analyses.[80] PAV can also be successfully used as both invasive and non-invasive ventilation.

PAV(+) unloads respiratory muscles, decreases work of breathing, and improves synchronicity by adapting to patient demand.[67,80] Sleep quality was shown to be improved, and randomized studies indicated both safety and faster weaning compared to conventional PSV. Despite partial unloading of respiratory muscles, respiratory muscle atrophy is unlikely to occur to the same degree as compared to controlled MV.

Like NAVA, PAV(+) depends on the preservation of the patient's respiratory drive. Neurological diseases and deep sedation may impair PAV(+) performance and will require an alternative mode. As PAV(+) involves pneumatic triggering, its inherent limitations are the same as of other pneumatically triggered ventilation modes. Dynamic hyperinsufflation and intrinsic PEEP may impair inspiratory cycling and leakage may cause auto-triggering. Because ventilatory demand may change as the respiratory situation worsens or improves, the patient on PAV must be monitored closely and settings adjusted accordingly. However, this limitation may be addressed with PAV+, where lung mechanics are assessed automatically to adjust the pressure support gain control. However, if compensation of elastance and resistance is too high, or in the case of over-assistance (high assist level), the PAV(+) system tends to *run away*, that is, the system supports self-generated flow towards the patient, which results in dynamic hyperinflation and impairing or even preventing expiration.[74] To avoid this, the ventilator-generated pressure must be lower than the pressure required to overcome the passive respiratory system properties. Practically, levels of assistance between 40% and 80% are recommended. In contrast to other modes of partial respiratory support, assist level in PAV does not directly relate to minute ventilation and oxygenation. In fact, high assist levels increase the risk of *runaway* tendency and may worsen gas exchange.[80] Whether specific benefits of PAV(+) translate into clinically relevant outcomes is still unclear and need to be evaluated in future research. Notably, there are no current standards for use of PAV(+).

Noisy Ventilation

Respiratory patterns are highly variable in healthy humans, but this variability may decrease with disease and age. The rationale of the so-called noisy pressure support ventilation (noisy PSV) is to restore variability by applying variable breathing patterns in combination with the advantages of spontaneous breathing in terms of pressure support ventilation.[81] Noisy PSV is a mode of partial ventilatory assist. Breaths are triggered pneumatically as in conventional PSV; however, tidal volumes vary randomly breath-by-breath within preset limits. In contrast to NAVA and PAV, variability in noisy PSV is thus extrinsic.

Noisy PSV is available in the *Infinity V500* ventilator (*Dräger*, Germany). Specific parameters to be adjusted are level of pressure support (*ΔPsupp*) and percentage of variation (0%–100%). Other settings include F_IO_2, CPAP level, ramp, and trigger threshold.

Noisy PSV has been extensively studied in experimental studies. In experimental ARDS, noisy PSV was shown to increase variability of breathing patterns, improve both oxygenation and ventilation–perfusion matching, and reduce lung inflammation compared to conventional PSV and pressure-controlled ventilation. Compared to conventional pressure-controlled ventilation, noisy PSV decreased tidal reaeration and hyperinflation as PSV did. In a small clinical trial, safety and feasibility of noisy PSV were demonstrated, as well as a decreased number of asynchrony events.

The basic physiologic rationale of noisy PSV is the recruitment of collapsed lung areas through intermittent application of higher airway pressures. Based on the non-linear pressure–volume curve of an injured lung, normally distributed variation of airway pressures and tidal volumes results in greater lung recruitment than de-recruitment. This dynamic effect may depend on presence, type, and extent of lung injury. However, experimental studies failed to show improved aeration with noisy PSV. Instead, a shift of perfusion from poorly to normally aerated regions was observed, which suggests recruitment of lung capillaries, improving ventilation–perfusion matching and oxygenation. Other physiologic mechanisms related to beneficial effects of noisy PSV are the presence of stochastic resonance, enhanced sinus arrhythmia, and an increased endogenous surfactant release. During variable ventilation, a coefficient of variation of 30%, which resembles the variable breathing patterns of healthy individuals, was shown to have greatest effect on lung function and respiratory mechanics.[82]

The benefits of noisy PSV on lung function and mechanics may depend on dynamic recruitment effects, which in turn are dependent on the presence and extent of lung injury. Thus, the beneficial effects of noisy PSV may be disease-specific, and theoretically less pronounced in the absence of lung injury. Noisy PSV is intended to recruit collapsed alveoli. However, if recruitment does not occur, intermittent tidal hyperinflation and overdistension in non-dependent lung regions may result. In contrast to PAV and NAVA, variability in noisy PSV is created randomly by the ventilator, which may promote asynchrony since tidal volumes do not relate to patient's inspiratory effort. Tidal volumes above 8 mL/kg PBW occur recurrently; however, in experimental studies at least, noisy PSV was not shown to aggravate lung injury in the short term. The role of noisy PSV in clinical practice remains unclear because large trials on clinical outcomes are not yet available. Noisy PSV is not a recommended primary mode of mechanical ventilation. A multicentre randomized controlled trial on the effects of noisy PSV during weaning is in progress and may help to better define the role of this innovative mode.

High-frequency Oscillatory Ventilation

High-frequency oscillatory ventilation (HFOV) represents a high-flow CPAP system, providing very high respiratory rates, that is, oscillations, with small tidal volumes (approx. 1–3 mL/kg PBW) at a relatively constant mean airway pressure (mP_{aw}). Technically, a column of gas is moved back and forth in the ventilatory circuit, which can be generated by either oscillators (mainly used in neonatal patients) or membrane diaphragms (for children and adult patients). In contrast to conventional mechanical ventilation, both inspiration and expiration phases of these small tidal volumes are active processes during HFOV.

HFOV is implemented in the *Sensormedics 3100B* ventilator (*Yorba Linda*, USA), the *Novalung Vision alpha* ventilator (Germany) or the *Metran R100* ventilator (Japan). Adjustable respiratory parameters include the frequency of oscillations (Hz), the amplitude of oscillations (mbar), F_IO_2, and the I:E ratio. Using the *Vision alpha* ventilator, mP_{aw} and cycle volume can be selected directly.

Before initiating HFOV, patent airways and an appropriate level of sedation must be ensured, while neuromuscular blocking agents may still be considered.[83] Depending on haemodynamic stability and level of hypoxaemia, some authors promote a recruitment manoeuvre before starting HFOV. Usual initial settings include an mP_{aw} of 5 cmH_2O above the value used during conventional mechanical ventilation (~25–30 cmH_2O) and an I:E ratio of 1:2 or 1:1 in more severe cases of hypoxaemia. In adult patients, the initial respiratory frequency is usually 5 Hz (300 breaths/min), but rates of 3–15 Hz, that is, 180–900 breaths/min, have been described. If the $paCO_2$ increases to unacceptable levels, the respiratory rate should be decreased, allowing more time for inspiration and, consequently, an increase in V_T. F_IO_2 can be initially set at 1.0 and gradually reduced to achieve adequate arterial oxygen saturation ($SpO_2 \geq 88\%$). If oxygenation does not improve, the mP_{aw} can be gradually increased in steps of 3–5 cmH_2O every 30–60 min and may be accompanied by a recruitment manoeuvre in an otherwise haemodynamically stable patient. To enhance ventilation and permit CO_2 elimination, the endotracheal tube cuff can be partially deflated. Generally, the use of a 5–8 cmH_2O cuff leak may be considered.[84] Failure to improve hypoxaemia or severe acidosis should prompt consideration of further measures, for example, prone position and extracorporeal lung support techniques. As a variant of HFOV, high-frequency percussive ventilation uses high-frequency sub-tidal volumes in combination with conventional low-frequency breathing. This mode has been claimed as particularly beneficial during ECMO use and weaning,[85] but evidence is weak. Weaning during HFOV is usually started with a reduction of F_IO_2 rather than mP_{aw}. Conventional ventilation can be resumed when F_IO_2 is 0.4 or lower and mP_{aw} is equal or less than 20 cmH_2O. Some ventilators, such as the *Novalung* device, allow spontaneous breathing during HFOV but do not provide patient-triggered pressure support. Therefore, direct extubation from HFOV is no common practice and may not be desirable.

In HFOV, tidal volumes are relatively small, that is, below anatomic dead space. However, oxygen transport to the alveoli is maintained mainly due to molecular diffusion of gas in the airways, while the F_IO_2 can be adjusted to ensure adequate oxygenation. Elimination of carbon dioxide is augmented by adequate minute ventilation, which mainly depends on tidal volume and frequency.[86] HFOV usually leads to a relatively high and constant mean airway pressure, which contributes to oxygen transport to the alveoli and contributes to prevent atelectasis. Furthermore, the small tidal volumes may reduce the risk of volutrauma.[84] Due to an increased mP_{aw}, a significant reduction of cardiac preload may occur with HFOV, requiring intravascular volume expansion (fluids) and use of vasoactive drugs. Barotrauma occurs more frequently during

HFOV than conventional mechanical ventilation, possibly leading to pneumothorax, which is suspected if hypotension and hypoxaemia develop suddenly. Obstruction of the endotracheal tube is a usual cause of hypercapnia during HFOV, which must be excluded when $paCO_2$ remains high despite adjustments of the ventilator settings.[87]

Current evidence on the risks and benefits of HFOV is contradictory. HFOV at least decreased VILI in experimental studies and improved oxygenation in some small clinical trials with severe ARDS patients. However, HFOV is not routinely used in adult ARDS, which is mainly the consequence of two clinical trials demonstrating no benefit or even harm. In 2013, the OSCILLATE study showed an increased mortality in ARDS patients treated with HFOV compared to conventional protective lung ventilation. The study was stopped early because of possible patient harm. Another study on HFOV (OSCAR) could not confirm these results. Of note, patients in the OSCILLATE trial received lower tidal volumes and higher PEEP levels than patients in the OSCAR trial, while in the OSCAR trial recruitment manoeuvres were not mandatory.[83] Taken together, both studies suggest that HFOV in early ARDS does not lower mortality rates. Therefore, there is no evidence to support the use of HFOV as first-line therapy during ARDS treatment.[85] However, both studies reported a small number of included patients, and their results might not be seen as reason for a blanket ban on HFOV in adults according to some authors. Indeed, HFOV may be indicated in certain emergencies.[83] However, rescue therapies including HFOV among others can be life-saving,[85] and it may serve as a rescue strategy in patients suffering from hypoxaemia, which is untreatable with conventional invasive mechanical ventilation.[85] Anyhow, the most adequate mP_{aw} for lung protection, which is able to avoid overdistension or atelectasis, as well as its future role, for example, in spontaneously breathing patients with and without ARDS, remains to be determined.[85] Rigorous trials are required to identify its optimal use.

Flow-controlled Ventilation

Flow-controlled ventilation (FCV) is a new mode of mechanical ventilation for surgical and intensive care patients, which differs substantially from others. While expiration is usually passive, both inspiration and expiration are controlled under FCV. During inspiration and expiration, flow is constant and inspiratory and expiratory phases directly follow each other. Accordingly, there are virtually no phases of zero airway flow, creating triangular airway pressure profiles. FCV is mainly intended to be applied using a special very thin cuffed endotracheal tube ('*Tritube*', *Ventinova Medical*, The Netherlands). This tube has an outer diameter of 4.4 mm and is equipped with the ventilation lumen, a cuff lumen, and a lumen for intratracheal pressure measurement. However, an adapter for standard endotracheal tubes is available, also allowing FCV in combination with double-lumen tube for thoracic surgery.

FCV is implemented in the *Evone* ventilator (*Ventinova Medical*, The Netherlands).

Adjustable settings include maximum inspiratory pressure (mbar), end-expiratory pressure (mbar), flow (L/min), IE, and FiO_2 (%). Of note, end-expiratory pressure can be as low as −10 mbar, representing negative end-expiratory pressure. In FCV, airway pressure changes linearly between the upper and lower airway pressure limits. Thereby, the size of tidal volume and the respiratory rate are consequences of setting pressures and flow. While the VT directly depends on the difference between the upper and lower airway pressure limits, the respiratory rate results from the airway flow with which airway pressure alternates between these limits. At given pressure limits, increasing airway flow increases respiratory rate and vice versa. Enlarging the difference between pressure limits at a given flow increases VT and vice versa. I:E should ideally be 1:1. Due to the high airway resistance associated with small-bore tube, spontaneous breathing should be prevented. However, for emergence from anaesthesia, it may be allowed by deflating the tube's cuff.

FCV has been studied in both experimental and clinical studies. Compared with conventional controlled ventilation, FCV attenuated lung injury and improved lung recruitment, pulmonary aeration, and gas exchange.[88,89] Improved ventilation efficiency may be mainly attributed to the controlled and linearized airway pressure decline during expiration. Furthermore, less energy is dissipated in the lungs due to the special flow and pressure profiles, especially when I:E is close to 1:1.[90] Apart from effects related to flow and airway pressure profiles, there are advantages related to the ultrathin tube, for example, in cases with critically obstructed airways as well as during laryngeal or tracheal surgery and tracheostomy.[91]

Future research is required to investigate the effects of FCV on clinical outcomes.

REFERENCES

1. Dolovich MB, Dhand R. Aerosol drug delivery: Developments in device design and clinical use. *Lancet*. 2011;**377**:1032–1045.
2. Ehrmann S, Roche-Campo F, Bodet-Contentin L, et al. Aerosol therapy in intensive and intermediate care units: Prospective observation of 2808 critically ill patients. *Intensive Care Med*. 2016;**42**:192–201.
3. Laube BL, Janssens HM, de Jongh FH, et al. What the pulmonary specialist should know about the new inhalation therapies. *Eur Respir J*. 2011;**37**:1308–1331.
4. Global Initiative for Asthma. Global Strategy for Asthma Management and Prevention, 2017. Available from www.ginasthma.org
5. Global Strategy for the Diagnosis, Management and Prevention of COPD, Global Initiative for Chronic Obstructive Lung Disease (GOLD) 2016. Available from: http://goldcopd.org
6. Mogayzel PJ, Naureckas ET, Robinson KA, et al. Cystic fibrosis pulmonary guidelines: Chronic medication for maintenance of lung health. *Am J Respir Crit Care Med*. 2013;**187**:680–689.
7. Flume PA, Mogayzel PJ, Robinson KA, et al. Cystic fibrosis pulmonary guidelines: Treatment of pulmonary exacerbation. *Am J Respir Crit Care Med*. 2009;**180**:802–808.
8. Mahoney BA, Smith WA, Lo DS, et al. Emergency interventions for hyperkalaemia. *Cochrane Database Syst Rev*. 2005;**18**:CD003235.
9. Ehrmann S, Chastre J, Diot P, et al. Nebulized antibiotics in mechanically ventilated patients: A challenge for translational research from technology to clinical care. *Ann Intensive Care 2017*. 2017;7:78.
10. Kalil AC, Metersky ML, Klompas M, et al. Management of adults with hospital-acquired and ventilator-associated pneumonia:

2016 clinical practice guidelines by the infectious diseases society of America and the American thoracic society. *Clin Infect Dis*. 2016;**63**:e61–111.
11. Ari A, Fink JB, Dhand R. Inhalation therapy in patients receiving mechanical ventilation: An update. *J Aerosol Med Pulm Drug Deliv*. 2012;**25**:319–332.
12. Abroug F, Ouanes-Besbes L, Fkih-Hassen M, et al. Prednisone in COPD exacerbation requiring ventilator support: An open-label randomized evaluation. *Eur Respir J*. 2014;**43**:717–724.
13. Luyt CE, Clavel M, Guntupalli K, et al. Pharmacokinetics and lung delivery of PDDS-aerosolized amikacin (NKTR-061) in intubated and mechanically ventilated patients with nosocomial pneumonia. *Crit Care*. 2009;**13**:R200.
14. Lu Q, Yang J, Liu Z et al. Nebulized ceftazidime and amikacin in ventilator-associated pneumonia cause by Pseudomonas aeruginosa. *Am J Respir Crit Care Med*. 2011;**184**:106–115.
15. Valachis A, Samonis G, Kofteridis DP. The role of aerosolized colistin in the treatment of ventilator-associated pneumonia: A systematic review and metaanalysis. *Crit Care Med*. 2015;**43**:527–533.
16. Solé-Lleonart C, Rouby JJ, Blot S, et al. Nebulization of antiinfective agents in invasively mechanically ventilated adults: A systematic review and meta-analysis. *Anesthesiology*. 2017;**126**:890–908.
17. Rello J, Solé-Lleonart C, Rouby JJ, et al. Use of nebulized antimicrobials for the treatment of respiratory infections in invasively mechanically ventilated adults: A position paper from the European society of clinical microbiology and infectious diseases. *Clin Microbiol Infect*. 2017;**23**:629–639.
18. Réminiac F, Vecellio L, Heuzé-Vourc'h N, et al. Aerosol therapy in adults receiving high flow nasal cannula oxygen therapy. *J Aerosol Med Pulm Drug Deliv*. 2016;**29**:134–141.
19. Réminiac F, Vecellio L, Loughlin RM, et al. Nasal high flow nebulization in infants and toddlers: An in vitro and in vivo scintigraphic study. *Pediatr Pulmonol*. 2017;**52**:337–344.
20. Resnier P, Mottais A, Sibiril Y, et al. Challenges and successes using nanomedicines for aerosol delivery to the airways. *Curr Gene Ther*. 2016;**16**:34–46.
21. Dugernier J, Reychler G, Wittebole X, et al. Aerosol delivery with two ventilation modes during mechanical ventilation: A randomized study. *Ann Intensive Care*. 2016;**6**:73.
22. Petitcollin A, Dequin PF, Darrouzain F, et al. Pharmacokinetics of high-dose nebulized amikacin in ventilated critically ill patients. *J Antimicrob Chemother*. 2016;**71**:3482–3486.
23. Zainudine BM, Biddiscombe M, Tolfree SE, et al. Comparison of bronchodilator responses and deposition patterns of salbutamol inhaled from a pressurized metered dose inhaler, as a dry powder and as a nebulised solution. *Thorax*. 1990;**45**:469–473.
24. Respaud R, Vecellio L, Diot P, et al. Nebulization as a delivery method for mAbs in respiratory diseases. *Expert Opin Drug Deliv*. 2015;**12**:1027–1039.
25. Youngren-Ortiz SR, Gandhi NS, Espana-Serrano L, et al. Aerosol delivery of siRNA to the lungs. Part 1: Rationale for gene delivery systems. *Kona*. 2016;**33**:63–85.
26. Hess DR, Fink JB, Venkataraman ST, et al. The history and physics of heliox. *Respir Care*. 2006;**51**:608–612.
27. Elleau C, Galperine RI, Guenard H, et al. Helium-oxygen mixture in respiratory distress syndrome: A double-blind study. *J Pediatr*. 1993;**122**:132–136.
28. Colnaghi M, Pierro M, Migliori C, et al. Nasal continuous positive airway pressure with heliox in preterm infants with respiratory distress syndrome. *Pediatrics*. 2012; **129**:e333–338.
29. Szczapa T, Gadzinowski J. Use of heliox in the management of neonates with meconium aspiration syndrome. *Neonatology*. 2011;**100**:265–270.
30. Martinon-Torres F, Rodriguez-Nunez A, Martinon-Sanchez JM. Nasal continuous positive airway pressure with heliox in infants with acute bronchiolitis. *Respir Med*. 2006;**100**:1458–1462.
31. Liet JM, Millotte B, Tucci M, et al. Noninvasive therapy with helium-oxygen for severe bronchiolitis. *J Pediatr*. 2005;**147**:812–817.
32. Kneyber MC, van Heerde M, Twisk JW, et al. Heliox reduces respiratory system resistance in respiratory syncytial virus induced respiratory failure. *Crit Care*. 2009;**13**(3):R71.
33. Katz A, Gentile MA, Craig DM, et al. Heliox improves gas exchange during high-frequency ventilation in a pediatric model of acute lung injury. *Am J Respir Crit Care Med*. 2001;**164**:260–264.
34. Winters JW, Willing MA, Sanfilippo D. Heliox improves ventilation during high frequency oscillatory ventilation in pediatric patients. *Pediatr Crit Care Med*. 2000;**1**:33–37.
35. Rodrigo G, Pollack C, Rodrigo C, et al. Heliox for nonintubated acute asthma patients. *Cochrane Database Syst Rev*. 2003;CD002884.
36. Rodrigo GJ, Rodrigo C, Pollack CV, et al. Use of helium-oxygen mixtures in the treatment of acute asthma: A systematic review. *Chest*. 2003;**123**:891–896.
37. Piva JP, Menna Barreto SS, Zelmanovitz F, et al. Heliox versus oxygen for nebulized aerosol therapy in children with lower airway obstruction. *Pediatr Crit Care Med*. 2002;**3**:6–10.
38. Kim IK, Phrampus E, Venkataraman S, et al. Helium/oxygen-driven albuterol nebulization in the treatment of children with moderate to severe asthma exacerbations: A randomized, controlled trial. *Pediatrics*. 2005;**116**:1127–1133.
39. Jolliet P, Tassaux D, Thouret JM, et al. Beneficial effects of helium:oxygen versus air:oxygen noninvasive pressure support in patients with decompensated chronic obstructive pulmonary disease. *Crit Care Med*. 1999;**27**:2422–2429.
40. Jolliet P, Tassaux D, Roeseler J, et al. Helium-oxygen versus air–oxygen noninvasive pressure support in decompensated chronic obstructive disease: A prospective, multicenter study. *Crit Care Med*. 2003;**31**:878–884.
41. Gerbeaux P, Gainnier M, Boussuges A, et al. Use of heliox in patients with severe exacerbation of chronic obstructive pulmonary disease. *Crit Care Med*. 2001; **29**:2322–2324.
42. Tassaux D, Jolliet P, Roeseler J, et al. Effects of helium-oxygen on intrinsic positive end-expiratory pressure in intubated and mechanically ventilated patients with severe chronic obstructive pulmonary disease. *Crit Care Med*. 2000;**28**:2721–2728.
43. Tassaux D, Gainnier M, Battisti A, et al. Helium-oxygen decreases inspiratory effort and work of breathing during pressure support in intubated patients with chronic obstructive pulmonary disease. *Intensive Care Med*. 2005;**31**:1501–1507.
44. Zapol WM, Kitz RJ. Buying time with artificial lungs. *N Engl J Med*. 1972;**286**:657–658.
45. Hill JD, O'Brien TG, Murray JJ, et al. Prolonged extracorporeal oxygenation for acute post-traumatic respiratory failure (shock-lung syndrome). *N Engl J Med*. 1972;**286**:629–34.
46. Zapol WM, Snider MT, Hill JD, et al. Extracorporeal membrane oxygenation in severe acute respiratory failure. A randomized prospective study. *JAMA*. 1979;**242**:2193–2196
47. Gattinoni L, Agostoni A, Pesenti A, et al. Treatment of acute respiratory failure with low-frequency positive-pressure

ventilation and extracorporeal removal of CO2. *Lancet.* 1980;**2**:292–294.
48. Peek GJ, Mugford M, Tiruvoipati R, et al. Efficacy and economic assessment of conventional ventilatory support versus extracorporeal membrane oxygenation for severe adult respiratory failure (CESAR): A multicentre randomised controlled trial. *Lancet.* 2009;**374**:1351–1363
49. Davies AR, Jones D, Bailey M, et al. Extracorporeal membrane oxygenation for 2009 influenza A(H1N1) acute respiratory distress syndrome. *JAMA.* 2009;**302**:1888–1895.
50. Patroniti N, Zangrillo A, Pappalardo F, et al. The Italian ECMO network experience during the 2009 influenza A(H1N1) pandemic: Preparation for severe respiratory emergency outbreaks. *Intensive Care Med.* 2011;**37**:1447–1457.
51. Combes A, Hajage D, Capellier G, et al. Extracorporeal Membrane Oxygenation for Severe Acute Respiratory Distress Syndrome. *N Engl J Med.* 2018;**378**:1965–1975.
52. Barbaro RP, MacLaren G, Boonstra PS, et al. Extracorporeal Life Support Organization. Extracorporeal membrane oxygenation support in COVID-19: An international cohort study of the Extracorporeal Life Support Organization registry. *Lancet.* 2020;**396**:1071–1078.
53. ELSO Adult Respiratory Failure Guidelines Extracorporeal Life Support Organization (ELSO) Guidelines for Adult Respiratory Failure ELSO Adult Respiratory Failure Guidelines. 2017. http://www.elso.med.umich.edu/guidelines.html
54. Pappalardo F, Pieri M, Greco T, et al. Predicting mortality risk in patients undergoing venovenous ECMO for ARDS due to influenza A (H1N1) pneumonia: The ECMOnet score. *Intensive Care Med.* 2013;**39**:275–281.
55. Schmidt M, Bailey M, Sheldrake J, et al. Predicting survival after extracorporeal membrane oxygenation for severe acute respiratory failure. The Respiratory Extracorporeal Membrane Oxygenation Survival Prediction (RESP) score. *Am J Respir Crit Care Med.* 2014;**189**:1374–1382.
56. Schmidt M, Zogheib E, Rozé H, et al. The PRESERVE mortality risk score and analysis of long-term outcomes after extracorporeal membrane oxygenation for severe acute respiratory distress syndrome. *Intensive Care Med.* 2013;**39**:1704–1713.
57. Hilder M, Herbstreit F, Adamzik M, et al. Comparison of mortality prediction models in acute respiratory distress syndrome undergoing extracorporeal membrane oxygenation and development of a novel prediction score: The PREdiction of Survival on ECMO Therapy-Score (PRESET-Score). *Crit Care.* 2017;**21**:301.
58. Roch A, Hraiech S, Masson E, et al. Outcome of acute respiratory distress syndrome patients treated with extracorporeal membrane oxygenation and brought to a referral center. *Intensive Care Med.* 2014;**40**:74–83.
59. Supady A, DellaVolpe J, Taccone FS, et al. Outcome prediction in patients with severe COVID-19 requiring extracorporeal membrane oxygenation—a retrospective international multicenter study. *Membranes (Basel).* 2021 Feb 27;**11**(3):170.
60. Brodie D, Bacchetta M. Extracorporeal membrane oxygenation for ARDS in adults. *N Engl J Med.* 2011;**365**:1905–1914.
61. Patroniti N, Bonatti G, Senussi T et al. Mechanical ventilation and respiratory monitoring during extracorporeal membrane oxygenation for respiratory support. *Ann Transl Med.* 2018;**6**:386
62. Amato MB, Meade MO, Slutsky AS, et al. Driving pressure and survival in the acute respiratory distress syndrome. *N Engl J Med.* 2015;**372**:747–755.
63. Paden ML, Conrad SA, Rycus PT, et al. ELSO Registry. Extracorporeal Life Support Organization Registry Report 2012. *ASAIO J.* 2013;**59**:202–210
64. Boyle AJ, Sklar MC, McNamee JJ, et al. International ECMO Network (ECMONet). Extracorporeal carbon dioxide removal for lowering the risk of mechanical ventilation: Research questions and clinical potential for the future. *Lancet Respir Med.* 2018;**6**:874–884.
65. Combes A, Fanelli V, Pham T, et al. European Society of Intensive Care Medicine Trials Group and the 'Strategy of Ultra-Protective lung ventilation with Extracorporeal CO2 Removal for New-Onset moderate to severe ARDS' (SUPERNOVA) investigators. Feasibility and safety of extracorporeal CO(2) removal to enhance protective ventilation in acute respiratory distress syndrome: The SUPERNOVA study. *Intensive Care Med.* 2019;**45**:592–600.
66. McNamee JJ, Gillies MA, Barrett NA, et al. Effect of lower tidal volume ventilation facilitated by extracorporeal carbon dioxide removal vs standard care ventilation on 90-day mortality in patients with acute hypoxemic respiratory failure: The REST randomized clinical trial. *JAMA.* 2021;**326**(11):1013–1023.
67. Singh PM, Borle A, Trikha A. Newer nonconventional modes of mechanical ventilation. *J Emerg Trauma Shock.* 2014;**7**:222–227.
68. Stock MC, Downs JB, Frolicher DA. Airway pressure release ventilation. *Crit Care Med.* 1987;**15**:462–6.
69. Mireles-Cabodevila E, Kacmarek RM. Should airway pressure release ventilation be the primary mode in ARDS? *Respir Care.* 2016;**61**:761–773.
70. Jain SV, Kollisch-Singule M, Sadowitz B, et al. The 30-year evolution of airway pressure release ventilation (APRV). *Intensive Care Med Exp.* 2016;**4**:11.
71. Andrews P, Habashi N. Airway pressure release ventilation. *Curr Probl Surg.* 2013;**50**:462–470.
72. Daoud EG, Farag HL, Chatburn RL. Airway pressure release ventilation: What do we know? *Respir Care.* 2012;**57**:282–292.
73. Lim J, Litton E, Robinson H, et al. Characteristics and outcomes of patients treated with airway pressure release ventilation for acute respiratory distress syndrome: A retrospective observational study. *J Crit Care.* 2016;**34**:154–159.
74. Tobin MJ, Mador MJ, Guenther SM, et al. Variability of resting respiratory drive and timing in healthy subjects. *J Appl Physiol.* Bethesda Md 1985. 1988;**65**:309–317.
75. Navalesi P, Longhini F. Neurally adjusted ventilatory assist. *Curr Opin Crit Care.* 2015;**21**:58–64.
76. Terzi N, Piquilloud L, Rozé H, et al. Clinical review: Update on neurally adjusted ventilatory assist—report of a round-table conference. *Crit Care Lond Engl.* 2012;**16**:225.
77. Stein H, Beck J, Dunn M. Non-invasive ventilation with neurally adjusted ventilatory assist in newborns. *Semin Fetal Neonatal Med.* 2016;**21**:154–161.
78. Gama de Abreu M, Belda FJ. Neurally adjusted ventilatory assist: Letting the respiratory center take over control of ventilation. *Intensive Care Med.* 2013;**39**:1481–1483.
79. Younes M. Proportional assist ventilation, a new approach to ventilatory support. Theory. *Am Rev Respir Dis.* 1992;**145**:114–120.
80. Valdez C, Sarani B. Proportional assist ventilation. *Curr Probl Surg.* 2013;**50**:484–488.
81. Gama de Abreu M, Spieth PM, Pelosi P, et al. Noisy pressure support ventilation: A pilot study on a new assisted ventilation mode in experimental lung injury. *Crit Care Med.* 2008;**36**:818–827.

82. Spieth PM, Carvalho AR, Güldner A, et al. Effects of different levels of pressure support variability in experimental lung injury. *Anesthesiology*. 2009;**110**:342–350.
83. Nguyen AP, Schmidt UH, MacIntyre NR. Should high-frequency ventilation in the adult be abandoned? *Respir Care*. 2016;**61**:791–800.
84. Derdak S. High-frequency oscillatory ventilation for acute respiratory distress syndrome in adult patients. *Crit Care Med*. 2003;**31**:S317–323.
85. Ng J, Ferguson ND. High-frequency oscillatory ventilation: Still a role? *Curr Opin Crit Care*. 2017;**23**:175–179.
86. Friesecke S, Stecher S-S, Abel P. High-frequency oscillation ventilation for hypercapnic failure of conventional ventilation in pulmonary acute respiratory distress syndrome. *Crit Care Lond Engl*. 2015;**19**:201.
87. Goffi A, Ferguson ND. High-frequency oscillatory ventilation for early acute respiratory distress syndrome in adults. *Curr Opin Crit Care*. 2014;**20**:77–85.
88. Schmidt J, Wenzel C, Spassov S, et al. Flow-controlled ventilation attenuates lung injury in a porcine model of acute respiratory distress syndrome: A preclinical randomized controlled study. *Crit Care Med*. 2020;**48**:e241–248.
89. Weber J, Schmidt J, Straka L, et al. Flow-controlled ventilation improves gas exchange in lung-healthy patients- a randomized interventional cross-over study. *Acta Anaesthesiol Scand*. 2020;**64**:481–488.
90. Barnes T, van Asseldonk D, Enk D. Minimisation of dissipated energy in the airways during mechanical ventilation by using constant inspiratory and expiratory flows—flow-controlled ventilation (FCV). *Med Hypotheses*. 2018;**121**:167–176.
91. Schmidt J, Günther F, Weber J, et al. Glottic visibility for laryngeal surgery: Tritube vs. microlaryngeal tube: A randomised controlled trial. *Eur J Anaesthesiol*. 2019;**36**:963–971.

PART 7

Care of the Ventilated Patient

23

Thromboprophylaxis

Emma Louise Hartley and Andrew Retter

KEY MESSAGES

- All critical care patients should have a venous thromboembolism risk assessment on admission to guide prophylaxis.
- Pharmacological prophylaxis with low molecular weight heparin is the preferred option resulting in a moderate reduction in mortality rate.
- Dose adjustment of pharmacological prophylaxis is required in extremes of weight and renal failure.
- Management of the hypercoagulable state in COVID 19 can be challenging.

CONTROVERSIES

- The role of mechanical prophylaxis versus low-molecular-weight heparin (LMWH) in non-critically and critically ill patients.
- The value of extended thromboprophylaxis in COVID-19 with a high risk of thrombosis without evidence of proven thrombosis.

FURTHER RESEARCH

- Optimal anticoagulation for critically ill patients with COVID-19.

Introduction

Venous thromboembolism (VTE), a largely preventable disease, is a major global health burden affecting over 2 in 1000 individuals annually.[1] Prior to the use of thromboprophylaxis, 59% of cases were related to hospital admission.[2] VTE risk assessment, a quality indicator from NHS England, encompasses a national screening programme on hospital admission. Subsequently, the number of deaths from VTE-related events within 90 days post discharge have shown a 20% reduction in the last 12 years.[3]

Critically ill patients are at high risk for VTE with 14% of post-mortem data showing massive or submassive pulmonary embolism.[4] Multiple risk factors exist often which predate admission. Additional risk factors acquired during admission include further immobilization, neuromuscular blockade, dialysis, vasopressors, and central venous catheterization.[5]

The UK National Institute for Clinical Excellence (NICE) recommend VTE risk assessment for all patients on admission to critical care to guide pharmacological prophylaxis.[6]

Current Accepted Practice

Pharmacological Prophylaxis with Heparin

All patients on admission to critical care should be assessed for the risk of VTE and bleeding to allow prescribing of pharmacological prophylaxis if not contraindicated. Daily review of prophylaxis should occur and more frequently if the condition of the patient is changing rapidly, to balance the risk of bleeding.[6] Pharmacological prophylaxis is continued during the in-hospital period with no requirement for extended duration treatment.[7]

Heparin—low-molecular-weight heparin (LMWH) or unfractionated heparin (UFH)—should be used as pharmacological prophylaxis in the critically care patient in preference to no anticoagulation.[7] The desirable consequences of LMWH outweigh the undesirable consequences of UFH and as such LMWH is recommended; however, alternative options may be required in renal and hepatic failure.[7]

Mechanical Prophylaxis

Mechanical prophylaxis refers to anti-embolism stockings (also termed graduated compression stockings (GCS)) or intermittent pneumatic compression (IPC) devices. In critically unwell patients not receiving pharmacological VTE prophylaxis, IPC or GCS are used. In acute stroke patients, GCS should not be offered with consideration given to IPC in those who are immobile.[6]

Anti-embolism stockings provide graduated compression to the calf; however, these should not be used in those with suspected or proven peripheral arterial disease, peripheral arterial bypass grafting, peripheral neuropathy, severe leg oedema, or any local skin condition[6]. Mechanical VTE prophylaxis should be considered for those in whom pharmacological prophylaxis is contraindicated and continued till the patient no longer has reduced immobility. Pharmacological VTE prophylaxis should be used over mechanical measures where possible with mechanical prophylaxis suggested over no VTE prophylaxis. Single prophylaxis with either mechanical or pharmacological measures is recommended over combined use[7] except in high-risk surgical patients.[8]

Aspirin and Direct Oral Anticoagulants (DOACs)

Aspirin plays a significant role in atherosclerotic disease in primary and secondary prevention, but it is less important in VTE prevention. It is associated with gastritis, haemorrhage, and a reduction in glomerular filtration, and therefore it is of high risk in the critically ill population. It results in a 25% reduction in rates of VTE, which is far less than associated with LMWH.[9]

VTE prophylaxis should still be considered for those who are already on antiplatelet agents for other conditions and for whom the risk of VTE outweighs the risk of bleeding. If the risk of VTE is high, then pharmacological prophylaxis should be used, and mechanical prophylaxis should be used if the risk of bleeding is high.[6]

LMWH should be used over DOACs for VTE prophylaxis in critical care. The caveat are patients with elective hip replacement surgery who receive either LMWH for 10 days followed by aspirin (75 or 150 mg) for a further 28 days, LMWH with anti-embolism stockings, or rivaroxaban (apixaban or dabigatran if contraindicated). Elective knee replacement guidelines are similar.[6]

Special Circumstances

If using pharmacological prophylaxis, a reduction in dose should occur in renal failure with preference for LMWH or UFH with reference to local protocols and multidisciplinary opinion. Renal failure is defined as an estimated glomerular filtration rate less than 30 mL/min/1.73 m^2.[6]

Thromboprophylaxis with LMWH is advised for those admitted to critical care with cancer. VTE prophylaxis is not offered to those receiving cancer-modifying treatments including radiotherapy, chemotherapy, or immunotherapy and who are mobile unless additional risk factors other than cancer are present (excluding myeloma and pancreatic cancer). The critical care patient as described above confers many additional risk factors for thromboembolism.

Many critically ill patients are at high risk for bleeding. Consideration should be given to pharmacological prophylaxis and contraindication in patients with active bleeding, underlying coagulopathy, thrombocytopenia ($<50 \times 10^9$/L), oral anticoagulation, or recent regional anaesthesia.

Evidence Base

Heparin for prevention of venous thromboembolism is associated with a probable reduction in absolute and relative mortality of PE and DVT without an increase in major bleeding based on systematic review data of randomized control trials.[10] LMWH, compared with UFH, has a moderate impact on mortality and VTE rate reduction with no difference in major bleeding rates. The mortality relative risk (RR) was 0.9 (95% CI: 0.75–1.08) and absolute risk reduction (ARR) was 24 fewer per 1000 (95% CI: 61 fewer to 19 more per 1000). In PE, the RR was 0.8 (95% CI: 0.44–1.46), with a baseline risk of 0.4%, ARR was 1 fewer per 1000 (95% CI: 2 fewer to 2 more per 1000).[10] The effect estimates favour LMWH use over UFH; however, the exact magnitude is unclear.[7] Extended duration of pharmacological prophylaxis has no effect on mortality and important relative effects but small absolute effects on VTE. There was an increased major bleeding rate; thus, harm is seen to outweigh net benefit.[11]

When comparing mechanical prophylaxis with pharmacological prophylaxis, there was little or no difference in mortality, a possible increase in PE and symptomatic DVT, but a reduction in major bleeding in systematic review of trauma patients and RCTs on critically ill medical patients.[7,12] However, there is low certainty about these estimated effects of pharmacological over mechanical prophylaxis and the resultant net benefit. Therefore, in patients who are at a very low risk, the burden of pharmacological prophylaxis may not be justified.

Using mechanical prophylaxis, compared with no prophylaxis, has little or no benefit on mortality (RR 0.93; 95% CI: 0.77–1.13; ARR 7 fewer per 1000; 95% CI: 24 fewer to 14 more per 1000), PE, or DVT rates when reviewing systematic review data incorporating trauma, medical, and stroke patients.[12,13] Adverse events include increased risk of falls, ulceration, and ischaemia, and although important they are not critical for decision-making. The small possible benefits outweigh the less important potential harm or burden, particularly in patients with a higher risk for VTE, who may have an increased ARR rate.

The addition of pharmacological to mechanical prophylaxis may reduce mortality (RR 0.50; 95% CI: 0.05–5.30; ARR 4 fewer per 1000; 95% CI: 8 fewer to 34 more per 1000), PE, and DVT, but the estimates are uncertain. The data used for this involved indirect evidence from trauma and stroke patients.[12,13] Major bleeding may be increased with combined therapy (RR 2.83; 95% CI: 0.30–26.7; ARR 51 more major bleeding events per 1000; 95% CI: 2 fewer to 720 more per 1000). Given the low certainty of the evidence, the risks associated with combined therapy outweigh the benefit and is therefore not recommended except in the high-risk surgical patient.

Limited evidence is available on IPC compared with GCS in VTE prophylaxis with only one RCT addressing the topic.[14] This study had few participants and a low number of events (1 death, 1 PE, and 3 DVTs), and as such the benefits of one option over the other cannot be ascertained. However, this is in contrast to acute stroke patients where GCS are associated with a reduction in the DVT rate but also harm from skin damage.[15] Use of IPC in this population has shown a reduction in the proximal DVT rate from 12.1% to 8.5% without the associated morbidity.[16]

Use of a DOAC (apixaban, rivaroxaban, or betrixaban) for prophylaxis probably has no impact on VTE-related mortality (RR 0.64; 95% CI: 0.21–1.98; ARR 0 fewer deaths per 1000; 95% CI: 1 fewer to 1 more per 1000) when compared to LMWH after review in three RCTs.[17] There is little impact on rates of VTE; however, an increased rate of major bleeding exists. Data was also analyzed whether extended DOAC use (30–42 days) versus non-DOAC in hospital prophylaxis provided any benefit. This resulted in no impact on mortality, a reduction in RR of PE, but again led to an increased risk of major bleeding (RR 1.99; 95% CI: 1.08–3.65). Given the increased risk of bleeding in both standard and extended durations, they are not recommended for VTE prophylaxis.

Physiology and Pharmacology

Unfractionated Heparin

Heparin, a sulphated polysaccharide, produces its anticoagulant effect by binding to antithrombin and potentiating its activity. This results in inactivation of a number of coagulation factors (thrombin,

Xa, IXa, Xia, and XIIa) and preventing fibrinogen converting to fibrin. There is often a variable anticoagulant response as heparin can bind to positively charged proteins, and therefore the monitoring of activated partial thromboplastin time (APTT) is required with frequent dose adjusting thereafter. The results of APTT can vary due to the different responsiveness of reagents to heparin, and therefore therapeutic ranges should be tailored accordingly. Standardization can be achieved by calibrating against an anti-Xa assay.[18]

Routes of administration include intravenously (IV) and subcutaneously (SC). With the use of a continuous IV infusion and bolus dose, the onset is immediate; however, in SC doses the anticoagulant effect is delayed for 1 h and peak plasma levels occur at 3 h.[18] It is metabolized through rapid saturable clearance and slow first-order mechanisms. Half-life is dependent on dosing, very short at lower doses with slower elimination at higher levels resulting in a longer half-life. Effects of UFH can be reversed with protamine.[18]

Heparin-induced thrombocytopenia (HIT) results from its binding to platelet factor 4 forming an antigen complex. IgG antibodies are formed, which bind with the antigen complex (Type 2 HIT) resulting in platelet activation and aggregation resulting in activation of the coagulation cascade and thrombosis.[19] The effect of HIT is greater with UFH than LMWH. Heparin should be stopped on confirmation of HIT and anticoagulation with a direct thrombin inhibitor instituted.

Heparin resistance occurs when high levels of heparin (>35,000 units/24 h) are required to achieve a therapeutic APTT. It can be related to antithrombin deficiency, increased heparin clearance, elevations in heparin binding proteins, or elevations in factor VIII. Management involves titrating to anti-Xa target levels (which has been shown to give lower heparin doses compared with APTT use even in heparin resistance), substitution to LMWH, and measurement of antithrombin III levels with replacement if deficient.[20]

LMWH

LMWH has a significantly smaller molecular weight compared to UFH and is derived from heparin by chemical or enzymatic depolymerization. It has a more predictable dose–response relationship and a longer half-life allowing once daily dosing. LMWH binds to antithrombin III inactivating factor Xa, with less ability to inactivate antithrombin than UFH. They are renally cleared with a prolonged half-life in patients with renal failure, therefore requiring a dose reduction. Laboratory monitoring is usually not required; however, in morbid obesity and renal failure the dose is difficult to determine. The anti-Xa assay (taken 4 h post dose) has been used in these cases to determine therapeutic levels.[18]

Mechanical Prophylaxis

The major benefits of IPC or GCS are the lack of requirement for systemic anticoagulation. IPCs rely on a pump that inflates and deflates air bladders periodically within a cuff that is around the limb. Variability exists with uniform or sequential inflation, different pressures, and can be for foot, calf, or whole leg. They squeeze blood from deep veins displacing it proximally preventing against stasis and DVT formation. On deflation of the pump, the veins will refill and the process repeats.[21]

GCS apply a constant pressure throughout the length of the limb, so reducing venous stasis, facilitating venous return, and maintenance of a reduced venous calibre, all reducing risk of DVT.[21] They provide the greatest degree of compression at the ankle with pressure reducing gradually up the stocking. Different degrees of compression are available.

Thromboprophylaxis in Covid-19 infection

COVID-19 coagulopathy is a distinct hypercoagulable disorder secondary to the SARS-CoV2 virus. It results from endothelial dysfunction, inflammation, and microvascular thrombi, leading to increased rates of thromboembolism. Thromboembolism is seen in up to 31% (95% CI: 20–41) of the critical care population, of which Computed tomography pulmonary angiogram (CTPA) and/or ultrasonography confirmed VTE in 27% (95% CI: 17%–37%) and arterial thrombotic events in 3.7% (95% CI: 0%–8.2%) despite prophylactic anticoagulation.[22] Given the increased risk of VTE, more aggressive thromboprophylaxis anticoagulant dosing is considered.

High-quality data in the form of randomized control trials does not exist for targeting venous thromboprophylaxis in this group; however, various international guidelines have been developed.[23] Therapeutic anticoagulation is not recommended for the prevention of thrombotic complications; however, intermediate dosing should be considered. Intermediate dose anticoagulation at double the standard prophylactic dose of LMWH is recommenced for the critical care of COVID-19 patients by the UK Intensive Care Society Guidelines.[24] LMWH or UFH can be used; however, LMWH is associated with some advantages, including once daily regimes and reduced incidence of HIT. Whichever regimen is chosen, careful consideration should be given to the competing risks of thrombosis and bleeding with adjustments made for extremes of weight, thrombocytopenia, and renal failure. In patients with AKI or creatinine clearance <15–30 mL/min, the use of UFH has been suggested.[23]

Mechanical prophylaxis should be considered in addition to pharmacological prophylaxis if no contraindication is present, which includes the use of IPC devices. Mechanical prophylaxis should be used alone when pharmacological prophylaxis is contraindicated.[23]

Controversies and Future Practice

The evidence available for interpreting the effect of venous thromboembolism prophylaxis and guideline formation is limited. The data analyzed for non-COVID-19 patients incorporates older studies that may not be relevant to the current critically ill population given changes in illness severity and length of stay. The current data provides little information with regard to benefit of mechanical prophylaxis with LMWH the preferred option.[7]

More studies are required to guide optimal dosing in the critically ill patients, particularly in those with different baseline risks, obesity, underweight patients, renal failure, and in COVID-19 disease. The baseline risk is important to assess in terms of bleeding and thrombosis risk, which may change over the critical care period and better inform decisions regarding mechanical and pharmacological prophylaxis.

The search continues for the ideal thromboprophylactic agent in this complex group of critically ill patients. Despite the risks associated with LMWH, the benefit far outweighs the harm and is currently the agent of choice.

REFERENCES

1. ISTH Steering Committee for World Thrombosis Day. Thrombosis: A major contributor to the global disease burden. *J Thromb Haemost*. 2014;**12**(10):1580–1590.
2. Heit JA, O'Fallon WM, Petterson TM, et al. Relative impact of risk factors for deep vein thrombosis and pulmonary embolism: A population-based study. *Arch Intern Med*. 2002;**162**(11):1245–1248.
3. NHS Outcomes Framework Indicators. Data set 5.1 deaths from venous thromboembolism (VTE) related events within 90 days post discharge from hospital. NHS Digital February 2022;3–11. https://digital.nhs.uk/data-and-information/publications/clinical-indicators/nhs-outcomes-framework/current/domain-5-treating-and-caring-for-people-in-a-safe-environment-and-protecting-them-from-avoidable-harm-nof/5-1-deaths-from-venous-thromboembolism-vte-related-events-within-90-days-post-discharge-from-hospital.
4. Berlot G, Calderan C, Vergolini A, et al. Pulmonary embolism in critically ill patients receiving antithrombotic prophylaxis: a clinical-pathologic study. *J Crit Care*. 2011;**26**(1):28–33.
5. Cook D, Crowther M, Meade M, et al. Deep venous thrombosis in medical-surgical critically ill patients: Prevalence, incidence, and risk factors. *Crit Care Med*. 2005;**33**(7):1565–1571.
6. National Institute for Health and Care Excellence. Venous thromboembolism in over 16s: Reducing the risk of hospital-acquired deep vein thrombosis or pulmonary embolism. 2018; 1–47. Clinical guideline NG89. www.nice.org.uk/guidance/ng89
7. Schunemann HJ, Cushman M, Burnett AE, et al. American Society of Hematology 2018 guidelines for management of venous thromboembolism: Prophylaxis for hospitalized and nonhospitalized medical patients. *Blood Adv*. 2018;**2**(22):3198–3225.
8. Anderson DR, Morgano GP, Bennett C, et al. American Society of Hematology 2019 guidelines for management of venous thromboembolism: Prevention of venous thromboembolism in surgical hospitalized patients. *Blood Adv*. 2019;**3**(23):3898–3944.
9. Watson HG, Chee YL. Aspirin and other antiplatelet drugs in the prevention of venous thromboembolism. *Blood Rev*. 2008;**22**(2):107–116.
10. Alhazzani W, Lim W, Jaeschke RZ, et al. Heparin thromboprophylaxis in medical-surgical critically ill patients: A systematic review and meta-analysis of randomized trials. *Crit Care Med*. 2013;**41**(9):2088–2098.
11. Hull RD, Schellong SM, Tapson VF, et al. Extended-duration venous thromboembolism prophylaxis in acutely ill medical patients with recently reduced mobility: A randomized trial. *Ann Intern Med*. 2010;**153**(1):8–18.
12. Barrera LM, Perel P, Ker K, et al. Thromboprophylaxis for trauma patients. *Cochrane Database Syst Rev*. **2013**(3):CD008303.
13. Naccarato M, Chiodo Grandi F, et al. Physical methods for preventing deep vein thrombosis in stroke. *Cochrane Database Syst Rev*. 2010(8) Aug 4;1–23:CD001922.
14. Salzman EW, Sobel M, Lewis J, et al. Prevention of venous thromboembolism in unstable angina pectoris. *N Engl J Med*. 1982;**306**(16):991.
15. Collaboration CT, Dennis M, Sandercock P, et al. Effectiveness of intermittent pneumatic compression in reduction of risk of deep vein thrombosis in patients who have had a stroke (CLOTS 3): A multicentre randomised controlled trial. *Lancet*. 2013;**382**(9891):516–524.
16. Collaboration CT, Dennis M, Sandercock PA, et al. Effectiveness of thigh-length graduated compression stockings to reduce the risk of deep vein thrombosis after stroke (CLOTS trial 1): A multicentre, randomised controlled trial. *Lancet*. 2009;**373**(9679):1958–1965.
17. Goldhaber SZ, Leizorovicz A, Kakkar AK, et al. Apixaban versus enoxaparin for thromboprophylaxis in medically ill patients. *N Engl J Med*. 2011;**365**(23):2167–2177.
18. Hirsh J, Warkentin TE, Shaughnessy SG, et al. Heparin and low-molecular-weight heparin: Mechanisms of action, pharmacokinetics, dosing, monitoring, efficacy, and safety. *Chest*. 2001;**119**(1 Suppl):64S–94S.
19. Franchini M. Heparin-induced thrombocytopenia: An update. *Thromb J*. 2005;**3**:14.
20. Lemmer JH, Jr., Despotis GJ. Antithrombin III concentrate to treat heparin resistance in patients undergoing cardiac surgery. *J Thorac Cardiovasc Surg*. 2002;**123**(2):213–217.
21. Morris RJ, Woodcock JP. Intermittent pneumatic compression or graduated compression stockings for deep vein thrombosis prophylaxis? A systematic review of direct clinical comparisons. *Ann Surg*. 2010;**251**(3):393–396.
22. Klok FA, Kruip M, van der Meer NJM, et al. Incidence of thrombotic complications in critically ill ICU patients with COVID-19. *Thromb Res*. 2020;**191**:145–147.
23. Flaczyk A, Rosovsky RP, Reed CT, et al. Comparison of published guidelines for management of coagulopathy and thrombosis in critically ill patients with COVID 19: Implications for clinical practice and future investigations. *Crit Care*. 2020;**24**(1):559.
24. Intensive Care Medicine Anaesthesia COVID-19 Guideline Development Group. Clinical guide for the management of critical care for adults with COVID-19 during the Coronavirus pandemic. Jointly published by The Faculty of Intensive Care Medicine, The Intensive Care Society, The Association of Anaesthetists and The Royal College of Anaesthetists. 28 October 2020. https://static1.squarespace.com/static/5e6613a1dc75b87df82b78e1/t/5f999cd5b3df86542e85d0ab/1603902680560/AdultCriticalCare-COVID-19-October2020.pdf

24

Fluid Balance

Hollmann D Aya and Maurizio Cecconi

KEY MESSAGES

- Fluid balance describes a pragmatic approach to monitor the total fluid status. Fluid overload is the percentage increase in body weight due to fluid and can be associated with organ dysfunction.
- Fluid balance is a relative measure taken from an uncalibrated zero point.
- Positive fluid balance has been associated with poor clinical outcomes in critical illness. However, it is unclear if this association is truly linked with the fluid balance or with other confounders.
- Fluid balance cannot be interpreted in isolation. Proactive strategies to achieve a negative balance should not compromise organ perfusion.

CONTROVERSIES

- The definition of 'fluid balance' as well as that of 'fluid overload' relies on the assumption that patients have a physiological neutral fluid balance on admission, which is often not the case.
- Fluid balance calculations are not always adjusted by non-measurable losses and are often inaccurate.
- Are poor outcomes associated with a positive fluid balance dependent on the type of fluid: colloids versus crystalloids or blood products?
- The timing of administration of fluids and outcomes is debated: early fluid resuscitation versus over a longer duration.
- Association between positive fluid balance and negative outcomes does not necessarily mean causality. Other confounders relate to the indication of fluid administration, for instance hypotension, hyperlactaemia, or oligoanuria; all of them also associated with poor outcomes. Furthermore, the exact mechanism that explains the deleterious effect of fluid overload is still unclear.

FURTHER RESEARCH

- Mechanisms underlying the deleterious effects of fluid overload on patient outcomes.
- The mechanisms that different fluid types have on the outcomes of fluid overload.

Introduction

Fluid therapy is one of the commonest interventions in intensive care units. The benefits of this therapy are well recognized, mainly in the context of resuscitation of patients in cardiovascular shock or in the process of haemodynamic optimization of patients after high-risk surgery. However, at certain point, fluid administration may become harmful. There is growing evidence that over-administration of intravenous fluid in critically ill patients is associated with poor outcomes. However, there is still uncertainty about the optimal dose, type and timing for fluid therapy, and duration of the effect of this intervention. For those reasons, the fluid balance is currently used at the bedside as a tool to monitor fluid administration and to avoid fluid overload and its undesired effects.

Current Accepted Practice

Definition of Fluid Balance

'Fluid balance' refers to the volume of fluid held in the body that represents the difference between the volume gained and lost during a defined period of time. The fluid balance chart is an input/output chart that documents everything a patient has taken (i.e. fluids ingested, enteral feeds, intravenous fluids, blood products, total parenteral nutrition and oral nutritional supplement drinks, and oral medication and intravenous medications) and what has been lost (i.e. nasogastric drainage, wound drains, vomit, rectal drainage, urine, and colostomy output) over a 24 h period.

Ideally, this information is crucial for fluid management, when considered alongside assessment of the cardiovascular system, oxygen requirements, presence of subcutaneous oedema, changes in body weight, and the subjective experience of the patient (feeling thirsty) when possible. In practice, this information is not always accurate and often ignores how well hydrated the patient was at baseline.

Fluid overload is defined by a percentage increase in body weight from day of admission and is associated with some degree of organ dysfunction such as pulmonary or peripheral oedema. A cut-off of

10% has been associated with increased mortality.[1] Fluid overload can be calculated as follows:

Fluid overload (%) = fluid balance (L)/admission body weight (kg) × 100.

Evidence Base

Acute Respiratory Distress Syndrome

There are several studies that suggest that a positive fluid balance is associated with acute lung injury (ALI) and acute respiratory distress syndrome (ARDS). Rosenberg et al.,[2] in a secondary analysis of a prospective cohort study, observed that negative cumulative fluid balance at day 4 of ALI is associated with significantly lower mortality, independent of severity of illness. Patients with fluid overload had more risk of respiratory failure, sepsis, and more ventilator days. Wiedemann et al.[3] reported the ARDSnet trial comparing two fluid-management strategies (conservative and liberal) in 1000 patients with ARDS. There was no mortality difference at 60 days (primary outcome). However, the conservative strategy improved the oxygenation index, the lung injury score, ventilator-free days (14.6 vs 12.1 days, $P < 0.001$), and length of stay in ICU (13.4 vs 11.2 days, $P < 0.001$) without increasing non-pulmonary organ failures.

Acute Renal Failure

Fluid overload is also associated with higher mortality in patients with acute kidney injury (AKI), adjusted for severity of illness. Bellomo and colleagues[4] studied the association between daily fluid balance and outcomes in 1453 critically ill patients receiving renal replacement therapy (RRT) in the RENAL study. Patients with negative fluid balance had lower severity of illness, were less likely to be hypotensive, and had lower APACHE and cardiovascular SOFA scores. Even so, after adjustment for these differences, a negative daily fluid balance portended markedly reduced risk of death at 90 days (adjusted odds ratio (OR) = 0.31; 95% CI: 0.24–0.43; $P < 0.0001$). These patients also had more days free of RRT, more ventilator-free days, and more ICU-free and hospital-free days compared to those with a positive fluid balance. Other studies have reported similar results. Payen et al.[5] in a secondary analysis of the sepsis occurrence in acute ill patients (SOAP) compared patients with and without AKI. AKI was defined by a renal sequential organ failure assessment score of 2 or greater, or by urine output under 500 mL/day. A total of 36% (1120 out of 3147) patients developed AKI, with 75% of episodes occurring within first 2 days of ICU admission. Average daily fluid balance was significantly higher in non-survivors than in survivors (1000 mL vs 150 mL; $P < 0.001$). The multivariable analysis reveals a 54% adjusted risk of death at 60 days in patients with AKI and a mean positive fluid balance (hazard ratio = 1.21; 95% CI: 1.13–1.28). Bouchard et al.[1] found that fluid overload at cessation of RRT was associated with increased risk death at 60 days even after adjustment for severity of illness and modality of dialysis (OR = 2.52; 95% CI: 1.55–4.08) in a post hoc analysis of the Program to Improve Care in Acute Renal Disease study. Grams et al.[6] reported that a positive fluid balance remained significantly associated with 60-day mortality (adjusted OR = 1.61 per L/d; 95% CI: 1.29–2.00), after adjusting for severity of illness, demographics, fluid strategy, mean daily central venous pressure and shock in patients from the Fluid and Catheter Treatment Trial (FACTT).

Sepsis

Fluid balance has also an impact in patients with sepsis. The management of patients with sepsis is mainly based on treating or eliminating the source of infection, the use of appropriate antimicrobial agents, and haemodynamic and other physiologic supportive measures. Pathophysiologically, sepsis results in a generalized systemic endothelial injury with increased capillary permeability, tissue oedema, and relative intravascular volume depletion in addition to vasodilation. Therapy of this syndrome includes the administration of relatively large amounts of fluid in an attempt to replete the intravascular space and stabilize the haemodynamics. Boyd et al.[7] conducted a retrospective review of the use of IV fluids during the first 4 days of care in 778 patients enrolled in the VASST study with septic shock and at least 5 mcg/min of noradrenaline. After correcting by age and the APACHE II score, a more positive fluid balance both at 12 h and at day 4 correlated significantly with increased mortality.

This evidence suggests that positive fluid balance is associated with higher mortality in septic shock. However, association does not confirm causality. Therefore, a logical question is: are those patients retaining fluid because they are dying, or they are dying because they are retaining fluids? In the first case, the therapeutic efforts should probably focus on the underlying cause of death, whereas, in the second case, efforts should be made to reverse fluid overload. In the trial reported by Wiedemann et al.,[3] no differences were found in mortality between conservative and liberal strategy of fluid administration in ARDS. Moreover, in a sub-study of this trial, Mikkelsen et al.[8] assessed the neuropsychological function at 2- and 12-month post-hospital discharge in survivors of ARDS. Out of 406 eligible survivors, they consented 213. They found that after adjustment for potential covariates, lower PaO_2 and enrolment in the conservative fluid-management strategy were independently associated with cognitive impairment at 12 months. A 'conservative' fluid strategy, then, may induce tissue hypoperfusion and long-term adverse outcomes. However, this study has limited external validity. Similarly, in a post hoc study of patients with traumatic brain injury recruited into the Saline versus Albumin Fluid Evaluation (SAFE) trial,[9] fluid resuscitation with albumin was associated with higher mortality rates than was resuscitation with saline. The albumin group received significantly less fluid than did patients in the saline group in the first 48 h, with a less positive fluid balance. Hjortrup et al.[10] assessed the effects of restricting resuscitation fluid (fluid challenges) after initial resuscitation. They randomized 151 adult patients with septic shock who had received initial fluid resuscitation. In the fluid restriction group, fluid boluses were permitted only if signs of severe hypoperfusion occurred, while in the standard care group, fluid boluses were permitted as long as circulation continued to improve. Although the fluid used for resuscitation was significantly reduced in the restriction group, there were no differences in terms of total fluid input or cumulative fluid balance. Similarly, patient-centred outcomes (such as death by day 90, ischaemic events in ICU, or worsening AKI) trended towards benefit with fluid restriction but non-significant statistically. Malbrain et al.[11] conducted a systematic review of the association between positive fluid balance and outcomes of critically ill patients. A restrictive fluid-management strategy was associated with a lower mortality compared to more liberal fluid strategy (24.7% vs 33.2%; OR = 0.42; 95% CI: 0.32–0.55; $P < 0.0001$). However, the interpretation of this meta-analysis is difficult, given the different types of studies selected.

Overall, there is not clear evidence that therapeutic interventions to reduce the fluid balance are effective in improving clinical outcomes.

Physiology and Pharmacology

Body fluid accounts for 55% of total body mass in women and 60% in men. Between 45% and 75% of this mass is water. Body fluid distributes in two compartments: intracellular fluid (ICF), which accounts for approximately 67% of total body fluid, and extracellular fluid (ECF), which accounts for 33% of total body fluid. The ECF is also distributed between the interstitial fluid (or extravascular volume) and plasma (intravascular volume). Interstitial fluid makes up 80% of the total ECF, which means that only about 7% of the total body fluid is in the intravascular space. Small volumes of ECF can also be found in cerebral spinal fluid, synovial fluid, and gastrointestinal secretions (saliva, gastric fluid, gall bladder, etc.).

ICF volume is mainly regulated by the cellular membrane, which allows some substances to diffuse freely while others require use of pumps across the membrane using active transport requiring adenosine triphosphate. Key electrolytes such as sodium, potassium, or calcium are moved across the cell membrane in this way.

However, most of fluid shifts occur in the ECF, which is divided by the capillary wall. This wall is composed of a unicellular layer of endothelial cells and is surrounded by a thin basement membrane on the outside of the capillary. Between endothelial cells, there are gaps called intercellular clefts. These are thin-slit curving channels through which fluid can circulate freely. The cleft is normally 6–7 nm wide, just slightly smaller than the diameter of an albumin protein. Vascular endothelial cells are protected from direct exposure to flowing blood by the glycocalyx, a highly hydrated mesh of membrane-associated glycosaminoglycans, glycoproteins, proteoglycans, and glycolipids. The glycocalyx structure on the luminal surface of microvascular endothelium is essential to prevent tissue oedema.[12]

The interstitial fluid has the same composition than plasma but much lower concentration of proteins. This interstitial space contains two major types of solid structures: collagen fibre bundles and proteoglycan filaments. The interstitial fluid is almost totally entrapped among the proteoglycan filaments and has the consistency of a gel. Occasionally, small rivulets of free fluid and small free fluid vesicles are also present. This free fluid is minimal in normal tissues. When a tissue develops oedema, this free fluid is expanded tremendously.

There are four primary forces that determine fluid movement through the capillary wall, also known as 'Starling forces':

1. The capillary hydrostatic pressure: which forces fluid outwards the capillaries.
2. The interstitial hydrostatic pressure: in loose subcutaneous tissue, this pressure is usually subatmospheric (about −3 mmHg); in tissues that are surrounded by capsules (i.e. kidneys, brain, and muscles), this pressure is positive.
3. The capillary plasma colloid osmotic pressure: which tends to force fluid inwards through the capillary membrane.
4. The interstitial fluid colloid osmotic pressure: which tends to force fluid outwards the capillary membrane.

Under normal conditions, all these forces are in a state of near-equilibrium: the amount of fluid filtering outwards form the arterial ends of capillaries equals almost exactly the amount of fluid returning to the circulation by absorption. The minimal difference is eventually returned to the circulation via the lymphatic system. The capillary filtration is also dependent on the permeability of the capillary wall (filtration coefficient), which varies among different tissues (minimal in brain, moderately large in subcutaneous tissue, large in the intestine, and very large in liver and kidney).[13]

From these concepts, it follows that small changes in the mean capillary pressure or in the capillary wall permeability will easily break the fine balance of the capillary filtration. The endothelial wall permeability and the oncotic pressure are variables not easy to manipulate. Hence, a negative fluid balance aims to reduce the intravascular volume, thus reducing the capillary hydrostatic pressure in order to get a net inwards flow through the capillary membrane. Then, the intravascular fluid can be eliminated by diuresis or RRT. The problem lies in the fact that a fluid balance is relative measure taken from an uncalibrated zero point. In other words, a neutral balance does not necessarily mean that the patient is euvolaemic. Hence, a parameter of intravascular filling independent of cardiac function has been investigated in intensive care patients: the mean systemic filling pressure (P_{msf}). This is the pressure in the cardiovascular system when there is no blood flow. Therefore, it depends on the intravascular volume and the total mean capacitance of the systemic vascular system. But when the heart is beating, the value of the P_{msf} is very close to the value of the pressure at venous side of the capillaries. P_{msf} has been investigated in critically ill patients, and values between 18 and 24 mmHg have been reported.[14,15] Several studies have investigated the effect of intravascular fluids on P_{msf}. A fluid challenge increases P_{msf} analogue (P_{msa}) similarly in fluid responders and non-responders, but this effect is transitory and returns to baseline in about 10 min.[16] In addition, the volumes used for a fluid challenge significantly affect the changes in the P_{msf} arm (a surrogate of the P_{msf}) and also the changes in cardiac output and the proportion of responders and non-responders.[17] Little is known about the impact of the values of P_{msf} in clinical outcomes of critically ill patients. Samoni et al.[18] proposed another way to measure fluid overload and hydration status using bioelectrical impedance vector analysis (BIVA) as a percentage of lean body mass. They observed a heterogeneous cohort of 125 patients admitted to intensive care. The cumulative fluid balance and the level of hydration were measured. Severe hyperhydration measured by BIVA was the only variable found to be significantly associated with ICU mortality (OR = 22.91; 95% CI: 2.38–220.07; $P < 0.01$). Regardless of the limitations of this study, it is a good example of how to use innovative technology to assess hydration and fluid overload in an objective fashion in critically ill patients.

Controversies and Future Practice

The association between a positive fluid balance with poor clinical outcomes is not exempt of controversy. There are several points that need to be addressed:

The definition of 'fluid balance' as well as that of 'fluid overload' relies on the assumption that patients were on a physiological neutral fluid balance on admission, which is often not the case. A 'positive' fluid balance may represent only returning to an euvolaemic state in an initially hypovolaemic patient.

Fluid balance calculations are not always adjusted by non-measurable losses, are often inaccurate, and do not provide information about the intravascular fluid state.

It is still unclear if the association of a positive fluid balance with poor outcomes depends on the specific type of fluid: different results could be observed using colloids rather than crystalloids or blood products.

The timing of administration of fluids is also a focus of debate. A positive fluid balance during the first 24 h of admission may have completely different consequences compared with the same fluid balance observed over a longer period of days.

Positive fluid balance can result from excessive fluid administration, oliguria, or both. This has important clinical consequences as oliguria may reflect AKI and may need RRT to correct the fluid imbalance. This represents a very important confounder in the association with clinical outcomes.

Association between positive fluid balance and negative outcomes does not necessarily mean causality. It is unclear if this association is truly linked with the fluid balance or if there are other confounders related to the indication of fluid administration, for instance hypotension, hyperlactaemia, or oligoanuria, all of them are also associated with poor outcomes. Furthermore, the exact mechanism that explains the deleterious effect of fluid overload is still unclear. Whether it is mediated by decreased oxygenation, by impairment of cellular membrane signalling, by decreased clearance of metabolism products, or other mechanisms requires further investigation.

Nevertheless, given the growing body of literature suggesting that 'excessive' fluid administration is associated with poor outcomes, especially at the time when organ ischaemia is not present or organ failure is already established, it seems reasonable reassessing the risk–benefit equation before prescription of further IV fluids. We would suggest keeping in mind two principles:

1. Fluid balance should never be interpreted in isolation but together with other clinical and biochemical information.
2. The use of proactive strategies to achieve a negative balance should be carefully implemented to avoid compromising organ perfusion.

REFERENCES

1. Bouchard J, Soroko SB, Chertow GM, et al. Program to Improve Care in Acute Renal Disease Study G. Fluid accumulation, survival and recovery of kidney function in critically ill patients with acute kidney injury. *Kidney Int.* 2009;**76**(4):422–427.
2. Rosenberg AL, Dechert RE, Network NNA, et al. Review of a large clinical series: Association of cumulative fluid balance on outcome in acute lung injury: A retrospective review of the ARDSnet tidal volume study cohort. *J Intensive Care Med.* 2009;**24**(1):35–46.
3. National Heart, Lung, and Blood Institute Acute Respiratory Distress Syndrome Clinical Trials Network, Wiedemann HP, Wheeler AP, et al. Comparison of two fluid-management strategies in acute lung injury. *N Engl J Med.* 2006; **354**(24):2564–2575.
4. Investigators RRTS, Bellomo R, Cass A, et al. An observational study fluid balance and patient outcomes in the Randomized Evaluation of Normal vs. Augmented Level of Replacement Therapy trial. *Crit Care Med.* 2012;**40**(6):1753–1760.
5. Payen D, de Pont AC, Sakr Y, et al. A positive fluid balance is associated with a worse outcome in patients with acute renal failure. *Crit Care.* 2008;**12**(3):R74.
6. Grams ME, Estrella MM, Coresh J, et al. Fluid balance, diuretic use, and mortality in acute kidney injury. Clin J Am Soc Nephrol. 2011;**6**(5):966–973.
7. Boyd JH, Forbes J, Nakada TA, et al. Fluid resuscitation in septic shock: A positive fluid balance and elevated central venous pressure are associated with increased mortality. *Crit Care Med.* 2011;**39**(2):259–265.
8. Mikkelsen ME, Christie JD, Lanken PN, et al. The adult respiratory distress syndrome cognitive outcomes study: Long-term neuropsychological function in survivors of acute lung injury. *Am J Respir Crit Care Med.* 2012;**185**(12):1307–1315.
9. Finfer S, Bellomo R, SAFE Study Investigators, et al. A comparison of albumin and saline for fluid resuscitation in the intensive care unit. *N Engl J Med.* 2004;**350**(22):2247–2256.
10. Hjortrup PB, CLASSIC Trial Group, Scandinavian Critical Care Trials Group, et al. Restricting volumes of resuscitation fluid in adults with septic shock after initial management: The CLASSIC randomised, parallel-group, multicentre feasibility trial. *Intensive Care Med.* 2016;**42**(11):1695–1705.
11. Malbrain ML, Marik PE, Witters I, et al. Fluid overload, de-resuscitation, and outcomes in critically ill or injured patients: A systematic review with suggestions for clinical practice. *Anaesthesiol Intensive Ther.* 2014;**46**(5):361–380.
12. van den Berg BM, Vink H, Spaan JA. The endothelial glycocalyx protects against myocardial edema. *Circ Res.* 2003;**92**(6):592–594.
13. Guyton AC. *Textbook of Medical Physiology.* 11th ed. Philadelphia: Elsevier Saunders; 2006.
14. Cecconi M, Aya HD, Geisen M, et al. Changes in the mean systemic filling pressure during a fluid challenge in postsurgical intensive care patients. *Intensive Care Med.* 2013;**39**(7):1299–1305.
15. Aya HD, Rhodes A, Fletcher N, et al. Transient stop-flow arm arterial-venous equilibrium pressure measurement: Determination of precision of the technique. *J Clin Monit Comput.* 2016 Feb;**30**(1):55–61. doi:10.1007/s10877-015-9682-y. Epub 2015 Mar 7.
16. Aya HD, Ster IC, Fletcher N, et al. Pharmacodynamic analysis of a fluid challenge. *Crit Care Med.* 2016; **44**(5):880–891.
17. Aya HD, Rhodes A, Ster IC, et al. Hemodynamic effect of different doses of fluids for a fluid challenge: A quasi-randomized controlled study. *Crit Care Med.* 2017 Feb;**45**(2):e161–e168. doi:10.1097/CCM.0000000000002067.
18. Samoni S, Vigo V, Resendiz LI, et al. Impact of hyperhydration on the mortality risk in critically ill patients admitted in intensive care units: Comparison between bioelectrical impedance vector analysis and cumulative fluid balance recording. *Crit Care.* 2016;**20**:95.

25

Sedation, Analgesia, and Paralysis

Yahya Shehabi and Maja M Green

KEY MESSAGES

- Clinical practice guidelines, albeit following comprehensive evidence reviews, share many limitations when applied to the management of individual patients.
- Novel coronavirus-induced respiratory failure (COVID-19) and the subsequent need for ventilatory support present significant challenges when applying the conventional approach to sedation management.
- Clinical trials comparing sedative agents and different sedation protocols do not show superiority of one agent or a particular sedation protocol over usual practice.
- Sedation intensity, proportionate to the complexity of mechanical ventilation, should be given to provide comfort and facilitate early weaning.
- Individual patient's symptom-oriented multimodal analgesia/sedation approach is preferred over a general protocol for all patients; one size does not fit all.
- Patient- and illness-related factors should be carefully considered in the choice of a specific sedative agent and a sedation depth for a specific clinical scenario.
- Moderate or deep sedation should only be provided for the shortest possible time when clinically indicated. Light sedation should be provided at the earliest clinically feasible time.

CONTROVERSIES

- Should patients needing complex ventilatory management, such as prone ventilation, be paralyzed? How is analgo-sedation best titrated in this context?
- Is there an ideal sedative agent to use? Should benzodiazepines be avoided?
- Despite recommendations by guidelines, why do clinicians continue to use deeper levels of sedation particularly in the early phase of critical illness?

FURTHER RESEARCH

- Evaluate the effect of age on relevant outcomes with different sedative agents such as dexmedetomidine and propofol.
- Evaluate the impact of targeted light sedation in prognostically enriched critically ill populations such as medical versus surgical and vasopressor-dependent versus non-shocked patients.
- What clinical outcomes should be used in future sedation trials? Is mortality the right outcome?

Introduction

Providing sedation and pain relief is an integral part of caring for critically ill patients to provide comfort, prevent distress, agitation, and facilitate therapeutic interventions. Published clinical practice guidelines recognize the need to optimize sedation and analgesic management to improve patient outcomes.[1,2,3] Different guidelines have focused on delivering effective analgesia, minimal sedation, and integrated patient-centred care.

The goals of sedation and analgesia in ventilated patient are as follows:

(1) Facilitate appropriate ventilatory support, and customize and adapt to the individual patient's requirements: to reduce ventilator dyssynchrony, allow a high positive end-expiratory pressure (PEEP) if needed, and to induce paralysis safely and/or tolerate prone ventilation.
(2) Maintain a comfortable, calm, and cooperative patient as much as is clinically feasible and whenever possible.
(3) Reduce emergence agitation and/or delirium with considered choice of sedatives and sedation depth.
(4) Facilitate liberation from mechanical ventilation and early access to physical and cognitive rehabilitation.

Supporting Evidence

Limitations of Clinical Practice Guidelines

Clinical practice guidelines, including the updated 2018 **P**ain, **A**gitation/**S**edation, **D**elirium, **I**mmobility (rehabilitation/mobilization), and **S**leep (disruption) (PADIS-2018) guidelines,[4] the Liberation from ICU approach[5] promoted by the Society of Critical Care Medicine, and the American Thoracic Society's Ventilation Liberation Guidelines,[6] provide the strongest evidence-based recommendations and suggestions for the management of pain and sedation in critically ill patients.

These guidelines, however, are not geared for individual patient management and lack the flexibility to individually optimize and manage pain and sedation needs at the bedside.

Clinicians often combine multiple analgesic and sedative agents to achieve the pain and sedation goals of individual patients. This is often highly effective and individually adapted. Clinical practice guidelines, however, make recommendations and/or suggestions for a single agent based on clinical trials, comparing one agent with another.[7,8]

While guidelines recommend light sedation for all patients, there is no universal consensus on what defines adequate sedation depth.[9] The optimal timing of sedation and pain assessments is also unknown. In addition, validated pain and sedation assessments are often subjective, especially in patients who cannot communicate and/or are deeply sedated.[10–12] Furthermore, the management of sedation in the early phase of mechanical ventilation remains challenging.[13,14]

Sedation and Analgesia with COVID-19

The coronavirus SARS-CoV$_2$-induced COVID-19 pandemic has presented new challenges in the application of clinical practice guidelines at the bedside. Not least because they reflect clinical trials conducted in stable and fully resourced systems. As such they do not easily apply, except as a general framework, in the COVID-19 pandemic.

Severe COVID-19-induced respiratory failure[15] has presented notable challenges related to analgesia and sedation and delirium management.

Patients with COVID-related respiratory distress often require long periods of mechanical ventilation, strict isolation with mortality often over 45%–50%.[16,17] The risk of aerosol viral transmission mandates the avoidance of sudden uncontrolled agitation which may result in self-extubation. Due to stretched nursing resources, usual standards of clinical sedation monitoring and rehabilitation have also been subject to variation. This might potentially result in longer and deeper than expected sedation than pre pandemic times.

These patients often need complex ventilatory management including the use of prone ventilation and/or neuromuscular blockade which is likely done with a deep level of sedation, to avoid ventilator dyssynchrony and potentially harmful early spontaneous breathing efforts.[18]

Sedation Trials and Limitations

Although light sedation has been recommended by different guidelines, most ICUs fail to provide light sedation, with majority of RCTs, showing often unnecessarily lengthy deep sedation.[19] Approaches to produce light sedation with calm, comfortable, and awake patients include protocolized sedation, sedation interruption, early goal directed sedation[20] and analgo/minimal sedation.[21]

Different sedation strategies have been tested in recently completed clinical trials (Table 25.1). A multicentre French study, the AWARE trial, compared usual care with an algorithm of over-sedation prevention using an escalating algorithm. With limitations such as a lack of systematic sedation monitoring and using only conventional sedatives, the study was terminated early for futility and inadequate power.[22] A multicentre trial of no sedation versus usual sedation practice failed to produce adequate separation in sedation level and improve survival or secondary outcomes such as ventilation-free days or delirium-free days.[23] Its limitations included the use of benzodiazepines in the control group and the open label design. The SPICE III trial tested the early dexmedetomidine sedation compared with usual care in patients ventilated for more than 24 h.[24] The difference in target sedation, although statistically significant, was probably not clinically important. The trial failed to show a superiority of early dexmedetomidine sedation on the primary outcome of overall mortality. Benefit, however, was observed in a sub-group of patients older than the cohort median age of 63.7 years. A Cochrane systematic review[25] suggested that sedation protocols when compared with usual care practice did not influence mortality or ventilation time and hospital length of stay.

The fundamental limitation of sedation trials is patients' heterogeneity. Sedation trials investigated a single agent or a specific sedation protocol with little attention to patient's individual needs and the dynamic nature of critical illness. Prognostic enrichment may be a necessary approach to consider for future trial design.

Table 25.1 Randomized clinical trials evaluating sedation practises in ICU

Trial name	Status	Country	Patients	Inclusion	Intervention	Comparator	Outcome
The A2B Trial (*n* = 1737)	Recruiting *NCT03653832*	United Kingdom	Ventilated ICU patients	Within 48 h of ventilation	Three-arm trial, dexmedetomidine and clonidine	Propofol	Time to extubation
SPICE III (*n* = 4000)	Completed and results published	ANZ, multicentre international	Ventilated ICU patients	Expected to ventilate >24 h	Early sedation with dexmedetomidine	Usual care	90-day mortality
MENDS II (*n* = 530)	Completed not published *NCT01739933*	US multicentre	Ventilated septic ICU patients	Mechanical ventilation	Dexmedetomidine	Propofol	Delirium and coma-free days
NONSEDA (*n* = 700)	Completed and results published	Scandinavia, multicentre	Ventilated ICU patients	Expected to ventilate >24 h	No sedation	Sedation with daily wake-up	90-day mortality
AWARE (*n* = 1180)	Completed and results published	France, multicentre	Ventilated ICU patients	Expected to ventilate >48 h	Prevention of over-sedation	Conventional sedation	90-day mortality
DESIRE (*n* = 203)	Completed and results published	Japan, single centre	Ventilated ICU patients	Expected to ventilate >24 h	Dexmedetomidine	Propofol	28-day mortality

Sources: Data from the following sources: The A2B: Alpha 2 Agonists for Sedation to Produce Better Outcomes from Critical Illness; SPICE III: early dexmedetomidine sedation in critically ill patients (NEJM 2019); MENDS II: Maximizing the Efficacy of Sedation and Reducing Neurological Dysfunction and Mortality in Septic Patients with Acute Respiratory Failure (results pending); NONSEDA: Non-sedation versus Sedation with a Daily Wake-up Trial in Critically Ill Patients Receiving Mechanical Ventilation (NEJM 2020); AWARE: Study of a Strategy to Prevent Over Sedation in Intensive Care Patients under Mechanical Ventilation (Ann Intensive Care 2018); DESIRE: Dexmedetomidine for Sepsis in ICU Randomized Evaluation Trial (JAMA 2017).

The lack of robust evidence for improved patient-centred outcomes has led to opinion-based approaches that lack high-level evidence, for example, The **A**wakening and **B**reathing **C**oordination, **D**elirium Monitoring and Management, and **E**arly Mobility (ABCDE)[26] and **e**arly **C**omfort using **A**nalgesia, minimal **S**edatives and maximal **H**uman Care (eCASH) concept.[27,28]

Nonetheless, while the above trials failed to show mortality benefit, earlier trials showed a shorter ventilation time and reduced delirium with the use of dexmedetomidine when compared with midazolam.[7] Other trials reported shorter time to extubation with dexmedetomidine compared with midazolam and propofol.[29] Trials in specific groups such as septic patients showed no benefits with dexmedetomidine over propofol[30] while a survival and other benefit was suggested in two meta-analyses of dexmedetomidine used in cardiac surgery.[31,32] Furthermore, age-dependent benefit has been shown in elderly patients treated with early dexmedetomidine sedation in the SPICE III trial.[24]

Small trials also showed that dexmedetomidine and quetiapine may shorten time to delirium resolution in ventilated and sedated patients.[33–35]

In the choice of which sedative/s to combine, factors to consider include patient's related ones such as age, prior use of opioids and/or antipsychotic agents, and co-morbidities. In addition, illness-related factors such as vasopressor dependency, medical versus post operative admission, and the need for specific interventions, such as targeted temperature management, neuromuscular blockade, prone ventilation, status epilepticus, severe burn, brain injury, extracorporeal support, and poor patient–ventilator synchrony, must be considered.

Treating clinicians and bedside caregivers dictate sedation depth, without established protocols that allow active consideration of all such factors to optimize individual sedation strategy. This often results in unnecessarily deep sedation, especially during the first crucial hours.[36,37]

Considering current knowledge and evidence, clinicians need to systematically consider multiple factors to help deliver optimal sedation at the right time for the right patient.

Pharmacology of Sedatives, Analgesics, and Paralytic Agents

Considering the factors mentioned, the choice of sedative agent/s can be an important determinant of relevant clinical outcomes such as sedation depth, time on mechanical ventilation, emergence agitation and delirium, and possibly mortality.[38,39] Table 25.2 provides a summary of relevant pharmacological factors that are important in the choice of sedative, analgesic and neuromuscular blockers,

Table 25.2 Sedative, paralytic, and analgesic agents in common use in ICU

Sedative agents	Peak effect (min)	Context sensitive $T_{1/2}$ (min)	Terminal half-life (h)	Usual dose	Main advantage	Main side effects	Special precautions
Propofol	1–2	Short, 3–10	5–7	25–100 μg/kg/min infusion	Short acting, no significant accumulation	Hypotension, apnoea	Avoid rapid bolus injection and avoid high dose
Midazolam	2–5, age and dose dependent	Prolonged, 40 to several hours	2–3	1–2 mg bolus; 0.5–10 mg/h infusion	Amnesia; deep sedation	Accumulation, hypotension	Avoid in renal impairment
Diazepam	5–7, age and dose dependent	Prolonged, 120 to several hours/days	20–40	5–10 mg bolus	Haemodynamic stability	Long elimination half-life	Infusion not recommended
Dexmedetomidine	45–60 without loading dose	Prolonged, up to 120 h	2–3	0.2–1.4 mcg/kg/h	Light sedation, minimal respiratory depression	Hypotension and bradycardia	No bolus injection, give through dedicated IV line
Paralytic agents							
Cis-atracurium	1–2, bolus	60–90, without reversal	1.5	0.1–0.4 mg/kg	Rapid onset of action	Safe	Nerve stimulator
Rocuronium	2–3, bolus	60–90, without reversal	1.5–2	0.6–1 mg/kg bolus; 10 μg/kg/min infusion	Short onset of action	Hypotension, allergy	Nerve stimulator
Pancuronium	3–4, bolus	120–360, without reversal	1–2.5	0.06–0.1 mg/kg bolus	Good for unstable patient	Tachycardia, hypertension	Not suitable for infusions
Analgesic agents							
Ketamine	3–5, dose and route dependent	40–60, intermediate	2.5–3	1–2 μg/kg/min infusion	Analgesia at low dose, sedative at high dose	Hypertension, tachycardia, and agitation	Avoid high dose; hallucination
Morphine	2–5, dose and route dependent	Intermediate, few hours	2–4	1–4 mg bolus; 1–10 mg/h infusion	Analgesia	Respiratory depression and tolerance	Accumulation; renal impairment
Fentanyl (and analogues)	2–3, dose and route dependent	Intermediate, few hours	2–5	25–100 μg bolus; 25–200 μg/h infusion	Analgesia	Bradycardia and respiratory depression	Accumulation and tolerance
Remifentanil	1, dose-dependent effects	Ultra-short, few minutes	0.2–0.3	0.025–0.2 μg/kg/min IV	Ultra-short onset/offset, analgesia	Respiratory depression and bradycardia	Tolerance
Non-steroidal agents	45–60	N/A	6	200–800 mg	No respiratory depression	Gastrointestinal and renal effects	Renal impairment
Paracetamol	30–45	N/A	8	0.5–4 g/day	Simple, reduce opiate needs	Liver damage	Avoid high dose

individually or as commonly used, in combination to provide the desired intensity of sedation to the right patient.

In a critical care setting, multimodal analgesia is frequent and usually opioid based. A recommendation to add low-dose ketamine if required is suggested.[40] Caution with the prescribed dose of ketamine should be used with known dose-dependent increase in side effects such as delirium and psychosis. Non-pharmacological measures and paracetamol should also be considered to reduce the overall opioid load. The use of non-steroidal anti-inflammatory drugs should only be considered with caution in view of renal injury and peptic ulcer provoking risks.

Paralytic agents are often administered to facilitate management of severe hypoxaemia. Administering paralytic agents eliminates the spontaneous breathing activity, allowing the tidal volume and inspired pressure to be controlled to desirable settings. It also facilitates special treatments such as prone positioning.[41] The absolute need for adequate sedation must be re-stressed with a recommendation for some regular external form of monitoring of its depth of sedation, clinically and with hypnogram tools such as bispectral analysis (BIS).

The provision of detailed pharmacology of sedative, analgesic, and paralytic agents is beyond the scope of this chapter; Table 25.1, however, provides basic and essential knowledge. Readers are referred to other recommended texts.

Practical Considerations and Algorithms

Managing Sedation and Analgesia

Comfort with minimal sedation and effective analgesia can be provided and is feasible for most patients.[27] If light sedation and analgesia do not achieve a calm and cooperative patient, then causes of failure should be corrected before deep sedation is considered. While the sedation algorithm is not prescriptive, it serves as a model for escalated targeted sedation and analgesia, goals of which are best achieved with frequent monitoring of sedation depth, analgesic efficacy, and screening for triggers of agitation and/or delirium.

There are several validated scales that are commonly used in the intensive care environment to assess pain, sedation, agitation, and delirium. Bedside caregivers and intensive care, clinicians are encouraged to use the scale they are most familiar with. This, however, should be used in a systematic approach rather than ad hoc and treatment should be titrated to achieve desired goals of sedation and analgesia.

To provide for increasing ventilation complexity and a variety of possible interventions, we provide a tailored practical algorithm (Figure 25.1) to facilitate the provision of low-, medium-, and high-intensity ventilation strategies in severe hypoxaemia.

Matching Intensity of Sedation and Ventilation Management

The principle behind the algorithm (Figure 25.1) is to obtain a calm, comfortable, and cooperative patient, facilitate early mobility and access to physical rehabilitation, allow communication and family engagement, and time orientation and sleep promotion. Patients breathing spontaneously but not ready for extubation can be managed with minimal or no sedation provided adequate pain relief is given. Patients who suffer ventilator dyssynchrony and need controlled ventilation with/without high PEEP may need moderate level of sedation. The dosages of sedative agents provided are only a guide and an individual patient tailored choice of agents and dose is highly recommended. On the other hand, patients with severe hypoxaemia treated with paralytic agents and/or prone positioning will need deeper level of sedation to prevent awareness, distress, and facilitate such treatments. It is recommended that sedation depth in these patients is monitored to deliver appropriate level of sedation and avoid unnecessary deep levels of sedation. In principle, regardless of the intensity of ventilation management, sedation level seen in general anaesthesia must be avoided.

A major principle of the intensity matched algorithm is the provision of early effective analgesia. In ventilated patients, opioids remain the cornerstone for pain management and tube tolerance. In some patients, escalated multimodal analgesia is needed.

It is suggested that pain and sedation assessments are done as per institutional routine (preferably every 4–6 h).

Managing Delirium and Agitation

Agitation and/or delirium in the context of mechanical ventilation and critical illness is relatively common. Despite years of research, no effective preventive strategies have been identified. Early recognition and management of modifiable triggers of agitation/delirium, such as pain, hyperthermia, hypoperfusion, infection and sepsis, electrolyte abnormalities, and lack of sleep, remains an essential component of any treatment bundle for hospitalized ICU patients. Non-pharmacological approach, however, such as mobilization, noise reduction, sleep promotion, and day–night orientation may offer some hope and is considered common sense good practice.

Nonetheless, the management of agitation/hyperactive delirium remains a clinician's challenge. Until recently, there was no evidence for pharmacologic treatment of agitation in ventilated patients. Dexmedetomidine reduced ventilation time and shortened time to resolution of agitation in mechanically ventilated critically ill patients.[33] This agent, however, is not suitable for the immediate control of agitated and/or combative patients, and rapidly acting agents such as midazolam and propofol should be used to gain immediate control of such patients. Injectable haloperidol, used to be a standard treatment in this situation, has been taken out of circulation in many countries due to risk of prolonged QT and ventricular tachycardia.

Figure 25.2 (MAD-A–Managing Agitation Delirium Algorithm) provides a guided step-by-step process to manage agitated delirium. The final pathway is to manage known and modifiable triggers and anticipate the likely cause.

Current and Future Research

Controversies and Unanswered Questions

Providing optimum sedation is one component of many treatments that critically ill patients receive during an intensive care stay, and so the individual contribution of the sedation choice to patient-centred outcomes is unknown. Nonetheless, sedation practice has moved towards the use of lighter sedation whenever clinically safe, better management of pain and delirium in patients with critical

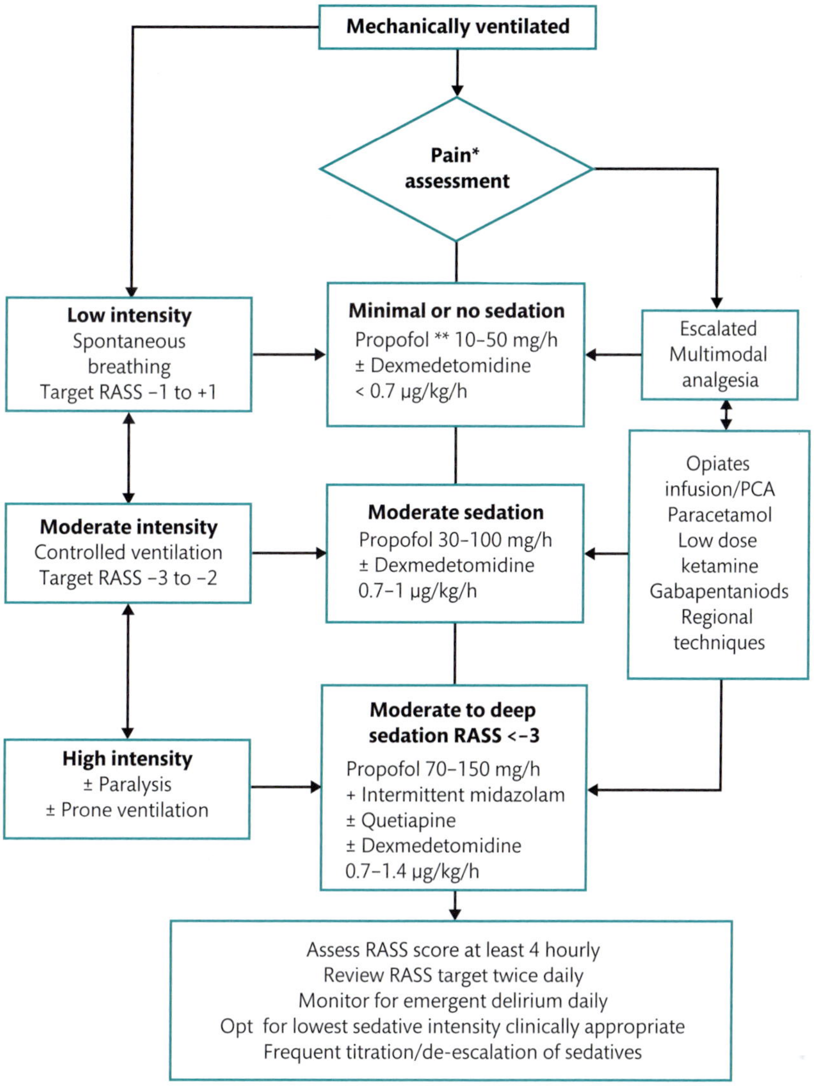

Figure 25.1 Symptom-oriented intensity matched sedation algorithm. Abbreviations: RASS: Richmond Agitation Sedation Scale (−5 is unresponsive to pain, −4 open eyes, move to physical stimulation, −3 open eyes to voice, −2 make eye contact <10 s, −1 make eye contact >10 s, 0 alert and calm, +1 restless, +2 agitated, +3 very agitated, and +4 combative) score.[11] *Pain assessment and adequate analgesia is given first. The default sedation target is light or minimal sedation. Clinicians determine the sedative intensity. **Propofol is the first line for titrated sedation with dexmedetomidine and/or quetiapine added as needed.

illness. Multiple systematic reviews,[42] however, suggest that the level of evidence for such practice is at best medium to low and mainly comes from observational studies.

The availability of rapid acting high affinity opioid such as remifentanil has opened the way to the concept of opioid-based sedation. While there is no data on the medium- or long-term outcomes of such an approach, so caution should be practised relying primarily on opioids to manage ventilated patients. Some proponents of analgo-sedation have recommended high-dose opioid. However, recent trials do not support this approach.[23] In the absence of high-level evidence, adherence to a rigid protocol is discouraged and individual patient approach would be preferred.

While many have suggested that the era of benzodiazepines, as sedative agents, in mechanically ventilated patients is over, midazolam remains an important and common agent in many parts of the world. Thus far, there is no high-level evidence from randomized trials to suggest that midazolam is associated with a worse patient-centred long-term outcome.

Similarly, deep sedation has been shown in many observational trials to be associated with poor long-term outcomes such as mortality. While this data suggests linkage, causality is not yet established, and studies of light sedation have failed to demonstrate beneficial outcomes apart from short-term ICU-related ones.

Future Research

To avoid heterogeneity in sedation trials, sedation strategies, comprising agent and intensity choice, need to be evaluated in prognostically enriched patient groups such as the elderly, medical versus surgical patients, and those with cardiovascular disease.

With almost all ICU sedation trials failing to show a mortality difference, the search for the appropriate relevant sedation-related long-term outcomes is important.

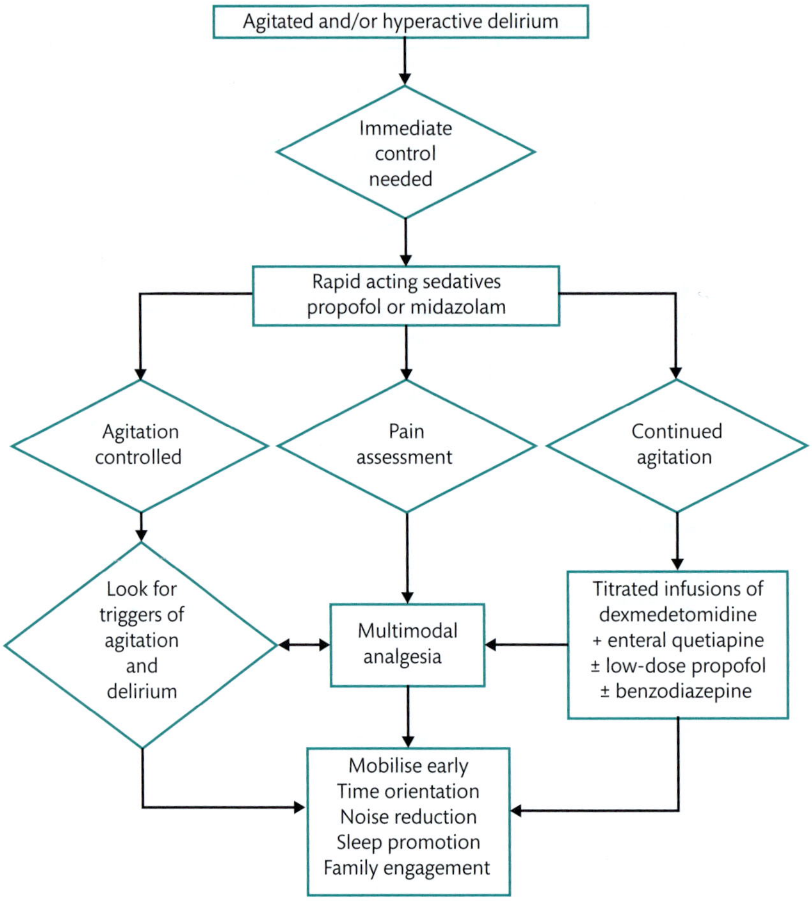

Figure 25.2 Management of agitation and delirium algorithm: MAD-A Algorithm. Control of hyperactive delirium should be promptly achieved with age-adjusted boluses of midazolam or propofol. Haloperidol could also be used, which is followed by specific anti-delirium agents such as dexmedetomidine and/or quetiapine with conventional sedatives reserved for control of breakthrough agitation. Review of pain relief and other triggers of delirium is imperative while non-pharmacological interventions are introduced as sedative medications are weaned.

Sedation strategies are usually delivered in a bundled approach. However, despite the popularity, there have been no prospective randomized trials into known common bundles such as the ABCDEF or eCASH.

REFERENCES

1. Barr J, Fraser GL, Puntillo K, et al. Clinical Practice Guidelines for the management of pain, agitation, and delirium in adult patients in the Intensive Care Unit. *Crit Care Med.* 2013;**41**:263–306.
2. Jacobi J, Fraser GL, Coursin DB, et al. Clinical practice guidelines for the sustained use of sedatives and analgesics in the critically ill adult. *Crit Care Med.* 2002;**30**:119–141.
3. Payen JF, Chanques G, Mantz J, et al. Current practices in sedation and analgesia for mechanically ventilated critically ill patients: A prospective multicenter patient-based study. *Anesthesiology*. 2007;**106**:687–695; quiz 891-2.
4. Devlin JW, Skrobik Y, Gélinas C, et al. Clinical practice guidelines for the prevention and management of pain, agitation/sedation, delirium, immobility, and sleep disruption in adult patients in the ICU. *Crit Care Med.* 2018;**46**:e825–e73.
5. Ely EW. The ABCDEF bundle: Science and philosophy of how ICU liberation serves patients and families. *Crit Care Med.* 2017;**45**:321.
6. Girard TD, Alhazzani W, Kress JP, et al. An Official American Thoracic Society/American College of Chest Physicians Clinical Practice Guideline: Liberation from mechanical ventilation in critically ill adults. Rehabilitation protocols, ventilator liberation protocols, and cuff leak tests. *Am J Respir Crit Care Med.* 2017;**195**:120–133.
7. Riker RR, Shehabi Y, Bokesch PM, et al. Dexmedetomidine vs midazolam for sedation of critically ill patients. A randomized trial. *JAMA*. 2009;**301**:489–499.
8. Jakob SM, Ruokonen E, Grounds RM, et al. Dexmedetomidine vs midazolam or propofol for sedation during prolonged mechanical ventilation: Two randomized controlled trials. *JAMA*. 2012;**307**:1151–1160.
9. Shehabi Y, Bellomo R, Kadiman S, et al. Sedation intensity in the first 48 hours of mechanical ventilation and 180-day mortality: A multinational prospective longitudinal cohort study. *Crit Care Med.* 2018;**46**:850–859.
10. Gélinas C, Fillion L, Puntillo KA, et al. Validation of the critical-care pain observation tool in adult patients. *Am J Crit Care.* 2006;**15**:420–427.
11. Sessler CN, Gosnell MS, Grap MJ, et al. The Richmond agitation-sedation scale: Validity and reliability in adult intensive care unit patients. *Am J Respir Crit Care Med.* 2002;**166**:17.
12. Ahlers SJ, van der Veen AM, van Dijk M, et al. The use of the Behavioral Pain Scale to assess pain in conscious sedated patients. *Anesth Analg.* 2010;**110**:127–133.

13. Balzer F, Weiß B, Kumpf O, et al. Early deep sedation is associated with decreased in-hospital and 2-years follow-up survival. *Crit Care*. 2015;**19**:197.
14. Shehabi Y, Bellomo R, Reade MC, et al. Early intensive care sedation predicts long-term mortality in ventilated critically ill patients. *Am J Respir Crit Care Med*. 2012;**186**:724–731.
15. Matthay MA, Aldrich JM, Gotts JE. Treatment for severe acute respiratory distress syndrome from COVID-19. *Lancet Respir Med*. 2020;**8**:433–434.
16. Zhou F, Yu T, Du R, et al. Clinical course and risk factors for mortality of adult inpatients with COVID-19 in Wuhan, China: A retrospective cohort study. *The Lancet*. 2020; **395**(10229):1054–1062.
17. Wunsch H. Mechanical ventilation in COVID-19: Interpreting the current epidemiology. *Am J Respir Crit Care Med*. 2020;**202**(1):1–4.
18. Gattinoni L, Chiumello D, Caironi P, et al. COVID-19 pneumonia: Different respiratory treatments for different phenotypes? *Intensive Care Medicine*. 2020;**46**(6):1099–1102.
19. Minhas MA, Velasquez AG, Kaul A, et al. Effect of protocolized sedation on clinical outcomes in mechanically ventilated intensive care unit patients: A systematic review and meta-analysis of randomized controlled trials. *Mayo Clin Proc*. 2015;**90**:613–623.
20. Shehabi Y, Bellomo R, Reade MC, et al. Early goal-directed sedation versus standard sedation in mechanically ventilated critically ill patients: A pilot study. *Crit Care Med*. 2013;**41**:1983–1991.
21. Strom T, Martinussen T, Toft P. A protocol of no sedation for critically ill patients receiving mechanical ventilation: A randomised trial. *Lancet*. 2010;**375**:475–480.
22. SRLF Trial Group. Impact of oversedation prevention in ventilated critically ill patients: A randomized trial—the AWARE study. *Ann Intensive Care*. 2018;**8**:93.
23. Olsen HT, Nedergaard HK, Strøm T, et al. Nonsedation or light sedation in critically ill, mechanically ventilated patients. *N Engl J Med*. 2020;**382**:1103–1111.
24. Shehabi Y, Howe B, Bellomo R, et al. Early sedation with dexmedetomidine in critically ill patients. *N Engl J Med*. 2019;**380**:2506–2517.
25. Aitken LM, Bucknall T, Kent B, et al. Protocol-directed sedation versus non-protocol-directed sedation in mechanically ventilated intensive care adults and children. *Cochrane Database Syst Rev*. 2018 Nov 12;**11**(11):CD009771.
26. Pandharipande P, Banerjee A, McGrane S, et al. Liberation and animation for ventilated ICU patients: The ABCDE bundle for the back-end of critical care. *Crit Care*. 2010;**14**:1.
27. Vincent JL, Shehabi Y, Walsh TS, et al. Comfort and patient-centred care without excessive sedation: The eCASH concept. *Intensive Care Med*. 2016;**42**:962–971.
28. Mehta S, Spies C, Shehabi Y. Ten tips for ICU sedation. *Intensive Care Med*. 2018 Jul;**44**(7):1141–1143.
29. Jakob SM, Ruokonen E, Grounds RM, et al. Dexmedetomidine for Long-Term Sedation Investigators. Dexmedetomidine vs midazolam or propofol for sedation during prolonged mechanical ventilation: Two randomized controlled trials. *JAMA*. 2012;**307**:10.
30. Kawazoe Y, Miyamoto K, Morimoto T, et al. Effect of dexmedetomidine on mortality and ventilator-free days in patients requiring mechanical ventilation with sepsis: A randomized clinical trial. *JAMA*. 2017;**317**:1321–1328.
31. Wang G, Niu J, Li Z, et al. The efficacy and safety of dexmedetomidine in cardiac surgery patients: A systematic review and meta-analysis. *PloS One*. 2018;**13**:e0202620.
32. Ji F, Li Z, Nguyen H, et al. Perioperative dexmedetomidine improves outcomes of cardiac surgery. *Circulation*. 2013:**127**(15):1576–1584.
33. Reade MC, Eastwood GM, Bellomo R, et al. Effect of dexmedetomidine added to standard care on ventilator-free time in patients with agitated delirium: A randomized clinical trial. *JAMA*. 2016;**315**:1460–1468.
34. Skrobik Y, Duprey MS, Hill NS, et al. Low-dose nocturnal dexmedetomidine prevents ICU Delirium. A randomized, placebo-controlled trial. *Am J Respir Crit Care Med*. 2018;**197**:1147–1156.
35. Devlin JW, Roberts RJ, Fong JJ, et al. Efficacy and safety of quetiapine in critically ill patients with delirium: A prospective, multicenter, randomized, double-blind, placebo-controlled pilot study. *Crit Care Med*. 2010;**38**:419.
36. Shehabi Y, Bellomo R, SAFE Study Investigators. Reply: Early deep sedation is often not justified. *Am J Respir Crit Care Med*. 2013;**187**:893.
37. Shehabi Y, Bellomo R, Mehta S, et al. Intensive care sedation: The past, present and the future. *Crit Care*. 2013;**17**:322.
38. Ferrell BA, Girard TD. Sedative choice: A critical decision. *Am J Respir Crit Care Med*. 2014;**189**:1295–1297.
39. Oldham M, Pisani MA. Sedation in critically ill patients. *Crit Care Clin*. 2015;**31**:563–587.
40. Wang L, Johnston B, Kaushal A, et al. Ketamine added to morphine or hydromorphone patient-controlled analgesia for acute postoperative pain in adults: A systematic review and meta-analysis of randomized trials. *Can J Anesth/J canadien d'anesthésie*. 2016;**63**:311–25.
41. Gattinoni L, Marini J. Prone positioning and neuromuscular blocking agents are part of standard care in severe ARDS patients: We are not sure. *Intensive Care Med*. 2015;**41**:2201–2203.
42. Jackson DL, Proudfoot CW, Cann KF, et al. A systematic review of the impact of sedation practice in the ICU on resource use, costs and patient safety. *Crit Care*. 2010;**14**:1.

26

Nutrition

Danielle E Bear and Zudin Puthucheary

KEY MESSAGES

- The provision of nutrition support to critically ill adults is an essential element of care and should be commenced within 24–48 h of admission to ICU.
- Under- and overfeeding should be avoided during ICU admission.
- Guideline recommendations for energy and protein dose should be followed.

CONTROVERSIES

- What is the most effective dose of energy and protein to reduce muscle wasting in critically ill adults?
- Should gastric residual volumes be monitored in all critically ill adults?
- Should indirect calorimetry be used to guide energy delivery in critically ill adults?

FURTHER RESEARCH

- What are the optimal energy and protein targets for critically ill patients?
- What impact does nutrition have on muscle wasting and functional recovery in critically ill patients?
- What is the best timing for enteral nutrition (continuous vs intermittent)?

Introduction

Nutrition in the critically ill patient has evolved over recent years from a supportive to a therapeutic intervention. Much data in the area of critical care nutrition is focused on reducing mortality; however, functional recovery post critical illness is a topic of increasing relevance as overall mortality rates decrease.

Current Accepted Practice

While there is limited consensus on most aspects of nutritional support,[1] experts agree that early feeding within the first 24–48 of ICU is beneficial.[2,3] The benefit of early enteral nutrition (EN) over parenteral nutrition (PN) has been challenged with the publication of the CALORIES Trial.[4] In this landmark study, early PN compared to EN did not alter mortality or infectious complications as previously reported.[5,6] However, the enteral route is preferred for early nutritional support.[2] A systematic review and meta-analysis reports that early EN does not alter mortality but reduces length of stay and infectious complications compared with early PN.[7] In order to achieve early feeding, protocols are recommended which take into account factors such as the route of feeding and management of gastric residual volumes (GRVs).[2,3]

Evidence Base

Nutritional Targets

Significant debate exists surrounding the optimum nutritional targets for critically ill patients. Current data does not extend past the first week of critical illness, where the recent trend is towards lower energy and higher protein targets. Additionally, there is a lack of translational science in the area and limited data on the optimal energy and protein targets to influence physical and functional recovery post discharge from the ICU.

As with other aspects of critical illness, patient heterogeneity as regards background nutritional status and response to feeding has not been accounted for until recently in data on nutritional targets. An ICU-specific nutrition risk score (NUTRIC) was developed to identify those who may benefit the most from meeting full nutrition targets[8] (Table 26.1). Initial validation data suggests that patients with a high score (5–9) who receive more nutrition have lower mortality rates than those with a low score (0–4). ICU-specific scoring is recommended in the ASPEN Guidelines[3] and may provide a useful tool for prioritization of patients for the use of early PN and those who require an individualized nutritional prescription to meet

Table 26.1 NUTRIC score for nutrition risk scoring in critical illness

NUTRIC score		
Variable	**Range**	**Points**
Age	<50 50–75 ≥75	0 1 2
APACHE II	<15 15 to <20 20–28 ≥28	0 1 2 3
SOFA	<6 6 to <10 ≥10	0 1 2
No. of co-morbidities	0–1 2+	0 1
Days from hospital to ICU admission	0 to <1 1+	0 1

Source: Adapted by permission from Springer Nature: Heyland DK, Dhaliwal R, Jiang X, et al. Identifying critically ill patients who benefit the most from nutrition therapy: The development and initial validation of a novel risk assessment tool. *Crit Care.* 2011;*15*(6):R268.

Table 26.2 Common equations for estimating energy requirements in critical care

Common equations for use in critical care	
Harris-Benedict	Males: (13.7516 × *W*) + (5.003 × *H*) − (6.755 × *A*)
	Females: 655.0955 + (9.5634 × *W*) + (1.8496 × *H*) − (4.6756 × *A*)
Ireton-Jones (1992)	(5 × *W*) − (10 × *A*) + (281 × sex) + (292 × trauma) + (851 × burn) + 1925
Ireton-Jones (1997)	(5 × *W*) − (11 × *A*) + (244 × sex) + (239 × trauma) + (840 × burn) + 1784
Penn State (1998)	(Harris-Benedict × 1.1) + (T_{max} × 140) + (VE × 32) − 5340 Uses actual body weight in non-obese and adjusted body weight (25%) in obese
Penn State (2003)	(Harris-Benedict × 0.85) + (T_{max} × 175) + (VE × 33) − 6344
Penn State (m)	(Mifflin-St Jeor × 0.96) + (T_{max} × 167) + (VE × 31) − 6212
ACCP	25 kcal × kg
Frankenfield	−11,000 − (VE × 100) + (BEE × 1.5) + (DOB dose × 40) + (*T* × 250) + (diagnosis of sepsis × 300)
Swinamer	(95 × BSA) − (6.4 × *A*) + (108 × *T*) + (24.2 × breaths/min) + (81.7 × VT) − 4349
Schofield	**Age / Males / Females** 19–29: 15.1 × *W* + 692 / 14.8 × *W* + 487 30–59: 11.5 × *W* + 873 / 8.3 × *W* + 846 60–74: 11.9 × *W* + 700 / 9.2 × *W* + 687 75+: 8.4 × *W* + 820 / 9.8 × *W* + 624
Henry	**Age / Males / Females** 10–18: 18.4 × *W* + 581 / 11.1 × *W* + 761 18–30: 16.0 × *W* + 545 / 13.1 × *W* + 558 30–60: 14.2 × *W* + 593 / 9.7 × *W* + 694 60–70: 13.0 × *W* + 567 / 10.2 × *W* + 572 70+: 13.7 × *W* + 481 / 10.0 × *W* + 577
Mifflin-St Jeor	Males: (10 × *W*) + (6.25 × *H*) − (5 × *A*) + 5
	Females: (10 × *W*) + (6.25 × *H*) − (5 × *A*) − 161
Faisy	(8 × *W*) + (14 × *H*) + (32 × VE) + (94 × *T*) − 4834

Notes:

BEE: basal energy expenditure (using Harris-Benedict); *W*: weight in kg; *H*: height in cm; *A*: age in years.

For sex, 1 is male, 0 is female; trauma present = 1; no trauma = 0; burns present = 1; no burns = 0.

T_{max}: maximum body temperature for last 24 h; VE: minute ventilation in L/min at time of measurement; kcal: calorie.

Diagnosis of sepsis = 1 for yes, 0 for no; DOB dose: dobutamine dose; *T*: body temperature; VT: tidal volume; BSA: body surface area.

nutritional targets. However, the latest update of the ESPEN guidance does not recommend a specific screening tool, but suggests that all patients admitted to the ICU for longer than 48 h should be considered at high nutrition risk.[2] Whichever guideline is followed, it is clear that a full nutrition assessment is imperative to the development of an appropriate feeding plan.

Energy

Energy provision in critical illness is a balance between over- and underfeeding, both being associated with detrimental effects. Provision of energy above resting energy expenditure has been shown to induce hypercapnia[9] that may increase ventilator time,[10] cause hyperglycaemia and hyperlipaemia, and may be responsible for increases in length of stay and infectious complications seen with PN, although the latter is contested.[4,7] In contrast, underfeeding is associated with increased infections, length of stay, ventilator time, and potentially mortality.[11,12] Underfeeding is more common than overfeeding, especially when EN only.[13]

Although indirect calorimetry is the gold standard for determining energy targets in critically ill patients, it is infrequently used due to cost, time, and intrinsic limitations, which include use with extracorporeal therapies, high oxygen requirement, and air leakage. For this reason, prediction equations (Table 26.2) are most frequently used to estimate energy targets. There is debate over the most accurate and appropriate of these, but the most widely used is the American College of Chest Physicians (ACCP), weight-based recommendation of 25 kcal/kg,[14] though it is both inaccurate and imprecise relative to indirect calorimetry[15] resulting in a high potential for significant under- or overfeeding. The modified Penn State equation has been reported as the most accurate equation to predict energy expenditure as it includes clinical variables such as temperature and minute ventilation.[16] Without the measured energy expenditure from indirect calorimetry, it is impossible to truly determine achievement (under or over) of nutritional targets. Even with indirect calorimetry, it remains unclear whether patients should be fed to the 100% of their predicted or measured energy expenditure, as endogenous glycolysis and lipolysis may contribute to the requirements in early critical illness by way of glucose and fat production.

Differences in body composition may provide some rationale for the inaccuracy of prediction equations as lean body mass is unaccounted for when weight alone is used. There is significant uncertainty surrounding the use of actual, ideal, or adjusted body weights in prediction equations, especially in the obese population. While it is generally accepted that actual body weight is appropriate with a normal BMI and those who are underweight, debate exists as regards the use of ideal or adjusted body weights in those who are overweight or obese; no consensus exists. However, ideal body weight has been repeatedly used in large feeding studies, reflecting the difficulty in obtaining an accurate actual body weight in clinical practice.[17,18] In practice, the weight (e.g. actual, ideal, or adjusted) used in the initial validation should be used appropriately in the chosen prediction equation.

Data suggests no benefit from feeding to target energy requirements relative to trophic feeding in patients with acute respiratory distress syndrome.[17] Additionally, critically ill patients randomized to target feeding (70%–100% of energy target) compared with permissive underfeeding (40%–60% of energy target) did not show any short-term clinical benefit.[19] Finally, the EPaNIC trial found a degree of harm when early PN (day 2) was used to supplement failing EN compared with commencing this on day 8.[18] Together, this data has led to the recent trend towards the provision of lower energy requirements over the first week of critical illness. Current practice, influenced by the very nature of ICU (delay in commencing EN, stepwise increase in EN, and feeding interruptions), already leads to significant underfeeding, and therefore prospective undertargeting of energy requirements may effectively lead to trophic feeding, which remains controversial.

Protein

Critical care nutrition has traditionally focused on the energy requirements during critical illness rather than protein. The possibility has been raised that failures of recent, large randomized controlled trials to show a benefit from nutrition are due to low protein provision. Protein is essential for muscle protein synthesis and therefore is the macronutrient most likely to impact on muscle wasting, though the most appropriate timing, route of delivery, schedule of delivery (e.g. continuous vs intermittent), and dose remain unclear.[20]

Clinical guidelines suggest providing a minimum of 1.2 g/kg/day and up to 2.5 g/kg/day for specific patient populations (Table 26.3),[2,3] including those receiving continuous renal replacement therapy where 1.5–1.7 g/kg/day is suggested.[2] These mainly observational recommendations relate to a survival benefit rather than a reduction in the loss of lean body mass or improvement in functional outcome. While higher doses of protein reduce nitrogen loss, this data remains difficult to interpret considering the inaccuracy of whole-body nitrogen balance measurement in critically ill patients. Additionally, a reduction in whole-body nitrogen loss may not necessarily be due to a reduction in the loss of lean body mass.

The potential beneficial effects of high protein intakes on muscle wasting have been challenged, either made no difference to muscle wasting[21] or indeed increased it.[22] This data suggests that the simple provision of additional protein may not be a useful strategy for reducing muscle loss and more data is required as regards macronutrient provision in critical illness.

Table 26.3 Recommended protein intakes in critically ill patients

Patient group	Protein target (g/kg)
General ICU	1.2–1.5
Continuous renal replacement therapy	1.5–1.7
Burns	1.5–2.0
Trauma	1.3–1.5
Obese	2.0–2.5 (ideal body weight)

Use of Parenteral Nutrition

PN has historically been utilized as a last resort in the critically ill due to the increased risk of infectious complications seen in older studies. This appears not to be the current concern. Moreover, underfeeding with EN alone, coupled with improvements in line care, has led to a change in the use of PN in the ICU. The presumed advantage of PN is accurate delivery of a known amount of prescribed nutrition. However, data on the beneficial effect of PN is conflicting. Therefore, the use of PN should be considered for each individual patient on the basis of nutrition risk (Table 26.1). In addition, care should be taken to avoid the overprovision of energy when providing either exclusive or supplemental PN as this may increase the risk of complications. When providing PN, care should be taken to monitor fluid balance, electrolytes, and blood sugar levels regularly as these may provide indications of metabolic tolerance.

Delayed Gastric Emptying

Aetiology

Delayed gastric emptying is one of the many manifestations of gastrointestinal (GI) intolerance in critical illness. Those who develop GI dysfunction have worse outcomes[23] and delayed gastric emptying leads to poor delivery of EN.[24] The causes are multifactorial and may include the aetiology of critical illness (e.g. surgical vs medical), severity of illness, use of narcotics, sedatives and/or vasopressors, hyperglycaemia, electrolyte abnormalities, and the feeding method (bolus vs continuous).[25]

GRVs are often used as a surrogate marker of delayed gastric emptying due to more accurate measures (e.g. scintigraphy, MRI, and ultrasound) proving unfeasible on the ICU.[26] Historically, high GRVs are used to predict risk of vomiting or regurgitation and subsequent development of ventilator-associated pneumonia (VAP) plus as an indicator of enteral feeding 'tolerance'. GRV has no association with risk of VAP, while being difficult to measure.[26] Nonetheless, 4–6 hourly GRV measurements are embedded in the practice of feeding the critically ill patient and current thresholds range from 100 to 500 mL, often dependent on personal choice or patient population. Others choose to use a percentage of the target feeding rate. The recent ASPEN Guidelines have recommended against measuring GRVs.[3] However, care must be taken with this approach in a surgical population in which limited data exists. High GRVs should not necessarily lead to automatic cessation of enteral feeding as this contributes to underfeeding, although concern regarding aspiration must clearly be considered. Rather, high GRVs should lead to consideration of alternative feeding strategies to optimize nutritional delivery and reduce the risk of complications.

Treatment of Delayed Gastric Emptying

Prokinetics are commonly used, though post-pyloric feeding and PN (full or supplementary) may be utilized in practice.[27] Erythromycin is a more effective prokinetic compared with metoclopramide; however, the latter is preferred due to concerns regarding antibiotic resistance.[28] Overall, the efficacy of prokinetics declines due to tachyphylaxis after 3 days as a single treatment or 6 days when used in combination.[28]

In order to reduce the incidence of underfeeding associated with delayed gastric emptying, the use of prophylactic prokinetics, as utilized in the PEP-uP Protocol,[29] has been suggested though safety data is lacking. Post-pyloric feeding may be a more effective treatment for persistent GI intolerance although robust definitive data is needed. Use of post-pyloric feeding compared with nasogastric feeding may reduce the incidence of pneumonia. However, delays in the placement of post-pyloric feeding tubes may limit feeding. For this reason, supplementary PN is often used in patients unable to meet nutritional targets secondary to GI intolerance. Supplementary PN may be best reserved for those in whom achieving nutritional targets are deemed very important.[30]

Conclusion

The provision of nutritional support to critically ill adults is an essential element of care. However, many uncertainties remain regarding the most appropriate dose of energy and protein and elements of feeding such as the measurement of GRVs. Future research should focus on the effect of nutrition support on muscle wasting and functional outcomes.

REFERENCES

1. Preiser JC, van Zanten ARH, Berger MM, et al. Metabolic and nutritional support of critically ill patients: consensus and controversies. *Crit Care*. 2015;**19**:35.
2. Singer P, Blaser AR, Berger MM, et al. ESPEN guideline on clinical nutrition in the intensive care unit. *Clin Nutr*. 2019;**38**(1):48–79.
3. McClave SA, Taylor BE, Martindale RG, et al. Guidelines for the provision and assessment of nutrition support therapy in the adult critically ill patient: Society of Critical Care Medicine (SCCM) and American Society for Parenteral and Enteral Nutrition (A.S.P.E.N.). *J Parenter Enteral Nutr*. 2016;**40**(2):159–211.
4. Harvey SE, Parrott F, Harrison DA, et al. Trial of the route of early nutritional support in critically ill adults. *N Engl J Med*. 2014;**371**:1673–1684
5. Gramlich L, Kichian K, Pinilla J, et al. Does enteral nutrition compared to parenteral nutrition result in better outcomes in critically ill adult patients? A systematic review of the literature. *Nutrition*. 2004;**20**:843–848.
6. Simpson F, Doig GS. Parenteral vs. enteral nutrition in the critically ill patient: A meta-analysis of trials using the intention to treat principle. *Intensive Care Med*. 2005;**31**:12–23.
7. Elke G, van Zanten AR, Lemieux M, et al. Enteral versus parenteral nutrition in critically ill patients: An updated systematic review and meta-analysis of randomized controlled trials. *Crit Care*. 2016;**20**(1):117.
8. Heyland DK, Dhaliwal R, Jiang X, et al. Identifying critically ill patients who benefit the most from nutrition therapy: The development and initial validation of a novel risk assessment tool. *Crit Care*. 2011;**15**(6):R268.
9. Lo HC, Lin CH, Tsai LJ. Effects of hypercaloric feeding on nutrition status and carbon dioxide production in patients with long-term mechanical ventilation. *J Parenter Enteral Nutr*. 2005; **29**(5):380–7
10. Klein CJ, Stanek GS, Wiles CE 3rd. Overfeeding macronutrients to critically ill adults: Metabolic complications. *J Am Diet Assoc*. 1998;**98**(7):795–806.
11. Villet S, Chiolero RL, Bollmann MD, et al. Negative impact of hypocaloric feeding and energy balance on clinical outcome in ICU patients. *Clin Nutr*. 2005;**24**:502–509.
12. Elke G, Wang M, Weiler N, et al. Close to recommended caloric and protein intake by enteral nutrition is associated with better clinical outcome of critically ill septic patients: Secondary analysis of a large international nutrition database. *Crit Care*. 2014;**18**:R2.
13. Alberda C, Gramlich L, Jones N, et al. The relationship between nutritional intake and clinical outcomes in critically ill patients: Results of an international multicenter observational study. *Intensive Care Med*. 2009;**35**:1728–1737.
14. Cerra FB, Benitez MR, Blackburn GL, et al. Applied Nutrition in ICU Patients: A consensus statement of the American College of Chest Physicians (ACCP). *Chest*. 1997;**111**:769–778.
15. Frankenfield D, Hise M, Malone A, et al. Prediction of resting metabolic rate in critically ill adult patients: Results of a systematic review of the evidence. *J Am Diet Assoc*. 2007;**107**(9):1552–1561.
16. Frankenfield DC, Coleman A, Alam S, et al. Analysis of estimation methods for resting metabolic rate in critically ill adults. *J Parenter Enteral Nutr*. 2009;**33**(1): 27–36.
17. National Heart, Lung, and Blood Institute Acute Respiratory Distress Syndrome (ARDS) Clinical Trials Network. Initial trophic vs full enteral feeding in patients with acute lung injury: the EDEN randomized trial. *JAMA*. 2012;**307**(8):795–803.
18. Casaer MP, Mesotten D, Hermans G, et al. Early versus late parenteral nutrition in critically ill adults. *N Engl J Med*. 2011;**365**:506–517.
19. Arabi YM, Aldawood AS, Haddad SH, et al. Permissive underfeeding or standard enteral feeding in critically ill adults. *N Engl J Med*. 2015;**372**(25): 2398–2408.
20. Bear DE, Wandrag L, Merriweather JL, et al. The role of nutritional support in the physical and functional recovery of critically ill patients: A narrative review. *Crit Care*. 2017;**21**(1):226.
21. Casaer MP, Langouche L, Coudyzer W, et al. Impact of early parenteral nutrition on muscle and adipose tissue compartments during critical illness. *Crit Care Med*. 2013;**41**(10):2298–2309.
22. Puthucheary ZA, Rawal J, McPhail M, et al. Acute skeletal muscle wasting in critical illness. *JAMA*. 2013;**310**:1591–1600.
23. Reintam A, Parm P, Kitus R, et al. Gastrointestinal failure score in critically ill patients: A prospective observational study. *Crit Care*. 2008;**12**:R90.
24. Rice TW, Swope T, Bozeman S, et al. Variation in enteral nutrition delivery in mechanically ventilated patients. *Nutrition*. 2005; **21**(7–8):786–792.
25. Deane A, Chapman MJ, Fraser RJ, et al. Mechanisms underlying feed intolerance in the critically ill: Implications for treatment. *World J Gastroenterol*. 2007; **13**:3909–3917.
26. Kar P, Jones KL, Horowitz M, et al. Measurement of gastric emptying in the critically ill. *Clin Nutr*. 2015;**34**(4):557–564.
27. Deane AM, Fraser RJ, Chapman MJ. Prokinetic drugs for feed intolerance in critical illness: current and potential therapies. *Crit Care Resusc*. 2009;**11**:132–143.
28. Nguyen NQ, Chapman M, Fraser RJ, et al. Prokinetic therapy for feed intolerance in critical illness: One drug or two? *Crit Care Med*. 2007;**35**:2561–2567.
29. Lee AY, Barakatun-Nisak MY, Airini IN, et al. Enhanced protein-energy provision via the enteral route in critically ill patients (PEP uP Protocol): A review of evidence. *Nutr Clin Pract*. 2016;**31**(1):68–79.
30. Bost RBC, Tjan DHT, van Zanten ARH. Timing of (supplemental) parenteral nutrition in critically ill patients: A systematic review. *Ann Intensive Care*. 2014;**4**:31.

27

Gastric Protection

Mette Krag, Morten Hylander Møller, Suveer Singh, and Matthew P Wise

KEY MESSAGES

- The prevalence of clinically important gastrointestinal bleeding in the intensive care unit (ICU) is ~2%–5%.
- Clinically important gastrointestinal bleeding in critically ill patients is reduced by proton pump inhibitors and histamine-2-receptor antagonists.
- Risk factors for gastrointestinal bleeding include severity of illness, circulatory support, renal replacement therapy, hepatic failure, and coagulopathy.
- Mortality is not affected by stress ulcer prophylaxis.
- Stress ulcer prophylaxis does not seem to increase the risk of nosocomial infections, clostridium difficile infection or myocardial ischaemia.

CONTROVERSIES

- Do proton pump inhibitors increase mortality in the most severely ill ICU patients?
- Is mechanical ventilation alone a risk factor for clinically important bleeding?
- Are all clinically relevant side effects from stress ulcer prophylaxis well characterized?
- If it is decided to use stress ulcer prophylaxis in a high-risk patient, what is the drug of choice?
- Should enteral feeding alter the decision to employ stress ulcer prophylaxis?

FURTHER RESEARCH

- Research on mortality in ICU patients with high disease severity receiving proton pump inhibitors is warranted.
- Additionally, randomized trials providing data on the association between enteral feeding and gastrointestinal bleeding and data on histamine-2-receptor antagonists versus placebo are lacking.

Introduction

Critically ill patients in the intensive care unit (ICU) are at risk of developing stress-related mucosal damage.[1] To prevent gastrointestinal (GI) bleeding in critically ill patients, stress ulcer prophylaxis (SUP) was introduced more than 40 years ago. Different agents for the prevention of GI bleeding have been used throughout the years. Initially, antacids and later sucralfate were the preferred agents, but with the introduction of histamine-2-receptor antagonists (H2RAs) the opportunity for intravenous administration became available. In a randomized clinical trial (RCT) from 1998, a significantly lower incidence of GI bleeding in patients receiving H2RA compared with sucralfate was reported.[2] Later on, proton pump inhibitors (PPIs) were introduced and today the vast majority of prescribed SUP is H2RA or PPI.[3] Today, SUP is recommended in international guidelines and is the standard of care in critically ill patients in ICUs worldwide.[4]

Pathophysiology of Stress-ulcer-associated Bleeding

The pathophysiology is not completely understood, but it has been hypothesized that stress ulcers are caused by decreased mucosal blood flow, ischaemia, and reperfusion injury—hence are less related to acid secretion than peptic ulcers. However, gastrin hypersecretion from parietal cells leading to acid secretion may play a role in specific patient populations (i.e. head injury) but not necessarily in other critically ill patient populations. Whether the presence of *Helicobacter pylori* infection contributes to stress ulceration is unclear.

Stress ulcerations during critical illness usually occur in the fundus and body of the stomach but may develop anywhere up to the ligament of Treitz (duodenojejunal flexure). Ulceration of the mucosal lining of the upper GI tract begins in the first hours following critical illness. Visible mucosal damage has been confirmed endoscopically in up to 90% of ICU patients after 3 days of admission, but the majority of these lesions remain superficial and asymptomatic.[5] However, some lesions may progress and erode

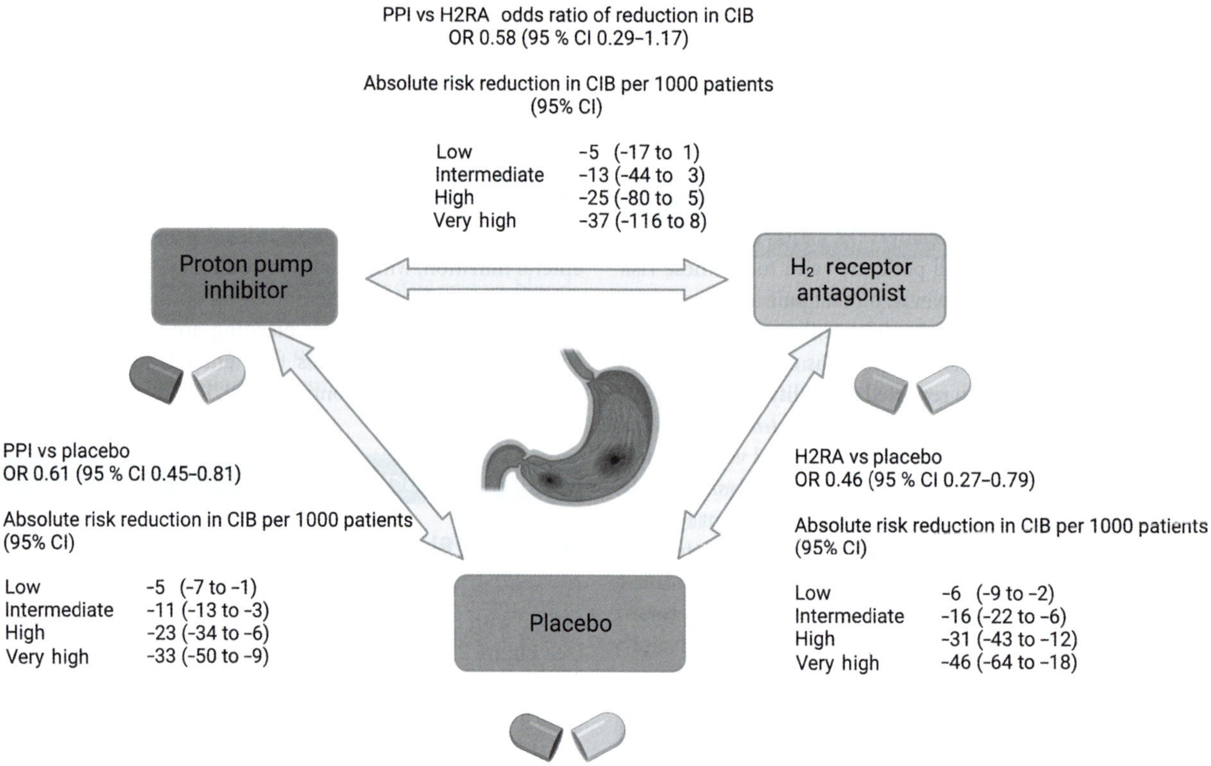

Figure 27.2 Effectiveness of proton pump inhibitors (PPI) and histamine receptor-2 (H_2RA) in reducing clinically important bleeding (CIB). Risk levels as defined in Figure 27.1.

Diagram by A Conway Morris created with BioRender.com. Data from Wang Y, et al., Efficacy and safety of gastrointestinal bleeding prophylaxis in critically ill patients: systematic review and network meta-analysis. *BMJ*. 2020;368:l6744.

significantly lower incidence of clinically important GI bleeding than those receiving sucralfate. No significant differences in length of stay in the ICU, incidence of ventilator-associated pneumonia (VAP), or mortality were reported. A systematic review comparing H2RA, sucralfate, and placebo ($n = 2814$) concluded that trial data was too flawed to draw conclusions on the preferred SUP agent and on whether to use SUP or not in general.[24]

Safety of Stress Ulcer Prophylaxis

Nosocomial Pneumonia

Acid suppressants increase the gastric pH, which can lead to overgrowth of bacteria in the stomach, particularly Gram-negative bacilli that originate in the duodenum (see Table 27.1). Oesophageal reflux and aspiration of gastric contents along the endotracheal tube may then lead to endobronchial colonization and/or VAP. An observational study from 2014 assessing 35,312 mechanically ventilated adult patients receiving either PPI or H2RA found an increased risk of pneumonia in patients receiving PPI as compared with those receiving H2RA.[11] However, high-quality RCTs and systematic reviews evaluating the risk of nosocomial pneumonia between different SUP agents have not been able to confirm this finding.[6,21,22,23]

Table 27.1 Evidence of SUP increasing the risk of infections

Pneumonia	Clostridium difficile
• PPI versus placebo: OR 1.39 (95% CI: 0.98–2.10) • Increase of 50/1000 pts • H2RA versus placebo: OR 1.26 (95% CI: 0.89–1.85) • Increase of 34/1000 pts	• PPI versus placebo: OR 0.82 (CI: 0.31–2.47) • Reduction of 3/1000 pts

CI: confidence interval.

Clostridium difficile Infection

As gastric acidity may be protective against infections, treatment with acid suppressants is hypothesized to increase the risk of enteric infections including *Clostridium difficile* infections (CDIs),[25] which is associated with increased mortality and excess length of ICU stay in critically ill patients.[8,26] Two large, low-risk-of-bias trials reported data on CDI: the SUP-ICU trial assessing PPI versus placebo ($n = 3350$)[6] and the PEPTIC trial assessing PPI versus H2RA ($n = 26982$).[23] In both trials, *Clostridium difficile* infection was rarely reported and none of the trials showed a significant difference between the intervention groups.

Cardiovascular Complications

An increased risk of cardiovascular events in patients receiving PPI has been suggested, and possible mechanisms leading to this have been investigated.[27] It has been hypothesized that the combination of clopidogrel and PPI results in increased risk of adverse cardiac events due to reduced efficacy of clopidogrel when combined with PPI, but data on this is ambiguous.[28] An observational study of

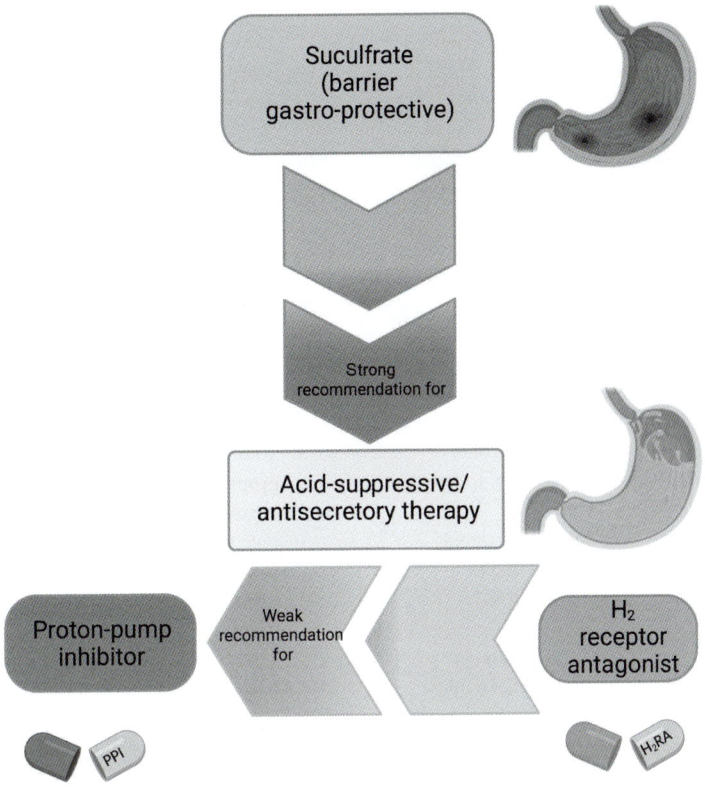

Figure 27.3 Graphical summary of the recommendations for the prescription of stress ulcer prophylaxis from gastrointestinal bleeding prophylaxis for critically ill patients: a clinical practice guideline.[9] Diagram by A Conway Morris created with BioRender.com.

Diagram by A Conway Morris created with BioRender.com. Data from Ye Z, Blaser AR, Lytvyn L, et al. Gastrointestinal bleeding prophylaxis for critically ill patients: a clinical practice guideline. *BMJ* 2020;368:l6722.

56,406 patients points at an increased risk of cardiovascular events in non-ICU patients treated with PPI independent of treatment with clopidogrel.[27] However, the quality of evidence on the association between PPI and cardiovascular events in critically ill patients is low with high risk of confounded results due to the observational design, and the results of the SUP-ICU trial did not confirm this.[6]

An Approach to Stress Ulcer Prophylaxis among Adult Critically Ill Patients

SUP have been widely and somewhat indiscriminantly used in critically ill patients for years, but research findings from recent years may have changed this. Results from large trials suggest that SUP reduce the risk of GI bleeding without any obvious effect on clinically important side effects, including nosocomial infections and myocardial ischaemia. This could suggest that SUP should be used in most critically ill patients. However, GI bleeding is a rare event also in patients not receiving prophylaxis (number needed to treat 59), and results from two large trials suggest possible increased mortality in the most severely ill patients receiving PPI.[6,23] Because the most severely ill patients also are those with the highest risk of developing stress ulceration and GI bleeding, the use of SUP and the choice of agent should be informed by an individual assessment on the risk of GI bleeding. Summary statements of suggested evidence-based recommendations are displayed in Figure 27.3.[9,21,22]

REFERENCES

1. Cook DJ, Griffith LE, Walter SD, et al. The attributable mortality and length of intensive care unit stay of clinically important gastrointestinal bleeding in critically ill patients. *Crit Care.* 2001;**5**:368–375.
2. Cook D, Guyatt G, Marshall J, et al. A comparison of sucralfate and ranitidine for the prevention of upper gastrointestinal bleeding in patients requiring mechanical ventilation. Canadian Critical Care Trials Group. *N Engl J Med.* 1998;**338**:791–797.
3. Krag M, Perner A, Wetterslev J, et al. Prevalence and outcome of gastrointestinal bleeding and use of acid suppressants in acutely ill adult intensive care patients. *Intensive Care Med.* 2015;**41**:833–845.
4. Krag M, Perner A, Wetterslev J, et al. Stress ulcer prophylaxis in the intensive care unit: An international survey of 97 units in 11 countries. *Acta Anaesthesiol Scand.* 2015;**59**:576–585.
5. Eddleston JM, Pearson RC, Holland J, et al. Prospective endoscopic study of stress erosions and ulcers in critically ill adult patients treated with either sucralfate or placebo. *Crit Care Med.* 1994;**22**:1949–1954.
6. Krag M, Marker S, Perner A, et al. Pantoprazole in patients at risk for gastrointestinal bleeding in the ICU. *N Engl J Med.* 2018;**379**:2199–2208.
7. Cook D, Heyland D, Griffith L, et al. Risk factors for clinically important upper gastrointestinal bleeding in patients requiring mechanical ventilation. Canadian Critical Care Trials Group. *Crit Care Med.* 1999;**27**:2812–2817.

8. Buendgens L, Bruensing J, Matthes M, et al. Administration of proton pump inhibitors in critically ill medical patients is associated with increased risk of developing Clostridium difficile–associated diarrhea. *J Crit Care.* 2014;**29**:696 e11–15.
9. Ye Z, Blaser AR, Lytvyn L, et al. Gastrointestinal bleeding prophylaxis for critically ill patients: A clinical practice guideline. *BMJ.* 2020;**368**:l6722.
10. Cook DJ, Fuller HD, Guyatt GH, et al. Risk factors for gastrointestinal bleeding in critically ill patients. Canadian Critical Care Trials Group. *N Engl J Med.* 1994;**330**:377–381.
11. Maclaren R, Reynolds PM, Allen RR. Histamine-2 receptor antagonists vs proton pump inhibitors on gastrointestinal tract hemorrhage and infectious complications in the intensive care unit. *JAMA Intern Med.* 2014;**174**:564–574.
12. Harvey SE, Parrott F, Harrison DA, et al. Trial of the route of early nutritional support in critically ill adults. *N Engl J Med.* 2014;**371**:1673–1684.
13. Kaukonen K-M, Bailey M, Suzuki S, et al. Mortality related to severe sepsis and septic shock among critically ill patients in Australia and New Zealand, 2000–2012. *JAMA.* 2014;**311**:1308–1316.
14. Granholm A, Krag M, Marker S, Alhazzani W, Perner A, Møller MH. Predictors of gastrointestinal bleeding in adult ICU patients in the SUP-ICU trial. *Acta Anaesthesiol Scand.* 2021 Jul;**65**(6):792–800.
15. Granholm A, Zeng L, Dionne JC, et al. Predictors of gastrointestinal bleeding in adult ICU patients: A systematic review and meta-analysis. *Intensive Care Med.* 2019;**45**:1347–1359.
16. Barletta JF, Lat I, Micek ST, et al. Off-label use of gastrointestinal medications in the intensive care unit. *J Intensive Care Med.* 2015;**30**:217–225.
17. Preslaski CR, Mueller SW, Kiser TH, et al. A survey of prescriber perceptions about the prevention of stress-related mucosal bleeding in the intensive care unit. *J Clin Pharm Ther.* 2014;**39**:658–662.
18. Frandah W, Colmer-Hamood J, Nugent K, et al. Patterns of use of prophylaxis for stress-related mucosal disease in patients admitted to the intensive care unit. *J Intensive Care Med.* 2013;**29**:96–103.
19. Marik PE, Vasu T, Hirani A, et al. Stress ulcer prophylaxis in the new millennium: A systematic review and meta-analysis. *Crit Care Med.* 2010;**38**:2222–2228.
20. Kantorova I, Svoboda P, Scheer P, et al. Stress ulcer prophylaxis in critically ill patients: A randomized controlled trial. *Hepatogastroenterology.* 2004;**51**:757–761.
21. Wang Y, Ye Z, Ge L, et al. Efficacy and safety of gastrointestinal bleeding prophylaxis in critically ill patients: Systematic review and network meta-analysis. *BMJ.* 2020;**368**:l6744.
22. Wang Y, Ge L, Ye Z, et al. Efficacy and safety of gastrointestinal bleeding prophylaxis in critically ill patients: An updated systematic review and network meta-analysis of randomized trials. *Intensive Care Med.* 2020;**46**:1987–2000.
23. Young PJ, Bagshaw SM, Forbes AB, et al. Effect of stress ulcer prophylaxis with proton pump inhibitors vs histamine-2 receptor blockers on in-hospital mortality among ICU patients receiving invasive mechanical ventilation: The PEPTIC randomized clinical trial. *JAMA.* 2020;**323**:616–626.
24. Messori A, Trippoli S, Vaiani M, et al. Bleeding and pneumonia in intensive care patients given ranitidine and sucralfate for prevention of stress ulcer: Meta-analysis of randomised controlled trials. *BMJ.* 2000;**321**:1103–1106.
25. Bavishi C, Dupont HL. Systematic review: The use of proton pump inhibitors and increased susceptibility to enteric infection. *Aliment Pharmacol Ther.* 2011;**34**:1269–1281.
26. Kwok CS, Arthur AK, Anibueze CI, et al. Risk of Clostridium difficile infection with acid suppressing drugs and antibiotics: Meta-analysis. *Am J Gastroenterol.* 2012;**107**:1011–1019.
27. Charlot M, Ahlehoff O, Norgaard ML, et al. Proton-pump inhibitors are associated with increased cardiovascular risk independent of clopidogrel use: A nationwide cohort study. *Ann Intern Med.* 2010;**153**:378–386.
28. Van Boxel OS, van Oijen MG, Hagenaars MP, et al. Cardiovascular and gastrointestinal outcomes in clopidogrel users on proton pump inhibitors: Results of a large Dutch cohort study. *Am J Gastroenterol.* 2010;**105**:2430–2436.

28

Mucus and Bronchopulmonary Clearance

Susannah Leaver and Jonathan Ball

KEY MESSAGES

- Airway surface liquid (ASL) covers the entire respiratory tract. Although mainly composed of water, other components include ions, proteins, and lipids, which change according to local function and play host to a vital microbiome.
- Together with the mucociliary escalator and cough reflex, ASL provides protection to the respiratory tract epithelium.
- Positive pressure ventilation affects the production, secretion, and composition of ASL.
- Assisting secretion clearance is a key intervention in the ICU.
- Many inhaled therapies are used to improve bronchopulmonary clearance and many without any evidence of benefit. While there is evidence of superiority for hypertonic saline over other mucolytics, this is not in the ventilated population.

CONTROVERSIES

- The control of the ionic concentration gradient in the luminal surface is incompletely understood.
- What constitutes a healthy and dysfunctional respiratory tract microbiome and how might we influence this?
- The role of air pollution and the climate emergency on lung and general health.

FURTHER RESEARCH

- Trials of the effectiveness of different mucolytics in ventilated patients.
- Comparative studies are addressing this.

Introduction

The human respiratory tract analyses, cleans, humidifies, and thermoregulates inspired gas, conveying it to within microns of our bloodstream thereby facilitating efficient diffusion of oxygen and carbon dioxide. On expiration, this gas conducting system reclaims some of the water and a little of the heat. The gas we inhale also contains microorganisms, particles, and toxic chemicals from which we are well protected by our epithelial defences.

Pathophysiology

The cellular architecture of the epithelial surface of the respiratory tract changes over its course from the nose and pharynx to the major conducting airways (trachea to the first 8–10 generations of cartilaginous bronchi); to the bronchioles (generations 10–15); to the respiratory bronchioles (generations 16–20); to the alveolar ducts (generations 20–23); and finally to the alveoli. The entire tract secretes a luminal, liquid barrier, the complex nature of which, in parallel with the structural changes of the epithelium, is adapted to local function.

This airway surface liquid (ASL) is 85%–97% water into which a complex and dynamically variable cocktail of ions, proteins, and lipids are secreted. The water is derived from plasma via the interstitium and passively follows an osmotic gradient into the airways. The control of this ionic osmotic gradient is both highly complex and incompletely understood. Airway epithelial cells express a very large number of ion channels and energy-dependent transporters on both their apical and basal surfaces creating the dynamic capacity for the epithelium to shift between a net secretory and net absorptive surface.[1,2] Indeed, as ASL is propelled proximally by the mucociliary escalator, there is net salt and water absorption (>90%) that is commensurate with the decreasing total cross-sectional area of the airways. Though these channels on respiratory epithelial cells include aquaporins (small, integral membrane proteins that facilitate water transport across cell membranes in response to osmotic gradients), they do not appear to play a major role in water transport except in the submucosal glands in the proximal airways.[3] The principal determinant of ASL volume is the lumen concentration of sodium chloride. This in turn is controlled by the active secretion of chloride and bicarbonate ions into the airway lumen (to increase water content), a process notably contributed to by the cystic fibrosis transmembrane conductance regulator or the absorption of sodium ions via epithelial sodium channels (to decrease water content). Notably, the mechanical stretch that results from tidal ventilation stimulates chloride and bicarbonate release and inhibits sodium absorption, thus stimulating airway hydration. Perhaps surprisingly, the pH of normal airway fluid is actively maintained at 7.0 and has a high buffering capacity, thereby neutralizing inhaled acids and alkalis and protecting the epithelium from toxic chemical exposure.

At the most distal extent of the respiratory tract, in the alveoli, the ASL is only ~0.1 μm thick and in addition to water contains surfactant, a complex phospholipid and protein mixture, that serves the vital function of reducing surface tension forces, thereby maximizing alveolar inspiratory compliance and minimizing expiratory collapse.[4] Surfactant dysfunction is a pathognomonic feature of acute respiratory distress syndrome and is covered in detail elsewhere.[5] Clearance of debris is affected by alveolar macrophages.

By contrast to the distal respiratory tract, in the proximal conducting airways the ASL is up to 10 μm thick. It is made up of two distinct layers: a primarily liquid/low viscosity peri-ciliary layer and above it, in contact with the luminal gas, a high viscosity/mucous gel layer, which may be continuous or form isolated rafts. The function of this mucous gel layer is to capture and neutralize the vast majority of the estimated 5–10,000 × 10^{10} particles we inhale daily. Normal proximal ASL is 97% water and contains ~3% solids made up of ~1% gel-forming mucins with the remainder being non-mucin proteins (antimicrobial, immunomodulatory, and protective molecules),[6] salts, lipids, and cellular debris. The mucins are a family of large (up to 3 × 10^6 D per monomer), highly anionic, glycoproteins (50%–90% carbohydrate) encoded by ~20 genes. Somewhat counterintuitively, only seven of the mucins are secreted from stored intra-cellular granules; the remainder are cell membrane bound and exhibit both structural functions and signal transduction properties. However, these membrane-bound mucins are released by cleavage near their transmembrane domain into the ASL by proteases or autocatalysis and account for ~10% of the mucous gel.[7]

Proximal airway geometry maximizes the impact of particles into this mucous gel by inducing turbulence and having a rapidly dichotomous branching structure that creates impact zones at bifurcations. In addition, as gas travels beyond the third generation, there is an exponential increase in the effective surface area causing a rapid deceleration in convectional gas flow, resulting in the gravitational drop out of suspended particles. The highly coordinated, in-plane beating of cilia across multiple cells of the epithelium then waft this particle-laden mucous gel layer proximally, the so-called mucociliary escalator, until it is passively swallowed and enters the gastrointestinal tract.[8] Larger aggregations of mucus may form and can trigger the cough reflex, which, subject to mechanical strength, should project the bolus well beyond the larynx.

The pseudostratified epithelium of the proximal, conducting airways, principally consists of a mosaic of ciliated and secretory cell types; the former being the majority though this is more so distally than proximally, as there is a progressive decline in overall mucus-secreting capacity with increasing airway generation. The putative explanation is that mucus secretion needs to be maximal in earlier airway generations where the majority of particle impaction occurs. Hence, these proximal generations have mucous glands and serous and goblet cells, the mid generations just have serous and goblet cells, and the later generations merely have Clara cells. Both ciliated and secretory cells have numerous microvilli that facilitate the transepithelial movement of fluid and electrolytes. Both cilia and microvilli are densely coated in highly negatively charged, membrane-bound mucins (MUC1, 4, 16, and 20). These project brush like resulting in near frictionless interactions between adjacent cilia and a strong osmotic pressure that traps water in the peri-ciliary layer forming a uniform surface just below the tips of the cilia. This mesh effectively excludes particles >25 nm. Like all of the other components of this intricate barrier defence system, the cilia beat frequency can be increased in response to changing conditions.[8]

In humans, the predominant mucins in the mucous gel layer of proximal ASL are MUC5AC (more proximally) and MUC5B (more distally). Both of these mucins form long single-chain homotypic polymers, which entangle into a mesh by non-covalent, calcium-dependent cross-linking. This mesh provides a physical barrier with pore sizes of ~500 nm, limiting penetration to small viruses with hydrophilic capsids. The glycan side chains trap very large quantities of water, and the resultant gel appears to act as a water reservoir for the peri-ciliary layer. In addition, these side chains help sequester microorganisms by acting as decoys for epithelial cell surface sugars.

Mucin production and secretion are regulated separately. Production is highly regulated at the transcriptional level with increases triggered by many pro-inflammatory stimuli with the ErbB receptor and interleukin-13 playing central roles in signal transduction. These exist on both the luminal and basal surfaces of secretory cells. Control of secretion differs between secretory cell types. Glands are controlled by cholinergic, adrenergic, and other neurohormonal signals via basal membrane receptors. By contrast, goblet cell secretion is dependent upon specific secretagogues, the most important of which appears to be luminal adenosine triphosphate (ATP), which acts via $P2Y_2$ receptors. ATP is continuously present at low levels in ASL, thereby ensuring basal levels of secretion. ATP is also released into the lumen as a consequence of mechanical deformation and exposure to a wide variety of mucosal irritants, thereby stimulating mucin secretion.

Mucin hypersecretion and/or dysregulation of ASL volume may increase the concentration of solids from 3% up to 15%, resulting in a more viscous, elastic, and adherent gel that is not easily cleared by the mucociliary escalator and is harder to expel by coughing. Inflammatory stimuli result in a dramatic increase in MUC5AC production (40–200 times) and a more modest increase (3–10 times) in MUC5B. This pathological mucus, usually produced and secreted in excessive quantities, causes mechanical obstruction to small- and medium-sized airways. Proximally this changes the microbiome, while distally it transforms the normally sterile environment into an excellent culture medium, especially for Staphylococcal species and environmental Gram-negative organisms.[9] This in turn stimulates an influx of inflammatory cells, in particular neutrophils. The resulting accumulation of host and microorganism deoxyribonucleic acid creates an even more viscous, elastic, and adherent sputum.

Though beyond the scope of this chapter, there is a rapidly emerging and critically important story of the lung microbiome (bacteria, viruses, fungi, and mycobacteria) and its role in airway physiology and lung diseases, both acute and chronic.[10,11]

The Negative Effects of Airway Conduits and Mechanical Ventilation (MV)

Placing a plastic tube into the trachea, thereby bypassing the nasopharynx and larynx, is an irritant to mechanical receptors, impairs the humidification and thermoregulation of inspired gas, disrupts the mucociliary escalator, and impedes the exit path of cough propelled sputum. Natural particle filtration, humidification, and thermoregulation of inspired gas is replaced by the delivery of medical gases and either by heat and moisture exchange filters or heated humidified circuits. In addition, the discomfort of the tube may necessitate sedative drugs that inhibit airway reflexes. The effects of positive pressure ventilation on the production, secretion, and composition of ASL are often subtle but may be profound and is thought to be influenced by both the fraction of inspired oxygen and the cumulative dose of mechanical energy delivered. The overall effect is often an increase in mucin production and secretion coupled with relative dehydration and the induction of airway inflammation.[12] Cumulatively, these effects place the patient at risk of retained, viscous secretions and subsequent predisposition to colonisation and infection. Prolonged MV will exacerbate all of these negative impacts and is frequently associated with muscle weakness and thus a weakened cough, with the resultant inability to generate an adequate peak cough flow/peak expiratory flow required to eliminate respiratory secretions.

Offsetting these negative effects is largely a matter of delivering optimal critical care including minimizing sedation, minimizing the mechanical stress of positive pressure ventilation (pressure limited, low tidal volume, optimized positive end-expiratory pressure, and minimized oxygen exposure), maximizing spontaneous breathing efforts, active weaning from MV at the earliest stages, early physical rehabilitation (during as well as after MV), timely bronchoscopic clearance of proximally impacted secretions, and adequate but not excessive hydration and nutrition. The value of antimicrobial stewardship and the potential benefits of therapies to re-establish a healthy microbiome must also be considered.

Specific Interventions to Improve Bronchopulmonary Clearance

Physiotherapy, Mechanical Devices, and Early Mobilization

This is addressed in detail in Chapter 30.

Mucoactive Agents

Numerous mucoactive agents are used to combat the deleterious effects of intubation and MV despite a lack of proven benefit. These work by modifying ASL production, secretion, and composition, and possibly the mucociliary escalator. Since there is limited data on the benefit of individual agents in mechanically ventilated patients, their effects have been extrapolated from their use in other respiratory conditions. Most agents are converted to aerosols by nebulization and placed in the ventilator circuit. Their efficacy is strongly influenced by many variables in this delivery process.[13]

Nebulized Hypertonic Saline (HS)

Nebulized HS (3%–14%) is an osmotic agent that transiently increases airway surface hydration by drawing water to the epithelial surface, thereby increasing ASL hydration and enhancing mucociliary clearance.[14] It is safe, inexpensive, and effective in improving sputum clearance in patients with cystic fibrosis, asthma, chronic bronchitis, and bronchiolitis, but there is a paucity of clinical trials looking at its use in adult ventilated patients.[15] There is however evidence of superiority over other nebulized mucolytic agents. In patients with cystic fibrosis, inhalation of nebulized HS (7%) for one year was associated with a reduction in the number of pulmonary exacerbations and increased lung function when compared to those receiving nebulized normal saline (0.9%).[16] When compared to normal saline, 3% HS, given to children with bronchiolitis, significantly reduced hospital admission.[17] HS also enhanced mucociliary clearance in patients with asthma, cystic fibrosis, and healthy controls when compared with 0.9% saline.[18,19] While there is anecdotal evidence of benefit in the intensive care population, large randomized controlled trials are required to determine its efficacy.

Nebulized Mannitol

Nebulized mannitol is postulated to improve mucus clearance through its osmotic properties. While there is no evidence for its use in ventilated populations, inhaled mannitol has been shown to improve lung function in cystic fibrosis patients.[20]

Dornase Alpha (DNAse–Pulmozyme)

Dornase alpha (DNAse—pulmozyme) is recombinant human deoxyribonuclease 1. DNA is released into the airway mucus by microorganisms and host neutrophils. When polymerized, DNA further increases mucus viscosity. Thus, reducing its concentration in airway secretions should reduce mucus viscosity. In patients with cystic fibrosis, nebulized dornase alpha reduced mucus viscosity and improved lung function.[21,22] Although used off-licence in critically ill ventilated patients, a Cochrane review found insufficient quality data to either support or refute its use when compared to placebo or hypertonic saline.[23]

N-acetylcysteine (NAC)

NAC, either oral or nebulized, is commonly used to improve sputum clearance. It is frequently nebulized in conjunction with a beta$_2$ agonist (see below) as it can induce bronchoconstriction. However, there is no evidence to support its use in any pathological condition or in mechanically ventilated patients.[24] Enteral carbocysteine has become as increasingly popular alternative and even adjunct to nebulized NAC,[25] but similarly lacks any evidence of benefit in mechanically ventilated patients.

Nebulized Beta$_2$ Agonists

Nebulized beta$_2$ agonists have pleiotropic effects on airway inflammation, epithelial and smooth muscle function, ASL production, secretion and composition, and ciliary function.[26,27] Some of these effects may be injurious[28,29] as can the systemic effects of this class of drugs.[30] Despite the absence of evidence to support their use in mechanically ventilated patients, there are prescribed frequently.[31] With the exception of patients with reversible bronchoconstriction, these agents have no role in improving bronchopulmonary clearance. Of note, there is arguably a stronger pharmacological case for using anti-muscarinic drugs,[32] but no trials have been performed in mechanically ventilated patients to inform rational administration. Similarly, the adjunctive use of inhaled corticosteroids has biological plausibility but has never been subjected to a randomized controlled trial (RCT) in mechanically ventilated patients.

Unfractionated Heparin

Unfractionated heparin has a number of therapeutic effects, including promotion of mucociliary clearance, antibacterial effects on common respiratory pathogens, and decreases sputum viscosity, making it a potential candidate for the prevention and treatment of pathogenic sputum. Trials to date have reported mixed results, but in patients with inhalational burns[33] and at risk of acute respiratory distress syndrome (ARDS),[34] there appears to be probable benefit and no harm.

REFERENCES

1. Toczylowska-Maminska R, Dolowy K. Ion transporting proteins of human bronchial epithelium. *J Cell Biochem.* 2012;**113**(2):426–432.
2. Hollenhorst MI, Richter K, Fronius M. Ion transport by pulmonary epithelia. *J Biomed Biotechnol.* 2011;**2011**:174306.
3. Verkman AS. Role of aquaporins in lung liquid physiology. *Respir Physiol Neurobiol.* 2007;**159**(3):324–330.
4. Parra E, Perez-Gil J. Composition, structure and mechanical properties define performance of pulmonary surfactant membranes and films. *Chem Phys Lipids.* 2015;**185**:153–175.
5. Nieman GF, Gatto LA, Habashi NM. Impact of mechanical ventilation on the pathophysiology of progressive acute lung injury. *J Appl Physiol (1985).* 2015;**119**(11):1245–1261.
6. Joo NS, et al. Proteomic analysis of pure human airway gland mucus reveals a large component of protective proteins. *PLoS One.* 2015;**10**(2):e0116756.
7. Widdicombe JH, Wine JJ. Airway gland structure and function. *Physiol Rev.* 2015;**95**(4):1241–1319.
8. Tilley AE, et al. Cilia dysfunction in lung disease. *Annu Rev Physiol.* 2015; 77:379–406.
9. Kelly BJ, et al. Composition and dynamics of the respiratory tract microbiome in intubated patients. *Microbiome.* 2016;**4**:7.
10. Invernizzi R, Lloyd CM, Molyneaux PL. Respiratory microbiome and epithelial interactions shape immunity in the lungs. *Immunology.* 2020;**160**(2):171–182.
11. Martin-Loeches I, Dickson R, Torres A, et al. The importance of airway and lung microbiome in the critically ill. *Crit Care.* 2020;**24**(1):537.
12. McCall MN, Illei PB, Halushka MK. Complex sources of variation in tissue expression data: Analysis of the GTEx lung transcriptome. *Am J Hum Genet.* 2016;**99**(3):624–635.
13. Ruickbie S, Hall A, Ball J. Therapeutic aerosols in mechanically ventilated patients. In: Vincent, J-L, ed. *In Annual Update in Intensive Care and Emergency Medicine 2011.* Berlin: Springer-Verlag; 2011:197–206.
14. Reeves EP, McCarthy C, McElvaney OJ, et al. Inhaled hypertonic saline for cystic fibrosis: Reviewing the potential evidence for modulation of neutrophil signalling and function. *World J Crit Care Med.* 2015;**4**(3):179–191.
15. Youness HA, et al. Dornase alpha compared to hypertonic saline for lung atelectasis in critically ill patients. *J Aerosol Med Pulm Drug Deliv.* 2012; **25**(6):342–348.
16. Elkins MR, et al. A controlled trial of long-term inhaled hypertonic saline in patients with cystic fibrosis. *N Engl J Med.* 2006;**354**(3):229–240.
17. Wu S, et al. Nebulized hypertonic saline for bronchiolitis: A randomized clinical trial. *JAMA Pediatr.* 2014;**168**(7):657–663.
18. Daviskas E, et al. Inhalation of hypertonic saline aerosol enhances mucociliary clearance in asthmatic and healthy subjects. *Eur Respir J.* 1996;**9**(4):725–732.
19. Robinson M, et al. Effect of increasing doses of hypertonic saline on mucociliary clearance in patients with cystic fibrosis. *Thorax.* 1997;**52**(10): 900–903.
20. Daviskas E, et al. Inhaled mannitol improves the hydration and surface properties of sputum in patients with cystic fibrosis. *Chest.* 2010;**137**(4):861–868.
21. Wagener JS, Kupfer O. Dornase alfa (Pulmozyme). *Curr Opin Pulm Med.* 2012;**18**(6):609–614.
22. Jones AP, Wallis C. Dornase alfa for cystic fibrosis. *Cochrane Database Syst Rev.* 2010(3):CD001127.
23. Claudius C, Perner A, Moller MH. Nebulised dornase alfa versus placebo or hypertonic saline in adult critically ill patients: A systematic review of randomised clinical trials with meta-analysis and trial sequential analysis. *Syst Rev.* 2015;**4**:153.
24. Masoompour SM, Anushiravani A, Tafaroj Norouz A. Evaluation of the effect of nebulized N-Acetylcysteine on respiratory secretions in mechanically ventilated patients: Randomized clinical trial. *Iran J Med Sci.* 2015;**40**(4):309–315.
25. Rahman I, MacNee W. Antioxidant pharmacological therapies for COPD. *Curr Opin Pharmacol.* 2012;**12**(3):256–265.
26. Bassford CR, Thickett DR, Perkins GD. The rise and fall of beta-agonists in the treatment of ARDS. *Crit Care.* 2012;**16**(2):208.
27. Salathe M. Effects of beta-agonists on airway epithelial cells. *J Allergy Clin Immunol.* 2002;**110**(6 Suppl):S275–281.
28. Peitzman ER, et al. Agonist binding to beta-adrenergic receptors on human airway epithelial cells inhibits migration and wound repair. *Am J Physiol Cell Physiol.* 2015;**309**(12):C847–855.
29. Patel M, Thomson NC. (R)-salbutamol in the treatment of asthma and chronic obstructive airways disease. *Expert Opin Pharmacother.* 2011;**12**(7):1133–1141.
30. Creagh-Brown BC, Ball J. An under-recognized complication of treatment of acute severe asthma. *Am J Emerg Med.* 2008;**26**(4):514 e1–3.
31. Chang LH, et al. Utilization of bronchodilators in ventilated patients without obstructive airways disease. *Respir Care.* 2007;**52**(2):154–158.
32. Meurs H, et al. A new perspective on muscarinic receptor antagonism in obstructive airways diseases. *Curr Opin Pharmacol.* 2013;**13**(3):316–323.
33. Lan X, et al. Nebulized heparin for inhalation injury in burn patients: A systematic review and meta-analysis. *Burns Trauma.* 2020;**8**:tkaa015.
34. Dixon B, et al. Nebulised heparin for patients with or at risk of acute respiratory distress syndrome: A multicentre, randomised, double-blind, placebo-controlled phase 3 trial. *Lancet Respir Med.* 2021;**9**(4):360–372.

29

Delirium and Sleep

Ahmed Al-Hindawi, Eli Rogers, and Marcela P Vizcaychipi

KEY MESSAGES

- Delirium is common among critically ill patients, occurring in up to 80% of patients.
- The causes of delirium are multifactorial but coalesce on common final pathways leading to the clinical manifestations.
- Structured validated tools such as CAM-ICU help detection.
- Treatment focuses on removing precipitating causes and non-pharmacological interventions. Pharmacological therapies can help control agitation but do not alter the underlying pathology, and in the case of benzodiazepines may paradoxically increase risk of delirium.

CONTROVERSIES

- Delirium is still considered a 'stand-alone' entity, while some evidence is emerging about initial signs as early manifestations of long-term cognitive brain disease.
- Hypoactive delirium seems to be under-recognized.
- Active assessment of delirium at admission to hospitals and perioperative care remains a non-essential clinical assessment and not part of standard clinical care.

FURTHER RESEARCH

- Research into non-medical interventions to prevent the development of delirium in hospitals.
- Active screening of risk factors for delirium on admission to hospitals, with the intention of identifying modifiable factors as part of a standard clinical approach.
- Use of bioinformatics and machine learning to identify clinical signs of delirium before it occurs.

Introduction

Delirium is defined as a transient, usually reversible, cause of cerebral dysfunction, and it manifests clinically with a wide range of neuropsychiatric abnormalities. It can occur at any age, but it occurs more commonly in patients who are elderly and have had prior compromised mental status.[1] This state can occur in any acutely unwell patient and those who are socially isolated, but older patients are often at risk as they have lower functional cognitive reserves to deal with pathological insults, such as surgery, sepsis, metabolic derangements, and burns.[2–5] The development of delirium in patients can be thought of in terms of organ failure. This metaphor has implications as data suggests that patients who develop delirium during their stay in hospital have increased mortality compared to patients who do not (Figure 29.1).[6,7] A conservative estimate of the incidence of delirium in acutely unwell patients is 20% and has been reported to be as high as 80%.[6,8]

Two phenotypic types of delirium occur: hyperactive and hypoactive delirium. Hyperactive delirium is heralded by overt physical and verbal agitation—this behaviour often draws attention and is what many healthcare professionals think of when delirium is defined, yet it only represents a small fraction (~5%) of the overall incidence of delirium. Hypoactive delirium is an inwards-reflective, physically and verbally depressed state that, due to its nature, often goes missed as patients draw little attention from nursing staff when it represents the overwhelming majority of patients.

The 5th edition of the Diagnostic and Statistical Manual of Mental Disorders (DSM-V) has simplified the diagnosis of delirium and specifically focuses on the fluctuating component to delirium. The National Institute of Clinical Excellence (NICE) 2019 Clinical Guideline 103 for the management of delirium suggests the use of Confusion Assessment Method (CAM) in ICU (CAM-ICU) for its high sensitivity, repeatability, objectivity, and ease of use.[9] Intensive care nurses are well positioned to operate this screening tool, and this should be performed daily to screen for temporal fluctuations suggestive of delirium.[10,11] Both the DSM-V and NICE place special emphasis on finding a cause once a diagnosis has been made.

Pathophysiology of Delirium

Sources differ upon the pathophysiology of delirium; it is caused by numerous aetiologies, yet the clinical presentation often appears similar in patients. The current prevailing concept unifying delirium research is that the many causes of delirium all trigger physiological

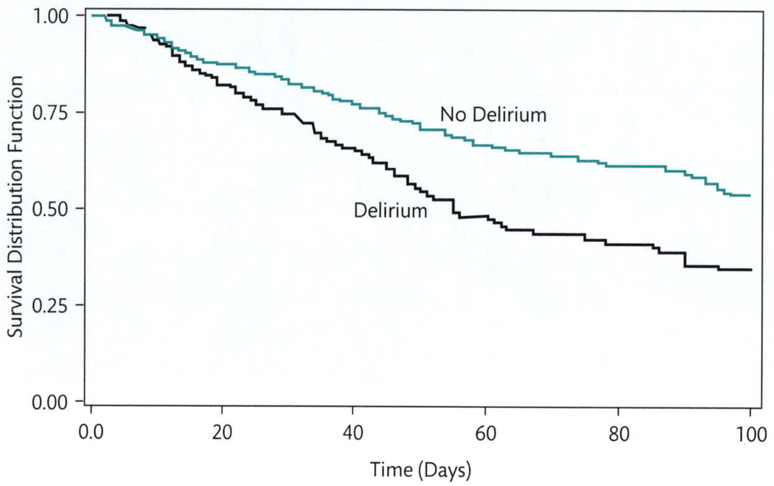

Figure 29.1 Mortality of patients with and without delirium demonstrating increased mortality of patient who suffer with delirium during their in-patient stay.[7] Diagram by A Conway Morris created with BioRender.com.

Reproduced *from Intensive Care Medicine*, Incidence, risk factors and consequences of ICU delirium, 33, 2007, pp. 66–73, Ouimet S, et al. With permission of Springer.

responses that eventually coalesce in a 'final common pathway' in the brain that causes the observed forms of delirium. There are several predominating theories for this final common pathway: neurotransmitter imbalance, neuroinflammation, and oxidative stress as illustrated in Figure 29.2.

The neurotransmitter hypothesis emphasizes the balance between cholinergic and dopaminergic pathways and suggests that delirium stems from a disruption of this neural balance.[12] The pathway systems are by nature opposing; acetylcholine represents an increase in neural excitation and dopamine representing a decrease, and disturbance of these pathways can lead to delirious effects. It has been shown, but remains controversial, that anticholinergic activity can be a predictor of hypoactive delirium and its severity[13] and further that hypercholinergic medications reverse this hypoactive

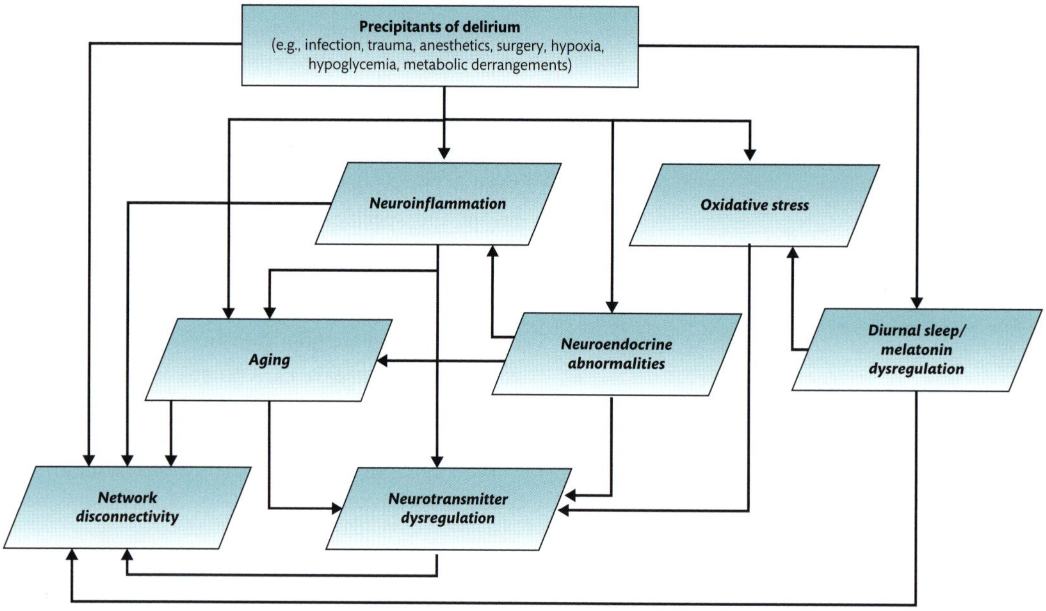

Figure 29.2 Interconnection of current aetiologic theories of delirium and their hypothesised interconnections. The primary and enduring theories, often complementary, are the neurotransmitter, neuroinflammatory, oxidative stress, and sleep dysregulation hypothesis.[15] Diagram by A Conway Morris created with BioRender.com.

Reprinted from *The American Journal of Geriatric Psychiatry*, 21(12), Maldonado JR. Neuropathogenesis of delirium: review of current etiologic theories and common pathways, pp. 1190–222. Copyright 2013, with permission from Elsevier and the American Association for Geriatric Psychiatry.

form of delirium. This has been supported further by evidence that dopamine-blocking medications too can ameliorate the symptoms of hypoactive delirium.[14] The cholinergic–dopaminergic balance has additionally been shown to interact with the glutaminergic and GABA-mediated pathways in the physiogenesis of delirium.[15]

The neuroinflammation hypothesis focuses upon the adverse effects of inflammation or trauma upon neural tissue and suggests that delirium may originate from inflammatory responses in the brain. It has been shown that stimulation of the peripheral nervous system can induce an inflammatory response that crosses the blood–brain barrier that can disrupt synaptic function, inducing delirium symptoms. The hypothesized pathway within the central nervous system begins with the activation of parenchymal cells, cytokines, and other proinflammatory mediators that are associated with adverse neurobehavioral and cognitive effects.[16] The increased presence of delirium in clinical settings could thus be attributed, in part, to infection or systemic response to trauma, the presence of foreign bodies, anaesthetics, or other situations that trigger the inflammatory cascade. It is through this method that SARS-CoV-2 is thought to cause delirium—it has been demonstrated that the virus causes direct central nervous system involvement.[17]

The oxidative stress hypothesis proposes that delirium stems from the adverse anoxic effects of hypoperfusion, namely that decreased oxidative energy production triggers cognitive dysfunction that presents as delirium. Studies have shown that oxidative stress, or conversely a deficiency of antioxidants, is associated with cognitive dysfunction, and further that delirious patients are significantly more likely to be poorly oxygenated, although this is correlative rather than causative.[18] The results are similar with other forms of oxidative stress, including sepsis and other infections.[15]

Additionally, it has been shown that there is an association between sleep and delirium; disruption of the normal sleep cycles and circadian rhythms is intertwined with the presence of delirium, and while a causation relationship has not been established, it is well known that the two are related.[19] Sleep deprivation exacerbates acute and pre-existing conditions, further disrupting homeostasis and magnifying organ dysfunction. Sleep disruptions heighten the physiological effects of neuroinflammation, neurotransmitter disruption, and oxidative stress, effectively aggravating the progression of the brain injury. For this reason, sleep deprivation is regarded as a key risk factor in the development of delirium and must be actively prevented by sleep quality monitoring to ensure proper recovery.

Polysomnography, a form of electroencephalography, has been used historically as a method of judging sleep depth, and thus as a tool to attempt to predict and prevent delirium. The association between these disruptions and observed delirium is currently a prominent topic of study, with further investigations into the interaction between medications and sleep in the development of delirium. Melatonin therapy by external administration is currently under investigation with the goal of restoration of circadian rhythms to promote proper sleep. Alternatively, noradrenaline, a common vasopressor used in ICU, has been linked to natural melatonin secretion; several studies have highlighted a potential antagonist effect while conflictingly others have demonstrated an agonistic effect. It is evident, however, that the use of adrenal catecholamines leads to disturbed pineal gland function and altered melatonin secretion, indicating a known influence of these medications upon sleep and thus delirium.[20,21] The use of sedatives (see Chapter 25) is additionally of particular interest in the ICU in controlling sleep; it is commonplace to give sedation and analgesic medications to critically ill patients, often to alleviate discomfort caused by injuries or interventions such as endotracheal tubes and mechanical ventilation. The research shows, however, that the usage of sedatives decrease both deep and rapid eye movement (REM) sleep and damages the restorative quality of the sleep that patients procure, thereby undermining its hypothesized delirium-controlling effects. The detailed influences upon sleep and delirium of specific treatments and known pharmacological interventions are described in later sections.[22]

In light of the conflicting and complimentary results of studies investigating the major hypotheses, it is most likely that a combination of neuroinflammation, neurotransmitter mediation, oxidative effects, and an association with REM sleep governs the development and pathophysiology of delirium.

Detection of Delirium

Detection of delirium is challenging—the lack of an encompassing definition creates heterogeneity in the diagnostic criteria. Thus, there has been varying efforts at applying the DSM-V definition of delirium into a scoring system that is sensitive and predictive of delirium. CAM-ICU is one such scoring system that emphasizes a temporally varying inattention and consciousness as it is central tenant for the diagnosis of delirium in ICU. It is simple to perform and has a high sensitivity for delirium.[23]

The Intensive Care Delirium Screening Checklist is another popular tool that has been superseded by CAM-ICU; its main drawback has been the emphasis on hyperactive delirium resulting in excellent sensitivities but with a specificity of 65%.[24]

The assessment test for delirium and cognitive impairment (A4T) is another important tool that has the benefit of including cognitive testing within its short questionnaire. Its short format allows for rapid assessment with favourable performance.

Predicting delirium prior to its development has also gathered some interest with the creation of the multiple scoring systems, with PRE-DELIRIC being of particular significance. The score was developed, and then re-calibrated, based on a large international cohort of ICU patients who found common denominators in their first day of their ICU stay for the development of delirium were namely severity of illness according to APACHE criteria, sedation, and morphine use. Its goodness of fit with true outcomes flattens out near the 0.4 mark indicating that its confidence of prediction falls above that mark. Nevertheless, it is helpful in identifying high-risk patients.[25,26] An easier-to-use linear model that does not require parameters from the first 24 h of a patient's ITU stay is the E-PRE-DELIRIC score.[27]

Further investigations into the cause of delirium could include polysomnography, a comprehensive multi-parameter test of sleep, specifically its depth and stages. The test involves instrumenting the patient looking for eye movements by electro-oculography, brain function by electroencephalography, muscular activity by electromyography, heart rhythms by electrocardiography, and respiratory function by peripheral pulse oximetry. Its use in the diagnosis of delirium is controversial as there is conflicting evidence on its specificity, but it is the most accurate test for lack of REM sleep as a cause of delirium.[28,29]

Pragmatically, often the patient's relatives are highly specific for any cognitive changes that would indicate the development of delirium prior to any positive test—a helpful hint that should be heeded.

Treatment of Delirium

Modifiable risk factors for the development of delirium are numerous but can be classified into patient specific and disease specific. Table 29.1 summarizes common modifiable risk factors that should be minimized. Emphasis should be places on ensuring as close to normal physiology as possible. Reducing dehydration and constipation, correcting hypoxia, ensuring that mobility by minimizing indwelling catheters, regular medication reviews, and ensuring adequate sleep are of paramount importance.

Initial management of delirium should be aimed at correcting the cause of delirium. If a medical condition has been the trigger of cause of delirium, then it is likely that the patient is going to continue to be delirious if the medical condition has not been treated. This is often difficult to correct immediately, but an exhaustive search of other causes should be performed, bearing in mind that there may be more than one precipitating cause.

There are several simple and non-pharmacological measures that should be employed at the hyperactive delirious patient. NICE recommends commencing with environmental de-escalation strategies, whether verbal or non-verbal. These include correcting sensory impairment with hearing aids or spectacles, clear precise communication, and frequent orientation strategies.[10]

Table 29.1 Summary of modifiable and non-modifiable risk factors for the development of delirium

Modifiable risk factors	Non-modifiable risk factors
Restraint • Physical • Urinary catheter • Intravenous lines • Monitoring	Age
Sleep disturbance	Genetic factors
Infection	Pre-existing cognitive decline • Dementia
Hypoxia	Pre-existing psychiatric illness • Depression and schizoaffective disorders specifically
Pain	Frailty
Use of steroids	
Severity of illness • Multiorgan failure • Mean arterial pressure at time of admission to ICU	
Dehydration	
Constipation	
Nutrition	
Polypharmacy	

Noise at night should be kept to a minimum, mimicking their normal environment. Simple adjuncts such as ear plugs have been shown to dramatically reduce the incidence of sleep deprivation and delirium.[30] It is emphasized that patients to be allowed nocturnal sleep with minimal interruptions, that efforts be made to reduce the impact and frequency of interventions that interfere with proper sleep, and that sedation be limited to the minimum necessary for patient comfort.

Sedation of the combative agitated delirious patient with benzodiazepines, such as midazolam and lorazepam, is often successful in the short term—patients are then compliant if not asleep and often do not cause problems. However, it has been demonstrated that sedation with benzodiazepines is associated with a 3.8-fold increase in the incidence of delirium—while the overt symptoms of hyperactive delirium are reduced, they often wake up more confused and more delirious once the effect of the benzodiazepine has worn off. Atypical antipsychotics, like haloperidol, are thus advocated for the control of agitation in delirium it not contraindicated. The Hope-ICU study, a randomized double-blinded placebo-controlled study, failed to demonstrate that prophylactic haloperidol increases delirium-free days while the MoDUS study failed to demonstrate a similar outcome from prophylactic lipid-soluble statins.[31,32]

The patient's relatives should be informed of the development of delirium. The American Delirium Society gives helpful guidance regarding delirium and its management and steps in which the relatives can help, for example, by bringing in objects that their relative recognizes.

Conclusion

Delirium is a fluctuating disease of cognition and inattention that is prevalent in the ICU setting with marked consequences. It is likely that a combination of neuroinflammation, neurotransmitter mediation, oxidative effects, and sleep dysregulation governs the development and physiogenesis of delirium.

Its prediction and diagnosis has been made simpler by helpful scoring systems that are easy to administer and are reliable. Treatment is aimed at finding the cause of the delirium, and removing exacerbators, while waiting for neurological recovery that could take days or weeks. The patient's relatives should be kept appraised of the developments and given guidance on the steps that they could do to aid recovery.

REFERENCES

1. Association AAP. *DSM-IV-TR: Diagnostic and Statistical Manual of Mental Disorders*. Washington, DC Am Psychiatr Assoc. 1994;143–147.
2. Holt-Lunstad J, Smith TB, Layton JB. Social relationships and mortality risk: A meta-analytic review. *PLoS Med*. 2010 Jul 27;7:e1000316
3. Palmu R. Mental disorders among burn patients. *Burns*. 2011;**36**:1072–1079.
4. Lundström M, Olofsson B, Stenvall M, et al. Postoperative delirium in old patients with femoral neck fracture: a randomized intervention study. *Aging Clin Exp Res*. 2007;**19**:178–186.

5. Meier-Ruge W, Hunziker O, Iwangoff P. Senile dementia: a threshold phenomenon of normal aging? A contribution to the functional reserve hypothesis of the brain. *Ann N Y Acad Sci.* 1991;**621**:104–118.
6. Lin S-M, Liu C, Wang C, et al. The impact of delirium on the survival of mechanically ventilated patients. *Crit Care Med.* 2004;**32**:2254–2259.
7. Ouimet S, Kavanagh BP, Gottfried SB, et al. Incidence, risk factors and consequences of ICU delirium. *Intensive Care Med.* 2007;**33**:66–73.
8. Pisani MA, Araujo KL, Van Ness PH, et al. A research algorithm to improve detection of delirium in the intensive care unit. *Crit Care.* 2006;**10**:R121.
9. Delirium: prevention, diagnosis and management in hospital and long-term care. London: National Institute for Health and Care Excellence (NICE); 2023 Jan 18. PMID: 31971702.
10. NICE. Delirium: prevention, diagnosis and management | Guidance and guidelines | NICE [Internet]. NICE; 2019;1–25 [cited 2021 Oct 17]. Available from: https://www.nice.org.uk/guidance/cg103
11. Association AP, others. *Diagnostic and Statistical Manual of Mental Disorders (DSM-5®).* American Psychiatric Pub; 2013.
12. Trzepacz PT. Delirium. Advances in diagnosis, pathophysiology, and treatment. *Psychiatr Clin North Am.* 1996 Sep;**19**(3):429–448.
13. Han L, McCusker J, Cole M, et al. Use of medications with anticholinergic effect predicts clinical severity of delirium symptoms in older medical inpatients. *Arch Intern Med.* 2001;**161**:1099–1105.
14. Trzepacz PT. Update on the neuropathogenesis of delirium. *Dement Geriatr Cogn Disord.* 1999;**10**:330–334.
15. Maldonado JR. Neuropathogenesis of delirium: Review of current etiologic theories and common pathways. *Am J Geriatr Psychiatry.* 2013;**21**:1190–1222.
16. Cerejeira J, Firmino H, Vaz-Serra A, et al. The neuroinflammatory hypothesis of delirium. *Acta Neuropathol.* 2010;**119**:737–754.
17. Kotfis K, Williams Roberson S, Wilson JE, et al. COVID-19: ICU delirium management during SARS-CoV-2 pandemic. *Crit Care.* 2020;**24**:176.
18. Egberts A, Fekkes D, Wijnbeld EH, et al. Disturbed serotonergic neurotransmission and oxidative stress in elderly patients with delirium. *Dement Geriatr Cogn Dis Extra.* 2015 Mar;**5**:450–458.
19. Watson PL, Ceriana P, Fanfulla F. Delirium: is sleep important? *Best Pract Res Clin Anaesthesiol.* 2012 Sep;**26**(3):355–366.
20. Bellapart J, Boots R. Potential use of melatonin in sleep and delirium in the critically ill. *Br J Anaesth.* 2012;**108**:572–580.
21. Marçola M, Carvalho-Sousa CE, Cecon E, et al. Dual effect of catecholamines and corticosterone crosstalk on pineal gland melatonin synthesis. *Neuroendocrinology.* 2017;**104**:126–134.
22. Pandharipande P, Ely EW. Sedative and analgesic medications: risk factors for delirium and sleep disturbances in the critically ill. *Crit Care Clin.* 2006 Apr;**22**(2):313–327, vii.
23. Ely EW, Inouye SK, Bernard GR, et al. Delirium in mechanically ventilated patients: Validity and reliability of the confusion assessment method for the intensive care unit (CAM-ICU). *JAMA.* 2001 May;**286**:2703–2710.
24. Bergeron N, Dubois MJ, Dumont M, et al. Intensive Care Delirium Screening Checklist: evaluation of a new screening tool. *Intensive Care Med.* 2001;**27**:859–864.
25. van den Boogaard M, Pickkers P, Slooter AJ, et al. Development and validation of PRE-DELIRIC (PREdiction of DELIRium in ICu patients) delirium prediction model for intensive care patients: observational multicentre study. *BMJ.* 2012;**9**;344:e420.
26. Van Den Boogaard M, Schoonhoven L, Maseda E, et al. Recalibration of the delirium prediction model for ICU patients (PRE-DELIRIC): A multinational observational study. *Intensive Care Med.* 2014;**40**:361–369.
27. Wassenaar A, van den Boogaard M, van Achterberg T, et al. Multinational development and validation of an early prediction model for delirium in ICU patients. *Intensive Care Med.* 2015;**41**:1048–1056.
28. Boesen HC, Andersen JH, Bendtsen AO, et al. Sleep and delirium in unsedated patients in the intensive care unit. *Acta Anaesthesiol Scand.* 2016;**60**:59–68.
29. Nakazawa Y, Yokoyama T, Koga Y, et al. Polysomnographic study of terminal sleep following delirium tremens. *Drug Alcohol Depend.* 1981;**8**:111–117.
30. Van Rompaey B, Elseviers MM, Van Drom W, et al. The effect of earplugs during the night on the onset of delirium and sleep perception: A randomized controlled trial in intensive care patients. *Crit Care.* 2012 **April**;16:R73.
31. Page VJ, Ely EW, Gates S, et al. Effect of intravenous haloperidol on the duration of delirium and coma in critically ill patients (Hope-ICU): A randomised, double-blind, placebo-controlled trial. *Lancet Respir Med.* 2013;**1**:515–523.
32. Page VJ, Casarin A, Ely EW, et al. Evaluation of early administration of simvastatin in the prevention and treatment of delirium in critically ill patients undergoing mechanical ventilation (MoDUS): A randomised, double-blind, placebo-controlled trial. *Lancet Resp Med.* 2017;**5**:727–737.

30

Physiotherapy

Bronwen Connolly and Paul Twose

KEY MESSAGES

- Physiotherapy in the intensive care unit (ICU) typically comprises both respiratory and physical rehabilitation management.
- Respiratory physiotherapy treatments enhance airway secretion clearance, optimize lung volume and improve oxygenation, reduce airway resistance and work of breathing, and minimize respiratory complications.
- Physical rehabilitation targets critical-illness-associated muscle wasting and weakness to enhance restoration of physical function.

CONTROVERSIES

- What is the effectiveness of respiratory physiotherapy in reducing the duration of mechanical ventilation and ICU length of stay?
- How early should mobilization commence and which patients benefit the most?
- What is the optimum dose of physical rehabilitation for improving long-term outcomes?

FURTHER RESEARCH

- Investigate optimal parameters, timing, and population for mechanical insufflation–exsufflation use in intubated patients.
- Determine appropriate 'dose', timing, and target responders of physical rehabilitation.
- Identify optimum training protocols for electrical muscle stimulation and the additional role of functional electrical stimulation.

Introduction

Physiotherapy is an integral component in the multi-professional management of critically ill patients. A primary aim of physiotherapy treatment in the intensive care unit (ICU) has traditionally been the respiratory management of mechanically ventilated patients. However, the importance of physical rehabilitation including early mobilization and exercise is increasingly recognized with greater awareness of post intensive care syndrome and the long-term effect of critical-illness-associated muscle wasting and weakness in ICU survivors. Combining respiratory and physical rehabilitation skillsets, physiotherapists actively contribute to ventilator and tracheostomy weaning as well as holistic rehabilitation programmes for critically ill patients.

Respiratory Physiotherapy Management

Patients who are ventilated are at risk of secretion retention, atelectasis, and ventilator-associated pneumonia. To manage this, respiratory physiotherapy aims to enhance airway secretion clearance, optimize lung volume and improve oxygenation, reduce airway resistance and work of breathing, and minimize respiratory complications.[1,2] Selection and progression of techniques employed by physiotherapists depend on clinical assessment of patients and the underlying respiratory pathophysiology.

Manual and Ventilator Hyperinflation

Both manual hyperinflation (MHI) and ventilator hyperinflation (VHI) increase lung volumes and mimic forced expirations to expel secretions.[3,4] MHI involves ventilator disconnection, slow inspiratory breaths delivered using a manual resuscitator bag to a peak airway pressure of 40 cmH_2O,[4] followed by an inspiratory hold of 2–3 s, and quick release of the bag to enhance expiratory flow. Inline pressure monitoring is recommended to avoid barotrauma.[2,5] Variability exists with regard to dosage and technique, yet there is evidence of benefit in pulmonary compliance, secretion clearance, airways resistance, and lung recruitment.[4,6–8] Precautions for MHI include cardiovascular instability, intra-aortic balloon pumps, or extracorporeal membrane oxygenation, and increased intracranial pressure. Contraindications include >10 cmH_2O positive end-expiratory pressure (PEEP), undrained pneumothoraces, and acute bronchospasm.[9] MHI can induce haemodynamic instability,[3] and ventilator disconnection can cause derecruitment and reduced oxygenation through loss of PEEP.

VHI avoids these adverse effects through delivery of steadily increasing ventilator volumes (typically in 200 mL increments) to a peak inspiratory pressure of 40 H_2O and a respiratory rate of 6–8 breaths.[4,10] VHI is generally performed in controlled modes (pressure or volume cycled), with prolonged inspiration, increased inspiratory flow rates, and generation of annular two-phase gas–liquid flow as observed in MHI to achieve effect.[11] No significant differences between VHI and MHI in secretion clearance, pulmonary compliance, oxygenation, and cardiovascular stability have been shown,[12] but avoidance of ventilator disconnection means that VHI may be more appropriate in patients at risk of clinical instability.

Positioning

A side-lying position with the affected region uppermost can enhance lung recruitment and facilitate gravity-assisted secretion drainage,[5,11] with further beneficial effect observed with inclusion of a head-down tilt (unless clinically contraindicated).[7] MHI and VHI are more effective when delivered in side-lying position.[7,10,13] In addition, regular turning into alternate lateral positions (to 45°), or delivery of respiratory physiotherapy (manual techniques and airways suctioning) delivered in either gravity-assisted or horizontal side-lying position, may reduce ventilator-associated pneumonia.[14,15]

Manual Techniques

Manual techniques include chest wall percussion, where rhythmic clapping performed during inspiration and expiration over focal chest areas creates energy waves that are transmitted through the airways to loosen secretions, and expiratory chest wall vibration, where the oscillatory effect produced enhances expiratory flow and secretion clearance. Caution is required as chest vibrations beyond functional residual capacity may cause derecruitment.[16] Evidence for effectiveness of expiratory vibrations is limited and is empirically used in conjunction with MHI and positioning.

Tracheal Suctioning

Tracheal suctioning for airway clearance is often accompanied by an installation of saline to assist with tenacious secretions, although this has limited efficacy.[17] Pre-oxygenation may be performed to reduce associated desaturation.

Table 30.1 The ICU Mobility Scale

Level	Classification
0	Nothing (lying in bed)
1	Sitting in bed and exercises in bed
2	Passively moved to chair (no standing)
3	Sitting over the edge of the bed
4	Standing
5	Transferring bed to chair
6	Marching on spot (at bedside)
7	Walking with the assistance of two or more people
8	Walking with the assistance of one person
9	Walking independently with a gait aid
10	Walking independently without a gait aid

Abridged from Hodgson *et al.*,[24] and with further detail on the definition of each classification.

Source: Adapted from Hodgson C, Needham D, Haines K, et al. Feasibility and inter-rater reliability of the ICU Mobility Scale. *Heart Lung: J Acute Crit Care*. 2014;43:19–24, Copyright 2014, with permission from Elsevier and The American Association of Heart Failure Nurses.

Mechanical Insufflation–Exsufflation

Mechanical insufflation–exsufflation (MI-E) is designed to augment the phases of cough, the main mechanism for secretion clearance. Inspiratory pressure (to ≈40 cmH_2O) is delivered to increase tidal volume, with a high negative force (to ≈−40 cmH_2O) applied on the final breath that enhances expiratory flow and augments secretion clearance by simulating the natural cough action. MI-E can be delivered via nose, mouth, or endotracheal or tracheostomy tube. Small-scale studies in critically patients have indicated benefit for increasing secretion clearance[18] as well as reducing reintubation rates during the post extubation ICU period.[19] However, further studies are needed to ensure generalizability of concomitant respiratory physiotherapy interventions and optimum MI-E protocols in intubated patients.

Physical Rehabilitation

Rehabilitation is the cornerstone for the management of post-critical illness morbidity.[20] Exercise-based or physical rehabilitation strategies aim to target the effects of intensive-care-unit-acquired weakness (ICUAW) and resulting physical and functional disability. In the United Kingdom, national guidelines and standards of care emphasize a seamless transition of rehabilitation delivery, commencing at ICU admission through to recovery in the community.[21,22] In the ICU, physical rehabilitation typically takes the form of early mobilization, but other adjuncts such as electrical muscle stimulation (EMS) and cycle ergometry can also be used.

Mobilization

Mobilization interventions promote patient movement over and above usual care to preserve or restore the integrity of musculoskeletal strength and function, whilst minimizing physical and functional impairment, as well as disability during recovery from critical illness.[23] Mobilization is characterized by a hierarchical progression of increasingly functional activities. These can be classified using non-linear scales such as the ICU Mobility Scale (Table 30.1) that record the highest level of activity achieved during a rehabilitation session or over the day.

Clinical reasoning and risk assessment determine which mobilization interventions to deliver with critically ill patients and when. This includes the assessments of illness severity, clinical stability, alertness, and cooperation of patients. Interventions should be individually tailored to patients with close monitoring of cardiorespiratory response. Strategies for unconscious patients include positioning, or electrical stimulation or passive cycle ergometry (see below). In awake patients, interventions may progress from active bed exercises (anti-gravity, with/without resistance) to out-of-bed mobilization such as sitting over the edge of the bed, marching on the spot, resistance training or active cycling, and walking.

Consensus recommendations regarding safety criteria for mobilizing mechanically ventilated patients are available,[25] and pooled data show very low levels of reported safety events occurring with mobilization interventions.[26] Short-term benefits are evident from physical rehabilitation delivered in the ICU, for example, improved quality of life, physical function, peripheral and respiratory muscle strength, reduced lengths of ICU and hospital stay, increased ventilator-free days, and reduced incidence of critical illness polyneuropathy/myopathy, but longer-term outcomes do not show improvement. However, methodological limitations (around target population, dose of intervention, accurate definitions of standard care in comparator groups, and consistent outcomes) necessitate further work.[27] The optimum dose of mobilization, in terms of frequency, intensity, type, and duration, remains undefined. Establishing the optimum timing is also a priority, within 48–72 h of mechanical ventilation some short-term clinical outcomes have been found to be improved.[28]

Adjuncts to Mobilization

Rehabilitation often relies on active participation from patients. Alternative therapeutic techniques are required in patients, where illness acuity, sedation, and/or reduced consciousness preclude volitional involvement. EMS (also known as neuromuscular electrical muscle stimulation) is one such technique, where intermittent stimuli are applied to superficial muscles via transcutaneous electrodes to induce muscle contraction with the aim of mitigating disuse atrophy. EMS can be applied to one more specific muscle groups. However, recent meta-analyses have shown discordant findings with regard to effects of EMS on clinical outcomes,[29,30] suggesting that future work is needed to determine optimum training protocols and short- and long-term effects.

Cycle ergometry (cycling performed at the ICU bedside using a specifically designed device) can be used passively (during periods of patient sedation and reduced consciousness), actively (through the patient's own effort), or active-assisted. Training protocols can be objectively set, for both upper (typically for active and active-assisted cycling) and lower limbs. A recent meta-analysis found cycling was safe, albeit without benefit on outcomes of physical function, duration of mechanical ventilation, length of stay, quality of life, or mortality.[31] However, more rigorously designed trials are recommended to investigate the therapeutic effect of cycling.[31]

EMS can be applied to several muscles simultaneously to enhance the performance of functional manoeuvres, such as cycling—termed 'functional electrical stimulation' (FES). One major recent randomized controlled trial comparing FES cycling to best practice standard care rehabilitation found no differences in outcomes.[32] Further research on the potential of FES cycling as a rehabilitation strategy is needed.

Conclusion

Physiotherapy in the ICU integrates both respiratory treatments and physical rehabilitation in the management of critically ill patients depending on individual patient assessment, with a broad range of techniques for selection across both elements available to physiotherapists. Aspects of both respiratory and rehabilitation practice require further investigation to inform the evidence base.

REFERENCES

1. Denehy L, Berney S. Physiotherapy in the intensive care unit. *Phys Ther Rev.* 2006;**11**(1):49–56.
2. Gosselink R, Bott J, Johnson M, et al. Physiotherapy for adult patients with critical illness: Recommendations of the European Respiratory Society and European Society of Intensive Care Medicine Task Force on Physiotherapy for Critically Ill Patients. *Intensive Care Med.* 2008;**34**:1188–1199.
3. Singer M, Vermaat J, Hall G, et al. Hemodynamic effects of manual hyperinflation in critically ill mechanically ventilated patients. *Chest.* 1994;**106**:1182–1187.
4. Berney S, Denehy L. A comparison of the effects of manual and ventilator hyperinflation on static lung compliance and sputum production in intubated and ventilated intensive care patients. *Physiother Res Int.* 2002;**7**:100–108.
5. Hodgson C, Denehy L, Ntoumenopoulos G, et al. An investigation of the early effects of manual lung hyperinflation in critically ill patients. *Anaesth Intensive Care.* 2000;**28**:255–261.
6. Hodgson C, Ntoumenopoulos G, Dawson H, et al. The Mapleson C circuit clears more secretions than the Laerdal circuit during manual hyperinflation in mechanically-ventilated patients: A randomised cross-over trial. *Aust J Physio.* 2007; **53**:33–38.
7. Berney S, Denehy L, Pretto J. Head-down tilt and manual hyperinflation enhance sputum clearance in patients who are intubated and ventilated. *Aust J Physio.* 2004;**50**:9–14.
8. Choi JS-P, Jones AY-M. Effects of manual hyperinflation and suctioning on respiratory mechanics in mechanically ventilated patients with ventilator-associated pneumonia. *Aust J Physio.* 2005;**51**:25–30.
9. Main E, Denehy L. *Cardiorespiratory Physiotherapy: Adults and Paediatrics*, 5th ed. Elsevier, UK; 2016.
10. Savian C, Paratz J, Davies A. Comparison of the effectiveness of manual and ventilator hyperinflation at different levels of positive end-expiratory pressure in artificially ventilated and intubated intensive care patients. *Heart & Lung.* 2006;**35**:334–341.
11. Denehy L. The use of manual hyperinflation in airway clearance. *Eur Respir J.* 1999, **14**:958–965.
12. Anderson A, Alexanders J, Sinani C, et al. Effects of ventilator vs manual hyperinflation in adults receiving mechanical ventilation: A systematic review of randomised clinical trials. *Physiotherapy.* 2015;**101**:103–110.
13. Dennis DM, Jacob WJ, Samuel FD. A survey of the use of ventilator hyperinflation in Australian tertiary intensive care units. *Crit Care Resusc.* 2010;**12**:262–268.
14. Mauri T, Berra L, Kumwilaisak K, et al. Lateral-horizontal patient position and horizontal orientation of the endotracheal tube to prevent aspiration in adult surgical intensive care unit patients: A feasibility study. *Respir Care.* 2010;**55**:294–302.
15. Ntoumenopoulos G, Presneill J, McElholum M, et al. Chest physiotherapy for the prevention of ventilator-associated pneumonia. *Intensive Care Med.* 2002;**28**:850–856.
16. Laws A, McIntyre R. Chest physiotherapy: A physiological assessment during intermittent positive pressure ventilation in respiratory failure. *Can Anaesth Soc J.* 1969;**16**:487–493.
17. Paratz JD, Stockton KA. Efficacy and safety of normal saline instillation: A systematic review. *Physiotherapy.* 2009;**95**:241–250.
18. Martínez-Alejos R, Martí JD, Li Bassi G, et al. Effects of mechanical insufflation-exsufflation on sputum volume in mechanically ventilated critically ill subjects. *Respir Care.* 2021 Sep;**66**(9):1371–1379. doi:10.4187/respcare.08641. Epub 2021 Jun 8. PMID: 34103385.
19. Gonçalves MR, Honrado T, Winck JC, et al. Effects of mechanical insufflation–exsufflation in preventing respiratory failure after extubation: A randomized controlled trial. *Crit Care.* 2012;**16**:R48.
20. Connolly B. Describing and measuring recovery and rehabilitation after critical illness. *Curr Op Crit Care.* 2015;**21**:445–452.
21. Guidelines for the Provision of Intensive Care Services, Edition 2. Available at http://wwwicsacuk/ICS/GuidelinesAndStandards/GPICS_2nd_Editionaspx 2019, Accessed 19/07/2019.

22. NICE: Rehabilitation after critical illness. NICE Clinical Guideline 83. *National Institute for Health and Care Excellence.* London, UK 2009;1–21. available at http://www.nice.org.uk/guidance/cg83.
23. Devlin JW, Skrobik Y, Gélinas C, et al. Clinical practice guidelines for the prevention and management of pain, agitation/sedation, delirium, immobility, and sleep disruption in adult patients in the ICU. *Crit Care Med.* 2018;**46**:e825–e873.
24. Hodgson C, Needham D, Haines K, et al. Feasibility and inter-rater reliability of the ICU Mobility Scale. *Heart Lung.* 2014;**43**:19–24.
25. Hodgson C, Stiller K, Needham D, et al. Expert consensus and recommendations on safety criteria for active mobilization of mechanically ventilated critically ill adults. *Crit Care.* 2014;**18**:658.
26. Nydahl P, Sricharoenchai T, Chandra S, et al. Safety of patient mobilization and rehabilitation in the ICU: Systematic review with meta-analysis. *Ann Am Thorac Soc.* 2017;**14**:766–777.
27. Connolly B, Denehy L. Hindsight and moving the needle forwards on rehabilitation trial design. *Thorax.* 2018;**73**:203–205.
28. Ding N, Zhang Z, Zhang C, et al. What is the optimum time for initiation of early mobilization in mechanically ventilated patients? A network meta-analysis. *PLoS ONE.* 2019;**14**(10):e0223151.
29. Liu M, Luo J, Zhou J, et al. Intervention effect of neuromuscular electrical stimulation on ICU acquired weakness: A meta-analysis. *Int J Nursing Sci.* 2020;7:228–237.
30. Zayed Y, Kheiri B, Barbarawi M, et al. Effects of neuromuscular electrical stimulation in critically ill patients: A systematic review and meta-analysis of randomised controlled trials. *Aust Crit Care.* 2020;**33**:203–210.
31. Takaoka A, Utgikar R, Rochwerg B, et al. The efficacy and safety of in-intensive care unit leg-cycle ergometry in critically ill adults. A systematic review and meta-analysis. *Ann Am Thorac Soc.* 2020;**17**(10):1289–1307.
32. Berney S, Hopkins RO, Rose JW, *et al.* Functional electrical stimulation in-bed cycle ergometry in mechanically ventilated patients: A multicentre randomised controlled trial. *Thorax.* 2021;**76**:656–663.

31

Human Factors

Christopher D Hingston

KEY MESSAGES

- Human error is common in healthcare and is a cause of significant morbidity and mortality globally. Understanding how this error may occur informs safer system design as well as root cause analysis, after an incident has occurred.
- Non-technical skills, which can be taught, trained, and assessed, may mitigate the effects of human error. These skills are of equal importance to the technical abilities and knowledge that have traditionally been sought.
- Promoting a flattened hierarchy and an open culture, where all staff are taught graded assertiveness techniques and encouraged to speak up when they identify problems, can trap minor errors, often before they can have significant consequences.

CONTROVERSIES

- Healthcare is delivered in a complex environment, and while human factor principles are gaining widespread acceptance, there remains a lack of high-quality evidence to support them.
- In order to have a significant impact on patient safety and outcomes, investment in human factors is required from individual to organizational levels. It is a scientific discipline and as such mandates the involvement of experts in the field to understand problems within healthcare systems, allowing solutions to be devised and implemented.

FURTHER RESEARCH

- The adoption of human factor principles in healthcare remains very much in its infancy compared to other high-risk industries. While a small number of studies have been able to show the benefits of good non-technical skills, particularly in the operating theatre environment, demonstrating significant benefits across large, complex healthcare organizations is likely to remain challenging. Many questions remain and research is urgently warranted if global patient harm due to human error is to be minimized.

Introduction

Healthcare professionals receive high levels of technical training associated with their roles. This results in excellent levels of clinical knowledge and expertise. Despite this considerable investment, ~10% patients admitted to hospital will suffer a serious adverse event.[1] In the United States of America, medical error is the third leading cause of death.[2] Critically ill patients admitted to the intensive care unit (ICU) experience, on average, 1.7 medical errors a day. Medication errors account for 78% of serious medical errors.[3] The burden on patients is obvious, but also economic consequences, such as increased length of hospital stay and litigation. The potential for error is likely higher in ICU, with many complex interventions being delivered by numerous healthcare professionals around the clock. Decades of research in other high-risk industries has found that human error is a significant factor in up to 80% accidents.

Human factors, also known as ergonomics, is the scientific discipline concerned with understanding the interaction of humans within the systems in which they operate, in order to optimize best performance. It considers both the physical and cognitive capabilities of individuals, as well as the organizational and cultural aspects of their environment. Although healthcare has been slow to embrace human factor principles, learning established in other industries is being adopted. Industrial psychologists have identified a set of non-technical skills (NOTECHS) that may be taught, trained, and assessed. NOTECHS, a group of cognitive and social skills, when used to complement the traditionally taught technical skills of medicine, can help to deliver safe and efficient healthcare. When these principles are applied to team training, it is often referred to as team resource management (TRM) training.

SHELL Model

The SHELL model (Figure 31.1) remains useful in understanding the broad concepts of human factors, including how, where, and why errors may occur.[4] It is especially helpful when considering the human factors that have contributed to harm or a near-miss, when undertaking root cause analysis. The individual lies at the centre of the model and is termed liveware. There are numerous influences on human performance and the corresponding likelihood of error. These include physical

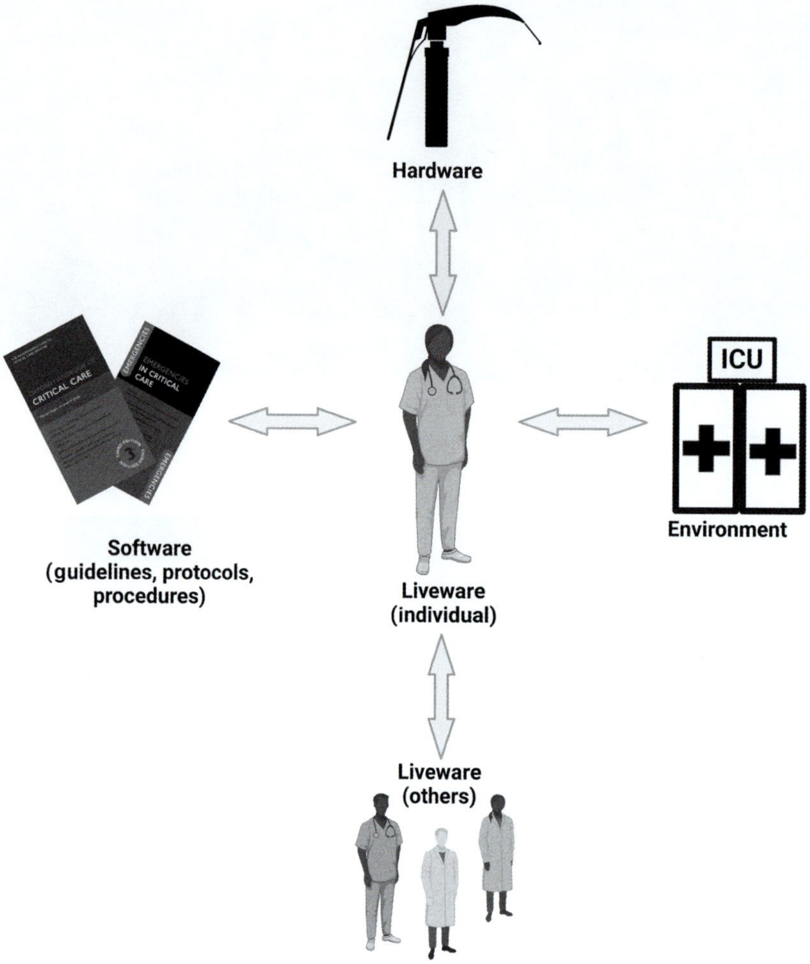

Figure 31.1 Representation of the SHELL model illustrating the concept of human factors and how individual performance is influenced by personal and external resources, as well as the environment.
Diagram by A Conway Morris created with BioRender.com. Data from Hawkins F.H. *Human factors in flight*. 2nd ed. Ashgate (Aldershot, UK); 1987.

size and shape, physical and emotional well-being, environmental tolerance, as well as clinical knowledge and skills. Acknowledging limitations within teams and taking steps to mitigate them are paramount to achieving optimal performance and ultimately minimizing risks.

Performance extends beyond intrinsic individual factors and there is recognition of the importance of external factors on the individual. The model describes liveware interactions with software, hardware, the environment, and other liveware; all of which may enhance or degrade individual performance.

Software–liveware interactions traditionally described the paper-based parts of the world, including rules, policies, guidelines, protocols, drug charts, and notes, to name a few. With digitalization and so much documentation, healthcare workers run the risk of errors of omission rather than commission, being unaware that a document exists. Technology brings benefits; for instance, an illegible script is a serious matter if vital information remains unintelligible or misinterpreted at a crucial moment.

Liveware–hardware interactions acknowledge how workplace technology, equipment, and devices may influence the capacity for error. It is hard to overstate the importance of careful product design in supporting safe practice. The manufacture of intuitive, user-friendly devices and equipment minimizes the possibility of user error. This aspect of the model relates to more than just the use of equipment. It might also encompass equipment malfunction, recognized or otherwise, as well as devices that may be missing or unavailable when required.

The liveware–environment aspect of the SHELL model identifies the limited physiological tolerance of humans. Personnel may be subject to various thermal stressors, particularly when using personal protective equipment. Less intuitive factors include lighting; if insufficient, as on a ward at night, clinical signs may be missed. Conversely, too much light may make ultrasound examination or fundoscopy challenging. The most significant environmental factor that can contribute to error in healthcare settings is noise. This is particularly common in larger teams responsible for managing resuscitation or deteriorating patients. Noise impedes effective communication and may inhibit important contributions from team members. The fundamental adage is to ensure that the team controls the environment, and that the environment does not control the team.

The final aspect of the SHELL model recognizes the importance of liveware–liveware interactions. This is a broad area covering communication, teamworking, hierarchies, and conflict management. It also includes local and organizational culture, which may be constructive or destructive. It is this aspect of the model that TRM training tends to focus upon and is discussed further.

Non-technical Skills

NOTECHS are a set of cognitive and inter-personal skills that have been identified in teams that perform well, but are often absent or lacking when adverse events are analyzed, despite each individual likely having the requisite technical abilities. Significant research has led to the development of various behavioural marker systems in order to better evaluate and train the NOTECH behaviours and skills that contribute to superior or substandard performance. While some differences exist between elements used in the assessment systems, they share more than they differ. Box 31.1 shows the taxonomy commonly used in the healthcare setting.[5]

Situational Awareness (SA)

Situational awareness is defined as the awareness of the elements in the environment, within a volume of time and space, the comprehension of their meaning, and the projection of their status into the near future. In essence, it comprises three components.

1. Physical perception using any or all of the senses (Perception).
2. Reliably understanding what these sensory inputs mean (Comprehension).
3. Projecting their meaning into the short-term future (Projection).

Good SA allows anticipation of likely next steps or events. High-performance teams will actively share SA in order to build further upon it. A shared mental model is thus formed by all. Any team member should be allowed to test this model if they perceive things differently. An open culture of permitting, and encouraging, team members to raise queries and concerns, with reciprocity and critical appraisal, is fundamental to the patient-centred goals. Teams demonstrating this behaviour identify and trap small errors more frequently, so avoid more significant errors. However, developing these behaviours may require significant cultural change, particularly where a perceived hierarchy exists. The aim is to foster a flattened hierarchy with an acceptable speak up culture. Multidisciplinary team training is needed. Skilled facilitator moderated simulation is well suited to this, identifying and providing feedback on both technical and non-technical skills. Team briefings and huddles prior to ward rounds or critical procedures promote SA. The surgical safety checklist is a low-cost example of how this style of intervention can reduce adverse patient outcomes.[6] Team briefings further build a positive team culture, sharing expectations of what is likely to happen and mentally rehearsing for when they do not. The latter helps to empower team members to intervene, particularly when critical events occur.

SA may take effort to obtain and maintain, depending on circumstances. Inadvertent failure at any of the three stages can result in it being rapidly lost. This is critical as good SA allows the practitioner to make better decisions. SA may be rapidly lost for many reasons, most commonly through distraction. In the busy clinical setting, interruptions are commonplace, in what has been termed the 'wicked environment'. When important decisions are being made, or critical interventions are taking place, it is essential that only directly relevant interruptions are permitted. In nursing, distractions have been recognized as a significant cause of drug administration errors. An effective intervention, which many hospitals have successfully implemented, is to issue the nurse with a tabard mandating that interruptions are not permitted during this important task. In aviation, the sterile cockpit rule is used at crucial phases of flight to allow only relevant communication. This same concept can be extended to healthcare during high-risk procedures or interventions. On occasion, SA may be lost when an individual becomes task fixated. This may be anticipated during events such as intubation, where the operator will be fixated on laryngoscopy. In order to maintain SA during this time, it is essential to explicitly delegate monitoring tasks to other team members. It is important that team members are mindful of others around them who may become task fixated and primed to interrupt if information is critical. In high-pressure situations, a 10-s 'timeout' every 10 min enables the team leader to update the team on progress, helping to maintain collective SA.

Box 31.1 Non-technical skill domains in healthcare [5]

Non-technical Skill Domains

- Situational awareness
- Decision making
- Communication
- Team working
- Leadership
- Managing stress
- Coping with fatigue

Decision-making

Significant progress has been made in understanding how humans make the 35,000 decisions required of them each day. The accepted paradigm on how decisions are made was developed by Nobel laureate Daniel Kahneman. He proposed that the brain has two systems of thinking. System 1 (fast thinking) is the largely unconscious and automated way in which humans operate the vast majority of time. System 2 (slow thinking) is conscious, rational thought, requiring far greater effort. Through repeated experience even complex system 2 thought patterns can become system 1 thinking. For the majority of the time, system 1 works well for the quantity of decisions that need to be made, but it does rely on numerous mental shortcuts or heuristics. These are prone to error and worse still, difficult to recognize. These are now recognized as inbuilt cognitive biases, of which well over 150 have been described. These are relevant to diagnostic error, which occurs in 5%–20% of physician–patient encounters. Common examples, to describe just a few, include *confirmation bias*, in which clinicians seek information to support a proposed diagnosis, ignoring facts that do not fit; *anchoring bias*, where once a diagnosis is made there is premature closure and no further questioning takes place; and *visceral bias*, where conclusions are influenced by personal feelings towards a patient. It is important that clinicians familiarize themselves with these biases and explicitly acknowledge the effect they have. Table 31.1 suggests a mnemonic that incorporates a number of strategies[7] to reduce diagnostic error.

Table 31.1 SWIPE acronym to recall strategies to avoid diagnostic error. Based on Trowbridge 2009.[7]

S	Systematic approach	Deliberately formulate a wide differential diagnosis using an anatomical or physiological approach
	Slow down	Use diagnostic time-outs to consider diagnostic accuracy
W	Why questions	Particularly relevant to why acute exacerbations of chronic diseases have occurred
I	Inconsistent data	Seek out data that does not fit
P	Pre-test probability	Use Bayesian theory to understand diagnostic testing
E	Embrace the zebras	Consider rare diagnosis or they will never be found
	Embrace your mistakes	Learn from and share previous errors

Communication

Communication is arguably the most important of the NOTECHS. The reported incidence of poor communication contributing directly to medical error varies widely from 30% to 70%, but it is likely more frequently implicated indirectly. Multiple opportunities exist for communication errors to occur, particularly during daily handover of care between shifts, but also between caring and consulting teams, interprofessional teams, and on transfer to other areas. Every interaction has the potential for the loss of information or transfer of misinformation. Checklists to aid structured handover have been shown to improve the process. An important obstacle to communication in the stressful environment of critical care is conflict. In one international point prevalence study, over 70% ICU staff reported conflict in the preceding week.[8] Nurse–physician conflict was the most common, followed by conflict between nurses, and then staff–relative conflicts. While well-managed conflict can lead to positive change, in this study, half of conflicts were perceived as serious or dangerous. Incivility has been clearly shown to directly impact upon diagnostic ability and result in a 12% decline in procedural performance, interestingly recipients of rudeness were unaware of this.[9] Furthermore, staff who witness incivility experience a fall in performance, and 75% patients will understandably view the organization less favourably. There remains much to be done to address this issue within healthcare, but the adage of focusing on 'what is right, not who is right' can go a long way to focusing disagreement constructively.

The practical difficulty of raising concerns, while avoiding conflict, has been recognized. The aviation industry has developed the PACE acronym (Box 31.2), a graded assertiveness technique. This advocates enquiry to ensure a proper understanding of the situation, and sharing concerns, and before challenging and escalating further. It should be noted that if an unsafe act were to occur, immediate intervention would be appropriate. While it takes practice, the use of PACE is well worth pursuing.

Box 31.2 An example of the PACE acronym being used to intervene

Graded Assertiveness: PACE

- **P** – Probe for a better understanding of what is going on and why
  "Jon, I was wondering why you didn't start Mrs Jones on any antibiotics?"
- **A** – Alert to abnormalities (why you are concerned)
  "Have you had a chance to see the bloods and CXR, it seemed to me that she might have a chest infection."
- **C** – Challenge the present strategy
  "Jon, I'm quite concerned as the history and investigations all suggest a chest infection. Delaying antibiotics will increase her likely mortality."
- **E** – Emergency warning of the current dangers and takeover situation
  "Dr White, I'm going to have to discuss the case with Dr Evans."

Teamwork and Leadership

Healthcare professionals are frequently drawn together to form ad hoc teams. The quality of teamwork within a system directly impacts upon patient outcomes, where patients receiving care from poor teams are five times as likely to experience complications or death.[10] A team relies on competent leadership but equally good followership. On a practical level, introducing team members, identifying individuals' skills and experience, responding to members that appear to be struggling, and debriefing after critical events are all markers of good team behaviours that are easy to implement.

Task Management

Prioritizing tasks that are important/urgent, over easy/non-urgent ones, is a key skill that healthcare professionals develop early in their careers. Equally important is considering task complexity so that they are delegated appropriately. In critical situations, it is easy to overload individuals with too many tasks. If the team is to perform well, this must be avoided, seeking extra help where needed and ensuring each team members' skills are used to best advantage.

Fatigue and Stress Management

Fatigue is defined as a physiological state of reduced mental or physical capacity which may develop due to lack of sleep or extended wakefulness, disrupted circadian rhythm, or increased workload. Healthcare culture now recognizes that long hours have a detrimental effect on performance. Even with changes in law to reduce total working hours the risk of fatigue remains, with work tempo, shift patterns, and disturbance of circadian rhythms presenting a challenge. Fatigued doctors make twice as many errors on a shift, posing a risk to patients. Healthcare workers endanger themselves, with an increase in needlestick injuries during night shifts, as well as numerous adverse physiological changes that are associated with long-term health sequelae. While acute fatigue is unavoidable, it is important to attenuate the effects through careful rota design, compulsory rest periods before and after shifts, as well as sufficient rest breaks.

Chronic workplace stress can result in burnout, a syndrome consisting of emotional exhaustion, depersonalization, and a diminished sense of personal achievement, driven primarily by workplace stressors. One-third of ICU team members are at high risk of burnout at any one time, and 50% physicians will experience it at some point in their career.[8] It too leads to increased medical error and reduced quality of care. The Maslach Burnout Inventory has been used to identify staff at risk. The most effective interventions to avoid burnout are at an organizational level and may be as simple as adjusting work patterns or intensity, but may necessitate altering whole team practices and ways of working. Interventions targeted at individuals, such as mindfulness or personal coping strategies, are less effective.[11]

Conclusion

Despite impressive advances in medical treatments, the greatest benefit that can be afforded to patients is to reduce iatrogenic harm. Medical error remains extremely commonplace and much of it is avoidable. Through the understanding of human factors and honing healthcare professionals' non-technical skills, this harm may be minimized, as has been demonstrated by other high-risk industries.

REFERENCES

1. Vincent C, Neale G, Woloshynowych M. Adverse events in British hospitals: Preliminary retrospective record review. *BMJ.* 2001;**322**:517–579.
2. Institute of Medicine (US) Committee on Quality of Health Care in America. *To Err is Human: Building a Safer Health System.* Washington (DC): National Academies Press (US); 1999.
3. Camiré E, Moyen E, Stelfox HT. Medication errors in critical care: Risk factors, prevention and disclosure. *Can Med Assoc J.* 2009;**180**(9):936–941.
4. Hawkins FH. *Human Factors in Flight.* 2nd ed. Ashgate (Aldershot, UK); 1987.
5. Flyn R. *Safety at the Sharp End. A Guide to Non-Technical Skills.* 1st ed. London: CRC Press; 2008.
6. Haynes AB, Weiser TG, Berry WR, et al. A surgical safety check-list to reduce morbidity and mortality in a global population. *N Engl J Med.* 2009;**360**(5):491–499.
7. Trowbridge RL. Twelve tips for teaching avoidance of diagnostic errors. *Med Teacher.* 2009; **30**(5):496–500.
8. Azoulay E, Timsit JF, Sprung CL, et al. Prevalence and factors of intensive care unit conflicts: The conflicus study. *Am J Respir Crit Care Med.* 2009;**180**(9):853–860.
9. Riskin A, Erez A, Foulk TA. The impact of rudeness on medical team performance: A randomized trial. *Pediatrics.* 2015;**136**(3):487–495.
10. Rosen MA, DiazGranados D, Dietz AS, et al. Teamwork in healthcare: Key discoveries enabling safer, high-quality care. *Am Psychol.* 2018;**73**(4):433–450.
11. Panagioti M, Panagopoulou E, Bower P, et al. Controlled interventions to reduce burnout in physicians: A systematic review and meta-analysis. *JAMA Intern Med.* 2017; **177**(2):195–205.

PART 8
Respiratory Infections

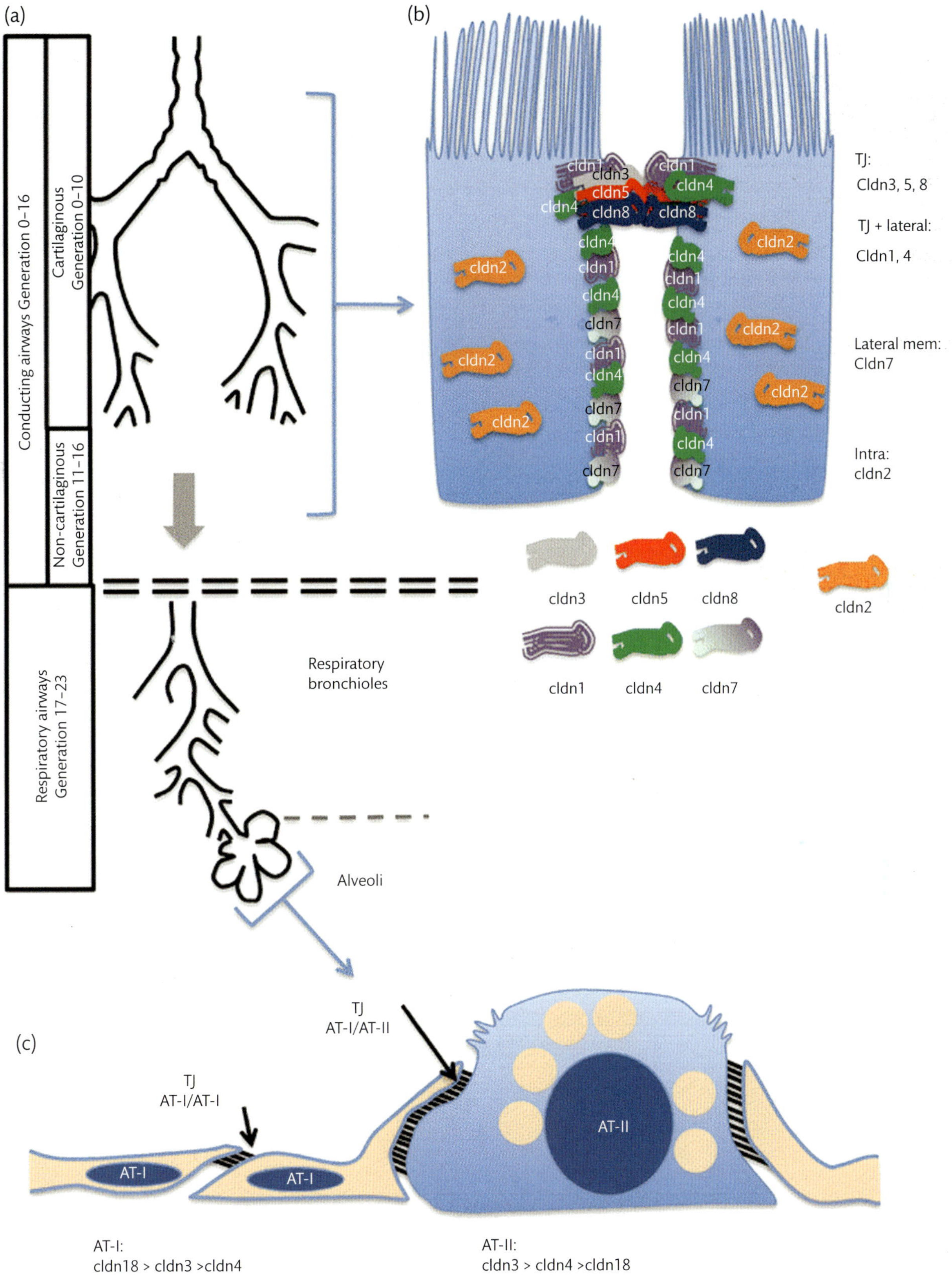

Figure 4.1 Function of epithelial cells: physical barrier and tight junctions. Organization of the airways and the airway epithelium. (a) The airways are subdivided into conductive and respiratory sections. The conductive airways contain cartilaginous and non-cartilaginous airways. The respiratory section constitutes the respiratory airways and the alveoli. (b) Scheme gives an overview of intracellular claudin (cldn) distribution in airway epithelial cells. The claudins predominantly localized at the tight junctions (TJ) (cldn3, 5, and 8), localized at the tight junctions and the lateral membrane (cldn1, 4), predominantly localized basolateral from the TJ (cldn7), and localized intracellular (cldn2) are depicted. (c) Scheme of the alveolar epithelium. The alveolar epithelium constitutes alveolar type I (AT-I) and type II (AT-II) cells. The tight junctions between adjacent AT-I cells are narrower than those between AT-I and AT-II cells. The most abundantly expressed claudins in AT-I and AT-II cells are cldn3, 4, and 18.

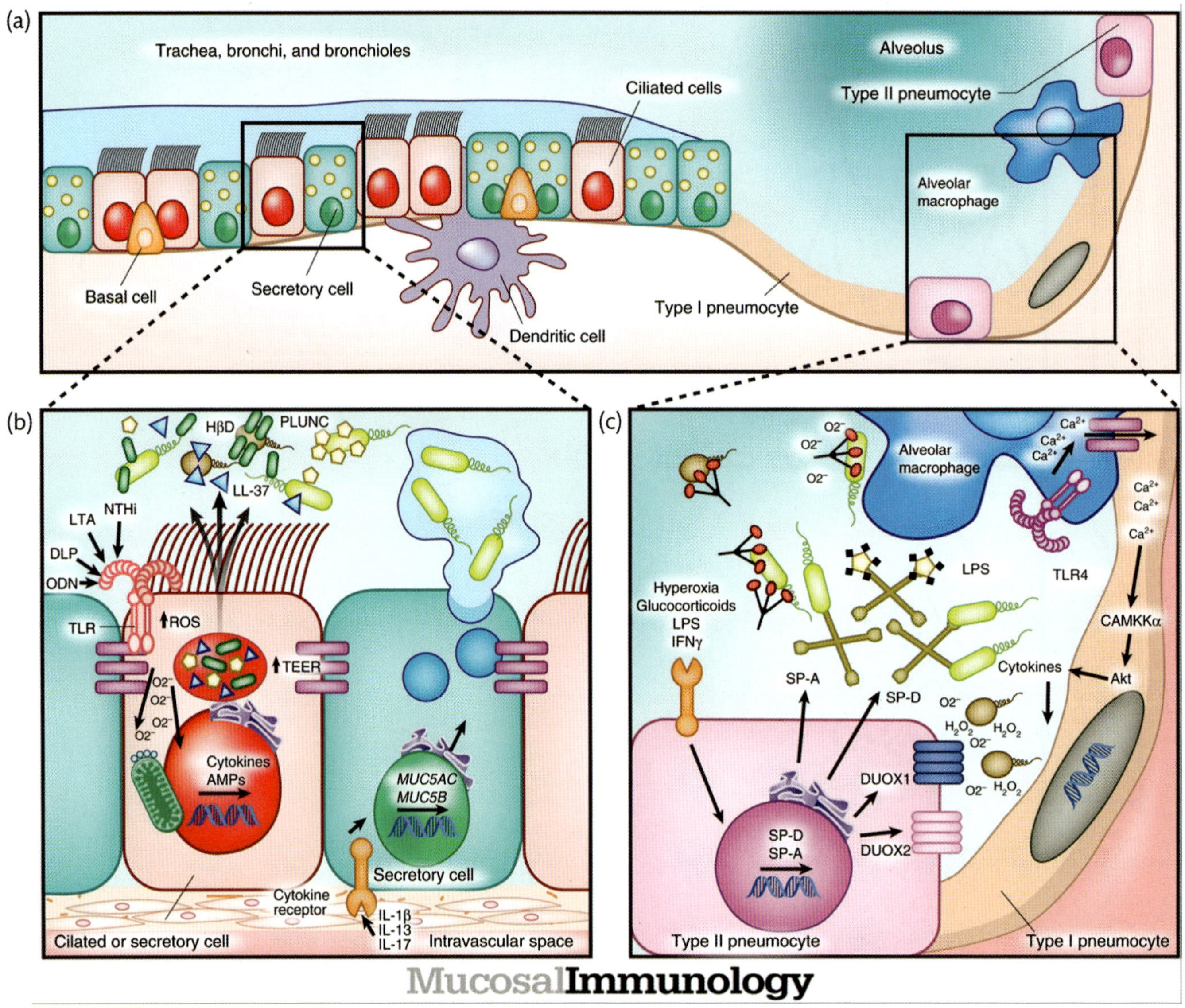

Figure 4.2 Epithelial cell function: inducible innate resistance. Inducible antimicrobial resistance mechanisms of lung epithelial cells. (a) Cells contributing to inducible epithelial airspace defence. (b) Inducible responses in the conducting airways. Pattern-recognition and cytokine receptors detect local danger signals in the conducting airways, responding with enhanced barrier and mucociliary functions to improve pathogen exclusion, increased production of microbicidal antimicrobial peptides and volatile species, and secretion of mediators of leucocyte recruitment and activation. (c) Inducible responses in the alveolar compartment. Epithelial cells in the gas exchange units of the lungs detect pathogen-associated molecular patterns, perceive stress signals and communicate with lung resident leukocytes, and respond through inducible modulation of barrier function, enhanced production of antimicrobial peptides, collectins and volatile species, and secretion of leucocyte-active cytokines. LTA, lipotechtoic acid; DLP, diacylated lipopeptides; HβD, human β-defensin; NTHi, non-typeable *Haemophillus influenza*; ODN, oligodeoxynucleotide; ROS, reactive oxygen species; SP, surfactant protein; TLR, Toll-like receptor; TEER, transepithelial electrical resistance.

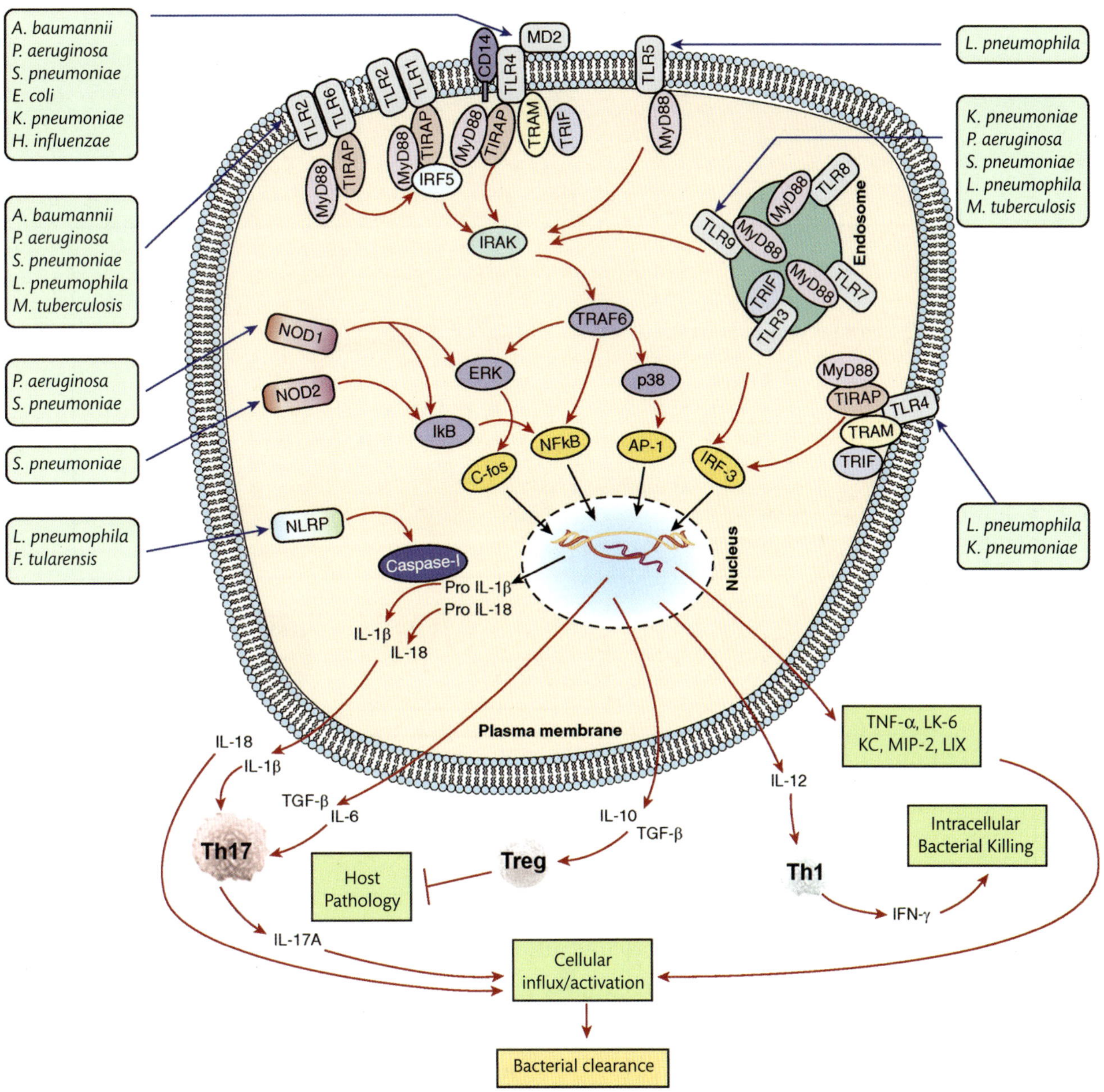

Figure 4.3 Signalling cascades on activation of pattern-recognition receptors by pulmonary pathogens. Plasma membrane–bound Toll-like receptors (TLRs) (TLR1, 2, 4, and 5) and endosome membrane–bound TLRs (TLR9) recognize bacteria in the lungs. After bacterial recognition, TLR2 (with TLR1 or 6), TLR4 (in association with MD-2 and CD14), TLR5, and TLR9 recruit MyD88, whereas TLR2 and TLR4 recruit both MyD88 and Toll-IL-1R domain-containing adapter protein (TIRAP). All of these TLRs activate IL-1 receptor–associated kinase (IRAK) after MyD88 recruitment, followed by recruitment of tumour necrosis factor receptor–associated factor 6 (TRAF6), ultimately resulting in activation of the transcription factor nuclear factor-kB (NF-kB) and mitogen-activated protein kinases (MAPKs). MAPK activation, in turn, results in the induction of transcription factors AP-1 and c-fos. In addition, TLR3 and TLR4 recruit the adaptor TIR-domain-containing adapter-inducing IFN-β (TRIF), ultimately leading to IRF3-mediated IFN-a/b and inducible nitric oxide synthase (iNOS) production through the intermediate signalling molecule TRAM, which is the bridging adaptor for TRIF-mediated signalling. In addition, pulmonary bacterial pathogens release ligands during infection that are recognized by nucleotide-binding oligomerization domains (NODs) and activate subsequent signalling pathways leading to NF-κB activation. Furthermore, when stimulated by ligands, the NOD-like receptor proteins (NLRP) induce activation of effector caspase-1, which cleaves the pro forms of IL-1β and IL-18. In turn, cytokine activation results in differentiation of naive T cells into Th1, Th17, or regulatory T cells (Tregs), thereby leading to pulmonary host defence or, in the case of Treg accumulation, resulting in host pathology. *A. baumannii, Acinetobacter baumannii; E. coli, Escherichia coli; F. tularensis, Francisella tularensis; H. influenzae, Haemophilus influenzae; K. pneumoniae, Klebsiella pneumoniae; L. pneumophila, Legionella pneumophila; M. tuberculosis, Mycobacterium tuberculosis; P. aeruginosa, Pseudomonas aeruginosa; S. pneumoniae, Streptococcus pneumoniae.*

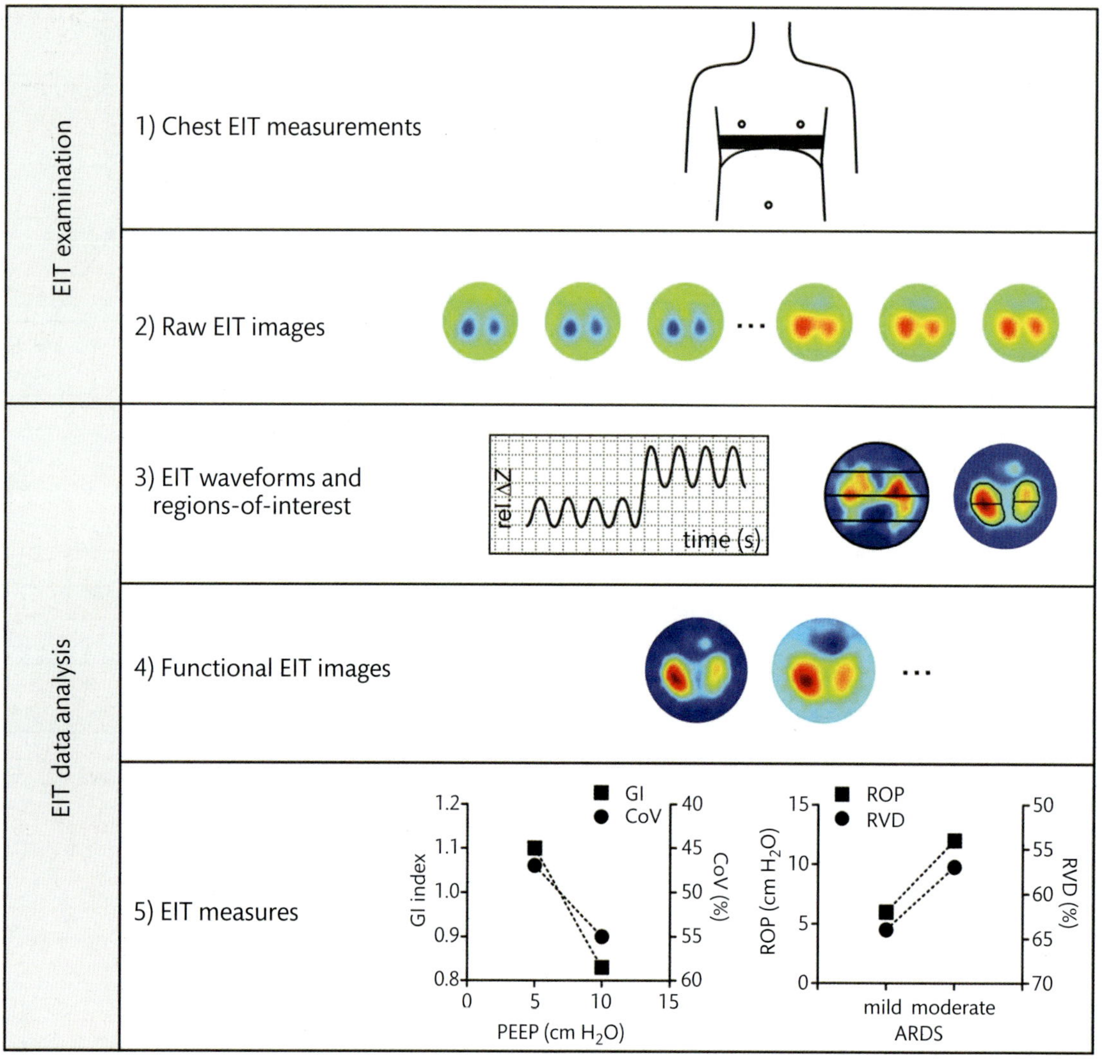

Figure 18.20 Schematic presentation of the chest EIT examination and data analysis. ARDS, acute respiratory distress syndrome; EIT, electrical impedance tomography; rel. ΔZ, relative impedance change; GI, global inhomogeneity index; CoV, centre of ventilation; PEEP, positive end-expiratory pressure; ROP, regional opening pressure; RVD, regional ventilation delay.

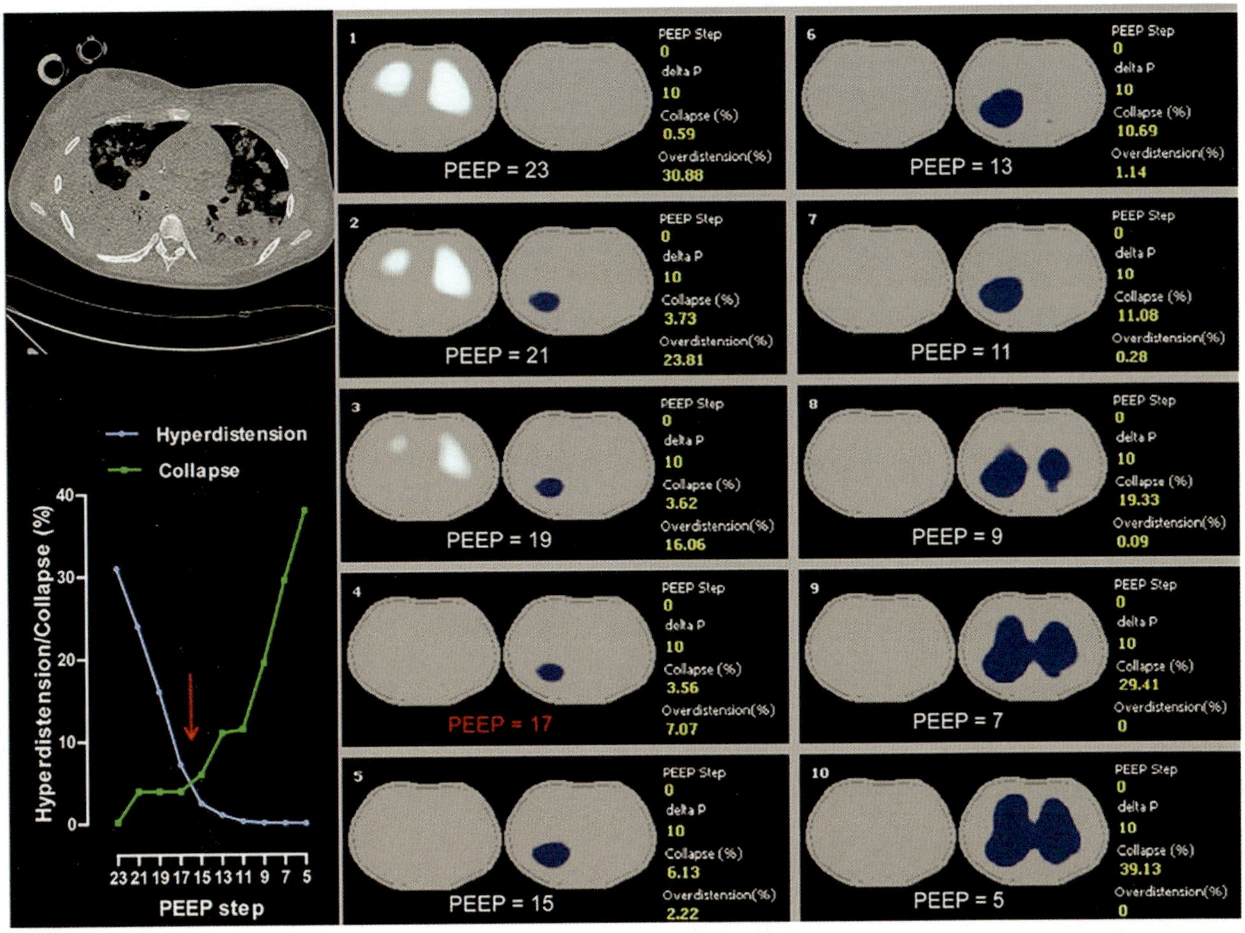

Figure 18.21 Using electrical impedance tomography (EIT) (Enlight, Timpel, Sao Paulo, Brazil) to assess the effect of decremental PEEP in a patient with severe ARDS (CT image, top left). Panels 1–10 show regional lung hyperdistention and collapse at each PEEP step in white and blue colours, respectively, obtained with the EIT electrode belt at the same level as the CT. The percentages of collapse and overdistension are provided at the right side of each panel and in the diagram (bottom left). With decreasing PEEP, hyperdistention fell (blue curve) and collapse rose (green curve). The crossover point between the curves is highlighted by the arrow. The corresponding PEEP step preceding the crossover shows the value of 17 cmH2O in red in panel 4.

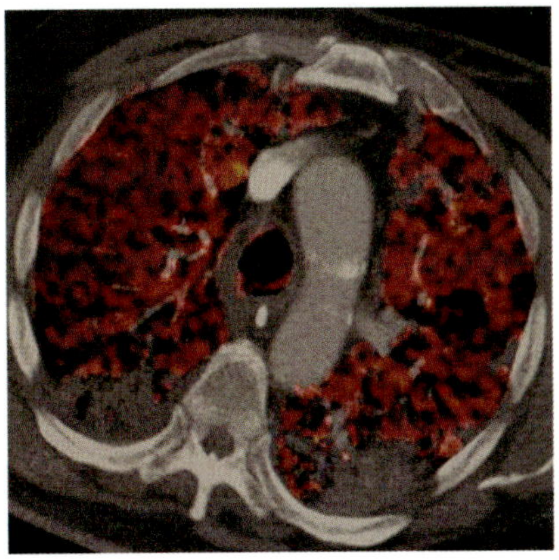

Figure 18.24 Dual-energy CT (DECT) pulmonary angiography in a Covid-19 patient with severe respiratory failure. (a) Maximal-intensity-projection CT images showing vascular tree-in-bud pattern in the upper lobes anterolaterally and (b) corresponding DECT blood volume colour map showing nodular decreased perfusion.

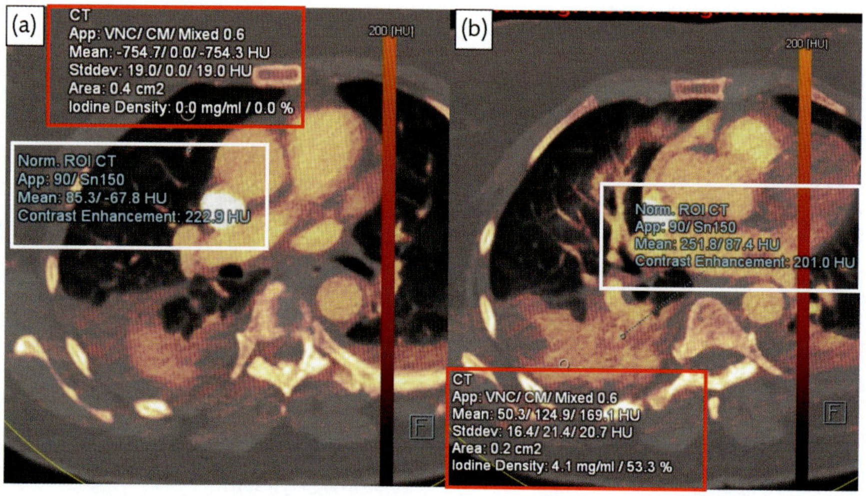

Figure 18.22 Dual-energy CT pulmonary angiography in a patient with ARDS. The images represent the combination of CT and iodine distribution images using dedicated, commercially available software (Liver VNC, Syngovia, Siemens, Forcheim, Germany). Dual-energy CT allows the calculation of specific materials within tissue, such as iodinated contrast within vessels and parenchyma, as a surrogate for perfusion. By first placing a region of interest (ROI) in a nearby artery to measure contrast enhancement (white rectangles), iodine density within a specific region can be measured in both mg/ mL and as a relative percentage of the total volume of iodine within the lung (red rectangles). The iodine density of 0 in the ventral, well-aerated lung (red rectangle in (a)) as compared to the iodine density of 4.1 mg/ mL, representing 53% of the iodine in the lung, within the dorsal, non-aerated lung (red rectangle in (b)) suggests that blood is being shunted through the non-aerated lung.

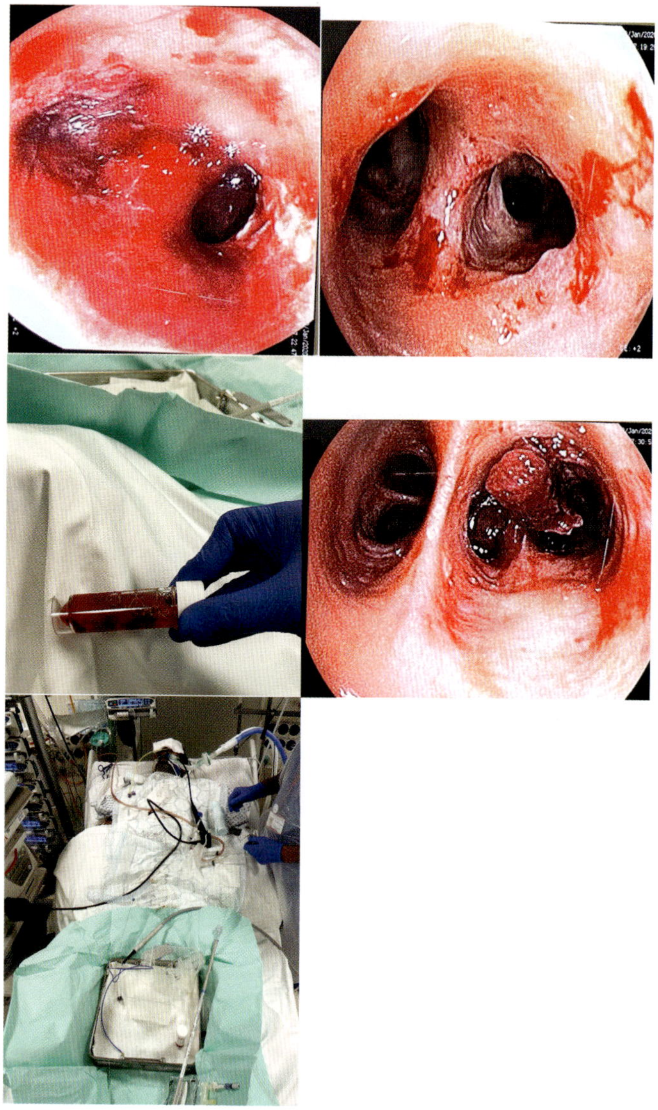

Figure 19.1 Cryoextraction.

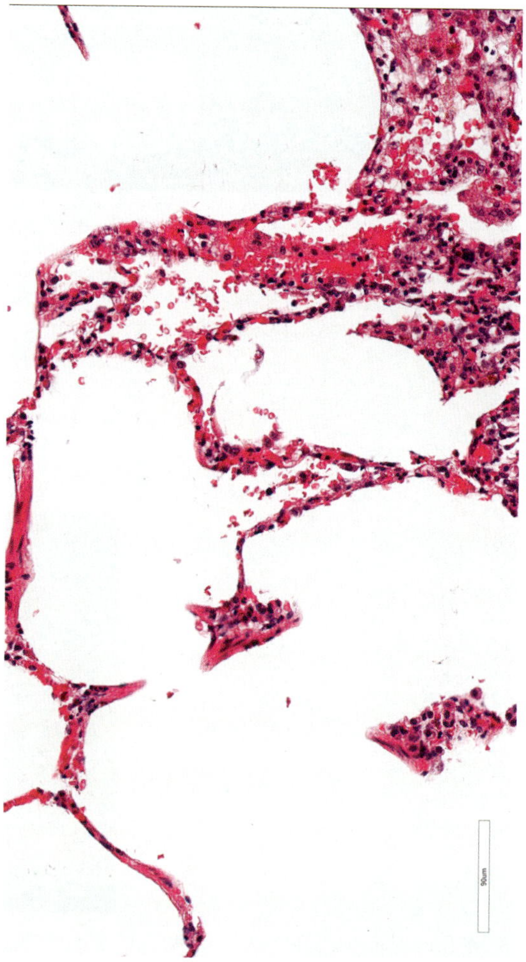

Figure 44.1 Most common pathologic finding in diffuse alveolar haemorrhage: pulmonary capillaritis: alveolar walls contain a neutrophilic infiltrate and there are red blood cells in the alveolar spaces along with focal haemosiderosis in macrophages (bottom right) (H&E 100×).

(d) (e)

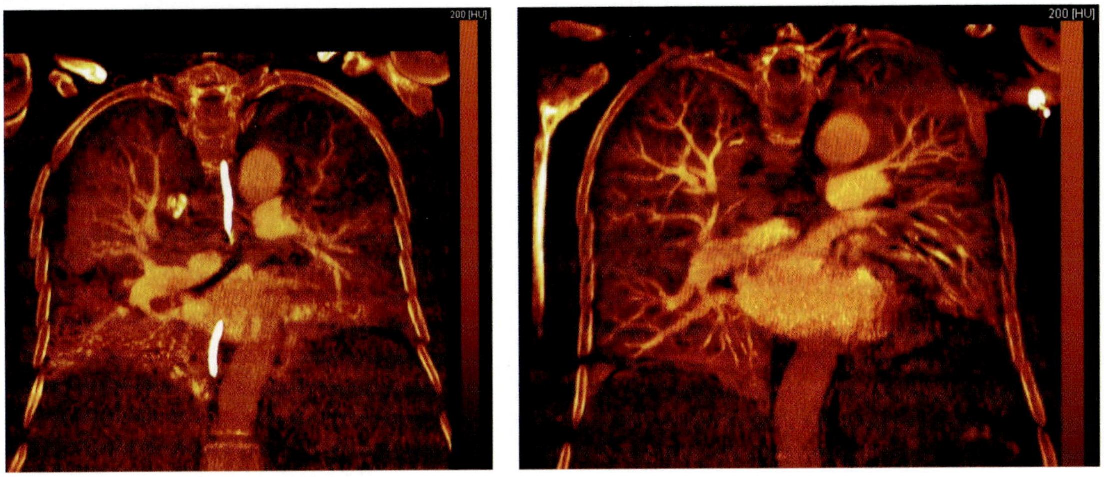

Figure 43.2 Image series from a patient with acute massive pulmonary embolism in the context of COVID-19 infection. Images courtesy of Dr Carole Ridge, Royal Brompton and Harefield Hospitals. (A) Axial CT pulmonary angiogram of patient with COVID pneumonitis and new hypotension. An occlusive filling defect in the left pulmonary artery is consistent with an acute pulmonary thrombus, and the main pulmonary artery is dilated. (B) Axial CT at the mid-cardiac level demonstrating right ventricular strain. The RV to LV ratio is 2.5 with marked straightening of the interventricular septum consistent with right ventricular strain. (C) Pulmonary angiogram. The patient underwent pulmonary thrombolysis using ultrasound assisted thrombolysis. Angiographic images confirm an occlusive left pulmonary artery thrombus. (D) Pre-thrombolysis dual-energy CT (DECT): coronal iodine map acquired with dual-energy CT demonstrates marked hypoenhancement of the left lung due to acute pulmonary artery thrombus. (E) Post-thrombolysis DECT: coronal iodine map 4 months after thrombolysis and anticoagulant therapy demonstrates improved left pulmonary iodine enhancement.

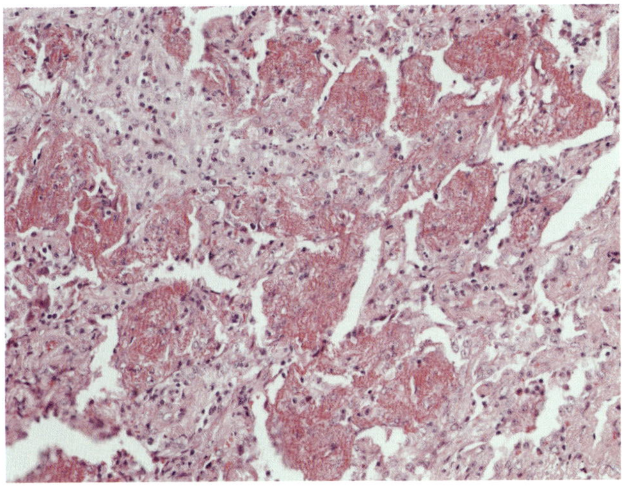

Figure 46.2 Photomicrograph of a Masson body composed of spindle-shaped fibroblasts in a loose matrix of immature connective tissue, typically forming intraluminal 'plugs' within alveolar ducts and sacs (200× magnification, H&E stain).

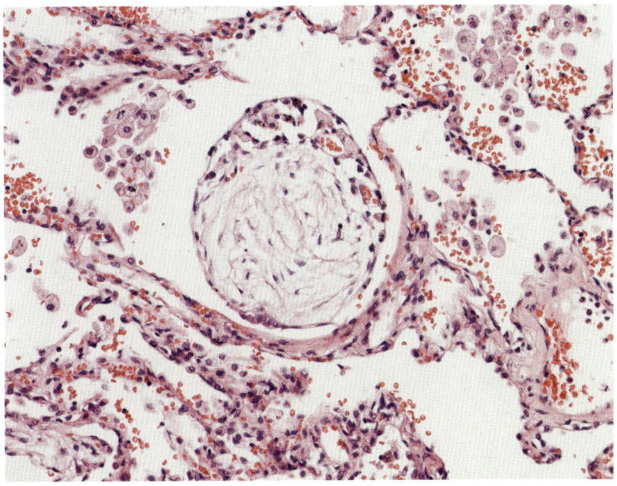

Figure 46.6 Photomicrograph of AFOP demonstrating intra-alveolar 'fibrin balls' and associated changes of organising pneumonia without obvious hyaline membrane formation (200× magnification, H&E stain).

Grade	Severity	Endobronchial features	Image
0	**No inhalation injury**	Absence of carbonaceous deposits, erythema, oedema, bronchorrhoea or obstruction	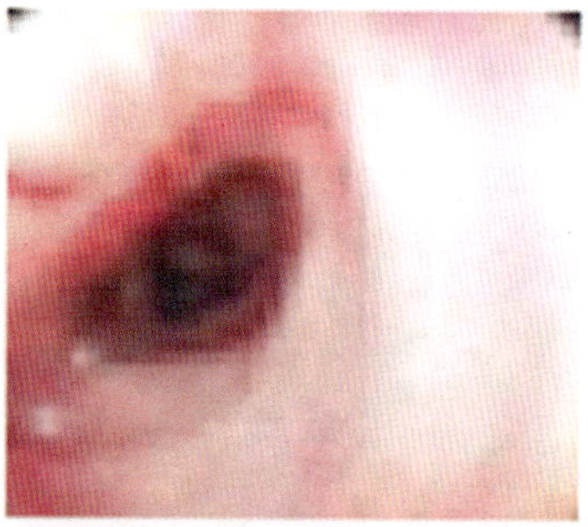
I	**Mild injury**	Minor or patchy areas of erythema, carbonaceous deposits in proximal or distal bronchi (any or combination)	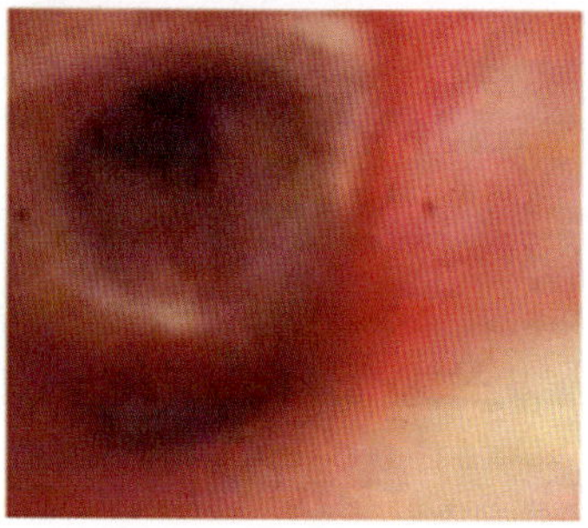
II	**Moderate injury**	Moderate degree of erythema, carbonaceous deposits, bronchorrhoea, with or without compromise of the bronchi (any or combination)	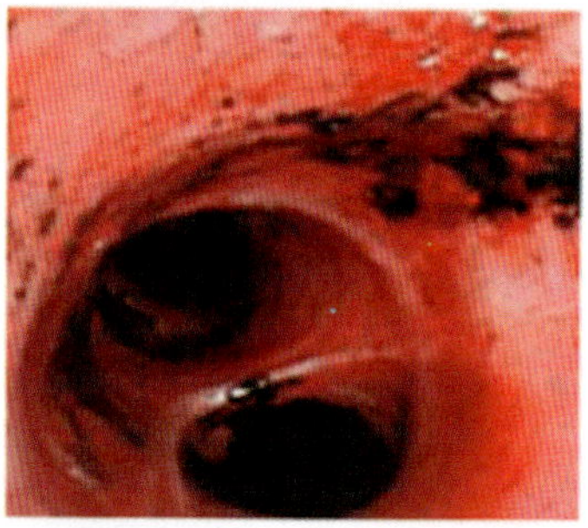
III	**Severe injury**	Severe inflammation with friability, copious carbonaceous deposits, bronchorrhoea, bronchial obstruction (any or combination)	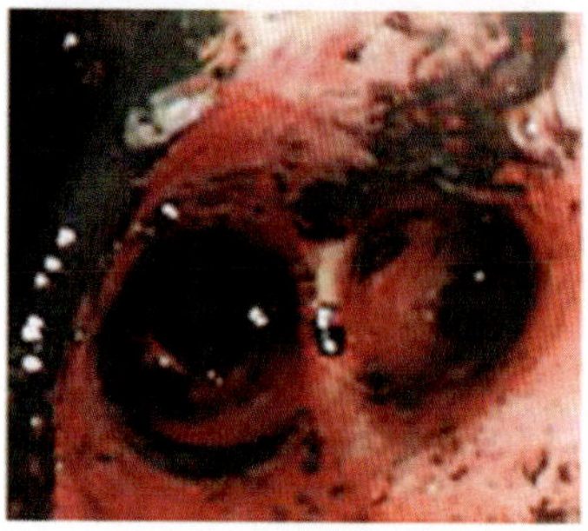
IV	**Massive injury**	Evidence of mucosal sloughing, necrosis, endoluminal obliteration (any or combination)	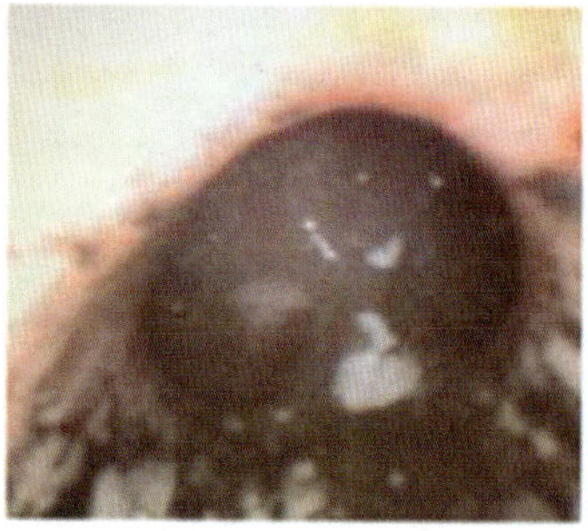

Figure 61.2 Abbreviated injury score.

32

Ventilator-associated Pneumonia

Vimal Grover and Suveer Singh

- VAP is highly prevalent (~10%–35%) and has a significant morbidity and attributable mortality (~10%–15%).
- Contamination of the lower airway by upper airway/gastro-oropharyngeal secretions is the primary aetiology.
- Standard definitions incorporate clinico-radiologico-microbiological parameters with or without respiratory physiological deterioration.
- Ventilator care bundles when implemented have been shown to reduce VAP rates in the ICU.

- The role of invasive sampling of the lower respiratory tract is uncertain but may help reduce antibiotic usage.
- Distinguishing tracheobronchitis from infected alveolar inflammation.
- Biomarkers such as interleukin-1β/interleukin-8 are accurate in 'ruling out' VAP but have not changed antibiotic prescribing practice thus far.
- The influence of behavioural factors and point-of-care tests in antibiotic stop decisions.
- Oral chlorhexidine is no longer considered part of VAP bundles due to association with potential harm.

- The development and implementation of biomarkers to change antibiotic prescribing.
- The influence of genetic predisposition to VAP development.
- The influence of PCR- and metagenomic-based point of of care platform tests on the accuracy of diagnosis, antibiotic stewardship and patient related outcomes.

Introduction

Ventilator-associated pneumonia (VAP) is a common nosocomial infection in intensive care. It is defined as a pneumonia that develops 48 h or more after insertion of an endotracheal tube (ETT or tracheostomy).[1] This definition serves to exclude lower-respiratory-tract infections that were developing prior to intubation. VAP develops in ~10%–35% of intubated patients and is influenced by the casemix and sample population.

The cumulative risk of developing VAP increases with duration of intubation, but the daily hazard rate decreases after day 5 (up to 3.3% daily hazard rate by day 5, 2.3% at day 10, and 1.3% at day 15). In the large multi-national EPIC III study, 60% of patients with infection had a respiratory tract as the site at the time the point-prevalence study was conducted. A significant number of these patients are likely to have had VAP, demonstrating its high prevalence.[2] Expression of incidence as a density (i.e. per 1000 ventilator days) provides some correction for duration of ventilation, and commonly reported rates vary from 1.2 to 17 per 1000 ventilator days.[3]

The absolute risk of VAP increases with days on a mechanical ventilator. It increases the costs of healthcare[4] and is responsible for a significant proportion of antimicrobial agent use in ICUs. Health economic model estimates suggest that a case of VAP adds nearly $40,000 to healthcare costs per patient in the USA. There is controversy as to the attributable mortality of VAP. This arises due to inclusion heterogeneity of casemix (medical, surgical, and mixed), biases associated with observational data, and variability in diagnostic criteria for VAP. A meta-analysis of eligible studies was not able to ascribe an accurate mortality estimate due to such heterogeneity. Furthermore, VAP rates may be affected by time-dependent factors; ICU discharge acts as a competing end point as such patients no longer contribute to the pool eligible to develop VAP. Models that utilize competing risks are still vulnerable to the effects of confounding due to their observational nature. Melsen et al. (2013) employed innovative methods to derive an attributable mortality of 13% (95% CI: 14%–38%).[5] In pre-defined subgroups, there appeared to be no attributable mortality from VAP in trauma patients (95% CI: 106%–45%), medical patients (95% CI: 41%–29%), or patients with APACHE II (Acute Physiology and Chronic Health Evaluation) scores <20 or > 30. In those patients with APACHE II scores 20–29, reflecting moderate severity of illness, the attributable mortality was 36% (95% CI: 29%–151%). In surgical patients, the figure was estimated to be 69% (95% CI: 8%–360%). Further analysis demonstrated that the VAP mortality risk was influenced by the increased risk of dying associated with an extended length of stay in ICU. More recent yet smaller observational studies suggest a similar but lower attributable mortality ~8.4%.[5] Thus, while there appears to be an attributable mortality associated with VAP, which varies with factors such as casemix, it is also apparent that a significant proportion of patients die with VAP rather than from it.

Aetiology of VAP

For VAP to develop, microorganisms need to enter and multiply in the lower respiratory tract, specifically the alveolar compartment. Colonization of the airways is possible, without infection. ETTs bypass innate defences of the upper respiratory tract (i.e. naso-oropharyngeal mucosal immunity, structural barriers, mucus, and humidification (Chapter 4)) while hindering the muco-ciliary escalator function. Sedation (by depressing the central respiratory drive to breathe), respiratory muscle weakness, and mechanical disadvantage (e.g. supine position, abdominal inactivity, and the presence of the tracheal tube) reduce effective cough and swallowing of secretions. Organisms present in the aerodigestive tract—the mouth (including dental plaque), sinuses, and upper gastrointestinal tract—collect in secretions that pool above the cuff. These organisms can migrate into the respiratory tract via micro-channels between the high-volume, low-pressure cuffs and the tracheal mucosa. From there, ventilator cycling blows the organisms more distally. Furthermore, organisms can also enter ETTs via the ventilator circuit and can form biofilms on the inside of the ETT to act as a further pool for lung contamination resulting in either colonization, tracheobronchitis, and/or parenchymal infection. The likelihood of VAP is also dependent on organism virulence and host immunity. Specifically, critically ill patients may develop acquired immune defects, the so-called immune hyporesponsiveness, predisposing to VAP.[6]

Pneumonia can occur in patients receiving non-invasive ventilation. Such patients are infrequently sedated and usually have intact laryngopharyngeal reflexes and cough. However, they can be impaired or restricted while the mask is in situ. Nevertheless, the rates of nosocomial pneumonia are reported to be less than those who have an ETT.[7]

Numerous types of microorganism can cause VAP. These include bacteria, viruses, or fungi. Likely organisms vary according to the duration of intubation as well as the profile of organisms present in individual ICUs and prior antibiotic administration. Geographical variations are notable. That said, the term 'ESKAPE', coined by Rice in 2008, accounts for ~80% of VAP isolates.[8] These are *Enterococcus faecium*, *Staphylococcus aureus*, *Klebsiella pneumoniae*, *Acinetobacter baumannii*, *Pseudomonas aeruginosa*, and *Enterobacter* species. *Escherichia coli* is not a common causative organism except in specific cases where faeco-oral transmission is likely. Enterococci including vancomycin-resistant Enterococci are also thought to be a rare cause of VAP despite increasing rates of colonization.

A further distinction between early- and late-onset VAP (within or after 96 h of ICU admission) has been suggested. In late-onset VAP, isolated bacteria are more likely to be multi-antibiotic resistant than antibiotic-sensitive. Prolonged hospital stays prior to intubation are more associated with late-onset VAP.

The role of viruses in VAP causation remains controversial (Chapter 34). Clearly, viral infection (e.g. influenza) can lead to secondary bacterial pneumonia. However, until the recent development of commercially available rapid diagnostic molecular isolation platforms, difficulty isolating viruses from the respiratory tract has prevented systematic study of any causative role.[9] More widespread use of viral molecular testing will bring with it the familiar challenges of identification, association, and causality.

Fungi are rarely thought to cause VAP. Candida is often detected in microbiological sampling of the airway tract, but this largely considered colonization rather than infection. Aspergillus species colonize too but may infect immunosuppressed patients. There are increasing reports of influenza-associated pulmonary aspergillosis in patients with acute respiratory distress syndrome (ARDS), who are otherwise not considered at risk for fungal pneumonia. Diagnosis requires a risk assessment with any evidence of tracheobronchitis and Aspergillus in respiratory tract samples and/or the presence of the galactomannan biomarker in BAL fluid or serum prompting suspicion of invasive fungal infection.[10] Furthermore Conway-Morris et al. (2009) detected pulmonary inflammatory cytokines in patients who only had candida present in bronchoalveolar lavage (BAL) samples. This was suggestive of infection rather than mere colonization and could indicate under-reporting of fungal infections.[11]

VAP should be differentiated from ventilator-associated tracheobronchitis (VAT). In the latter, there are many similar features (cough, fever, and purulent secretions), but persistent parenchymal changes are absent from the chest X-ray. Interpretation becomes more complex when lung imaging is already abnormal, thus masking developing parenchymal abnormalities, particularly subtle changes. VAT may be an intermediate process that develops prior to VAP and can prolong duration of mechanical ventilation. Recent evidence from the most comprehensive observational multicentre study so far of 2960 patients in Europe and South America revealed an incidence of 11% for VAT and 12% VAP. VAT progressed to VAP in 12% of patients. Those treated with appropriate antibiotics were significantly less likely to progress to VAP than with inappropriate antibiotics (8% vs 29%, odds ratio 0.21 (95% CI: 0.11–0.41)). Mortality was significantly higher in patients with VAP (40%) than those with VAT or no infection (29% and 30%, respectively).[12]

Risk Factors for VAP Development

Risk factors for developing VAP may be considered fixed or modifiable. Fixed factors include male gender, chronic obstructive pulmonary disease, age >60 years, greater illness severity, neurosurgery, and admission with a low Glasgow Coma Scale (GCS) or head injury. Modifiable factors include the use of gastric-ulcer prophylaxis, supine positioning, reintubation and the need for prolonged mechanical ventilation, enteral feeding, aspiration, low cuff pressures, sinusitis, and the presence of ARDS. These factors can be considered independently for their role in promoting VAP. There is a common final pathway into which all these factors contribute—the increased risk of micro-aspiration of orogastric contents into the lower respiratory tract. Intubation may inoculate the respiratory tract and the risks of this increase with reintubation, as does mortality.

Gastro-prophylaxis (stress-ulcer prophylaxis (Chapter 27)) is used routinely in ICU patients (see the section 'Prevention of VAP').

Its aim is to reduce the risk of gastrointestinal bleeding that occurs with the stress of critical illness. The consequence of its use is to raise the stomach pH, thereby promoting the growth of aerobic Gram-negative bacilli in the digestive tract. Nasogastric tubes used for enteral feed can predispose to sinusitis, and enteral feeding can increase the risk of regurgitation and aspiration. Supine positioning may contribute to an increased risk of aspirating gastric contents (see the section 'Prevention of VAP' for further detail).

Diagnosis of VAP

Timely and accurate diagnosis of VAP is crucial but remains the subject of much debate. In patients who are infected, early administration of antimicrobials is lifesaving. However, in patients who do not have infections such as VAP but are treated with empirical antibiotics, there is the attendant risk of development of *Clostridium difficile*–associated diarrhoea/colitis, other side effects, and encouragement of antimicrobial resistance. Ideally, a rapid test with high diagnostic accuracy (highly sensitive and specific) to enable reliable rule-in and rule-out of VAP should be available (Chapter 14).

By conventional microbiological standards, microorganisms may take 48–72 h for identification. A Gram stain will provide limited information more quickly. False-negative results (failure to detect an infection that is present) may occur due to inadequate microbiological sampling, prior antimicrobial treatment, or infection with culture-negative organisms. False-positive results (diagnosing VAP in the absence of actual infection) occurs with sampling of organisms colonizing the proximal airways.

There is currently no universally agreed *practical* gold standard for the diagnosis of VAP. The historical gold standard is the examination of histopathological specimens to detect infected inflammation in the alveoli of lung parenchyma. This relies on post-mortem examination, thereby underestimating sensitivity by skewing towards the severe end of the VAP clinical spectrum. Even within this 'gold standard' there is variability in the reporting of specimens by pathologists. One lesson learnt from the examination of such specimens is that VAP is a multifocal disease. This is in keeping with the concept of mechanical ventilation propagating organisms into multiple areas of the respiratory tract. Its significance is that microbiological sampling has to occur at the correct site to avoid a false-negative result.

As a result of this uncertainty, there have been several attempts at creating diagnostic criteria for VAP. These utilize a combination of clinical, radiological, and microbiological features to identify VAP.

Clinical features have been adopted from criteria used to diagnose community-acquired pneumonia and hospital-acquired pneumonia. They include cough, dyspnoea, and auscultatory changes such as wheeze or crackles, fever, altered white cell count (raised or reduced), worsening gas exchange, and purulent secretions. Most of these features can occur in non-infective pneumonia mimics such as traumatic pulmonary contusions, pulmonary embolism, pulmonary oedema, and ARDS. As assessed against histopathology, fever had a sensitivity of 67% and specificity of 65% for VAP diagnosis. Purulent secretions had reasonable sensitivity (83%) but low specificity (42%)—approximating to a 1 in 6 chance of a false-positive result; white cell count changes had 77% sensitivity and 58% specificity. Therefore, single clinical features do not have great utility in diagnosing VAP.

The presence of new infiltrates on a chest X-ray has a sensitivity of 92% but at the expense of poor specificity (33%), and while this indicates a high risk of falsely diagnosing VAP, the absence of new infiltrates makes VAP unlikely. Wunderink et al. (1992) compared different radiological features with the histopathological gold standard.[13] The theme was that features with high sensitivity had lower specificity and vice versa. Alveolar infiltrates had sensitivity and specificity of 88% and 27%, respectively. Air bronchograms suggestive of consolidation were 83% sensitive but 58% specific overall. These were subdivided into single bronchograms (17% sensitive/96% specific) and multiple ones (67% sensitive/62% specific). Fissure abutment had as high a specificity (96%) as single air bronchograms but poor sensitivity (6%). Tests with high specificity can be used for ruling-in pathology.

Attempts have been made to combine potentially diagnostic features. Johanson's criteria[14] comprised new or progressive changes on chest X-ray, along with two or more of: fever (>38 °C), raised or low white cell count, and the presence of purulent secretions. In another such study, sensitivity was 69% and specificity was 75%.

In addition to the clinical criteria outlined above, microbiological sampling may aid both the identification of an organism and the diagnosis of infection.

Specimen acquisition can occur in the following ways:

- *Tracheobronchial aspirate (TBA)*: An in-line suction catheter is inserted through the ETT or tracheostomy, and secretions are suctioned. Such secretions are present in the proximal airways and may not reflect organisms present in the distal airways. Moreover, TBA may detect organisms colonizing the trachea and bronchi.
- *Non-directed bronchial lavage*: A sterile suction catheter is introduced via the ETT and lodged distally. 20 mL of saline is instilled and gently aspirated back. There is a loss of yield, with approximately 2–3 mL of fluid returned (the remainder is absorbed by the respiratory mucosa). There is a possibility of contamination of the catheter as it is introduced via the ETT. Furthermore, it is difficult to direct the catheter. It mostly enters the right lung.
- *Non-directed protected specimen brush (PSB)*: The sampling apparatus (a catheter with a distal brush) is protected from airway organisms by an outer sheath. The sheath with the inner sampling tube is inserted via the ETT; the brush is then advanced further (avoiding contamination) and sampling occurs, before withdrawing the brush back into the sheath before removal. The PSB cannot be guided to a defined area of lung with accuracy blindly, but this can be achieved via bronchoscopy.
- *Mini-bronchoalveolar lavage (mini-BAL)*: Similar to the PSB, there is an outer sheath. Once this has been introduced into the airways, an inner catheter is passed and lodged distally. There is no brush, but saline is instilled in aliquots and the aspirate obtained reflects sampling from more distal airways. Once again, the sampled area cannot be directed accurately.
- *BAL*: A fibreoptic bronchoscope (Chapter 19) is directed to the area of interest (identified from a new or progressive infiltrate on chest X-ray). If there is widespread shadowing, the right middle lobe may be sampled due to ease of lodging the bronchoscope there. Saline is instilled and suctioned into an attached sputum

trap. Directed PSB sampling can also be achieved via the working channel of the bronchoscope.

Overall, the ease of sampling reduces, but the ability to direct samples to distal airways increases from (i) to (v). These methods have been compared to the histopathological gold standard. TBA had 69% sensitivity/92% specificity for VAP diagnosis. PSB had 22%–36% sensitivity/50%–77% specificity. When used for Gram stain of organisms, mini-BAL had 56% sensitivity/89% specificity. The utility of BAL when compared with this gold standard depends upon the culture method employed (the presence of intracellular organisms on Gram stain, BAL neutrophil level, or $\geq 10^4$ colony forming units/mL (cfu/mL)). Sensitivity varied from 11% to 100% and specificity from 45% to 100%.[15]

Bronchoscopy more than other techniques (due to the duration of the procedure) can result in loss of positive end-expiratory pressure (PEEP) and a temporary derangement in gas exchange. Compared to BAL, non-invasive techniques tend to overestimate the true incidence of VAP, and the use of BAL can reduce antibiotic use by 21%.

Respiratory cultures may be assessed by semi-quantitative or qualitative culture. Using standard operating procedures for sample processing, a threshold for organism growth is set to reduce the likelihood detecting colonizing rather than infecting organisms. For BAL and mini-BAL, $\geq 10^4$ cfu/mL is used. For PSB $\geq 10^3$ cfu/mL is the threshold and for TBA $\geq 10^5$ cfu/mL is the threshold (reflecting more proximal sampling with a higher risk of sampling colonizing organisms). Qualitative culture divides growth into none/light/moderate and heavy. A positive culture is defined by moderate or heavy growth. There is controversy as to whether semi-quantitative is superior to qualitative culture. The Centers for Disease Control (CDC) consider semi-quantitative ($\geq 10^4$ cfu/mL) growth and qualitative microbiology to be equal in their recent VAP definition.

Surveillance Definitions and Scoring Systems for VAP Diagnosis

The need to compare VAP rates over time and between units has driven the development of diagnostic definitions, including those set out by the CDC/National Healthcare Safety Network (NHSN) and European Centre for Disease Prevention and Control (ECDC). These are intended for surveillance and reporting purposes rather than bedside diagnostic use. The clinical pulmonary infection score (CPIS) combines radiological, clinical, and microbiological factors and was designed for bedside clinical use.

CDC/NHSN Definition for HAP

This definition (Table 32.1) is limited by the fact that it applies to all HAP, which incorporates VAP. It combines clinical and radiological features, omitting microbiology. It was compared with BAL microbiology in nearly 300 patients with a sensitivity of 84% and a specificity of 69%.[16] One caveat for the BAL microbiology is that a $\geq 10^5$ cfu/mL threshold was used for positivity rather than $\geq 10^4$ cfu/mL. This definition has been criticized for not including deterioration in lung physiology or oxygenation and for having too many subjective elements.

Table 32.1 The CDC/NHSN definition of hospital-acquired pneumonia diagnosed by clinico-radiological criteria

Chest X-ray signs	Two serial chest X-rays with at least one feature: • New or progressive *and* persistent infiltrate • Cavitation • Consolidation
Clinical features	At least one of the following: • Fever (temperature >38°C) in the absence of another cause • Low white cell count (<4.0 × 10^9 cells/L) or raised white cell count (>12.0 × 10^9 cells/L) • For adults >70 years of age, altered mental status with no other cause responsible And ≥2 of the following: • New onset of purulent sputum or change in sputum character • Increased respiratory secretions or increased requirements for suction • New onset or worsening cough, or dyspnoea, or tachypnoea • Bronchial breath sounds or rales • Worsening gas exchange, for example, (PaO_2/F_iO_2) ≤ 240 mmHg increased oxygen requirement or increased ventilatory demand

Note: Microbiological confirmation is not required. This definition does not specifically apply to ventilator-associated pneumonia (VAP), which is a subset of patients with HAP.
Source: Adapted from Horan T, Andrus M, Dudeck M. CDC/NHSN surveillance definition of healthcare-associated infection and criteria for specific types of infections in the acute care setting. *Am J Infect Control.* 2008;36(5):309–332, Copyright 2008, with permission from Elsevier and the Association for Professionals in Infection Control and Epidemiology.

Ventilator-associated Events (VAEs)

Arising from critiques of the previous HAP definition, and use of VAP as a quality and performance indicator in US ICUs, the CDC published new VAP surveillance criteria in 2013, and updated since then most recently in January 2021, aiming to reduce diagnostic variability and allow effective benchmarking of VAP rates. Removal of chest radiographic criteria, due to concerns about subjective reporting, is one of the more controversial components.

The new classification focuses on deteriorations in patients receiving mechanical ventilation (Figure 32.1). In order for a so-called VAE to occur, there has to be a period of stable or improving ventilation before deterioration. A ventilator-associated condition (VAC) occurs if the clinical worsening is sustained for 2 or more days. This serves to exclude transient events, such as atelectasis, that resolve quickly and do not impact further on a patient's progress. Sustained deteriorations may be pulmonary or non-pulmonary; pulmonary causes include pneumonia, pulmonary oedema, and ARDS.

VACs are identified as infection-related (IVAC) if the patients have VAC and an abnormal temperature or white cell count and have been given antibiotics for at least 4 days. Additionally, possible pneumonias are defined if there are purulent secretions and/or pathogenic bacteria identified. If either of these is present (secretions or bacteria), the IVAC is denominated as a 'possible pneumonia'. Pathogenic bacteria can be identified in the microbiology sample, via histopathology, pleural fluid culture, or tests for Legionella.

ECDC Criteria

The ECDC surveillance criteria identify VAP using radiological, clinical, and microbiological features.[17] There are five categories

Patient nas a baseline period of stability or improvement on the ventilator, defined by ≥ 2 calender days of stable or decreasing daily minimum* FiO_2 or PEEP values. The baseline period is defined as the 2 calendar days immediately preceding the first day of increased daily minimum PEEP or FiO_2.
*Daily minimum defined by lowest value of FiO_2 or PEEP during a calender day that is maintained for > 1 hour.

⇩

After a period of stability or improvement on the ventilator, the patient has at least one of the following indicators of worsening oxygenation:
1) Increase in daily minimum* FiO_2 of ≥ 0.20 (20 points) over the daily minimum FiO_2 of the first day in the baseline period, sustained for ≥ 2 calender days.
2) Increase in daily minimum* PEEP values of ≥ 3 cmH_2O over the daily minimum PEEP of the first day in the baseline period[1], sustained for ≥ 2 calender days.
*Daily minimum defined by lowest value of FiO_2 or PEEP during a calendar day that is maintained for > 1 hour.
[1]Daily minimum PEEP values of 0.5 cmH_2O are considered equivalent for the purposes of VAE surveillance.

⇩

Ventilator-Associated Condition (VAC)

⇩

On or after calendar day 3 of mechanical ventilation and within 2 calendar days before or after the onset of worsening oxygenation, the patient meets both of the following criteria:
1) Temperature > 38°C or < 36°C, **OR** while blood cell count ≥12,000 cells/mm^3 or ≤ 4,000 cells/mm^3.
AND
2) A new antimicrobial agent(s) (see Appendix for eligible antimicrobial agents) is started and is continued for ≥ 4 qualifying antimicrobial days (QAD).

⇩

Infection-related Ventilator-Associated Complication (IVAC)

⇩

On or after calendar day 3 of mechanical ventilation and within 2 calendar days before or after the onset of worsening oxygenation, ONE of the following criteria is met **(taking into account organism exclusions specified in the protocol)**:

1) Criterion 1: Positive culture of one of the following specimens, meeting quantitative or semi-quantitative thresholds† as outlined in protocol, without requirement for purulent respiratory secretions:
   - Endotracheal aspirate, ≥ 10^5 CFU/ml or corresponding semi-quantitative result
   - Bronchoalveolar lavage, ≥10^4 CFU/ml or corresponding semi-quantitative result
   - Lung tissue, ≥ 10^4 CFU/g or corresponding semi-quantitative result
   - Protected specimen brush, ≥ 10^3 CFU/ml or corresponding semi-quantitative result
2) Criterion 2: Purulent respiratory secretions (defined as secretions from the lungs, bronchi, or trachea that contain ≥ 25 neutrophils and ≤ 10 squamous epithelial cells per low power field [lpf, ×100])† **PLUS** organism identified from one of the following specimens (to include qualitative culture, or quantitative/semi-quantitative culture without sufficient growth to meet Criterion #1):
   - Sputum
   - Endotracheal aspirate
   - Bronchoalveolar lavage
   - Lung tissue
   - Protected specimen brush
3) Criterion 3: One of the following positive tests:
   - Organism identified from pleural fluid (where specimen was obtained during thoracentesis or initial placement of chest tube and NOT from an indwelling chest tube)
   - Lung histopathology, defined as: 1) abscess formation or foci of consolidation with intense neutrophil accumulation in bronchioles and alveoli; 2) evidence of lung parenchyma invasion by fungi (hyphae, pseudohyphae, or yeast forms); 3) evidence of infection with the viral pathogens listed below based on results of immunohistochemical assays, cytology, or microscopy performed on lung tissue
   - Diagnostic test for *Legionello* species.
   - Diagnostic test on respiratory secretions for influenza virus, respiratory syncytial virus, adenovirus, parainfluenza virus, rhinovirus, human mettapneumovirus, coronavirus

†If the laboratory reports semi-quantitative results, those results must correspond to the quantitative thresholds. Refer to Table 2 and 3.

⇩

Possible Ventilation-Associated Pneumonia (PVAP)

Figure 32.1 Centres for disease control criteria for ventilator-associated condition (VAC), infective ventilator-associated condition (IVAC), and possible ventilator-associated pneumonia (pVAP). From NHSN, CDC.[18]

Reproduced from National Healthcare Safety Network. Ventilator-associated event, January 2023. Centres for Diseaese Control. Available (with no fee) from https://www.cdc.gov/nhsn/pdfs/pscmanual/10-vae_final.pdf.

of VAP (PN1–4) depending on the quality of sampling and the microbiological method used or the absence of positive microbiology (PN5). PN1 represents high-quality sampling (i.e. BAL) and quantitative microbiology; PN2 with lesser quality sampling, higher contamination risk, and so a higher quantitative threshold; PN3 with non-respiratory tract samples; and PN4 with sputum/lower-respiratory-tract culture with non-quantitative microbiology. PN5 uses only radiological and clinical criteria to diagnose VAP. The ECDC criteria allow ICUs to monitor infection rates over time. However, unless identical microbiological methods are used, benchmarking between units is difficult. For instance, the use of BAL rather than TBA led to a four-fold reduction in measured VAP in one report. With ECDC criteria, the threshold for positive microbiology for TBA is ≥10^6 cfu/mL rather than ≥10^5 cfu/mL.

Clinical Pulmonary Infection Score

CPIS was created and validated by Pugin et al.[19] and uses six categories covering systemic (temperature and peripheral blood white cell count) and pulmonary (tracheal secretions, oxygenation, lung radiography, and microbial culture) inflammation. A score greater than 6 was deemed diagnostic of VAP. In their analysis on 28 patients with quantitative microbiology as the gold standard, the sensitivity was 93% and specificity was 100%. If a histopathological rather than microbiological gold standard was used, the sensitivity fell to 72%–77% and specificity to 42%–85%, depending on which cut-off score was used. Using BAL as a gold standard, the sensitivity and specificity were 30%–89% and 17%–80%. Clearly altering the cut-off level (the CPIS score used to define VAP) as well as the method of microbiological analysis altered the diagnostic performance of the scoring system. Moreover, a number of the individual criteria used to summate the score are subject to inter-individual variation. Schurink et al. (2004) measured the agreement level (kappa value) as 0.14–0.18—which is low, for individuals calculating the CPIS in a series of 52 patients. Overall, the sensitivity and specificity of CPIS appear to be 60%–89% and 42%–85%, respectively.[20]

Overall, there are a variety of methods and scoring system for diagnosing VAP. It is likely that the methods will have high concordance in cases of 'absent' or 'definite' VAP (e.g. high CPIS). In cases where there is possible VAP (a 'grey' area), there is likely to be more variability between diagnostic methods depending on the sampling method and diagnostic standard used.

Biomarkers in VAP

The delays inherent in conventional microbiological diagnosis of VAP, as well as the variation in diagnostic definitions alluded to, have led to the investigation of biomarkers for more accurate and rapid diagnosis (Chapter 16). For VAP, a satisfactory biomarker should allow rapid diagnosis and monitoring of infection and prognostication.

Morrow and de Lemos[21] proposed that an ideal biomarker should

- be easy and quick to measure,
- add new information compared with existing tests or markers (such as a higher sensitivity or specificity), and
- assist the clinician in decision-making (e.g. starting or stopping antibiotics).

Other features of an ideal VAP biomarker are the presence of a cost-effective and validated assay, the ability to rapidly track the development and resolution of infection, and the high-quality evidence of patient outcome improvement from biomarker-guided antimicrobial therapy.[22] To date, no such ideal has been achieved.

Challenges in VAP biomarker work include frequent small, single-centre studies, using variable gold standards for diagnosis, thus rendering comparisons difficult. Finding a single infection-specific biomarker seems unlikely given the complexity and redundancy of inflammatory pathways. Furthermore, the diagnosis of infection requires it to be distinguished from non-infectious inflammatory mimics (e.g. surgery and trauma). Both processes ultimately lead to a complex network of processes associated with cell damage and the release of common sets of pro- and anti-inflammatory cytokines and other biologically active mediators (i.e. endocrine, neurohormonal, and coagulation). While host biomarkers may signal infection, finding pathogen-specific signatures has proven even more challenging. Therefore, while biomarkers could potentially influence commencement or cessation of antimicrobials, stewardship would still require microbiological identification of the pathogen. The site of biomarker sampling may also be relevant: a marker from the peripheral blood (e.g. C-reactive protein, or CRP) will not indicate the site of an infection—here additional clinical, radiological, and microbiological criteria will be required to determine a diagnosis of VAP.

The most promising and/or widely used biomarkers include CRP, procalcitonin (PCT), cytokines, and the triggering receptor expressed on myeloid cells-1 (TREM-1).

C-reactive Protein

CRP was discovered by Tillett and Francis as a pentameric protein capable of precipitating the fraction C component of pneumococcus. It is released from the liver as an acute phase protein in response to acute inflammation. It can activate complement, binding to receptors such as phosphocholine on dead cells (apoptotic or necrotic) as well as bacteria. It has a half-life of 19 h, and its serum level is only dependent on production.

Povoa et al. measured CRP in a prospective medical/surgical ICU cohort as part of the BioVAP studies. For the subset of patients with VAP, the sensitivity and specificity were 87.5% and 86.1% at a cut-off level of >96 mg/L. If pyrexia was added to CRP, specificity increased but sensitivity fell. The rate of change of CRP, its highest value, and persistence at day 6 were associated with VAP prediction and outcomes[23]

Given that serum CRP levels may increase with non-infective inflammatory states, as well as infections at other sites, Linssen et al. (2008) utilized a high-sensitivity assay to assess BAL fluid levels of CRP. It was compared with a microbiologically proven VAP as the gold standard. However, in this study of 117 patients, BAL CRP did not discriminate between VAP and non-VAP.[24]

Overall, serum levels of CRP, their peak, and lack of rate of decline can potentially aid in the diagnosis of VAP, where other sites of infection are unlikely.

Procalcitonin

Under conditions of health, PCT, a 116 amino acid polypeptide, is synthesized and secreted by the C-cells of the thyroid. Once cleaved, it releases calcitonin, katacalcin, and an N-terminal fragment (NProCT). PCT is secreted in basal conditions in small quantities (<0.05 ng/mL) and has a half-life of 24 h. However, with systemic sepsis, PCT is produced in larger amounts from differentiated and parenchymal cells. Its serum levels can reach 1000 ng/mL as this form of PCT is not cleaved. Its function remains unknown. If PCT is administered to animals with sepsis in supraphysiological amounts, mortality increases. Anti-PCT antibodies diminish the severity of sepsis suggesting PCT may have an immunomodulatory role. PCT is measured either semi-quantitatively (<0.5, 0.5–2, 2–10, or > 10 ng/mL) or quantitatively.

PCT is raised in post-surgical states, post-cardiac arrest, trauma, renal failure, burns, and following transplant rejection. With regard to serum levels of PCT, it remains unclear as to its utility in diagnosing VAP. Studies have provided conflicting results as to whether absolute levels or changes are associated with pneumonia development. Serum PCT are not specific to the site of infection, but its level may correlate with the severity of pneumonia. Pulmonary levels of PCT have been measured but with poor diagnostic performance.[24]

Overall, PCT does not appear to be a good *diagnostic* biomarker for VAP. However, its role may be in prognostication and antimicrobial de-escalation. Stolz et al. randomized 101 patients in a multicentre trial to PCT-guided de-escalation or to conventional antibiotic therapy. PCT-guided antibiotic use was lower (13 antibiotic-free days alive 28 days after VAP onset compared with 9.5 in the control arm). ICU length of stay and duration of mechanical ventilation and mortality were no different between the groups.[25] PCT levels may also prognosticate, with falling levels predictive of survival and a failure-to-fall reflective of an increased mortality risk.

Triggering Receptor Expressed on Myeloid Cells-1

TREM-1 is present as two isoforms, surface TREM-1 and soluble TREM-1 (sTREM-1). Surface TREM-1 is present on the surface membrane of neutrophils and monocytes. Activation of this receptor leads to pro-inflammatory cytokine release and neutrophil degranulation. TREM-1 amplifies the immune response to extracellular but not intracellular infection. sTREM-1 is either cleaved from the cell surface by metalloproteinases or directly synthesized.

sTREM-1 has been measured in blood and the lungs (e.g. BAL fluid). There is conflicting evidence as to its utility as an adjunctive diagnostic biomarker for VAP. Combining pulmonary surface TREM-1 and plasma sTREM-1 as part of a biomarker panel does improve diagnostic accuracy,[26] but prospective studies demonstrating influence on patient-focused outcomes are lacking.

Cytokines

Pro-inflammatory and anti-inflammatory cytokines are present in both the plasma and pulmonary compartments; their levels change with infectious and non-infective inflammation. Measurement of plasma and pulmonary cytokines and the relevance of their compartmentalization by analyzing the ratio of pulmonary to plasma levels have been studied in VAP. In particular, IL-1β and IL-8 are raised in the lung in VAP. Grover et al. (2014) assessed the utility of IL-1β as part of a combination of soluble and cell surface biomarkers in serum and BAL to positively diagnose VAP; it did not have sufficiently high accuracy alone.[26] However, IL-1β and IL-8 together had a high negative predictive value at a cut-off level of < 10 pg/mL in BAL samples.[11] This provided a very low post-test probability of VAP (2.8%) in patients with suspected VAP who fell below the cut-off.

The utility of this combination of IL-1β and IL-8 to exclude VAP (i.e. an analogy to the plasma D dimer as a 'rule-out' test for venothromboembolic disease) was demonstrated in a prospective multicentre study (VAPrapid) of 150 patients (53 with VAP diagnosed by quantitative microbiology). The IL-1β/IL-8 combination was confirmed as having excellent rule-out performance in VAP.[27] Despite this performance, it did not influence clinician decision-making with no change in antibiotic-free days due to factors separate from the test's accuracy. While IL-1β/IL-8 have the best diagnostic performance to date, none of these tests have proven ability to alter initial antibiotic prescribing nor survival outcomes.

The Impact of COVID-19

Ventilated patients with COVD-19 are at high risk of deterioration. The development of VAP can compound the respiratory failure, characterized by clinic-radio-pathological processes such as a lymphocytic pneumonitis, severe pulmonary microangiopathy and ARDS (see Chapter 35). The extent of superadded infection is not definitively confirmed but appears to be elevated. Concerns regarding aerosolization risks of bronchoscopic sampling and persistently raised inflammatory markers may encourage broad spectrum anti-infectives for longer courses. While prompt recognition and treatment is vital, so too is an appropriate stop time. The incidence of VAP may have increased following the liberal use of dexamethasone, together with increased use of other immunomodulatory therapies. Safe practice guidance for bronchoscopy has been published to aid its use in COVID.[28] Of increasing importance, demonstrated during the COVID pandemic, are point-of-care PCR-based multi-panel platforms that provide rapid identification of several viruses, bacteria, and common resistance patterns. Whether their use in the diagnosis of VAP leads to improved antibiotic stewardship programmes is the subject of current research.

Prevention of VAP

Measures to prevent VAP require a multifaceted, evidence-based approach that incorporates aetiology and pathogenesis of the disease, risk reduction strategies, and surveillance. International guidelines from the UK, Europe, and USA emphasize key aspects using graded recommendations with largely similar statements and relatively small differences.[29]

The ventilator care bundle consists of a set of evidence-based measures to prevent the development complications of ventilation, including VAP. The current components include elevation of the head of the bed, daily sedation interruption and assessment of the readiness to extubate, stress-ulcer prophylaxis, subglottic suction, and venous thromboembolism prevention. Until recently, use of oral chlorhexidine was recommended. This is no longer the case in light of emerging evidence to suggest potential harm. Standard effective oral care including teeth brushing is the replaced standard.

Reduction in the Duration of Mechanical Ventilation

VAP is an exposure-dependent condition; measures aimed at reducing duration of mechanical ventilation can minimize exposure time for VAP development. Standardized weaning protocols, incorporating weaning readiness assessments, (i.e. appropriate sedation holds and re-titration), and daily spontaneous breathing trials for extubation readiness consistently demonstrate success in reducing days on ventilation. However, early (6–8 days) versus late (13–15 days) tracheostomy does not alter VAP incidence.

Reduction in Respiratory Tract Microbial Burden

Reintubation of patients (~10%–18%) increases the risks of airway contamination and VAP. In ventilated patients, dental plaque build-up harbours bacteria in biofilms. Mechanical disruption with toothbrushing can dislodge this or prevent its formation. Studies of the use of selective digestive tract decontamination (SDD), selective oral decontamination (SOD), and oral chlorhexidine have been conducted to assess their efficacy in VAP prevention. SDD involves the application of oral and enteral antibiotics that are not enterally absorbed, with or without parenteral antibiotics. The reported outcome benefits of SDD, including a significant reduction in lower-respiratory-tract infection, are negated by poor uptake by clinicians due to concerns over the development of antimicrobial resistance; this is not supported by any consistent evidence.

SOD only involves topical oral antibiotics rather than enteral and/or parenteral. It appears to be superior to oral chlorhexidine use; the latter may indeed be harmful. The beneficial effect of chlorhexidine antiseptic in previous trials may be due to differential effects seen in cardiac surgical and non-cardiac patients. While chlorhexidine may be beneficial in patients undergoing cardiac surgery, in the non-cardiac surgical population there is a signal towards harm and its routine use is no longer recommended in the US guidelines, although no recommendation is made in European guidelines.

Elevation of the head of the bed reduces the risk of aspiration. The optimal angle remains under debate, with a supine position most likely to result in aspiration, compared with a 45° angle. However, such a high position is rarely achieved in practice. A target of 30° is recommended.

While stress-ulcer prophylaxis reduces the risk of gastrointestinal bleeding, there are concerns that the raised gastric pH encourages the growth of VAP-causative organisms. Aspiration, enhanced by establishing enteral feeding, potentially increases the risk of VAP,[29] although this risk was not found in recent RCTs on the topic (Chapter 27).

Routine use of prophylactic antibiotics to prevent VAP has been studied with potential reductions in VAP development but without an associated improvement in outcome. Currently, the use of prophylactic antibiotics is not recommended.

ETT Modifications and Ventilator Tubing

Endotracheal and tracheostomy tubes can incorporate a posterior port to allow subglottic suction of secretions, reducing the burden of micro-aspiration beyond the cuff. Suction may be manual and intermittent or automated and continuous. In patients who are already being treated with the ventilator bundle of care, the additive use of subglottic suction may reduce early VAP, length of stay, and antibiotic use but not late VAP or mortality.

The ETT cuff shape and material has been modified over recent years in an attempt to reduce leakage between the cuff and tracheal mucosa. Conventional polyvinylchloride cuff shapes (symmetrical) may be formed of excess material, allowing longitudinal folds to develop and facilitate leakage. Tapered cuffs have been employed to minimize this, as has polyurethane (PU), to reduce the thickness of the cuff while maintaining physical strength, thereby reducing fold formation. Cuff pressures are also important, with studies suggesting suboptimal pressures are prevalent and contribute to micro-aspiration. Regular or continuous measurement can be useful in this regard, although not proven. The evidence base suggests the potential advantage of such PU-tapered cuff ETTs with subglottic suction in reducing the risk of early VAP, particularly in higher risk groups such as cardiac surgical patients. However, tapered tube design appears to potentially increase risk.[30] Nevertheless, despite definitely promising and theoretically advantageous technological advances, further randomized trials of effectiveness in VAP reduction and health economic evaluation are required before their place as a key established component of VAP bundles occurs.

Silver-coated ETTs have been advocated for the reduction of VAP. The release of silver ions over time reduces biofilm formation owing to its antimicrobial properties. A Cochrane review suggested that silver-coated ETT may reduce VAP development but had very few eligible studies.[31]

With regard to the ventilator circuit, closed suction is recommended to minimize breaks to the circuit. Frequent routine changes of the ventilator tubing are best avoided as studies suggest that VAP rates are higher; instead, changing when contaminated or once-weekly as a routine is recommended.[29]

Concluding Remarks

VAP has a reported incidence of ~10%–35%, prolongs the duration of mechanical ventilation, increases the costs of healthcare and antimicrobial use, and has an attributable mortality of approximately 13% depending on the clinical setting. It is caused by aspiration of microorganisms past the cuff of the ETT into the airway, where ventilator cycling propels it distally to infect a susceptible host. Local tracheobronchitis and/or more distal infection may then ensue. Diagnosis of VAP does not have a unified definition but incorporates established elements of clinical, microbiological, physiological or radiographic deterioration, and involves differentiation from colonization or tracheobronchitis. There are a variety of methods of microbiological sample acquisition and analysis, with directed sampling and quantitative microbiology potentially reducing false-positive rates. Biomarkers such as IL-1β/IL-8 and newer point-of-care rapid molecular diagnostic platforms hold promise in refuting (or diagnosing) VAP, but studies of their impact on clinical decision-making, particularly behaviours around antimicrobial prescribing, are at an early stage. Prevention of VAP is crucial to avoid the harm associated with the condition and involves targeting all aspects of the VAP aetiological pathway, while the implementation of bundles of care using standard protocols and surveillance reduces VAP rates.

REFERENCES

1. NICE. PSG002 Technical patient safety solutions for prevention of ventilator-associated pneumonia in adults: Guidance. *NICE Guidelines*. 2008.
2. Vincent J-L, Sakr Y, Singer M, et al. Prevalence and outcomes of infection among patients in Intensive Care Units in 2017. *JAMA*. 2020;**323**(15):1478–1487.
3. Skrupky LP, McConnell K, Dallas J, et al. A comparison of ventilator-associated pneumonia rates as identified according to the National Healthcare Safety Network and American College of Chest Physicians criteria. *Crit Care Med*. 2012;**40**(1):281–284.
4. Kollef MH, Hamilton CW, Ernst FR. Economic impact of ventilator-associated pneumonia in a large matched cohort. *Infect Control Hosp Epidemol*. 2012;**33**(3):250–256.
5. Melsen WG, Rovers MM, Groenwold RHH, et al. Attributable mortality of ventilator-associated pneumonia: A meta-analysis of individual patient data from randomised prevention studies. *Lancet*. 2013; **13**(8): 665–671.

6. Conway Morris A, Anderson N, Brittan M, et al. Combined dysfunctions of immune cells predict nosocomial infection in critically ill patients. *Br J Anaesthesia*. 2013;**111**(5):778–787.
7. Girou E, Schortgen F, Delcaux C, et al. Association of noninvasive ventilation with nosocomial infections and survival in critically ill patients. *JAMA*. 2000;**284**(18):2361–2367.
8. Sandiumenge A, Rello J. Ventilator-associated pneumonia caused by ESKAPE organisms: Cause, clinical features, and management. *Curr Opin Pulm Med*. 2012 May;**18**(3):187–193.
9. Luyt CE, Combes A, Nieszkowska A, et al. In: Torres A, Ewig S, eds. Chapter 11. Viral VAP. *Nosocomial Pneumonia and Ventilator-Associated Pneumonia*. European Respiratory Society. 2011; **53**:113–121.
10. Loughlin L, Hellyer TP, Lewis White P, et al. Pulmonary Aspergillosis in patients with suspected ventilator-associated pneumonia in UK ICUs. *Am J Respir Crit Care Med*. 2020;**202**(8):1125–1132.
11. Conway Morris A, Kefala K, Wilkinson TS, et al. Diagnostic importance of pulmonary interleukin-1 beta and interleukin-8 in ventilator-associated pneumonia. *Thorax*. 2009;**65**(3):201–207.
12. Martin-Loeches I, Povoa P, Rodríguez A, et al. Incidence and prognosis of ventilator-associated tracheobronchitis (TAVeM): A multicentre, prospective, observational study. *Lancet Respir Med*. 2015 Nov;**3**(11):859–868.
13. Wunderink RG, Woldenberg LS, Zeiss J, et al. The radiological diagnosis of autopsy proven ventilator-associated pneumonia. *Chest*. 1992;**101**:458–463.
14. Johanson WGJ, Pierce AK, Sanford JP, et al. Nosocomial respiratory infections with gram-negative bacilli. The significance of colonization of the respiratory tract. *Ann Intern Med*. 1972;**77**:701–706.
15. Chastre J, Fagon J-Y. Ventilator-associated pneumonia. *Am J Respir Crit Care Med*. 2002;**165**(7):867–903.
16. Horan T, Andrus M, Dudeck M. CDC/NHSN surveillance definition of healthcare-associated infection and criteria for specific types of infections in the acute care setting. *Am J Infect Control*. 2008;**36**:309–332.
17. Plachouras D, Lepape A, Suetens C. ECDC definitions and methods for the surveillance of healthcare- associated infections in intensive care units. *Int Care Med*. 2018;**44**(12):2216–2218.
18. National Healthcare Safety Network. Ventilator-associated event, January 2023. Centres for Disease Control. Available from https://www.cdc.gov/nhsn/pdfs/pscman ual/10-vae_final.pdf
19. Pugin J, Auckenthaler R, Mili N, et al. Diagnosis of ventilator-associated pneumonia by bacteriologic analysis of bronchoscopic and nonbronchoscopic 'blind' bronchoalveolar lavage fluid. *Am Rev Respir Dis*. 1991;**143**:1121–1129.
20. Schurink CA, Van Nieuwenhoven CA, Jacobs JA, et al. Clinical pulmonary infection score for ventilator-associated pneumonia: Accuracy and inter-observer variability. *Intensive Care Med*. 2004;**30**(2):217–224.
21. Morrow DA, de Lemos JA. Benchmarks for the assessment of novel cardiovascular markers. *Circulation*. 2007;**115**:949–952.
22. Grover V, Soni N, Kelleher P, et al. Biomarkers in the diagnosis of ventilator-associated pneunonia. *Curr Resp Med Rev*. 2012;**8**(3):184–192.
23. Póvoa P, Martin-Loeches I, Ramirez P, et al. Biomarker kinetics in the prediction of VAP diagnosis: Results from the BioVAP study. *Ann Intensive Care*. 2016; Dec;**6**(1):32.
24. Linssen CF, Bekers O, Drent M, et al. C-reactive protein and procalcitonin concentrations in bronchoalveolar lavage fluid as a predictor of ventilator-associated pneumonia. *Ann Clin Biochem*. 2008 May;**45**(Pt 3):293–298.
25. Stolz D, Smyrnios N, Eggimann P, et al. Procalcitonin for reduced antibiotic exposure in ventilator-associated pneumonia: A randomised study. *Eur Respir J*. 2009;**34**(6): 1364–1375.
26. Grover V, Pantelidis P, Soni N, et al. A Biomarker panel (bioscore) incorporating monocytic surface and soluble TREM-1 has high discriminative value for ventilator-associated pneumonia: A prospective observational study. *PLoS ONE*. 2014;**9**(10): e109686.
27. Hellyer TP, Mcauley DF, Walsh TS, et al. Biomarker-guided antibiotic stewardship in suspected ventilator-associated pneumonia (VAPrapid2): A randomised controlled trial and process evaluation. *Lancet Respir Med*. 2020;**8**:182–191.
28. Luo F, Darwiche K, Singh S, et al. Performing bronchoscopy in times of the COVID-19 pandemic: Practice statement from an International Expert Panel. *Respiration*. 2020;**99**(5):417–422.
29. Hellyer TP, Ewan V, Wilson P, et al. The Intensive Care Society recommended bundle of interventions for the prevention of ventilator-associated pneumonia. *J Intensive Care Soc*. 2016;**17**:238–243.
30. Rouzé A, Jaillette E, Poissy J, et al. Tracheal tube design and ventilator-associated pneumonia. *Respir Care*. 2017;**62**:1316–1323.
31. Tokmaji G, Vermeulen H, Muller MC, et al. Silver-coated endotracheal tubes for prevention of ventilator-associated pneumonia in critically ill patients. *Cochrane Database Syst Rev*. 2015;**12**(8):CD009201.

33

Bacterial Pneumonia

David R Woods and Ricardo J José

- Predicted mortality and risk of requiring critical care admission should be assessed for all patients using a validated scoring system.
- Empiric antibiotic regimens should take into account local guidelines and ecology.
- Risk factors for resistant organisms in both community- and hospital-acquired pneumonia (HAP) should be considered when selecting empiric regimens.
- In severe community-acquired pneumonia, macrolides have a proven immunomodulatory role. Only corticosteroids, recently have yet demonstrated similar benefit.
- With the exception of infection caused by ***Pseudomonas aeruginosa***, short antibiotic courses of 5–7 days should be standard even in critical care.
- Novel diagnostic techniques may in the future allow point-of-care or rapid laboratory-based confirmation of diagnosis, causative pathogen and phenotypic antibiotic susceptibility, and predict risk of deterioration.

- Single or combination empiric antibiotic regimens for HAP in critical care—US guidance recommends Gram-positive agents added to dual Gram-negative cover for patients at increased risk of mortality or resistant organisms. Elsewhere progressively more rationalized regimens are recommended.
- Routine broadening of the empiric antibiotic spectrum in critically unwell patients with pneumonia does not improve clinically relevant outcomes.

- The role of non-antibiotic antibacterial therapies such as lytic bacteriophage therapy. This utilizes naturally occurring viruses that infect specific bacteria, replicate, and induce bacterial lysis.
- The impact of newer or alternative immunomodulatory agents other than corticosteroids or Azithromycin on bacterial pneumonia. These include statins, aspirin, intravenous immunoglobulin, activated protein C, recombinant tissue factor pathway inhibitor, plasma-derived antithrombin III, recombinant thrombomodulin, and sivelestat.
- Confocal laser endomicroscopy delivers fluorescent-labelled ligands to the distal respiratory tract via the bronchoscope working channel, which are then detected by a multi-core fibre attached to a laser scanning proximal light source, also inserted via the working channel. This may allow observation of the evidence of distal respiratory infectious organisms and interactions with the host immune system.
- Precision mucosal sampling techniques have been developed to analyze the respiratory metabolome. Their role in rapid diagnostics requires further evaluation.
- The role of molecular infection biomarkers and quantitative polymerase chain reaction (PCR) as part of point-of-care tests for rapid diagnostics improves outcomes and antibiotic stewardship.

Introduction

Bacterial pneumonia is defined as alveolar and lung parenchymal inflammation due to infection by a bacterial pathogen. This typically manifests with infective symptoms including but not limited to cough productive of purulent sputum, dyspnoea, hypoxia, and pyrexia. It correlates clinically with bronchial breath sounds, radiological evidence of new pulmonary infiltrates, and often raised blood markers of inflammation. Community-acquired pneumonia (CAP) refers to an infection contracted outside of a hospital setting, whereas hospital-acquired pneumonia (HAP) defines an infection developing at least 48 h following hospitalization and not incubating at the time of admission. Some definitions include pneumonia developing within 10 days of hospital discharge as HAP.

HAP can be divided into early onset, within 5 days of hospital admission, and late onset beyond this. Non-intensive care unit (ICU)-acquired pneumonia may have a different ecology, and so can be distinguished from HAP developing on the ICU among non-ventilated patients. Ventilator-associated pneumonia (VAP), developing at least 48 h after initiation of invasive mechanical ventilation, is discussed previously.

Healthcare-associated pneumonia (HCAP) described pneumonia in patients exposed to a variety of healthcare settings other than acute hospital admission or within 90 days of an acute admission. The microbiological aetiology does not differ from CAP with no significant increase in the rate of resistant organisms, yet guidelines targeting HCAP lead to a higher rate of inappropriate broad-spectrum antibiotic use. Thus, while it may identify a cohort at increased risk of poor outcomes, it is unhelpful in guiding management, and currently such patients are considered to have CAP.

CAP has an annual incidence in Europe and the USA ranging between 1 and 2.5 per 1000 adults, increasing with older age, particularly 65 years and above, and male sex.[1,2] Pneumonia accounts for a significant proportion of the intensive care case mix, varies depending on resources and admission thresholds. In the UK in 2018–2019, 5.2% of patients with CAP required admission to ICU and over 20,000 ICU admissions had a primary or secondary diagnosis of pneumonia, representing 12.2% of all ICU admissions.[2,3] Overall, lower respiratory tract infections remain a major cause of mortality causing 3 million deaths worldwide in 2016, more than double that for example of road traffic accidents,[4,5] with mortality being as high as 35% among the ICU cohort.[1]

The microbiological profile of CAP and HAP has evolved over time. Even when microbiological testing is advised and undertaken, no pathogen is identified in up to 63.3% of cases though the figure is lower in ICU with better access to lower respiratory tract sampling (Table 33.1).[1,6] *Streptococcus pneumoniae* remains the most commonly identified pathogen in both CAP overall and among patients admitted to ICU. Atypical bacteria account for 7%–20% of CAP. They are intracellular, more difficult to isolate, and often require a different antibiotic strategy. Despite the perceived relative mildness of atypical infections, Table 33.1 demonstrates that the prevalence of the majority of common organisms is similar comparing the overall and ICU cohorts.

Table 33.1 Microbiological aetiology (percentage) of microbiologically positive community-acquired pneumonia

	United Kingdom (all cases)[a]	Global (non-ICU admission)[b]	Global (ICU admissions)[b]
Typical bacteria			
Streptococcus pneumoniae	42.1	43	42
Haemophilus influenzae	12.3	5	3
Staphylococcus spp.	2.6	2	2
Moraxella catarrhalis	0.8		
Atypical bacteria			
Legionella spp.	9.1	8	8
Chlamydophila spp.	5.9	3	3
Mycoplasma pneumoniae	5.3	3	2
Coxiella burnetii	0.3	2	1
Gram-negative bacteria			
Pseudomonas aeruginosa		4	5
Enterobacteriaceae	2.6	2	1
Other			
Respiratory viruses	18.6	12	4
Polymicrobial		13	22

Note: ICU: intensive care unit.

Source: Data from [a]Welte T, Torres A, Nathwani D. Clinical and economic burden of community-acquired pneumonia among adults in Europe. *Thorax*. 2012;67:71–79; and [b]Cillóniz C, Cardozo C, García-Vidal C. Epidemiology, pathophysiology, and microbiology of community-acquired pneumonia. *Ann Res Hosp*. 2018;2:1.

Traditionally nosocomial and drug-resistant pathogens have emerged in CAP, including *Pseudomonas aeruginosa*, extended-spectrum β-lactamase-producing (ESBL) *Enterobacteriaceae*, methicillin-resistant *Streptococcus aureus* (MRSA)—termed 'PES pathogens'—and *Acinetobacter baumannii*. These account for up to 7% of microbiologically positive CAP, have a high prevalence of antibiotic resistance, and require a different antibiotic strategy.[1] They have a more aggressive clinical phenotype, associated with increased rates of ICU admission, complications, and mortality (Table 33.2).

Among HAP, community-acquired pathogens are more likely to be responsible for early HAP, whereas *Staphylococcus* and Gram-negative bacteria become more prevalent in late HAP (Table 33.3). The prevalence of resistant organisms, both resistant strains such as MRSA and intrinsically resistant bacteria like *A baumannii*, varies worldwide.[7]

Current Practice

Community-acquired Pneumonia

Management of CAP is influenced by a number of national and international guidelines.[8–12] Those from the UK, Europe, and the USA are summarized in Figure 33.1. This outlines an approach to assessing and managing such patients in a hospital setting, and in particular patients at risk of requiring intensive care. Information pertaining to community management is omitted.

Diagnosis should be based on presentation with an acute illness with indicative symptoms and signs of infection and, in hospital, confirmed with a chest radiograph demonstrating compatible new infiltrate(s). Alongside clinical assessment, a stratification tool should be used to improve decision-making in several aspects of care.

The British Thoracic Society (BTS) and National Institute for Health and Care Excellence (in England and Wales) recommend using the CURB-65 score (discussed below). The American Thoracic Society (ATS) and Infectious Diseases Society of America (IDSA) recommend the Pneumonia Severity Index (PSI; Figure 33.2). Both assess 30-day mortality and are used to assist decision-making surrounding need for hospital admission.

Neither score performs well in predicting severe community-acquired pneumonia (SCAP), usually defined as the presence of at least one organ failure requiring intensive care support, or in predicting need for intensive care. Although not included in guidelines, the SMART-COP score (Figure 33.3) is validated and performs well for this purpose. Alternatively, different prediction rules are suggested (listed within Figure 33.1).

Decisions regarding ICU admission can also be supported by general or sepsis-specific illness severity predictors, such as the National Early Warning Score 2 and the quick Sepsis-related Organ Failure Score (qSOFA), and by assessments of frailty and physiological reserve, such as the Clinical Frailty Scale. However, decisions should not be based solely on scoring systems and clinical judgement is paramount.

Table 33.2 Characteristics of community-acquired resistant Gram-negative bacterial pneumonia

Organism	Microbiological features	Geographical variation	Risk factors	Clinical features
Pseudomonas aeruginosa	High intrinsic antibiotic resistance Biofilm formation	Low prevalence in Australia	Structural lung disease Smoking exposure to aerosolized contaminated water Prior hospitalization or antibiotic use	*S. aureus* and *C. albicans* co-infection Mortality up to 20%–50%, though lower among community-acquired cases than nosocomial
Klebsiella pneumoniae	Increasing prevalence of ESBL expression	High prevalence in Asia	Female sex Alcoholism Diabetes mellitus	Bacteraemia, septic shock and respiratory failure, common Necrotizing pneumonia Mortality up to 30%–50%
Staphylococcus aureus MRSA PVL+SA	PVL+ seen in MRSA and MSSA	Low but rising prevalence	COPD Smoking Intravenous drug abuse Prodromal viral illness Prior antibiotics	Necrotizing or haemorrhagic pneumonia Toxic shock Skin lesions and necrosis Mortality up to 10%–35% (MRSA), 40%–75% (PVL+)
Acinetobacter baumanii	Lower resistance from community-acquired isolates compared to nosocomial Ceftriaxone resistance common	Higher prevalence in Asia-Pacific region Low prevalence in the UK and USA	Warm and humid months Alcoholism Diabetes mellitus Chronic lung disease	Fulminant presentation with respiratory failure and shock Mortality up to 40%–60%
Stenotrophomonas maltophilia	High intrinsic antibiotic resistance Increasing trimethoprim-sulfamethoxazole resistance		Chronic lung disease Immunodeficiency Corticosteroids Prior hospitalization, mechanical ventilation, or antibiotics	Haemorrhagic pneumonia Mortality up to 30%–40%

S. aureus: *Staphylococcus aureus*; *C. albicans*: *Candida albicans*; ESBL: extended-spectrum β-lactamases; MRSA: methicillin-sensitive *Staphylococcus aureus*; PVL+(SA): Panton-Valentine leucocidin positive (*Staphylococcus aureus*); MSSA: methicillin-sensitive *Staphylococcus aureus*; COPD: chronic obstructive pulmonary disease; UK: United Kingdom; US: United States of America.

All admitted patients should have blood cultures, sputum culture, pneumococcal urinary antigen, and *Mycoplasma pneumoniae* polymerase chain reaction (PCR) on a respiratory tract sample where possible. Patients with severe pneumonia should also have *Legionella pneumophila* urinary antigen, *Chlamydia pneumoniae* antigen and/or PCR, and extended atypical PCRs on invasive respiratory samples where possible. The presence of a significant pleural effusion should warrant early assessment and consideration of a diagnostic aspirate progressing to drainage if there are features of pleural infection. Patients requiring mechanical ventilation should have a lower respiratory tract sample sent for microbiology; ERS/ESCMID suggest bronchoalveolar lavage (BAL) as the preferred method.

Table 33.3 Microbiological aetiology of microbiologically positive hospital-acquired pneumonia

	United Kingdom (%)	United States (%)	Global (%)
Staphylococcus aureus MRSA MSSA	21.9 4.4 17.5	25.2 11.3 13.9	22.8 8.9 13.9
Pseudomonas spp.	11.9	21.0	21.0
Klebsiella spp.	10.3	14.2	15.0
Escherichia spp.	10.9	6.0	7.2
Acinetobacter spp.	0.5	2.9	5.3
Streptococcus spp.	6.2	5.4	5.1
Enterobacter spp.	5.3	4.6	4.6
Serratia spp.	6.1	4.2	4.0
Stenotrophomonas spp.	1.7	3.9	3.5
Haemophilus spp.	13.4	4.2	3.4

Note: MRSA: methicillin-resistant *Staphylococcus aureus*; MSSA: methicillin-sensitive *Staphylococcus aureus*.

Source: Data from the SENTRY antimicrobial surveillance database for 2013–2019 (https://sentry-mvp.jmilabs.com/).

Choice of antimicrobial therapy is influenced by the assessment of severity and involves empiric antibiotic regimens. In the absence of contraindications, a non-pseudomonal β-lactam combined with a macrolide is indicated for severe pneumonia, whereas monotherapy omitting the macrolide can be considered in non-severe cases unless there is specific concern for an atypical pathogen. In North America, combination therapy is preferred for all admitted patients. Although macrolides can be used as monotherapy in patients with non-severe disease and penicillin allergy, in severe disease a respiratory fluoroquinolone is an appropriate alternative. The specific choice of drug(s) will vary locally according to local ecology and resistance patterns.

Regimens should be modified where there is concern regarding potentially resistant organisms based on relevant risk factors (listed within HAP algorithm; Figure 33.4). As all *P. aeruginosa* will require non-standard antibiotic therapy, it is worth considering the specific risk factors for infection with this pathogen (Figure 33.5). These can be combined into one of a number of specific scoring systems to assess the risk of a multi-resistant organism causing CAP, including the PES score (Figure 33.6) and the Drug Resistance in Pneumonia (DRIP) Score (Figure 33.7).

Concern for a resistant Gram-negative should prompt broadening of the β-lactam to a broad-spectrum antipseudomonal β-lactam. Initial monotherapy is appropriate, though ERS/ESCMID recommend dual therapy with either ciprofloxacin or an aminoglycoside.

	BTS/NICE†	ERS/ESCMID	ATS/IDSA
Diagnosis	Clinical suspicion: acute illness ≤21 days with cough and ≥1 of fever, sputum, dyspnoea, wheeze or chest pain Supportive clinical signs Confirmed by new infiltrate(s) on CXR for all attending hospital		
Admission	**CURB-65** 0–1: Consider discharge ≥2: Consider admission	**CRB** ≥1: Consider admission *CRP and PCT may have a role*	**PSI** ≤70: Consider discharge 71–90: May need admission >90: Consider admission
ICU or Intermediate Care Unit Admission	**CURB-65** ≥3: Consider need for ICU	Severe, defined by one of two rules: Consider need for ICU • Acute respiratory failure • Septic shock • Extension of CXR infiltrates • Severely decompensated comorbidities ≥2 of: • Systolic bp <90 mmHg • P/f <33.3 kPa • ≥2 lobes involved on CXR • Mechanical ventilation • Vasopressor support >4 h	Severe, defined by **2007 IDSA/ATS Criteria**: Consider need for ICU ≥1 major criterion: • Vasopressor support • Mechanical ventilation *or* ≥3 Minor criteria: • RR ≥30 /min • P/F <33.3 kPa • Multilobar infiltrates • Confusion/disorientation • Uraemia >7.1 mmol/L • Leucopaenia <4 ×10^9/L • Thrombocytopaenia <100 ×10^9/L • Hypothermia <36°C • Hypotension requiring aggressive fluid resuscitation
Microbiology	**CURB 0–1:** • No routine sampling **CURB-65≥2:** • Blood cultures ×1 • Sputum gram stain and MCS if no prior Abx or failing to improve • Pneumococcal urinary Ag • Consider *legionella* urinary Ag if specific risk factors • *Mycoplasma* PCR (sputum or URT swab) **CURB-65≥3**; as above plus: • Sputum gram stain and MCS • *Legionella* urinary Ag • *Chlamydophila* Ag and/or PCR on invasive respiratory samples • Atypical PCRs if available, else consider paired serology **Additionally:** • Early diagnostic thoracentesis if associated pleural effusion *Within 4 h of diagnosis, or 1 h if shock*	**All admitted patients:** • Blood cultures ×2 • Sputum gram stain and MCS • Pneumococcal urinary Ag • Pneumococcal qPCR (sputum and blood), if already on Abx • *Legionella* urinary Ag • Atypical PCRs ± IgM, if available **Additionally:** • Diagnostic thoracentesis if 'significant' pleural effusion • Bronchoscopy in non-resolving pneumonia where gas exchange allows - BAL preferred - Bronchoscopic protected specimen brush or quantitative endotracheal aspirate are alternatives • Consider transthoracic needle aspiration *only* in severely unwell patients with focal infiltrate and otherwise non-diagnostic samples *Immediately after diagnosis, within 1h if shock*	**Severe by 2007 IDSA/ATS Criteria:** • Sputum gram stain and MCS* • Blood cultures x1* • Pneumococcal urinary Ag • *Legionella* urinary Ag **Or if empirical or previous treatment for MRSA or Pseudomonas, or hospitalised with IV Abx within 90 days*

Figure 33.1 Algorithm for management of adults hospitalised with community-acquired pneumonia, adapted from national and international guidelines.

†United Kingdom guidelines presented as a composite of the BTS and NICE guidelines, which are broadly complementary. Empirical antibiotic recommendations are as per NICE as this is most recently published.

Data from Lim et al. BTS guidelines for the management of community acquired pneumonia in adults: update 2009. *Thorax* 2009;64:iii1–iii55; NICE Clinical Guideline 191: Pneumonia in adults: diagnosis and management. 2014; NICE Pneumonia (community-acquired): antimicrobial prescribing. 2019; Woodhead et al. Guidelines for the management of adult lower respiratory tract infections – Summary. *Clin Microbiol Infect* 2011;17(Suppl. 6):1–24; and Metlay et al. Diagnosis and Treatment of Adults with Community-acquired pneumonia: An Official Clinical Practice Guideline of the American Thoracic Society and Infectious Diseases Society of America. *Am J Resp Crit Care Med* 2019;200(7):e45–67.

BTS: British Thoracic Society; NICE: National Institute for Health and Care Excellence (England and Wales); ERS: European Respiratory Society; ESCMID: European Society of Clinical Microbiology and Infectious Diseases; ATS: American Thoracic Society; IDSA: Infectious Diseases Society of America; CXR: chest radiograph; CURB-65: community-acquired pneumonia risk stratification score based on the presence of confusion, urea, respiratory rate, blood pressure, and age; CRB: community-acquired pneumonia risk stratification score modified from CURB-65 excluding urea and age; PSI: pneumonia severity index; CRP: C-reactive protein; PCT: procalcitonin; ICU: intensive care unit; P/F: ratio of arterial oxygen partial pressure to fraction of inspired oxygen; MCS: microscopy, culture, and sensitivity; Ag: antigen; PCR: polymerase chain reaction; URT: upper respiratory tract; qPCR: quantitative polymerase chain reaction; BAL: bronchoalveolar lavage; IV: intravenous; Abx: antibiotics; PO: per os; IVOS: intravenous to oral switch review; PVL: Panton-Valentine leucocidin; MDR: multi-drug-resistant (defined as resistance to at least one agent within at least three antimicrobial categories); ESBL: extended-spectrum β-lactamase; MRSA: methicillin-resistant *Staphylococcus aureus*; piptazobactam: piperacillin-tazobactam; RSV: respiratory syncytial virus; GCSF: granulocyte-colony stimulating factor; LMWH: low molecular weight heparin; NIV: non-invasive ventilation; CPAP: non-invasive continuous positive airway pressure; COPD: chronic obstructive pulmonary disease; ARDS: acute respiratory distress syndrome.

Empirical Antibiotics	**CURB 0-1:** • amoxicillin PO • penicillin allergy: doxycycline or clarithromycin PO **CURB-65 2:** • amoxicillin ± clarithromycin PO *if atypical suspected* • penicillin allergy: doxycycline *or* clarithromycin PO **CURB-65 ≥3:** • co-amoxiclav PO/IV *plus* clarithromycin PO/IV • penicillin allergy: levofloxacin PO/IV *recommended duration **5 days** for all* *if IV, review IVOS at 48 hours*	**Non-severe:** *one of* • aminopenicillin/β-lactamase inhibitor ± macrolide • non-antipseudomonal cephalosporin ± macrolide • respiratory fluoroquinolone • penicillin G ± macrolide **Severe:** *one of* • non-antipseudomonal third generation cephalosporin *plus* macrolide • respiratory fluoroquinolone ± non-antipseudomonal 3rd generation cephalosporin *recommended duration **≤8 days*** *consider PCT to guide* *initial therapy IV and review IVOS*	**Non-severe:** *one of* • β-lactam *or* non-antipseudomonal third generation cephalosporin *or* ceftaroline *plus* macrolide • respiratory fluoroquinolone • β-lactam *or* non-antipseudomonal third generation cephalosporin *or* ceftaroline *plus* doxycycline **Severe:** *one of* • β-lactam *plus* macrolide • β-lactam *plus* respiratory fluoroquinolone *do not use PCT to guide initial Abx* *recommended duration **≥5 days** guided by validated measure of clinical stability*
Resistant Organusms	**PVL+*Staphylococcus aureus*** strongly suspected or confirmed: • empirical antibiotics as above • *plus* IV linezolid *plus* IV clindamycin *plus* IV rifampicin *Review previous results including colonisation with MDR bacteria*	Severe with risk factors for ***Pseudomonas aeruginosa***: • antipseudomonal cephalosporin *or* acylureidopenicillin/β-lactamase inhibitor *or* meropenem *plus* • ciprofloxacin • *or* macrolide *plus* aminoglycoside Risk factors for **gram-negative enteric bacterium, especially ESBL**, without risk of *P. aeruginosa*: • ertapenem may be used	Locally-validated risk factors for **MRSA**: • IV vancomycin *or* linezolid Locally-validated risk factors for ***Pseudomonas aeruginosa***: • piptazobactam *or* cefepime *or* ceftazidime *or* aztreonam *or* meropenem *or* imipenem
Aspiration		Suspect if pneumonia follows a witnessed aspiration or if known risk factors **Non-severe:** *one of* • β-lactam/β-lactamase inhibitor • clindamycin • IV cephalosporin *plus* PO metronidazole • moxifloxacin **Severe:** *one of* • clindamycin *plus* cephalosporin • cephalosporin *plus* metronidazole	Do not routinely add anaerobic cover unless abscess or empyema is suspected
Viral		Consider influenza and RSV PCRs during the winter season	Influenza rapid PCR when community circulation Oseltamivir for all positive patients admitted to hospital Continue standard empirical Abx
Adjuncts	Venous thromboembolism prophylaxis Corticosteroids not recommended GCSF not recommended Nutritional support in prolonged illness Airways clearance if indicated	LMWH if in respiratory failure Corticosteroids not recommended Management of septic shock is supportive	Do not routinely use corticosteroids Consider corticosteroids in refractory septic shock

Figure 33.1 Continued

NIV/CPAP	NIV/CPAP not routinely indicated If considered, must be within critical care with immediate access to intubation	Can consider NIV in patients with COPD and ARDS	
Complications	Re-investigate non-response at 72 h with bloods and CXR Early effective pleural drainage for frank empyema or fluid pH <7.2 Consider uncommon respiratory pathogens in presence of lung abscess May need prolonged Ab × ≤6 weeks ± surgical drainage	Non-response ≤72 h: consider antimicrobial resistance or virulent organism Non-response >72 h: consider and investigate for complication	
Follow Up	23-valent pneumococcal vaccination Influenza vaccination as per guidelines Smoking cessation advice Repeat CXR at 6 weeks only if persistent symptoms or signs or higher risk (age >50, smokers)	23-valent pneumococcal vaccination	No follow up imaging if symptoms resolve in 5–7 days

Figure 33.1 Continued

Concern for MRSA should prompt the addition of a glycopeptide agent. Panton-Valentine leucocidin positive *S. aureus* (either methicillin-sensitive or methicillin-resistant) warrants the addition of a combined regimen including linezolid and clindamycin for toxin suppression. Complex cases should be discussed with a microbiologist.

Antibiotics must be started as soon as possible after presentation and within 1 h in patients who are septic: those with evidence of infection-associated organ dysfunction, defined by an increase of two or more in the Sequential Organ-Failure Assessment (SOFA) score or predicted by the presence of at least two qSOFA criteria.[13] As with any infection, principles of antimicrobial stewardship apply. Microbiology results and clinical response should be reviewed, and antibiotic regimens narrowed, adjusted, or converted from intravenous to enteral whenever possible. Generally, where there is good clinical response, a short course of 5–7 days of antibiotics is appropriate. As yet, biomarkers including C-reactive protein (CRP) and procalcitonin (PCT) have not demonstrated superiority to clinical judgement in determining need for and

Demographics	Comorbidities	Clinical Assessment	Investigations
Male: **age in years**	Neoplasia: **+30**	Confusion: **+20**	Arterial pH <7.35: **+30**
Female: **age in years -10**	Liver disease: **+20**	Respiratory rate ≥30: **+20**	Urea ≥11 mmol/L: **+20**
Nursing home resident: **age in years +10**	Congestive heart failure: **+10**	Systolic bp <90 mmHg: **+20**	Sodium <130 mmol/L: **+20**
	Cerebrovascular disease: **+10**	Heart rate ≥125 bpm: **+15**	Glucose ≥14 mmol/L: **+10**
	Renal disease: **+10**	Temperature <35 or ≥40°C: **+15**	Haematocrit <0.30: **+10**
			Pleural effusion present: **+10**
			p_aO_2 <8 kPa: **+10**

Risk Class (total points)		30-day Mortality	Recommended Disposition
I	(<50 points)	0.1 %	Outpatient
II	(51–70 points)	0.6 %	Outpatient
III	(71–90 points)	2.8 %	Consider brief inpatient assessment
IV	(91–130 points)	8.2 %	Inpatient
V	(>130 points)	29.2 %	Inpatient

Figure 33.2 Pneumonia severity index (PSI). Pneumonia severity index (also referred to as the 'Pneumonia Patient Outcomes Research Team' (PORT) score) for predicting mortality and appropriateness for outpatient management in community-acquired pneumonia in adults.

Reproduced from Fine et al. A prediction rule to identify low-risk patients with community-acquired pneumonia. *N Engl J Med* 1997;336:243–50 (Mass Medical Society).

+2	**S**ystolic blood pressure: <90mmHg
+1	**M**ultilobar involvement on CXR
+1	**A**lbumin <35 g/l
+1	**R**espiratory rate: Age ≤50 years: rate ≥25 /min Age >50 years: rate ≥30 /min
+1	**T**achycardia: ≥125 bpm
+1	**C**onfusion (new onset)
+2	**O**xygen: Age ≤50 years: p_aO_2 <9.3 kPa *or* SpO_2 ≤93 % *or* P/F <44.4 kPa *(if on O_2)* Age >50 years: p_aO_2 <8 kPa *or* SpO_2 ≤90 % *or* P/F <33.3 kPa *(if on O_2)*
+2	**P** arterial pH: <7.35

Total Points	Risk of needing intensive respiratory or vasopressor support
0–2	Low
3–4	Moderate (1 in 8)
5–6	High (1 in 3)
≥7	Very high (2 in 3)

Figure 33.3 SMART-COP score. SMART-COP score for predicting need for intensive respiratory or vasopressor support in community-acquired pneumonia in adults. CXR: chest radiograph; p_aO_2: arterial oxygen partial pressure; SpO_2: peripheral oxygen saturation; *P/F*: ratio of arterial oxygen partial pressure to fraction of inspired oxygen.

Adapted from Charles PGP, et al., SMART-COP: A Tool for Predicting the Need for Intensive Respiratory or Vasopressor Support in Community-Acquired Pneumonia. *Clinical Infectious Diseases* 2008;47:375–84, by permission of the Infectious Diseases Society of America.

duration of antibiotics, but trends in these biomarkers can be a useful adjunct.

In terms of adjunctive management, appropriate venous-thromboembolism prophylaxis is warranted for all patients. Corticosteroids are not recommended routinely but can be considered in associated refractory septic shock. Non-invasive ventilation is not routinely advised but where considered should be provided in a critical care area with immediate access to escalation. Patients not responding within 48–72 h should be reassessed, including a review of their antibiotic regimen and investigation for possible complications including pleural infection or abscess formation.

Hospital-acquired Pneumonia

Aspects of the national and international guidelines relevant to non-ventilator-associated HAP are summarized in Figure 33.4.[9,14–16] Risk assessment for a resistant organism, which is more likely than in CAP, is vital. This is influenced by the duration of admission prior to onset of infection, background rate of resistant organisms in the setting to which the patient was admitted, prior use of broad-spectrum antibiotics, co-morbidities including structural lung disease and immunosuppression, and known colonization with a relevant organism. Resistant organisms are more likely to cause severe HAP, and therefore critically unwell patients are relatively more likely to be infected with a resistant organism.

Non-invasive respiratory samples should be collected for microbiological testing wherever possible. In patients who require endotracheal intubation, further samples should be obtained at this point, ranging from an endotracheal aspirate to a BAL as deemed appropriate.

In patients admitted for between 3 and 5 days, adjudged to have a non-severe HAP and at low risk of a resistant organism, the commonest causes are likely to be *S. pneumoniae* and methicillin-sensitive *S. aureus*. Such patients can initially be treated with β-lactam monotherapy. In severe HAP or those at increased risk of resistant Gram-negative organisms, this should be escalated to monotherapy with a broad-spectrum antipseudomonal β-lactam or a respiratory fluoroquinolone. In critically unwell patients, consideration should be given to dual antipseudomonal cover from two different antibiotic classes (for example cephalosporin or carbapenem plus aminoglycoside). Patients at risk of MRSA should have a glycopeptide antibiotic or linezolid added to the empirical regimen.

Immunocompromised Patients

Patients with significant underlying immunodeficiency are not adequately covered by these general guidelines. Such patients are at increased risk of community- and hospital-acquired resistant organisms, but also at increased risk of pulmonary infection due to non-bacterial pathogens and specific opportunistic bacteria including *Nocardia* species, *Mycobacterium tuberculosis*, and non-tuberculous mycobacteria. Presentations may be atypical, and a higher index of suspicion is required both of pneumonia and of an underlying resistant organism.

In view of this and the specific antimicrobial regimens dictated by a number of these organisms, cross-sectional imaging and invasive diagnostics including BAL, and where relevant thoracentesis and lymph node sampling, should be considered. All patients should be discussed with their parent specialist as well as with respiratory and microbiology or infectious diseases teams. Management of opportunistic infections in immunocompromised hosts is discussed elsewhere.[17–20]

Evidence Base

Severity Scoring Systems

The most used and referenced are PSI (Figure 33.2) and CURB-65.[21,22] Both predict 30-day mortality. The PSI aims to identify low mortality risk patients who may be candidates for outpatient management.

Comparisons of PSI against CURB-65 yield varying results, but they appear comparable overall. The components of the CURB-65 score are Confusion, elevated Urea, elevated Respiratory rate, low systolic Blood pressure, and age over 65. These components are additively scored, with three or more points indicating a high (22%) mortality. The CURB-65 is appealing in its simplicity and easy scoring at the bedside and uses several components also present in the PSI score. Both scores, however, have limitations. There is often

	NICE	ERS/ESICM/ESCMID/ALAT	IDSA/ATS
Diagnosis	Clinical suspicion: new fever, purulent sputum, leucocytosis, worsening oxygenation New infiltrate(s) on CXR ≥48 h since admission and not incubating at time of admission Not mechanically ventilated		
Severity	**Clinical assessment** of severity No validated tool	ICU specific risk score (eg **APACHE II**) High mortality risk considered >15%	**High mortality risk** *Includes:* • Septic shock • Mechanical ventilation
Assessment for Resistant Organisms	**MDR organism** risk factors: • Onset >5 days after admission • Relevant comorbidity (including severe respiratory disease, immunosuppression) • Recent use of broad-spectrum Abx • Colonisation with MDR organism • Recent contact with health or social care setting pre-admission	**MDR organism** risk factors: • Hospital setting with a background rate of MDR organisms ≥25% • Previous antibiotic use • Recent hospital admission >5 days • Colonisation with MDR organism	**MRSA** risk factors: • Prior IV abx within 90 days • Admitted to a unit with >20% or unknown rate of MRSA amongst *S aureus* isolates • High mortality risk **Resistant gram-negative bacteria, including *P aeruginosa***, risk factors: • Prior IV Abx within 90 days • Structural lung disease • High mortality risk
Microbiology	Non-invasive respiratory sample in all patients where possible	If intubated, distal quantitative, proximal quantitative or proximal qualitative respiratory samples	Non-invasive respiratory sample If intubated, semi-quantitative endotracheal aspirate
Empirical Antibiotics	**Onset within 3–5 days of admission:** • Consider following guidelines for CAP **Non-severe and low MDR organism risk:** • Co-amoxiclav (PO if possible) • Penicillin allergy: doxycycline *or* cefalexin *or* co-trimoxazole *or* levofloxacin **Severe or increased MDR organism risk:** *IV monotherapy with one of* • Piptazobactam • Ceftazidime *or* ceftriaxone *or* cefuroxime • Meropenem • Ceftazidime/avibactam • Levofloxacin **MRSA** *Add in* • Vancomycin *or* teicoplanin *or* linezolid	**Low mortality and MDR organism risk:** *IV monotherapy with one of* • Ertapenem • Ceftriaxone *or* cefotaxime • Moxifloxacin *or* levofloxacin **High MDR and/or >15% mortality risk *without* septic shock:** • Single broad-spectrum gram-negative agent • ± MRSA cover **High MDR and/or >15% mortality risk *with* septic shock:** • Dual broad-spectrum gram-negative antipseudomonal agent • ± MRSA cover	**Low mortality and MDR organism risk:** *IV monotherapy with one of* • Piptazobactam • Cefepime • Levofloxacin • Imipenem *or* meropenem **Low mortality but high MRSA risk:** • One of the agents above • *Plus* vancomycin *or* linezolid **High mortality risk or IV Abx within 90 d:** *IV dual therapy with two of* • Piptazobactam *or* cefepime *or* ceftazidime *or* imipenem *or* meropenem • Levofloxacin *or* ciprofloxacin • Amikacin *or* gentamicin *or* tobramycin • Aztreonam *Plus* vancomycin *or* linezolid
Stewardship	Start within 4 hours of diagnosis or within 1 hour if septic shock If clinically stable, start oral where able Else review IVOS within 48 h Adjust regimens to local antibiograms and patient microbiology results 5-day duration for all patients if response	Adjust regimens to local antibiograms and patient microbiology results 7–8 day duration if no immunodeficiency, cystic fibrosis or necrotising pneumonia If CPIS ≤6 at diagnosis and 72 h, do not routinely continue Abx Do not use biomarkers to guide duration except if: initial inappropriate Abx, severe immunocompromise, highly resistant organism, second line Abx required	Adjust regimens to local antibiograms and patient microbiology results Dose based on weight and drug levels and consider extended/continuous infusions 7-day duration if response Do not use PCT or CRP to decide on starting Abx Use PCT with clinical criteria to review stopping Abx Do not use CPIS to decide on starting or stopping Abx

Figure 33.4 Algorithm for management of adults with non-ventilator-associated hospital-acquired pneumonia, adapted from national and international guidelines.

NICE: National Institute for Health and Care Excellence (England and Wales); ERS: European Respiratory Society; ESICM: European Society of Intensive Care Medicine; ESCMID: European Society of Clinical Microbiology and Infectious Diseases; ALAT: Latin American Thoracic Association; IDSA: Infectious Diseases Society of America; ATS: American Thoracic Society; CXR: chest radiograph; ICU: intensive care unit; APACHE II: Acute Physiology and Chronic Health Evaluation II scoring system for measuring severity of illness in adult patients admitted to intensive care; MDR: multi-drug-resistant (defined as resistance to at least one agent within at least three antimicrobial categories); Abx: antibiotics; MRSA: methicillin-resistant *Staphylococcus aureus*; IV: intravenous; *S. aureus*: *Staphylococcus aureus*; *P. aeruginosa*: *Pseudomonas aeruginosa*; CAP: community-acquired pneumonia; PO: per os; piptazobactam: piperacillin-tazobactam; IVOS: intravenous to oral switch; CPIS: clinical pulmonary infection score to assess for hospital-acquired/ventilator-associated pneumonia based on temperature, white cell count, tracheal secretions, oxygenation, chest radiograph appearances, and culture result; PCT: procalcitonin; CRP: C-reactive protein.

Data from NICE Guideline 139: Pneumonia (hospital-acquired): antimicrobial prescribing. 2019; Torres et al. International ERS/ESICM/ESCMID/ALAT guidelines for the management of hospital-acquired pneumonia and ventilator-associated pneumonia. *Eur Respir J* 2017;50:1700582; and Kalil et al. Management of Adults With Hospital-acquired and Ventilator-associated Pneumonia: 2016 Clinical Practice Guidelines by the Infectious Diseases Society of America and the American Thoracic Society. *Clin Infect Dis* 2016;63(5):e61–111.

- Prior *P aeruginosa* infection/colonization*
- Prior tracheostomy
- Bronchiectasis
- Very severe COPD (FEV_1 ≤30%)
- Intensive respiratory and/or vasopressor support

* *Conveys highest risk and should prompt consideration of antipseudomonal antibiotic therapy*

Figure 33.5 Risk factors for community-acquired *Pseudomonas aeruginosa* pneumonia.

P. aeruginosa: *Pseudomonas aeruginosa*; COPD: chronic obstructive pulmonary disease; FEV_1: forced expiratory volume in one second.

Adapted from Restrepo et al. Burden and risk factors for Pseudomonas aeruginosa community-acquired pneumonia: a multinational point prevalence study of hospitalised patients. *Eur Respir J* 2018;52:1701190 (ERS publications).

a difference in which patients are stratified as high risk by each, and a significant number are misclassified as low risk but go on to have poor outcomes. In particular, the performance of both is poorer at extremes of age.

In predicting ICU admission, PSI and CURB-65 have a low pooled sensitivity of just 48% and 49%, respectively.[23] In contrast, at a threshold of three or more,[25] the IDSA/ATS minor criteria have an area under the receiver-operator characteristic curve (AUROC) of 0.85 for ICU admission and 0.85 for mechanical ventilation and SMART-COP have 0.85 and 0.83, respectively.[24] All are comparable for predicting mortality. In patients under 50 years, SMART-COP is again able to better predict need for invasive ventilation or vasopressor support with an AUROC of 0.87.[25]

In HAP, general intensive care severity scales such as the Acute Physiology And Chronic Health Evaluation II Score and definitions of high mortality risk such as the presence of septic shock or need for mechanical ventilation suffer from the same limitations as noted for tools in CAP in that they are of limited applicability at the bedside and identify patients already requiring intensive care support, respectively.

Antibiotic Regimens in Community-acquired Pneumonia

Reviewing the effect of widespread uptake of antibiotic therapy in 1964 demonstrated a mortality reduction from bacteraemic *S. pneumoniae* pneumonia from 84% to 17%.[26] Conversely, initial escalated empirical therapy for CAP may in fact increase mortality, as well as increase the length of hospital stay, and the risk of renal failure, *Clostridium difficile* infection, and secondary isolation of resistant and Gram-negative organisms. The potential disadvantages extend further, including the economic burden and importantly the effects on antimicrobial resistance.

In the UK, relatively narrow-spectrum antibiotic use in CAP is supported by the low clinically relevant antibiotic resistance rates among the common pathogens. In other regions, however, this is not the case. Considering non-meningitis European Committee on Antimicrobial Susceptibility Testing 2019 breakpoints, the prevalence of in vitro penicillin resistance in *S. pneumoniae* isolated in CAP patients is just 0.4% in the UK. In comparison, 61.7% and 53.2% of US isolates are susceptible to penicillin and azithromycin, respectively, and just 38.9% and 4.3% of Chinese isolates are susceptible to penicillin and erythromycin, respectively.[7] This reinforces the need to consider local ecology and guidelines in determining empiric regimens.

S. pneumoniae β-lactam resistance has however fallen since introduction of the pneumococcal vaccine, as a result of reduced nasal carriage of resistant serotypes. Interestingly, in clinical practice, resistance neither appears to be associated with treatment failure nor poorer clinical outcomes, and β-lactam monotherapy has been shown to be non-inferior to combination with a macrolide in hospitalized adults with non-severe CAP.

While in vitro resistance to penicillin among *Haemophilus influenzae* isolated in CAP patients is high at around 30%, and culture rates are low suggesting lesser in vivo significance. Macrolide- and cephalosporin-resistant *H. influenzae* is rare.[7]

β-Lactams are inactive against atypical organisms causing CAP because of their intracellular nature or lack of cell wall. Although macrolide-resistant *M. pneumoniae* has emerged in Asia, for example in China where erythromycin resistance has been noted in

Age 40–65 years	+1
Age >65 years	+2
Male	+1
Previous antibiotic use within 1 month	+2
Chronic respiratory disorder	+2
Chronic renal disease	+3
Impaired consciousness or evidence of aspiration	+2
Fevers or shivers	−1

≤1: Low risk of resistant organism
Usual empiric antibiotics for CAP3

2–4: Medium risk of resistant organism
Assess individual risk and microbiology

≥5: High risk of resistant organism
Follow local/national guidelines
Consider empirical treatment of resistant organisms

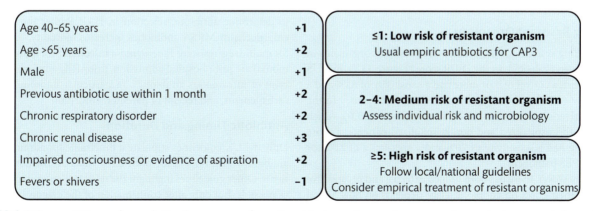

Figure 33.6 PES score. PES score for predicting the presence of a multi-resistant organism causing community-acquired pneumonia (named for *Pseudomonas aeruginosa*, extended-spectrum β-lactamase-producing *Enterobacteriaceae*, and methicillin-resistant *Staphylococcus aureus*) and suggested antimicrobial strategy.

CAP: community-acquired pneumonia; MRSA: methicillin-resistant *Staphylococcus aureus*.

Data from Prina et al. Risk Factors Associated with Potentially Antibiotic-Resistant Pathogens in Community-Acquired Pneumonia. *Ann Am Thorac Soc.* 2015;12(2):153–60 and Cillóniz et a. Multidrug Resistant Gram-Negative Bacteria in Community-Acquired Pneumonia. *Crit Care* 2019;23:79.

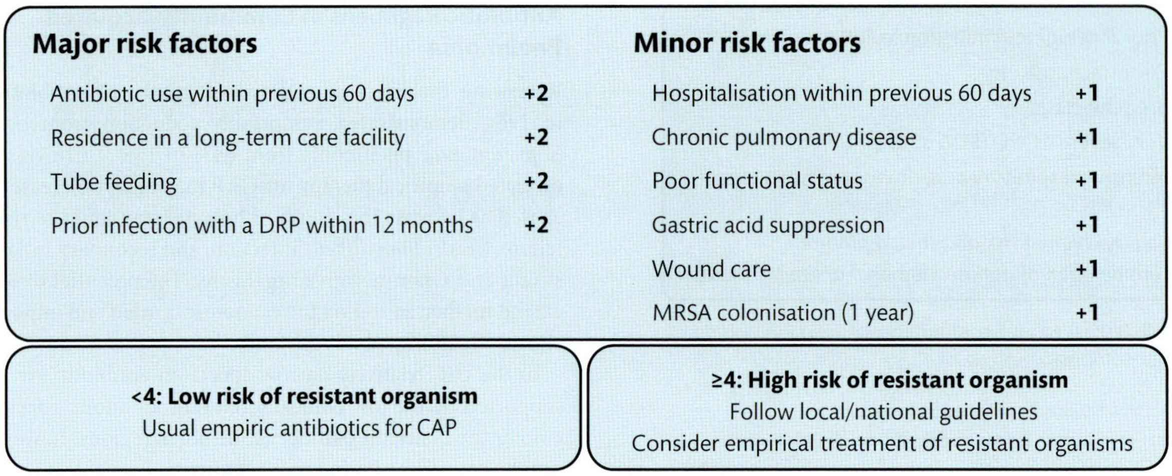
Major risk factors
Antibiotic use within previous 60 days +2
Residence in a long-term care facility +2
Tube feeding +2
Prior infection with a DRP within 12 months +2
Minor risk factors
Hospitalisation within previous 60 days +1
Chronic pulmonary disease +1
Poor functional status +1
Gastric acid suppression +1
Wound care +1
MRSA colonisation (1 year) +1
<4: Low risk of resistant organism
Usual empiric antibiotics for CAP
≥4: High risk of resistant organism
Follow local/national guidelines
Consider empirical treatment of resistant organisms

Figure 33.7 Drug resistance in pneumonia (DRIP) score. DRIP score for predicting multi-resistant organisms in community-acquired pneumonia and suggested antimicrobial strategy.

DRP: drug-resistant pathogen; MRSA: methicillin-resistant *Staphylococcus aureus*.

up to 69% of CAP cases, this remains rare in Europe and America. *L. pneumophila* and *C. pneumoniae* remain widely sensitive to both macrolides and fluoroquinolones.

Macrolides have a role in the management of CAP as immunomodulators, beyond their antimicrobial effects against both typical and atypical organisms. Among CAP patients admitted to ICU, the addition of a macrolide to the antibiotic regimen significantly reduces mortality, independent of the presence of a macrolide-resistant organism. At metanalysis, the pooled risk ratio for mortality with macrolide use in the ICU cohort is 0.75 (95% confidence interval: 0.58–0.96; $p = 0.02$).[27] Such benefit is confined to critically ill patients admitted to ICU, reflecting increased prevalence of a hyperinflammatory endotype and increased baseline likelihood of poor outcomes among this cohort.

ICU admission in CAP is not in itself a risk factor for resistant organisms. In the majority of critically ill patients, the routine use of escalated antibiotic regimens is not indicated. Indeed, where ICU admission alone prompted empirical addition of anti-MRSA therapy, 30-day mortality actually increased.[28]

Predicting Resistant Organisms

Several scoring systems for the prediction of resistant organisms in CAP have been evaluated. In the DRIP score (Figure 33.7), in a US patient cohort, a cut-off of 4 or more had a sensitivity of 82% and a specificity of 81% for predicting drug-resistant pathogens.[29] In the Spanish derivation cohort for the PES score (Figure 33.6), which included both hospitalized and non-hospitalized patients, a score of 5 or more had a sensitivity of 70% and a specificity of 71% for predicting PES pathogens.[30]

Overall, however, there has been limited external and prospective validation. Their effect on antibiotic usage depends on how liberal or conservative empiric broad-spectrum antibiotic regimens are. Management algorithms based on scoring systems, while improving on HCAP criteria, have yet to be shown to improve clinical outcomes or antimicrobial stewardship. Currently, the role for these scores is in supporting the decision not to broaden the spectrum of empirical antibiotics in a patient assessed to be at low risk for a resistant organism.

Antibiotic Regimens in HAP

As in CAP, empiric antibiotic regimens in HAP should reflect the local ecology and antibiogram alongside patient-specific risk factors. The general combined prevalence of *S. aureus* and Gram-negative organisms in this cohort (Table 33.3) warrants appropriately targeted antibiotics even when risk factors for resistance are low. While IDSA/ATS recommend dual Gram-negative cover in patients with risk factors for *P. aeruginosa* or other Gram-negative infections, there is a paucity of evidence supporting this.[17] This is further explored in the 'Controversies and Future Directions' section.

The only consistently identified risk factor for resistant organisms in HAP is prior receipt of intravenous antibiotics. Using this criterion in isolation will however miss a proportion of patients with infection due to a resistant organism. Although it has been suggested that MRSA colonization may predict isolation from respiratory samples, there is no data supporting the use of screening results to determine antibiotic selection in HAP. Rather the addition of empirical anti-MRSA antibiotics increases mortality.[28] Risk factors for multidrug-resistant *P. aeruginosa* infection (not limited to pneumonia) are prior hospital admission, prior ICU admission, prior receipt of intravenous antibiotics, in particular fluoroquinolones or carbapenems, and receipt of parenteral nutrition.

Antibiotic Timing and Duration

Only the UK guidelines stipulate a timeframe for administration of antibiotics—within 4 h for both CAP and HAP in non-septic patients. Other guidelines highlight the need to give antibiotics as soon as possible, but only after confirmation of the diagnosis and appropriate assessment, so as to limit inappropriate use of antibiotics. While there is a clear rationale for early administration of antibiotics, supportive data is inconsistent for CAP and lacking for HAP.

In sepsis, the Surviving Sepsis Campaign requires antibiotic administration within 1 h. Retrospective database analyses have shown a linear increase in mortality for every hour of delay in antibiotic administration from hospital presentation. While this risks being an arbitrary timepoint in the clinical course, a similar linear increase in mortality was noted when using onset of fluid-refractory hypotension as the reference timepoint in a cohort with sepsis defined by the systemic inflammatory response syndrome criteria coupled with a clinical suspicion of infection.[31]

The quality and biological plausibility of these data have been robustly challenged. They are heavily adjusted, which is appropriate since sicker patients may be recognized earlier and therefore receive antibiotics earlier. However, given the retrospective nature, they struggle to account for timing and appropriateness of other aspects of early resuscitation and management.

A prespecified analysis of septic patients managed with goal-directed therapy targeting either central venous saturations or lactate showed no association between mortality and time between hospital presentation or onset of fluid-refractory shock and antibiotic administration.[32] Similarly, prospective studies in patients with shock and Gram-negative bacteraemia, respectively, identified degree of initial physiological derangement and failure to ameliorate this with resuscitation as risk factors for mortality rather than timing or appropriateness of antibiotic administration.

These conflicting results reflect the challenges encountered in many trials including critically ill patients. Such patients should continue to receive antibiotics as early as possible. Antimicrobial stewardship dictates appropriate microbiological sampling should be undertaken wherever possible prior to administration of an appropriate antibiotic regimen following national guidelines and local antibiograms and considering the most likely source of infection and patient factors. As stressed by the Surviving Sepsis Campaign, other aspects of resuscitation and monitoring must be applied with as much vim. Furthermore, management of suspected sepsis must not preclude expedient investigation and management of alternative or concurrent causes of critical illness.

Longer antibiotic courses increase risk of adverse effects and development of secondary infection with a resistant organism and have cost and length of stay implications and impact on local ecology. While short courses are routinely used, patient factors such as clinical response, development of complications including pleural infection or abscess, and the presence of underlying structural lung disease or immunocompromise influence this decision.

Several studies in uncomplicated CAP have demonstrated short courses of antibiotics to be as effective as longer courses. While these include patients labelled as having severe pneumonia, they universally exclude patients admitted to ICU prior to randomization. There is unfortunately limited published data evaluating antibiotic duration in patients admitted to ICU.

Protocolized discontinuation of antibiotics according to clinical criteria from day 5 onwards compared to physician-dictated duration of antibiotics achieved a separation of antibiotic duration of 5 and 10 days, respectively.[33] There was no difference in any outcome measure including resolution of signs and symptoms at 30 days, in-hospital and 30-day mortality, inpatient complications, ICU admission, and length of hospital stay. The median duration of antibiotics in the intervention arm was equal to the shortest permitted, confirming that clinical criteria are effective in supporting decisions to discontinue antibiotics.

Similarly, a retrospective review of patients with severe CAP as stratified by CURB-65 assessed cohorts treated for 7 days and for a mean of 12 days. It demonstrated no difference in 30-day mortality, requirement for mechanical ventilation or vasopressor support, or development of complications.[34]

There is similarly limited direct evidence for antibiotic duration in patients with HAP admitted to ICU. A review of the few studies exploring the question in VAP showed no effect on 28-day mortality of 7–8-day courses versus 10–15-day courses of antibiotics.[35] Shorter courses reduced the occurrence of further VAP due to multi-resistant organisms. As the acuity and mortality of non-ventilator-associated HAP is generally less than VAP and the microbiological profile comparable, it is not unreasonable to extrapolate this data.

The dogma of prolonged antibiotics in the presence of structural lung disease or specific organisms, notably *P. aeruginosa*, is not well explored in the literature. Among ICU patients, this is considered in a study comparing defined antibiotic durations for management of VAP.[36] Patients infected with non-fermenting Gram-negative bacteria managed with 8 rather than 15 days of antibiotics had unchanged mortality, duration of mechanical ventilation, and length of ICU stay. However, the shorter duration was associated with a significant increase in both relapse and superinfection.

The potential for biomarkers, most prominently CRP and PCT, to modify the duration of antibiotics is limited by the increasing acceptance of shorter courses as the norm. Biomarker trials do however corroborate the evidence for shorter duration of antibiotics even among critically unwell patients.

Two studies use a PCT fall ≥80% to <0.5 μg/L as a prompt to consider stopping antibiotics as compared to standard of care with antibiotic duration determined by guidelines and physicians.[37,38] Both consider critically ill patients admitted with infection to ICU, with a predominance of pneumonia and a proportion septic. A reduction in the duration of antibiotics from 10 to 7 and from 7 to 5 days was achieved, respectively. In both trials, there was no difference in mortality, reinfection or requirement for further antibiotics, or length of ICU or hospital stay.

In fact, in the latter study, PCT-guided antibiotics significantly reduced mortality at 28 days and 1 year. A similar effect is noted in a metanalysis of PCT-guided antibiotic use for respiratory infections of all acuity.[39] Duration of antibiotics and associated side effects, but also 30-day mortality, were reduced. These mortality benefits may be related to reduced antibiotic-associated adverse effects, reduced risk of acquiring a multi-resistant organism, increased consideration given to alternative aetiologies in the setting of an unexpectedly low PCT, or potential for escalation of management in the setting of a notably elevated PCT.

Biomarkers have potential roles beyond this and should form part of the re-evaluation at 72 h in patients not responding adequately. Ratio of admission to day 3 CRP differentiates survivors from non-survivors and may help to predict adequacy of empiric antibiotics in patients in whom an organism is isolated.[40,41] Admission CRP >100 mg/L and moreover failure to fall by ≥50% by day 4 predict development of pleural infection or pulmonary abscess.[25]

Furthermore, in CAP biomarkers can improve the prognostic value of the scoring systems discussed above. Combining PSI and CURB-65 with CRP at a cut-off of 250 mg/L improves prediction of 30-day mortality. Integration of PCT >2.0 ng/mL and serum lactate >2.0 mmol/L with CURB-65 improves prediction of need for ICU.

Admission PCT correlates with risk of needing invasive respiratory or vasopressor support with a linear increase to a plateau of 22% for PCT ≥10 ng/mL.[42] Combined with any of these biomarkers, the predictive ability of the ATS/IDSA criteria, PSI, or SMART-COP improves.

Pharmacology

The goal of antimicrobial therapy is to achieve adequate drug concentrations at the site of infection to result in killing of bacteria without toxicity or significant adverse events. This is achieved by maintaining drug levels above the minimum inhibitory concentration (MIC) or minimal bactericidal concentration in either a time- or concentration-dependent manner.

Antimicrobials can be classified according to solubility. β-Lactams (including penicillins, cephalosporins, carbapenems, and monobactams), glycopeptides, and aminoglycosides are hydrophilic and have a small volume of distribution but are unable to passively diffuse through the plasma membranes of eukaryotic cells and are therefore inactive against intracellular pathogens and are renally eliminated. In contrast, macrolides, quinolones, tetracyclines, and linezolid are lipophilic antibiotics and have a large volume of distribution, can diffuse across eukaryotic plasma cell membranes, are active against intracellular pathogens, and are first metabolized by the liver.[43]

Antimicrobials such as β-lactams, linezolid, and clindamycin have an optimal effect when the concentration is greater than the MIC in a time-dependent manner ($T >$ MIC). To optimize efficacy, these antimicrobials are given in frequent doses that keep the concentration above MIC for >90% of the time ($T >$ MIC 90%) or by administering prolonged or continuous infusions to keep the concentration above the MIC all the time ($T >$ MIC 100%). The optimal effect of aminoglycosides, metronidazole, and fluoroquinolones occurs at the peak concentration (C_{max}), and the prolonged post-antibiotic effect of these antimicrobials allows for less frequent dosing. Vancomycin, tetracyclines, macrolides, and tigecycline have their best effect when the concentration is kept above MIC for a prolonged period ($T >$ MIC) but also at the peak concentration (C_{max}) and therefore are usually administered at higher doses and frequent intervals. Importantly, therapeutic drug monitoring should be carried out where available and for antimicrobials where there is a concentration–toxicity relationship (including aminoglycosides and glycopeptides).

During sepsis, including from CAP, many physiological changes impact drug pharmacokinetics. These include increased cardiac output, redistribution of fluid between intravascular and extravascular compartments, and reduced circulating albumin levels. This is particularly important for hydrophilic drugs where higher than standard doses (loading doses) may be needed to ensure optimal concentrations at the infection site from the first dose. Furthermore, highly protein-bound antimicrobials (for example teicoplanin or ertapenem) may be underdosed in the presence of hypoalbuminaemia. If patients develop renal or hepatic impairment, elimination of drugs is reduced and accumulation increased, potentially leading to toxicity. In contrast, renal replacement therapy may enhance drug clearance. This is particularly the case for β-lactams, aminoglycosides, quinolones, and glycopeptides.

Controversies and Future Directions

Antibacterial Strategies

In HAP, US guidelines suggest combination antibiotic regimens with a Gram-positive agent added to dual Gram-negative cover for patients at increased risk of mortality or resistant organisms. Elsewhere progressively more rationalized regimens are recommended. UK guidelines advise broad-spectrum Gram-negative monotherapy for such patients with a narrower definition of increased risk of resistant organisms. The decision to include MRSA cover is separated (Figure 33.4).

The main justification for combination empiric regimens is the increased likelihood of adequate coverage in the context of relatively high rates of resistance. This is particularly relevant in HAP in critical care—for example considering *P. aeruginosa*, single-antibiotic susceptibility rates are lower both in respiratory isolates and among the ICU cohort. The proposed rationale for definitive use, as opposed to de-escalation in accordance with the antibiogram, includes the potential for antimicrobial synergy and a protective effect on the emergence of resistance. Conversely, the likelihood of toxicity and drug interactions may increase.

While the prevalence and multidrug resistance rates of *P. aeruginosa* and *Klebsiella* species, the commonest two Gram-negative organisms isolated in HAP, may be lower in the UK compared to Europe and North America, they remain significant (Table 33.4). Local guidelines in the UK most frequently recommend piperacillin-tazobactam followed by amoxicillin-clavulanate for severe HAP. Susceptibility to these single agents among microbiologically positive HAP in the UK is just 82.9% for piperacillin-tazobactam against *P. aeruginosa* and 84.6% and 72.9%, respectively, against *Klebsiella* species.[7]

In Gram-negative and *P. aeruginosa* sepsis, in vitro susceptibility to empiric combination regimens is associated with lower mortality risk. However, there is limited contemporary data assessing this in HAP. One study surprisingly showed appropriate initial antibiotics not to be associated with mortality.[44] One consideration is that aminoglycosides, which are commonly added to a β-lactam in combination regimens and which have best in vitro synergism, reach relatively poor lung tissue concentrations at appropriate plasma levels.

Among patients admitted to ICU with HAP with a mean APACHE II score of 23, upfront use of carbapenem and vancomycin combination therapy failed to improve mortality at any measured timepoint

Table 33.4 Multidrug resistance rates in microbiologically positive hospital-acquired pneumonia

	Pseudomonas aeruginosa		*Klebsiella spp.*	
	Prevalence (%)	MDR rate (%)	Prevalence (%)	MDR rate (%)
United Kingdom	11.9	1.3	10.3	0.4
Europe	20.8	6.3	15.2	4.9
North America	20.7	4.9	14.2	1.8

Note: Comparison of MDR prevalence in the two Gram-negative pathogens most commonly responsible for hospital-acquired pneumonia. MDR: multidrug resistant (defined as resistance to at least one agent within at least three antimicrobial categories).

Source: Data from the SENTRY antimicrobial surveillance database for 2013–2019 (https://sentry-mvp.jmilabs.com/).

or length of ICU stay but increased the subsequent isolation of resistant organisms.[45] The majority of patients in the control arm received combination therapy with piperacillin-tazobactam plus ciprofloxacin or an aminoglycoside however, which in fact resulted in improved Gram-negative cover. Patients with MRSA pneumonia though fared the same in both arms, with vancomycin failing to improve outcomes. Again, routine broadening of the empiric antibiotic spectrum in critically unwell patients with pneumonia does not improve clinically relevant outcomes.

Although new agents have a role in the management of CAP and HAP, no new antibiotic classes relevant to pneumonia have been discovered since linezolid was approved in 2000. In an era where antibiotic resistance is a mounting concern, interest in alternative antibacterial therapies has grown. Chief among these, lytic bacteriophage therapy utilizes naturally occurring viruses that infect specific bacteria and replicate and induce bacterial lysis.[46] There is a body of evidence for their use from countries and periods in which antibiotics were less available, for example Soviet-era Russia. Although there are increasing preclinical data, clinical experience of bacteriophages in cases of infection with resistant organisms remains isolated to case reports. These do, however, demonstrate their potential efficacy and tolerability—for example, a case of post-lung cancer resection *P. aeruginosa* pneumonia and bronchopleurocutaneous fistula, in which the patient had deteriorated and the organism developed increasing resistance with sequential antibiotics, responded well to a cocktail of bacteriophages administered intravenously and via nebulization.[47]

Immunomodulatory Strategies

As much of the morbidity and mortality in severe pneumonia, particularly CAP, can be attributed to exaggerated hyperinflammatory host responses, many potential therapies targeting this have been explored. Beyond macrolides, discussed in the 'Evidence Base' section, the most commonly used group of drugs is corticosteroids.

The role of corticosteroids in the adjunctive management of septic shock is not discussed here. Trials exploring corticosteroid use in adults with bacterial CAP without sepsis have yielded varying results, hampered in part by disparate inclusion criteria, steroid regimens, antimicrobial management, and outcome measures. The most recent Cochrane metanalysis concludes corticosteroids reduce mortality in adults with severe CAP but not in those with non-severe CAP. This reports a reduction in early clinical failure, time to clinical cure, length of hospital stay, and development of complications including respiratory failure and acute respiratory distress syndrome (ARDS), shock, lung abscess, and pleural involvement.

Such headline results require deeper evaluation, however. Excluding the five small trials in which a total of just 154 patients received corticosteroids and the risk of bias for allocation concealment was unclear, corticosteroids demonstrated no impact on mortality. Only one remaining study, by Confalonieri in 2005, found a signal towards a mortality benefit with no deaths out of 23 patients in the hydrocortisone arm in ICU, in hospital or at 60 days. The placebo arm in-hospital mortality was 30%, comparable to that predicted by APACHE II scores.

In contrast, Blum et al. in 2015 found prednisolone reduced time to clinical stability and length of hospital stay in 392 patients with all severities of CAP but observed no difference in mortality. The CAP-related mortality was low at 1%–2%, and the average PSI scores place the cohorts at low to moderate risk. Trials have been criticized for clinical end points in which fever resolution and fall in CRP form key components as these can be isolated effects of corticosteroids, though this study is less susceptible to such shortcomings.

Other trials have looked to enrich the study population by attempting to capture an inflammatory cohort. Torres et al. in 2015 showed patients with SCAP defined by 1998 ATS criteria or PSI Class V and with admission CRP >150 mg/L receiving methylprednisolone had a lower rate of treatment failure. However, this was solely due to radiographic progression beyond 72 h with no statistically significant clinical correlate. No mortality difference was noted. Among other shortcomings, only a third of patients were actually in PSI Class V, and fewer than a quarter received a macrolide as part of their antibiotic regimen.

Looking beyond corticosteroids and macrolides, a range of immunomodulatory agents with a potential role either in primary management of CAP or management of associated ARDS or sepsis have been identified. These include statins, aspirin, intravenous immunoglobulin, activated protein C, recombinant tissue factor pathway inhibitor, plasma-derived antithrombin III, recombinant thrombomodulin, and sivelestat. However, trials have so far failed to demonstrate a significant benefit.[48]

In the CIGMA trial, there is a signal of increased ventilator-free days in patients with elevated CRP and PCT and low immunoglobulin M (IgM) managed with IgM-enriched intravenous immunoglobulins. GM-CSF is known to play a key role in innate immunity in the lungs, and its therapeutic role in pulmonary alveolar proteinosis is recognized. While there has perhaps been greater interest in its role in the management of viral pneumonitis, preclinical work on GM-CSF for bacterial pneumonia has translated into limited clinical experience suggesting nebulization may improve oxygenation and outcomes in ARDS secondary to pneumonia.[49] Prospective studies are awaited. Further putative agents including neutrolysing pneumolysin, mesenchymal stem cells, and agents targeting pattern recognition receptors and protease-activated receptors have largely yet to move beyond preclinical study.[48]

Novel Diagnostics

Advances in diagnostics might improve the robustness of a diagnosis of pneumonia, enable individualized antimicrobial selection, and benefit antimicrobial stewardship. An aspirational investigation or group of investigations would allow rapid point-of-care confirmation of the diagnosis of pneumonia, the organism, and the antimicrobial susceptibility such that if indicated the appropriate antimicrobial regimen can be started directly and expediently following presentation.

Confocal laser endomicroscopy delivers fluorescent-labelled ligands to the distal respiratory tract via the bronchoscope working channel, which are then detected by a multi-core fibre attached to a laser scanning proximal light source, also inserted via the working channel. This has already been demonstrated in humans to be sensitive and specific in detecting lung cancer in vivo. Ligands have been developed which enable the detection of bacteria in ex vivo models.

This is limited by the need for bronchoscopy. One solution that overcomes this is the analysis of exhaled breath volatile organic compounds, which may be produced by the body or pathogen during a pathophysiological process. Detection can be using laboratory techniques including gas chromatography and mass spectrometry or a point-of-care nanosensor array termed an eNose. These can distinguish pneumonia from controls in VAP, detect *P. aeruginosa* colonization in children with cystic fibrosis, and differentiate groups of and individual organisms in ex vivo analysis of BAL fluid.

Precision mucosal sampling techniques have also been developed to analyze the respiratory metabolome. A synthetic absorptive matrix (SAM) can be deployed to the nasal mucosa, termed nasosorption. This is better tolerated than nasopharyngeal aspirates (NPA) or nasal swabs and can be repeated during evolution of an infection. The SAM can also be deployed via the bronchoscope working channel, termed bronchosorption. Both techniques procure more concentrated samples compared to NPA or BAL, resulting in a greater sensitivity. Similarly, bronchial microsampling uses an absorbent probe to sample distal airways via the bronchoscope working channel. Only licensed in Japan, this improves yield versus BAL for metabolomic sampling and enables microbiome sampling by both culture and molecular diagnostics.

Existing molecular diagnostics employ PCR to identify specific microbial DNA, for example the GeneXpert system. While still requiring a specimen to be obtained, molecular diagnostics are not dependent on culturing an organism and therefore reduce time to diagnosis and improve sensitivity particularly in patients already on antibiotics.

Multiplex PCR uses a range of primers to simultaneously screen for a larger number of organisms. Broad range assays evaluate a target region, for example 16S ribosomal RNA for bacteria or 18S ribosomal RNA for fungi, referencing a genetic library and therefore can detect most described pathogens. Increasing the sensitivity in this way inevitably reduces the specificity for distinguishing active infection from colonization. However, quantitative PCR can achieve similar results to quantitative culture in this regard. Retrospective studies have suggested such tools have the potential to alter management, though robust prospective data confirming this and demonstrating an impact on outcomes is awaited. Cost and throughput currently limits widespread use.

Whereas laser endomicroscopy and exhaled breath analysis may facilitate diagnosis and pathogen identification, neither gives information on antimicrobial susceptibility. Genotypic resistance can be rapidly assessed with molecular diagnostics where specific resistance genes have been identified. Beyond this, tracking of nanomotion oscillations using electrical transduction or atomic force microscopy, which can distinguish viable from non-viable pathogens and where a signature nanomotion pattern has been determined to even identify the organism, can be used to assess phenotypic antibiotic susceptibility more rapidly than culture techniques.

Biomarkers

The post hoc identification of a cohort who might benefit from IgM-enriched intravenous immunoglobulins in the face of the overall negative CIGMA trial reinforces the need for study population enrichment. In ARDS, latent class analysis has enabled post hoc distinction of a hyperinflammatory subphenotype or endotype which can be achieved with a small number of variables not including CRP. Moreover, re-analyzing trials stratified by these endotypes has identified novel outcomes. Less than overwhelming results utilizing CRP and PCT to target immunomodulation in CAP may simply reflect that these parameters do not adequately distinguish the hyperinflammatory endotype.

The limitations of CRP and PCT in pneumonia are discussed in the 'Evidence Base' section. An array of potential novel biomarkers has been evaluated, primarily focusing on improving diagnosis and prognosis and predicting need for admission or ICU.[50] Higher levels of the pro-inflammatory cytokines, interleukin-6 and tumour necrosis factor alpha (TNFα), and the hormokine proadrenomedullin correlate with increased mortality in CAP. TNFα levels are also higher in CAP patients requiring mechanical ventilation, developing ARDS, or developing an acute kidney injury.

These biomarkers are non-specific and can be elevated in various inflammatory states. In contrast, at ICU admission, the ratio of expression of the Fas apoptotic inhibitory molecule 3 gene (*FAIM3*) and the placenta-specific 8 gene (*PLAC8*) has been shown to distinguish patients with CAP from those with mimics including aspiration and exacerbations of chronic obstructive pulmonary disease, asthma, and heart failure.[51] Similarly, a wider assessment of the transcriptome in septic patients admitted to ICU identified a distinct signature in pneumonia compared to faecal peritonitis.[52]

None of these tests has yet been adequately validated for use as prospective tools that can influence management or outcome in CAP. However, there is potential for a tool combining a number of biomarkers alongside physiological indices to confirm CAP diagnosis including in patients admitted to ICU with shock or ARDS, identify patients likely to deteriorate following admission and therefore benefit from ICU admission, and identify the hyperinflammatory endotype potentially benefitting from immunomodulation.

REFERENCES

1. Cillóniz C, Cardozo C, García-Vidal C. Epidemiology, pathophysiology, and microbiology of community-acquired pneumonia. *Ann Res Hosp.* 2018;**2**:1.
2. Lim WS, Lawrence H. British Thoracic Society National Audit Report: Adult Community Acquired Pneumonia Audit 2018–2019. *Br Thorac Soc Rep.*; 10.1–13 (https://www.brit-thoracic.org.uk/quality-improvement/clinical-audit/national-adult-community-acquired-pneumonia-audit-201819/)
3. Intensive Care National Audit & Research Centre. Key statistics from the Case Mix Programme—adult, general critical care units 1 April 2018 to 31 March 2019, https://onlinereports.icnarc.org (2019).
4. World Health Organization. The top 10 causes of death, https://www.who.int/en/news-room/fact-sheets/detail/the-top-10-causes-of-death (2018, accessed March 17, 2020).
5. José RJ. Respiratory infections: A global burden. *Ann Res Hosp.* 2018;**2**:12-undefined.
6. Welte T, Torres A, Nathwani D. Clinical and economic burden of community-acquired pneumonia among adults in Europe. *Thorax.* 2012;**67**:71–79.
7. JMI Laboratories. SENTRY Antimicrobial Surveillance, 1997 https://sentry-mvp.jmilabs.com/app/sentry-public/adhoc (accessed March 16, 2020).
8. Lim WS, Baudouin S, George R, et al. British Thoracic Society guidelines for the management of community acquired pneumonia in adults: Update 2009. *Thorax.* 2009;**64**:iii1–iii55.
9. Woodhead M, Aliyu S, Ashton C, et al. NICE Clinical Guideline 191: Pneumonia in adults: Diagnosis and management, https://www.nice.org.uk/guidance/cg191 (2014).
10. National Institute for Health and Care Excellence. NICE: Pneumonia (community-acquired): Antimicrobial prescribing. London; 2019.

11. Woodhead M, Blasi F, Ewig S, et al. Guidelines for the management of adult lower respiratory tract infections—summary. *Clin Microbiol Infect.* 2011;**17**:1–24.
12. Mandell LA, Wunderink RG, Anzueto A, et al. Infectious Diseases Society of America/American Thoracic Society consensus guidelines on the management of community-acquired pneumonia in adults. *Clin Infect Dis.* 2007;**44**:S27–72.
13. Singer M, Deutschman CS, Seymour CW, et al. The Third International Consensus definitions for sepsis and septic shock (Sepsis-3). *JAMA.* 2016;**315**:801.
14. National Institute for Health and Care Excellence. Pneumonia (hospital-acquired): Antimicrobial prescribing NICE guideline. London, www.nice.org.uk/guidance/ng139 (2019, accessed May 23, 2020).
15. Torres A, Niederman MS, Chastre J, et al. International ERS/ESICM/ESCMID/ALAT guidelines for the management of hospital-acquired pneumonia and ventilator-associated pneumonia. *Eur Respir J.* 2017;**50**:1700582-undefined.
16. Kalil AC, Metersky ML, Klompas M, et al. Management of Adults with Hospital-acquired and Ventilator-associated Pneumonia: 2016 Clinical Practice Guidelines by the Infectious Diseases Society of America and the American Thoracic Society. *Clin Infect Dis.* 2016;**63**:e61–e111.
17. José RJ, Brown JS. Opportunistic bacterial, viral and fungal infections of the lung. *Medicine (United Kingdom).* 2016;**44**:378–383.
18. Restrepo A, Clark NM. Nocardia infections in solid organ transplantation: Guidelines from the Infectious Diseases Community of Practice of the American Society of Transplantation. *Clin Transplant.* 2019; **33**:e13509-undefined.
19. National Institute for Health and Care Excellence. *Tuberculosis. NICE Guideline 33.* London, https://www.nice.org.uk/guidance/ng33 (2016;1–107).
20. Haworth CS, Banks J, Capstick T, et al. British Thoracic Society guidelines for the management of non-tuberculous mycobacterial pulmonary disease (NTM-PD). *Thorax.* 2017;**72**:ii1–ii64.
21. Fine MJ, Auble TE, Yealy DM, et al. A prediction rule to identify low-risk patients with community-acquired pneumonia. *N Engl J Med.* 1997;**336**:243–250.
22. Lim WS, van der Eerden MM, Laing R, et al. Defining community acquired pneumonia severity on presentation to hospital: An international derivation and validation study. *Thorax.* 2003;**58**:377–382.
23. Chalmers JD, Mandal P, Singanayagam A, et al. Severity assessment tools to guide ICU admission in community-acquired pneumonia: Systematic review and meta-analysis. *Intensive Care Med.* 2011;**37**:1409–1420.
24. Chalmers JD, Taylor JK, Mandal P, et al. Validation of the Infectious Diseases Society of America/American Thoracic Society minor criteria for intensive care unit admission in community-acquired pneumonia patients without major criteria or contraindications to intensive care unit care. *Clin Infect Dis.* 2011;**53**:503–511.
25. Chalmers JD, Singanayagam A, Hill AT. Predicting the need for mechanical ventilation and/or inotropic support for young adults admitted to the hospital with community-acquired pneumonia. *Clin Infect Dis.* 2008;**47**:1571–1574.
26. Austrian R, Gold J. Pneumococcal bacteremia with especial reference to bacteremic pneumococcal pneumonia. *Ann Intern Med.* 1964;**60**:759–776.
27. Sligl WI, Asadi L, Eurich DT, et al. Macrolides and mortality in critically Ill patients with community-acquired pneumonia: A systematic review and meta-analysis. *Crit Care Med.* 2014;**42**:420–432.
28. Jones BE, Ying J, Stevens V, et al. Empirical anti-MRSA vs standard antibiotic therapy and risk of 30-day mortality in patients hospitalized for pneumonia. *JAMA Intern Med.* 2020;**180**:552–560.
29. Webb BJ, Dascomb K, Stenehjem E, et al. Derivation and multicenter validation of the drug resistance in pneumonia clinical prediction score. *Antimicrob Agents Chemother.* 2016;**60**:2652–2663.
30. Prina E, Ranzani OT, Polverino E, et al. Risk factors associated with potentially antibiotic-resistant pathogens in community-acquired pneumonia. *Ann Am Thorac Soc.* 2015;**12**:153–160.
31. Kumar A, Roberts D, Wood KE, et al. Duration of hypotension before initiation of effective antimicrobial therapy is the critical determinant of survival in human septic shock. *Crit Care Med.* 2006;**34**:1589–1596.
32. Puskarich MA, Trzeciak S, Shapiro NI, et al. Association between timing of antibiotic administration and mortality from septic shock in patients treated with a quantitative resuscitation protocol. *Crit Care Med.* 2011;**39**:2066–2071.
33. Uranga A, Espana PP, Bilbao A, et al. Duration of antibiotic treatment in community-acquired pneumonia: A multicenter randomized clinical trial. *JAMA Intern Med.* 2016;**176**:1257–1265.
34. Choudhury G, Mandal P, Singanayagam A, et al. Seven-day antibiotic courses have similar efficacy to prolonged courses in severe community-acquired pneumonia—a propensity-adjusted analysis. *Clin Microbiol Infect.* 2011;**17**:1852–1858.
35. Pugh R, Grant C, Cooke RPD, et al. Short-course versus prolonged-course antibiotic therapy for hospital-acquired pneumonia in critically ill adults. *Cochrane Database Syst Rev.* 2015;CD007577.
36. Chastre J, Wolff M, Fagon JY, et al. Comparison of 8 vs 15 days of antibiotic therapy for ventilator-associated pneumonia in adults: A randomized trial. *JAMA.* 2003;**290**:2588–2598.
37. Bouadma L, Luyt C-E, Tubach F, et al. Use of procalcitonin to reduce patients' exposure to antibiotics in intensive care units (PRORATA trial): A multicentre randomised controlled trial. *Lancet.* 2010;**375**:463–474.
38. de Jong E, van Oers JA, Beishuizen A, et al. Efficacy and safety of procalcitonin guidance in reducing the duration of antibiotic treatment in critically ill patients: A randomised, controlled, open-label trial. *Lancet Infect Dis.* 2016;**16**:819–827.
39. Schuetz P, Birkhahn R, Sherwin R, et al. Serial procalcitonin predicts mortality in severe sepsis patients: Results from the multicenter procalcitonin MOnitoring SEpsis (MOSES) Study. *Crit Care Med.* 2017;**45**:781–789.
40. Coelho L, Póvoa P, Almeida E, et al. Usefulness of C-reactive protein in monitoring the severe community-acquired pneumonia clinical course. *Crit Care.* 2007;**11**:R92.
41. Bruns AHW, Oosterheert JJ, Hak E, et al. Usefulness of consecutive C-reactive protein measurements in follow-up of severe community-acquired pneumonia. *Eur Respir J.* 2008;**32**:726–732.
42. Self WH, Grijalva CG, Williams DJ, et al. Procalcitonin as an early marker of the need for invasive respiratory or vasopressor support in adults with community-acquired pneumonia. *Chest* 2016;**150**:819–828.

43. Pea F, Viale P. Bench-to-bedside review: Appropriate antibiotic therapy in severe sepsis and septic shock—does the dose matter? *Crit Care.* 9;**13**:214.
44. Sangmuang P, Lucksiri A, Katip W. Factors associated with mortality in immunocompetent patients with hospital-acquired pneumonia. *J Global Inf Dis.* 2019;**11**:13.
45. Kim JW, Chung J, Choi SH, et al. Early use of imipenem/cilastatin and vancomycin followed by de-escalation versus conventional antimicrobials without de-escalation for patients with hospital-acquired pneumonia in a medical ICU: A randomized clinical trial. *Crit Care.* 2012;**16**:R28.
46. Chang RYK, Wallin M, Lin Y, et al. Phage therapy for respiratory infections. *Adv Drug Deliv Rev.* 2018;**133**:76–86.
47. Maddocks S, Fabijan AP, Ho J, et al. Bacteriophage therapy of ventilator-associated pneumonia and empyema caused by pseudomonas aeruginosa. *Am J Respir Crit Care Med.* 2019;**200**:1179–1181.
48. Woods DR, José RJ. Current and emerging evidence for immunomodulatory therapy in community-acquired pneumonia. *Ann Res Hosp.* 2017;**1**:33–undefined.
49. Herold S, Hoegner K, Vadász I, et al. Inhaled granulocyte/macrophage colony–stimulating factor as treatment of pneumonia-associated acute respiratory distress syndrome. *Am J Respir Crit Care Med.* 2014;**189**:609–611.
50. Karakioulaki M, Stolz D. Biomarkers in pneumonia—beyond procalcitonin. *Int J Mol Sci.* 2019;**20**:2004.
51. Scicluna BP, Klein Klouwenberg PMC, van Vught LA, et al. A molecular biomarker to diagnose community-acquired pneumonia on intensive care unit admission. *Am J Respir Crit Care Med.* 2015;**192**:826–835.
52. Burnham KL, Davenport EE, Radhakrishnan J, et al. Shared and distinct aspects of the sepsis transcriptomic response to fecal peritonitis and pneumonia. *Am J Respir Crit Care Med.* 2017;**196**:328–339.
53. Metlay JP, Waterer GW, Long AC, et al. Diagnosis and treatment of adults with community-acquired pneumonia: An official clinical practice guideline of the American Thoracic Society and Infectious Diseases Society of America. *Am J Resp Crit Care Med.* 2019;**200**(7):e45–67.

34

Viral Pneumonias

Jordi Rello, Eleonora Bunsow, and Leonel Lagunes

- Respiratory viruses are a major cause of community-acquired pneumonia and can lead to severe community-acquired pneumonia (CAP) with intensive care unit (ICU) admission.
- The tendency to develop severe infections is influenced by the virus, the immune status of the host, and the development of secondary bacterial infections.
- Molecular diagnostics for viral infections have revolutionized our understanding of this area.

CONTROVERSIES

Should detection of reactivated herpesvirade (herpes simplex, cytomegalovirus) in the lungs of mechanically ventilated patients prompt treatment with anti-viral agents?

The role of anti-viral therapy and adjunctive immunomodulatory therapy in viral pneumonia requires well-conducted clinical trials.

Introduction

Pneumonia is one of the leading causes of hospitalization and death in children and adults worldwide. The highest incidence is observed among children under 5 and among adults older than 65 years. In 2015, according to the World Health Organization (WHO), pneumonia killed an estimated of 922,000 children under the age of 5 years, representing 15% of all deaths of children under that age.[1] Mortality in adult population ranges from 2% to 14%; however, in elderly and patients admitted to intensive care unit (ICU) this percentage can rise up to 40%.[2] The reported annual incidence of community-acquired pneumonia (CAP) requiring hospitalization is 24.8 cases per 10,000 adults in the USA. Approximately, 20%–40% of patients with CAP needed hospitalization with 20%–30% developing severe CAP (SCAP), requiring treatment in ICUs, with a third of these patients needing mechanical ventilation.[3] The economic costs of pneumonia in the USA alone are estimated to exceed US$17 billion per year.[3]

Through standard microbiological tests, it is possible to identify the etiologic agent of CAP in only 30%–50% of cases. This shows the limited effectiveness of microbiological tests in diagnosis. However, the introduction of newer tests, such as nucleic acid amplification techniques, has significantly improved the ability to detect multiple viral pathogens revealing viral pathogens in a high percentage of CAP.[4–6]

Viral Pneumonia

Viral infections are commonly associated with upper respiratory tract infection (URTI), ranging from asymptomatic or common cold to sinusitis and acute otitis media.[7–10] The influenza pandemic in 2009 confirmed the importance of influenza virus A (H1N1) in the development of pneumonia. Besides influenza, the role of other viruses, such as respiratory syncytial viruses (RSVs), rhinoviruses (RVs), and coronavirus among others, are also well recognized. Severe acute respiratory syndrome (SARS-CoV-2), the agent responsible for COVID-19, is covered in detail in Chapter 35.

At the extremes of ages, young children and elderly adults, viral pneumonia is more frequent. It has been estimated that about 200 million cases of viral CAP occur each year. In addition to the major impact on health already mentioned, the economic impact of viral respiratory tract infection (VRTI) is high. It is estimated that the total annual expenditure (including direct and indirect costs) of non-influenza-related VRTI in the USA, is more than US$40 billion. The total economic costs of influenza epidemics in the USA are higher, representing an amount of US$87.1 billion each year. One of the important factors in respiratory viral illnesses is their seasonality. Influenza virus, coronavirus, human metapneumovirus (hMPV), and RSV are more frequent during winter months, finding greater diversity in tropical areas. However, RV is circulating in the population throughout the year, with seasonal peaks in the spring and autumn, and parainfluenza virus (PIV) is more frequent from autumn to spring.

Many viruses have been implicated in the development of viral pneumonia, including both respiratory viruses and non-respiratory viruses. Within the respiratory virus group, the major pathogens are influenza viruses A, B, and C; RSVs; RVs; hMPVs; PIV types 1, 2, 3, and 4 (PIVs); human bocaviruses (hBoVs); coronaviruses (CO229E, OC43, NL63, HKU1, SARS, MERS, and SARS-CoV-2); adenoviruses; enteroviruses; hantaviruses; and coxsackie viruses. Non-respiratory viruses include varicella zoster virus; human herpesvirus; and cytomegalovirus (CMV) and Epstein-Barr (EBV) virus among others which are well known causes of pneumonia, mainly in adults and immunocompromised patients, and are considered in the section 'Herpesvirade Pneumonia and Viral Reactivation'.

Severe Viral Pneumonia

Viruses are identified in 36%–62% of SCAP. The frequency of individual viruses varies according to the study, although RV (23.6%–57.7%), PIV (20.8%–27.1%), and RSV (13.9%–27.1%) are the most frequently detected. Influenza, hMPV, and adenovirus were also identified, albeit less frequently. It is therefore apparent that viruses beyond influenza should be considered in SCAP, and multiplex polymerase chain reaction (PCR) tests directed towards a range of viruses become standard.

Viral Pneumonia in Immunosuppressed Patients

New treatments prolong survival of transplanted patients and human immunodeficiency virus (HIV) patients, creating a group who are vulnerable to pneumonia arising from both respiratory and non-respiratory viruses. Whilst the pathogenic role of CMV is well established in this population, the advent of widespread PCR testing has implicated RSV, influenza virus, adenovirus, PIV, hMPV, and coronaviruses in the development of severe pneumonia in these patients. The precise virus involved varies to some extent with the cause of the underlying immune impairment. In haematopoietic cell transplant (HCT) patients, RSV is the most frequently detected virus (30% of patients with respiratory infections) with a high associated mortality (6.5%–26.7%). In patients with HCT and RSV, treatment with ribavirin should not be delayed as without treatment mortality may rise to 80%. In solid organ transplant recipients, the incidence and mortality of respiratory viruses is lower than in HCT and depends on the transplanted organ, with highest incidences and mortality in lung transplant. In HIV patients, severe respiratory infections due to respiratory viruses have also been described. However, the epidemiology differs from transplant patients, for example RSV is not a frequent cause of CAP in hospitalized adults with HIV, with only a few cases reported.[11,12] After highly active antiretroviral therapy, hospitalization attributable to influenza infection decreased drastically, from 48 per 1000 persons/year in 1995 to 5 per 1000 person/year during 1996–1999, also mortality decreased. However, despite these improvements and routine vaccination, influenza remains a substantial threat to patients with HIV.

Diagnosis

Diagnosis of respiratory infection has improved radically in the last decade. The use of viral culture and immunofluorescence assays led to many false negatives and delayed results. PCR is more sensitive than the classic microbiological methods, increasing the number of viruses detected in respiratory samples and also reducing time to result.[13,14] With a time frame of hours, results can now readily impact on clinical decision making. However, the results obtained in PCR do not always imply active virus replication, and differentiation of asymptomatic carriage versus infection requires correlation with the clinical presentation. Although rapid antigen tests are increasingly available, these do not cover all viruses, and their lower test performance requires confirmatory testing with PCR.

Clinical Manifestation, Radiologic Findings, and Laboratory

Differentiating bacterial and viral pneumonia clinically is challenging. Respiratory viral infections usually follow seasonal patterns, although several viruses can be co-circulating at specific times of the year. It has been suggested by some authors that viral pneumonias have less fever and more upper respiratory symptoms than bacterial pneumonia. The Center for Disease Control (CDC) and the European CDC launched a surveillance system based on the influenza-like illness (ILI): a syndrome that alerts for possible outbreaks, based on acutely presenting clinical manifestations such as fever or feverishness, malaise, headache, myalgia, and at least one of the following three respiratory symptoms: cough, sore throat, and shortness of breath. This approach has led to clinical implications in some centres, where every patient with ILI in 'flu season' receives anti-virals until viral pneumonia has been ruled out.

Other features may point towards viral pneumonia, for instance pregnant women who require ICU care for respiratory failure are more likely to have influenza-viral pneumonia than matched non-pregnant women.

Radiological investigations are non-specific, and may range minimal changes to bilateral consolidation, and do not reliably distinguish between viral or bacterial infections. Super-added issues in ICU, including fluid overload and mechanical ventilation, further reduce the specificity of radiology in sCAP.

Laboratory findings, such as lower leucocyte counts and lower C-reactive protein, have been suggested as distinguishing features of viral rather than bacteria pneumonia, and higher procalcitonin is indicative of bacterial infection but lacks sensitivity at presentation. However, neither radiological nor laboratory parameters have sufficient performance to confidently differentiate viral from bacterial infection, and to further complicate matters, co-infection with bacteria is common. The key to diagnosis lies with microbiological confirmation of the pathogen.

Prevention and Treatment

In healthy non-severe adults, neuraminidase inhibitors demonstrated a less than 1-day reduction in influenza symptoms but reduction in complications and antimicrobial use.[15] In contrast, in immunocompromised patients, neuraminidase inhibitors are demonstrated to reduce symptom duration by days, hospitalizations, and mortality. In the case of (rare) suspicion of oseltamivir resistance, balantavir or amantadines can be used. Intravenous zanamivir provides a parental alternative in cases of resistance. In RSV, ribavirin has been approved by the Food and Drug Administration (FDA) for RSV treatment. It is more frequently used in immunocompromised patients; however, data are limited with contradictory results.

Only influenza and COVID-19 have effective vaccines, and the influenza vaccine should be repeated annually to cover antigenic drift and strain emergence; whether such measures are required for COVID-19 will become apparent over time. The search for vaccines against RSV and hMPV is ongoing. For RSV, Palivizumab, a monoclonal antibody against the fusion glycoprotein of RSV, is used to prevent RSV infection in premature infants.

Although antibiotics have no role in the treatment of viral infections, where co-infection occurs, which is common in influenza, or secondary hospital-acquired infections, they are clearly indicated.

Specific Respiratory Viruses

Influenza Virus

Influenza viruses (family Orthomyxoviridae) are enveloped negative-strand RNA viruses with segmented genomes containing 7–8 gene segments. The family includes five genera: influenza virus A, influenza virus B, influenza virus C, thogotovirus, and isavirus. Influenza A and B viruses have a similar structure, whereas influenza C is more divergent. Influenza A viruses (IAVs) had a significant risk of zoonotic infection, host switch, and the generation of pandemics. IAVs are covered with projections of three proteins: haemagglutinin (viral receptor-binding protein and fusion protein), neuraminidase (required for cleavage of neuramic acids on host cells), and matrix 2 (M2). The most prevalent serotype (H1N1) has been among us since at least the 1918 pandemic. The 'Spanish flu' that killed almost 50 million people has been linked by genomic reconstruction to an IAV H1N1.[16] This serotype occurred seasonally until 2009 when the pandemic strain 2009/A/H1N1 swept the globe. Critical illness in the 2009 pandemic arose most commonly in adults with a median age of 40 years, being uncommon in those older than 65 years. Poor outcomes from H1N1 virus infection have been recorded in neonates, pregnant women, and individuals with morbid obesity, immunocompromise, or serious co-morbidities. A comparison between features of infection arising from influenza and the novel coronavirus, SARS-CoV-2 (see below), is set out in Table 34.1, and risk factors are compared in Figure 34.1.[17]

Respiratory Syncytial Virus

RSV is an enveloped RNA virus B that belongs to the *Paramyxoviridae* family, and it is classified into two antigenic groups, A and B.[18] The role of RSV in lower respiratory tract infections in infants and young children is well described, but it also has been identified as an important cause of viral pneumonia in the adult population. Annual hospitalizations arising from RSV infection are estimated in 25.4 per 10,000 in adults aged >65 years[19] and is responsible, in the USA, for approximately 11,000 deaths per year. Mortality rises to more than 70% in patients >75 years old.[20]

The clinical manifestations of RSV pneumonia in adults are very similar to other viral pneumonias. However, compared with influenza viruses some signs and symptoms are more common in RSV including wheezing, rhinorrhoea, lower fever, and greater likelihood of patient age ≥65 years or immunocompromise.

Rhinovirus

RVs are members of the genus enterovirus of the *Picornaviridae* family. Until a few years ago, only two groups of RVs (A and B) were known. However, new molecular techniques and genotyping led to the discovery of a third kind of RV (RV-C) having distinct structural and biological characteristics. Among the three species, more than 160 different genotypes are known. The RV is commonly

Table 34.1 Selected comparisons between influenza virus and SARS-CoV-2

Parameter	Influenza virus	SARS-CoV-2
Receptor usage	Sialic acid	ACE2
Viral surface protein processing	Haemagglutinin processing by trypsin-like proteases	Spike protein processing by host proteases, including TMPRSS2, cathepsin L and furin, neuropilin 1
Cellular tropism	Respiratory epithelial cells: types I and II alveolar epithelial cells; ciliated cells	Respiratory epithelial cells: type II alveolar epithelial cells, ciliated cells and secretory cells; sustentacular and horizontal basal cells of the olfactory epithelium Intestinal epithelial cells; endothelial cells; renal parenchymal cells
Tissues affected and pathology	Upper respiratory tract; lower respiratory tract (severe cases)	Upper respiratory tract; lower respiratory tract; intestinal tract; cardiovascular or endothelial system; kidneys; nervous system
Viral recognition in airway epithelial cells	TLR3; RIG-I; ZBP1	TLR3; RIG-I; MDA5
Site of viral replication	Nuclear	Cytoplasmic
Viral evasion of initial host response	NS1; PB2; PB1-F2	NSP1; ORF6; NSP13; others? (extrapolated from other coronaviruses)
Extrapulmonary complications	Limited; cardiac: myocarditis (rare); neurological: encephalitis (rare)	Extensive; olfactory: anosmia; endothelial: thrombosis; neurological: stroke, encephalitis, neuropsychiatric; gastrointestinal: nausea, vomiting, diarrhoea
Viral evolution and antigenicity	Antigenic shift; antigenic drift	Antigenic drift?
Prior immunity	Previous infection; vaccination; subtype specificity	No specific SARS-CoV-2 immunity prior to late 2019–2020; protective immunity from other human coronaviruses unclear; vaccination started December 2020

MDA5, melanoma differentiation-associated 5; NS1, nonstructural protein 1; PB2, polymerase basic protein 2; RIG-I, retinoic acid-inducible gene I; SARS-CoV-2, severe acute respiratory syndrome coronavirus 2; TLR3, Toll-like receptor 3; TMPRSS2, transmembrane serine protease 2; ZBP1, Z-DNA binding protein 1.

Source: Reprinted by permission from Springer Nature: Flerlage T, Boyd DF, Meliopoulos V, et al. Influenza virus and SARS-CoV-2: Pathogenesis and host responses in the respiratory tract. *Nat Rev Microbiol.* 19(7):425–441. Copyright 2021.

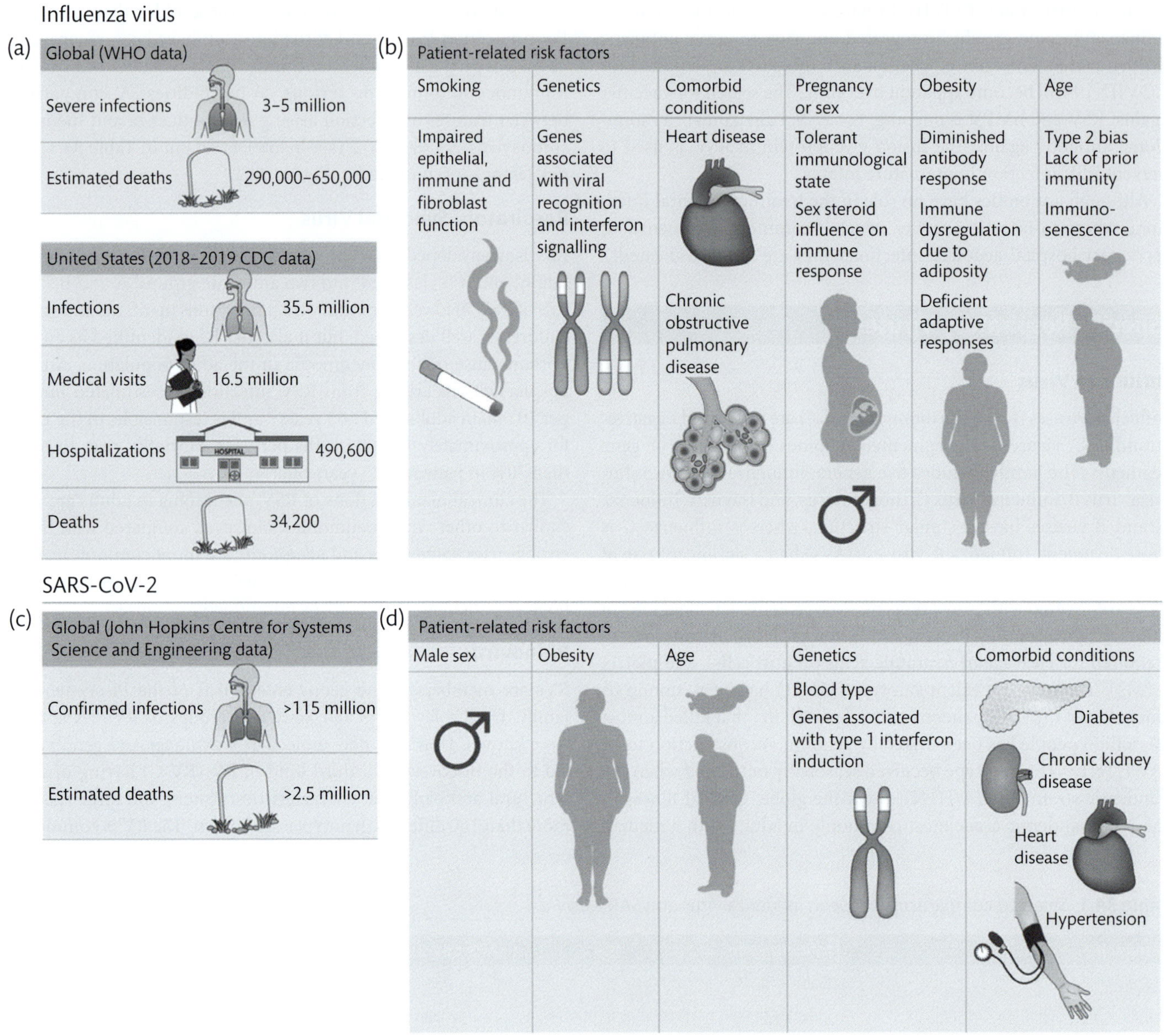

Figure 34.1 Patient-related risk factors for severe influenza and SARS-CoV-2 infections. Adapted from Flerlage et al.[17] Estimates of influenza burden from WHO and CDC respectively, and SARS-CoV-2 from Johns Hopkins data. Type 2 bias is bias towards type 2/Th2 immune responses.

associated with URTI, usually associated with the common cold and is therefore considered the most common human infectious agent worldwide.[21,22] They can also cause a wide range of respiratory diseases, playing an important role in the development of infections of the lower respiratory tract infection, including pneumonia.

The relationship between RV species and clinical disease in adults is unclear; whilst some authors have found worse outcomes segregate to RV-A and RV-B, other studies do not support this.

Human Metapneumovirus

HMPV is an enveloped RNA virus that also belongs to the *Paramyxoviridae* family, *Metapneumovirus* genus in the *Pneumovirinae* subfamily.[23] Two genotypes of hMPV have been identified, A and B.[24] It was isolated for first time in 2001 in the Netherlands from 28 young children with respiratory tract infections.

The metapneumovirus hospitalization rate in adults older than 65 years old is 22.1/10,000.[25] Clinical presentation is very similar to other respiratory viruses in the adult population, and it is difficult to make the diagnosis based only on clinical presentation. In general, patients with hMPV have nasal congestion, cough, and rhinorrhoea in approximately 75%. Compared with influenza virus, patients with hMPV were older, had more cardiovascular disease, were more often smokers, had lower fever (mean temperature 37.8 ∘C), and more wheezing.[25,26] Walsh et al. reported that 13% of the patients with hMPV were admitted to ICU with a mortality rate of 6.6%.

Coronavirus (Including MERS-CoV and SARS-CoV)

Coronaviruses are RNA viruses. In the mid-1960s, the first two human coronavirus (HCoV) were discovered and named 229E and OC43. After that, five more human coronavirus strains were identified: NL63, HKU1, SARS-CoV, and recently MERS-CoV and SARS-CoV-2 (see Chapter 35).

Human coronaviruses 229E and OC43 are very common in the elderly. In general, patients present upper respiratory symptoms. A hospital cohort showed that patients admitted with OC43 spend more days in the hospital, needed more ICU with mechanical ventilation, and showed more pulmonary infiltrates on chest radiographs than those with 229E. Human coronavirus OC43 together with VNL63 and HKU1 was associated with lower respiratory tract infection in adult population with high rate of co-infection with other respiratory viruses (38%–42%). Human coronavirus 229E was more frequently detected in immunocompromised.

SARS-CoV and Middle East Respiratory Syndrome Coronavirus (MERS-CoV) caused severe respiratory infection with high mortality relative to other CoVs. The SARS-CoV pandemic started in China in November 2002 and lasted until July 2003, with rapid spread around the world affecting 26 countries. A total of 8098 patients with 774 deaths (10%) were reported during the pandemic. Mortality rose up to 50%, commonly in elderly with co-morbidities. The disease started with fever, myalgia, non-productive cough, diarrhoea, and chills or rigor. After these influenza-like symptoms, the disease can progress to mild respiratory symptoms or to a moderate–severe variant with dyspnoea and hypoxia requiring mechanical ventilation in approximately 25% of subjects. Chest radiographs vary, at the beginning of the disease with subtle peripheral pulmonary infiltrates to progressive multifocal airspace disease. The diagnosis is with serology and RT-PCR: if the first sample has a negative result with high suspicion of SARS, a second sample should be analysed because sensitivity of RT-PCR can be low at the beginning and could be false negative. MERS-CoV was isolated for the first time in June 2012 in Saudi Arabia from a patient who died with severe respiratory disease. As of May 2016, the WHO has been notified of 1728 laboratory-confirmed cases of infection with MERS-CoV in 27 different countries with a mortality rate of 36.1% (624 deaths); however, the mortality rate can rise above 70%, especially in patients with co-morbidities. Clinical presentation is very similar to SARS-CoV, starting with fever, cough, myalgia, and gastrointestinal symptoms including diarrhoea and vomiting progressing rapidly to pneumonia and in a high percentage developed acute respiratory distress syndrome (ARDS), multi-organ failure, and death. Findings on chest X-ray are similar as in viral pneumonia or ARDS, especially affecting lower lung zones. Camels are the reservoir for MERS-CoV, although the transmission is most frequently from person to person in close contact. Diagnosis is through RT-PCR; although serology and culture are available, these two techniques are slow and need trained personal. Therapy is primarily supportive. COVID-19 is covered in detail in Chapter 35.

Parainfluenza

Parainfluenza are RNA viruses that also belong to the family *Paramyxoviridae*, divided into four serotypes, numbered 1–4. They are responsible for URTI, croup, bronchiolitis, and pneumonia in young children. In the USA, they represent the second most common cause of hospitalization for acute respiratory infection, with PIV-3 the most important pathogens.[27,28] The most severe disease is seen in the elderly and immunocompromised, especially among recipients of haemopoietic stem cell transplantation.

Other Respiratory Viruses

Other respiratory viruses that have been associated to viral pneumonia are human bocavirus, adenovirus, and human enterovirus D68 (EV-D68).

Human Bocavirus

hBoV is a DNA virus that belongs to the *Parvoviridae* family, discovered in 2005. Four subtypes have been identified, named from 1 to 4. HBoV1 is most frequently associated with respiratory infections, in contrast to hBoV2–4, was isolated in the gastrointestinal tract and probably associated with acute gastroenteritis.[29,30] The role of bocavirus in the development of pneumonia and acute otitis media has been studied mainly in paediatric population.[31,32] Severe pneumonia has been described in immunocompromised adults, but the role of this virus in immunocompetent adult population is not clear. No specific treatment exists beyond supportive measures.

Adenovirus

Adenovirus is also a DNA virus with over 50 serotypes linked to a broad range of infections. Adenovirus disease ranges from mild illness, such as URTI, conjunctivitis, or pharyngitis, to severe illness, including meningitis, gastroenteritis, and pneumonia. Adenovirus has been described as a cause of severe pneumonia in patients under immunosuppressive regimens.[33] However, adenovirus pneumonia is also reported in immunocompetent adults.[34] Serotypes 3, 4, 7, and 21 are most commonly associated with CAP in immunocompetent adults. Patients present with fever, cough, and dyspnoea whilst diarrhoea is relatively rare (10%). A high percentage of patients with adenoviral pneumonia requires intubation (67%) with a mortality rate of 24%.

Human Enterovirus D68

EV-D68 is an RNA virus member of human enterovirus D, genus *Enterovirus*, and *Picornaviridae* family. It is associated with acute respiratory infections, mostly in children but can also be seen in adults. From August 2014 to January 2015, an outbreak of enterovirus D68 affected the USA, with a total of 1153 confirmed cases by the CDC and 14 patients died. This was in the context of an increased number of EV-68 infections reported around the world in the recent years and a growing association with severe respiratory disease. Most of the publications concerning this virus relate to paediatric populations. In adults, EV-D68 was detected in 0.44% of patients hospitalized with CAP; no specific symptoms were described, with patients presenting with cough and difficulties in breathing.

Herpesvirade Pneumonia and Viral Reactivation

Several members of the *Herpesvirade* family of viruses, including varicella zoster virus (VZV) (human alphaherpesvirus 3), herpes simplex virus (HSV), cytomegalovirus (CMV), and EBV, can cause viral pneumonitis. Although rare, pneumonia from these viruses typically occurs as a result of primary infection in immunocompromised hosts, such as those following solid organ or bone marrow transplantation. Herpesvirade develop latent infection, residing in host cells (neurons for HSV and VZV, bone marrow progenitors for CMV, and epithelial cells and lymphocytes for EBV) and can reactivate following acute illness or stress.

Diagnosis of viral pneumonia arising from these viruses is complicated by their frequent reactivation and shedding in critically ill patients, who often have concomitant alveolar infiltration from other causes such as ARDS. Histological confirmation of infection, with viral inclusion bodies and multi-nucleated giant cells, is seldom feasible as it requires invasive tissue biopsy.

Observational studies have shown herpesvirade detection in the lower respiratory tract between 20% and 40% of mechanically ventilated patients. Although there is an association between viral detection and mortality, this is confounded by severity of illness. Whether the detection of herpesvirade in the respiratory secretions of mechanically ventilated patients should prompt treatment with anti-viral drugs remains uncertain, with a notable lack of high-quality studies to inform practice.[35] With the advent of routine molecular diagnostics that cover herpesvirade, the frequency of such detections is almost certain to increase. Which patients, if any, would benefit from anti-viral treatment for reactivated herpesvirade is unclear. Detection of viraemia in addition to pulmonary detection may prompt treatment by clinicians, especially in the case of cytomegalovirus. However, for now, the treatment of such patients remains empiric and should be guided by their immune status and the absence of other detectable pathogens.

Conclusion

Viral pathogens are a major cause of SCAP, and their role is increasingly appreciated following the advent of widespread PCR testing. Although clinical and radiological features may point towards viral infection, these lack specificity for viral versus bacterial infection and diagnosis has to rest on molecular viral detection. There are limited anti-viral options, and most care is supportive, focusing on limiting iatrogenic injury and treating secondary or coexisting bacterial infection. Whilst the role of low-dose steroids for COVID-19 pneumonia requiring supplementary oxygen or mechanical ventilation is favourable, their role in other viral pneumonias remains uncertain or even deleterious (influenza) due to the increase in replication and prolongation of viral shedding. That said, we are in a period of new antiviral agents through emerging structural molecular biological technology. Together with the development of adaptive platforms of clinical research design, the chance of effective antiviral therapies for SCAP are foreseeable.

REFERENCES

1. WHO. World Health Organization [Internet]. World Health Organization. [cited 2021 Jan 19]. Available from: https://www.who.int
2. Niederman MS. Community-acquired pneumonia: The U.S. perspective. *Semin Respir Crit Care Med.* 2009;**30**(2):179–188.
3. File TM, Marrie TJ. Burden of community-acquired pneumonia in North American adults. *Postgrad Med.* 2010;**122**(2):130–141.
4. Wu X, Wang Q, Wang M, et al. Incidence of respiratory viral infections detected by PCR and real-time PCR in adult patients with community-acquired pneumonia: A meta-analysis. *Respiration.* 2015;**89**(4):343–352.
5. Karhu J, Ala-Kokko TI, Vuorinen T, et al. Lower respiratory tract virus findings in mechanically ventilated patients with severe community-acquired pneumonia. *Clin Infect Dis.* 2014;**59**(1):62–70.
6. Gadsby NJ, Russell CD, McHugh MP, et al. Comprehensive Molecular Testing for Respiratory Pathogens in Community-Acquired Pneumonia. *Clin Infect Dis.* 2016;**62**(7):817–823.
7. Winther B. Rhinovirus infections in the upper airway. *Proc Am Thorac Soc.* 2011;**8**(1):79–89.
8. Savolainen-Kopra C, Blomqvist S, Kilpi T, et al. Novel species of human rhinoviruses in acute otitis media. *Pediatr Infect Dis J.* 2009;**28**(1):59–61.
9. Pavia AT. What is the role of respiratory viruses in community-acquired pneumonia? What is the best therapy for influenza and other viral causes of community-acquired pneumonia? *Infect Dis Clin North Am.* 2013;**27**(1):157–175.
10. Ruuskanen O, Lahti E, Jennings LC, et al. Viral pneumonia. *Lancet.* 2011;**377**(9773):1264–1275.
11. Cunha BA, Syed U, Hage JE. Respiratory syncytial virus (RSV) community-acquired pneumonia (CAP) in a hospitalized adult with human immunodeficiency virus (HIV) mimicking influenza A and *Pneumocystis (carinii) jiroveci* pneumonia (PCP). *Heart Lung.* 2012;**41**(1):76–82.
12. Gupta A, Mody P, Gupta S. A case of respiratory syncytial virus infection in an HIV-positive adult. *Case Rep Infect Dis.* 2012;**2012**:267028.
13. Talbot HK, Falsey AR. The diagnosis of viral respiratory disease in older adults. *Clin Infect Dis.* 2010;**50**(5):747–751.
14. Templeton KE, Scheltinga SA, Beersma MFC, et al. Rapid and sensitive method using multiplex real-time PCR for diagnosis of infections by influenza a and influenza B viruses, respiratory syncytial virus, and parainfluenza viruses 1, 2, 3, and 4. *J Clin Microbiol.* 2004;**42**(4):1564–1569.
15. Tejada S, Jansson M, Solé-Lleonart C, et al. Neuraminidase inhibitors are effective and safe in reducing influenza complications: Meta-analysis of randomized controlled trials. *Eur J Intern Med.* 2021 Apr;**86**:54–65.
16. Taubenberger JK, Hultin JV, Morens DM. Discovery and characterization of the 1918 pandemic influenza virus in historical context. *Antivir Ther.* 2007;**12**(4 Pt B):581–591.
17. Flerlage T, Boyd DF, Meliopoulos V, et al. Influenza virus and SARS-CoV-2: Pathogenesis and host responses in the respiratory tract. *Nat Rev Microbiol.* 2021 Jul;**19**(7):425–441.
18. Falsey AR, Walsh EE. Respiratory syncytial virus infection in adults. *Clin Microbiol Rev.* 2000;**13**(3):371–384.
19. Mullooly JP, Bridges CB, Thompson WW, et al. Influenza- and RSV-associated hospitalizations among adults. *Vaccine.* 2007;**25**(5):846–855.
20. Matias G, Taylor R, Haguinet F, et al. Estimates of mortality attributable to influenza and RSV in the United States during 1997–2009 by influenza type or subtype, age, cause of death, and risk status. *Influenza Other Respir Viruses.* 2014;**8**(5):507–515.
21. Mäkelä MJ, Puhakka T, Ruuskanen O, et al. Viruses and bacteria in the etiology of the common cold. *J Clin Microbiol.* 1998;**36**(2):539–542.
22. Royston L, Tapparel C. Rhinoviruses and respiratory enteroviruses: Not as simple as ABC. *Viruses.* 2016 Jan 11;**8**(1):16.
23. van den Hoogen BG, Bestebroer TM, Osterhaus ADME, et al. Analysis of the genomic sequence of a human metapneumovirus. *Virology.* 2002;**295**(1):119–132.

24. Papenburg J, Carbonneau J, Isabel S, et al. Genetic diversity and molecular evolution of the major human metapneumovirus surface glycoproteins over a decade. *J Clin Virol.* 2013;**58**(3):541–547.
25. Widmer K, Griffin MR, Zhu Y, et al. Respiratory syncytial virus- and human metapneumovirus-associated emergency department and hospital burden in adults. *Influenza Other Respir Viruses.* 2014;**8**(3):347–352.
26. Walsh EE, Peterson DR, Falsey AR. Human metapneumovirus infections in adults: Another piece of the puzzle. *Arch Intern Med.* 2008;**168**(22):2489–2496.
27. Counihan ME, Shay DK, Holman RC, et al. Human parainfluenza virus-associated hospitalizations among children less than five years of age in the United States. *Pediatr Infect Dis J.* 2001;**20**(7):646–653.
28. Weinberg GA, Hall CB, Iwane MK, et al. Parainfluenza virus infection of young children: Estimates of the population-based burden of hospitalization. *J Pediatr.* 2009;**154**(5):694–699.
29. Chow BDW, Ou Z, Esper FP. Newly recognized bocaviruses (HBoV, HBoV2) in children and adults with gastrointestinal illness in the United States. *J Clin Virol.* 2010;**47**(2):143–147.
30. Arthur JL, Higgins GD, Davidson GP, et al. A novel bocavirus associated with acute gastroenteritis in Australian children. *PLoS Pathog.* 2009;**5**(4):e1000391.
31. Fry AM, Lu X, Chittaganpitch M, et al. Human bocavirus: A novel parvovirus epidemiologically associated with pneumonia requiring hospitalization in Thailand. *J Infect Dis.* 2007;**195**(7):1038–1045.
32. Meriluoto M, Hedman L, Tanner L, et al. Association of human bocavirus 1 infection with respiratory disease in childhood follow-up study, Finland. *Emerg Infect Dis.* 2012;**18**(2):264–271.
33. Weigt SS, Gregson AL, Deng JC, et al. Respiratory viral infections in hematopoietic stem cell and solid organ transplant recipients. *Semin Respir Crit Care Med.* 2011;**32**(4):471–493.
34. Clark TW, Fleet DH, Wiselka MJ. Severe community-acquired adenovirus pneumonia in an immunocompetent 44-year-old woman: A case report and review of the literature. *J Med Case Rep.* 2011;**5**:259.
35. Hagel S, Scherag A, Schuierer L, et al. Effect of antiviral therapy on the outcomes of mechanically ventilated patients with herpes simplex virus detected in the respiratory tract: A systematic review and meta-analysis. *Crit Care.* 2020;**24**:584.

35

COVID-19 in the Intensive Care Unit: Epidemiology, Pathophysiology, Respiratory Management, Haemodynamic Support, Renal Support, Pharmacological Treatments, and Superinfection

Jonathon P Fanning, Gianluigi Li Bassi, Patricia Rieken Macedo Rocco, Lorenzo Ball, Antonio Messina, Marlies Ostermann, Matteo Bassetti, and Daniele Roberto Giacobbe

35.1 **Epidemiology of COVID-19 in the Intensive Care Unit**

Jonathon P Fanning and Gianluigi Li Bassi

- Coronavirus disease 2019 (COVID-19) has placed substantial burden on patients and healthcare systems worldwide.
- A small proportion of COVID-19 patients require hospitalization, and among those up to 20% develop critical illness and require intensive care unit admission. This percentage is significantly lower in those vaccinated against SARS-CoV-2.
- Estimated case fatality rate in mechanically ventilated COVID-19 patients approximates 40–50% and varies among different geographical regions. This percentage is significantly lower in those vaccinated against SARS-CoV-2.
- There is evidence that mortality in critically ill COVID-19 intensive care unit (ICU) patients has declined over time, likely due to improved clinical care and evidence-based treatment.
- High-level heterogeneity limits conclusions derived by pooling results across studies due to differences in illness severity, thresholds for mechanical ventilation, ICU admission/triage criteria, clinical practices, and resource constraints, as well as timing differences relative to surges, rapidly changing social behaviours, and the lack of standardized reporting.

- Explore outcomes and the burdens on healthcare services before and after national initiatives around COVID-19 are implemented, most importantly related to vaccines.
- Post-exposure prophylaxis therapies and their effect in influencing infection rates and/or severity in vaccinated and non-vaccinated individuals.
- The impact of variation in global distribution and implementation of vaccination programmes on outcomes and future threats of SARS-CoV-2.
- The impact of the burden of COVID-19 on healthcare services and staff, its regional variation, and the most effective models of care.

Introduction

Coronavirus disease 2019 (COVID-19) is the infectious disease caused by SARS-CoV-2, a novel beta coronavirus that was declared a pandemic by the World Health Organisation on 11 March 2020, after 118,000 cases and 4291 deaths were reported across 114 countries. Tremendous burdens have subsequently been placed on patients and international healthcare services, especially intensive care units (ICUs). To date, over 203 million cases and 4.3 million COVID-19-associated deaths have been reported worldwide.[1] Updated post pandemic data will likely supercede this chapter. The impact of COVID infection in vaccinated and unvaccinated survivors is the subject of extensive international research.

Use of Intensive Care Resources

Approximately 20% of unvaccinated SARS-CoV-2-infected patients require hospitalization,[2] 15%–20% of these requiring admission to an ICU.[3,4] Such severely ill patients often develop severe pneumonia and acute respiratory distress syndrome (ARDS), the latter diagnosed in 40%–96% of patients admitted to ICUs and its severity strongly associated with mortality risk. Heterogeneous figures regarding the use of invasive mechanical ventilation (IMV) have been reported in COVID-19 patients in ICUs, varying from 20% to 100%.[5] Such variability likely reflects temporal trends in ICU resources throughout the pandemic and changes in those who were intubated as clinical practice has evolved.

Illness Severity

Respiratory symptoms and fever are the most common symptoms at admission. Patients with dyspnoea, a respiratory rate ≥30 breaths/min, oxygen saturation ≤93%, and/or arterial partial pressure of oxygen/oxygen (PaO_2/FiO_2) concentration ≤300 mmHg are generally considered to have 'severe' illness.[6] Progression to respiratory failure requiring IMV or other organ failure, including shock, requires admission to ICU. However, conventional severity scoring inadequately reflects the acute severity of COVID-19 ICU patients, and the distribution of ICU patients with COVID-19 across more severe PaO_2/FiO_2 categories, combined with greater mortality, indicates a higher degree of acute respiratory disease than seen with other viral pneumonias. The pathophysiological differences with other viral pneumonitides may explain some of these differences.

Outcomes

Mortality in COVID-19 ICU patients has varied from 25% to 50%, consistent with the severity of ARDS and associated complications. Survival has improved with evidence-based treatments, as the pandemic has progressed, though higher rates persist in resource-limited settings.[7] Among patients requiring IMV, the case fatality rate (CFR, the proportion of the population dying within a specific time period) has been heterogeneous. Indeed, meta-analyses of currently available evidence estimate the CFR as 45% (95% CI: 39%–52%),[8] but 56% when the analysis is restricted to patients with known hospital outcomes. These figures in mechanically ventilated patients are higher than with other viral pneumonias and previous outbreaks of severe respiratory infections, including SARS-CoV in 2003 (reported CFR = 45%–58%), Middle East respiratory syndrome (60%–74%), and H1N1 influenza (24.2%–26.5%). The duration of intensive care and supportive therapies are clinically relevant outcomes. However, from a statistical perspective, estimating these durations is challenging since episodes are time-dependent and potentially multiple, and determined by the competing, terminal events of discharge-alive and death. Within this limitation, ICU stays typically are longer than other surgical/medical populations requiring IMV, ranging from ~7 to 20 days; COVID-19 ICU patients are also more likely to require organ support and for longer periods of time.

Risk Factors Associated with Severity and Outcomes

Knowledge regarding baseline patient characteristics and risk factors associated with ICU and hospital mortality is evolving.[9]

Demographic Factors

Key demographic, co-morbidity, and clinical variables have proven associations with both an individual's risk of infection and propensity for critical illness/risk of dying once infected. Relative to historical and non-COVID-19 viral pneumonia patients, critically ill COVID-19 patients are disproportionately from non-white racial/ethnic groups (only partially attributable to co-morbidities and social circumstances) and more likely to be from deprived areas, male, or obese. Among those critically ill with COVID-19, the two most notable, consistent, statistically significant demographic differences between survivors and non-survivors is age >50, ranging from a hazard risk of death of 2.63 (95% CI: 2.06–3.35) in patients 50–59 years old to 11.0 (8.9–13.8) in patients over 80.[10] Male gender also increases mortality risk, consistent with the well-established observation that infectious respiratory diseases generally are more severe and associated with greater mortality in men. This said, the influences of older age and maleness on mortality appear more pronounced with COVID-19 than with other respiratory infections.

Co-morbidities

Most co-morbidities are associated with an increased risk of critical illness from COVID-19, including cardiovascular disease, diabetes, respiratory disease (i.e. severe asthma), obesity, prior haematological malignancy or recurrent other cancer, kidney, liver and neurological disease, and autoimmune conditions. The most common and consistently reported co-morbidities are arterial hypertension and obesity. Interestingly, while premorbid health is always of prognostic significance in the critically ill, those with COVID-19 are less likely to have needed assistance with ADLs or have serious co-morbidities prior to hospitalization than historical and non-COVID viral-pneumonia ICU patients.

Geographic and Temporal Considerations

The overall CFR in the most-severe COVID-19 patients requiring IMV varies widely among continents, ranging from 36% (24%–48%) to 52% (19%–85%). Higher CFR was reported in earlier epicentres, secondary to the resource challenges faced in the pandemic's initial stages, resulting in unfavourable healthcare provider to patient ratios, and low rates of life-saving and labour-intensive interventions.[4] Conversely, triaging patients with co-morbidities, specifically in settings with ventilator/ICU bed shortages, may have contributed to lower CFRs, with younger and less-frail patients prioritized and older, frailer patients dying without ICU or IMV support. Mortality has declined in COVID-19 ICU patients over time,[11] likely secondary to improved care, greater clinical experience, and more evidence guiding treatment.

Overall, COVID-19 has placed greater burdens on critical-care services than other viral pneumonias though the extent of this burden has varied as the pandemic has waxed and waned. Future research efforts must continue to explore outcomes and the burdens on healthcare services before and after national initiatives around COVID-19 are implemented, most importantly related to vaccines.

35.2 Pathophysiology

Patricia Rieken and Macedo Rocco

- Development and progression of COVID-19 may be associated with the following mechanisms: (1) direct virus-induced cytotoxicity in ACE2-expressing cells, (2) dysregulation of the renin–angiotensin–aldosterone system because of virus-mediated ACE2 downregulation, (3) dysregulation of immune responses, (4) endothelial cell injury and thrombo-inflammation, and (5) tissue fibrosis.
- COVID-19 is a systemic disease involving different organs and pathophysiological functions.
- Understanding inter-individual variability in COVID-19 enables a precision medicine approach against SARS-CoV-2 infection and COVID-19 pathology.

- Characteristics of virus–host interactions involving SARS-CoV-2 are different and their primary role in the evolution of the severity of the disease are unknown.
- The different potential pharmacological approaches to COVID-19 should be better elucidated, being different treatments competitive each other.
- The optimized precision medicine approach against COVID-19 infection has yet to be defined although newer evidenced-based therapeutic successes are emerging rapidly.

- Pathophysiological mechanisms leading to different organ dysfunctions and severity require better elucidation to develop targeted treatments for prevention and cure.

Viral Cell Invasion

Although the recovery rate of COVID-19 is high, this infectious disease remains a significant global health issue.[12] SARS-CoV-2 uses the human angiotensin-converting enzyme 2 (ACE2) cell surface protein as a receptor to enter cells[13] and transmembrane serine protease 2 contributes to SARS-CoV-2 cell entry by cleaving the viral spike protein into a conformational form necessary for membrane fusion. The virus surface spike glycoprotein (S-protein) is a key determinant of the viral–host range and contains two domains, S1 and S2, which are separated by a protease cleavage site. A successful host cell invasion by the virus involves direct binding of the virus S1 receptor-binding domain to the host ACE2 peptidase extracellular domain, exposing the S1–S2 inter-domain protease site, which upon cleavage by host proteases leads to S2-mediated virus–host cell membrane fusion. Neutrophil elastase also has an important role in SARS-CoV-2 infection because it has a cleavage site near the S1–S2 subunits.[14]

Viral-Host Interactions and Immunopathology

Many characteristics of virus–host interactions involving SARS-CoV-2 remain unknown; however, the development and progression of COVID-19 may be associated with the following mechanisms: (1) direct virus-induced cytotoxicity in ACE2-expressing cells, (2) dysregulation of the renin–angiotensin–aldosterone system as a result of virus-mediated ACE2 downregulation, (3) dysregulation of immune responses, (4) endothelial cell injury and thrombo-inflammation, and (5) tissue fibrosis.[15]

Pulmonary Pathology

COVID-19 presents a heterogeneous clinical spectrum from no symptoms to multiple organ dysfunction syndrome.[16] Lungs are the organ most affected by SARS-CoV-2 infection, and pneumonia is the most frequent and serious clinical manifestation observed in cases of severe COVID-19. The expression of ACE2 is higher in the nasopharynx than in alveolar tissue, thus explaining initiation of SARS-CoV-2 infection in the upper respiratory tract.[17] ACE2 expression in the nasopharynx is lower in children than in adults, which seems to be associated with age-related differences in developing COVID-19.[18] Autopsies of the lungs have shown neutrophil and mononuclear cell infiltration, diffuse alveolar damage with alveolar oedema and hyperplasia of type II epithelial cells, hyaline membrane and thrombus formation, as well as fibrosis.

Endothelial dysfunction has been found in several patients with COVID-19 and may be attributed to (1) the effects of SARS-CoV-2 in the endothelium because ACE2 is also expressed in smooth muscle cells and in the arterial and venous endothelium of several organs; (2) hypoxia due to pulmonary dysfunction, leading to reduced blood flow and vasoconstriction; and (3) production of pro-inflammatory mediators.[19] Increased levels of thrombin, tissue factor V and VIII, and fibrinogen, combined with the formation of neutrophil extracellular traps, may result in coagulation dysfunction and increased risk of systemic macro- and micro-thrombosis.[20]

Extrapulmonary Pathology

The heart is also susceptible to SARS-CoV-2 because ACE2 is highly expressed in cardiomyocytes and pericytes, the latter leading to capillary endothelial dysfunction.[16] Moreover, the association of systemic and local inflammation with hypoxia may lead to myocardial injury.

Several patients also developed acute kidney injury (AKI) because ACE2 is expressed in kidney tissue.[21] In addition to direct kidney damage by SARS-CoV-2, the increased systemic inflammatory process, and the use of anti-viral agents may also cause nephrotoxicity.[16]

Gastrointestinal dysfunction may be caused by direct damage due to increased expression of ACE2 in the luminal surface of intestinal epithelial cells, as well as diffuse endothelial cell inflammation of the small intestine and mesenteric ischemia.[19] The liver can be affected in several individuals with COVID-19 because cholangiocytes express ACE2, which make them susceptible to direct virus-induced cytotoxicity. Moreover, liver damage can be related to systemic inflammation and the use of drugs, the mechanisms of which require clarification.[15]

Neurologic dysfunction has been reported with increasing frequency in cases of COVID-19.[16,22] ACE2 is expressed in olfactory bulb cells, neurons, astrocytes, and oligodendrocytes; therefore, the virus may disseminate rapidly through important brain areas once the olfactory epithelium is infected. SARS-CoV-2 may also infect the cerebral vascular endothelium and cross the blood–brain barrier via infected leukocytes, thus migrating into the central nervous system.

The progression and severity of COVID-19 has been correlated with age, race, ethnicity, sex, the expression pattern of ACE2 receptor, as well as individual immune regulation.[23] Thus, understanding inter-individual variability might enable a precision medicine approach against COVID-19 infection.

35.3 Respiratory Management

Lorenzo Ball

- COVID-19 can cause pneumonia with hypoxemic respiratory failure, requiring varying degrees of respiratory support.
- COVID-19 and ARDS from other causes have distinct pathophysiological traits that must be considered when delivering respiratory support.

- The role of higher PEEP levels should be clarified in COVID-19.
- The best type of non-invasive respiratory support is matter of debate, as are the criteria for respiratory support escalation.

- Randomized trials should clarify the optimum ventilatory and weaning strategy of patients receiving IMV for COVID-19-related pneumonia.
- Criteria for intubation should be better studied, especially for patients receiving non-invasive respiratory support.
- Accurate and clinically useful predictive tools for success or failure of non-invasive oxygen/ventilation therapies, incorporating assessment of work of breathing, gas exchange, and other relevant parameters.

Introduction

Respiratory support is the cornerstone of clinical management of COVID-19 patients.[24,25] Severe COVID-19 pneumonia often meets the Berlin criteria for acute respiratory distress syndrome (ARDS) (see Chapter 21). However, when matched by extent of lung involvement to ARDS control patients, COVID-19 patients had higher respiratory system compliance and lower PaO_2/FiO_2 ratio.[26] The extent of radiological ground-glass attenuation with preserved elastance is an important determinant of hypoxia.[27] These distinct pathophysiological traits must be considered when delivering respiratory support to patients with COVID-19.

Oxygen Therapy

Conventional oxygen therapy is the first-line treatment of hypoxaemia and is indicated when SpO_2 is <93% on room air. Various devices including nasal canulae, face mask, and reservoir face masks are used, with a target SpO_2 of 92%–94%/PaO_2 >60 mmHg/8 kPa. As hypoxia is not always accompanied by dyspnoea, regular monitoring of oxygen saturations is vital. Conventional oxygen therapy delivers low flow, unable to fulfil the requirements of patients with respiratory distress and increased peak inspiratory flow. When the inspiratory flow exceeds the oxygen delivery supplied by the interface, the patient will entrain room air resulting in a low fraction of inspired oxygen (FiO_2). In this context, heated-humidified high-flow nasal cannulas (HFNCs) present some advantages for delivering oxygen (see Chapter 7). HFNCs have been used extensively in COVID-19 and avoided intubation in selected patients.[28] Nonetheless, signs of respiratory distress, use of accessory muscles, respiratory rate above 25–28/min, and persistent hypoxaemia are signs of treatment failure during conventional and high-flow oxygen therapy, when non-invasive positive pressure respiratory support or IMV should be considered.

Non-invasive Positive Pressure Respiratory Support

Both continuous positive airway pressure (CPAP) and bilevel non-invasive positive pressure ventilation (NIPPV) are options for treating acute hypoxemic respiratory failure (see Chapters 8 and 9). Their role in the management of ARDS is debated; however, the COVID-19 pandemic has boosted the use of these respiratory support strategies, allowing delivery of ventilation outside of the intensive care unit.[29] These measures may represent the ceiling of care in patients to whom ICU admission is declined and be used as bridge to invasive ventilation in the case of shortage of ICU beds. Both CPAP and NIPPV can be delivered through face masks and helmets. The latter were extensively used during the COVID-19 pandemics, especially in Europe, for their better tolerability and the potential for reducing environmental viral dispersion.[30] A recent randomized trial showed that, compared to HFNC, helmet NIPPV resulted in a similar number of days free of respiratory support and lower intubation rates in COVID-19 patients.[31] A dedicated ventilator is required to deliver NIPPV, while CPAP can be administered with a high-flow generator only. Typical levels of CPAP applied range from 10 to 15 cmH_2O, while inspiratory pressures up to 25 cmH_2O are applied in NIPPV. Indeed, evidence emerging from the recovery RS study favours CPAP over HFNC in the pre-ICU setting. While concerns regarding HFNC-delivered oxygen have centred around risks of aerosolization and the quantity of oxygen required compared to CPAP or NIPPV, the field is evolving as more and perhaps better quality emerges through large adaptive platform trials. With that in mind, and recognizing that all these modalities have often complimentary roles in the treatment strategy of patients with COVID-19-associated acute respiratory failure, a management framework guide for clinicians has been produced by the UK National Health Service (Figure 35.1).

Invasive Mechanical Ventilation

There are no randomized controlled trials (RCTs) investigating the best ventilator settings in COVID-19; therefore, most recommendations

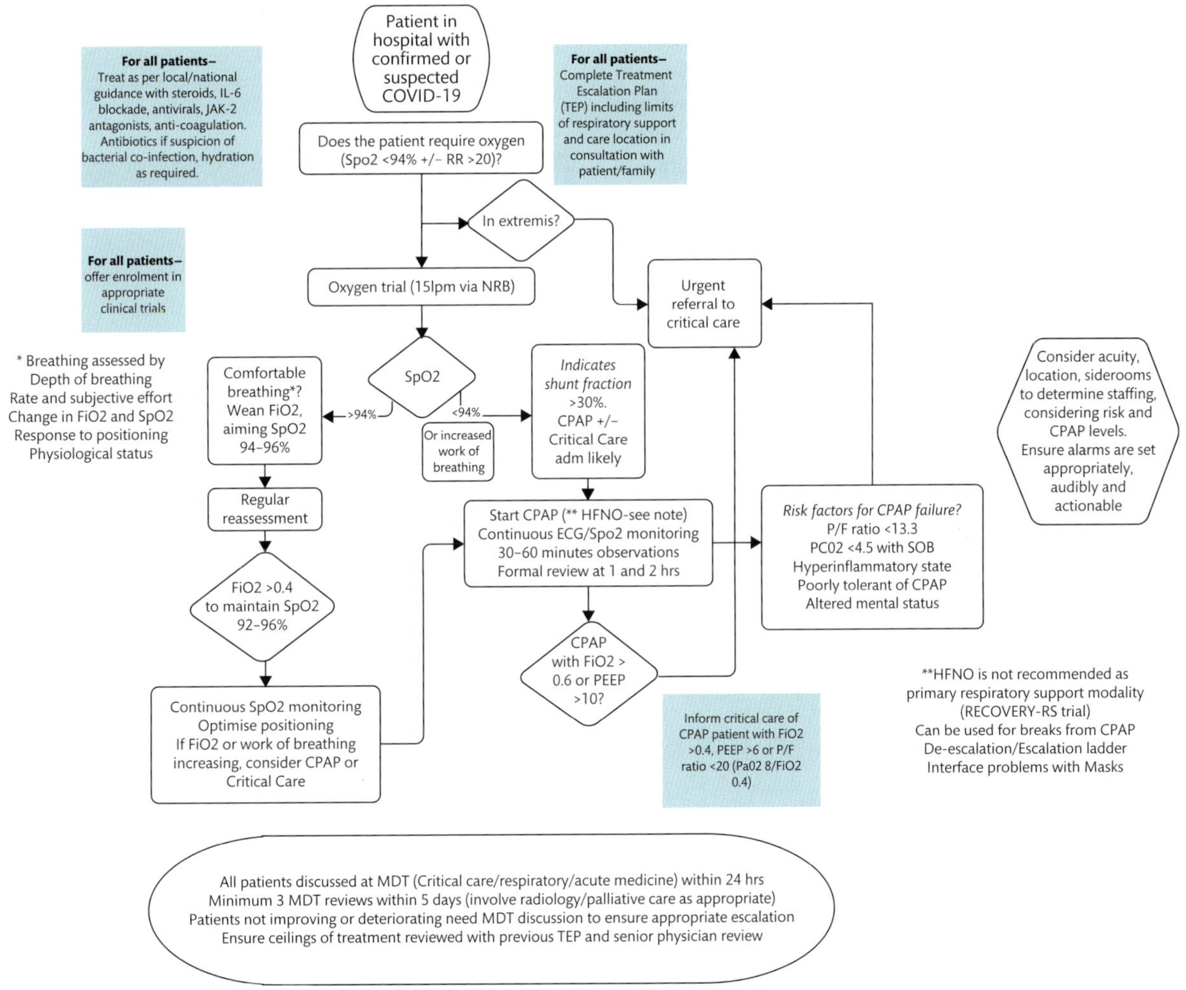

Figure 35.1 Pathways for patients presenting to hospital with suspected or confirmed COVID-19 respiratory infection. This is guidance pertinent to patients in the UK National Health Service within England and taken from NHS London Critical Care Cell–CPAP and Respiratory Failure Guidance for COVID-19 Dec 2021. It is subject to change as ongoing evidence emerges. ACC, adult critical care; ARU, acute respiratory unit; TEP, treatment escalation plan; MDT, multi-disciplinary team. CPAP, continuous positive airway pressure; HFNO, high-flow nasal oxygen.

From NHSE-I Guidance: PAP and Respiratory Failure. Adapted from University College Hospitals COVID guidelines.

are derived from ARDS studies with tidal volumes of 6 mL/kg predicted body weight recommended. Slightly higher tidal volumes could be tolerated in the subgroup of patients with relatively higher compliance, provided that this does not result in high driving pressure (plateau-PEEP), which should be ideally kept below 14 cmH_2O. As in ARDS, the optimum PEEP remains uncertain (see Chapter 21) with limited evidence for any particular PEEP strategy. PEEP-induced alveolar recruitment in COVID-19 was heterogeneous,[32] limited in most patients and resulted in worse respiratory system compliance.[33] For these reasons, PEEP levels in COVID-19 should be limited to those strictly necessary to maintain sufficient oxygenation targets, namely PaO_2 above 60 mmHg or SpO_2 above 90%–92%.

Role of Rescue Therapies

Prone positioning has a proven role in mortality reduction in ARDS although it remains underused. It has found widespread adoption in COVID-19, with often dramatic effects on oxygenation despite limited impact on respirator mechanics. Although the evidence base for inhaled nitric oxide, prostaglandins, and almitrine are weak, they may improve oxygenation by improving perfusion of aerated areas. Extracorporeal membrane oxygenation (ECMO) is reserved for those unresponsive to simpler rescue measures, consistent with severe ARDS, or in those with complications preventing optimal ventilatory support. Careful selection for veno-venous ECMO has provided favourable outcomes but not universally (see Chapter 22.3).[34] Extracorporeal CO_2 removal is less invasive, although remains an unproven therapy.

35.4 Haemodynamic Support

Antonio Messina

- The guidelines for haemodynamic support during the COVID-19 are based upon those in non-COVID critically ill patients. No alternative specific strategy is suggested.
- COVID-19-related manifestations of cardiac dysfunction are broad and still without known unique features. Echocardiographic patterns are non-specific, particularly in intubated critically ill patients.
- The chronic effects of COVID-19 infection on the cardiovascular system are not yet well understood; they may increase the risk of chronic heart dysfunction in those patients who recovered from the acute phase even without clinically relevant cardiac symptoms.

- The prevalence of shock caused by COVID-19 infection has also been reported with high variability (from 1% to 35%) due to variation in selected cohorts, the severity of illness, and the definition adopted to identify haemodynamic instability.
- COVID-19-related biochemical cardiac injury is not necessarily linked to cardiac-dysfunction-associated haemodynamic instability and/or shock.
- Most echocardiographic pathological patterns in critically ill patients are non-specific and often transient and hence of questionable clinical significance in the acute phase in haemodynamically stable patients.

- New-onset chronic heart failure is a key concern for those patients who recovered from the COVID-19 infection. The prevalence and degree of chronic cardiac dysfunction is an open field of research.
- Studies to investigate whether sustained inflammation could increase the risk of arrhythmias, myocardial fibrosis, and, potentially, chronic heart dysfunction, even in milder disease.

Introduction

Despite the prevalent lung tropism associated with prominent functional and morphological features,[35] it is clear that COVID-19 infection may trigger a multi-systemic disease involving different organs,[36–38] including the heart. There are several possible patterns of cardiovascular dysfunction associated with COVID-19: signs of direct inflammatory (myocarditis) or ischemic (infarction) insult, hypovolemia (due to sustained fever and dehydration), right ventricular (RV) dysfunction related to the effects of mechanical ventilation and/or pulmonary embolism, or, eventually, cardiovascular dysfunction due to superimposed hospital-acquired sepsis.[35,39–41]

Goals of Therapy

Guidelines adopted during the COVID-19 crisis regarding optimal haemodynamic support did not suggest any specific strategy in these patients since all the recommendations have been based upon guidelines in non-COVID critically ill patients.[42] The main goal of management for shock or haemodynamic instability in patients with COVID-19 is to optimize arterial pressure and cardiac output in the context of severe lung injury needing prolonged mechanical ventilation and associated with increased risk of microvascular thrombosis and/or pulmonary embolism. The main recommendations regarding the haemodynamic support may be summarized as follows[42]:

- Acute fluid resuscitation should be based on the administration of buffered/balanced crystalloids over either unbalanced crystalloids, colloids, or albumin.
- The responsiveness to fluid administration should be assessed by means of using dynamic parameters, skin temperature, capillary refilling time, and/or lactate levels over static parameters to assess fluid responsiveness.
- Cardiovascular support should be achieved by administering norepinephrine as the first-choice vasopressor. Target pressure should be then obtained by adding either vasopressin (up to 0.03 units/min) or epinephrine if high levels of norepinephrine are required. Patients receiving vasopressors should have an arterial catheter placed.
- Clinically evident cardiac dysfunction and persistent hypoperfusion despite adequate fluid loading and the use of vasopressor agents should be managed by using dobutamine with cardiac output trend measurements.

Cardiac Assessment

One of the most controversial points regarding the haemodynamic findings and, accordingly, support of COVID-19 patients is related to the assessment of cardiac abnormalities. In fact, on the one hand, COVID-19-related biochemical cardiac injury has been reported with significant variability in several cohort studies[42]; on the other hand, the exact clinical significance of elevated biomarkers is unknown and not necessarily related to a cardiac dysfunction causing hemodynamic instability and/or shock. Moreover, the prevalence of shock itself caused by COVID-19 infection has also been reported with high variability (from 1% to 35%) due to variation in selected cohorts, the severity of illness, and the definition adopted to identify the haemodynamic instability.[42] The pathophysiologic mechanisms of cardiovascular impact in COVID-19 include cardiac complications directly related to myocardial involvement (favoured by pre-existing systemic disease) or secondary to pulmonary damage, leading to a broad spectrum of left and RV diastolic dysfunction.[39,40] These patterns may be associated or not with biochemical damage.[43]

Critical-care echocardiography has been widely used in the COVID-19 crisis.[44] It has identified different phenotypes of acute ventricular dysfunction (right or left) requiring prompt specific interventions as well as secondary diastolic impairments, potentially affecting the weaning process.[45]

A large systematic review has recently appraised the echocardiographic findings in hospitalized and, predominantly, ICU COVID-19 patients.[45] The authors reported normal echocardiographic examination in about 50% of enrolled subjects. Moreover, the largest contributory study of this metanalysis (enrolling about one-third of the overall number of patients) showed that the majority of subjects had non-specific patterns of ventricular dysfunction.[46] Moreover, in the majority of the studies, the left ventricle systolic function has been reported as normal. Finally, a proper assessment of LV diastolic dysfunction in this population of patients was lacking and the potential role of this pattern on the mortality left unclear.[45]

RV dysfunction is a key component of COVID-19-related ARDS. For this reason, along with the increased risk of thromboembolic complications in this setting and with the impact of mechanical ventilation on the right heart, serial echocardiographic assessment of RV function has proven clinically helpful in the titration of fluid therapy, thoracic pressure adjustments, and pharmacological (including short-term inhaled nitric oxide) support of this subgroup of COVID-19-related critically ill patients.[47,48] In certain patients with very severe RV dysfunction, combinations of inotropes, selective pulmonary vasodilators, and other pharmaceutical agents for pulmonary hypertension (i.e. sildenafil, prostacyclin, and antithrombotic techniques) have been tried with appropriate haemodynamic monitoring and expert multispecialty supervision. However, there is no universal or generalized strategy for these cases.

Myocarditis

Heart involvement is, as previously said, multifactorial and mostly related to lung dysfunction, mechanical support, and amplified thrombogenesis. However, the effect of COVID-19 myocardial involvement has also been demonstrated in less severe clinical forms involving healthy individuals. In fact, a study conducted on young professional athletes recovering after COVID-19 without the need for hospitalization showed that a non-negligible number (15%) had evidence of myocarditis on cardiac magnetic resonance.[39]

Data from endomyocardial biopsies and autopsies suggests that virus-mediated myocarditis may not be common in COVID-19. However, this virus has shown a unique affinity for the ACE2 receptor, which is found on cells in the lungs, heart, and other organs and on endothelial cells lining the body's blood vessels. In this context, the systemic inflammation originating from the infected systemic vessels, and not a direct myocyte infection, may explain most myocardial injury findings among patients hospitalized with COVID-19. Again, the recovery of these complex cytokine-mediated pathways is still not understood.

New-onset chronic heart failure is one of the concerns for those patients who recover from the COVID-19 infection. In fact, right or left ventricular abnormalities (especially the diastolic dysfunction) recover in the majority of survivors of severe COVID-19 within a year. But this is not universal. The sustained inflammation could increase the risk of arrhythmias, and heart failure even among patients with milder infections, leading to myocardial fibrosis and, potentially, chronic heart dysfunction in the following decades. This remains a matter of important speculation that numerous large studies internationally (e.g. PHOSP-COVID UK) aim to address.

35.5 **Renal Support**

Marlies Ostermann

- Kidney replacement therapy (KRT) provision during the COVID-19 pandemic can be challenging due to a high number of patients needing KRT, shortage of machines and consumables, supply problems, reduced filter life, and shortage of trained staff.
- There is no universal solution for KRT provision in COVID-19. Alternative KRT modalities should be considered and regular adjustments of the KRT protocol may be necessary.
- An anticoagulation escalation strategy is essential to prolong filter life and reduce waste.
- A strong Critical Care–Nephrology relationship is vital to overcome challenges in KRT provision.
- Local, regional, and national systems for coordination of KRT emergency provision need to be established.

- COVID-19 is a pro-inflammatory prothrombotic condition. Inflammatory molecules, damage-associated molecular patterns, pathogen-associated molecular patterns, and viral particles contribute to the immunoinflammatory response in critically ill patients with COVID-19.
- Whether a specific KRT modality or anticoagulation method is superior in patients with COVID-19-associated AKI is unknown.
- It has been recommended to develop a registry of patients with severe COVID-19-associated AKI to study whether variations in clinical practice relating to KRT use and circuit performance affect clinical outcomes.

- Many healthcare agencies have authorized emergency use of various extracorporeal blood purification techniques, including haemoperfusion, adsorption, plasma exchange, and continuous renal replacement therapy (CRRT) with special membranes to remove inflammatory molecules and viral particles.
- Prospective RCTs are also needed to investigate whether the use of extracorporeal blood purification techniques is associated with improved outcomes, including the prevention and mitigation of AKI and other organ failures.

Indications for Kidney Replacement Therapy

AKI is a common complication of COVID-19 and kidney replacement therapy (KRT) may be needed.[49] Outside a surge situation, there is no evidence that KRT should be managed differently from patients with AKI in the context of other illnesses (Box 35.1). Indications, modality, dose, and anticoagulation strategies should follow current consensus recommendations.[50] However, in situations with a rapid increase in ICU demand, the provision of KRT may be challenged for a variety of reasons: high number of patients with severe AKI or end-stage kidney disease requiring KRT, supply problems, limited availability of consumables, reduced KRT performance, and shortage of staff. In this case, there is no universal solution, and adjustments have to be made based on the most urgent needs and challenges. In 2020, recommendations for KRT provision during a pandemic were developed with the aim to outline some general principles and provide guidance on how to maximize the number of patients receiving KRT[51] (Box 35.1).

Modalities of Kidney Replacement Therapy

During periods where the KRT demand exceeds usual availability, all potential modalities should be considered, including continuous renal replacement therapy (CRRT), intermittent haemodialysis (IHD), prolonged intermittent renal replacement therapy (PIRRT), and acute peritoneal dialysis (PD).[52–54] The potential advantages and disadvantages of these different techniques are outlined in Table 35.1. The final choice is often determined by the availability of machines and consumables, the infrastructure (for instance, existence of permanent water supply suitable for IHD), and the availability of appropriately trained staff to deliver KRT safely. If logistically feasible, early transition from CRRT to IHD with online-generated dialysate,

Table 35.1 Advantages and disadvantages of different KRT modalities in COVID-19

Modality	Advantages in COVID-19	Disadvantages in COVID-19
IHD	• Widely available • Allows use of same machine for several patients per day	• Less effective in reaching daily fluid balance • Requires trained dialysis staff
PIRRT (using IHD or CRRT machines)	• Allows use of one machine for several patients per day • Uses higher blood flows that may reduce risk of circuit clotting	• Less familiar • Potential need for systemic anticoagulation • Drug dosing is challenging
CRRT	• Achieves steady-state control of solutes and acid–base status • Allows better management of fluid status • No need for additional staff (i.e. renal dialysis nurse)	• Requires one machine per patient per day • Need for trained staff • Requires anticoagulation • Dependent on consumables
Acute PD	• No concerns about circuit clotting • No need for vascular access • Low risk of haemodynamic instability	• Less familiar • Potentially challenging in prone position • Risk of peri-catheter leaks • Requires expertise to insert catheter into peritoneal cavity • Need for trained staff • Dependent on consumables

Note: CRRT, continuous renal replacement therapy; IHD, intermittent haemodialysis; KRT, kidney replacement therapy; PD, peritoneal dialysis; PIRRT, prolonged intermittent renal replacement therapy.

Source: Adapted from Nadim MK, Forni LG, Mehta RL, et al. COVID-19-associated acute kidney injury: Consensus report of the 25th Acute Disease Quality Initiative (ADQI) Workgroup. *Nat Rev Nephrol.* 2020;16:747–764. Adapted under the terms of the Creative Commons Attribution 4.0 International License (http://creativecommons.org/licenses/by/4.0/).

Box 35.1 Recommendations for KRT provision during a pandemic

If resources are adequate

- It is recommended that the provision of KRT follows existing guidelines.
- The decision to initiate KRT should be based on the overall condition and prognosis of the patient, not on isolated urea or creatinine values.
- Timing of KRT initiation, vascular access site, and modality of acute KRT should be based on patient needs, local expertise, and the availability of staff and equipment.
- The dose of KRT should be based on current recommendations and be adjusted in response to changes in clinical, physiological, and/or metabolic status.
- Premature circuit clotting can interrupt KRT sessions and substantially affect the dose delivered. This complication may require the KRT prescription to be adjusted.
- If CRRT is used, it is recommended to monitor circuit life and to implement strategies to reduce the risk of circuit clotting.

If resources are limited

- Where potentially life-threatening complications of AKI are developing, such as fluid overload, hyperkalaemia, metabolic acidosis or severe uraemia, careful medical management using diuretics, potassium binding resins, and bicarbonate may be considered to temporize or potentially avoid the need for KRT in selected patients. Each case should be assessed by a senior nephrologist and/or intensivist.
- Where complications of AKI are refractory to medical therapy or become life-threatening, KRT should be started urgently unless a decision has been made not to escalate therapy.

Modality

- Modality choice may be affected by the supply of disposable materials (dialyzer filters, circuits, dialysis solutions, and anticoagulation medications), machine availability, and the availability of appropriately trained staff to operate machines and safely deliver KRT.
- All KRT modalities should be considered in COVID-19-associated AKI, but clinicians should be aware of the implications of KRT modality on fluid balance and pharmacokinetics.
- The selection of modality should be based on patient needs, local expertise, and availability of staff and equipment.
- In the event of limited machine availability, consider shorter durations of IHD or use of CRRT machines for PIRRT.
- Advantages of PIRRT or IHD include a reduced need for anticoagulation and shorter duration of therapy sessions, thereby optimizing machine and human resources to increase the number of patients who can receive KRT per day.
- If IHD or CRRT machine availability is limited, consider the use of acute PD.

Dose

- The dose of RRT should be prescribed at the beginning of the KRT session following local protocols. It should be reviewed regularly and tailored to the needs of the patient.
- There is no evidence for clinical benefit from enhanced doses of KRT in COVID-19 patients.
- Lower than usual flow rates should be considered once metabolic control has been achieved, especially if there is concern about the availability of consumables.
- If shorter durations of IHD or PIRRT are prescribed or required, fluid removal targets and KRT dose should be adjusted to achieve acceptable fluid balance targets and metabolic control.

Anticoagulation

- It is recommended that patients with COVID-19-associated AKI receive anticoagulation agents during extracorporeal KRT.
- KRT circuit performance should be closely monitored to ensure maximal circuit patency as the initial anticoagulation strategy may not be effective in all patients.
- Emphasis should be placed on best choice of site and length of vascular access to optimize circuit patency.
- It is recommended that centres establish a stepwise escalation and/or alternative plans for KRT anticoagulation.

Other supportive measures

- Patients treated with acute KRT should receive standard enteral nutrition as long as there are no significant electrolyte abnormalities or fluid overload refractory to KRT.
- In patients receiving acute KRT, medications should be reviewed regularly and adjusted as necessary.

General organization

- A coordinated response to an increase in KRT demand and/or supply chain failure at an organizational, regional, and national level is needed to deliver effective therapy to the greatest number of patients.

Note: AKI, acute kidney injury; IHD, intermittent haemodialysis; KRT, kidney replacement therapy; PD, peritoneal dialysis; PIRRT, prolonged intermittent renal replacement therapy.

Source: Data from Nadim MK, Forni LG, Mehta RL, et al. COVID-19-associated acute kidney injury: Consensus report of the 25th Acute Disease Quality Initiative (ADQI) Workgroup. *Nat Rev Nephrol.* 2020;16:747–764.

or urgent PD in selected patients, may help reduce CRRT demand. Conditions may change quickly so that adjustments may have to be made on a regular basis and often without much warning. Sudden supply failures and limited availability of consumables, including dialysis fluid, represent a major challenge. Potential solutions to maintain KRT capacity include the application of IHD (provided access to online-generated dialysate is available), the use of acute PD, and in-house production of dialysis fluid.[55] Close monitoring of KRT performance and filter life is particularly important to reduce waste and to optimize the use of KRT resources (Box 35.1). These measures, coupled with local, regional, and national multi-centre collaboration, and a corresponding increase in trained medical and nursing staff may avoid downstream rationing of care and save lives during the peak of a pandemic.[56] Many healthcare agencies have authorized emergency use of various extracorporeal blood purification techniques, including haemoperfusion, adsorption, plasma exchange, and CRRT with special membranes to remove inflammatory molecules and viral particles.[56,57] However, these techniques have not yet been formally studied in this patient population. Future trials should measure the ability of extracorporeal blood purification methods to remove target molecules, including assessment of their kinetics, to confirm the pathophysiological rationale for their use in critically ill patients with COVID-19. Prospective RCTs are also needed to investigate whether the use of extracorporeal blood purification techniques is associated with improved outcomes, including the prevention and mitigation of AKI and other organ failures.

35.6 Pharmacological Treatment and Superinfections

Matteo Bassetti and Daniele Roberto Giacobbe

- The pharmacological approach to COVID-19 is generally based on anti-viral and anti-inflammatory drugs, reflecting the intention to counteract the two different components that may participate to organ damage: (i) the virus and (ii) a dysregulated host response to the virus.
- Anti-viral, anti-inflammatory, anti-dysregulated host response, and anti-coagulant agents have been proposed as possible pharmacological tools in patients with COVID-19.
- A crucial aspect of the pharmacological approach to critically ill patients with COVID-19 is the treatment of bacterial and fungal superinfections.

- Alternative agents/dosages to the recommended dexamethasone 6 mg/d are also reasonably expected to provide benefits, but the related evidence currently stems from smaller RCTs or remains inconclusive.
- From a theoretical standpoint, it is reasonable to suppose that higher dosages of prophylactic anti-coagulants (sometimes called enhanced dosages) may be beneficial in selected subgroups of critically ill patients with COVID-19. This is suggested prior to but not in the ICU. Thus, the role of enhanced thromboprophylaxis, beyond standard prophylaxis or therapy for confirmed thrombosis, is not proven and still to be clarified.
- The use of antibiotics in critically ill patients with COVID-19 and suspected but not proven bacterial co-infection remains controversial, with a judicious use being ultimately suggested coupled with improvements in the diagnostics of bacterial infections in patients with COVID-19.

- To understand whether future anti-viral agents may have a role in the treatment of critically ill patients with COVID-19.
- To further compare the efficacy of different steroid agents and of different steroid dosages in critically ill patients with COVID-19.
- To understand how to prevent/reduce the development of nonreversible pulmonary fibrosis in survivors from severe COVID-19 pneumonia.
- The role of post-exposure prophylactic agents in reducing infection rates and/or disease severity following exposure to infection in those vaccinated or not.

Introduction

From a therapeutic perspective, a peculiar aspect of SARS-CoV-2 is its rapid worldwide spread. Indeed, this initially implied a complete lack of high-level evidence on any possible pharmacological treatment for COVID-19, with administration of anti-viral and anti-inflammatory treatment being based on compassionate or off-label uses on most occasions.[58] Subsequently, results from large RCTs have become available, which have allowed a more solid, evidence-based approach to the pharmacological treatment of COVID-19 in the critically ill patient, although grey areas deserving further study still remain.

Pharmacological Management of COVID-19

The pharmacological approach to COVID-19 is generally based on anti-viral and anti-inflammatory drugs, reflecting the intention to counteract the two different components that may participate to organ damage: (i) the virus and (ii) a dysregulated host response to the virus. Furthermore, anti-coagulant agents are administered for preventing or treating thrombotic complications connected to the disease pathophysiology. A summary of the results from pertinent RCTs is available in Table 35.2, whereas a narrative brief presentation of agents employed for the treatment of critically ill patients with COVID-19 is provided in the following paragraphs. Clearly, the rapidly evolving evidence base for therapeutic successes pre and with hospital implies the need to review the most updated evidence sources, which is beyond this chapter.

Anti-viral Agents

Among anti-viral agents, the nucleotide analogue remdesivir was extensively studied during the first year of the pandemic. While on the one hand a possible favourable impact on mortality has been reported in patients with COVID-19 requiring supplementary oxygen/non-invasive ventilation (conditionally supporting the use of remdesivir), on the other hand the results of the ACTT-1 and SOLIDARITY RCTs consistently showed a lack of effect in patients on IMV, in whom the use of remdesivir is thus currently not recommended.[59,60] No other marketed anti-viral agents, or agents with in vitro anti-viral activity, are currently recommended for the treatment of critically ill patients with COVID-19 because either of lack of results from large RCTs or lack of efficacy in large RCTs. Of note, neutralizing monoclonal antibodies are currently recommended in outpatients at risk of disease progression and seronegative patients admitted to hospital or ICU. Newer anti-viral agents such as molnupiravir and nirmatrevir/ritonavir have also demonstrated proven benefit in at-risk patients in outpatient settings, but in critically ill patients at a later stage in the disease they are not currently recommended.

Anti-inflammatory Agents

Regarding anti-inflammatory agents, at the beginning of the pandemic the use of steroids was highly controversial due to previous conflicting evidence on their efficacy stemming from small experiences in patients with severe MERS-CoV and SARS-CoV-1 infections and concerns regarding the possible persistence of viraemia

Table 35.2 Pharmacological treatment of COVID-19 in critically ill patients requiring invasive mechanical ventilation

Drug	Mechanism of action/ purpose	Results from large RCTs	Key messages/controversies
Remdesivir (not recommended)	• Adenosine analogue that binds to RNA-dependent RNA polymerase, acting as an RNA chain terminator	• In the subgroup of ventilated patients in open-label SOLIDARITY RCT, the 28-day mortality was 43% (98/524) and 38% (71/233) in remdesivir and standard care arms, respectively (OR 1.20, with 95% CI from 0.80 to 1.80), whereas in the double-blind ACTT-1 RCT, in the subgroup of invasively ventilated patients, the 28-day mortality was 22% (28/131) and 19% (29/154) in remdesivir and placebo arms, respectively (OR 1.13, with 95% CI from 0.57 to 2.23)[59,60]	• While a possible favourable effect of remdesivir, despite without a large effect size, cannot be ruled out in non-invasively ventilated patients with COVID-19 requiring supplemental oxygen, no favourable effect of remdesivir has been registered in invasively ventilated critically ill patients with COVID-19, and remdesivir is thus not recommended in this population
Steroids (recommended)	• Reduction of the host inflammatory response through interaction with glucocorticoids receptors	• The beneficial effect on mortality of dexamethasone (6 mg/d for up to 10 days) in the RECOVERY RCT was apparently more marked in the subgroup of patients receiving invasive mechanical ventilation (29% [95/324] versus 41% [283/683] in dexamethasone and usual care arms, respectively: rate ratio 0.64, with 95% CI from 0.51 to 0.81)[61] • Other studies have explored the possible role of hydrocortisone, methylprednisolone, or other dexamethasone dosages in critically ill patients with COVID-19, with either conflicting or encouraging but preliminary results	• Up to now, the more strikingly RCT-derived protective effect from mortality in critically ill patients with COVID-19 has been observed after the administration of dexamethasone 6 mg/d for up to 10 days • Alternative agents/dosages to dexamethasone 6 mg/d are also reasonably expected to provide benefit, although the related evidence currently stems from smaller RCTs or remains inconclusive
Tocilizumab (conditionally recommended)	• Humanized monoclonal IgG1 antibody that inhibits both membrane-bound and soluble IL-6 receptors	• In the REMAP-CAP RCT, 353, 48, and 402 patients were assigned to tocilizumab, sarilumab (also inhibiting IL-6), and standard care, respectively. Patients were enrolled within 24 h after starting organ support in ICU. In a Bayesian analysis, cumulative ORs for organ support-free days were 1.64 (with 95% credible interval from 1.25 to 2.14) and 1.76 (with 95% credible interval from 1.17 to 2.91) for tocilizumab and sarilumab, respectively, as compared to standard care (with posterior probabilities of superiority to standard care higher than 99.9% and of 99.5%, respectively). With regard to 90-day survival, the HR for IL-16 inhibitors versus standard care was 1.61 (with 95% credible interval from 1.25 to 2.08), with a posterior probability of superiority higher than 99.9%[63] • In the RECOVERY RCT (in which subjects with progressive COVID-19 and CRP ≥75 mg/L were considered for enrolment), the patients receiving invasive mechanical ventilation at baseline in tocilizumab and standard care arms were 268/2022 (13%) and 294/2094 (14%), respectively. In the entire cohort, tocilizumab was associated with reduced 28-day mortality (31% [621/2022] versus 35% [729/2094]: risk ratio 0.85, with 95% CI from 0.76 to 0.94). In patients receiving invasive mechanical ventilation at baseline, mortality was 49% (131/268) and 51% (149/294) in tocilizumab and usual care arms, respectively (risk ratio 0.94, with 95% CI from 0.74 to 1.18). In subgroup analyses, consistent results were observed in patients with progressive disease previously treated with steroids[62]	• The recommendation for tocilizumab is conditional, with administration within 24 h of organ support initiation in ICU to be considered for patients with increased inflammatory markers and with a progressive disease who do not respond to steroid treatment • Administration of tocilizumab should be avoided in patients with severe immunosuppression or in patients with contraindications (risk of gastrointestinal perforation; increased of transaminases >5 times the upper limit of normal; low platelet count)
Anti-coagulants (recommended)	• Reduction of the risk of micro-thrombosis and macro-thrombosis connected to endothelial injury and prothrombic status	• In the INSPIRATION RCT, the primary efficacy end point (a composite of venous or arterial thrombosis, treatment with extracorporeal membrane oxygenation, or mortality within 30 days) was registered in 46% and 44% of patients in intermediate dosage (enoxaparin, 1 mg/kg daily) versus standard thromboprophylaxis (enoxaparin 40 mg/d) arms, respectively (absolute risk difference 1.5%, with 95% CI from −6.6% to 9.8%). Major bleeding occurred in 2.5% and 1.4% of patients in intermediate and standard thromboprophylaxis arms, respectively. Severe thrombocytopenia was more frequent in the intermediate dosage arm (2.2% versus 0%: risk difference 2.2%, with 95% CI from 0.4% to 3.8%)[65] • Combined REMAP-CAP, ACTIV-4, and ATTACC RCTs, median organ support-free days and hospital survival were comparable between therapeutic dosage (with unfractionated or low molecular weight heparin) and local standard thromboprophylaxis arms, respectively, with major bleeding occurring in 3.1% and 2.4% of patients in therapeutic dosage and standard thromboprophylaxis arms, respectively[64]	• While it is clear that prophylaxis with anti-coagulants is necessary (and that anti-coagulant therapy is necessary in patients with thrombotic complications), selected subgroups of patients in intensive care that may benefit from intermediate/therapeutic versus standard dosages for prophylactic purposes are still to be delineated

CI, confidence interval; COVID-19, coronavirus disease 2019; CRP; C-reactive protein; HR, hazard ratio; ICU, intensive care unit; OR, odds ratio; RCT, randomized controlled trial.

and its consequences. Then, after some encouraging results from observational studies in patients with COVID-19 but limited by non-negligible confounding, the results from the open-label adaptive platform RECOVERY RCT showed a remarkable benefit of intravenous dexamethasone (6 mg once daily for up to 10 days) versus standard care with respect to the primary end point of 28-day mortality, especially in critically ill patients.[61] Alternative agents/dosages to dexamethasone 6 mg/d are also reasonably expected to provide benefits, although the related evidence currently stems from smaller RCTs or remains inconclusive. Higher doses in those without an expected clinical response have been suggested to possibly be effective in a portion of patients but only in a multidisciplinary setting without evidence base or current knowledge of the optimal timing and benefit risk in the short or medium term. Another agent counteracting a dysregulated host response that has been proven efficacious in selected critically ill patients with COVID-19 is tocilizumab (or the lesser used sarilumab), a monoclonal antibody inhibiting the pro-inflammatory cytokine interleukin 6 (IL-6). The timeline of the use of tocilizumab in critically ill patients with COVID-19 during the course of the pandemic is somewhat peculiar, with an initial widespread off-label use at the beginning, a subsequent avoidance based on lack of efficacy suggested in the first released RCTs, and then a resurgence of use in selected subgroups of critically ill patients (e.g. administration within 24 h organ support initiation in patients with worsening condition despite previous steroid treatment) based on the results of the REMAP-CAP and RECOVERY RCTs.[62,63] Other agents counteracting the host response (e.g. baricitinib, chloroquine/hydroxychloroquine, tofacitinib, colchicine, and anakinra) have been currently proven either efficacious/inefficacious in non-critically ill patients with COVID-19 or inefficacious in critically ill patients with COVID-19, and their use is thus not recommended in critically ill patients with COVID-19 at the time of writing. With regard to anti-coagulant agents, while it is clear that therapeutic dosages should be used for treating thrombotic complications, the use of prophylactic versus therapeutic dosages for the prevention of thrombotic complications in critically ill patients with COVID-19 is still debated. Recently, an analysis of three different RCTs (REMAP-CAP, ACTIV-4, and ATTACC) has been published, showing no additional benefits in ICU patients with COVID-19 receiving therapeutic dosages of anticoagulants versus standard local thromboprophylaxis. By contrast, in those moderately sick patients outside ICU, therapeutic dose heparin increased the probability of survival to hospital discharge with reduced organ support, albeit at increased bleeding risk 1.9% versus 0.9%.[64]

This is in line with the lack of additional benefits in critically ill patients with COVID-19 of intermediate versus prophylactic dosages of anti-coagulants registered in the INSPIRATION RCT.[65] From a theoretical standpoint, it is reasonable to suppose that higher dosages (for prophylactic purposes, sometimes called enhanced) may be beneficial in selected subgroups

Table 35.3 Key concepts and controversies in the approach to superinfections in critically ill patients with COVID-19

Domain	Key concepts/controversies
CABP in critically ill patients with COVID-19	• At hospital admission, the possible radiological presentation of COVID-19 pneumonia as unilateral or bilateral consolidative pulmonary lesions makes it difficult to distinguish between viral pneumonia and coexistence of viral pneumonia and bacterial co-infection/superinfection, thereby possibly prompting useless antibacterial treatments with consequent risks of toxicity and resistance selection. On the other hand, it cannot be excluded that delaying antibacterial treatment in critically ill patients who truly have CABP could unfavourably influencing prognosis. This complex topic is still a matter of debate, with improved diagnostics (both phenotypical and molecular) and collection of specimens (blood and respiratory specimens) for microbiological analysis before initiation of empirical antibacterials likely being crucial for better delineating selected patients that may benefit from antibacterial therapy (or from non-initiation/early discontinuation of antibacterial therapy).
HABP/VABP/BSI in critically ill patients with COVID-19	• Like classical ICU populations, also COVID-19 patients should be considered at risk for developing BSI, HABP, or VABP. An important difference with classical populations is the administration of anti-inflammatory agents for the treatment of COVID-19 pneumonia, which may mitigate the increase of serum inflammatory markers, rendering it more difficult to recognize the superimposed infectious process. Up to now, no specific, consistent distribution of causative agents has been demonstrated in critically ill COVID-19 patients with superimposed BSI/HABP/VABP, with Gram-positive bacteria and Gram-negative bacteria alternatively reported as the predominant aetiology in different observational studies.
Invasive mould diseases in critically ill patients with COVID-19	• Prevalence of CAPA has been variably reported from 0% to 33% in critically ill patients with COVID-19, likely reflecting the presence of a true prevalence heterogeneity but also the diagnostic difficulties surrounding this entity. Indeed, serum fungal markers are of limited value and there are no specific radiological lesions, with recognition being also hampered by the concomitant presence of pulmonary lesions connected to the baseline viral disease. In this scenario, bronchoscopy remains fundamental, both to recognize possible *Aspergillus* tracheobronchitis and for collecting bronchoalveolar lavage fluid specimens for culture and galactomannan dosage, lateral flow tests, and molecular tests. Specific diagnostic criteria for CAPA and approaches to CAPA in critically ill patients are available in the literature.[14,16] Another possible invasive fungal disease in critically ill patients with COVID-19 is mucormicosis, especially reported, but not only, from low- and middle-income countries.[70] The most common presentations are rhino-orbito-cerebral mucormycosis and pulmonary mucormycosis, with microbiological diagnostic confirmation being highly recommended. Glycaemic control, reduction/discontinuation of steroid treatment, rapid evaluation for surgical debridement, and antifungal therapy are the cornerstones of a proper multidisciplinary approach to mucormycosis in COVID-19 critically ill patients.
Reactivation of CMV, HSV, and VZV infections in critically il patients with COVID-19	• While increases in the blood and lower respiratory tract viral loads of CMV, HSV, and VZV have been widely reported, whether this is truly an expression of systemic disease with organ damage needing anti-viral treatment has still to be clearly established. Although it appears reasonable to consider specific anti-viral treatment when responsibility of viral reactivation for a superimposed organ damage is probable according to the disease course, further evidence is urgently needed to correctly guide the management of possible viral reactivations in critically ill patients with COVID-19.

CABP, community-acquired bacterial pneumonia; CAPA, COVID-19-associated pulmonary aspergillosis; CMV, cytomegalovirus; COVID-19, coronavirus disease 2019; HABP, hospital-acquired bacterial pneumonia; HSV, herpes simplex virus; ICU, intensive care unit; VABP, ventilator-associated bacterial pneumonia; VZV, varicella-zoster virus.

of moderately sick patients with COVID-19, perhaps at a stage where the antithrombin III levels and other co-factors for heparin, as well as intrinsic fibrinolytic mechanisms, are still more effective than at the later stage of critical illness. These uncertainties are nonetheless still to be clearly delineated.

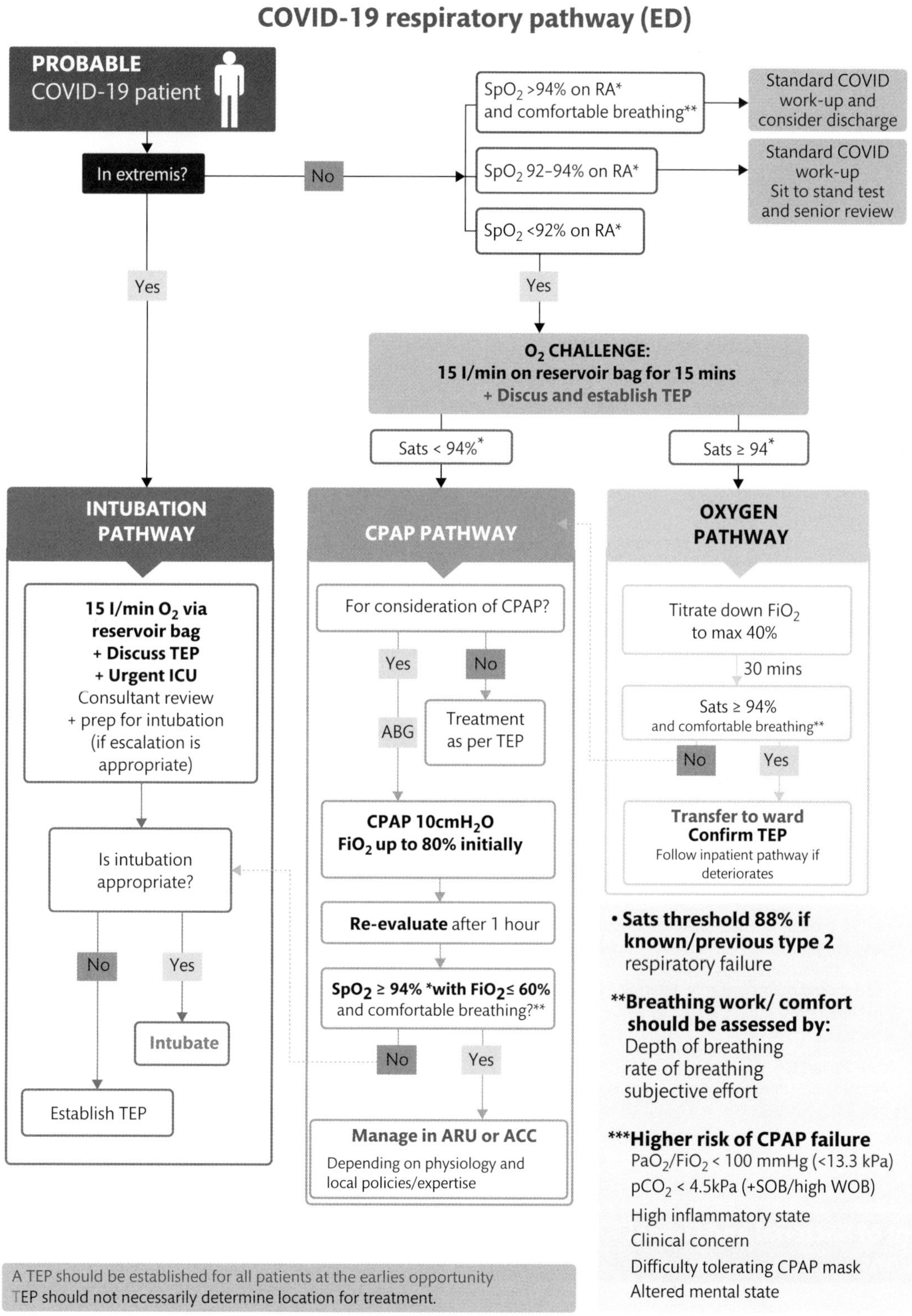

Adapted from University College London Hospitals COVID guidelines

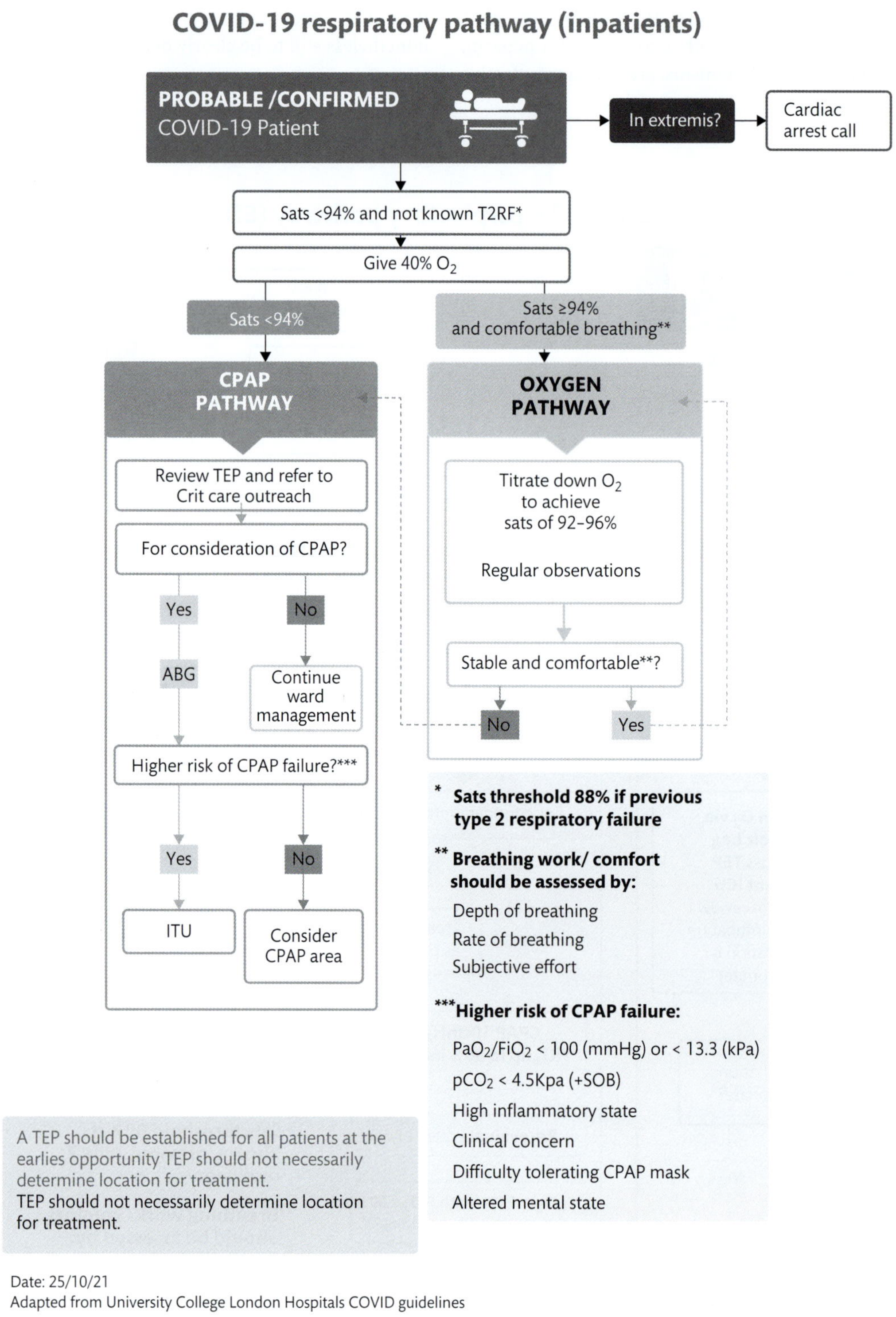

Management of Bacterial and Fungal Superinfections

An additional crucial aspect of the pharmacological approach to critically ill patients with COVID-19 is the treatment of bacterial and fungal superinfections. In comparison to the standard approach to these infectious processes in classical ICU populations, some particular aspects should be highlighted when dealing with COVID-19 patients: (i) some specific COVID-19 superinfections, like COVID-19-associated pulmonary aspergillosis, have been described and are increasingly being understood in their clinical, laboratory, and radiology characteristics to improve their recognition,[66] while reports of mucormycosis in India have been reported; (ii) the possible absent or reduced increase in classical laboratory markers (e.g. C-reactive protein) of bacterial and fungal infections in critically ill patients treated with anti-inflammatory agents (e.g. tocilizumab) should raise awareness and suspicion about non-classical presentations of superinfections in COVID-19 patients.[67] The utility of fungal markers such as beta D glucan and galactomannan has been advocated in this regard, for diagnosis and monitoring adjuncts to clinical response. Against this backdrop, antibiotic and diagnostic stewardship will play a critical role. Indeed, clinic skills in recognizing subtle clinical presentations of superinfections combined with optimal laboratory diagnostic support (through both phenotypical and molecular diagnostics) are crucial for differentiating the manifestation due to the underlying viral disease and the superimposed bacterial or fungal infections, thereby allowing an appropriate yet selected use of antibacterial and antifungals agents. Since development and spread of antibiotic and antifungal resistance in critically ill patients with COVID-19 has been reported from many parts of the world,[68,69] judicious use of antibiotic and antifungal agents in critically ill patients with COVID-19 is likely essential for avoiding as much as possible an excessive selective pressure for antimicrobial resistance, together with adequate infection-control measures. A summary of key concepts and controversies in the therapeutic approach to superinfections in critically ill patients with COVID-19 is available in Table 35.3.

REFERENCES

1. COVID-19 Map—Johns Hopkins Coronavirus Resource Center [Internet] 2020. Available from: https://coronavirus.jhu.edu/map.html
2. Wu Z, McGoogan JM. Characteristics of and important lessons from the coronavirus disease 2019 (COVID-19) outbreak in China: Summary of a report of 72314 cases from the Chinese Center for Disease Control and Prevention. *JAMA*. 2020;**323**:1239–1242.
3. Richardson S, Hirsch JS, Narasimhan M, et al. Presenting characteristics, comorbidities, and outcomes among 5700 patients hospitalized with COVID-19 in the New York City Area. *JAMA*; 2020;**323**:2052–2059.
4. Grasselli G, Pesenti A, Cecconi M. Critical care utilization for the COVID-19 outbreak in Lombardy, Italy: Early experience and forecast during an emergency response. *JAMA*. 2020;**323**:1545–1546.
5. Wunsch H. Mechanical ventilation in COVID-19: Interpreting the current epidemiology. *Am J Respir Crit Care Med*. 2020;**202**:1–4.
6. COVID-19 Clinical management: Living guidance [Internet]. [cited 2021 Aug 10]. Available from: https://www.who.int/publications/i/item/WHO-2019-nCoV-clinical-2023.1
7. African COVID-19 Critical Care Outcomes Study (ACCCOS) Investigators. Patient care and clinical outcomes for patients with COVID-19 infection admitted to African high-care or intensive care units (ACCCOS): A multicentre, prospective, observational cohort study. *Lancet*. 2021;**397**:1885–1894.
8. Lim ZJ, Subramaniam A, Ponnapa Reddy M, et al. Case fatality rates for patients with COVID-19 requiring invasive mechanical ventilation. A meta-analysis. *Am J Respir Crit Care Med*. 2021;**203**:54–66.
9. Scientific Evidence for Conditions that Increase Risk of Severe Illness | COVID-19 | CDC [Internet]. [cited 2021 Aug 10]. Available from: https://www.cdc.gov/coronavirus/2019-ncov/science/science-briefs/underlying-evidence-table.html
10. Docherty AB, Harrison EM, Green CA, et al. Features of 20 133 UK patients in hospital with covid-19 using the ISARIC WHO Clinical Characterisation Protocol: Prospective observational cohort study. *BMJ*. 2020;**369**:m1985.
11. COVID-ICU Group on behalf of the REVA Network and the COVID-ICU Investigators. Clinical characteristics and day-90 outcomes of 4244 critically ill adults with COVID-19: A prospective cohort study. *Intensive Care Med*. 2021;**47**:60–73.
12. Geerts JM, Kinnair D, Taheri P, et al. Guidance for health care leaders during the recovery stage of the COVID-19 pandemic: A consensus statement. *JAMA Netw Open*. 2021;**4**:e2120295.
13. Ou X, Liu Y, Lei X, et al. Characterization of spike glycoprotein of SARS-CoV-2 on virus entry and its immune cross-reactivity with SARS-CoV. *Nat Commun*. 2021;**11**:1620.
14. Bhattacharyya C, Das C, Ghosh A, et al. SARS-CoV-2 mutation 614G creates an elastase cleavage site enhancing its spread in high AAT-deficient regions. *Infect Genet Evol*. 2021;**90**:104760.
15. Lopes-Pacheco M, Silva PL, Cruz FF, et al. Pathogenesis of multiple organ injury in COVID-19 and potential therapeutic strategies. *Front Physiol*. 2021;**12**:593223.
16. Robba C, Battaglini D, Pelosi P, et al. Multiple organ dysfunction in SARS-CoV-2: MODS-CoV-2. *Expert Rev Respir Med*. 2020;**14**:865–868.
17. Sungnak W, Huang N, Becavin C, et al. SARS-CoV-2 entry factors are highly expressed in nasal epithelial cells together with innate immune genes. *Nat Med*. 2020;**26**:681–687.
18. Bunyavanich S, Do A, Vicencio A. Nasal gene expression of angiotensin-converting enzyme 2 in children and adults. *JAMA*. 2020;**323**:2427–2429.
19. Varga Z, Flammer AJ, Steiger P, et al. Endothelial cell infection and endotheliitis in COVID-19. *Lancet*. 2020;**395**:1417–1418.
20. Barnes GD, Burnett A, Allen A, et al. Thromboembolism and anticoagulant therapy during the COVID-19 pandemic: Interim clinical guidance from the anticoagulation forum. *J Thromb Thrombolysis*. 2020:**50**:72–81.
21. Fan C, Lu W, Li K, et al. ACE2 expression in kidney and testis may cause kidney and testis infection in COVID-19 patients. *Front Med (Lausanne)*. 2020;**7**:563893.
22. Battaglini D, Santori G, Chandraptham K, et al. Neurological complications and noninvasive multimodal neuromonitoring in critically ill mechanically ventilated COVID-19 patients. *Front Neurol*. 2020;**11**:602114.
23. Benetti E, Tita R, Spiga O, et al. ACE2 gene variants may underlie interindividual variability and susceptibility to COVID-19 in the Italian population. *Eur J Hum Genet*. 2020;**28**:1602–1614.
24. Robba C, Battaglini D, Ball L, et al. Distinct phenotypes require distinct respiratory management strategies in severe COVID-19. *Respir Physiol Neurobiol*. 2020;**279**: 103455
25. Marini JJ, Gattinoni L. Management of COVID-19 respiratory distress. *JAMA*. 2020;**323**:2329–2330.
26. Chiumello D, Busana M, Coppola S, et al. Physiological and quantitative CT-scan characterization of COVID-19 and typical

ARDS: A matched cohort study. *Intensive Care Med.* 2020; **46**:2187–2196.

27. Ball L, Robba C, Herrmann J, et al. Lung distribution of gas and blood volume in critically ill COVID-19 patients: A quantitative dual-energy computed tomography study. *Crit Care.* 2021; **25**:214.
28. Zucman N, Mullaert J, Roux D, et al. Prediction of outcome of nasal high flow use during COVID-19-related acute hypoxemic respiratory failure. *Intensive Care Med.* 2020; **46**:1924–1926.
29. Amirfarzan H, Cereda M, Gaulton TG, et al. Use of helmet CPAP in COVID-19—a practical review. *Pulmonology.* 2021;**27**:413–422.
30. Cabrini L, Landoni G, Zangrillo A. Minimise nosocomial spread of 2019-nCoV when treating acute respiratory failure. *Lancet* 2020;**395**:685.
31. Grieco DL, Menga LS, Cesarano M, et al. Effect of helmet noninvasive ventilation vs high-flow nasal oxygen on days free of respiratory support in patients with COVID-19 and moderate to severe hypoxemic respiratory failure: The HENIVOT randomized clinical trial. *JAMA.* 2021;**325**:1731–1743.
32. Mauri T, Spinelli E, Scotti E, et al. Potential for lung recruitment and ventilation-perfusion mismatch in patients with the acute respiratory distress syndrome from coronavirus disease 2019. *Crit Care Med.* 2020;**48**:1129–1134.
33. Ball L, Robba C, Maiello L, et al. Computed tomography assessment of PEEP-induced alveolar recruitment in patients with severe COVID-19 pneumonia. *Crit Care.* 2021;**25**: 81.
34. Barbaro RP, MacLaren G, Boonstra PS, et al. Extracorporeal membrane oxygenation support in COVID-19: An international cohort study of the Extracorporeal Life Support Organization registry. *Lancet.* 2020;**396**:1071–1078.
35. Grasselli G, Tonetti T, Protti A, et al. Pathophysiology of COVID-19-associated acute respiratory distress syndrome: A multicentre prospective observational study. *Lancet. Resp Med.* 2020;**8**:1201–1208.
36. Wiersinga W.J, Rhodes A, Cheng AC, et al. Pathophysiology, transmission, diagnosis, and treatment of coronavirus disease 2019 (COVID-19): A review. *JAMA.* 2020;**324**: 782–793.
37. Varga Z, Flammer AJ, Steiger P, et al. Endothelial cell infection and endotheliitis in COVID-19. *Lancet.* 2020;**395**:1417–1418.
38. Sultan S, Altayar O, Siddique SM, et al. AGA institute rapid review of the gastrointestinal and liver manifestations of COVID-19, meta-analysis of international data, and recommendations for the consultative management of patients with COVID-19. *Gastroenterology.* 2020;**159**:320–334.e327.
39. Guo T, Fan Y, Chen M, et al. Cardiovascular implications of fatal outcomes of patients with coronavirus disease 2019 (COVID-19). *JAMA Cardiology.* 2020;**5**:811–818.
40. Knight DS, Kotecha T, Razvi Y, et al. COVID-19: Myocardial injury in survivors. *Circulation.* 2020;**142**:1120–1122.
41. Martin L, Derwall M, Al Zoubi S, et al. The septic heart: Current understanding of molecular mechanisms and clinical implications. *Chest.* 2019;**155**:427–437.
42. Alhazzani W, Moller MH, Arabi YM, et al. Surviving Sepsis Campaign: Guidelines on the management of critically ill adults with Coronavirus Disease 2019 (COVID-19). *Intensive Care Med.* 2020;**46**:854–887.
43. Chapman AR, Bularga A, Mills NL. High-sensitivity cardiac troponin can be an ally in the fight against COVID-19. *Circulation.* 2020;**141**:1733–1735.
44. Messina A, Greco M, Cecconi M. What should I use next if clinical evaluation and echocardiographic haemodynamic assessment is not enough? *Curr Op Crit Care.* 2019; **25**:259–265.
45. Messina A, Sanfilippo F, Milani A, et al. COVID-19-related echocardiographic patterns of cardiovascular dysfunction in critically ill patients: A systematic review of the current literature. *J Crit Care.* 2021;**65**:26–35.
46. Dweck MR, Bularga A, Hahn RT, et al. Global evaluation of echocardiography in patients with COVID-19. *European Heart Journal—Cardiovascular Imaging.* 2020;**21**: 949–958.
47. Malas MB, Naazie IN, Elsayed N, et al. Thromboembolism risk of COVID-19 is high and associated with a higher risk of mortality: A systematic review and meta-analysis. *EClinicalMedicine.* 2020;**29**:100639.
48. Mondal S, Quintili AL. Thromboembolic disease in COVID-19 patients: A brief narrative review. *J Intensive Care.* 2020 Sep 14;**8**:70.
49. Ostermann M, Lumlertgul N, Forni LG, et al. What every Intensivist should know about COVID-19 associated acute kidney injury. *J Crit Care.* 2020;**60**:91–95.
50. Lameire N, Kellum JA. Contrast-induced acute kidney injury and renal support for acute kidney injury: A KDIGO summary. *Crit Care.* 2013;**17**:205.
51. Nadim MK, Forni LG, Mehta RL, et al. COVID-19-associated acute kidney injury: Consensus report of the 25th Acute Disease Quality Initiative (ADQI) Workgroup. *Nat Rev Nephrol.* 2020;**16**:747–764.
52. Chua HR, MacLaren G, Choong LH, et al. Ensuring sustainability of continuous kidney replacement therapy in the face of extraordinary demand: Lessons from the COVID-19 pandemic. *Am J Kidney Dis.* 2020;**76**:392–400.
53. Sourial MY, Sourial MH, Dalsan R, et al. Urgent peritoneal dialysis in patients with COVID-19 and acute kidney injury: A single-center experience in a time of crisis in the United States. *Am J Kidney Dis.* 2020;**76**:401–406.
54. Fisher R, Clarke J, Al-Arfi K, et al. Provision of acute renal replacement therapy, using three separate modalities, in critically ill patients during the COVID-19 pandemic. An after action review from a UK tertiary critical care centre. *J Crit Care.* 2021;**62**:190–196.
55. Lumlertgul N, Tunstell P, Watts C, et al. In-house production of dialysis solutions to overcome challenges during the coronavirus disease 2019 pandemic. *Kidney Int Rep.* 2021;**6**:200–206.
56. Ronco C, Bagshaw SM, Bellomo R, et al. Extracorporeal blood purification and organ support in the critically ill patient during COVID-19 pandemic: Expert review and recommendation. *Blood Purif.* 2021;**50**:17–27.
57. Ronco C, Reis T, Husain-Syed F. Management of acute kidney injury in patients with COVID-19. *Lancet Resp Med.* 2020;**8**:738–42.
58. Bassetti M, Pelosi P, Robba C, et al. A brief note on randomized controlled trials and compassionate/off-label use of drugs in the early phases of the COVID-19 pandemic. *Drugs Context.* 2020;**9**:2020-5-2.
59. Beigel JH, Tomashek KM, Dodd LE, et al. Remdesivir for the treatment of Covid-19—final report. *N Engl J Med.* 2020;**383**:1813–1826.
60. WHO Solidarity Trial Consortium, Pan H, Peto R, et al. Repurposed antiviral drugs for Covid-19—interim WHO solidarity trial results. *N Engl J Med.* 2021;**384**:497–511.
61. Group RC, Horby P, Lim WS, et al. Dexamethasone in hospitalized patients with Covid-19. *N Engl J Med.* 2021;**384**:693–704.
62. RECOVERY Collaborative Group. Tocilizumab in patients admitted to hospital with COVID-19 (RECOVERY): A randomised, controlled, open-label, platform trial. *Lancet.* 2021;**397**:1637–1645.

63. REMAP-CAP Investigators, Gordon AC, Mouncey PR, et al. Interleukin-6 Receptor Antagonists in Critically Ill Patients with Covid-19. *N Engl J Med.*2021;**384**:1491–1502.
64. REMAP-CAP Investigators; ACTIV-4a Investigators; ATTACC Investigators. Therapeutic anticoagulation with heparin in critically ill patients with Covid-19. *N Engl J Med.* 2021;**385**:777–789
65. INSPIRATION Investigators, Sadeghipour P, Talasaz AH, et al. Effect of intermediate-dose vs standard-dose prophylactic anticoagulation on thrombotic events, extracorporeal membrane oxygenation treatment, or mortality among patients with COVID-19 admitted to the intensive care unit: The INSPIRATION randomized clinical trial. *JAMA.* 2021;**325**:1620–1630.
66. Koehler P, Bassetti M, Chakrabarti A, et al. Defining and managing COVID-19-associated pulmonary aspergillosis: The 2020 ECMM/ISHAM consensus criteria for research and clinical guidance. *Lancet Infect Dis.* 2021;**21**:e149–e162.
67. Giacobbe DR, Battaglini D, Ball L, et al. Bloodstream infections in critically ill patients with COVID-19. *Eur J Clin Invest.* 2020;**50**:e13319.
68. Magnasco L, Mikulska M, Giacobbe DR, et al. Spread of carbapenem-resistant gram-negatives and *Candida auris* during the COVID-19 pandemic in critically ill patients: One step back in antimicrobial stewardship? *Microorganisms.* 2021;**9**:95.
69. Son HJ, Kim T, Lee E, et al. Risk factors for isolation of multi-drug resistant organisms in coronavirus disease 2019 pneumonia: A multicenter study. *Am J Infect Control.* 2021 Oct;**49**(10):1256–1261.
70. Rudramurthy SM, Hoenigl M, Meis JF, et al. ECMM/ISHAM recommendations for clinical management of COVID-19 associated mucormycosis in low- and middle-income countries. *Mycoses.* 2021;**64**:1028–1037.

36

Pleural Infection

Loïc Lang-Lazdunski

- The incidence of pleural infection is increasing worldwide. All patients with a pleural effusion and sepsis or pneumonia should have adequate imaging and a diagnostic pleural aspiration.
- Intercostal chest tube drainage is recommended for purulent effusions and for those cases where pleural fluid pH is less than 7.20.
- The bacteriology of pleural infection may differ significantly from the one of pneumonia. Further, bacteria involved in community-acquired pleural infection and hospital-acquired infections differ. Appropriate antibiotic strategies should recognize these differences.
- The combination of tPA and DNase is the only proven intrapleural therapy significantly improving outcomes in patients whose tube drainage alone is inadequate.
- Patients failing to improve clinically after 5 days of maximal medical management should be referred to a thoracic surgeon for consideration of thoracoscopic debridement of empyema. Late referral significantly increases the risk of thoracotomy.

- Is there an optimal size of chest tube for drainage of the pleural space? Current evidence suggests that small-bore tubes should now be considered as first line.
- Comparison of video-assisted thoracic surgery (VATS) against the combination of intrapleural tPA and DNAse in the treatment of pleural infection. The mid-term complications of surgery must also be taken into consideration.

- The exact role and timing of surgery remains controversial. The role of early thoracoscopic debridement should be evaluated in a large randomized controlled trial.

Introduction

Pleural infection is a common complication of pneumonia, affecting approximately 80,000 patients per year in the USA and UK alone.[1–4] Pleural infection significantly increases the morbidity and mortality associated with pulmonary infections, with a mortality rate in adults approaching 20%.[1–4] The incidence of pleural infection appears to be increasing globally, across all age ranges. However, pleural infection is more common in paediatric and elderly populations. Pleural infection is more common in men than in women, and its incidence is higher in patients with diabetes mellitus, chronic lung disease, rheumatoid arthritis, or those with a history of alcohol and substance abuse.[1] Staphylococcal-related infections are generally associated with longer hospital stays and higher in-hospital mortality. The increasing incidence of aerobic Gram-negative bacteria found in ICU patients, antibiotic resistance, and high mortality associated with empyema in ICU patients (>40% in some series) is a major concern. This chapter summarizes recent advances in the management of pleural infections including recently published evidence and the latest clinical guidelines. Pleural tuberculosis will not be covered in this chapter.

Physiology and Bacteriology

Initially, pleural fluid accumulates in the pleural cavity due to increased permeability of the pleural membranes in response to inflammation. Fluid moves into the pleural space due to locally increased capillary vascular permeability, activation of immune response (e.g. neutrophil migration), and release of proinflammatory cytokines (e.g. Il-6, Il-8, and TNF-α).[1] At early stage, pleural fluid has a normal glucose level (>40 mg/dL) and pH (>7.20) and is sterile. This is a simple parapneumonic effusion, defined as an exudative pleural fluid collection, free flowing, and without evidence of bacterial infection or white cell activity. It is most likely type of effusion to resolve without pleural drainage. A Complicated parapneumonic effusion refers to a pleural fluid collection resulting from bacterial pneumonia, lung abscess, or bronchiectasis, where there is biochemical evidence of early bacterial invasion and fibrinous septations. Empyema is defined as a purulent fluid collection in the pleural space. Although pneumonia remains the most common cause of pleural infection, lung abscess, bronchopleural fistula, oesophageal perforation, post-surgical infections, aspiration, penetrating chest trauma, and subphrenic abscess may also result in empyema. Iatrogenia (repeated pleural aspirations or drainage) represent a non-exceptional cause of pleural infection in patients with malignant or chronic pleural effusion.

There are classically three stages in the evolution of pleural infection. *Stage 1* is the *exudative stage* where only a small amount of free fluid is present in the pleural space. *Stage 2* is the *fibrino-purulent stage*, characterized by higher neutrophil count and fibrin deposition. At this stage, it is common for pleural fluid to be loculated. *Stage 3* is the organized stage where fibroblasts grow into the pleural membranes and produce a thick pleural peel causing lung trapping and preventing lung re-expansion. This process is driven by mediators such as platelet-derived growth factor and transforming growth factor beta. At this stage of 'organized empyema', chest tube drainage and intrapleural fibrinolytics are likely to fail and surgery is often the only valid therapeutic option. Classically, stage 3 is observed after 3 weeks from the onset of pleural infection. However, there is marked inter-individual variation and approximately 50% of patients do not have fibrous pleural scarring even 3 weeks after the onset of pleural infection.

Bacteriology

Streptococcus pneumoniae, *S. pyogenes*, and *Staphylococcus aureus* are the organisms traditionally associated with pleural infection.[2,5–7] Additionally, the *S. milleri* group consisting of *S. anginosus*, *S. intermedius*, and *S. constellatus* are part of the normal human flora which become significant in the setting of pleural infection, accounting for 30%–50% of adult cases of community-acquired empyema. *S. aureus* is more commonly seen in the older, hospitalized patient with co-morbidities. It is often associated with cavitation and abscess formation, with empyema present in up to 25% of adult cases. Increasing numbers of cases of empyema caused by community-acquired multi-resistant *S. aureus* (MRSA) are being reported, and this pathogen should be considered in the appropriate setting of both community- and hospital-acquired empyema. Anaerobic bacteria significantly contribute to pleural infection, being identified as the sole or co-pathogen in 25%–76% of cases. The importance of differentiating community-acquired empyema from hospital-acquired empyema is crucial as the latter often has a different bacteriology. Organisms such as MRSA, *Enterobacteriaceae*, and anaerobes are more prevalent in nosocomial empyema. Awareness of local prevalence and antimicrobial sensitivities is essential to guide clinical decisions and antibiotic selection. Identification of the causative pathogen(s) in pleural infection can be difficult, with the microbiological diagnosis remaining elusive in up to 40% of cases despite standard pleural fluid culture.[1,6] The yield of causative organisms can be significantly increased by the use of bacterial nucleic acid amplification.[6,8] In the MIST-1 study, a microbiological diagnosis was achieved in 58% of patients, with a further 16% achieving diagnosis using nucleic acid amplification techniques (bacterial DNA polymerase chain reaction). Interestingly, only 12% of patients had positive blood cultures.[9]

Atypical Bacterial, Fungal, and Parasitic Infections

Pleural diseases due to atypical organisms are uncommon. The majority of these infections are considered opportunistic and are more commonly observed in immuno-suppressed patients (e.g. AIDS, malignancies, immunosuppression, and transplant).[10]

Viral Infections

Viruses such as adenovirus, hantavirus, cytomegalovirus, herpes virus, hepatitis, Epstein-Barr virus, and arbovirus can cause pleural effusions. Those effusions are usually small and in general pleural fluid is not aspirated for diagnosis. These effusions are commonly exudates showing lymphocytic predominance. Most of them resolve spontaneously.[10] During the COVID-19 pandemic, SARS-CoV-2 infection has represented a common cause of pleural effusion and empyema in critically patients with sometimes atypical microbiology.[11]

Current Accepted Practice

Diagnosis

Clinical Presentation

Clinical presentations can range from severe sepsis to a relatively indolent presentation with low-grade fever and weight loss. A high index of suspicion is required for the diagnosis of pleural infection. Patients may simply present with a pleural effusion on chest X-ray in the setting of pneumonia. Patients may also present with fever, pleuritic chest pain, cough, purulent sputum, and dyspnoea. Of note, the absence of pleuritic pain does not exclude pleural infection. Further, no specific clinical feature accurately predicts the need for pleural drainage. Needle aspiration of a pleural effusion is generally required to find out whether the pleural space is infected or not[12] (Figure 36.1).

Imaging

Chest X-ray

Chest X-ray has long been the initial radiologic investigation for the assessment of a chest infection or pleural effusion. Chest X-ray will usually show a pleural effusion with or without lung parenchyma abnormalities. Pleural effusions may be bilateral, the larger usually on the side primarily affected by pneumonia. In the setting of complex effusions, septations and air fluid levels may be apparent.[13–14]

Pleural Ultrasound

The last decade has seen a significant trend to employ pleural ultrasound (US) at the bedside to assess for the presence of pleural effusion in patients with suspected or proven pleural infection. The advent of affordable and portable ultrasound has made bedside procedures possible in hospital rooms, emergency departments, intensive care units, and surgical theatres. Pleural ultrasound is fast, safe, and effective in confirming the presence of pleural fluid, loculations, pleural peel, and in localizing the optimal site for diagnostic tap and therapeutic intervention (chest tube insertion and thoracoscopic debridement).[15–18]

Computed Tomography (CT)

Pleural effusions are commonly detected on CTs performed for the assessment of pneumonia. In terms of diagnosis and planning of intervention, contrast-enhanced thoracic CT with correct timing of contrast injection allowing better definition of the pleural abnormalities is the imaging investigation of choice at most centres. Chest CT allows not only the assessment of the pleura itself but chest tube

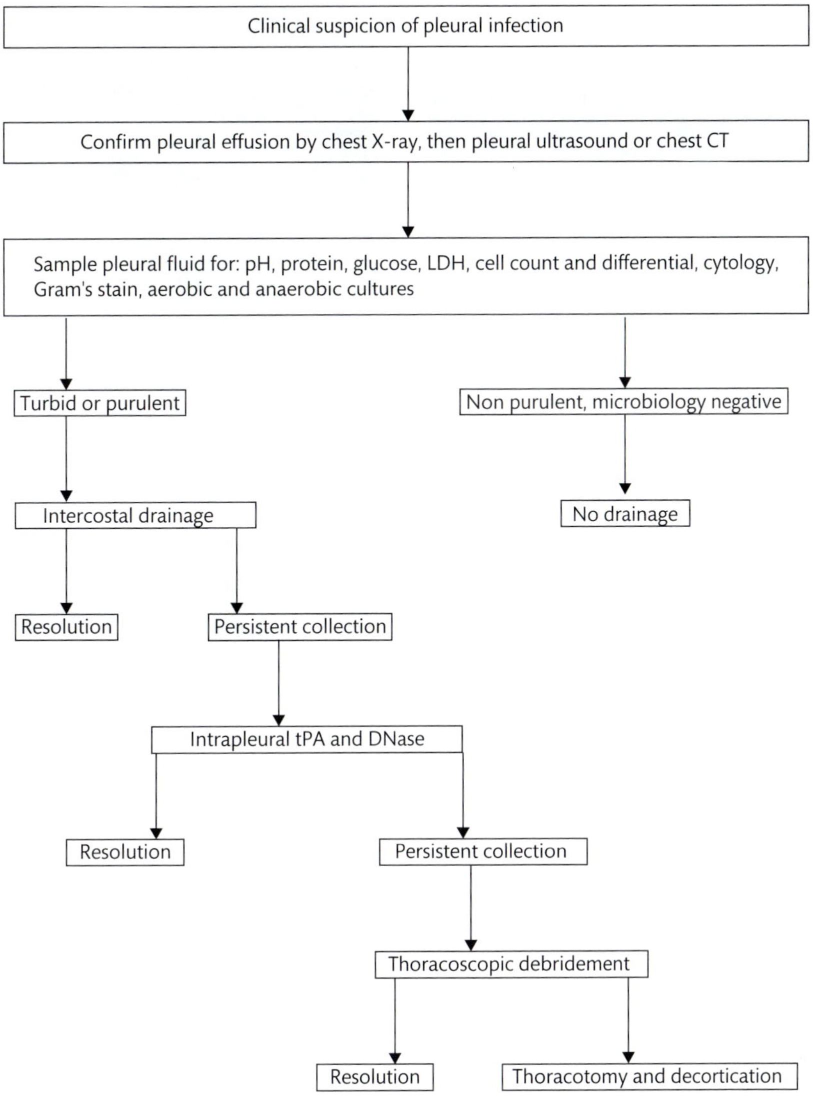

Figure 36.1 Algorithm for the diagnosis and management of pleural infection.

position, presence and degree of loculations, lung parenchymal changes, endobronchial lesions, and differentiation of lung abscess from loculated empyema.[19]

Magnetic Resonance Imaging (MRI)

MRI is not routinely used for the assessment of pleural infection, though it has been shown to allow assessment of complex loculated effusions and demonstrate chest wall involvement. Use of MRI minimizes radiation from contrast media and is therefore a valid alternative to CT especially in young patients who require repeated imaging.

Thoracentesis

Thoracentesis remains a key procedure in the diagnosis and management of pleural infection. Current guidelines advise sampling of effusions >10 mm in depth associated with pneumonia, chest trauma, or recent thoracic surgery with features of sepsis. Image guidance (US or CT) has been shown to decrease the risk of complication including organ perforation in pleural fluid sampling. Pleural ultrasound improves the accuracy of aspiration site selection. Simple marking of a site for pleural sampling away from the location of the actual procedure is no better than 'blind' aspiration. Moreover, the ability of clinicians to use pleural ultrasound themselves allows real-time visualization of pleural anatomy and identification of dangers during thoracentesis such as solid organs (liver, spleen, and heart), intercostal vessels, and consolidated lung.

Pleural Fluid Analysis and Biomarkers of Infection

Routine tests on pleural fluid include pH, protein, lactate dehydrogenase (LDH), cell count and differential, glucose and cytology, cultures for bacteria, mycobacteria, and fungi. Pleural fluid must be properly handled and submitted to diagnostic laboratories in appropriate volume and containers. Samples for cell counts and differentials must be collected in anticoagulated tubes otherwise the total white blood cell (WBC) count will be artifactually lowered.[20] Sending fluid in blood culture bottles increases culture yields.[21] Gross inspection of the colour and odour of pleural fluid may suggest a specific diagnosis (putrid smelling pus suggests anaerobic infection). The pH of physiologic pleural fluid is >7.60 because carbon dioxide diffuses freely across pleural membranes, but bicarbonates

Table 36.1 Comparison of pleural fluid characteristics in relation to stage of pleural infection

	Simple parapneumonic effusion	Complicated parapneumonic effusion	Empyema
Appearance	Clear or turbid	Cloudy	Pus
Biochemistry	pH >7.30 LDH may be elevated Glucose >60 mg/dL	pH <7.20 LDH >10,000 IU/L Glucose <35 mg/dL	N/A
Cell count	Neutrophils usually <10,000/μL	Neutrophils >10,000/μL	N/A
Gram's stain/ culture	Negative	May be positive	May be positive

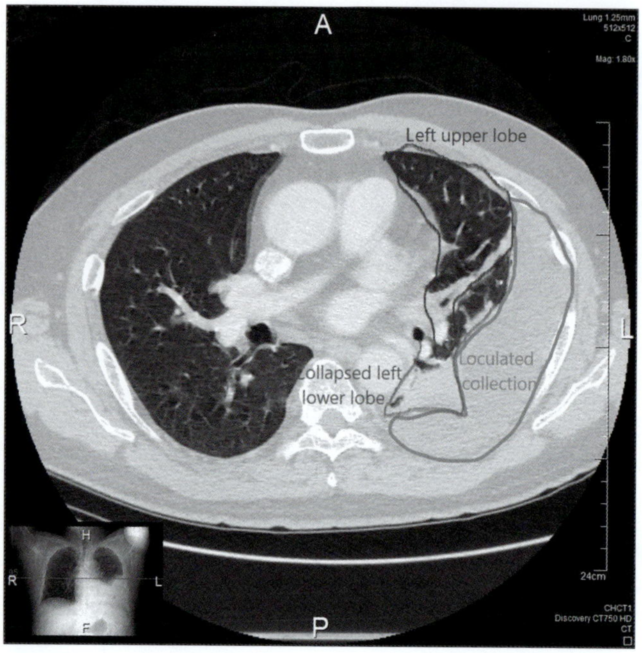

Figure 36.2 Chest computed tomography scan in a patient with complicated parapneumonic effusion. There is a large complex pleural effusion visible at the left base causing collapse of left lower lobe. Pneumonic changes are visible in the left lower lobe.

anions are retained and accumulate in normal pleural fluid. Pleural fluid pH should always be measured if pleural infection is suspected, except in the case of frank pus where at least chest tube drainage is always indicated.[12] A blood gas analyzer should be used as litmus paper is unreliable in the assessment of pleural pH. The method of sample collection is important, as confounding factors, such as local anaesthetic or air in the sampling syringe, or prolonged time between sample collection and processing, have been shown to artificially alter sample pH.[22–23] Pleural fluid protein, glucose, and LDH concentration can also aid characterization of pleural fluid and determine management, and together with microbiological culture, should be requested on initial samples.[20,24] Whilst protein concentration can contribute to confirming an effusion as an exudate, it does not have value in determining the need for tube drainage of an effusion versus less invasive management.[24] Pleural fluid cytology and assessment for acid fast bacilli should be performed as clinically indicated. A predominance of polynuclear cells is expected in bacterial pleural infection. Alternative aetiologies should be discussed if the effusion is not neutrophil-dominant.[1] Newer biomarkers have been assessed to examine their efficacy in diagnosing pleural effusions secondary to bacterial infection and to prognosticate on the likelihood of these effusions becoming complicated. Those include C-reactive protein (CRP), procalcitonin, tumour necrosis factor-alpha, myeloperoxidase, soluble triggering receptor expressed on myeloid cells (sTREM-1), and liposaccharide-binding protein.[24] None of these markers is superior to the classically accepted markers of pleural fluid pH <7.20 or pleural fluid glucose <60 mg/dL.[24] (Table 36.1)

Evidence-based Management

Based on studies demonstrating that effusions less than 1 cm (from parietal pleura to visceral pleura) would resolve with antibiotic therapy alone and not require further intervention, current guidelines recommend the sampling of parapneumonic effusions with a thickness ≥10 mm.[1,12,26] However, parapneumonic effusions are often loculated and the assessment of thickness on chest X-ray is therefore problematic. Hence, pleural US or CT, particularly in the setting of lower lobe consolidation, is now considered the mainstay imaging modalities for parapneumonic effusions. Use of real-time pleural ultrasound by trained operators has been shown to improve the safety of sampling effusions, with reported reductions in iatrogenic pneumothorax compared to 'blind' pleural aspirations by more than 50%.[15–16] Real-time pleural US has been incorporated into diagnostic algorithms in most pleural guidelines. It is sensitive in detecting small volumes of fluid and may detect loculations not obvious on CT[12] (Figures 36.2–36.4).

Multiple approaches can be considered when treating a patient with pleural infection, ranging from antibiotics alone to thoracotomy and decortication. The initial optimal management is determined by the answers to several key questions: should the pleural space be drained? How urgently it should be drained? How it should be drained? Should intrapleural adjunct therapy be used? The initial imaging and results of the pleural fluid sampling, appearance, and pH provide the earliest information determining the need for formal chest tube insertion and continuous drainage. Frank pus, regardless of other determinants, warrants immediate drainage of any pleural collection. Other features recommending drainage include positive Gram stain, positive culture, and pleural fluid pH <7.20 or glucose <60 mg/dL.[1,12]

Patient's fitness and general condition (nutritional status), associated co-morbidities, and age often influence the therapeutic approach. Adequate nutritional support, corrections of metabolic abnormalities, and treatment of associated co-morbidities are essential to optimize medical therapy (e.g. equilibration of diabetes, treatment of heart failure, and physiotherapy to avoid sputum retention).

Recently, a clinical score (RAPID) based on five variables (renal, age, purulence, infection source, and dietary factors) was validated to identify and stratify patients at risk of poor outcome at presentation.[27] Patients were stratified into low risk (0–2), medium risk (3–4), or high risk (5–7) of poor outcomes including death at 3 months, need for surgical intervention at 3 months, or increased length of

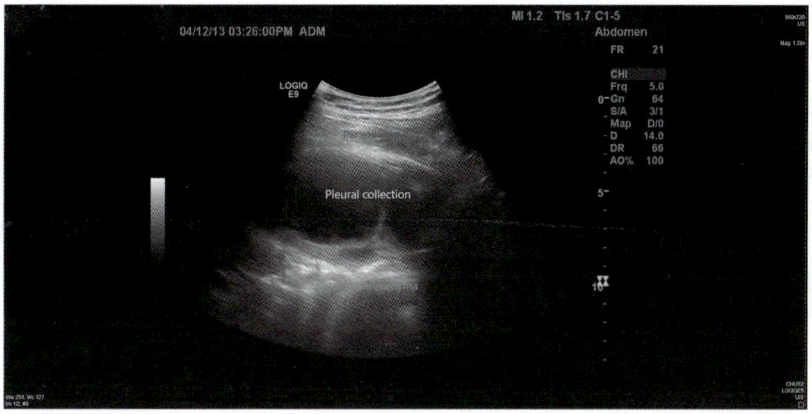

Figure 36.3 Pleural ultrasound in a patient with complicated parapneumonic effusion. Ultrasound scan showing a complex multi-loculated effusion in a patient with parapneumonic empyema.

stay in hospital. Age, urea, albumin, hospital-acquired infection, and non-purulence predicted poor outcome. Longer in-hospital stay was associated with increasing RAPID score.

Observation

The American College of Chest Physicians guidelines outline four categories of pleural fluid collection in the setting of infection.[28] These range from <1 cm effusions through to empyema as determined by radiological features, pH, Gram stain, culture, and the presence of pus. Only category 1 effusions (very low risk), described as minimal and free flowing and <1 cm, are considered safe for observation without diagnostic sampling. Category 2 (low risk) effusions (≥10 mm but <1/2 hemithorax, pH >7.2 and negative Gram stain and culture) may be observed without formal drainage. Category 3 (moderate risk) effusions (large but free flowing effusions, loculated effusions, or effusions with thickened parietal pleura; or pH <7.2; or positive Gram stain or culture) and category 4 (empyema) effusions should be drained urgently due to the associated risk of poor outcome. It is important to note that these recommendations can serve as a useful guide but are mainly based on expert opinion and supported by limited evidence.

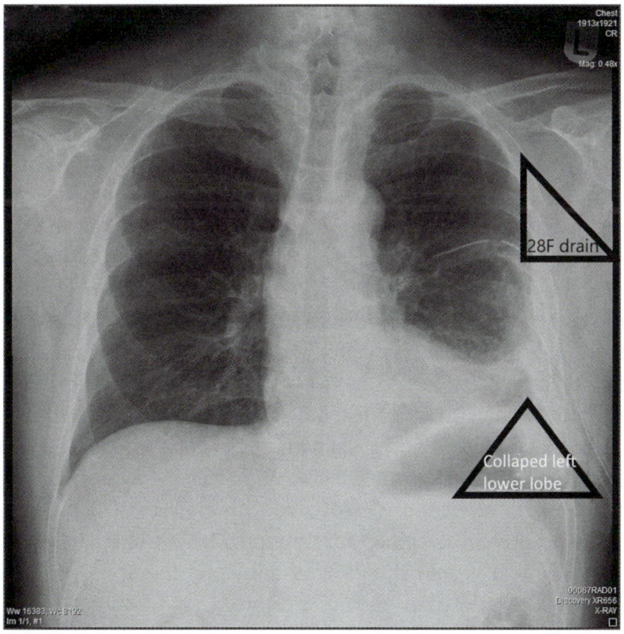

Figure 36.4 Chest X-ray of patient after videothoracoscopic debridement of empyema. This study shows a large drain in situ (28F) following videothoracoscopic debridement of a large left parapneumonic empyema. There is no residual pleural collection, but poor expansion of the left lower lobe is still present.

Antibiotics

All patients with suspected pleural infection should receive appropriate antibiotic cover following thoracocentesis and review of pleural fluid analysis. The initial antibiotherapy should be based on local prescribing guidelines and resistance patterns and adapted as soon as possible to Gram's stain results and cultures. In patients with community-acquired pleural infection and positive pleural cultures, 50% of cases are reported to be due to penicillin-sensitive streptococci, with the remainder due to organisms that are penicillin-resistant, such as staphylococci and *Enterobacteriaceae*. Approximately 25% of community-acquired pleural infections include anaerobic bacteria and 40% will have negative pleural cultures. Therefore, empiric antibiotic choice should cover common community-acquired bacterial pathogens and anaerobic bacteria.[2,29] Penicillins, penicillins with beta-lactamase inhibitors, cephalosporins, and fluoroquinolones all have good penetration in pleural tissues. Metronidazole and clindamycin also penetrate well and cover anaerobic bacteria. Aminoglycosides have poor pleural penetration and may be less effective in the acidic environment of the pleural space during infection.[1,2] In the setting of hospital-acquired pleural infection, antibiotic selection should also cover MRSA and anaerobic bacteria. The combination of a carbapenem or antipseudomonal penicillin and an agent active against MRSA (e.g. vancomycin or Linezolid) is required.[1–2]

Duration of antibiotic therapy is based on a combination of clinical response, bacteriology when available, and inflammatory marker (CRP) response. Radiological changes can persist for weeks after clinical improvement and should not be the sole criteria for continuation of therapy nor would that be an indication of treatment failure. The exact timing of switch from intravenous to oral antibiotic therapy is not clearly defined, but at least 1 week of intravenous therapy followed by 1–3 weeks of oral therapy as appropriate—based on clinical response—is generally used. Of course, adequate nutrition is essential as well as correction of associated co-morbidities (e.g. heart failure, renal failure, diabetes, and vitamin deficit).

Thoracentesis

The risk of complications in pleural infections is decreased by minimizing the number of interventions. Therefore, initial thoracentesis should be therapeutic as well as diagnostic if possible. The reasoning behind this is that if fluid is drained and does not re-accumulate, the patient may not require further invasive treatment. Alternatives include insertion of a small-bore catheter or a therapeutic thoracentesis.[16,18] These approaches have not been directly compared in prospective studies. Further management will depend on initial fluid findings and clinical progress.

Chest Tube Drainage

Recent publications have emphasized the frequency of complications during interventional pleural procedures.[15–18] Guidelines exist for insertion of chest tubes as do safety protocols and web-based simulations. Whenever possible, imaging guidance should be used, and adequate supervision by an experienced operator is essential. Historically large bore tubes (>20 Fr) have been used for the drainage of pleural infection with minimal evidence-based support of superiority. Recent evidence suggests that small-bore chest tubes (≤14 Fr) may be as effective and better tolerated due to less pain.[30] Chest tubes should be placed on an underwater seal and ideally on suction to improve drainage and promote lung re-expansion. Failure of successful drainage with a small-bore tube often results from multiple loculations in the pleural cavity. Rather than immediate insertion of a larger tube, consideration should be given to repeated imaging of the pleural space, insertion of additional small-bore drains, intrapleural therapy, or surgery. There are no absolute criteria stating how long a drain should be kept in the pleural space, but in clinical practice chest drains are removed when the patient is clinically better, when inflammatory markers have returned to normal level (essentially WBC and CRP), when there is no residual pleural effusion on chest X-ray, and when daily drainage is <50 mL.

Intrapleural Therapy

In the past two decades, multiple studies and randomized trials have examined the role of administration of intrapleural fibrinolytics (streptokinase and urokinase) in improving drainage of loculated pleural effusions.[3,9] Most of these studies were uncontrolled or had significant limitations. A large randomized control study examined the efficacy of intrapleural streptokinase (250,000 IU twice daily for 3 days) compared to saline. This study did not show a difference in length of hospitalization, mortality or need for surgery, and radiographic outcomes between the two groups, and sub-group analyses did not show any benefits from the use of intrapleural streptokinase.[9] A recent meta-analysis found no mortality benefit with intrapleural fibrinolytics alone.[31] The Multicenter Intrapleural Sepsis Trial-2 (MIST-2) showed that the combination of tPA and DNase (but not the individual agents alone) resulted in improved radiological appearance, decreased surgical referral at 3 months, and reduced in-hospital stay significantly compared to placebo, without excessive adverse events.[3] Serious complications are uncommon, but pain can occur, especially with the first injection. Severe bleeding requiring transfusion is rare (<2%). Treatment is contraindicated in those with recent thoracic surgery, significant bleeding diathesis, or bronchopleural fistula. Recently, a randomized controlled trial showed that pleural irrigation with normal saline could significantly increase pleural fluid drainage and reduce referrals for surgery versus chest tube drainage alone in patients with pleural infection.[32] Future studies need to define if intrapleural therapy is best used in every patient or be reserved for those who have failed standard medical management.

Surgery

Surgery remains an option when medical therapy is inadequate. Current guidelines suggest surgery should only be recommended in patients with a residual pleural collection and persistent sepsis despite adequate antibiotic therapy and drainage.[28,33,34] In considering the role for surgery, it should be remembered that the majority of patients with pleural infection can be managed with antibiotics and chest tube drainage. Only 18% of patients in the MIST-1 trial failed this approach and only 11% in MIST-2 trial.[3,9] In the MIST-2 trial, 96% of patients receiving intrapleural tPA and DNase were successfully treated without surgery.[9] Two small randomized clinical trials in adults comparing first-line videothoracoscopic debridement with medical treatment (chest tube drainage with or without intrapleural fibrinolytics and antibiotics) failed to show a survival advantage from early surgical intervention, although surgery resulted in shorter hospital stay.[35–36] A large retrospective trial looking at 4424 patients with pleural infection concluded that surgical therapy offered a lower risk of death after adjustment for age, sex, and co-morbidities.[34] In stage 3 empyema, evidence suggests that surgery remains the only valid option. Thus, only adequate surgical decortication can remove pleural peel and adequately re-expand the lung. Historical studies stated that this goal can only be achieved through thoracotomy. However, evidence accumulated over the past two decades suggests that adequate debridement of the pleural cavity and full decortication can be achieved by video-assisted thoracic surgery (VATS) with equivalent outcomes.[33] In paediatric empyema, a large meta-analysis and systematic review of the literature comparing operative versus non-operative management suggested that primary surgical therapy is associated with a lower risk of treatment failure, a lower in-hospital mortality rate, length of stay, duration of tube drainage, and duration of antibiotic therapy.[37] However, the potential mid-term and long-term effects of surgery should be weighted carefully.[38] Intercostal neuralgia is most common following VATS or thoracotomy, and the occurrence of chronic chest pain must be studied properly in randomized trials. In the absence of a large randomized study, many paediatric physicians still believe that VATS should not be offered upfront and that intrapleural fibrinolytic therapy should remain the first-line approach.[39] Finally, in the rare scenario of uncontrolled pleural sepsis despite multiple surgical drainages, or where the lung has been destroyed through an underlying infection (necrotizing pneumonia, previous extensive tuberculosis, or widespread bronchiectasis), a valid therapeutic option is to perform an open window thoracostomy.[40] This procedure can prove a life-saving option even in frail patients, by eliminating durably the source of sepsis. Recent experiences suggest that mini-vacuum-assisted closure therapy could represent a good option in frail or debilitated patients in poor general condition.[41]

Controversies and Future Practice

The optimal size of chest tube for drainage of the pleural space remains controversial, and evidence suggests that small-bore tubes should now be considered as first line.

To date, no trials have compared VATS against the combination of intrapleural tPA and DNAse in the treatment of pleural infection. Several randomized controlled trials are actively recruiting patients in Europe and North America. The mid-term complications and cost of surgery must also be taken into consideration.

The exact role and timing of surgery remains controversial, but patients failing medical therapy should be referred to a thoracic surgeon without delay for consideration of early thoracoscopic drainage to avoid thoracotomy and decortication. The role of early thoracoscopic debridement should be evaluated in a large randomized controlled trial.

REFERENCES

1. Corcoran JP, Rahman NM. Effusions from infections: Parapneumonic pleural effusion and empyema. In: Light RW, Lee YCG, eds. *Textbook of Pleural Diseases*. 3rd ed. CRC Press; 2016:295–330.
2. Rosenstengel A, Lee YCG. Pleural infection-current diagnosis and management. *J Thoracic Dis*. 2012;**4**:186–193.
3. Rahman NM, Maskell NA, West A, et al. Intrapleural use of tissue plasminogen activator and DNase in pleural infection. *N Engl J Med*. 2011;**365**:518–526.
4. Davies CW, Kearney SE, Gleeson FV, et al. Predictors of outcome and long-term survival in patients with pleural infection. *Am J Respir Crit Care Med*. 1999;**160**:1682–1687.
5. Lisboa T, Waterer GW, Lee YC. Pleural infection: Changing bacteriology and its implications. *Respirology*. 2011;**16**:598–603.
6. Foster S, Maskell NA. Bacteriology of complicated parapneumonic effusions. *Curr Opin Pulm Med*. 2007;**13**:319–323.
7. Burgos J, Lujan M, Falcó V, et al. The spectrum of pneumococcal empyema in adults in the early 21st century. *Clin Infect Dis*. 2011;**53**:254–261.
8. Maskell NA, Batt S, Hedley EL, et al. The bacteriology of pleural infection by genetic and standard methods and its mortality significance. *Am J Respir Crit Care Med*. 2006;**174**:817–823.
9. Maskell NA, Davies CW, Nunn AJ, et al. UK Controlled trial of intrapleural streptokinase for pleural infection. *N Engl J Med*. 2005;**352**:865–874.
10. Teixeira LR, Vargas FS. Effusions from atypical infections. In: Light RW, Lee YCG, eds. *Textbook of Pleural Diseases*. 3rd edition. CRC Press; 2016:343–352.
11. Glendening J, Koroscil M. A report of fungal empyema following recovery of severe SARS-CoV-2 infection. *Chest*. 2020;**158**(4):A566.
12. Davies HE, Davies RJ, Davies CW. BTS Pleural Disease Guideline Group Management of pleural infection in adults: British Thoracic Society Pleural Disease Guideline 2010. *Thorax*. 2010;**65**:ii41–ii53.
13. Brixey AG, Luo Y, Skouras V, et al. The efficacy of chest radiographs in detecting parapneumonic effusions. *Respirology*. 2011;**16**:1000–1004.
14. Rahman NM, Gleeson FV. New directions in the treatment of infected pleural effusion. *Clin Radiol*. 2006;**61**:719–722.
15. Koenig SJ, Narasimhan M, Mayo PH. Thoracic ultrasonography for the pulmonary specialist. *Chest*. 2011;**140**:1332–1341.
16. Duncan DR, Morgenthaler TI, Ryu JH, et al. Reducing iatrogenic risk in thoracentesis: Establishing best practice via experiential training in a zero-risk environment. *Chest*. 2009;**135**:1315–1320.
17. Diacon AH, Brutsche MH, Solèr M. Accuracy of pleural puncture sites: A prospective comparison of clinical examination with ultrasound. *Chest*. 2003;**123**:436–441.
18. Wrightson JM, Fysh E, Maskell NA, et al. Risk reduction in pleural procedures: Sonography, simulation and supervision. *Curr Opin Pulm Med*. 2010;**16**:340–350.
19. Raj V, Kirke R, Bankart MJ, et al. Multidetector CT imaging of pleura: Comparison of two contrast infusion protocols. *Br J Radiol*. 2011;**84**:796–799.
20. Heffner JE. Pleural fluid analysis. In: Light RW, Lee YCG, eds. *Textbook of Pleural Diseases*. 3rd ed. CRC Press; 2016:153–173.
21. Menzies SM, Rahman NM, Wrightson JM, et al. Blood culture bottle culture of pleural fluid in pleural infection. *Thorax*. 2011;**66**:658–662.
22. Cheng DS, Rodriguez RM, Rogers J, et al. Comparison of pleural fluid pH values obtained using blood gas machine, pH meter, and pH indicator strip. *Chest*. 1998;**114**:1368–1372.
23. Rahman NM, Mishra EK, Davies HE, et al. Clinically important factors influencing the diagnostic measurement of pleural fluid pH and glucose. *Am J Respir Crit Care Med*. 2008;**178**:483–490.
24. Porcel JM. Pleural fluid tests to identify complicated parapneumonic effusions. *Curr Opin Pulm Med*. 2010;**16**:357–361.
25. Porcel JM, Vives M, Cao G, et al. Biomarkers of infection for the differential diagnosis of pleural effusions. *Eur Respir J*. 2009;**34**:1383–1389.
26. Skouras V, Awdankiewicz A, Light RW. What size parapneumonic effusions should be sampled? *Thorax*. 2010;**65**:91.
27. Rahman NM, Kahan BC, Miller RF, et al. A clinical score (RAPID) to identify those at risk for poor outcome at presentation in patients with pleural infection. *Chest*. 2014;**145**:848–855.
28. Colice GL, Curtis A, Deslauriers J, et al. Medical and surgical treatment of parapneumonic effusions: An evidence-based guideline. *Chest*. 2000;**118**:1158–1171.
29. Teixeira LR, Villarino MA. Antibiotic treatment of patients with pneumonia and pleural effusion. *Curr Opin Pulm Med*. 1998;**4**:230–234.
30. Rahman NM, Maskell NA, Davies CW, et al. The relationship between chest tube size and clinical outcome in pleural infection. *Chest*. 2010;**137**:536–543.
31. Cameron R, Davies HR. Intra-pleural fibrinolytic therapy versus conservative management in the treatment of adult parapneumonic effusions and empyema. *Cochrane Database Syst Rev*. 2008;**2**:CD002312.

32. Hooper CE, Edey AJ, Wallis A, et al. Pleural irrigation trial (PIT): A randomised controlled trial of pleural irrigation with normal saline versus standard care in patients with pleural infection. *Eur Respir J*. 2015;**46**:456–463.
33. Scarci M, Abah U, Solli P, et al. EACTS expert consensus statement for surgical management of pleural empyema. *Eur J Cardiothorac Surg*. 2015;**48**:642–653.
34. Farjah F, Symons RG, Krishnadasan B, et al. Management of pleural space infections: A population-based analysis. *J Thorac Cardiovasc Surg*. 2007;**133**:346–351.
35. Bilgin M, Akcali Y, Oguzkaya F. Benefits of early aggressive management of empyema thoracis. *ANZ J Surg*. 2006;**76**:120–122.
36. Wait MA, Sharma S, Hohn J, et al. A randomized trial of empyema therapy. *Chest*. 1997;**111**:1548–1551.
37. Avansino JR, Goldman B, Sawin RS, et al. Primary operative versus nonoperative therapy for pediatric empyema: A meta-analysis. *Pediatrics*. 2005;115(6):1652–1659.
38. Furrer M, Rechsteiner R, Eigenmann V, et al. Thoracotomy and thoracoscopy: Postoperative pulmonary function, pain and chest wall complaints. *Eur J Cardiothorac Surg*. 1997;**12**:82–87.
39. Paraskakis E, Vergadi E, Chatzmichael A. Bouros. Current evidence for the management of paediatric parapneumonic effusions. *Curr Med Res Opin*. 2012;**28**:1179–1192.
40. Molnar TF. Current surgical treatment of thoracic empyema in adults. *Eur J Cardiothorac Surg*. 2007;**32**:422–430.
41. Sziklavari Z, Ried M, Neu R, et al. Mini-open vacuum-assisted closure therapy with instillation for debilitated and septic patients with pleural empyema. *Eur J Cardiothorac Surg*. 2015;**48**:e9–16. doi: 10. 1093/ejcts/ezv186.

37

Fungal Respiratory Infections

Matteo Bassetti, Alessia Carnelutti, and Elda Righi

Key Messages

- Diagnoses of invasive fungal infections have increased over decades and are associated with high mortality rates.
- Immunocompromised and critically ill patients represent patient populations at risk for fungal infections.
- *Candida* spp. and *Aspergillus* spp. are the most common pathogens causing invasive fungal infections.
- Aspergillosis and *Pneumocystis jiroveci* pneumonia represent severe forms of lung infections.
- The diagnosis of invasive fungal infections can be challenging; nonculture-based methods can facilitate the management of high-risk patients.
- Timely and appropriate antifungal treatment is paramount in the management of invasive fungal infections.
- Relatively new antifungals (e.g. triazoles and echinocandins) are available and have been used in the treatment of invasive fungal infections.

- Nonculture diagnostic tests: the roles of beta-d-glucan and galactomannan.
- The value of fluconazole in candidemia: still a good option?
- Diagnosis of aspergillosis in non-neutropenic critically ill patients: discrimination between infection and colonization.
- Duration of prophylaxis for *Pneumocistis jiroveci* pneumonia in non-HIV patients.

- Use of algorithms based on risk factors and nonculture diagnostic methods for the diagnosis of invasive fungal diseases.
- Development of resistance to echinocandins in *Candida* spp.
- Efficacy of new antifungal therapies (isavuconazole) for the treatment of aspergillosis.
- Large randomized trials to establish the efficacy of combination therapies for the treatment of invasive fungal infections.

Introduction

Invasive fungal infections (IFIs) are life-threatening diseases characterized by high mortality rates, especially among critically ill and immunocompromised patients.[1] Risk factors for IFIs are represented by impairment of defence mechanisms (e.g. lymphocyte dysfunction, drug-induced immunosuppression, and presence of invasive devices such as intravascular catheters) along with prolonged hospitalizations and broad-spectrum antimicrobial therapies.[2] The increasing complexity of medical care, the advent of more potent chemotherapeutic regimens, and the increasing number of solid organ (SOT) and haematopoietic stem cell transplant (HSCT) recipients have contributed to the rise of IFIs over the past years.[2]

Overall, *Candida* spp. and *Aspergillus* spp. represent the leading cause of IFIs.[3] Among others, *Pneumocystis jiroveci* can cause severe pneumonia in immunocompromised patients, and *Cryptococcus neoformans* is responsible for pulmonary and cerebral localization of infections.[3] Endemic fungal pathogens (e.g. *Histoplasma capsulatum*, *Coccidioides immitis*, *Blastomyces dermatitidis*, *Paracoccidioides brasiliensis*, and *Sporothrix schenckii*) can cause lung and/or systemic involvement in immunocompetent and immunocompromised hosts although their incidence is usually restricted to defined geographic locations. Opportunistic fungal organisms, such as Mucor species, are less commonly isolated and may cause pneumonia, sinuses, and/or central nervous system infections in patients with immune defects (e.g. haematological malignancies).[3]

The diagnosis of fungal infections, especially pneumonia, can be challenging and is often made on a presumptive basis. Nonculture-based diagnostic tests for fungal infections represent a non-invasive diagnostic tool that has been used more often to help in therapeutic decisions.

In critically ill and immunocompromised patients, the prognosis often depends on the severity of the underlying disease or is linked to a change in factors affecting the immune status. The spectra of diseases and risk factors associated with the most common fungal infections, candidiasis and aspergillosis, are manifold. While aspergillosis usually causes severe pulmonary disease in immunocompromised patients, Candida is not recognized as a cause of primary lung infection, as supported by autopsy studies.[4] The colonization of the lower respiratory tract with Candida, however, can occur in critically ill patients with dysbiosis. Its association with poor outcomes is still unclear.[4]

Here, we review the clinical characteristics and therapeutic aspects of infections caused by *Candida* spp., *Aspergillus* spp., *Pneumocystis jiroveci*, and *Cryptococcus neoformans*.

Candidiasis

Candida spp. represents the fourth most frequently isolated pathogen in nosocomial bloodstream infections.[5] Risk factors for candidemia include neutropenia, broad-spectrum antibiotic therapy, gastrointestinal surgery, and total parenteral nutrition.[2] Candida attributable mortality in the intensive care unit (ICU) can be as high as 40%–50%. Although the critically ill are among the most at risk of Candida infections, rates are rising among patients on general wards.[6] In recent years, the epidemiology of *Candida* spp. distribution has changed, with reductions in the relative frequency of *albicans* (CA) compared to non-*albicans* (NAC) species. The increase in NAC species presents challenges to antifungal treatment; *C. krusei* and *C. glabrata* are resistant to fluconazole, while *C. parapsilosis* can be difficult to eradicate because of its biofilm production and higher MICs for echinocandins.[2,7] The choice of an adequate and timely antifungal treatment for severe candidiasis, however, is paramount and has a direct impact on patients' mortality.[2]

Imperfect tests for Candida infections can contribute to delayed antifungal treatment; blood cultures remain the essential investigation for candidemia but are characterized by low sensitivity and prolonged time to positivity (>72 h from the time of blood sample collection). For this reason, guidelines recommended a pre-emptive, diagnosis-based approach including patients' risk factors along with serological techniques (e.g. beta-D-glucan (BDG) and mannan–antimannan), reducing antifungal exposure, and avoiding therapy delays.[8] The definitive choice of the antifungal strategy is based on several factors, including patient characteristics, renal and hepatic function, haemodynamic stability, local of Candida ecology (e.g. NAC proportion), availability of serological tests, and infection site (see Table 37.1).

Various classes of antifungals are used to treat Candida infections, including azoles (fluconazole and voriconazole), echinocandins (caspofungin, micafungin, and anidulafungin), and polyenes (amphotericin B, liposomal, and lipid complex formulations). Due to toxicity (especially nephrotoxicity), amphotericin B deoxycholate is no longer recommended nor are itraconazole and posaconazole due to paucity of data proving efficacy.[8] The use of echinocandins as first-line treatment for candidemia, especially in critically ill patients, has been recommended due to favourable safety profiles, fungicidal activity, broader spectrum of activity, and reduced drug–drug interactions. Liposomal (L-AmB) and lipid complex amphotericin B are considered as alternatives in the targeted treatment of candidemia. Voriconazole is not recommended as a first-line therapy for candidemia due to reduced tolerability, IV formulation renal toxicity, and frequent drug–drug interactions, but its use could be considered as an alternative to other therapies or as step-down therapy for *C. krusei* or voriconazole-susceptible *C. glabrata*. Despite the emphasis given to newer molecules, fluconazole remains a well-tolerated antifungal agent displaying significantly lower costs compared to echinocandins and polyenes. In ICU, fluconazole is often used in clinically stable patients with CA or *C. parapsilosis* infections and in de-escalation therapy. In order to avoid organ involvement, the current guidelines for candidemia recommend a 14-day treatment after blood culture negativity along with ophthalmologic fundus examination to exclude disseminated endocular infection and trans-oesophageal echocardiography to rule out endocarditis.[8] Due to the risk of biofilm production, persistent infections, and resistance selection, central venous catheters should be removed in the case of candidemia although there are yet no data from randomised, controlled trials.

Aspergillosis

Aspergillus spp. is a ubiquitous filamentous fungus able to produce small spores (conidia) that can be aerosolized and inhaled by humans.[9] Conidia are usually rapidly eliminated, but alterations of host immune system can favour pathogen invasiveness resulting in a wide spectrum of clinical syndromes. Pulmonary involvement, however, often represents the main presentation of aspergillosis.[9] *Aspergillus fumigatus* is involved in up to 90% of human infections and is characterized by production of very small conidia and rapid replication, whereas other species (e.g. *A. niger*, *A. flavus*, and *A. terreus*) account for a minority of cases.

Clinical manifestations of aspergillosis depend on the interplay between the fungus and host immune system, resulting in a wide variability of clinical syndromes that may evolve one into another depending on the degree of immunosuppression.

Invasive aspergillosis (IA), characterized by angioinvasion and hyphae dissemination to lungs and other organs (e.g. brain, skin, or eyes), usually occurs in severe immunocompromised hosts such as HSCT recipients, patients with prolonged neutropenia, or those receiving high-dose steroids.[10] IA is characterized by a rapid clinical course presenting with cough, chest pain, haemoptysis, and fever and progressing to respiratory failure often associated with multi-organ failure. Radiological findings typically associated with IA include the 'halo' sign (a rim of ground-glass opacity that surrounds a nodule), the 'air crescent' sign (a cavitated lesion with an intracavitary mass and a surrounding rim of air), and lung cavities.[9]

Table 37.1 Antifungals used for the treatment of candidemia according to various patient characteristics

Characteristic / Drug	Previous therapy with an azole	Shock	Severe renal failure	Hepatic failure
Fluconazole	Not recommended	Not recommended	Not recommended	Not recommended
Echinocandins	Recommended	Recommended	Recommended	Recommended
Lip-AmB	Recommended	Recommended	Not recommended	Moderate recommendation
Voriconazole	Moderate recommendation	Moderate recommendation	Only oral formulation	Not recommended

Lip-AmB: lipid-formulation of amphotericin B.

It should be noted, however, that clinical and radiological manifestations are influenced by the degree of immunosuppression and can be non-specific when the 'classic' risk factors are lacking, for example in non-neutropenic critically ill patients. In this setting, the most common presentation of IA is refractory fever despite antibiotic treatment, generally associated with worsening of lung function evolving over several days or weeks, with alterations of CT scan ranging from nodular patterns to bilateral pulmonary infiltrates, with typical radiological findings evidenced only in a minority of cases. Overall, IA is associated with high mortality rates, exceeding, in some reports, 90% among HSCT recipients and critically ill patients.[11] Chronic forms of aspergillosis, such as chronic pulmonary aspergillosis—which includes subacute IA, chronic cavitary pulmonary aspergillosis, and aspergilloma, usually affect patients with underlying respiratory disease rather than immunocompromised patients, including previously treated tuberculosis, atypical mycobacterial infection, chronic obstructive pulmonary disease (COPD), bronchiectasis, fibrocavitatory sarcoidosis, and lung cancer.[12] In these patients, clinical presentation often occurs with constitutional symptoms (weight loss, sweats, and anorexia), chronic productive cough, shortness of breath, chest pain, and haemoptysis. Lung cavities with or without an aspergilloma, infiltrates, nodules, and various degrees of lung or pleural fibrosis are the most common radiological findings.[12,13] In patients with hypersensitivity to *Aspergillus*, repeated inhalation may result in allergic bronchopulmonary aspergillosis, typically leading to asthma exacerbations and, if untreated, the development of bronchiectasis and chronic pulmonary disease.[13]

Over time, the incidence of IA has increased worldwide, primarily due to the progressive expansion of patient populations with immune deficits.[12] Overall, approximately 8.8% of HSCT recipients develop IFIs; of these, 80% of cases are caused by *Aspergillus* spp. The progressive advances in medical care have, however, led to an expansion of patient populations at risk for IA. Among patients admitted to ICU, for example, IA is an emerging problem often associated with delayed diagnosis and inadequate antifungal treatment. In this setting, incidence widely varies across studies, ranging between 0.017% and 17%.[14] Aspergillosis represents the most common missed infectious disease diagnosed at autopsy. Among critically ill patients, COPD and high-dose steroids have been recognized as independent risk factors for both respiratory tract colonization with *Aspergillus* spp. and development of IA.[10] Solid organ transplantation, decompensated liver cirrhosis, prolonged use of steroids or T-cell immunosuppressive treatment (i.e. infliximab or alemtuzumab), solid malignancies, HIV infection with CD4 count <50 cells/μL, and concomitant H1N1 or COVID-19 respiratory infection are also recognized risk factors for the development of IA in non-neutropenic patients.[15,16]

During the Severe Acute Respiratory Syndrome-Coronavirus 2 (SARS-CoV-2) pandemic, an increasing number of cases of COVID-19-associated pulmonary aspergillosis (CAPA) has been published.[16] CAPA has been associated with increased mortality rates, ranging between 16% and 25%, compared with patients without evidence for aspergillosis, particularly in the setting of ICU. However, whether SARS-CoV-2 represents an independent risk factor for the development of CAPA or additional risk factors (e.g. use or corticosteroids) play a pivotal role the risk of disease progression is still unclear. The diagnosis of CAPA is challenging, but in the setting of SARS-CoV-2 pneumonia the presence of multiple pulmonary nodules or cavitation should raise the suspicion of CAPA and further investigations for pulmonary aspergillosis, mainly represented by the detection of galactomannan (GM) antigen in bronchoalveolar lavage (BAL) fluid, should be considered.

The diagnosis of aspergillosis can be challenging. The National Institute of Allergy and Infectious Diseases Mycoses Study Group (EORTC/MSG) criteria for the diagnosis proved that probable and possible IFIs—originally designed for cancer and HSCT patients—appear inadequate for the diagnosis of IA in non-neutropenic critically ill population.[10,17] The reasons for this include the absence of typical risk factors for IA in ICU patients, causing a low grade of suspicion, the lack of specificity of clinical and radiological findings, and the challenge of discriminating between colonization and infection when *Aspergillus* spp. is recovered from respiratory tract cultures. For these reasons, a new category of 'putative' aspergillosis has been introduced. According to this algorithm, in critically ill patients a case of *Aspergillus*-positive endotracheal aspirate culture is considered a probable IA in presence of compatible signs and symptoms, abnormal radiological findings, and either host risk factors or BAL positivity on direct microscopy or cultures.[17] The bronchoscopic appearances of invasive tracheobronchitis are typical. Similar to Candida infections, nonculture-based diagnostic tests, in particular GM, have been introduced for the diagnosis of Aspergillus. GM is a component of the cell wall of *Aspergillus* released during tissue invasion and has been demonstrated to be useful for the diagnosis of IA from serum or BAL in severely immunocompromised and critically ill patients. However, sensitivity and specificity of GM greatly vary according to patients' characteristics and degree of immunosuppression. Nowadays, plasma GM is considered a useful diagnostic tool only in neutropenic patients as it has low sensitivity in non-neutropenic ICU patients. Conversely, GM determination in BAL has been found to be highly sensitive and specific also in non-neutropenic critically ill patients, with a sensitivity and specificity of 88% and 87% for 0.5 unit cut-off value, respectively.[19] BDG is a pan-fungal serum assay (with the exception of *Cryptococcus* spp. and *Mucor* spp.) and has been reported to have an overall sensitivity of 90% and a specificity of 85% for a cut-off value of 80 pg/mL in haematologic patients with IA and similar diagnostic accuracy in non-neutropenic critically ill patients.[20,21] False-positive results have been described in the case of concomitant administration of beta-lactams, albumin, immunoglobulins, dialysis, and use of gauzes.

Antifungal therapy for IA includes three classes of active antifungals: triazoles (itraconazole, posaconazole, voriconazole, and isavuconazole), polyenes, and echinocandins.[17,22]

Current guidelines recommend voriconazole as first-line treatment (Table 37.2).[22,23] Most common adverse events associated with voriconazole include neurotoxicity, alteration of liver enzymes, and cutaneous reactions. Therapeutic drug monitoring of voriconazole is strongly recommended in order to reduce the risk of adverse events and optimize its efficacy, considering the potential for wide plasmatic variability caused by genetic factors and drug–drug interactions. Isavuconazole also represents a valid option for IA treatment and is characterized by fewer drug-drug interactions and toxicity compared to voriconazole. Liposomal amphotericin B and echinocandins represent possible alternative regimens, but—compared to voriconazole—can only be administered intravenously. Combination therapy of voriconazole plus an echinocandin or amphotericin B should be considered only as salvage treatment in selected cases, but evidence

Table 37.2 Drugs of choice and alternative drugs for invasive fungal infections

Pathogen	First-line treatment	Alternative
Aspergillus spp.	Voriconazole Isavuconazole	Lip-AmB Posaconazole (salvage) Caspofungin (salvage)
Pneumocystis jiroveci	Trimethoprim/sulfamethoxazole + prednisone if PaO_2 <70 mmHg for 21 days	Primaquine + clindamycin Pentamidine IV Echinocandins
Cryptococcus spp.	*Localized pulmonary disease* Fluconazole *Disseminated (meningitis and pneumonia)* Lip-AmB + flucytosine	Voriconazole Posaconazole

Lip-AmB: lipid-formulation of amphotericin B.

comes from small studies and case series and further investigations are required in order to establish the potential advantages of this approach in comparison with monotherapy. Newer nebulised azoles are in development such as opeloconazole. Caspofungin monotherapy represents the first choice in the fever-driven approach, which consists of the empiric prescription of an antifungal treatment in neutropenic patients receiving chemotherapy for cancer or HSCT and presenting with fever despite parenteral antibacterial treatment ≧96 h, aiming to the reduction of incidence of IA.[24]

Pneumocystis jiroveci Pneumonia (PJP)

Pneumocystis jiroveci (previously known as *P. carinii*) is a ubiquitous pathogen that usually causes asymptomatic infections in immunocompetent subjects.[3] In immunocompromised patients, *P. jiroveci* reactivation (or, less commonly, reinfection) causes severe pneumonia with mortality rates up to 50% (PJP).[3]

Although less common since the introduction of highly active antiretroviral therapy (HAART), PJP is a common opportunistic infection in patients with HIV/AIDS, especially for those with a CD4 T-cell count below 200 cells/mm^3 or high viral loads. PJP can also cause severe infections in patients with haematologic diseases, transplants recipients, or receiving immunosuppressive therapy (e.g. corticosteroids), although the incidence in these patient populations is reduced with the use of antimicrobial prophylaxis.[25] PJP can also occur in patients who are not immunocompromised, often those on longer term corticosteroids.[25]

Clinical presentation of PJP often starts with high fever, cough, shortness of breath, and progresses to severe hypoxia.[25] Typical radiographic findings are characterized by bilateral, coalescent interstitial pulmonary infiltrates showing a 'ground-glass' appearance. Microbiological diagnosis consists in the demonstration of *P. jiroveci* cysts in patients' BAL. An alternative test for the diagnosis of PJP is the use BDG, especially in patients with low number of cysts such as non-HIV patients. A meta-analysis analyzing about 400 cases of PJP reported BDG average sensitivity and specificity of 94.8% and 86.3%, respectively.[26] A negative result of serum BDG is sufficient for ruling out PJP, due to the high negative predictive value, but only in HIV-positive patients.[27] Quantitative PCR in BAL represents an alternative diagnostic tool for PJP, but the method is not standardized and no algorithm is available to distinguish between colonization and infection so far.

Mortality rates in patients with PJP can vary from 5% to 50% depending on the disease severity and patient's risk factors. Older age, low albuminemia, low alveolar–arterial oxygen gradient (<50 mmHg), and treatment delay have been associated with mortality.[25,28] Trimethoprim–sulfamethoxazole (TMP–SMX) administered for 21 days represents the first-choice treatment for *Pneumocystis* pneumonia (Table 37.2).[28] Since *P. jiroveci* lacks ergosterol in the cell wall, antifungals (except echinocandins) are not effective.[28] Corticosteroids are recommended in association with antibiotics in patients with severe forms (PaO_2 < 70 mmHg) and have been associated with lower respiratory failure and mortality rates compared to patients non-receiving corticosteroids.[28] TMP–SMX is also indicated for PJP prophylaxis in HIV-infected adults with T CD4 cell count below 200 cells/mmc and in HIV-negative patients receiving immunosuppressive medications such as corticosteroids (e.g. >20 mg of prednisolone for >8 weeks) or recipients of SOT or HSCT.

Cryptococcosis

Cryptococcus neoformans is a ubiquitous environmental encapsulated fungus that colonizes the lungs after inhalation and can cause life-long latent infection. Reactivation can occur in immunocompromised patients.[29] Isolated pulmonary disease usually presents with clinical features, such as cough, fever, shortness of breath, and pleuritic pain, often with multiple cavitated nodules at pulmonary CT scan.[29] In severely immunocompromised patients, *C. neoformans* can disseminate to the central nervous system (causing cryptococcal meningitis), bones, and skin.[29,30] Cryptococcal meningitis presentation ranges from mild to severe symptoms, with headache, fever, nausea, vomiting, visual alterations, and seizures. Skin involvement may present with purpura, vesicles, nodules, abscesses, ulcers, granulomas, pustules, or cellulitis.[30] The sensitivity and specificity of cryptococcal antigen in cases of meningitis have been reported to be >90% both in cerebrospinal fluid and serum, whereas in isolated pulmonary disease cryptococcal antigen has been detected in only 80% of cases in serum.[31] The positivity of cerebrospinal fluid cultures for *Cryptococcus* is always diagnostic for cryptococcal meningitis, while the isolation of *Cryptococcus* from respiratory samples can be either expression of infection or colonization. Current guidelines recommend different therapeutic approaches according to disease severity and body site involved.[32] In the case of meningitis, severe pneumonia or disseminated disease, lipid formulations of amphotericin B, alone or in association with flucytosine, are recommended as initial regimen, followed by long-term fluconazole (Table 37.2).[32] In isolated pulmonary involvement with mild clinical symptoms, fluconazole is the drug of choice, administered for at least 6 months. In severe immunocompromised patients, pulmonary involvement is associated with meningitis in approximately 20% of cases; thus, lumbar puncture in these cases is strongly recommended.[32]

REFERENCES

1. Blot SI, Vandewoude KH. Estimating attributable mortality of candidemia: Clinical judgement vs matched cohort studies. *Eur J Clin Microbiol Infect Dis.* 2003;**22**:132–133.
2. Pappas PG. Invasive candidiasis. *Infect Dis Clin North Am.* 2006;**20**(3):485–506.

3. Kontoyiannis DP, Marr KA, Park BJ, et al. Prospective surveillance for invasive fungal infections in hematopoietic stem cell transplant recipients, 2001–2006: Overview of the Transplant-Associated Infection Surveillance Network (TRANSNET) Database. *Clin Infect Dis.* 2010;**50**:1091–1100.
4. Meersseman W, Lagrou K, Spriet I, et al. Significance of the isolation of Candida species from airway samples in critically ill patients: A prospective, autopsy study. *Intensive Care Med.* 2009;**35**:1526–1531.
5. Wisplinghoff H, Bischoff T, Tallent SM, et al. Nosocomial bloodstream infections in US hospitals: Analysis of 24,179 cases from a prospective nationwide surveillance study. *Clin Infect Dis.* 2004;**39**:309–317.
6. Bassetti M, Molinari MP, Mussap M, et al. Candidaemia in internal medicine departments: The burden of a rising problem. *Clin Microbiol Infect.* 2013;**19**:E281–284.
7. Keighley C, Garnham K, Harch SAJ. et al. Candida auris: Diagnostic Challenges and Emerging Opportunities for the Clinical Microbiology Laboratory. *Curr Fungal Infect Rep.* 2021;**15**,116–126.
8. Cornely OA, Bassetti M, Calandra T, et al. ESCMID* guideline for the diagnosis and management of Candida diseases 2012: Non-neutropenic adult patients. *Clin Microbiol Infect.* 2012;**18**(Suppl 7):19–37.
9. Segal BH. Aspergillosis. *N Engl J Med.* 2009;**360**:1870–1884.
10. De Pauw B, Walsh TJ, Donnelly JP, et al. Revised definitions of invasive fungal disease from the European Organization for Research and Treatment of Cancer/Invasive Fungal Infections Cooperative Group and the National Institute of Allergy and Infectious Diseases Mycoses Study Group (EORTC/MSG) Consensus Group. *Clin Infect Dis.* 2008;**46**:1813–1821.
11. Bitar D, Lortholary O, Le Strat Y, et al. Population-based analysis of invasive fungal infections, France, 2001–2010. *Emerg Infect Dis.* 2014;**20**:1149–1155.
12. Smith NL, Denning DW. Underlying conditions in chronic pulmonary aspergillosis including simple aspergilloma. *Eur Respir J.* 2011;**37**:865–872.
13. Kosmidis C, Denning DW. The clinical spectrum of pulmonary aspergillosis. *Thorax.* 2015;**70**:270–277.
14. Baddley JW, Stephens JM, Ji X, et al. Aspergillosis in Intensive Care Unit (ICU) patients: Epidemiology and economic outcomes. *BMC Infect Dis.* 2013;**13**:29.
15. Taccone FS, Van den Abeele AM, Bulpa P, et al. Epidemiology of invasive aspergillosis in critically ill patients: Clinical presentation, underlying conditions, and outcomes. *Crit Care.* 2015:**19**;7.
16. Koheler P, Bassetti M, Chakrabarti A, et al. Defining and managing COVID-19-associated pulmonary aspergillosis: The 2020 ECMM/ISHAM consensus criteria for research and clinical guidance. *Lancet Infect Dis.* 2021(6):e149–e162.
17. Bassetti M, Righi E, De Pascale G, et al. How to manage aspergillosis in non-neutropenic intensive care unit patients. *Crit Care.* 2014;**18**:458.
18. Blot SI, Taccone FS, Van den Abeele AM, et al. AspICU Study Investigators. A clinical algorithm to diagnose invasive pulmonary aspergillosis in critically ill patients. *Am J Respir Crit Care Med.* 2012;**186**:56–64.
19. Meersseman W, Lagrou K, Maertens J, et al. Galactomannan in bronchoalveolar lavage fluid: A tool for diagnosing aspergillosis in intensive care unit patients. *Am J Respir Crit Care Med.* 2008;**177**:27–34.
20. Lahmer T, Rasch S, Schnappauf C, et al. Comparison of Serum Galactomannan and 1,3-Beta-D-glucan determination for early detection of invasive pulmonary aspergillosis in critically ill patients with hematological malignancies and septic shock. *Mycopathologia.* 2016;**181**(7–8):505–511.
21. Acosta J, Catalan M, del Palacio-Pérez-Medel A, et al. Prospective study in critically ill non-neutropenic patients: Diagnostic potential of (1,3)-β-D-glucan assay and circulating galactomannan for the diagnosis of invasive fungal disease. *Eur J Clin Microbiol Infect Dis.* 2012;**31**:721–731.
22. Walsh TJ, Anaissie EJ, Denning DW, et al. Infectious Diseases Society of America. Treatment of aspergillosis: Clinical practice guidelines of the Infectious Diseases Society of America. *Clin Infect Dis.* 2008;**46**:327–360.
23. Patterson TF, Thompson GR 3rd, Denning DW, et al. Executive Summary: Practice Guidelines for the Diagnosis and Management of Aspergillosis: 2016 Update by the Infectious Diseases Society of America. *Clin Infect Dis.* 2016 Aug 15;**63**(4):433–442.
24. European Society of Clinical Microbiology and Infectious Diseases (ESCMID) Fungal Infection Study Group (EFISG). 2021. https://www.escmid.org/research_projects/study_groups/efisg/
25. Thomas CF, Jr., Limper AH. Pneumocystis pneumonia. *N Engl J Med.* 2004;**350**:2487–2498.
26. Karageorgopoulos DE, Qu JM, Korbila IP, et al. Accuracy of β-D-glucan for the diagnosis of *Pneumocystis jirovecii* pneumonia: A meta-analysis. *Clin Microbiol Infect.* 2013;**19**(1):39–49.
27. Li WJ, Guo YL, Liu TJ, et al. Diagnosis of pneumocystis pneumonia using serum (1-3)-β-D-Glucan: A bivariate meta-analysis and systematic review. *J Thorac Dis.* 2015;**7**:2214–2225.
28. Limper AH, Knox KS, Sarosi GA, et al. An official American Thoracic Society statement: Treatment of fungal infections in adult pulmonary and critical care patients. *Am J Resp Crit Care Med.* 2011;**183**:96–128.
29. Lacomis JM, Costello P, Vilchez R, et al. The radiology of pulmonary cryptococcosis in a tertiary medical center. *J Thorac Imaging.* 2001;**16**:139–148.
30. Sloan DJ, Parris V. Cryptococcal meningitis: Epidemiology and therapeutic options. *Clin Epidemiol.* 2014;**6**:169–182.
31. Binnicker MJ, Jespersen DJ, Bestrom JE, et al. Comparison of four assays for the detection of cryptococcal antigen. *Clin Vaccine Immunol.* 2012;**19**:1988–1990.
32. Perfect JR, Dismukes WE, Dromer F, et al. Clinical practice guidelines for the management of cryptococcal disease: 2010 Update by the Infectious Diseases Society of America. *Clin Infect Dis.* 2010;**50**:291–322.

38

Mycobacterial Infections

Christopher Orton, Hannah Jarvis, and Onn Min Kon

- Sampling to confirm a diagnosis and to provide drug sensitivity is a key aim even in paucibacillary and extrapulmonary disease.
- Rapid polymerase chain reaction (PCR) may provide a more timely diagnosis of TB and also allow for identification of drug resistance.
- In cases with uncertain absorption, isoniazid and rifampicin should be given IV with other second-line drugs.

- The timing, triggers, combination of agents, and duration of treatments for non-tuberculous mycobacterial disease undergo evolving guideline recommendations.

- Non-sputum-based molecular biomarker tests for accurate rapid diagnosis of active tuberculosis.

Introduction

The *Mycobacterium* genus comprises over 150 Gram-negative, rod-shaped bacilli encompassing the mycobacterium tuberculosis complex (*M. tuberculosis*, *M. Africanum*, *M. bovis*, and *M. microti*) and the non-tuberculous mycobacteria (NTM). Tuberculosis (TB), the clinical manifestation of the mycobacterium tuberculosis complex infection, is by far the most clinically relevant, but NTM infection is now being increasingly identified in the developed world.

TB is a leading cause of death worldwide, causing an estimated 1.4 million deaths globally in 2019.[1] It remains relevant to developed countries given the significant issues of global migration patterns, drug resistance, the human immunodeficiency virus (HIV) pandemic, and iatrogenic immune suppression.

Whilst only 3% of TB inpatient cases require critical care admission,[2] the in-hospital mortality for such patients is high at up to 68.7%.[3] Pulmonary involvement is typical but extrapulmonary disease may present acutely in nearly any organ system, mimicking other infectious or non-infections processes. Acute respiratory distress syndrome (ARDS) is the most common reason for critical care involvement, accounting for 81.1% of TB patient admissions to a low-incidence, western European intensive care units (ICUs).[2] Multi-organ failure, cardiac arrest, septic shock, toxicity from anti-tuberculous medication, and neurological deterioration secondary to tuberculous meningitis are other important sequelae requiring invasive organ support.

TB is a treatable disease with timely identification and initiation of therapy vital in providing the best outcomes. TB patients requiring critical care input often present additional challenges, including the difficulty in obtaining microbiological confirmation and the provision of effective anti-tuberculous treatment in the context of poor absorption and frequently encountered multi-organ dysfunction.

Diagnosis

The gold standard of TB diagnosis is culture confirmation, ensuring diagnostic certainty and also providing drug susceptibility. Samples should ideally be sent for culture prior to treatment initiation, but particularly in non-pulmonary TB a positive culture can be difficult to achieve given difficulties with route of sampling and the paucibacillary nature of some presentations (e.g. TB meningitis). Even in the setting of extrapulmonary disease, an attempt to identify pulmonary tuberculosis (PTB) (e.g. CT thorax) is worthwhile considering as this compartment is generally more accessible. A wide range of tissue and fluid samples can undergo microbiological examination, but all should be assessed by an auramine or Ziehl Neilsen stain and cultured for a minimum of 6 weeks. The desire to achieve culture confirmation must however be balanced against the need for early initiation of treatment which has been associated with improved survival, especially in the context of severe disease.[4]

Molecular methods such as the polymerase chain reaction (PCR)–based Xpert® MTB/RIF and Xpert Ultra probe are increasingly used as they are superior to the smear test and in addition allows rapid identification of rifampicin resistance, a marker of potential MDR-TB disease.[1,5]

An expectorating patient with suspected PTB should provide at least three sputum samples for mycobacterial culture. Sputum samples that demonstrate a positive auramine reading are described as 'smear positive', classifying the patient as highly infectious. If negative and in an intubated patient, non-directed tracheal aspirates can be sent, whilst directed bronchoscopic lavage should be considered where insufficient microbiological sampling has been obtained. Pleural aspirates should also be sent for mycobacterial culture.

Respiratory isolation in a negative pressure room (with at least 12 air changes per hour) should be enforced for all patients with suspected PTB, especially in those with 'Smear positive' disease. When a ventilation circuit is not closed, respiratory protection with the use of N-95 or higher-level respirator mask by staff is recommended. Repeated sputum analysis stratifies infectivity and the response to treatment. Most patients with fully sensitive smear positive disease are rendered non-infectious by 2 weeks, but in the intensive care setting. with less reliable drug absorption and more intensive respiratory secretions, a persistent positive smear will generally mean isolation should continue.

ARDS (see Chapter 21) is commonly encountered in ICU patients with PTB, particularly in those receiving mechanical ventilation. Established mechanical ventilation strategies such as lower tidal volumes and conservative fluid management may be appropriate. ARDS is potentially over-diagnosed in this cohort as confluent tuberculous bronchopneumonia is a radiological mimic.[6]

Extrapulmonary TB is often paucibacillary, and histological or cytological analysis is therefore more significant with the identification of lymphocytic effusion or caseating granulomas consistent with a diagnosis of TB. A lumbar puncture is crucial in identifying tuberculous meningitis as diagnosis is initially based on typical cerebrospinal fluid findings—raised protein, lymphocyte predominance, and reduced glucose. Positive CSF culture ultimately offers confirmation, and the use of the Xpert® MTB/RIF and also Xpert Ultra probe has been shown to be comparable with microscopy.[5,6] Urine culture may be useful in disseminated, miliary TB.[6] Blood cultures are known to be useful in diagnosing miliary TB in HIV sufferers, with mycobacteraemia proportional to CD4 count.[6]

Interferon gamma release assays (IGRAs) have been developed principally for the diagnosis of latent TB infection. IGRAs are highly specific for the diagnosis of TB infection as they measure interferon gamma release triggered by TB antigens using ex vivo stimulation. As the antigens are more specific to *Mycobacterium tuberculosis* infection and are not found in BCG vaccines, cross-reactivity with immunization or most NTM infections are avoided. IGRAs should be used cautiously as active TB cannot be distinguished from latent infection, and a negative result cannot be used to rule out active disease given only a moderately high sensitivity.[6] Similarly the tuberculin skin test is frequently negative in the most severely affected by TB, and although may indicate prior infection with TB, it is less specific given cross-reactivity with the BCG vaccine and NTM.

Radiology (Chapter 18) is often crucial in supporting the diagnosis of TB prior to microbial confirmation. Chest radiographs classically demonstrate apical consolidation with cavitation (Figure 38.1) although plain films can reveal any consolidative pattern, mediastinal lymphadenopathy, effusion, or be entirely unremarkable. Bronchiectatic airways or calcification may be indicative of previous TB infection. Atypical features are common in the elderly or immunocompromised as radiological findings are dependent on the host's immune response. Cross-sectional imaging should be considered for atypical cases as the identification of intrathoracic cavities, mediastinal nodes, effusions, as well as extrapulmonary disease sites allows for targeted microbiological sampling. CT can help differentiate the 'tree in bud' and centrilobular nodules found in active disease (Figure 38.2) from long-standing fibrotic changes. MRI is useful in CNS disease. PET-CT may have a role in the identification of occult disease sites for sampling.

Ultimately, it may not be possible to achieve microbiological validation of TB in an appropriate clinical timeframe. Raised clinical suspicion based on a history, epidemiological risk factors (e.g. recent TB contact), supportive radiology, and cytological/biochemical analysis of fluid results will often therefore lead to a decision to treat. Ensuring that all possible sampling for culture material has occurred prior to treatment initiation maximizes the chance

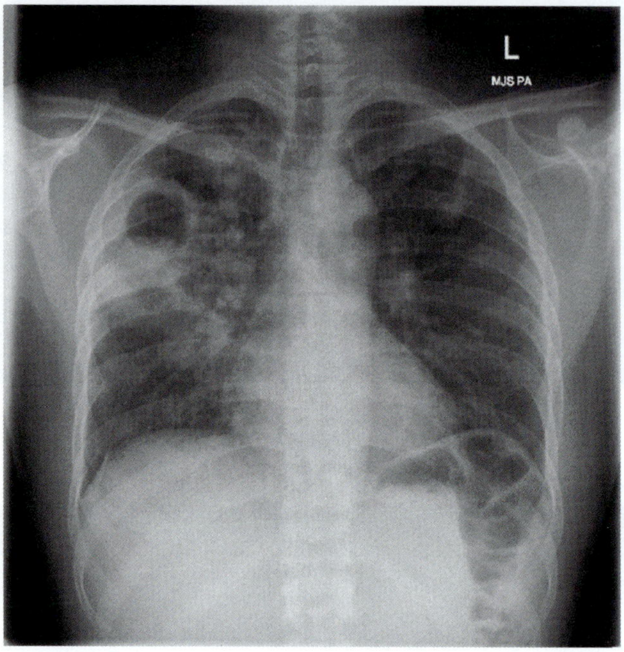

Figure 38.1 Chest radiograph demonstrating a right apical cavity with bilateral upper zone infiltrates.

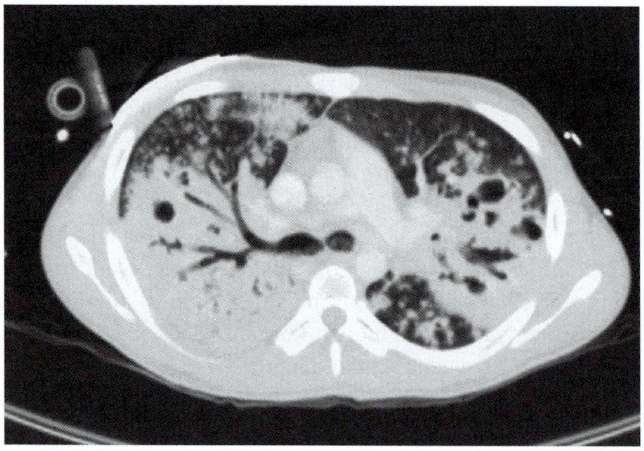

Figure 38.2 CT thorax demonstrating bilateral 'tree-in-bud' and confluent TB bronchopneumonia in an intubated and ventilated patient.

of subsequent validation and the provision of drug sensitivities. Culture confirmation, the central aim of TB diagnosis, was only achieved in 61% of UK TB cases notified in 2019.[7] The proportion of PTB cases with confirmatory culture (74.2%) was significantly higher than for extrapulmonary disease (44.5%).[11] 10.8% of all TB isolates are resistant to at least one first-line antibiotic with 1.3% demonstrating multi-drug-resistant TB (MDR-TB).[11]

Treatment and Side Effects

Timely identification and initiation of treatment is paramount in the treatment of TB. Retrospective review of patient outcomes in two Western European ICUs with severe active PTB demonstrated a 26% 30-day mortality, with a time of greater than 1 month from symptom onset to treatment found to be an independent predictor of mortality (OR 3.49).[8]

Aggressive antibiotic treatment is supported as secondary respiratory infection occurs in 67%, with 59% developing a nosocomial pneumonia in one German cohort.[9] Other ICU-related complications included pneumothorax in 14%, ARDS in 13.8%, acute renal failure in 12.1%, and multiple organ failure in 3.4%.[2] The need for mechanical ventilation in respiratory failure cause by TB is high and independently associated with an increased risk of mortality.[10] Whilst the use of non-invasive ventilation strategies may ameliorate some of the complications associated with mechanical ventilation, there is a limited evidence base to support its use, which may relate to concerns regarding the aerosolization of infection.[11]

Standard quadruple therapy with rifampicin, isoniazid, pyrazinamide, and ethambutol forms the basis of anti-tuberculous treatment.[12] Regimes should consist of a minimum of three antimicrobial agents to reduce the risk of developing mycobacterial drug resistance. Rifampicin and isoniazid are the central bactericidal backbone of the regime but are associated with potential hepatotoxicity. Pyrazinamide and ethambutol are renally excreted with dose adjustments required with a glomerular filtration rate of less than 30 mL/min/1.73 m^2. Ethambutol is associated with potential optic nerve toxicity, and visual testing is indicated prior to commencing treatment, preventing its use in ventilated, sedated patients. The risk of isoniazid related peripheral neuropathy is reduced with supplementation with pyridoxine. Second- and third-line drugs including moxifloxacin, amikacin, linezolid, clofazimine, and meropenem with clavulanate are reserved for cases of drug intolerance or resistance.[9]

Patients in the ICU setting present specific challenges with high rates of hepatic and renal dysfunction, necessitating caution with anti-tuberculous medication (Figure 38.3). Furthermore, routine practices such as visual acuity testing are not feasible in the critically unwell patient. Enteral absorption may be uncertain with increased drug level monitoring pragmatic as sub-therapeutic drug levels are associated with treatment failure and drug resistance. For such cases or in the sedated patient, an initial parenteral regime could consist of rifampicin, isoniazid, and moxifloxacin. Pyrazinamide can be given through a naso-gastric tube. Secondary bacterial co-infection is common, so a low threshold is required for initiation of broad-spectrum antibiotics.[2] Therapeutic drug monitoring is available for rifampicin, isoniazid, ethambutol, moxifloxacin, levofloxacin, and amikacin.

The risk of developing hepatotoxicity may be increased with older age, alcohol excess, HIV, or hepatitis co-infection. UK guidance suggests that cessation of anti-tuberculous medication should occur with a 3–5-fold increase in transaminases or a rise in bilirubin.[13] A relatively non-hepatotoxic regime should be substituted, such as levofloxacin or moxifloxacin and amikacin with continuation of ethambutol. Rifampicin and isoniazid are then sequentially reintroduced once liver-function tests are back to baseline.[8]

There are several important drug interactions between rifampicin and drugs commonly used in intensive care including morphine, fentanyl, and midazolam.[11] In addition, anti-retroviral therapies can interact with rifampicin and specialist advice is recommended in cases of TB/HIV co-infection. In general, rifampicin should not be administered with any of the protease inhibitors or other approved non-nucleoside reverse transcriptase inhibitors (NNRTIs) apart from efavirenz—due to alterations in levels of the drugs or

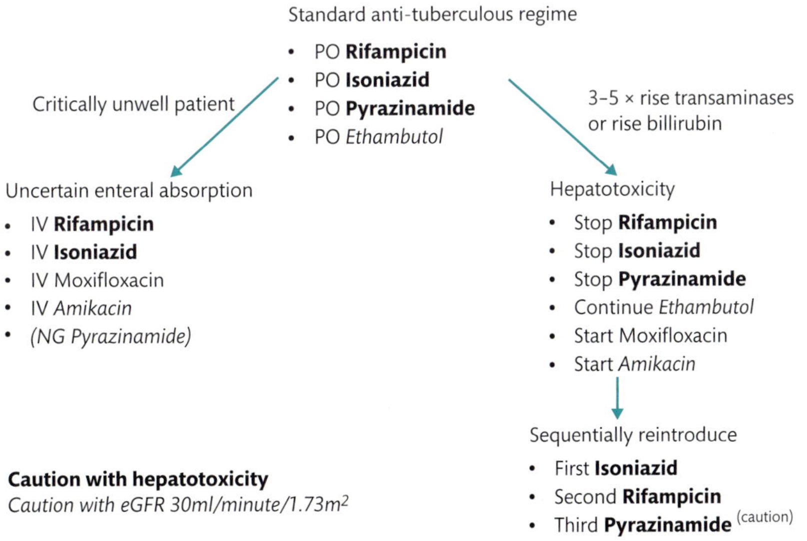

Figure 38.3 Treatment algorithm for TB in patients with uncertain parenteral absorption and hepatotoxicity.

side effects such as liver toxicity. An alternative approach is to use rifabutin in place of rifampicin.[14]

High-dose dexamethasone or prednisolone with gradual withdrawal has been shown to have a role in TB meningitis and pericardial disease. For meningeal disease, starting dexamethasone concomitantly with anti-tuberculous intravenous treatment is recommended at a dose of 0.3 mg/kg/day where GCS is 15 and at a dose of 0.4 mg/kg/day where GCS is reduced.[11] In pericardial disease, starting prednisolone 60 mg/day and withdrawing over 2–3 weeks is advised to reduce the speed of fluid re-accumulation although the evidence for utilizing this routinely is still unclear.[11]

A paradoxical reaction in TB is defined as a clinical or radiological worsening of pre-existing TB lesions or the development of new lesions, in a patient receiving anti-tuberculous medication that initially improved with treatment. Most cases are mild and transient, but significant morbidity and death have been reported. Paradoxical reactions are likely related to an abnormal immune response or reconstitution of the immune system and hence the incidence is higher in patients with HIV co-infection.[15] Concomitant use of steroids (or other immunomodulators) may be necessary if such reactions are significant.

NTM are frequent colonizers in chronic respiratory disease but may be a primary pathogen in the immunosuppressed/HIV co-infection patient. In HIV, disseminated MAI may be the cause of severe disease. Treatment initially consists of rifampicin/rifabutin, ethambutol, and clarithromycin/azithromycin with prolonged courses necessary.

Controversies and Future Practice

MDR-TB defined as a resistance to rifampicin and isoniazid remains a persistent concern in the management of the disease. In the UK, in 2019, 1.3% of newly reported TB cases were multi-drug resistant. In the UK, PCR testing of primary samples to identify rifampicin resistance is recommended for all patients with culture confirmed TB with full drug sensitivity testing if resistance to rifampicin is identified.[11] If rifampicin resistance is detected, then the patient should be treated as per an MDR-TB protocol with at least five agents to which the mycobacterium should be sensitive.[12]

New agents such as Bedaquiline and Delamanid are now available to aid the fight against MDR-TB. Identification of a biomarker-based, low-cost, non-sputum-based test remains as an important priority for the medium term. Further biomarker work to identify markers of treatment success remains a long-term goal.[16]

REFERENCES

1. World Health Organisation (WHO). Global TB report 2020. 2020.
2. Erbes R, Oettel K, Raffenberg M, et al. Characteristics and outcome of patients with active pulmonary tuberculosis requiring intensive care. *Eur Resp J*. 2006;**27**(6):1223–1228.
3. Otu A, Hasmi M, Mukhtar A, et al. The critically ill patient with tuberculosis in intensive care: Clinical presentations, management and infection control. *J Crit Care*. 2018;**45**:184–196.
4. Kethireddy S, Light RB, Mirzanejad Y, et al. Mycobacterium tuberculosis septic shock. *Chest*. 2013;**144**:474–482.
5. Park M, Kon OM. Use of Xpert MTB/RIF and Xpert Ultra in extrapulmonary tuberculosis. *Expert Rev Anti Infect Ther*. 2021;**19**:65–77.
6. Hagan G, Nathani N. Clinical review: Tuberculosis on the intensive care unit. *Crit Care*. 2013 *17*, 240.
7. Public Health England. Tuberculosis in England: 2020 report. Public Health England, London; 2020.
8. Zahar JR, Azoulay E, Klement E, et al. Delayed treatment contributes to mortality in ICU patients with severe active pulmonary tuberculosis and acute respiratory failure. *Intensive Care Med*. 2001;**27**:513–520.
9. Horsburgh CR, Barry CE, Lange C. Treatment of Tuberculosis. *N Engl J Med*. 2015;**373**:2149–2160.
10. Balkema CA, Irusen EM, Taljaard JJ, et al. Tuberculosis in the intensive care unit: A prospective observational study. *Int J Tuberc Lung Dis*. 2014;**1**:824–830.
11. Passi NN, Buckley J. Tuberculosis on the intensive care unit. *Br J Hosp Med (Lond)*. 2018;**79**:142–147.
12. Tuberculosis NICE guideline Published: 13 January 2016 nice.org.uk/guidance/ng33
13. Ramappa V, Aithal GP. Hepatotoxicity related to anti-tuberculosis drugs: Mechanisms and management. *J Clin Exp Hepatol*. 2013;**3**:37–49.
14. Havlir DV, Getahun H, Sanne I, et al. Opportunities and challenges for HIV care in overlapping HIV and TB epidemics. *JAMA*. 2008;**300**:423–430.
15. Bloch S, Wickremasinghe M, Wright A, et al. Paradoxical reactions in non-HIV tuberculosis presenting as endobronchial obstruction. *Eur Resp Rev*. 2009;**18**:295–298.
16. Pai M, Schito M. Tuberculosis diagnostics in 2015: Landscape, priorities, needs, and prospects. *J Infect Dis*. 2015;**211**:S21–28.

39

Travellers' Pneumonia

Dhruva Chaudhry, Pawan Kumar Singh, and Manjunath B Govindagoudar

- Globalization of infections through international travel has made travel medicine increasingly relevant.
- Pneumonia among travellers is an infrequent but important cause of fever and morbidity.
- Destination, trip duration and timing, local exposures, age, sex, and co-morbidity are important risk factors affecting outcome.
- H1N1, SARS, MERS, currently COVID-19, and future emerging infections of significance pose global threats and need ongoing vigilance at least at the clinical level.
- Infection control measures and personal protection are crucial when dealing with travellers' pneumonias to reduce transmission.

- The effectiveness of rapid diagnostic test and trace symptoms for the prevention of cluster infections in fellow travellers during air, land, or sea travel.
- What is the most effective set of measures that will minimize the risk of the spread of infection after travel and prevent the disruption of travel, as demonstrated during the COVID-19 pandemic.

- Accessible and accurate rapid diagnostic point-of-care tests (POCTs) of infection that prevent the need to isolate.
- Development of effective antiviral agents that will reduce illness and transmission risks at the point of diagnosis.
- The creation of universal vaccines within structural biology that will enable rapid vaccine production for future emerging zoonotic infectious agents that may cause travellers' pneumonia.

Introduction

Travel medicine requires specialist knowledge, awareness of local disease epidemiology, and dedicated clinical services to meet the health needs of the increasing number of travellers. International travellers may be affected by several infectious diseases. Several health concerns have been highlighted among travellers such as gastrointestinal manifestations, neurological diseases, respiratory problems, and systemic illnesses. Travellers may be impacted by such diseases while acting as vectors for spread of infection. However, pneumonia is a rare cause for travellers seeking medical care. Literature focusing on pneumonia among travellers is limited, making the prevalence of specific aetiologies of travellers' pneumonia highly variable.

Epidemiology

The epidemiology of infections among travellers depends upon the areas visited, indigenous infections, and their local prevalence. More than 600 million people travel annually and 15%–50% of those experience health problems related to travel.[1] Diarrhoea represents half to two-thirds of these conditions, followed by respiratory tract infection (RTI; 14%–31%), fever (12%–15%), and skin complaints (12%).[2] In a study by Steffen et al., the estimated incidence of acute febrile RTI was 1261 per 100,000 travellers for a stay of 1 month in a developing country, that is, an attack rate of 1.26%.[2] A similar study in Nepal found the prevalence of RTI to be 17.55% and pneumonia to be 0.46%.[3] Pneumonia may not be the common focus of infections but is an important cause of fever among returning travellers[4–6] (Table 39.1). The majority of these patients acquire pneumonia, especially due to influenza during the months of November through April in the northern hemisphere and from April to October in the southern hemisphere. Most patients improve with outpatient care. However, the mortality from pneumonia among returning travellers was 1% in a Canadian study (3/309 deaths).[7] With the current COVID-19 pandemic, the travel history has become far more important. Several guidelines have been adopted by various countries to screen as well as quarantine travellers with or without symptoms.

Aetiology

The pathogens causing respiratory infection in travellers are similar to those in non-travellers. The data including COVID-19 pandemic

Table 39.1 Respiratory diagnoses reported in the Geosentinel Global Emerging Infections Surveillance Network Database from November 1997 to September 2001

Diagnosis	N = 1719
URTI	1177
LRTI	693
Bronchitis	349 (20.3)
Pneumonia	232 (13.5)
Influenza	96 (5.6)
Legionairre's disease	2 (0.12)
Pleurisy	14 (0.81)

Note: URTI, upper respiratory tract infection; LRTI, lower respiratory tract infection.
Source: Data from Freedman DO, Kozarsky PE, Weld LH, et al. GeoSentinel: The global emerging infections sentinel network of the International Society of Travel Medicine. *J Travel Med.* 1999;6(2):94–98.

is lacking, but commonly it is believed that bacterial pneumonia comprises around 50% of all travel-associated pneumonias.[4,6] Moreover, travellers are also exposed to pulmonary diseases attributed to other fungal pathogens that are endemic to the visited destination (Table 39.2). Malaria, dengue, and tuberculosis represent the most commonly reported overall infections among travellers. The syndrome of eosinophilic pneumonias is caused by several parasitic infections such as tropical pulmonary eosinophilia, Katayama syndrome, Loeffler's syndrome, paragonimiasis, echinococcosis, toxocariasis, etc. Endemicity of fungal infections such as histoplasmosis, coccidiomycoses, and blastomycoses is a concern for migrants and visitors to South America, the Southern USA, and parts of Central, West, and Southern Africa (coccidiomycosis flourishes in desert to semi-desert conditions, histoplasmosis is found in humid, tropical climates with temperatures of 20–30 °C, whereas blastomycosis is common near river valley of Mississippi and apart from similar areas in central America). Respiratory diseases due to tick bites, chiggers bite, and zoonotic infections are also common in tropics. Viral agents causing respiratory diseases and pneumonias have put air travel under scrutiny because of high attack rates, which was recently observed in COVID-19 pandemic and prior pandemics. Recently, outbreaks of influenza (H1N1 2009), severe

Table 39.2 Common aetiological agents causing travel related pneumonias

Bacterial pneumonia	*Streptococcus pneumoniae*, *Staphylococcus aureus* including MRSA, *Mycoplasma pneumonia*, *Legionella pneumophila*, *Coxiella burnetti*, *Leptospira* sp., *Mycobacterium tuberculosis*, and *Haemophilus influenza*
Viral pneumonia	Influenza virus, dengue, SARS-CoV-1 and 2, MERS-CoV, and pulmonary renal syndrome (Hanta virus)
Fungal pneumonia	Histoplasmosis (*Histoplasma capsulatum*), blastomycosis (*Blastomyces dermatidis*), coccidiomycosis (*Coccidiodes immitis*), Paracoccidiomycosis (*Paracoccidioides brasiliensis*), and *Pneumocystis jiroveci*
Parasitic infections	Schistosomiasis (*Shistosoma hemotobium*), tropical pulmonary eosinophilia (Wuccheria, Brugia), paragonimiasis (*Paragonimus westermanii*), strongyloidosis (strongyloides), Toxocariasis (*Toxocara canis*), pulmonary hydatid cyst, (*Echinococcus* spp.)
Protozoa	Malaria (plasmodium)

Table 39.3 Risk factors associated with acquisition of pneumonia in travellers

Factors associated with risk of pneumonia among travellers	
Age	More than 40 years
Sex	Male
Trip duration	Prolonged duration (more than 30 days)
Type of travel	Peace corps and healthcare workers
Co-morbidities	Diabetes mellitus, chronic renal disease, immuno-compromised state, heart failure, obesity, etc.

acute respiratory syndrome (SARS) and Middle East respiratory syndrome (MERS) by coronaviruses (2003 and 2012), and 2019–2020 pandemic of SARS-CoV-2 with its variants in latest avatar raised the issues of global health security and safety of travellers. In addition to the safety of travellers, it has also brought into notice the risk of transmission by them and subsequent spread in their countries of visit or origin.

Individual risk factors such as co-morbidities, age, duration and timing of trip, and type of travel are important details that can influence the outcome for pneumonia during travel. Age more than 40 years, the presence of co-morbidities such as diabetes, heart failure, and renal failure have been associated with increased risk of lower RTIs.[5] Compared with shorter trips, the travel duration of more than 30 days was associated with an increased risk of influenza and lower RTI. Persons visiting Central Asia and Indian subcontinent during the autumn months (September to November) are at high risk of acquisition of lower RTIs and bronchitis[5] (Table 39.3).

Transmission

The inhalation route of transmission for several infections is a major area of concern due to high acquisition rates leading to an exponential spread of airborne infections especially in closed spaces. Influenza, coronavirus, tuberculosis, anthrax, histoplasmosis, coccidiomycoses, etc. are spread through inhalational route. Legionella infection is primarily transmitted through aerosols and aspiration of contaminated water while using spas and swimming pools during stay in resorts and hotels or in cruise ships. Transmission of zoonotic diseases primarily occurs through contact with infected animals or their excretions and rarely human to human: pulmonary Hanta virus (rodents), tularaemia (rabbits and hares), leptospirosis (rats), Q-fever (sheep and goats), and MERS-COV (dromedary camels).[8] SARS-CoV-2 now is well established to spread through aerosols and droplets. Rickettsial infections are transmitted by tick bite while Tsutsugamushi fever is transmitted by chiggers, larvae of the mite family Trombiculidae. Most airborne transmission is by aerosol generation and hence requires relatively closer and prolonged contact. Fomite-associated transmissions have been implicated for the spread of infections, but their true contribution to the outbreaks are not known.

Diagnosis

A detailed clinical history regarding travel destination, duration of travel, type and timing of trip (business, leisure, adventure, etc.), food habits while on trip, unprotected sex, use of spas/swimming pools/rivers or lakes during a stay, as well as age, co-morbidity, and vaccination status of the returned traveller is most important.

The common presenting symptoms include fever, cough, sore throat, shortness of breath, sputum production, and haemoptysis. Fever is usually associated with headache and myalgia especially in viral infections. Cough may be dry or associated with sputum production. Extrapulmonary manifestations such as nausea, diarrhoea, abdominal pain (legionella), and skin rash/eschar (rickettsiosis/scrub typhus) may be present and point towards a specific aetiology. The clinical course may be indolent as in mycobacterial infection, histoplasmosis, melioidosis and schistosomiasis, or fulminant leading to respiratory failure as in SARS-CoV-1 and 2, MERS-CoV, and H1N1 influenza pneumonitides. Patients of COVID-19 infection may have loss of smell, taste, diarrhoea, as well as transient conjunctivitis.

Thorough clinico-radio-laboratory investigations are required to find the aetiological agent not only for treatment but also for surveillance purposes. Special tests will require a high index of clinical suspicion. Despite these, microbiological diagnosis is not possible in all the cases, and empirical management based on an epidemiological profile and clinical features may be required (Figure 39.1).

Specific Infections

Tuberculosis

Acquiring TB infection is usually defined as conversion from a negative to a positive tuberculin skin test (TST), or a positive TST in a child. Foreign travel has been identified as a risk factor for a positive TST in studies.[9,10] BCG naive status, travel to countries with high incidence of TB, duration of travel, and conditions requiring prolong and close contact with TB-infected persons such as healthcare workers, peace corps volunteers, etc. have been cited as independent risk factors.[10,11] Infection with TB during air travel has been documented, but the overall risk is low.[12]

The World Health Organization (WHO) guidelines recommend that long-term travellers (greater than 3 months) travelling from low- to high-incidence countries should have TSTs pre- and post-travel. Newly acquired infection should be treated accordingly. BCG vaccination is considered to be of limited use in travellers with the exception of infants under 6 months and young children and healthcare workers.[13] There is currently no established role for interferon gamma release assays to determine seroconversion in frequent travellers from low to high prevalence countries of tuberculosis.

Legionnaire's Disease (LD)

LD was first identified during an outbreak of *Legionella pneumophila* among travellers attending the 1976 American Legion convention in Philadelphia.[14] Whirlpool spas have been identified as sources of LD in hotels and cruise ships in several studies.[15,16] Pontiac fever is an acute self-limiting manifestation of infection by *Legionella pneumophila*, without respiratory features. Features of LD include fever, non-productive cough, headache, myalgias, rigors, dyspnoea, diarrhoea, and delirium.[17] Neurological and gastrointestinal manifestations in a patient with pneumonia must call for investigating for LD. Alveolar infiltrates on imaging are sensitive for LD but have limited specificity.[18] Several working groups have been formed for collecting data on LD and forming guidelines.[19]

In recent years, the understanding of LD has improved substantially, and new diagnostic and treatment strategies have been introduced.[19] Laboratory testing is necessary for the confirmation of outbreaks. Urinary antigen test (UAT) detection and serology testing are rapid detection tests and are easily available in high-incidence countries. The UAT has 70%–95% sensitivity for the most prevalent serogroup 1, and up to 99% specificity, but may miss other serotypes. Respiratory culture is also recommended if possible. PCR if available is highly sensitive and specific (95%–99%, >99% respect). Four-fold increases in serology are considered diagnostic.

Levofloxacin and azithromycin are preferred for treatment because they are bactericidal, achieve high intracellular concentrations with lung tissue, and are active against all *Legionella* species that cause human infection. Alternatives include ciprofloxacin, moxifloxacin, clarithromycin, roxithromycin, and doxycycline

Influenza

Influenza is a highly contagious acute respiratory disease and has been causing epidemics and pandemics throughout the centuries. Primary influenza virus pneumonia is uncommon but carries a high case fatality rate. Influenza outbreaks have been described frequently in travellers on board ships and aircraft, where conditions are ideal for rapid transmission due to enclosed space and close contacts. International travel is important in influenza epidemiology as it is a major factor in the intercontinental spread of new antigenic variants of influenza viruses. An outbreak of A/Sydney/05/97 (H3N2) influenza on a cruise ship, which introduced this antigenic variant to both the USA and Canada in 1997, is a historical example.[20] There are three types of influenza viruses: A, B, and C. Type A causes widespread epidemics and pandemics, type B is associated with regions and epidemics, and type C is associated with sporadic cases. The clinical picture consists of an abrupt onset fever with malaise, headache, sore throat, myalgia, coryza, and a dry cough lasting 2–5 days. The clinical features in children and in the elderly may differ in some aspects, and children may present with febrile convulsions, conjunctivitis, and croup.

Historically, influenza has caused the greatest number of pandemics.[21] Recent pandemics include H5N1 and H7N9, both avian strains of influenza A and the pandemic of H1N1 (2009). Because of high transmissibility rate, not only tourists and travellers but the healthcare staff involved in care of infected travellers are also at high risk. For the treatment of patients with severe influenza, oseltamivir is the preferred agent; peramivir or zanamir may be used for patients who cannot tolerate oral or inhaled agents.

SARS and MERS

The recent influential coronavirus-related disease among humans includes the severe acute respiratory syndrome coronavirus (i.e. SARS-CoV) pandemic in 2003 and Middle East respiratory syndrome (i.e. MERS-CoV) in 2012.[22,23]

SARS spreads by droplet transmission or direct person-to-person through close contact.[24] While the pattern of transmission of MERS-CoV remains unclear, hypotheses include frequent zoonotic transmissions with limited subsequent human-to-human transmission. Evidence suggests that the dromedary camel is a reservoir for the MERS-CoV. The clinical picture of SARS and MERS appears to

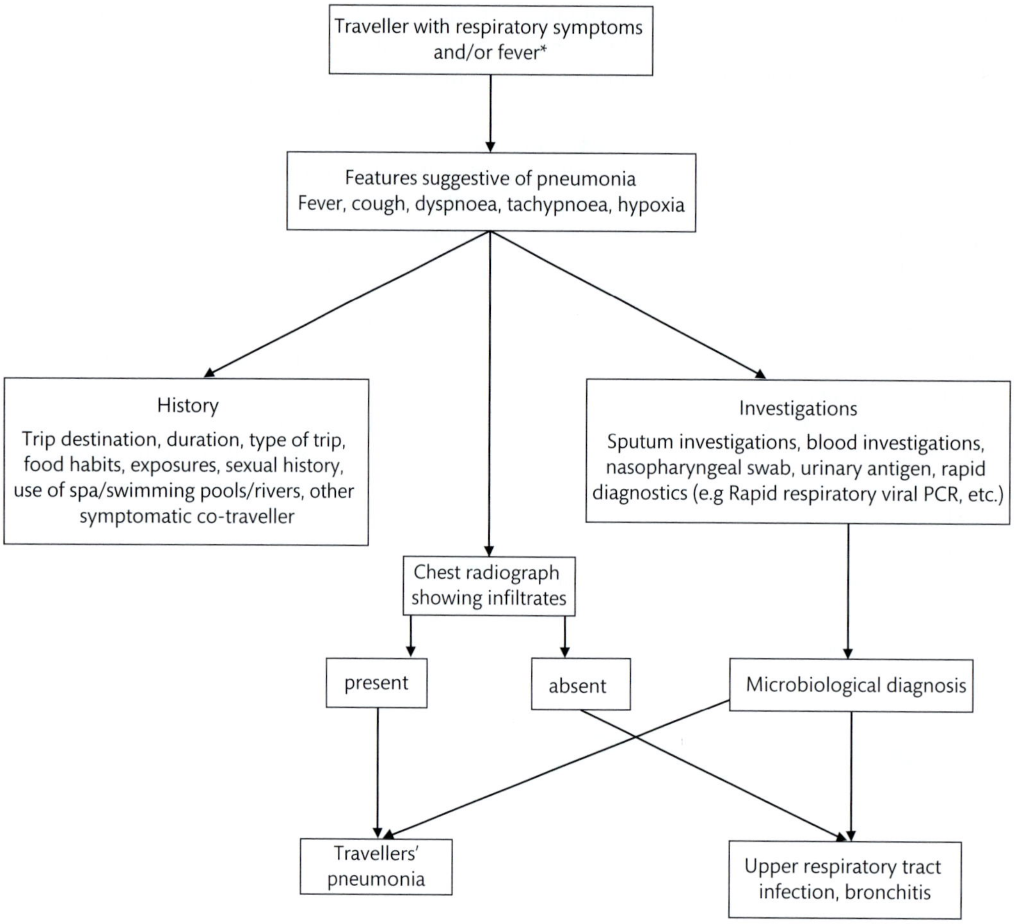

Figure 39.1 Approach to a returned traveller with respiratory symptoms. *Consider isolation, infection control measures, PPE, and early liaison with local public health/microbiology.

be similar. In 2003, SARS-CoV caused higher rates of infections in healthcare settings and affected healthier and younger persons with WHO estimated 10%–15% overall case fatality rate.[25]

MERS-CoV has emerged in the Middle East where religious mass gatherings take place in Saudi Arabia every year and potentially contribute to the international spread. The Saudi Ministry of Health in 2014 recommended that elderly people, above 65 years of age, and those with chronic diseases, pregnant women, and children (under 12 years) coming for Hajj and Umrah should postpone the performance of the Hajj and Umrah. Even after the pandemic, several sporadic cases continue to be reported in the Middle East.

COVID-19 Disease

COVID-19 originated in the Wuhan territory of China but spread across the world in a matter of few weeks. Being caused by a variant of coronavirus, SARS-CoV-2, the clinical picture is largely similar to SARS. Patients present with fever, malaise, and body aches. A significant proportion of subjects develop breathlessness and hypoxia. Rare manifestations such as myocarditis, encephalitis, and hepatitis have also been reported.[26] The various drugs repurposed for the management of COVID-19 disease have been anti-retroviral drugs, anti-parasitic drugs, anti-HCV drugs, as well as anti-influenza drugs although the quality of evidence for their use is still low.[27] Evidence generation lagged behind significantly to the spread of virus, but the early use of steroids was shown to reduce mortality in one of the landmark trials. The overall mortality in India and most of the developing countries has been relatively low (below 3%). High-risk groups have been people with co-morbidities, obesity, and the elderly. Currently, there have been over 20 vaccines under trial or in marketing phase for COVID-19. This is further discussed in Chapter 35 on COVID-19.

Role of Critical Care in Emerging Global Infections

Infections such as H1N1 influenza, SARS, and MERS may have a fulminant course and often require intensive care unit (ICU) admission and ventilator support in view of hypoxemic respiratory failure and hemodynamic monitoring. High-flow nasal oxygenation, invasive mechanical ventilation with low tidal volume strategy, and extra corporeal membrane oxygenator (ECMO) played important roles in the management of H1N1 pandemic in 2009.[28] ECMO emerged as an important treatment/salvage modality during this pandemic, with a high number of patients ventilated critically ill patients.[29] In contrast, during the SARS outbreak, up to 20% of SARS patients required intensive care admission for respiratory failure and cardiopulmonary monitoring. Despite high transmissibility, the proportion of and absolute numbers of critically ill patients were low. Non-invasive ventilation was widely used and able to prevent intubation and mechanical ventilation in two-thirds of severe cases. Various global agencies have issued standard care practice guidelines for surge in cases of viral pneumonia during pandemics.

Tropical infections such as malaria, scrub typhus, and leptospirosis are characterized by multisystem involvement. Bacterial pneumonia that are caused by highly virulent strains may progress to acute respiratory distress syndrome and severe sepsis/septic shock necessitating ICU admission.

Infection Control and Personal Protection

Breaking the human-to-human transmission cycle remains the cornerstone of infection control practices, especially infections with high transmissibility like influenza (H1N1), SARS, MERS, and SARS-CoV-2. Hand hygiene is a major component of standard precautions and one of the most effective methods to prevent transmission of pathogens associated with healthcare. It was estimated that the probability of SARS infection was 6% per shift among nurses in Toronto which was attributed to hand-to-hand transmission.[30] In addition to hand hygiene, the use of personal protective equipment (PPE), especially the mask covering the entry points of nose and mouth, should be guided by risk assessment and the extent of contact anticipated with blood and body fluids or pathogens. PPE includes clean gloves, fluid-resistant gown, mask and eye protection, or a face shield. Source control measures, such as respiratory hygiene/cough etiquette, developed during the SARS outbreak are now considered part of standard precautions. Ensuring safe waste management of products contaminated with blood, body fluids, and secretions and excretions as clinical waste in accordance with local regulations also plays a significant role in infection control.

Conclusion

With increase in international travel, infectious agents are migrating frequently and changing the epidemiology of airborne infectious diseases in particular. Respiratory infection including pneumonia in returned travellers is an important cause for healthcare seeking. Risk of contracting the infections depends on destination, trip duration, type of trip, etc., and the host factors such as age, gender, and co-morbid conditions. Aetiology of pneumonia in returned travellers is diverse and requires an index of clinical suspicion with the appropriate, sometimes special, testing. Critical care management is supportive and predominantly for respiratory failure. Respiratory infections due to H1N1, SARS, MERS, and SARS-CoV-2 have posed a global threat and need constant reconnaissance of travellers. Infection control measures and PPE should be deployed while treating these highly infectious diseases. Specific treatments are available for influenza viruses and relevant bacterial pneumonias.

REFERENCES

1. Bruni M, Steffen R. Impact of travel-related health impairments. *J Travel Med.* 1997;**4**(2):61–64.
2. Steffen R, Rickenbach M, Wilhelm U, et al. Health problems after travel to developing countries. *J Infect Dis.* 1987;**156**(1):84–91.
3. Hochedez P, Vinsentini P, Ansart S, et al. Changes in the pattern of health disorders diagnosed among two cohorts of French travelers to Nepal, 17 years apart. *J Travel Med.* 2004;**11**(6):341–346.
4. Doherty JF, Grant AD, Bryceson AD. Fever as the presenting complaint of travellers returning from the tropics. *Q J Med.* 1995;**88**(4):277–281.
5. Freedman DO, Kozarsky PE, Weld LH, et al. GeoSentinel: The global emerging infections sentinel network of the international Society of Travel Medicine. *J Travel Med.* 1999;**6**(2):94–98.
6. Parola P, Soula G, Gazin P, et al. Fever in travelers returning from tropical areas: Prospective observational study of 613 cases hospitalised in Marseilles, France, 1999–2003. *Travel Med Infect Dis.* 2006;**4**(2):61–70.
7. MacPherson DW, Guérillot F, Streiner DL, et al. Death and dying abroad: The Canadian experience. *J Travel Med.* 2000;**7**(5):227–233.
8. Zumla A, Dar O, Kock R, et al. Taking forward a 'One Health' approach for turning the tide against the Middle East respiratory syndrome coronavirus and other zoonotic pathogens with epidemic potential. *Int J Infect Dis.* 2016;**47**:5–9.
9. Saiman L, San Gabriel P, Schulte J, et al. Risk factors for latent tuberculosis infection among children in New York City. *Pediatrics.* 2001;**107**(5):999–1003.
10. Houston S. Tuberculosis risk and prevention in travelers—what about BCG? *J Travel Med.* 1997;**4**(2):76–82.
11. Cobelens FG, van Deutekom H, Draayer-Jansen IW, et al. Risk of infection with Mycobacterium tuberculosis in travellers to areas of high tuberculosis endemicity. *Lancet.* 2000;**356**(9228):461–465.
12. Rieder HL. Risk of travel-associated tuberculosis. *Clin Infect Dis.* 2001;**33**(8):1393–1396.
13. Ponce C, Dolea C. The World Health Organisation (WHO) and International Travel and Health: New collaborative, evidence-based and digital directions. *Travel Med Infect Dis.* 2019;**27**:1.
14. Fraser DW, Tsai TR, Orenstein W, et al. Legionnaires' disease: Description of an epidemic of pneumonia. *N Engl J Med.* 1977;**297**(22):1189–1197.
15. Jernigan DB, Hofmann J, Cetron MS, et al. Outbreak of Legionnaires' disease among cruise ship passengers exposed to a contaminated whirlpool spa. *Lancet.* 1996;**347**(9000):494–499.
16. Thomas DL, Mundy LM, Tucker PC. Hot tub legionellosis. Legionnaires' disease and Pontiac fever after a point-source exposure to Legionella pneumophila. *Arch Intern Med.* 1993;**153**(22):2597–2599.
17. Ricketts K, Joseph CA, Yadav R. Travel-associated Legionnaires disease in Europe in 2008. *Euro Surveill.* 2010;**15**(21):19578.
18. Macfarlane JT, Miller AC, Roderick Smith WH, et al. Comparative radiographic features of community acquired Legionnaires' disease, pneumococcal pneumonia, mycoplasma pneumonia, and psittacosis. *Thorax.* 1984;**39**(1):28–33.
19. Carratalà J, Garcia-Vidal C. An update on Legionella. *Curr Opin Infect Dis.* 2010;**23**(2):152–157.
20. Saunders-Hastings PR, Krewski D. Reviewing the history of pandemic influenza: Understanding patterns of emergence and transmission. *Pathogens.* 2016;**5**(4):66.
21. Lai S, Qin Y, Cowling BJ, et al. Global epidemiology of avian influenza A H5N1 virus infection in humans, 1997–2015: A systematic review of individual case data. *Lancet Infect Dis.* 2016;**16**(7):e108–e18.
22. Lee N, Hui D, Wu A, et al. A major outbreak of severe acute respiratory syndrome in Hong Kong. *N Engl J Med.* 2003;**348**(20):1986–1994.

23. Zaki AM, van Boheemen S, Bestebroer TM, et al. Isolation of a novel coronavirus from a man with pneumonia in Saudi Arabia. *N Engl J Med*. 2012;**367**(19):1814–1820.
24. Yu IT, Wong TW, Chiu YL, et al. Temporal-spatial analysis of severe acute respiratory syndrome among hospital inpatients. *Clin Infect Dis*. 2005;**40**(9):1237–1243.
25. Donnelly CA, Ghani AC, Leung GM, et al. Epidemiological determinants of spread of causal agent of severe acute respiratory syndrome in Hong Kong. *Lancet*. 2003;**361**(9371):1761–1766.
26. Kwok KO, Huang Y, Tsoi MTF, et al. Epidemiology, clinical spectrum, viral kinetics and impact of COVID-19 in the Asia-Pacific region. *Respirology*. 2021;**26**(4):322–333.
27. Awadasseid A, Wu Y, Tanaka Y, et al. Effective drugs used to combat SARS-CoV-2 infection and the current status of vaccines. *Biomed Pharmacother*. 2021;**137**:111330.
28. Noah MA, Peek GJ, Finney SJ, et al. Referral to an extracorporeal membrane oxygenation center and mortality among patients with severe 2009 influenza A (H1N1). *JAMA*. 2011;**306**(15):1659–1668.
29. Webb SA, Pettilä V, Seppelt I, et al. Critical care services and 2009 H1N1 influenza in Australia and New Zealand. *N Engl J Med*. 2009;**361**(20):1925–1934.
30. Huang F, Armando M, Dufau S, et al. Covid-19 outbreak and health care worker behavioral change toward hand hygiene practices. *J Hosp Infect*. 2021;**111**:27–34.

40

Pharmacology of Anti-infective Drugs in Critical Illness

Vanya Gant

- Changes in PK/PD parameters influence drug concentration and capacity to achieve therapeutic effect.
- Pathophysiological variations in critically ill patients can affect PK/PD parameters, especially with hydrophilic agents.
- Continuous infusion of antibiotics optimizes time-dependent antibiotic effect as it ensures that the antibiotic concentrations exceed pathogen MIC for a longer period of time.
- Critically ill patients are at higher risk of treatment failure in the context of increasing infections with multi-drug-resistant microorganisms, if the modified PK characteristics are not considered.
- Therapeutic drug monitoring (TDM) is occasionally recommended for patients with severe infections.

- Too few data are available for correlates of therapeutic ranges and bacterial killing for many anti-infective drugs.
- The field is complicated by the constantly shifting sands of emerging antibiotic resistance.

- We need new antibiotics/enzyme inhibitor combinations to treat multi-drug-resistant microorganisms.
- The impact of ECMO and other extracorporeal circuits on antimicrobial plasma concentrations and how to adjust for them.

Introduction

Concepts and Definitions

Pharmacokinetics (PK, derived from Ancient Greek *pharmakon* 'drug' and *kinetikos* 'moving, putting in motion') characterizes all those elements of an individual drug's journey through the organism to which or whom it is administered through the different stages of absorption, distribution, metabolism, and excretion. All these elements impact the final concentration within the blood and target tissues.[1]

We describe important PK concepts in Table 40.1. Changes in any of these parameters affect drug concentration and therapeutic efficacy (in the case of antibiotics, antibiotic-induced bacterial kill or stasis; bactericidal, bacteriostatic, respectively).[2]

Pharmacodynamics (PD) refers to the relationship between drug concentration at the site of action and the resulting effect. Different factors determine the efficacy of a drug: antibiotic concentration at

Table 40.1 Pharmacokinetic terms and alterations in critical illness

Pharmacokinetic parameter	Definition	Changes in critically ill patients
Volume of distribution (V_d)	Drug-specific theoretical constant that relates serum drug Concentration to the amount of drug in the body	Increased in acute inflammatory phase (capillary leak and fluid shifts)
Half-life ($T_{1/2}$)	Time required for the serum concentration to be reduced by half, assuming first-order elimination	Increased (renal or hepatic dysfunction)
Maximum concentration (C_{max})	Maximum or peak concentration after a single dose	Decreased (↑V_d, hypermetabolic states)
Minimum concentration (C_{min})	Minimum (or trough) concentration just before the next dose	Increased (renal or hepatic dysfunction)
Area under the curve (AUC)	Represents the total drug exposure (in blood and body) over time (24-h period)	Decreased (↑V_d, hypermetabolic states) Increased (renal or hepatic dysfunction)

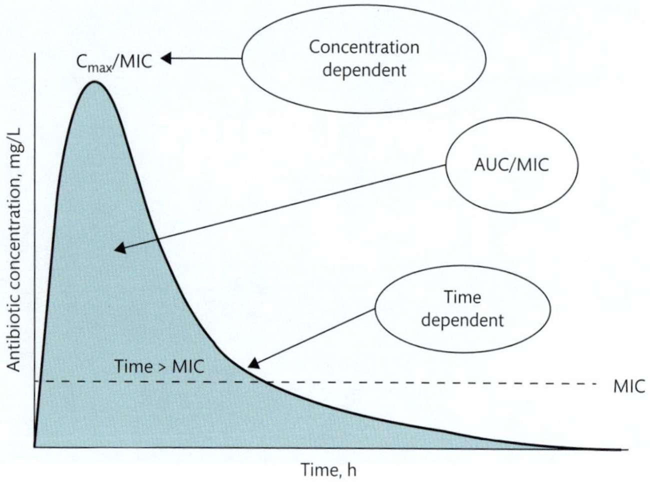

Figure 40.1 Relationship between pharmacokinetic and pharmacodynamic parameters.

the site of infection, microbial load, the minimum inhibitory concentration (MIC) for the pathogen, and the post-antibiotic effect (PAE; time required to resume normal growth following antibiotic exposure). The MIC is the lowest concentration necessary to inhibit the growth of the pathogen in vitro by 90%. The relationship between MIC and achievable antibiotic concentration in a tissue determines the resultant antibiotic action.[2]

Three PD parameters commonly used to predict antibiotic efficacy are (1) the ratio of maximum serum concentration to the MIC (C_{max}/MIC), (2) the ratio of the area under the plasma concentration versus time curve (AUC) versus MIC (AUC/MIC), and (3) the duration of the dosing interval that plasma concentrations exceed the MIC (T > MIC)[3] (Figure 40.1).

Anti-infective agents can be classified into two main categories from their PK/PD features. Concentration-dependent antibiotics such as aminoglycosides are those whose killing is determined by C_{max} or peak concentration relative to the pathogen MIC (C_{max}/MIC ratio). In contrast, beta-lactams are time-dependent antibiotics, and their effect is produced by the duration of time (T) that antibiotic concentrations exceed pathogen MIC (T > MIC). Some antibiotics such as glycopeptides or fluoroquinolones show mixed PD. Killing here relates to both antimicrobial concentration and time greater than MIC (AUC/MIC ratio). While the same principles relating to the need for adequate concentrations of antifungals to be present for effective fungal killing, the situation is in some ways less straightforward, as there are not only radically different classes of antifungal agents but also very considerable variation in the structures and properties of such agents within any one class.[4] Fungal infections are further discussed in Chapter 37.

Special Issues in the Critically Ill Patients

PK/PD parameters can be affected in critically ill patients due to changes in fluid distribution and homeostasis, hypoalbuminaemia, changes in renal clearance, changes in organ function, and the use of extracorporeal circuits.[5]

Table 40.2 Classification of antibiotics in terms of solubility

	Hydrophilic agents	Lipophilic agents
Characteristics	Smaller V_d Renal clearance Increased clearance in severe sepsis Distribution mainly in extracellular space	Larger V_d Hepatic clearance More likely to penetrate deep tissues Active against intracellular microorganisms
Examples	Beta-lactams Aminoglycosides Glycopeptides Daptomycin	Fluoroquinolones Macrolides Linezolid Rifampicin Metronidazole Tetracyclines

Solubility characteristics of the antibiotics (hydrophilic vs lipophilic) and organism-specific behaviours (such as intra vs extracellular pathogens) are also additional factors to be considered in the context of critical illness (Table 40.2). These are considered in more detail in the next section.

Pharmacological Considerations in Critical Illness

Fluid Shifts and Alterations in the Volume of Distribution

Patients with sepsis and particularly septic shock develop vasodilatation and increased vascular permeability leading to capillary leakage. This phenomenon is characterized by a fluid shift from the intravascular compartment to the interstitial space, resulting in hypotension requiring large volumes of resuscitation fluids and therefore an increased volume of distribution (V_d).[4] Interventions such as mechanical ventilation, extracorporeal membrane oxygenation (ECMO), or plasma exchange increase the V_d and will specifically decrease hydrophilic antibiotics' plasma concentrations. Some pathologies leading to increased V_d are pleural effusion, mediastinitis, and advanced liver disease. Conversely, lipophilic antibacterial and antifungal concentrations are not as affected by these fluid shifts as they have by their very nature a larger initial V_d.

Plasma Protein Binding

Serum albumin concentration is an important factor when prescribing antibiotics in critically ill patients. Hypoalbuminaemia is particularly important in the context of hydrophilic drugs that are highly protein-bound and have a renal clearance pathway. Low albumin is associated with an increase in the unbound fraction of antibiotic, in turn leading to an increase in the drug's V_d and accordingly decreased serum concentrations. Uraemia, acidosis, low pH, heparin, and some other drugs may additionally decrease serum protein binding ability.

Highly protein-bound antibiotics include ceftriaxone, teicoplanin, ertapenem, and daptomycin. These drugs may achieve a very high initial C_{max}—but subsequently fail to maintain sufficient concentration above the MIC, requiring shorter dosing intervals and/or higher doses.

Changes in Renal Clearance

Critically ill patients may present in different stages of acute kidney injury, with normal renal function or even augmented renal clearance (ARC). ARC is the result of an increased blood flow to major organs, mainly due to the effect of fluid loading, the use of vasoactive agents, and the underlying inflammatory response. ARC is defined as creatinine clearance >130 mL/min and typically occurs in younger males with trauma, sepsis, pancreatitis, or burns.

Depending on their bacterial killing characteristics, the action of some antibiotics will be more affected than others. Time-dependent antibiotics are very susceptible to the influence of ARC as their effect depends on maintaining adequate plasma concentration throughout the dosing interval.

Changes in Organ Function Scores

Sepsis can depress myocardial contractility, reducing organ perfusion, and a subsequent abrupt loss of kidney function. Renal function in critically ill patients can change significantly, rapidly, and even briefly. Many additional and sometimes necessary drugs such as furosemide, vancomycin, and gentamicin can also add to nephrotoxicity.

Acute liver injury may be caused by infection-associated cholestasis or hepatocellular injury, ischaemic hepatitis, haemolysis, or direct damage from hepatotoxic drugs[5,6] (Table 40.3). Additionally, alterations in blood flow also affect hepatic drug metabolism; increased blood flow will lead to increased hepatic metabolism and conversely hepatic impairment will result in accumulation of those antibiotics metabolized by the liver throughout reduced clearance.

Antibiotics to be avoided (if at all possible) in liver disease are chloramphenicol (higher risk of bone marrow suppression), erythromycin, tetracyclines, nitrofurantoin, and combination standard antituberculous therapy.[7,8]

Extracorporeal Circuits—Renal Replacement Therapy (RRT) and ECMO

There exist several modalities of RRT, such as continuous venovenous hemofiltration (CVVHF), hemodiafiltration, intermittent haemodialysis (IHD), and sustained low-efficiency dialysis. Antibiotic clearance greatly varies across different RRT modalities, making correct antimicrobial dosage more challenging in patients under continuous RRT.

During CVVHF, antibiotic plasma concentration will mainly depend on renal clearance and the protein-binding properties of the drug. Accordingly, hydrophilic antibiotics with high renal clearance and low protein binding will be removed very efficiently. Some notable exceptions exist: ceftriaxone and (flucl)oxacillin, although hydrophilic, are characterized by primary biliary elimination; levofloxacin and ciprofloxacin, although lipophilic, are renally cleared. Other variables affecting drug clearance include the timing and flow rates of RRT, filter /membrane material, and surface area. Antibiotics during RRT should be individualized to the patient according to specific RRT modality and the characteristics. One easy rule is to administer antibiotics after each IHD cycle.

ECMO is a highly invasive intervention in patients with cardiorespiratory failure that has shown to increase the V_d for certain drugs such as meropenem or ceftriaxone in ex vivo studies and in neonates. Some exceptionally lipophilic drugs such as voriconazole are sequestered in the ECMO circuit, mainly due to adsorption to tubing and ECMO membranes. However, this cannot be extrapolated to other lipophilic anti-infectives and more research needs to be done to quantify the impact of ECMO on PK/PD parameters. Of note, these patients also often require CVVHF. Here, therapeutic drug monitoring (TDM) and individualized regimens appear pragmatic as we await better evidence.[8]

Table 40.3 Anti-infective agents causing hepatotoxicity

Hepatocellular injury	Cholestatic injury	Fulminant hepatic failure
Chloramphenicol Clindamycin Penicillin G, amoxicillin, and oxacillin Trimethoprim–sulfamethoxazole Isoniazid Amphotericin Triazole antifungals (except fluconazole) Ciprofloxacin	Erythromycin, clarithromycin Cephalosporins Penicillin G, amoxicillin, cloxacillin, amoxicillin-clavulanic acid, Flucloxacillin Nitrofurantoin Trimethoprim–sulfamethoxazole 5-fluorocytosine Caspofungin	Sulphonamides Trimethoprim–sulfamethoxazole PAS (*para*-aminosalicylic acid)

Strategies to Optimize Treatment in Critically Ill Patients

There are two main approaches to optimizing antimicrobial treatment in critically ill patients: (a) altered administration techniques such as once-daily dosing or prolonged infusion and/or (b) dose adjustment guided by TDM.

Altered Administration Techniques

The relentless rise in infections with increasingly resistant organisms in patients with altered drug PK characteristics has generated multiple PK studies that apply dosing simulations aiming to optimize anti-infective regimens for maximum efficacy.[9,10]

PK/PD-based dosing has changed the way aminoglycosides are prescribed from thrice to once daily, improving the safety and efficacy of these antimicrobials.

Multiple studies investigating β-lactams suggest that prolonging duration of infusion, or as a continuous infusion, increases the likelihood of achieving PK/PD targets. This approach is important in situations where there is a high risk of therapeutic failure because of patient or pathogen characteristics.[10]

Continuous infusion of vancomycin reduces the total daily dosage and therefore diminishes the risk of nephrotoxicity. It also results in a faster time to consistent therapeutic concentrations; this may be vital in the context of severe infections with resistant microorganisms. Furthermore, from a practical perspective, blood for plasma concentrations can be taken at any time.

These concepts can be implemented in critically ill patients when the MIC data are available.[10,11]

Therapeutic Drug Monitoring

There is extensive evidence for frequent sub-therapeutic exposure from standard doses of different antibiotic classes. TDM was initially used to minimize toxicities, but in critically ill patients it is being increasingly used to optimize dosing.[11]

It is feasible and reasonably widely available for aminoglycosides, glycopeptides, and some antifungal agents.

Peak serum levels are traditionally obtained with the third dose or after dose adjustment and then trough levels are (and should be, for aminoglycosides) subsequently assessed. Trough concentrations need to be checked 30 min before the next dose and peak concentrations 30–45 min after the end of intravenous infusion of the drug (ideally through a different venous access).[3] There is no point measuring peak doses with aminoglycosides when these are administered once a day; trough levels are however essential.

Pharmacokinetics and Pharmacodynamics of Frequently Used Antimicrobials in Critically Ill Patients

Beta-lactams

The β-lactam antibiotics include penicillins, cephalosporins, and carbapenems. Due to their low toxicity, high therapeutic ratio, and broad-spectrum activity, they are very often the first-line treatment for critically ill patients.

β-Lactams bind to penicillin-binding proteins within the bacterial cell membrane, leading to osmotic pressure-induced bacterial cell death. They are generally hydrophilic in nature and display time-dependent antimicrobial activity. The most significant parameter to determine efficacy is $T >$ MIC as antibiotic concentrations just below the MIC are completely ineffective. This necessitates a close and necessary knowledge of the half-life ($T_{1/2}$) of the β-lactam antibiotics as regards their serum concentration.[12]

Penicillins

- *Benzylpenicillin*: While the half-life of penicillin G in normal humans is very fast (approximately 30–50 min), its disappearance from the blood is very significantly slowed in patients with severe hepatic and renal dysfunction.

Penicillin/β-lactamase Inhibitor Combinations

- *Amoxicillin-clavulanic acid*: Extra-renal elimination of clavulanic acid is much more rapid than that for amoxicillin, and the elimination $T_{1/2}$ of amoxicillin increases six-fold in patients with severe renal failure. Ideally, the two drugs need independent dosage, but this is not possible with fixed combinations. The use of this drug combination in patients with GFR <30 mL/min is not recommended.
- *Piperacillin-tazobactam* is very commonly used for the treatment of nosocomial infections, especially when infection with *Pseudomonas aeruginosa* is suspected. The $T >$ MIC can be maximized by administration as a prolonged or continuous infusion. Morbidly obese patients may require upwardly adjusted dosage for treating severe infections with pathogens with high MICs [13].

Cephalosporins

- *Ceftriaxone*: It is slowly eliminated by the kidneys, probably due to high protein binding (about 95%), and is mostly excreted in the bile. The dose of ceftriaxone does not need to be adjusted in patients receiving CVVHF.
- *Ceftazidime and Cefepime*: Dosage reduction (by spacing out the doses rather than reducing each dose) is necessary in patients with renal impairment. Pharmacokinetics in critically ill patients receiving CRRT remain very difficult to model and predict in view of the multiple variables affecting their clearance. Dosage should be 'personalized' whenever possible in conjunction with relevantly qualified pharmacists.

Carbapenems

- *Meropenem*: This is primarily eliminated unchanged in the urine. Meropenem dosage in adults with renal impairment is based on creatinine clearance. Probenecid competes with meropenem for active tubular secretion. This can lead to a 33%–38% increase in the $T_{1/2}$ of meropenem with increases in subsequent systemic exposure of up to 56%. Meropenem may in addition reduce valproic acid plasma concentrations to sub-therapeutic levels.
- *Imipenem/cilastatin*: This fixed drug combination should be avoided, if possible, because of the very different PK/PD characteristics of its constituents.

Aminoglycosides

Aminoglycosides inhibit bacterial growth by inhibiting protein synthesis via irreversible binding to the 30S ribosomal subunit of susceptible bacteria. They are used commonly against multi-drug-resistant Gram-negative organisms.

Aminoglycosides exhibit concentration-dependent bactericidal activity with an important PAE, whereby organisms take time to 'recover' even though the drug itself has been eliminated. A C_{max}/MIC ratio of ≥10 results in faster clinical improvement in patients with Gram-negative infections. Dosage is based on ideal weight.

TDM is recommended in the context of critically ill patients with severe infections.[7,8]

- *Gentamicin*: Once-daily administration enhances the bacterial killing effect with high peak drug concentration as well as leading to a prolonged PAE of perhaps as much as 12 h. Gentamicin (like all aminoglycosides) is (by modern standards) capable of causing very significant toxicity, some of it irreversible. For this reason, these highly effective drugs should be reserved for the very sick or where no safer alternative exists. These should be used for more than 5 days only in exceptional circumstances. In addition, they are nephrotoxic in their own right caused by a direct effect on the renal cortex and can produce tubular necrosis at high concentrations. This can be highly relevant for patients whose illness may drive renal dysfunction and AKI in its own right. While it is also accepted there is a (cumulative) dose relationship with what is most often only partly irreversible ototoxicity, this does not absolve gentamicin from being implicated in ototoxicity despite consistently 'safe' peak and trough levels. In addition, several rare genetic mutations are known to be associated with irreversible damage after a single dose of this class of drugs.
- *Amikacin* is almost completely eliminated in an active unchanged form. If the duration of therapy is less than 7 days, once-daily administration of amikacin produces lower incidence of nephropathy than the traditional 12-h modality. Amikacin has a similar propensity to cause ototoxicity to gentamicin, and to date there are no 'safe' aminoglycosides.
- Accordingly, aminoglycosides are capable of both excellent therapeutic activity and considerable toxicity, some of it irreversible. This balance of risk and efficacy must always be carefully considered for all patients, based on their individual circumstances.

Glycopeptides

Glycopeptides bind rapidly and irreversibly to the cell wall of susceptible bacteria and inhibit cell wall synthesis. They display mixed PK/PD characteristics with time-dependent killing activity relying on AUC/MIC rate; in addition, they are large molecules, which may limit their ability to achieve high enough concentrations in poorly vascularized tissues. AUC/MIC calculations are difficult to apply at the bedside in an individual critically ill patient, so serum trough concentration is used as a surrogate.

- *Vancomycin*: Patients in ICU usually require higher doses of vancomycin as V_d is higher and clearance is variable. Renal function, APACHE score, age, and serum albumin are the main factors implicated in drug clearance variability. Due to high variability in vancomycin plasma concentrations, TDM is essential to guide correct vancomycin dosage.
- *Teicoplanin*: This is a highly protein-bound antibiotic eliminated predominantly by the kidneys. There is wide inter-patient variability in critically ill patients with renal impairment. Accordingly, higher loading and maintenance doses with trough level TDM (which is not easily accessible) in critically ill patients are suggested. In practice, the former is easy to enact (teicoplanin having a high therapeutic ratio). HD does not increase the clearance of teicoplanin so in patients treated with this modality there is no need for extra doses.

Fluoroquinolones

Fluoroquinolones inhibit DNA gyrase and topoisomerase, resulting in ultimately lethal double-stranded DNA damage. Due to exceptional tissue penetration and its original, excellent activity against the vast majority of the Gram-negative *Enterobacteriaceae*, ciprofloxacin has been seen as a good alternative to treat severe infections in penicillin-allergic patients. Unfortunately, the very wide and often unjustified prescription of this agent has driven an inexorable rise in antibiotic resistance, and many, if not most, UK institutions now can no longer use fluoroquinolones empirically because of unacceptable rates of de novo resistance in *Enterobacteriaceae*. Few countries apart from those in Scandinavia are now any better off.

- *Ciprofloxacin*: HD removes only about 2% of the given dose and therefore there is no need for a supplemented dose post-haemodialysis.
- *Levofloxacin*: It has little clearance by HD. CVVHF might have enhanced clearance of levofloxacin, but once-daily dose is enough to maintain adequate levels.

Other Classes of Antibacterials

- *Colistin*: This old drug, originally left behind because of toxicity and the advent of 'better' antibiotics, is now undergoing a renaissance as 'better' drugs become useless through antibiotic resistance. It changes the permeability in the outer membrane and hence rapid cell death. It should be reserved for cases infected with multi-drug-resistant organisms. In practice, the drug is reasonably well tolerated for short periods of time by most; reversible renal impairment and neurotoxicity are its main drawbacks. New dose guidelines mandate a 9MU loading dose followed by 3MU tds. TDM is recommended for PK/PD target achievement and mitigation of toxicity—but is not widely available. Colistin is relatively unaffected by RRT regimens, although falls short of a blanket recommendation in this respect as CRRT regimens and equipment vary so widely.
- *Linezolid* is used in the context of multi-drug-resistant Gram-positive organism infections. It binds to the 50S ribosomal subunit and inhibits bacterial protein synthesis. It is removed by haemodialysis; the dose should be given after the dialysis. Despite being removed during CVVHF, no dose adjustment is recommended.
- *Daptomycin* disrupts bacterial cell membrane function. It requires reduction of the dose in the context of renal impairment, HD, or CVVHF. It does not need to be adjusted in the context of obesity.

Antifungal Agents

These agents have been found to be increasingly necessary in the context of ICU, at least partly driven by an increasingly immunosuppressed casemix, the propensity for fungi to act as replacement flora and 'step into the bacterial microbiome void' left by the widespread destruction of normal bacterial flora by broad antibiotics, and their propensity for infecting those with long intravenous lines, cancer, and those on total parenteral nutrition. ICU clinicians in general are less familiar with their properties than they are with antibacterial agents, however.

Azoles

The currently licensed prototypic azoles include *fluconazole*, *itraconazole*, *voriconazole*, *posaconazole*, and *isavuconazole*. All but fluconazole are lipophilic, with large V_ds. Accordingly, they may behave very differently in typically dynamic ICU situations. Most ICU fungal infection, however, are due to *Candida* species and fungemia. Assessment of antifungal sensitivities for invasive isolates is crucial here; as fluconazole, if it can be used, has excellent tissue penetration and has the most favourable toxicity profile. Specialist advice for the other azoles is necessary—as not all may achieve local tissue concentrations rapidly, if at all. The triazoles voriconazole and isavuconazole have excellent anti-aspergillus activity and are frequently first line in suspected or proven invasive pulmonary aspergillosis. Finally, apart from fluconazole, these agents have very considerable and complex interactions with hepatic cytochrome enzymes, either inducing, inhibiting, or a combination of both. This in turn results in literally hundreds of highly clinically relevant drug interactions, making their safe use only possible with essential specialist pharmacist and clinical microbiologist input, tailored to individual patients' other therapies.

Echinocandins

This class of agents, which include *anidulofungin*, *caspofungin*, and *micafungin*, has found favour in the context of ICU because of their very favourable toxicity profile, relative lack of important drug interactions, and undoubted efficacy against almost all clinically relevant strains of *Candida*, while having fungostatic but not fungicidal activity against aspergillus and no effect on other clinically relevant moulds. They differ very considerably in their PK/PD characteristics, however. Anidulafungin for example has no recognized excretion pathway and is thought to slowly disintegrate within tissues to non-active metabolic products. They also exhibit different tissue penetration characteristics, and we recommend that any proposed use beyond line-associated *Candida* fungemia should be discussed with both suitably experienced pharmacists and microbiologists.

Liposomal Amphotericin Preparations

Several lipid/*amphotericin* preparations emerged as candidate antifungal agents for use in the ICU setting. Most have been found deficient in terms of efficacy and clinical outcomes; some have very limited data to recommend them and are not recommended. *Ambisome*™, however, remains an effective alternative for the treatment of invasive mould infections, increasingly recognized in ICUs because of necessary highly immunosuppressive therapies. Again, dosage and duration of therapy should be discussed with suitably qualified pharmacists and microbiologists as this agent's pharmacological PK/PD characteristics are quite unique.

Treatment Failure and Antibiotic Resistance

Infections in the ICU are increasingly often caused by multi-drug-resistant organisms, prompting increasingly stringent, judicious use of this class of drugs to reduce selective pressure on sensitive strains.

The MIC is a critical factor of the PK/PD relationship, which defines the drug exposure necessary to ensure a patient achieves a plasma concentration associated with maximal efficacy. In addition, when modified PK characteristics are not considered, critically ill patients will be at higher risk of treatment failure.

Individualized dosage regimens based on TDM and altered administration techniques should be supported by appropriately qualified pharmacists together with frequent microbiology input relating to MIC estimation, and interpretation and sensitivity patterns combined with stringent infection control measures represent the cornerstones of optimal clinical outcomes and control of the spread of multi-resistant organisms.

REFERENCES

1. McKenzie C. Antibiotic dosing in critical illness. *J Antimicrob Chemother.* 2011 Apr;**66**(Suppl 2):ii25–31.
2. Roberts JA, Abdul-Aziz MH, Lipman J, et al. International Society of Anti-Infective Pharmacology and the Pharmacokinetics and Pharmacodynamics Study Group of the European Society of Clinical Microbiology and Infectious Diseases. Individualised antibiotic dosing for patients who are critically ill: challenges and potential solutions. *Lancet Infect Dis.* 2014 Jun;**14**(6):498–509.
3. Petrosillo N, Drapeau CM, Agrafiotis M, et al. Some current issues in the pharmacokinetics/pharmacodynamics of antimicrobials in intensive care. *Minerva Anestesiol.* 2010 Jul;**76**(7):509–524.
4. Droege ME, Van Fleet SL, Mueller EW. Application of antibiotic pharmacodynamics and dosing principles in patients with sepsis. *Crit Care Nurse.* 2016 Apr;**36**(2):22–32. doi:10.4037/ccn2016881. PMID: 27037336.
5. Periáñez-Párraga L, Martínez-López I, Ventayol-Bosch P, et al. Drug dosage recommendations in patients with chronic liver disease. *Rev Esp Enferm Dig.* 2012 Apr;**104**(4):165–184. doi:10.4321/s1130-01082012000400002. PMID: 22537365.
6. Verbeeck RK. Pharmacokinetics and dosage adjustment in patients with hepatic dysfunction. *Eur J Clin Pharmacol.* 2008 Dec;**64**(12):1147–1161.
7. Verbeeck RK. Pharmacokinetics and dosage adjustment in patients with hepatic dysfunction. *Eur J Clin Pharmacol.* 2008 Dec;**64**(12):1147–1161.
8. Amarapurkar DN. Prescribing medications in patients with decompensated liver cirrhosis. *Int J Hepatol.* 2011;**2011**:519526.
9. Jager NG, van Hest RM, Lipman J, et al. Therapeutic drug monitoring of anti-infective agents in critically ill patients. *Expert Rev Clin Pharmacol.* 2016 Jul;**9**(7):961–979.
10. Wong G, Sime FB, Lipman J, et al. How do we use therapeutic drug monitoring to improve outcomes from severe infections in critically ill patients? *BMC Infect Dis.* 2014 Nov 28;**14**:288.
11. Blot SI, Pea F, Lipman J. The effect of pathophysiology on pharmacokinetics in the critically ill patient—concepts appraised by the example of antimicrobial agents. *Adv Drug Deliv Rev.* 2014 Nov 20;77:3–11.
12. Gonçalves-Pereira J, Póvoa P. Antibiotics in critically ill patients: A systematic review of the pharmacokinetics of β-lactams. *Crit Care.* 2011;**15**(5):R206.
13. Awissi D, Beauchamp A, Hébert E, et al. Pharmacokinetics of an extended 4-hour infusion of piperacillin-tazobactam in critically ill patients undergoing continuous renal replacement therapy. *Pharmacotherapy.* 2015 Jun;**35**(6):600–607.

PART 9

Critical Care Management of Pulmonary Diseases and Other Respiratory Manifestations

41

Chronic Obstructive Pulmonary Disease

Andrea Carsetti and Simone Bazurro

KEY MESSAGES

- Chronic obstructive pulmonary disease (COPD) is characterized by persistent respiratory symptoms and airflow limitation (post-bronchodilator $FEV_1/FVC < 0.70$).
- The most common precipitating causes of an acute exacerbation of COPD (AECOPD) are respiratory tract infections (viral or bacterial infections).
- Medical therapy includes short-acting inhaled beta$_2$-agonists, inhaled anticholinergics, systemic corticosteroids, and antibiotics if bacterial infection is suspected.
- Non-invasive ventilation (NIV) is indicated to treat respiratory acidosis.
- Criteria for invasive mechanical ventilation should be promptly recognized.

CONTROVERSIES

- The role of ECCO2R needs to be established.

FURTHER RESEARCH

- Further prospective evidence is needed for proper patient selection and to demonstrate the theoretical advantages of ECCO2R as a rescue therapy, either to prevent intubation, or as an adjunct to NIV, or for liberation from mechanical ventilation.

Introduction

Chronic obstructive pulmonary disease (COPD) is characterized by persistent respiratory symptoms and airflow limitation that is due to airway and/or alveolar abnormalities usually caused by significant exposure to noxious particles or gases.[1]

It is a major cause of chronic morbidity and mortality worldwide representing the fourth leading cause of death in the world.

The following are risk factors for COPD:

- Tobacco smoke
- Indoor air pollution
- Occupational exposures
- Outdoor air pollution
- Genetic factors
- Ageing and female gender
- Lung growth and development alteration
- Socioeconomic status
- Asthma and airway hyper-reactivity
- Chronic bronchitis
- Infections

COPD should be considered in any patient who refers dyspnoea, chronic cough, or sputum production, and/or a history of exposure to risk factors for the disease. Spirometry is needed for diagnosis. A post-bronchodilator ratio between forced expiratory volume (FEV_1) and forced vital capacity (FVC) less than 0.70 ($FEV_1/FVC < 0.70$) confirms the presence of persistent airflow limitation.[1]

The classification of airflow limitation severity in COPD is shown in Figure 41.1. However, it is recognized that airflow limitation alone is an imperfect measure of disease severity in COPD, and the most recent update of the Global Initiative for Chronic Obstructive Lung Disease (GOLD) report uses a combination of spirometric measures, symptoms, and frequency of exacerbations to grade COPD. Grading is given as spirometric (GOLD) class (Figure 41.1) with an A–D score determined by severity of symptoms and frequency and severity of exacerbations, as an example a patient with severe impairment of airflow with heavy symptomatic burden and frequent exacerbations would be graded GOLD grade 4, group D.

An acute exacerbation of COPD (AECOPD) is defined as an acute worsening of respiratory symptoms that results in additional therapy.[1] It is defined as

- mild: treated with short-acting bronchodilators (SABDs) only;
- moderate: treated with SABDs plus antibiotics and/or oral corticosteroids;
- severe: hospitalization is required.

Severe exacerbations may also be associated with acute respiratory failure. The most common precipitating causes are respiratory

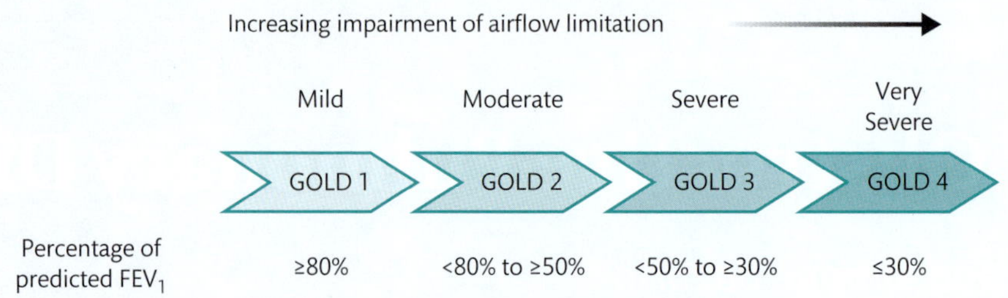

Figure 41.1 Classification of airflow limitation severity (based on post-bronchodilator FEV_1) in patient with FEV_1/FCV <0.70. FEV_1, forced expiratory volume in one second; FVC, forced vital capacity.
Diagram by A Conway Morris created with BioRender.com.

tract infections (viral or bacterial infections). Occasionally, exacerbations are caused by air pollution or other environmental factors. Other concurrent conditions need to be excluded (e.g. pulmonary embolism, pneumothorax, and congestive heart failure).

Pathophysiology

Chronic inflammation is responsible for repeated injury and repair and causes pathological changes in the airways, lung parenchyma, and pulmonary vasculature.[2] Mucus gland hypertrophy and goblet cell metaplasia can be seen in central airways. In more peripheral airways, characteristic changes are smooth muscle hypertrophy, peri-bronchial fibrosis, and luminal occlusion by mucus. Support for non-cartilaginous airways can be lost with structural changes to the alveoli. Oxidative stress and excess of proteinases are characteristic features of inflammation in COPD. The destruction of elastin, due to protease–antiprotease imbalance, can result in emphysema. Inflammatory mediators released from macrophages, neutrophils and lymphocytes in peripheral airways, lung parenchyma, and pulmonary vessels mediate other structural changes. Repeated injury may lead to excessive production of muscle and fibrous tissue in the airway wall, contributing to airway narrowing and increased airway resistance.[3] These changes are responsible for

- airflow limitation and gas trapping,
- gas exchange abnormality,
- mucus hypersecretion,
- pulmonary hypertension.

Pulmonary hypertension develops late in COPD due to hypoxic vasoconstriction of small pulmonary arteries resulting in structural changes (intimal hyperplasia and smooth muscle hypertrophy/hyperplasia).[4]

Expiratory resistance is greatly increased in patients with COPD.[5] The loss of elastin support of the airway produces a dynamic narrowing of the small airways during expiration, reducing maximum flow (expiratory flow limitation). When the time for exhalation is less than the minimum time required to reach the relaxation volume of the respiratory system, dynamic hyperinflation occurs. During AECOPD, expiratory flow limitation is worsened by bronchospasm, increased mucus production, and mucosal oedema. Tachypnoea also contributes to increasing dynamic hyperinflation by reducing the time for exhalation. Whilst acute worsening of dynamic hyperinflation has some positive effects, limiting dynamic airway narrowing during expiration and increasing elastic recoil generating intrinsic positive end-expiratory pressure (iPEEP),[6] it also has other detrimental effects. Firstly, the patient must develop a negative pressure equal to iPEEP to initiate inspiratory flow.[7] Secondly, dynamic hyperinflation worsens the length–tension relationship of respiratory muscles impairing their function.[8] Finally, dynamic hyperinflation increases end-expiratory lung volume that reduces lung compliance, increases the work of breathing, and causes alveolar overdistention.

Altered distribution of ventilation–perfusion ratios (*V*/*Q*) is a common cause of hypoxaemia during exacerbations.[9] In some patients, hypercapnia can be worsened by excessive administration of supplemental oxygen. This phenomenon can be related to decrease hypoxic ventilatory response during oxygen administration, loss of hypoxic vasoconstriction with increased dead space and worsening in *V*/*Q*, and Haldane effect (oxygenation of blood in the lungs displaces CO_2 from haemoglobin).

Initial Assessment and Management

The severity of exacerbation can be defined according to the patient's clinical signs:[10]

- No respiratory failure: respiratory rate (RR) 20–30 breaths per minute (bpm), no use of accessory respiratory muscles, no changes in mental status, hypoxaemia improved with supplemental oxygen (FiO_2 28%–35%), and no increase in $PaCO_2$.
- Non-life-threatening acute respiratory failure: RR >30 bpm; using accessory respiratory muscles, no change in mental status, hypoxaemia improved with supplemental oxygen (FiO_2 28%–35%), and $PaCO_2$ increased compared with baseline or elevated 50–60 mmHg.
- Life-threatening acute respiratory failure: RR >30 bpm, using accessory respiratory muscles, acute changes in mental status, hypoxaemia not improved with supplemental oxygen or requiring FiO_2 >40%, $PaCO_2$ increased compared with baseline or elevated >60 mmHg (8 kPa), or the presence of acidosis (pH < 7.25).

Co-morbidities are common in patients with COPD, and exacerbations must be differentiated from other conditions such as acute coronary syndrome, congestive heart failure, pulmonary embolism, and pneumonia.

During acute hypercapnic respiratory failure (AHRF) in patients with exacerbation of COPD, oxygen should be titrated to achieve a saturation of 88%–92%.[11]

Box 41.1 Initial management of acute exacerbation COPD

Assess severity of symptoms, ABG, and chest X-ray
Administer supplemental oxygen (SaO_2 88%–92%)
Short-acting inhaled beta$_2$-agonists with short-acting anticholinergics
- Albuterol (Salbutamol) 2.5–5 mg q20 min for three doses nebulized
- Ipratropium 500 mcg q20 min for three doses nebulized

Consider corticosteroids (prednisolone 40 mg)
Consider antibiotics
Consider thromboembolism prophylaxis
Identify and treat associated conditions

ABG: arterial blood gas; SaO_2: arterial oxygen saturation.

Initial medical therapy includes short-acting inhaled beta$_2$-agonists with short-acting anticholinergics.[12] Systemic corticosteroids can be helpful to improve lung functions, oxygenation, and recovery. They should be administered for 5–7 days.[13] Intravenous methylxanthines (theophylline or aminophylline) are not recommended during acute exacerbation as they can produce significant side effects.[14] Antibiotics may be considered when signs of bacterial infection are present, in particular in the case of increased sputum volume and purulence and in patients requiring mechanical ventilation (invasive or non-invasive).[15] Initial management of AECOPD is summarized in Box 41.1. The GOLD report suggested criteria for intensive care unit (ICU) admission[1] are severe dyspnoea not responding to initial treatment, altered mental status, persistent or worsening hypoxaemia or respiratory acidosis despite treatment, and haemodynamic instability or need for imminent invasive ventilation.

Non-invasive Ventilation (NIV)

NIV should be started when pH <7.35 and $PaCO_2$ >45 mmHg (6 kPa) persist despite initial medical management (see Chapters 8 and 9 for further details on NIV).[16] There is no lower limit of pH below which an NIV trial is contraindicated. However, the failure rate of NIV is higher when pH is <7.25 and the patient should be managed in an appropriate area (high dependency unit (HDU)/ICU) to guarantee prompt tracheal intubation and invasive mechanical ventilation (IMV) if required. Continuing NIV despite a patient's deterioration increases mortality.

The GOLD report indications for NIV include respiratory acidosis ($PaCO_2$ of >6.0 kPa with pH <7.35) and severe dyspnoea or evidence of respiratory muscle fatigue or hypoxaemia despite appropriate supplemental oxygen. Contraindications are set out in Box 41.2 respectively. In the presence of relative contraindications, patients should be managed in HDU/ICU to guarantee early recognition of NIV failure and need for IMV. Continuous monitoring of oxygen saturation and intermittent measurement of $PaCO_2$ and pH are indicated during NIV. ECG monitoring is suggested in the case of tachycardia (>120 bpm), dysrhythmia, and a history of cardiomyopathy. Arterial blood gas (ABG) measurement is needed prior to starting NIV to quantify the severity of respiratory failure. Chest radiography should not delay the initiation of NIV in case of severe acidosis but should be performed to identify any causative conditions and/or complications. Other investigations including full blood count, renal function tests, ECG, and echocardiography are helpful to rule out concomitant reversible factors contributing to AHRF.

Box 41.2 Contraindication for non-invasive ventilation

Absolute
Severe facial deformity
Facial burns
Fixed upper airways obstruction
Vomiting/severe upper gastrointestinal bleeding

Relative
pH <7.15 (pH < 7.25 and additional adverse feature)
GCS < 8
Confusion/agitation
Cognitive impairment
Excessive secretions

GCS: Glasgow coma scale.

Pressure support and pressure control ventilation are both effective in AECOPD. Initial NIV set-up is summarized in Box 41.3. A full-face mask should be the first type of interface used.

An improvement in pH and RR within 1–2 h predicts a successful outcome.[17,18] On the other hand, a worsening of physiological parameters requires clinical review, change of interface, adjustment of ventilator settings, and careful consideration of endotracheal intubation and IMV. Common reasons for NIV failure are excessive mask leak, inadequate pressure support, and ventilator–patient asynchrony. Before considering NIV to have failed, it is important to check common technical issues and ventilator settings.

Time on NIV should be maximized in the first 24 h.[16] Thereafter, time on NIV can be gradually reduced with increasingly prolonged periods of self-ventilation during the day, whilst continuing with NIV overnight. $PaCO_2$ monitoring guides the weaning process. NIV is usually discontinued when pH is normalized with $PaCO_2$ <45 mmHg (6 kPa) and improvement of patient's condition. However, normalization of $PaCO_2$ may not be possible in patients with chronic hypercapnia.

Box 41.3 NIV set-up

Initial pressure settings
EPAP 3 cmH_2O (or higher if OSA)
IPAP 15 cmH_2O (20 cmH_2O if pH <7.25)
Up-titrate IPAP to 20–30 cmH_2O over 10–30 min to achieve adequate tidal volume
Review work of breathing by clinical assessment, pH, and $paCO_2$ within 30–60 min and adjust
IPAP should not exceed 30 cmH_2O or EPAP 8* cmH_2O without expert review
Backup rate
16–20
I:E ratio
1:2 to 1:3
Inspiratory time
0.8–1.2 s

*Possible need of EPAP >8 cmH_2O: severe OHS (BMI >35), oppose intrinsic PEEP in severe airflow obstruction.

BMI: body mass index; EPAP: expiratory positive airway pressure; I:E: inspiratory: expiratory; IPAP: inspiratory positive airway pressure; OHS: obesity hypoventilation syndrome; OSA: obstructive sleep apnoea.

Box 41.4 Indication for invasive mechanical ventilation in acute exacerbation of COPD from BTS/ICS guidelines

Imminent respiratory arrest
Severe respiratory distress
Failure of or contraindications to NIV
Persisting pH <7.15 or deterioration in pH despite NIV
Depressed consciousness (GCS < 8)

Note: GCS: Glasgow coma scale; NIV: non-invasive ventilation.

Source: Data from Davidson AC, Banham S, Elliott M, et al. BTS/ICS guideline for the ventilatory management of acute hypercapnic respiratory failure in adults. *Thorax*. 2016;71(Suppl 2):ii1–35.

Invasive Mechanical Ventilation

Indications for IMV in AECOPD are summarized in Box 41.4. There is insufficient evidence to support the use of absolute values of pH or $PaCO_2$ as intubation criteria.[19] However, IMV should be considered when pH is <7.25 and is indicated when pH is <7.15 after initial management. IMV should be considered if acidosis persists or worsens after NIV trial. Initial setting for IMV is shown in Box 41.5. The aim of mechanical ventilation is to decrease respiratory distress, reduce dynamic hyperinflation, and improve respiratory acidosis and hypoxaemia. Airflow obstruction promotes hyperinflation. It can be complicated by barotrauma, impaired gas exchange, and patient discomfort. The first approach to reduce iPEEP involves prolonging expiratory time and shortening the inspiratory time, so reducing the minute volume.[20] This can lead to alveolar hypoventilation. However, in AECOPD, rapid restoration of normal PaO_2 and $PaCO_2$ is not imperative. Careful setting of external PEEP (ePEEP) is important as it can improve expiratory airflow, limit dynamic hyperinflation, and improve alveolar ventilation.[21] Setting ePEEP at 50%–80% of iPEEP is recommended.[22] In patients allowed to breathe spontaneously, iPEEP represents a pressure load that must be overcome to trigger the ventilator. Appropriate ePEEP is also able to counterbalance this threshold load, improving patient–ventilator synchrony.[23] ePEEP should never be set higher than iPEEP.

When all acute conditions have been treated and patient stabilized, a weaning process from mechanical ventilation can be started. Spontaneous breathing trial should be conducted using a pressure support of 5–8 cmH_2O rather than T-piece or continuous positive airway pressure (CPAP) alone.[24] Post-extubation NIV is recommended in patients at high risk for extubation failure (patients with hypercapnia, COPD, congestive heart failure, or other serious co-morbidities).[24]

Box 41.5 Initial setting for invasive mechanical ventilation

Tidal volume
  6–8 mL/kg
Respiratory rate
  10–15 bpm
I:E ratio
  1:2 to 1:4
Oxygenation
  SaO_2 88%–92%
Acid-base
  pH 7.2–7.4

I:E: inspiratory:expiratory; SaO_2: arterial oxygen saturation.

Extra-corporeal Carbon Dioxide Removal (ECCO2R)

The use of ECCO2R has emerged as a potentially important adjunct to the management of patients with AECOPD in the ICU setting. It is further discussed in Chapter 22. The literature awaits results of ongoing randomized controlled trials to demonstrate its theoretical advantages, although side effects such as bleeding remain higher than desirable[25]. Two fundamentally different scenarios are reported. Firstly, the setting in the awake patient, it may be used to avoid intubation as an alternative to NIV in those intolerant or not responding to NIV. There is observational historical case-matched evidence of CO_2 reduction and prevention of intubation in up to 56% of patients but with bleeding in up to one-third.[25]. Secondly, it may be used in the weaning phase of ventilation as an adjunct to liberate patients from ventilation or even to prevent potentially injurious ventilatory settings by controlling the hypercarbia. The role of ECCO2R therapy in this patient group will be defined in the coming years.[26]

REFERENCES

1. Global initiative for chronic obstructive lung diseases. Global strategy for the diagnosis, management, and prevention of chronic obstructive pulmonary disease (2023 report). 2023. (available from https://goldcopd.org/2023-gold-report-2/)
2. Hogg JC, Timens W. The pathology of chronic obstructive pulmonary disease. *Annu Rev Pathol.* 2009;**4**(1):435–459.
3. McDonough JE, Yuan R, Suzuki M, et al. Small-airway obstruction and emphysema in chronic obstructive pulmonary disease. *N Engl J Med.* 2011;**365**(17):1567–1575.
4. Sakao S, Voelkel NF, Tatsumi K. The vascular bed in COPD: Pulmonary hypertension and pulmonary vascular alterations. *Eur Respir Rev.* 2014;**23**(133):350–355.
5. Paredi P, Goldman M, Alamen A, et al. Comparison of inspiratory and expiratory resistance and reactance in patients with asthma and chronic obstructive pulmonary disease. *Thorax.* 2010;**65**(3):263–267.
6. Somfay A, Porszasz J, Lee SM, et al. Dose-response effect of oxygen on hyperinflation and exercise endurance in nonhypoxaemic COPD patients. *Eur Respir J.* 2001;**18**(1):77–84.
7. Jubran A, Tobin MJ. Pathophysiologic basis of acute respiratory distress in patients who fail a trial of weaning from mechanical ventilation. *Am J Respir Crit Care Med.* 1997;**155**(3):906–915.
8. Laghi F, Tobin MJ. Disorders of the respiratory muscles. *Am J Respir Crit Care Med.* 2003;**168**(1):10–48.
9. Barberà JA, Roca J, Ferrer A, et al. Mechanisms of worsening gas exchange during acute exacerbations of chronic obstructive pulmonary disease. *Eur Respir J.* 1997;**10**(6):1285–1291.
10. Celli BR, Barnes PJ. Exacerbations of chronic obstructive pulmonary disease. *Eur Respir J.* 2007;**29**(6):1224–1238.
11. Austin MA, Wills KE, Blizzard L, et al. Effect of high flow oxygen on mortality in chronic obstructive pulmonary disease patients in prehospital setting: Randomised controlled trial. *BMJ.* 2010;**341**:c5462–c5462.
12. Celli BR, MacNee W. ATS/ERS Task Force. Standards for the diagnosis and treatment of patients with COPD: A summary of the ATS/ERS position paper. *Eur Respir J.* 2004;**23**(6):932–946.

13. Leuppi JD, Schuetz P, Bingisser R, et al. Short-term vs conventional glucocorticoid therapy in acute exacerbations of chronic obstructive pulmonary disease: The REDUCE randomized clinical trial. *JAMA*. 2013;**309**(21):2223–2231.
14. Barr RG, Rowe BH, Camargo CA. Methylxanthines for exacerbations of chronic obstructive pulmonary disease: Meta-analysis of randomised trials. *BMJ*. 2003;**327**(7416):643.
15. Woodhead M, Blasi F, Ewig S, et al. Guidelines for the management of adult lower respiratory tract infections. *Eur Respir J*. 2005;**26**(6):1138–1180.
16. Davidson AC, Banham S, Elliott M, et al. BTS/ICS guideline for the ventilatory management of acute hypercapnic respiratory failure in adults. *Thorax*. 2016;**71**(Suppl 2):ii1–35.
17. Plant PK, Owen JL, Elliott MW. Non-invasive ventilation in acute exacerbations of chronic obstructive pulmonary disease: Long term survival and predictors of in-hospital outcome. *Thorax*. 2001;**56**(9):708–712.
18. Confalonieri M, Garuti G, Cattaruzza MS, et al. A chart of failure risk for noninvasive ventilation in patients with COPD exacerbation. *Eur Respir J*. 2005;**25**(2):348–355.
19. Pierson DJ. Indications for mechanical ventilation in adults with acute respiratory failure. *Respir Care*. 2002;**47**(3):249–262–265.
20. Tuxen DV, Lane S. The effects of ventilatory pattern on hyperinflation, airway pressures, and circulation in mechanical ventilation of patients with severe air-flow obstruction. *Am Rev Respir Dis*. 1987;**136**(4):872–879.
21. Kondili E, Alexopoulou C, Prinianakis G, et al. Pattern of lung emptying and expiratory resistance in mechanically ventilated patients with chronic obstructive pulmonary disease. *Intensive Care Med*. 2004;**30**(7):1311–1318.
22. Ranieri VM, Giuliani R, Cinnella G, et al. Physiologic effects of positive end-expiratory pressure in patients with chronic obstructive pulmonary disease during acute ventilatory failure and controlled mechanical ventilation. *Am Rev Respir Dis*. 1993;**147**(1):5–13.
23. Guerin C, Milic-Emili J, Fournier G. Effect of PEEP on work of breathing in mechanically ventilated COPD patients. *Intensive Care Med*. 2000;**26**(9):1207–1214.
24. Ouellette DR, Patel S, Girard TD, et al. Liberation from mechanical ventilation in critically ill adults: An Official American College of Chest Physicians/American Thoracic Society Clinical Practice Guideline. *Chest*. 2017;**151**(1):166–180.
25. Braune S, Sieweke A, Brettner F, et al. The feasibility and safety of extracorporeal carbon dioxide removal to avoid intubation in patients with COPD unresponsive to noninvasive ventilation for acute hypercapnic respiratory failure (ECLAIR study): Multicentre case-control study. *Intensive Care Med*. 2016 Sep;**42**(9):1437–1444. doi: 10.1007/s00134-016-4452-y.
26. Combes A, Auzinger G, Capellier G, et al. ECCO2R therapy in the ICU: Consensus of a European round table meeting. *Crit Care*. 2020 Aug 7;**24**(1):490. doi: 10.1186/s13054-020-03210-z.

42

Asthma

Mara Ricci, Giovanni Carmine Iovino, Lucrezia Mincione, Ivan Dell'atti, and Salvatore Maurizio Maggiore

KEY MESSAGES

- Asthma is characterized by inflammation of the distal airways, leading to reversible airflow restriction and impaired pulmonary function.
- Exacerbations may be triggered by many factors, but the principles of management remain to reduce bronchoconstriction, decrease inflammation, and improve gas exchange.
- Management of severe exacerbations in ICU consists of medical therapy and optimized ventilatory support.
- Careful attention to mechanical ventilator settings is key to avoiding worsening dynamic hyperinflation, its consequences, and barotrauma.

CONTROVERSIES

- The role and timing of non-invasive ventilation (NIV) in acute severe asthma is uncertain.

FURTHER RESEARCH

- The interaction between asthma and viral infections, and optimal management of both.
- The timing and optimal use of NIV in acute severe asthma.

Introduction

Asthma is a heterogeneous clinical syndrome characterized by recurring episodes of reversible airflow obstruction due to bronchial hyper-reactivity in susceptible subjects. It may evolve towards a gradual decay of respiratory function and an irreversible remodelling of the airways. Acute episodes of bronchoconstriction of different severity, even life-threatening, may complicate asthma.

Epidemiology

Asthma is the most common chronic respiratory disorder in the world,[1] affecting about 300 million people. Its prevalence is approximately 5%–10% in Europe and has increased during the last decade. Approximately 10% of asthmatic patients have severe life-threatening exacerbations requiring intensive care unit (ICU) admission in 2%–20% of cases and mechanical ventilation in 4%.[2]

Aetiology

In genetically predisposed subjects, a severe asthma attack can be triggered by various conditions including inhaled allergens (i.e. *Dermatophagoides pteronyssinus*, arthropods, moulds, yeasts, and animal proteins), food allergens, drugs, occupational sensitizers (isocyanates and wheat flour), infections, pollution, gastroesophageal reflux, exercise, cold air, and smoking. More than half of asthma exacerbations are related to viral infections.

Pathophysiology

Asthma is a chronic inflammatory disorder of the respiratory system characterized by reversible airway hyper-reactivity that can lead to irreversible airway remodelling. Inflammation occurs in airways of different calibre, from bronchi to bronchioles, with different degrees of obstruction. Inflammatory cells (T-helper cells, lymphocytes, eosinophils, neutrophils, and mast cells), mediators (histamine, IgE, PAF, IL4, IL5, IL13, IL17, IL12, and IL23), and airway cells are involved in the process.[3] A trigger can thus activate type 2 inflammatory cascade, with the release of mediators and histamine from mast cells, lymphocytes type 2 (T_H2), and granulocytes. High concentration of cytokines (such as IL-4, IL-5, IL-13, and IL-9), released by lymphocytes, promotes oedema, hyper-responsiveness of airway, and increased secretions. Eosinophils play a central role in the inflammatory response

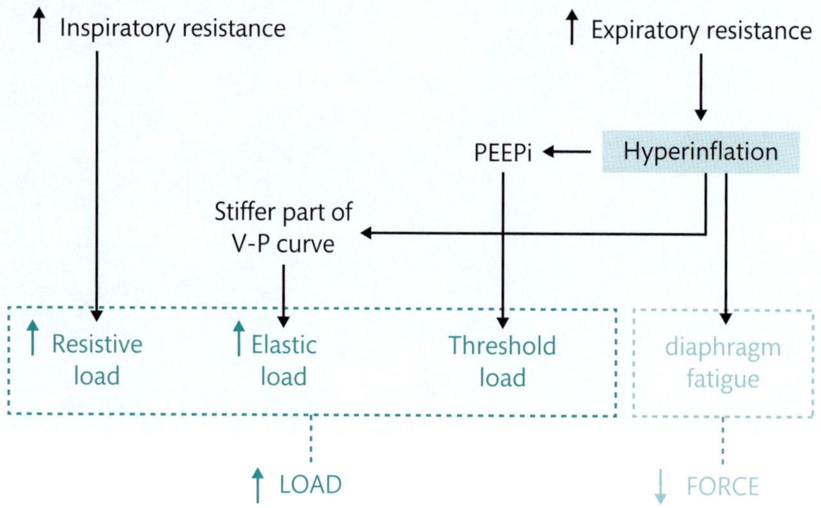

Figure 42.1 Pathophysiology of acute asthma, leading to acute respiratory failure. Asthma is characterized by an increase in airway resistance to gas flow. Increase in inspiratory resistance leads to an increase in resistive load. Increase in expiratory resistance causes dynamic hyperinflation and generation of intrinsic positive end-expiratory pressure that constitutes a threshold load for starting inspiratory flow and decreases the force-generating capacity of the diaphragm due to its flattening. In addition, hyperinflation causes a shift of tidal ventilation on the upward, stiffer part of the volume–pressure curve of the respiratory system that, in turn, increases the elastic load. The imbalance between the increased load on the respiratory muscles and the decreased respiratory muscle's force leads to alveolar hypoventilation and hypercapnic respiratory failure up to the respiratory arrest.

of asthma by releasing a series of mediators, such as leukotriene C4 and PAF.[3] In addition, neutrophil infiltration, more than eosinophils, is associated with more severe and uncontrolled asthma. Allergic asthma is activated by recognition of an IgE–allergen complex by mast cells from at least the second contact with it.

Permanent remodelling follows a long period of bronchoconstriction through hypertrophy and hyperplasia of smooth muscle cells and goblet cells and the deposition of collagen with thickening of airway walls. Airway obstruction may be spontaneously or pharmacologically reversible, but it can become irreversible over the period of many years.

Chronic and exacerbated asthma are characterized by predominantly expiratory airflow resistance, which can lead to dynamic hyperinflation during severe attacks. Incomplete exhalation, driven by reduced airflow and increased respiratory rate, leads to 'gas trapping' and the generation of intrinsic or auto-PEEP (PEEPi).[4] The vicious cycle of increased work of breathing through needing to overcome PEEPi, distended lungs moving onto less advantageous segments of the pressure–volume curve, and impaired diaphragmatic function are illustrated in Figure 42.1. Gas exchange is further impaired by ventilation/perfusion (V_A/Q) mismatch,[5] leading to hypoxaemia. V_A/Q mismatch is driven by several mechanisms, including alveolar hypoventilation and hyperinflation-driven alveolar hypertension and alveolar capillary collapse, the latter phenomenon then worsened by hypoxic pulmonary vasoconstriction.

Classification

Classification of asthma severity is set out in Table 42.1, covering factors such as symptomatic and functional burden, nocturnal features, and spirometric measures (forced expiratory volume in the first second (FEV_1) or daily variability of peak expiratory flow (PEF)). Control of symptoms allows classification of therapeutic response (Box 42.1).[6]

Severe uncontrolled asthma is defined as asthma that requires treatment with high-dose inhaled corticosteroids (ICS) and long-acting β_2 receptor agonist (LABA) or leukotriene modifier/theophylline for the previous year or systemic corticosteroids (CS) for ≥50% of the previous year to prevent it from becoming uncontrolled or that remains uncontrolled despite this therapy. Patients with severe uncontrolled asthma are at high risk of developing severe asthmatic exacerbations, also named 'status asthmaticus', a life-threatening condition that does not respond to the repetitive administration of short-acting inhaled β_2 adrenergic receptor agonists (SABA).[7]

Table 42.1 Classification of asthma by severity

Persistent asthma	Mild	Moderate	Severe
Symptoms	>1 time a week But <1 time a day	Daily, attacks affect activity	Continuous, limited physical activity
Nocturnal symptoms	>2 times a month	>1 time week	Frequent
FEV1 or PEF	>80% predicted or variability 20%–30%	60%–80% predicted or variability >30%	<60% predicted or variability >30%

Box 42.1 Definition of severe uncontrolled asthma

Uncontrolled asthma

(1) Poor symptom control.
(2) Frequent severe exacerbations: two or more rescue courses of systemic corticosteroids in the previous year for three or more days.
(3) Serious exacerbations: at least one hospitalization, ICU stay, or mechanical ventilation in the previous year.
(4) Airflow limitation: pre-bronchodilator and FEV1 <80% predicted (with reduced FEV1/FVC defined as less than the lower limit of normal).
(5) Controlled asthma that worsens on tapering of high doses of inhaled corticosteroids or systemic corticosteroids (or additional biologic agents).

Note: At least one of the five items defines uncontrolled asthma. FVC: forced volume vital capacity.

Source: Adapted with permission of the © ERS 2022. Chung KF, Wenzel SE, Brozek JL, et al. International ERS/ATS guidelines on definition, evaluation and treatment of severe asthma. *Eur. Resp. J.* 2014;43(2):343–373; DOI: 10.1183/09031936.00202013.

Clinical Features

Patients with a severe asthmatic attack have a rapid and sudden onset syndrome including cough, shortness of breath, wheeze, and dyspnoea often referred as chest tightness or pain of differing degrees of severity and combinations. These symptoms can be intermittent and generally worse at night. The most severe patients present with acute respiratory failure (ARF), which is typically a type II respiratory failure (hypercapnic) caused by alveolar hypoventilation. These patients have severe dyspnoea, talk in incomplete sentences, and have a rapid shallow breathing with use of accessory muscles. During life-threatening attack, cyanosis, gasping, exhaustion of respiratory muscles, and reduced consciousness occur. Physical examination reveals tachycardia (often >120 beats/min), tachypnoea (often >30 breaths/min), pulsus paradoxus (decrease in systolic arterial pressure by >25 mmHg on inspiration), hypoxaemia (SaO_2 <90% or PaO_2 <60 mmHg), and loud wheezes then silent chest due to the absence of inspiratory airflow in the presence of marked dynamic hyperinflation.[8] In imminent respiratory arrest, wheeze disappears, alongside bradycardia, bradypnea, somnolence, and diaphoresis until respiratory arrest.

Diagnosis

Diagnosis of asthma exacerbation is principally based on clinical tests. Arterial blood gases (ABGs), spirometry, and chest X-ray can help mostly in determination of the severity and responsiveness to treatment. Patient evaluation must be completed with a rapid and complete history including previous hospitalizations or emergency department access, ICU admission, current therapy, and co-morbidities. This assessment should not, however, delay intervention.[8]

ABG analysis may show normo- or hypercapnia and hypoxaemia despite a high respiratory rate. Respiratory acidosis is commonly due to patient exhaustion, inadequate alveolar ventilation, and/or an increase in dead space caused by an ineffective, compensatory rapid, shallow breathing pattern. Metabolic acidosis may coexist due to an increase in lactic acid, related to increased work of breathing, tissue hypoxia, and treatment with high dose of β_2 receptor agonists.

Assessment of spirometry before and after treatment can be useful in evaluating severity and response to therapy, but more severely affected patients may be unable to perform effective spirometry. There is a correlation between serial functional trajectories of spirometry and severity of asthma attack which can be useful to detect severe or even life-threatening exacerbations.[9]

Chest X-ray is not crucial for diagnosis. It can, however, demonstrate associated respiratory conditions (e.g. pneumonia), assess indirect signs of overdistention (e.g. diaphragm flatting), and exclude complications (e.g. pneumothorax).

Several pathologies can mimic asthma exacerbation. These include paroxysmal vocal cord dysfunction, tracheal lesions, laryngospasm, presence of foreign bodies in the airway, diffuse panbronchiolitis, COPD exacerbations, croup, cardiogenic oedema ('cardiac asthma'), aortic arch abnormalities, rhinosinus disease, and severe gastroesophageal reflux.

Treatment

Key issues in the management of severe asthma are (1) increase in alveolar ventilation, (2) resting the respiratory muscles, and (3) minimizing dynamic hyperinflation. Critical care management of asthma may be considered as non-ventilator or ventilatory management.

Non-ventilatory Management

Oxygen

Oxygen therapy is standard care for acute asthma attack. Recommendations are SaO_2 >93% and >95% in high-risk populations (pregnant women and with ischaemic heart disease).[9] As hypoxaemia is often mild, low O_2 flow (2–4 L/min via nasal cannulae or face mask) may be sufficient.[9] Oxygen-driven nebulizers with using higher O_2 flow (10–12 L/min) aid delivery of nebulized drugs to the small calibre airways. Caution must be placed during oxygen therapy, and a close monitoring of O_2 saturation is necessary to avoid carbon dioxide retention, especially in severe airway obstruction and chronically hypercapnic patients.[10]

Drugs

The objectives of medical therapy for severe asthma are

- decreasing bronchoconstriction,
- reducing inflammation, and
- improving patient–ventilator interaction.

Bronchodilation

Bronchodilation can be achieved by administering inhaled short-acting beta$_2$ agonists (SABA) and short-acting muscarinic antagonists. These drugs can be administered using either metered-dose inhaler or nebulizer. Inhaled drug therapies are further discussed in Chapter 22. Although intravenous beta-agonists appear to offer little benefit in acute asthma,[11] they may play a role when small airway obstruction prevents conduction of inhaled drug and may provide an earlier clinical response.

Corticosteroids

Corticosteroids reduce inflammation and increase the number and sensitivity of β_2 adrenergic receptors but do not have a direct bronchodilatory effect. They can be administered through oral, inhalation, or intravenous routes and produce their effect on lung function within 6–12 h. High-dose ICS are preferable because of local vasoconstriction and can be added to inhaled beta-agonists, leading to a decrease in oedema formation and plasma exudation, improving bronchodilatory effects.

Sedation

Sedation is used to improve comfort, safety, and patient–ventilator synchrony in mechanically ventilated patients. Various agents may be used, including propofol that has bronchodilator properties. Alongside sedatives, opioids help achieve sedation, amnesia, and respiratory-driven suppression. Morphine can exacerbate bronchospasm, and therefore Fentanyl and Remifentanil are preferred. Ketamine is considered an attractive alternative because of its sympathomimetic and bronchodilator properties. Dexmedetomidine, an α_2-agonist, can be useful for sedation in patients requiring non-invasive ventilation (NIV).[12] If adequate sedation is difficult to obtain and/or extreme patient–ventilator asynchrony occurs, respiratory muscle paralysis should be considered.

Magnesium Sulphate

Magnesium sulphate ($MgSO_4$) can have therapeutic effects through modulation of smooth muscle contractions and the inhibition of calcium release from the sarcoplasmic reticulum. In addition, cyclic adenosine monophosphate-dependent protein and adenylate cyclase are among the many enzymes that require magnesium for their function. This may explain why magnesium may potentiate the action of β_2-agonists.[13] Overall, the effects of magnesium administrations are bronchodilation and attenuation of the neutrophil respiratory burst in acute severe asthma and a global improvement of pulmonary function. The use of $MgSO_4$ is part of guidelines for severe asthma in hospital, that is, adults with FEV_1 <25%–30% predicted with symptoms and/or who fail to respond within 1 h to initial treatment manifesting refractory hypoxaemia. Currently, the recommended dose is 2 g intravenously over 20 min.[8,9] The role of nebulized $MgSO_4$ is still unclear, but it may bring benefits when isotonic solution of $MgSO_4$ is used as the diluent for inhaled salbutamol. Adverse effects are flushing, fatigue, and pain at the site of infusion; hypermagnesaemia has been described in patients with kidney failure or in elderly patients with small bowel hypomobility.

Ventilatory Management

Endotracheal Intubation

Immediate intubation should be performed when patients with severe acute asthma show signs of respiratory muscle fatigue, neurological obtundation, or respiratory arrest.[14] Airway obstruction not responsive to therapy, respiratory rate >40 breath/min, silent chest despite respiratory effort, and persistent respiratory or lactic acidosis are additional trigger factors to institute invasive ventilation.[15] High level of $paCO_2$ or respiratory acidosis alone is not necessarily an indication for intubation. Several studies demonstrated a potential detrimental effect of intubation and mechanical ventilation, potentially leading to increased mortality in these patients.[15] Therefore, a strategy combining a trial of NIV with pharmacological therapy has been suggested in an ICU setting with a rescue plan for intubation.[16]

Ventilator Settings

The primary goal of mechanical ventilation in intubated patients with severe asthma is minimizing dynamic hyperinflation. Minute ventilation is an important determinant of lung hyperinflation. Reducing minute ventilation limits hyperinflation, intrinsic PEEP, and their negative effects (barotrauma and hypotension).[4,14] To achieve this minimal ventilation, a strategy of permissive hypercapnia should be used, limiting tidal volume to 6–7 mL/kg and respiratory rate to 10–14 breaths/min, thus prolonging the expiratory time beyond 4 s.[14] Acute exacerbations of asthma can lead to respiratory failure requiring ventilatory assistance. NIV may prevent the need for endotracheal intubation in selected patients. For patients who are intubated and undergo mechanical ventilation, a strategy that prioritizes avoidance of ventilator-related complications over correction of hypercapnia was first proposed 30 years ago and has become the preferred approach. Excessive pulmonary hyperinflation is a major cause of hypotension and barotrauma. An appreciation of the key determinants of hyperinflation is essential to rational ventilator management. Standard therapy for patients with asthma undergoing mechanical ventilation consists of inhaled bronchodilators, corticosteroids, and drugs used to facilitate controlled hypoventilation. Nonconventional interventions, such as heliox, general anaesthesia, bronchoscopy, and extracorporeal life support, have also been advocated for patients with fulminant asthma but are rarely necessary. Immediate mortality for patients who are mechanically ventilated for acute severe asthma is very low and is often associated with out-of-hospital cardiorespiratory arrest before intubation. However, patients who have been intubated for severe asthma are at increased risk for death from subsequent exacerbations and must be managed accordingly in the outpatient setting.[9] Using a high inspiratory flow rate (≥60–70 L/min) during volume assist-control ventilation can decrease the inspiration–expiration ratio and prolong expiration. Applying external PEEP below intrinsic PEEP can help to improve expired volumes and reduce work of breathing during assisted ventilation without increasing the risk of barotrauma.

Hypercapnia

A rise of dead space secondary to alveolar overdistension in severe asthmatic patients and the application of a 'hypoventilation strategy' will lead to hypercapnia. This is generally well tolerated in status asthmaticus, and the related complications are uncommon. Indeed, attempts to restore normocapnia can worsen alveolar hyperinflation and overdistension. Although rare, potentially severe consequences of hypercapnia are increased intracranial pressure and cardiac arrhythmias. Therefore, appropriate considerations are required. Alkalinizing therapy with slow infusion of sodium bicarbonate has been recommended if pH is less than 7.15–7.2[17] although not generally used in modern management algorithms.

Respiratory Monitoring

To minimize lung hyperinflation and prevent barotrauma and their detrimental hemodynamic consequences, it is important to monitor parameters of respiratory mechanics during mechanical ventilation, including end-inspiratory plateau pressure (P_{plat}), peak airway pressure, intrinsic PEEP, and end-inspiratory lung volume (see Chapter 11). *Plateau pressure* represents average end-inspiratory alveolar pressure and can assess lung hyperinflation during mechanical ventilation. The aim is to keep it <30 cmH_2O to minimize the risk of barotrauma and hypotension (though the pressure in some pulmonary units might still be higher because of heterogeneous impairment in lung mechanics). Accurate measurement of plateau pressure requires an end-inspiratory pause of around 0.5 s in asthma, and shorter may overestimate plateau pressure. *Peak pressure* depends on end-expiratory pressure, resistive pressure (related to airway resistance and to inspiratory flow), and on elastic pressure (related to delivered tidal volume and to lung elastance). Peak pressure can be useful to track changes in the mechanical properties of the respiratory system but is a poor estimate for end-inspiratory alveolar pressure and cannot be used to monitor the degree of lung hyperinflation. *Intrinsic PEEP* (PEEPi) can be used to monitor lung hyperinflation and to assess the risk of barotrauma and hypotension. Early airway closure at low respiratory rate, highly compliant ventilatory circuit, and short end-expiratory pause (under 2–3 s) may lead to underestimation of intrinsic PEEP. In contrast, expiratory muscle activity during expiration can overestimate its value. *End-inspiratory lung volume* is the sum of tidal volume and the volume trapped because of dynamic hyperinflation. In mechanically ventilated, paralysed patients, it is measured as the total amount of gas exhaled during a prolonged expiration (60 s). This is a good index of lung hyperinflation, and it is useful to predict ventilator-related complications (barotrauma and hypotension).[18]

Non-invasive Positive Pressure Ventilation (NIPPV)

Use of NIPPV in acute severe asthma remains a debated topic. This technique of ventilation provides several theoretical advantages for improving lung function with a marginal benefit in reduction of respiratory rate. NIPPV offloads fatiguing respiratory muscles resulting from bronchial obstruction and hyperinflation and improves gas exchange (Chapters 8 and 9).[19] These beneficial effects translate into less intubation if NIPPV is applied early,[20] thus avoiding the risk of intubation-related complications and ventilator-associated pneumonia. Globally, there is a reduction of number of hospital admissions and length of ICU and hospital stay.[21] However, the absence of data regarding a beneficial effect on survival and the need of more consistent studies preclude making a strong recommendation regarding the use of NIPPV for acute asthma.[22] NIV is widely used in the acute care setting for ARF across a variety of aetiologies. The European Respiratory Society/American Thoracic Society recommendations for the clinical application of NIV are based on the most current literature.[22] The guideline committee was composed of clinicians, methodologists, and experts in the field of NIV. The committee developed recommendations based on the Grading, Recommendation, Assessment, Development, and Evaluation (GRADE) methodology for each actionable question. The GRADE Evidence to Decision framework in the guideline development tool was used to generate recommendations. A number of topics were addressed using technical summaries without recommendations, and these are discussed in the supplementary material. This guideline committee developed recommendations for 11 actionable questions in a population–intervention–comparison–outcome (PICO) format, all addressing the use of NIV for various aetiologies of ARF. The specific conditions where recommendations were made include exacerbation of chronic obstructive pulmonary disease, cardiogenic pulmonary oedema, de novo hypoxaemic respiratory failure, immunocompromised patients, chest trauma, palliation, post-operative care, weaning, and post-extubation. This document summarizes the current state of knowledge regarding the role of NIV in ARF. Evidence-based recommendations provide guidance to relevant stakeholders.[22] Low levels of inspiratory pressure support (5–7 cmH_2O) and PEEP (3–5 cmH_2O) are the preferable starting parameters of NIPPV. Subsequent increase of inspiratory pressure support (2 cmH_2O every 15 min) can be made to decrease respiratory rate <25 breaths/min, whilst ensuring inspiratory peak pressure <25 cmH_2O. Inspiratory trigger sensitivity should be set to decrease the work of breathing and to enhance patient's comfort whilst avoiding autotriggering. Expiratory trigger value is generally set at 40% of peak inspiratory flow with ±10% variations according to the inspiratory time. To optimize patient's comfort and work of breathing, pressure ramp should be sufficiently steep.

High-flow Nasal Oxygen Therapy (HFNO)

HFNO can deliver high flow (up to 70 L/min) of heated and humidified gas at a controlled concentration of oxygen through a special nasal cannula or other interfaces (including for tracheostomy) (see Chapter 7). It is indicated as respiratory support in patients with mild-moderate hypoxemic respiratory failure.[23] Its use has some theoretical benefits, such as effective CO_2 clearance, better alveolar ventilation, and reduced work of breathing. As compared to conventional oxygen therapy, HFNO show in fact at least similar clinical efficacy in terms of improving oxygenation and reducing respiratory rate and heart rate. Furthermore, HFNO can potentially reduce airway inflammation and improve mucociliary function compared with inhalation of dry and cold gases.

Helium-Oxygen (HeO_2)

Helium is insoluble, inert, gas with low density and high kinematic viscosity. As a result of the lower density, helium has a larger binary diffusion coefficient for carbon dioxide when compared with ambient air. Furthermore, helium converts some areas of turbulent flow to laminar flow, enhancing both convective and diffusive forces and effectively recruiting low V/Q units. The use of HeO_2 in patients with acute severe asthma is not part of routine care, but it may be considered for patients who do not respond to standard therapy. HeO_2 can also be used as an adjuvant therapy for aerosol treatments by improving lung diffusion of aerosolized particles. Although clinical trials have not shown superiority of HeO_2 over air–O_2 during NIPPV in terms of intubation rate, a subset of patients at higher risk of NIPPV failure might benefit from the use of HeO_2.[24] This is further discussed in chapter 22.

Coronavirus Disease 2019 and Asthma

Coronavirus disease 2019 (COVID-19) is a pandemic illness caused by severe acute respiratory syndrome coronavirus 2 (SARS-CoV-2) (Chapter 35). The virus has respiratory tropism and causes various clinical manifestations including acute respiratory distress syndrome. Asthmatic patients do not appear over-represented among COVID-19 patients.[25] However, large data sets are emerging, and the evidence evolves. For instance, those on a combination of inhaled steroids, a LABA and an additional controller are at increased risk of critical care, from a large UK cohort (ISARIC4).[26] This also suggests a seemingly protective effect for those over 50 years with asthma who had inhaled steroids in the 2 weeks prior to admission with COVID-19 compared to non-asthmatics. Small studies with asthmatic subgroups of COVID-19 patients have shown similar outcome in terms of ICU admission and mortality as non-asthmatic COVID-19 patients.[25] There is a lower expression of angiotensin-converting enzyme-2 receptor of SARS-CoV-2 in airway cells of patients with asthma and a decrease in eosinophils count as a consequence of down-regulation of type 2 inflammatory response, which is responsible of asthma exacerbation. In asthmatic patients with COVID-19, recent guidelines recommend continuing both oral and inhaled corticosteroid therapy, which may also have a protective role against the progression of COVID-19.[27]

REFERENCES

1. Bahadori K, Doyle-Waters MM, Marra C, et al. Economic burden of asthma: A systematic review. *BMC Pulm Med.* 2009;**9**:24.
2. Pendergraft TB, Stanford RH, Beasley R, et al. Rates and characteristics of intensive care unit admissions and intubations among asthma-related hospitalizations. *Ann Allergy Asthma Immunol.* 2004;**93**:29–35.
3. Lambrecht BN, Hammad H, Fahy JV. The cytokines of asthma. *Immunity.* 2019;**50**:975–991.
4. Tuxen DV, Lane S. The effects of ventilatory pattern on hyperinflation, airway pressures, and circulation in mechanical ventilation of patients with severe air-flow obstruction. *Am Rev Respir Dis.* 1987;**136**:872–879.
5. Ballester E, Reyes A, Roca J, et al. Ventilation-perfusion mismatching in acute severe asthma: Effects of salbutamol and 100% oxygen. *Thorax.* 1989;**44**:258–267.
6. Chung KF, Wenzel SE, Brozek JL, et al. International ERS/ATS guidelines on definition, evaluation and treatment of severe asthma. *Eur Respir J.* 2014 Feb;**43**(2):343–373. Erratum in: *Eur Respir J.* 2014 Apr;43(4):1216. Dosage error in article text.
7. Scoggin CH, Sahn SA, Petty TL. Status asthmaticus. A nine-year experience. *JAMA.* 1977;**238**:1158–1162.
8. British Thoracic Society and SIG. Network. British guidelines on management of asthma. July 2019.
9. Global Initiative for Asthma, Global Strategy for Asthma Management and Prevention. 2021.
10. Chien JW, Ciufo R, Novak R, et al. Uncontrolled oxygen administration and respiratory failure in acute asthma. *Chest.* 2000;**117**:728–733.
11. Travers A, Jones AP, Kelly K, et al. Intravenous beta2-agonists for acute asthma in the emergency department. *Cochrane Database Syst Rev.* 2001;**2**:CD002988.
12. Takasaki Y, Kido T, Semba K. Dexmedetomidine facilitates induction of noninvasive positive pressure ventilation for acute respiratory failure in patients with severe asthma. *J Anesth.* 2009;**23**:147–150.
13. Cydulka RK. Why magnesium for asthma? *Acad Emerg Med.* 1996;**3**:1084–1085.
14. Leatherman J. Mechanical ventilation for severe asthma. *Chest.* 2015;**14**:1671–1680.
15. Brenner B, Corbridge T, Kazzi A. Intubation and mechanical ventilation of the asthmatic patient in respiratory failure. *J Emerg Med.* 2009;**37**:S23–34.
16. Murase K, Tomii K, Chin K, et al The use of non-invasive ventilation for life-threatening asthma attacks: Changes in the need for intubation. *Respirology.* 2010;**15**:714–720.
17. Feihl F, Perret C. Permissive hypercapnia. How permissive should we be? *Am J Respir Crit Care Med.* 1994;**15**:1722–1737.
18. Oddo M, Feihl F, Schaller MD, et al. Management of mechanical ventilation in acute severe asthma: Practical aspects. *Intensive Care Med.* 2006;**32**:501–510.
19. Nava S, Hill N. Non-invasive ventilation in acute respiratory failure. *Lancet.* 2009;**374**:250–259.
20. Althoff MD, Holguin F, Yang F, et al. Noninvasive ventilation use in critically ill patients with acute asthma exacerbations. *Am J Respir Crit Care Med.* 2020;**202**:1520–1530.
21. Lim WJ, Mohammed Akram R, Carson KV, et al. Non-invasive positive pressure ventilation for treatment of respiratory failure due to severe acute exacerbations of asthma. *Cochrane Database Syst Rev.* 2012;**12**:CD004360.
22. Rochwerg B, Brochard L, Elliott MW, et al. Official ERS/ATS clinical practice guidelines: Non-invasive ventilation for acute respiratory failure. *Eur Respir J.* 2017;**50**:1602426.
23. Rochwerg B, Einav S, Chaudhuri D, et al The role for high flow nasal cannula as a respiratory support strategy in adults: A clinical practice guideline. *Intensive Care Med.* 2020;**46**:2226–2237.
24. Maggiore SM, Richard JC, Abroug F, et al. A multicenter, randomized trial of noninvasive ventilation with helium-oxygen mixture in exacerbations of chronic obstructive lung disease. *Crit Care Med.* 2010;**38**:145–151.
25. Beurnier A, Jutant EM, Jevnikar M, et al. Characteristics and outcomes of asthmatic patients with COVID-19 pneumonia who require hospitalisation. *Eur Respir J.* 2020;**56**:200187.
26. Bloom CI, Drake TM, Docherty AB, et al. Risk of adverse outcomes in patients with underlying respiratory conditions admitted to hospital with COVID-19: A national, multicentre prospective cohort study using the ISARIC WHO Clinical Characterisation Protocol UK. *Lancet Respir Med.* 2021;**9**(7):699–711.
27. COVID-19: GINA Answers to Frequently Asked Questions on Asthma Management 2020 (https://ginasthma.org/covid-19-gina-answers-to-frequently-asked-questions-on-asthma-management/).

43

Thromboembolic Disease

Caroline Patterson and Derek Bell

KEY MESSAGES

- Critically ill patients have an increased susceptibility to VTE as a result of individual and situation-associated risk factors.
- VTE risk assessment is recommended for all patients admitted to the intensive care unit (ICU), and most patients should receive thromboprophylaxis. Bleeding risk may outweigh the benefits of prophylactic anticoagulation.
- A diagnosis of DVT during ICU admission has a negative effect on patient outcomes, and even small pulmonary emboli may be life threatening in patients with reduced cardiopulmonary reserve.

CONTROVERSIES

- Monitoring clinical effectiveness of low-molecular-weight heparin (LMWH) thromboprophylaxis using anti-factor Xa levels is more challenging in critically unwell patients, and inadequate dosing is a potential risk. Unfractionated heparin (UFH), LMWH, and mechanical thromboprophylaxis differ in efficacy and safety, and the prophylaxis recommended for certain subgroups of critically ill patients may differ.

FURTHER RESEARCH

- A randomized controlled trial in which routine DVT screening is performed in addition to an optimized thromboprophylaxis regimen would provide information to guide future clinical practice.
- The role of tailored thromboprophylaxis in critically ill patients, and especially in those at the extremes of body weight with renal insufficiency and taking antiplatelet agents, has yet to be clearly defined.
- The potential role for low-dose systemic or catheter-directed thrombolysis in patients without haemodynamic compromise is also uncertain.

Introduction

Venous thromboembolism (VTE) encompasses deep vein thrombosis (DVT) and pulmonary embolism (PE). There is concern that VTE may be underdiagnosed in critically ill patients and many diagnoses occur post-mortem.[1]

Frequency of VTE

The prevalence of (a) symptomatic DVT from admission to 48 h on intensive care unit (ICU) is 3.5%–6%.[2,3]

The incidence of DVT during ICU admission is reported as ~10% for medical–surgical ICU patients, despite thromboprophylaxis, and up to 65.8% of VTE occurs in patients receiving prophylaxis for >80% of the time.[4,5] Twenty to thirty percent of untreated calf vein DVTs are said to extend into the thigh, where they present a 40%–50% risk for PE.[6] Proven DVT progresses to PE in 11.5% of mechanically ventilated patients despite thromboprophylaxis.[7] Pulmonary emboli are often asymptomatic. In the PROTECT study, PE was diagnosed in 19% of patients but clinically silent in 60% of these.[3] Pooled autopsy studies indicate a PE prevalence of 7%–27% among critically ill patients; death occurring in 0%–12%.[8]

Risk Factors for VTE

VTE occurs in the presence of at least one of three aetiological factors—blood flow disruption, vascular endothelial injury, and hypercoagulability, eponymously known as Virchow's triad.

Predisposing factors for VTE in critical care patients include personal or family history of VTE and premorbid dialysis-dependent renal failure.[8] Others include advanced age, illness, injury, trauma, and recent surgery. During ICU admission, further risk factors are prolonged immobility (exacerbated by sedation), mechanical ventilation, central venous catheterization (particularly femoral), renal support, platelet transfusion, and vasopressors. Thus, activation of the coagulation cascade in critical illness, with defective inhibition of coagulation and attenuation of fibrinolysis seen during mechanical ventilation, increases the likelihood of VTE.

VTE Screening and Diagnosis

At present there is no consensus on the best method of VTE screening and prevention in critically ill patients. History and physical examination lack reliability,[9] while clinical prediction rules (e.g. Wells prediction rule and revised Geneva scoring system) are not validated in the ICU. D-dimer levels and tests of molecular hypercoagulability (activated protein C resistance ratio, prothrombin mutation, protein C, protein S, antithrombin, anticardiolipin antibody, and lupus anticoagulant) are not predictive of DVT in ICU.[9] The usefulness of troponin and B-type natriuretic peptide as diagnostic tests is also limited.

Focused bilateral compression ultrasound (CUS) (assessing compressibility of the common femoral and popliteal veins) is the recommended imaging modality for DVT detection in critically ill patients.[10]

Lower limb CUS is highly sensitive and specific for proximal DVT. Diagnostic accuracy is reduced in asymptomatic patients and those with isolated distal or recurrent DVT.[11] False-positive results may occur with positive end-expiratory pressure (PEEP) and with large central venous catheters that impede blood flow and mimic thrombus.

Routine ultrasound screening for DVT is not recommended in ICU patients due to a lack of evidence supporting improved outcomes or cost effectiveness versus appropriate thromboprophylaxis.[12]

Non-specific clinical signs that should raise suspicion of PE in mechanically ventilated patients include tachycardia, hypotension, hypoxia or hypocarbia, and unexplained weaning failure and unexplained pyrexia (arising from pulmonary infarction, necrosis, haemorrhage, atelectasis, or local inflammation).

Computed tomography pulmonary angiogram (CTPA) allows visualization of the pulmonary arteries to the subsegmental level and is the first-line imaging modality for the confirmation of PE, with a sensitivity of 83% and a specificity of 96%.[13] CTPA allows quantitative assessment of clot burden, ventricular dimensions as surrogates of right ventricular dysfunction (RVD), risk stratification in PE, and mimics of PE. CTPA does come with the hazards of iodinated contrast, ionizing radiation, and patient transfer.

Transthoracic echo (TTE) is not sufficiently sensitive for the diagnosis of PE, missing >50% of angiography proven PEs. Its role in critically ill patients is as a tool to risk stratify patients with proven embolism. RVD is an independent and powerful predictor of early death following PE[14] but may be due to concomitant cardiorespiratory disease.

Trans-oesophageal echo (TOE) allows better visualization of the proximal pulmonary arteries than TTE. In a prospective study of ICU patients with suspected PE, the sensitivity of TOE for the detection of proximal embolism was 84% with specificity 84%. Although sensitivity was adequate for emboli in the main or right pulmonary artery, it was limited for left proximal or lobar emboli and inferior to CTPA for distal PE.[15]

In mechanically ventilated ICU patients with clinically suspected PE, CTPA is therefore the preferred diagnostic imaging modality. In haemodynamically unstable patients, when CTPA is not possible, bedside TTE may support a diagnosis, with the caveat of potential false-negative result. Additional bilateral CUS of the lower limbs may be warranted to look for DVT.[16]

The adoption of single-photon emission computed tomography for the diagnosis of PE in critically ill patients is limited by low sensitivity, a high proportion of inconclusive scans, and limited availability. Magnetic resonance angiography is not recommended for ruling out PE.

Clinical Significance of VTE

DVT is associated with prolonged ICU and hospital length of stay (7.28 days and 11.2 days, respectively) and trends towards increased mortality.[17] DVT increases the risk of PE in critically ill patients and potentially worse outcomes in those with limited cardio-respiratory reserve.[8] Secondary haemodynamic compromise can occur 24–48 h after acute PE.

Treatment of VTE

European Society of Cardiology guidelines propose a risk stratification model to determine therapeutic management of PE based on the cumulative prognostic value of clinical data, imaging features of RVD, circulating biomarkers of myocardial injury and RVD, and the presence of co-morbidity.[16]

Treatment of High-risk PE

Patients with PE and haemodynamic instability should be considered high-risk. Haemodynamic instability in this context is defined as (1) cardiac arrest, (2) obstructive shock (SBP < 90 mmHg or the requirement for inotropic support) with end organ hypoperfusion, or (3) persistent hypotension (SBP < 90 mmHg or a pressure drop >40 mmHg for >15 min without another cause).

Administration of supplemental oxygen is indicated to maintain SaO_2 <90%. Correction of hypoxaemia may not be possible without simultaneous pulmonary reperfusion. PEEP should be applied with caution.

Intravenous anticoagulation with a weight-adjusted dose of unfractionated heparin (UFH) should be initiated without delay in patients with suspected high-risk PE. Treatment with systemic thrombolysis should be administered in the absence of contraindications. Systemic thrombolysis leads to faster improvements in pulmonary obstruction, pulmonary artery pressure, and pulmonary vascular resistance than UFH alone.

Meta-analysis of thrombolysis trials indicates a significant reduction in the combined outcome of mortality and recurrent PE with thrombolysis but at the cost of a 9.9% rate of severe bleeding and a 1.7% rate of intracranial haemorrhage.[18]

Accelerated administration of recombinant tissue-type plasminogen activator (rtPA; 100 mg over 2 h) is recommended over prolonged infusions of first-generation thrombolytic agents (e.g. streptokinase and urokinase).

In the event of cardiac arrest attributed to acute PE, cardiopulmonary resuscitation should be continued for at least 60–90 min after thrombolysis has been administered because of cases of successful resuscitation at this point.

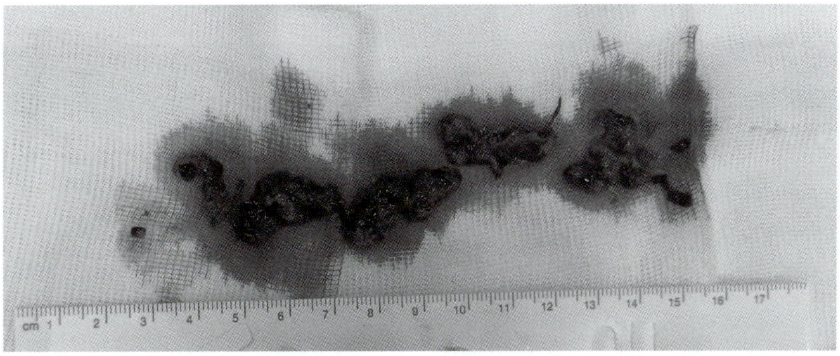

Figure 43.1 Thrombectomy: Aspirated clot using vacuum-assisted catheter thrombectomy performed on a patient with acute pelvic deep venous thrombosis. Image courtesy of Dr Carole Ridge, Royal Brompton and Harefield Hospitals.

Image courtesy of Dr Carole Ridge, Royal Brompton and Harefield Hospitals.

Unsuccessful thrombolysis is reported in 8% of patients with high-risk PE.[19] In the event of high bleeding risk, or failure of systemic thrombolysis, catheter-directed thrombolysis, catheter-assisted thrombus removal or surgical embolectomy can be considered (Figures 43.1 and 43.2).

Published case series of surgical embolectomy report perioperative mortality between 4% and 59%. Advanced age, pre-surgical cardiac arrest, and pre-surgical thrombolytic therapy are associated with worse outcomes.[20]

Veno-venous or veno-arterial extracorporeal membrane oxygenation (ECMO) is increasingly used for haemodynamic support in high-risk PE patients and may be used to facilitate stabilization for surgical embolectomy.

After haemodynamic stabilization of the high-risk patient, anticoagulation treatment is continued as per intermediate- or low-risk PE patients.

For those patients with acute VTE who are treated with anticoagulants, inferior vena cava (IVC) filter placement does not appear to reduce recurrent PE, including fatal PE, and is not recommended.[21]

Treatment of Intermediate/Low-risk PE

In the absence of haemodynamic instability at presentation, further risk stratification of PE is recommended. The Pulmonary Embolism Severity Index (PESI), which integrates PE severity and co-morbidity, is one of the most extensively validated prediction tools, and a simplified version of the PESI (sPESI) has been shown to be non-inferior to the PESI in predicting 30-day mortality.

For normotensive patients, those with an sPESI of 0 or PESI I–II should be considered low risk. Patients with any of (1) sPESI ≥1, (2) RVD, or (3) elevated cardiac biomarkers should be considered intermediate–low risk, and those with sPESI ≥1 and both RVD and elevated cardiac biomarkers should be considered intermediate–high risk.[16]

Prompt initiation of anticoagulation in non-high-risk patients with confirmed VTE is recommended to reduce symptoms, rates of recurrent VTE, and death, but treatment must be balanced against the risk of major bleeding.

If anticoagulation is initiated parenterally, subcutaneous, weight-adjusted low-molecular-weight heparins (LMWHs) (e.g. Dalteparin, Tinzaparin, and Enoxaparin) or a selective factor Xa inhibitor (e.g. fondaparinux) are recommended over UFH as they are associated with a lower risk of major bleeding and heparin-induced thrombocytopenia. UFH is recommended for patients with serious renal impairment (creatinine clearance (CrCl) ≤ 30 mL/min).

Novel oral anticoagulants (NOACs, e.g. Dabigatran, Rivaroxaban, Apixiban, and Edoxaban) are recommended over vitamin K antagonists (VKAs, e.g. warfarin) for the initial and long-term treatment of VTE in patients without cancer. In patients with so-called cancer-associated thrombosis, LMWH is recommended. If choosing a VKA, oral treatment should overlap with parenteral anticoagulation until a therapeutic international normalised ratio (INR) is achieved.[16]

Fondaparinux, DOACs, or VKAs should not be used in pregnant patients with suspected or proven PE. UFH and LMWH do not cross the placenta and are safer during pregnancy.

Systemic thrombolysis should not be routinely administered as primary treatment for intermediate- or low-risk PE but may be considered as a rescue treatment for patients who develop haemodynamic compromise despite anticoagulation.

Prophylaxis of VTE

The details of thromboprophylaxis are addressed in Chapter 23. As such, the key points are alluded to here. Thromboprophylaxis is associated with a reduction in mortality in critically ill patients.[22] While a number of strategies are used, LMWHs are the most widely adopted drugs for this purpose and are the agent advised in guidelines such as those from the UK National Institute of Health and Care Excellence (NICE).[23] Monitoring LMWH through the measurement of anti-Xa activity can be helpful in patients with reduced CrCl. Critically ill patients with normal renal function demonstrate significantly lower anti-Xa levels in response to LMWH than ward-based medical patients. Compared with general ward patients, critically ill patients may require greater doses of thromboprophylaxis to achieve adequate protection although the role of monitoring anti-Xa levels for prophylaxis remains uncertain.

Where bleeding risk is high or anticoagulation is contra-indicated, mechanical prophylaxis, ideally with both graduated compression stockings and intermittent pneumatic compression devices, can be used. IVC filters are not recommended for routine first-line use but may have a role in carefully selected patients who cannot be managed in other ways.

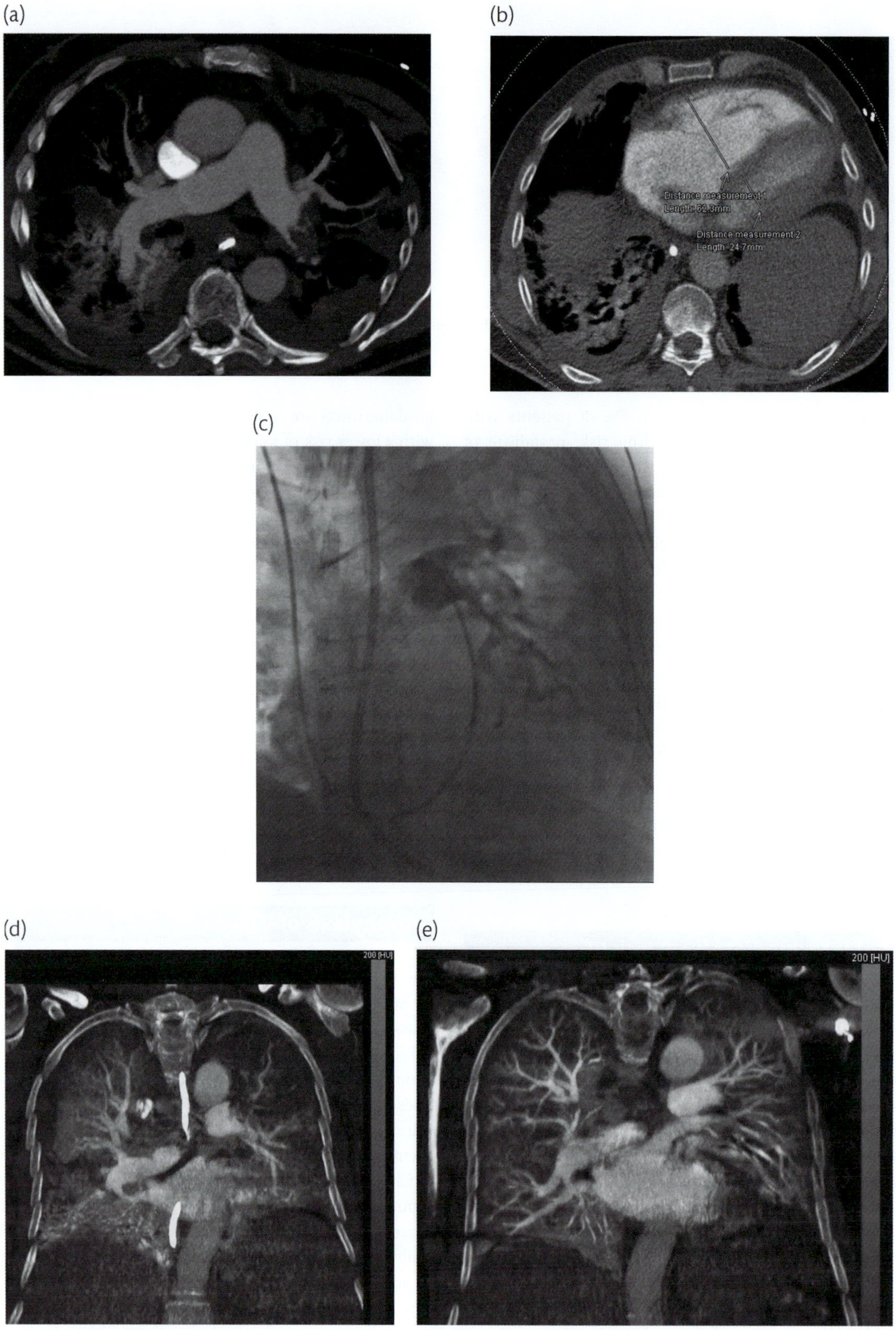

Figure 43.2 Image series from a patient with acute massive pulmonary embolism in the context of COVID-19 infection. Images courtesy of Dr Carole Ridge, Royal Brompton and Harefield Hospitals. (A) Axial CT pulmonary angiogram of patient with COVID pneumonitis and new hypotension. An occlusive filling defect in the left pulmonary artery is consistent with an acute pulmonary thrombus, and the main pulmonary artery is dilated. (B) Axial CT at the mid-cardiac level demonstrating right ventricular strain. The RV to LV ratio is 2.5 with marked straightening of the interventricular septum consistent with right ventricular strain. (C) Pulmonary angiogram. The patient underwent pulmonary thrombolysis using ultrasound assisted thrombolysis. Angiographic images confirm an occlusive left pulmonary artery thrombus. (D) Pre-thrombolysis dual-energy CT (DECT): coronal iodine map acquired with dual-energy CT demonstrates marked hypoenhancement of the left lung due to acute pulmonary artery thrombus. (E) Post-thrombolysis DECT: coronal iodine map 4 months after thrombolysis and anticoagulant therapy demonstrates improved left pulmonary iodine enhancement. See plate section.
Images courtesy of Dr Carole Ridge, Royal Brompton and Harefield Hospitals.

Coronavirus Disease 2019 (COVID-19)

Derangement of haemostasis with hypercoagulability is well recognized in patients with COVID-19 (see Chapter 35 for more details on COVID-19).

The incidence of PE in critically ill COVID-19 patients has been reported to be as high as 33.3% despite standard prophylactic anticoagulation.[24]

Thromboprophylaxis is currently recommended for all patients with suspected or confirmed COVID-19 admitted to hospital. The data around therapeutic anticoagulation and higher dose prophylaxis for patients without proven VTE remains uncertain. While some studies have shown benefit in patients outside of critical care,[25] this does not appear to translate into benefit for patients needing non-invasive or invasive respiratory support despite this latter group being at highest risk of thromboembolic disease.[26] There is insufficient evidence at present to support high-dose prophylaxis or treatment dose anticoagulation for critically ill patients without a suspected or documented VTE.[27]

Clinical trials to evaluate different anticoagulants and the role of antiplatelet agents as well as use of post-discharge thromboprophylaxis for patients with severe COVID-19 are ongoing.

In conclusion, thromboembolic disease remains a significant threat to critically ill patients, and while prophylaxis can reduce this risk it does not eliminate it. A high index of suspicion is required for pulmonary thromboembolism, where the diagnostic modality of choice is CTPA. Thrombolysis should be used in cases of high-risk PE without contra-indications, but for lower-risk PE and DVTs, the mainstay of treatment is anticoagulation.

REFERENCES

1. Perkins GD, McAuley DF, Davies S, et al. Discrepancies between clinical and post-mortem diagnoses in critically ill patients: An observational study. *Crit Care*. 2003;7: R129–R132.
2. Geerts WH, Bergqvist D, Pineo GF, et al. Prevention of venous thromboembolism: American College of Chest Physicians Evidence-Based Clinical Practice Guidelines (8th Edition). *Chest*. 2008;**133**(6 Suppl):381S–453S.
3. PROTECT Investigators for the Canadian Critical Care Trials Group and the Australian and New Zealand Intensive Care Society Clinical Trials Group, Cook D, Meade M, et al. Dalteparin versus unfractionated heparin in critically ill patients. *N Engl J Med*. 2011;**364**:1305–1314.
4. Cook D, Crowther M, Meade M, et al. Deep venous thrombosis in medical–surgical critically ill patients: Prevalence, incidence, and risk factors. *Crit Care Med*. 2005;**33**:1565–1571.
5. Patel R, Cook DJ, Meade MO, et al. Burden of Illness in venous Thrombo-Embolism in Critical care (BITEC) Study Investigators; Canadian Critical Care Trials Group. Burden of illness in venous thromboembolism in critical care: A multicenter observational study. *J Crit Care*. 2005;**20**:341–347.
6. Kakkar VV, Howe CT, Flanc C, et al. Natural history of postoperative deep-vein thrombosis. *Lancet*. 1969;**2**: 230–232.
7. Ibrahim EH, Iregui M, Prentice D, et al. Deep vein thrombosis during prolonged mechanical ventilation despite prophylaxis. *Crit Care Med*. 2002;**30**:771–774.
8. Cook D, Crowther M, Meade M, et al. venous thrombosis in medical–surgical ICU patients: Prevalence, incidence and risk factors. *Crit Care*. 2003; 7(Suppl 2): P111.
9. Crowther MA, Cook DJ, Griffith LE, et al. Deep venous thrombosis: Clinically silent in the intensive care unit. *J Crit Care*. 2005;**20**:334–340.
10. Frankel HL, Kirkpatrick AW, Elbarbary M, et al. Guidelines for the appropriate use of bedside general and cardiac ultrasonography in the evaluation of critically ill patients—part I: General ultrasonography. *Crit Care Med*. 2015;**43**:2479–2502.
11. Guyatt GH, Akl EA, Crowther M, et al. American College of Chest Physicians Antithrombotic Therapy and Prevention of Thrombosis Panel Executive summary: Antithrombotic Therapy and Prevention of Thrombosis, 9th ed: American College of Chest Physicians Evidence-Based Clinical Practice Guidelines. *Chest*. 2012;**141**(2 Suppl):7S–47S.
12. Sud S, Mittmann N, Cook DJ, et al. Canadian Critical Care Trials Group; E-PROTECT Investigators. Screening and prevention of venous thromboembolism in critically ill patients: A decision analysis and economic evaluation. *Am J Respir Crit Care Med*. 2011;**184**:1289–1298.
13. Stein PD, Fowler SE, Goodman LR, et al. PIOPED II Investigators. Multidetector computed tomography for acute pulmonary embolism. *N Engl J Med*. 2006 1;**354**:2317–2327.
14. Sanchez O, Trinquart L, Colombet I, et al. Prognostic value of right ventricular dysfunction in patients with haemodynamically stable pulmonary embolism: A systematic review. *Eur Heart J*. 2008;**29**:1569–1577.
15. Vieillard-Baron A, Qanadli SD, Antakly Y, et al. Transesophageal echocardiography for the diagnosis of pulmonary embolism with acute cor pulmonale: A comparison with radiological procedures. *Intensive Care Med*. 1998;**24**:429–433.
16. Konstantinides SV, The Task Force for the diagnosis and management of acute pulmonary embolism of the European Society of Cardiology (ESC). 2019 ESC Guidelines for the diagnosis and management of acute pulmonary embolism developed in collaboration with the European Respiratory Society (ERS): The Task Force for the diagnosis and management of acute pulmonary embolism of the European Society of Cardiology (ESC). *Eur Respir J*. 2019;**54**:1901647.
17. Malato A, Dentali F, Siragusa S, et al. The impact of deep vein thrombosis in critically ill patients: a meta-analysis of major clinical outcomes. *Blood Transfus*. 2015;**13**:559–568.
18. Marti C, John G, Konstantinides S, et al. Systemic thrombolytic therapy for acute pulmonary embolism: a systematic review and meta-analysis. *Eur Heart J*. 2015;**36**:605–614.
19. Meneveau N, Séronde MF, Blonde MC, et al. Management of unsuccessful thrombolysis in acute massive pulmonary embolism. *Chest*. 2006;**129**:1043–1050.
20. Pasrija C, Kronfli A, Rouse M, et al. Outcomes after surgical pulmonary embolectomy for acute submassive and massive pulmonary embolism: A single-center experience. *J Thorac Cardiovasc Surg*. 2018;**155**:1095–1106.e2.
21. Kearon C, Akl EA, Ornelas J, et al. Antithrombotic therapy for VTE disease: CHEST guideline and expert panel report. *Chest*. 2016;**149**:315–352.
22. Ho KM, Chavan S, Pilcher D. Omission of early thromboprophylaxis and mortality in critically ill patients: A multicenter registry study. *Chest*. 2011;**140**:1436–1446.
23. NICE guideline [NG89] Venous thromboembolism in over 16s: Reducing the risk of hospital-acquired deep vein thrombosis or pulmonary embolism. Published: 21 March 2018 Last updated: 13 August 2019.

24. Klok FA, Kruip M, van der Meer NJM, et al. Confirmation of the high cumulative incidence of thrombotic complications in critically ill ICU patients with COVID-**19**: An updated analysis. *Thromb Res*. 2020;**191**:148–150.
25. REMAP-CAP Investigators; ACTIV-4a Investigators; ATTACC Investigators. Therapeutic anticoagulation with heparin in critically ill patients with Covid-19. *N Engl J Med*. 2021 **26**;385:777–789.
26. ATTACC Investigators; ACTIV-4a Investigators; REMAP-CAP Investigators. Therapeutic anticoagulation with heparin in noncritically ill patients with Covid-19. *N Engl J Med*. 2021 **26**;385:790–802.
27. Cuker A, Tseng E, Nieuwlaat R, et al. American Society of Hematology 2021 guidelines on the use of anticoagulation for thromboprophylaxis in patients with COVID-19. *Blood Adv*. 2021;**5**:872–888.

44

Pulmonary Haemorrhage

Vasilis Kouranos

KEY MESSAGES

- Diffuse alveolar haemorrhage should always be considered in patients presenting with prominent cough, haemoptysis, acute shortness of breath, and bilateral new pulmonary infiltrates in chest X-ray.
- Bronchoscopy with bronchoalveolar lavage can often establish the diagnosis when haemosiderin macrophages are identified.
- Lung biopsy may often be required to establish the diagnosis in the absence of typical findings in the conventional diagnostic tests. Kidney biopsy may also be considered when pulmonary–renal syndrome is identified.
- Multi-disciplinary approach and integration of clinical information from careful clinical history, available imaging, blood tests, bronchoalveolar lavage data, and often biopsy specimen is necessary in order to reach a confident and valid clinical diagnosis.
- Given the lack of evidence-based treatment, management is mainly empirical. In the acute setting, the management focuses on respiratory support and the correction of abnormalities in the coagulation cascade. Corticosteroids and immunosuppressive agents are commonly used as first-line therapy to treat the underlying condition. The role of plasma exchange remains unclear as empirical treatment option.

CONTROVERSIES

- Establishing an early and confident diagnosis of diffuse alveolar haemorrhage (DAH) is often challenging. Given the acute nature of the disease and often fast progression, there is limited room for diagnostic tests and other investigations, while early immunosuppressive treatment can mask the underlying cause.
- The use of high dose of immunosuppressive treatment (especially corticosteroids) seems to change the disease's natural history and prevent life-threatening respiratory failure leading to mechanical ventilation in most immune-mediated cases of DAH. Nonetheless, it can lead to clinical deterioration in non-immune-mediated causes such as heart failure and infections. Careful clinical history and examination with often limited but crucial diagnostic tests (echocardiography and BAL) are mandatory.
- It is unclear whether DAH in the context of bone marrow transplant is an immune-mediated phenomenon or not.
- The extent and duration of plasma exchange as an intervention relies on the patient's clinical response and potential underlying cause.

FURTHER RESEARCH

- Studies in refractory ANCA-associated vasculitis would provide information regarding the exact level and type of immunosuppression that should be used in patients failing to respond to conventional corticosteroid therapy.
- Studies comparing patients with empirical management as opposed to those with histological confirmation of the disease could show when and whether a lung biopsy should be considered in the context of DAH.

Introduction

Diffuse alveolar haemorrhage (DAH) is a potentially catastrophic complication of numerous underlying immune-driven and non-immune-driven conditions.[1] Irrespective of the underlying condition and its pathogenesis, the predominant pathohistological finding is blood leakage in the alveoli, usually at multiple sites. DAH often remains a diagnostic and therapeutic challenge as it may manifest in various ways and is frequently life threatening. The presenting clinical picture varies, but episodes of haemoptysis, pulmonary infiltrates on chest imaging, hypoxia, and progressive respiratory failure are the most commonly reported manifestations. A multi-disciplinary approach is often key to reaching a confident diagnosis and management plan. Different terminologies have been used in the past for this condition including intrapulmonary haemorrhag-e, diffuse pulmonary haemorrhage, pulmonary alveolar haemorrhage, pulmonary capillary haemorrhage, alveolar bleeding, or microvascular pulmonary haemorrhage. In this chapter, we review the causes, clinical features, diagnostic criteria, treatment, and prognosis of DAH with a specific focus on the most common case scenarios.

Pathogenesis

DAH is associated with the injury to the lung microvasculature including the capillaries, arterioles, and venules lining around the alveoli.[2] Several categorizations have been reported. From a clinical perspective,[3] DAH can be (a) immune-mediated (antineutrophil cytoplasmic antibody (ANCA)-associated vasculitis or in the context of connective tissue disease), (b) congestive heart failure associated, and (c) miscellaneous (wide range of different causes: infection, trauma, clotting disorder, drugs, malignancy, and haematopoietic stem cell transplantation), and idiopathic (no specific cause identified). When reviewing the histopathology of patients with DAH,[2] the evidence include (a) DAH associated with vasculitis or capillaritis, (b) bland DAH without evidence of capillaritis or vasculitis, and (c) DAH clearly associated with another process or clinical condition such as diffuse alveolar damage, lymphangioleiomyomatosis, drug-induced lung injury, metastatic tumour to the lungs, and mitral stenosis.

Pulmonary capillaritis is the most frequent underlying histologic finding described in patients with DAH (Figure 44.1). The predominant features include extensive intra-alveolar haemorrhage and necrotizing pulmonary endothelitis. Neutrophils usually infiltrate the interalveolar and peribronchiolar septal vessels (pulmonary interstitium), leading to impairment of the alveolocapillary barrier and anatomic disruption of the capillaries (even necrosis of the capillary walls). Loss of the integrity of the alveolar-capillary basement membrane results in leakage of red blood cells and neutrophils into the alveolar space and the interstitium. Haemosiderin-laden macrophages then accumulate within the alveolar spaces and interstitium. Their presence usually indicates prior episodes of alveolar haemorrhage. Neutrophil death and fragmentation, with subsequent release of the intracellular proteolytic enzymes and reactive oxygen species, results in the development and progression of inflammation. Pulmonary capillaritis is associated with systemic vasculitides, connective tissue disorders, immune complex-mediated disorders, and post-transplant haemorrhages representing a clear target for immunosuppressive treatment.

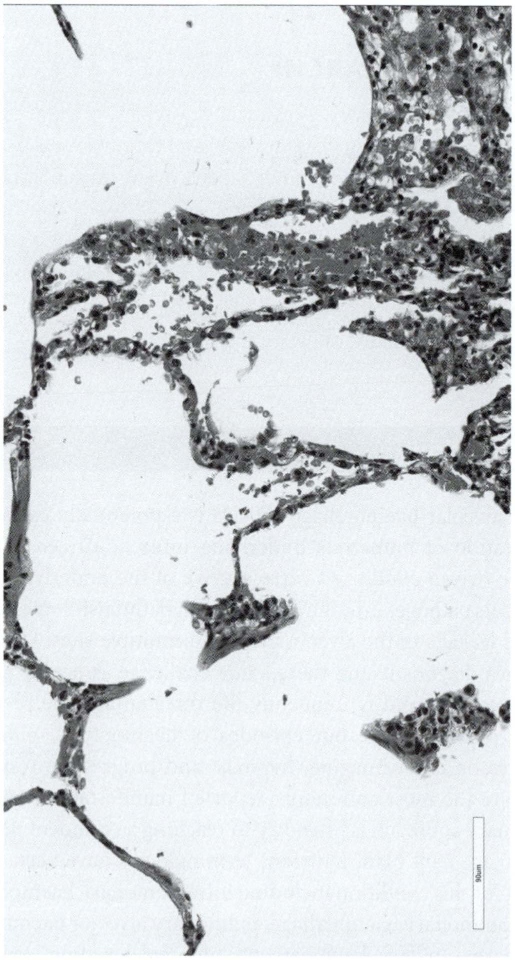

Figure 44.1 Most common pathologic finding in diffuse alveolar haemorrhage: pulmonary capillaritis: alveolar walls contain a neutrophilic infiltrate and there are red blood cells in the alveolar spaces along with focal haemosiderosis in macrophages (bottom right) (H&E 100×). See plate section.

In bland DAH, there is no evidence of inflammation of the pulmonary vessels (capillaries, venules, and arterioles) despite the 'leaking blood'. The epithelial lesions are usually microscopic and are scattered geographically. This pattern is usually observed in drug-induced DAH, systemic lupus erythematosus (SLE), disseminated intravascular coagulation, cardiac originated DAH (mitral stenosis or mitral regurgitation), and infections such as HIV or infective endocarditis.

DAH is frequently reported in patients with the acute respiratory distress syndrome (ARDS) (see Chapter 21). ARDS is characterized by formation of an intra-alveolar hyaline membrane, interstitial oedema with minimal inflammation, and, at times, 'secondary' DAH. In this category, DAH is caused by processes other than pulmonary vascular inflammation or direct extravasation of red cells. Diffuse alveolar damage, the primary lesion in ARDS, is characterized by interstitial and intra-alveolar oedema, capillary congestion, microthrombi, epithelial necrosis and sloughing, the presence of fibrinous exudates in alveolar air spaces, and hyaline membrane formation. ARDS, cytotoxic drugs, radiation treatment, SLE, and cocaine inhalation have been associated with diffuse alveolar damage resulting in DAH.

Epidemiology

Epidemiological data regarding the most common cause of DAH are limited given the rarity of the condition. Immune-driven DAH is usually associated with capillaritis or endotheliitis.[4] Systemic necrotizing vasculitides (principally microscopic polyangiitis (MPA) and granulomatous polyangiitis (GPA) (or Wegener's granulomatosis)) account for the majority of cases of auto-immune DAH. Other causes of auto-immune DAH include anti-glomerular basement membrane (anti-GBM) antibody disease, connective tissue diseases (primarily SLE), exogenous agents (e.g. trimellitic anhydride and isocyanates), or drugs (e.g. D-penicillamine, propylthiouracil, etc.). Idiopathic pulmonary haemosiderosis is not associated with any renal or extra-pulmonary component and seems to be more common in children. In a 28-year retrospective cohort of patients presenting with DAH,[5] immune-mediated causes including vasculitis, anti-GBM disease, and other connective tissue disease were identified in 36% of patients (35/97). Heart (left ventricular systolic or diastolic impairment) failure and valvular heart disease accounted

Table 44.1 Causes of diffuse alveolar haemorrhage

Immune mediated—usually associated with capillaritis	
Anti-GBM disease/Goodpasture's syndrome	
ANCA-associated vasculitis	Granulomatous polyangiitis or Wegener's granulomatosis (GPA)
	Microscopic polyangiitis (MPA)
	Eosinophilic granulomatous polyangiitis or Churg–Strauss syndrome (EGPA)
	Pauci-immune GN
Idiopathic rapidly progressive GN	
Idiopathic pauci-immune pulmonary capillaritis	
Connective tissue diseases	Systemic lupus erythematosus
	Anti-phospholipid syndrome
Henoch–Schönlein purpura/IgA nephropathy	
Hypo-complementeric urticarial vasculitis	
Acute lung-graft rejection	
Non-immune-mediated	
Immunocompromised status	Bone marrow transplant
	HIV
Exogenous agents or drugs	Cocaine
	Trimellitic anhydride
	Isocyanates
	D-Penicillamine
Coagulopathy	Anticoagulants, antiplatelet agents, or thrombolytics
Cardiac disease	Heart failure
	Mitral valve stenosis or regurgitation
Infection	Invasive aspergillosis, CMV infection, legionellosis, and HSV infection
ARDS	
Idiopathic pulmonary haemosiderosis	

Abbreviations: GBM, glomerular basement membrane; ANCA, antineutrophil cytoplasmic antibody; GN, glomerulonephritis; Ig, immunoglobulin; ARDS, acute respiratory distress syndrome; CMV, cytomegalovirus; HSV, herpes simplex virus.

for approximately one-fourth of the cases. Similarly, among critically ill patients with DAH,[6] vasculitis accounted for 19% (7/37) of all cases. DAH can also complicate bone marrow transplantation either as an immune or non-immune-mediated phenomenon. Causes are set out in Table 44.1.

Clinical Manifestations/Diagnostic Tools

The clinical presentation of DAH is highly variable and ranges from asymptomatic radiographic abnormalities to severe life-threatening respiratory failure.[1,7] Even though the majority of patients experience a variable degree of haemoptysis, approximately one-third of all patients with DAH are lacking this symptom because the total alveolar volume is large and can absorb large amounts of blood, without extending more proximally into the airways. Symptoms can either be lung dominant and reflect alveolar bleeding alone including dyspnoea, cough, and chest pain or include a variety of systemic disease features such as fever, skin rash, ocular, sinus, nasal or ear symptoms, haematuria, mononeuritis multiplex, inflammatory arthritis, and muscle weakness. The early recognition of systemic disease symptoms may be critical in reaching an early and accurate diagnosis of the underlying condition and requires a high degree of clinical suspicion.

A careful history including review of systems, review of exposures, and past medical history as well as a comprehensive physical examination is critically important for the characterization of any underlying causes of DAH and especially systemic underlying diseases. Anaemia and/or decreasing haemoglobin values are usually identified in laboratory studies as a marker of intrapulmonary blood loss. Pulmonary–renal syndrome is usually defined when there is concomitant DAH and concurrent glomerulonephritis (GN).[8] The vast majority of these cases is attributable to immune-mediated causes, most frequently ANCA-associated vasculitis or Goodpasture (anti-GBM antibody syndrome). On the other hand, there is no common renal involvement in patients with DAH associated with bone marrow transplantation and infections in immunosuppressed patients. Findings consistent with GN warrant a prompt and aggressive evaluation that sometimes include percutaneous renal biopsy. Features of common causes of DAH are set out in Table 44.2.

Imaging

Chest radiography may show new, old, or both new and old patchy or diffuse bilateral alveolar infiltrates, often with a batwing appearance[9] (Figure 44.2). However, focal and even unilateral patterns indistinguishable from pneumonia may occur. Recurrent episodes of haemorrhage may often result in interstitial lung disease changes including reticulation and rarely traction bronchiectasis or honeycombing. Chest high-resolution computed tomography provides additional information to support a diagnosis of DAH[10] (Figure 44.3). Focal or diffuse areas of ground glass opacification and/or consolidation are usually described, which are expected to resolve within a few days to weeks after the alveolar bleeding control. The resolution of this process is slower than that of the infiltrates related to pulmonary oedema but faster than the disappearance of the inflammatory/infectious radiological changes observed in pneumonias. A 'crazy-paving' pattern has been reported in some cases following the resolution of the acute haemorrhage which is characterized by interlobular and intralobular septal thickening mixed with geographical ground glass opacification. Additional radiological abnormalities may be attributable to many of the underlying systemic disorders or represent infectious complications related to systemic immunosuppression. Some of these findings include cavitating pulmonary nodules and masses and large airway inflammation and stenosis due to granulomatous inflammation in GPA, fibrosis and bronchiectasis in MPA, airway inflammation and inflammatory infiltrates in Eosinophilic granulomatous polyangiitis (EGPA), and pleural effusions in SLE.

Table 44.2 Features in most common causes of DAH and treatment options

Specific condition	Frequency	Diagnostic features	Serological features	Treatment
GPA	33% pulmonary capillaritis	GN, sinusitis, multiple cavitary pulmonary infiltrates, and granulomatous inflammation	c-ANCA	Corticosteroids, MTX, AZA, cyclophosphamide, and Rituximab
EGPA	Rare	Asthma, eosinophilia, cutaneous lesions, mono- or polyneuropathy, and cardiac involvement	p-ANCA	Corticosteroids, MTX, AZA, cyclophosphamide, Rituximab, and Mepolizumab
MPA	50%	GN, fever, myalgia, and arthralgia	p-ANCA	Corticosteroids, MTX, AZA, cyclophosphamide, and Rituximab
Goodpasture syndrome	Very common	Smokers and pulmonary-renal syndrome	Anti-GBM	Plasmapheresis plus immunosuppression
SLE	10% DAH	Fever, arthralgia, and rash	ANA, anti-ds-DNA, and reduced compliment	Corticosteroids, MTX, AZA, cyclophosphamide, Rituximab, Tocilizumab, and Tofacitinib?
Idiopathic pulmonary haemosiderosis	All patients	Bland haemorrhage	No antibodies	Immunosuppression?

Laboratory Tests

Laboratory studies typically include full blood count with differential, ESR, CRP, coagulation studies, serum creatinine and urea, ANCA testing (by indirect immunofluorescence (c-ANCA and p-ANCA) and antigen-specific ELISA (PR3- and MPO-ANCA)), anti-GBM antibodies, anti-nuclear antibodies (ANA), anti-cyclic citrullinated peptide antibodies, rheumatoid factor, anti-phospholipid antibodies, creatine kinase, urinalysis for microscopic haematuria, red cell casts, and proteinuria and urine drug screen.

Pulmonary Function Tests

A transient, reversible increase in the diffusing capacity for carbon monoxide (DLCO) has been previously reported in patients with DAH.[11] This increase is attributed to the enhanced uptake of carbon monoxide by extra-vascular blood. However, DLCO measurements are not routinely used to evaluate patients with suspected DAH because there are usually no baseline DLCO values to compare and the acute disease presentation precludes such investigations.

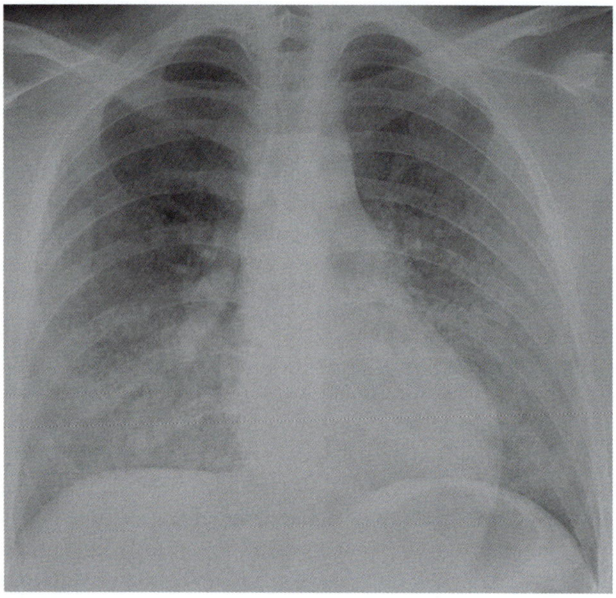

Figure 44.2 Chest X-ray in a patient with non-immune mediated DAH (cocaine user).

Bronchoalveolar Lavage

The purpose of bronchoscopy with bronchoalveolar lavage (BAL) is primarily to confirm the presence of intra-alveolar blood, exclude the large airways as a source of bleeding, and rule out infection. The detection of greater than 20% haemosiderin-laden macrophages among all alveolar macrophages provides support for a diagnosis of DAH.[12,13] Such findings may be detectable in the BAL fluid weeks to months after the disease development, while in cases of acute haemorrhage, increasingly bloody BAL returns may precede. The presence of haemosiderin-laden macrophages should fit in the clinical scenario it is commonly seen in patients with diffuse alveolar damage. The diagnostic yield of bronchoscopy is usually higher if the procedure is performed within 48 h from original presentation especially since empirical treatment may often be used. BAL specimens should always be sent for routine bacterial, mycobacterial, fungal, and viral stains and cultures, as well as for Pneumocystis stains.

Biopsy

Since the majority of established diagnostic criteria for pulmonary vasculitis, for example, the American College of Rheumatology criteria for GPA,[14] do require the histological confirmation of vascular inflammation by tissue biopsy, tissue transbronchoscopic (TBBx) or surgical lung biopsies are often required to confirm the diagnosis histologically. Compared to TBBx, surgical lung biopsies are associated with a higher diagnostic yield for pulmonary vasculitis given the fact that a larger amount of tissue is surgically and not blindly extracted and reviewed. Capillaritis was present in 17%–43% of surgical lung biopsies in patients with GPA.

Diagnostic Approach

The list of underlying aetiology of DAH is very broad. A careful history and physical examination are mandatory for the evaluation of these patients. Due to the relatively non-specific nature of the clinical–radiological signs and symptoms of DAH, additional laboratory tests, bronchoscopy with BAL and even a biopsy are frequently required to accurately diagnose and optimally manage patients with DAH.[12]

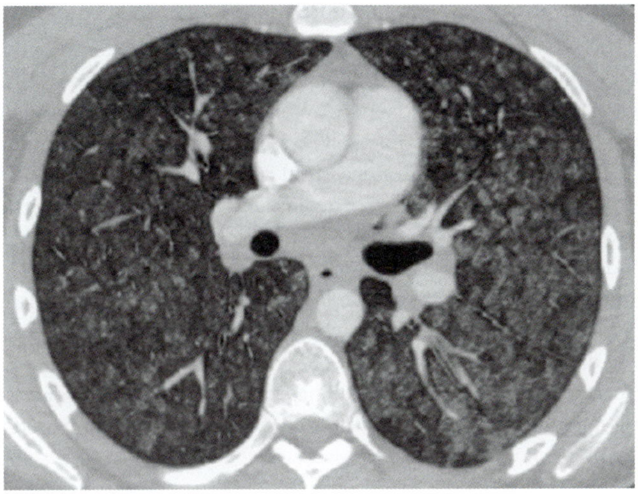

Figure 44.3 HRCT imaging in a patient with non-immune mediated DAH (cocaine user).

Once the diagnosis of DAH is considered highly likely, the clinician must ascertain whether an underlying cause is present since this would eventually affect the management decisions. Serologic studies may prove important although the results may not be available in a manner timely enough to guide immediate management. When a pulmonary–renal syndrome is suggested by accompanying haematuria or renal dysfunction, anti-GBM antibody and ANCA levels should definitely be checked. Tests for complement fractions C3 and C4, anti-double-stranded DNA, and anti-phospholipid antibodies should be ordered if an underlying condition such as SLE or anti-phospholipid antibody syndrome is suspected. If the underlying cause remains elusive after a thorough clinical evaluation that includes imaging studies, serologic studies, and bronchoscopy, then surgical biopsy should be considered. The exact targeted organ for the biopsy would be decided depending on the level of suspicion. Lung biopsy is often performed with video-assisted thoracoscopy, especially when disease is lung dominant (i.e. in idiopathic pulmonary haemosiderosis). The role of surgical lung biopsy in the diagnosis of DAH remains controversial in an acute setting.[15] The risks of a biopsy are excessive in patients with severe DAH and respiratory failure. Post-operative complications such as infection and air leaks may also be exacerbated by immunosuppressive agents often used. Therefore, lung biopsy may be useful in non-critically ill patients with suspected DAH after multi-disciplinary review of all ancillary studies, kidney biopsy, and BAL are non-diagnostic. Renal biopsy specimens should also undergo immunofluorescence staining, which may reveal linear deposition of immunoglobulins and immune complexes along the basement membrane in patients with Goodpasture syndrome or of granular deposits in patients with SLE. In patients with ANCA-associated capillaritis, immune complexes are usually lacking.

Treatment of DAH

DAH is associated with high morbidity and mortality and therefore requires prompt and aggressive multi-disciplinary management. The mortality exceeds 50%, especially in patients requiring intensive care unit (ICU) admission despite treatment offered.[6,15] As a general rule, there is no standard treatment for DAH given the diversity of the potential causes. It is crucial to identify and treat the underlying cause of the DAH. The main principles of treatment are the following:

(1) Supportive care including circulation and ventilatory support and transfusion when required. The ventilatory support ranges from simple oxygen supplementation to mechanical ventilation. Due to the fast progression of the disease, patients can present with acute type I respiratory failure and ARDS, when high levels of supplementary oxygen and positive end-expiratory pressure (PEEP) are often needed to maintain acceptable oxygenation. There is no consensus on the ideal mechanical ventilation settings in DAH, but often high PEEP levels have been used to tamponade the alveolar bleeding and maintain open airways.

(2) Treatment of underlying disease includes intensive immunosuppressive treatments to control disease activity, plasmapheresis to remove autoantibodies, and antivirals or antibiotics for infection-associated pulmonary haemorrhages. High-dose corticosteroids are usually started promptly to control the inflammatory activity, alongside with any targeted treatment for underlying disease. Corticosteroids have been considered as part of standard therapy for all the immune-mediated DAH focusing on reducing acute inflammatory responses such as lung alveolar epithelial swelling, thrombotic microangiopathy, and increased inflammatory cells and cytokines. The role of other immunosuppressive regimen in immune-mediated DAH syndromes needs to be individualized and is discussed later in specific disorders.

(3) Rapid and effective local haemostasis. Coagulopathy in all patients with DAH should be closely monitored and accordingly corrected. Commonly accepted targets are platelet counts more than 50,000/mL and a prothrombin time-international normalized ratio less than 1.5. Depending on the causes, platelet transfusions, vitamin K supplementation, cryoprecipitates, and fresh frozen plasma should be supplemented. Various prothrombotic treatments including antifibrinolytics, particularly lysine analogues, tranexamic acid (TXA) and epsilon aminocaproic acid (EACA), thrombin, and FVIIa have been used for DAH to stop the bleeding. TXA prevents conversion of plasminogen into plasmin, inhibiting fibrinolysis and stabilizing blood clots. In addition to intravenous use, intrapulmonary or aerosolized TXA has been used for DAH. TXA therapy has failed to show significant effect on reducing bleeding-associated mortality in patients with haematologic malignancies but also increased risk of post-operative seizures and showed limited efficacy in profound and recurrent bleeding.

Corticosteroids

Traditionally, systemic high-dose intravenous corticosteroids (500 mg to 1 g/day of intravenous methylprednisolone for 3 days) are recommended to treat DAH, even while pursuing a diagnostic workup. Delaying pulse therapy in a critically ill patient for even a few hours maybe catastrophic. Nonetheless, the main challenge when using high-dose immunosuppressive therapy is the risk of underlying infection. Rapid resolution of bleeding can occur, often within 24–72 h of initiation of therapy. The exact dose is still not also well defined. One study investigating the dose effect of corticosteroids for DAH suggested that patients treated with low-dose methylprednisolone (<250 mg/day) had a significantly lower ICU mortality rate compared to the patients treated with medium-dose (250–1000 mg/day) or high-dose (>1000 mg/day) methylprednisolone, and overall mortality did not differ by the doses of corticosteroids.[16] Following the 3-day pulse, corticosteroids (dose of methylprednisolone 60–120 mg per day or equivalent) should be continued for a few weeks until control of the bleeding and extra-pulmonary manifestations has been achieved. The tapering dose of corticosteroids following intravenous treatment is usually adjusted on a patient-by-patient basis according to the clinical characteristics, the extent of imaging abnormalities, and the clinical suspicion/confidence of the underlying aetiology. Cyclophosphamide or other immunosuppressive agents should be withheld until a specific diagnosis mandating treatment with these agents has been substantiated since the specific therapeutic regimen is dictated by the underlying disorder.

Plasmapheresis

Plasmapheresis is a central component of therapy for Goodpasture disease. Its role as routine treatment in other disorders has not yet been clarified. Nonetheless, plasmapheresis may have an adjunctive role especially in patients with DAH and severe renal insufficiency and in patients with severe or progressive DAH refractory to corticosteroids or immunosuppressive agents. Each exchange involves 1–1.5 times the total plasma volume and is replaced with albumin or fresh frozen plasma to eliminate autoreactive antibodies or triggering factors rapidly. Although anecdotal evidence reported excellent patient outcomes and safety, long-term follow-up data or matched analyses to compare the efficacy of plasmapheresis to methylprednisolone have failed to show significant benefits. The current evidence-based guidelines recommend using plasmapheresis in ANCA-associated vasculitis patients with DAH presenting with hypoxemic respiratory failure requiring either high-flow supplemental oxygen or mechanical ventilation.[17] In that setting, plasmapheresis together with immunosuppressive therapy has been associated with more rapid disappearance of anti-GBM antibodies and improved renal function than treatment with immunosuppressive agents alone. Although the performance of plasma exchange ranges between daily and every other day for a maximum of 2–3 weeks, the exact extent and duration of plasma exchanges are unclear and should be guided by the patient's clinical response. Immunosuppressive therapy is required to inhibit antibody production and rebound hyper-synthesis that may occur following discontinuation of plasma exchange. Either cyclophosphamide (2 mg/kg per day) or azathioprine (2 mg/kg per day), combined with prednisone (1 mg/kg per day), have been used.[18] Most experts favour oral cyclophosphamide over azathioprine, but studies comparing these agents have not been performed.

Rituximab, a chimeric monoclonal antibody targeting CD20, has been used as an alternative effective immunosuppressive regimen in GPA and other ANCA-associated vasculitis.[19] Antibody-mediated modification and/or depletion of ANCA-producing CD20(+) plasma cells is a proposed mechanism for Rituximab to decrease autoantibody production and to control disease activity. Although most of the studies have been limited in numbers, Rituximab is considered to be an effective therapeutic option for DAH in connective tissue disease or auto-immune disorders. In one study, Rituximab was used on a compassionate use basis for patients with refractory ANCA-associated vasculitis and successful treatment outcomes were reported. Comparison between Rituximab and cyclophosphamide pulse therapy for ANCA-associated vasculitis showed a similar efficacy.[19] A randomized trial comparing the effect of combination therapies of glucocorticoids plus Rituximab (375 mg/m^2 once weekly for 4 weeks) and glucocorticoids plus cyclophosphamide (2 mg/kg/day) also demonstrated comparable efficacy of Rituximab for the remission induction in severe ANCA-associated vasculitis, and Rituximab showed a better effectiveness for recurrent disease, major renal disease, or alveolar haemorrhage. Even for long-term remission, Rituximab has shown significantly longer remission duration and improved overall survival when compared to azathioprine maintenance.

REFERENCES

1. Collard HR, King TE Jr, Schwarz MI. Diffuse alveolar hemorrhage and rare infiltrative disorders of the lung. In: Broaddus VC, Mason RJ, Ernst JD, et al. eds. *Murray & Nadel's Textbook of Respiratory Medicine*. 6th ed. New York: Elsevier; 2016:1207–1220.
2. Travis WD. Pathology of pulmonary vasculitis. *Semin Respir Crit Care Med*. 2004; **25**:475–482.
3. Schwarz MI, Brown KK. Small vessel vasculitis of the lung. *Thorax*. 2000;**55**:502–510.
4. Watts RA, Lane SE, Bentham G, et al. Epidemiology of systemic vasculitis: A ten-year study in the United Kingdom. *Arthritis Rheum*. 2000;**43**:414–419.
5. de Prost N, Parrot A, Picard C, et al. Diffuse alveolar haemorrhage: Factors associated with in hospital and long-term mortality. *Eur Respir J*. 2010; **35**(6):1303–1311.
6. Rabe C, Appenrodt B, Hoff C, et al. Severe respiratory failure due to diffuse alveolar hemorrhage: Clinical characteristics and outcome of intensive care. *J Crit Care*. 2010; **25**(2):230–235.
7. De Lassence A, Fleury-Feith J, Escudier E, et al. Alveolar hemorrhage. Diagnostic criteria and results in 194 immunocompromised hosts. *Am J Respir Crit Care Med*. 1995; **151**(1):157–163.
8. Cordier JF, Cottin V. Alveolar hemorrhage in vasculitis: Primary and secondary. *Semin Respir Crit Care Med*. 2011;**32**(3):310–321.
9. Castaner E, Alguersuari A, Gallardo X, et al. When to suspect pulmonary vasculitis: Radiologic and clinical clues. *Radiographics*. 2010; **30**(1):33–53.
10. Hansell DM. Small-vessel diseases of the lung: Ct-pathologic correlates. *Radiology*. 2002;**225**(3):639–653.
11. Ewan PW, Jones HA, Rhodes CG, et al. Detection of intrapulmonary hemorrhage with carbon monoxide uptake. Application in goodpasture's syndrome. *N Engl J Med*. 1976; **295**(25):1391–1396.
12. De Lassence A, Fleury-Feith J, Escudier E, et al. Alveolar hemorrhage. Diagnostic criteria and results in 194 immunocompromised hosts. *Am J Respir Crit Care Med*. 1995; **151**(1):157–163.
13. Maldonado F, Parambil JG, Yi ES, et al. Haemosiderin-laden macrophages in the bronchoalveolar lavage fluid of patients with diffuse alveolar damage. *Eur Respir J*. 2009;**33**(6):1361–1366.
14. Chung SA, Langford CA, Maz M, et al. 2021 American College of Rheumatology/Vasculitis Foundation guideline for the management of antineutrophil cytoplasmic antibody-associated vasculitis. *Arthritis Rheumatol*. 2021 Aug;**73**(8):1366–1383.

15. Papiris SA, Manali ED, Kalomenidis I, et al. Bench-to-bedside review: Pulmonary–renal syndromes—an update for the intensivist. *Crit Care*. 2007;**11**(3):213.
16. Rathi NK, Tanner, AR, Dinh A, et al. Low-, medium- and high-dose steroids with or without aminocaproic acid in adult hematopoietic SCT patients with diffuse alveolar hemorrhage. *Bone Marrow Transplant*. 2015;**50**:420–426.
17. Szczepiorkowski ZM, Winters JL, Bandarenko N, et al. Guidelines on the use of therapeutic apheresis in clinical practice—evidence-based approach from the Apheresis Applications Committee of the American Society for Apheresis. *J Clin Apher.* 2010;**25**: 83–177.
18. Walsh M, Merkel PA, Peh CA, et al. Plasma exchange and glucocorticoids in severe ANCA-associated vasculitis. *N Engl J Med*. 2020;**382**:622–631.
19. Stone JH, Merkel PA, Spiera R, et al. Rituximab versus cyclophosphamide for ANCA-associated vasculitis. *N Engl J Med*. 2010;**363**:221–232.

45

Pulmonary Hypertension and Cor Pulmonale

Laura C Price, S John Wort, and Simon J Finney

KEY MESSAGES

- Pulmonary hypertension (PH) occurs frequently in critically ill patients, as part of several intensive care unit (ICU) syndromes, and, less commonly, as a primary cause for ICU admission. The presence of PH, especially when associated with right ventricular (RV) dysfunction or failure (cor pulmonale), is associated with increased mortality in all settings.

CONTROVERSIES

- Is RV dysfunction a bystander of severe acute respiratory distress syndrome ARDS (group 3 PH) or is it independently associated with mortality? As such, should PH and RV dysfunction be treatment targets?
- Does COVID-19 pneumonitis as a cause of ARDS have a different, more pulmonary vascular, phenotype than non-COVID phenotypes?

FURTHER RESEARCH

- In acute pulmonary embolism (PE), RV supportive approaches are increasingly important. Future studies will be important to understand their role.

Definitions

Pulmonary hypertension (PH) is defined as a mean pulmonary arterial pressure (mPAP) ≥25 mmHg as measured by right-heart catheterization (RHC).[1] It should be emphasized that echocardiographic measurements derived from the tricuspid regurgitant jet estimate RV *systolic* pressures (RVSPs) not *mean* pulmonary arterial pressures as measured by RHC. Pre-capillary or pulmonary arterial hypertension (PAH) is defined when the pulmonary capillary occlusion or wedge pressure (PCWP) is less than or equal to 15 mmHg, whereas a PCWP above 15 mmHg describes elevated left atrial pressure, usually due to left-sided heart disease (Table 45.1).

Cor pulmonale encompasses acute or acute-on-chronic RV dysfunction and failure. Long-standing elevation in pulmonary arterial pressure results in the RV becoming hypertrophic in response to the high afterload. Conversely, acute rises in pulmonary vascular resistance (PVR) will usually not be associated with an RVSP over 50 mmHg, as the failing RV is naive to increased afterloads.

A pulmonary hypertensive crisis is a feared complication with an acute increase in PVR and right-sided pressure, equalization of PVR and systemic vascular resistance (SVR) causing RV ischaemia, and a fall in cardiac output (CO) with systemic hypotension. PH crises can be precipitated by stimuli including pain, tracheal suctioning, hypoxia, and acidosis, and can occur in the post-operative setting as well as during intercurrent illnesses such as lung infection.

Classification of PH

PH is grouped according to similar pathophysiology and response to advanced PH therapies (Table 45.2).[2] Group 1 PH (PAH) is the previous 'primary PH' grouping and encompasses several subtypes including PAH associated with congenital heart disease, connective tissue diseases, and idiopathic PAH. Group 2 PH is left-sided heart disease, group 3 PH is lung disease (group 3 PH), and group 4 is chronic thromboembolic PH (CTEPH). A crucial reason to accurately diagnose the subtype of PH is the response to PAH advanced therapies. In group 2 PH patients, pulmonary vasodilators can precipitate pulmonary oedema as pulmonary blood flow increases against a fixed elevation in pulmonary venous pressure.

Aetiology of PH in ICU

Some examples of acute and chronic PH that may be encountered in ICU are described (Table 45.3). By far the most common causes of PH are groups 2 and 3, which may be in combination, and it is important to distinguish group 1 or 4 PH from these as therapies

Table 45.1 Definitions of pulmonary hypertension and right ventricular dysfunction

RHC Normal ranges	**Pre-capillary PH (groups 1,3,4,5)**	**Post-capillary PH, group 2**
RAP (4-8)mmHg mPAP (<20)mmHg PCWP (<15)mmHg DPG* (<7)mmHg CO (4-5) litres/min PVR (<3) Wood units	Normal or raised mPAP≥25mmHg PCWP≤15mmHg, 'normal' - CO variable PVR >3 WU	Normal or raised mPAP≥25mmHg PCWP>15mmHg, raised *Isolated post-capillary PH:* *DPG<7mmmHg ± PVR≤3WU* *Post- and pre-capillary PH:* *DPG≥7mmHg ± PVR >3 WU*
Echo signs of PH Peak TR velocity (m/s) • *If ≤2.8, PH unlikely* • *If 2.9-3.4, look at additional signs* • *If >3.4, PH likely*	**Additional echo signs of PH** Short PvAct <80ms PA diameter>25mm RV dilatation ± dysfunction Flattened intraventricular septum Right atrial area (> 18cm^2) IVC decreased inspiratory collapse Pericardial effusion	**Features of group 2 PH** Echo features of group 2 PH: LV systolic dysfunction LV diastolic dysfunction *Left atrial dilatation* *Septal e/e'* Clinical features of HFpEF: *Hypertension, obese, diabetic, AF, ischaemic heart disease*

PH is defined at right-heart catheterization (RHC, upper panels) by mPAP ≥25 mmHg in stable resting patients. At echocardiography (echo), PH is suggested by TR velocity (v) exceeding 2.8 m/s, which using the simplified Bernoulli equation (RVSP = $4v^2$ + RAP mmHg) gives an estimated RV systolic pressure (RVSP) >40 mmHg (noting that this value increases with age by 0.4 mmHg/year). PH also shortens the acceleration time across the pulmonary valve (PvAcT) due to the presence of high pulmonary vascular resistance (PVR), also seen in ventilated patients and in lung disease. The severity of PH may depend on the chronicity (see 'definitions' section), with the resulting RV dysfunction in any setting crucial to detect, with echo extremely useful to assess this (lower boxes), as well as clinical markers of shock, including lactataemia and end organ dysfunction (liver, renal, and gut). Assessment of cardiac output at RHC is useful to calculate, with PVR = mPAP − PCWP/cardiac output. Further calculations are useful to classify subtypes of group 2 PH according to the level of pre- and post-capillary PH, where the diastolic PA pressure gradient (dPAP-PCWP) remains <7 mmHg in cases of passive elevation of pressures in isolated post-capillary pressure, whereas diastolic pressure gradient (DPG) ≥7 mmHg in cases with an additional reactive pre-capillary component.

Abbreviations: PH, pulmonary hypertension; mPAP, mean pulmonary arterial pressure; dPAP, diastolic pulmonary arterial pressure; RHC, right-heart catheterization; m/s, metres per second; PCWP, pulmonary capillary wedge pressure; RVSP, right ventricular systolic pressure; TR, tricuspid regurgitation; RV, right ventricular; RAP, right atrial pressure; CO, cardiac output; PVR, pulmonary vascular resistance; DPG, diastolic pressure gradient; PvAct, pulmonary valve acceleration time; IVC, inferior vena cava; LV, left ventricular; HFpEF, heart failure with preserved ejection fraction; AF, atrial fibrillation.

Table 45.2 Updated clinical classification of pulmonary hypertension

PH Group	Subtypes of PH within group
Group 1, PAH	Heritable PAH: BMPR2; ALK-1, ENG, SMAD9, CAV1, KCNK3; Unknown. Associated with: Congenital heart diseases (*helpful sub-classification available*) Connective tissue diseases (especially scleroderma, SLE, mixed connective tissue disease), HIV infection, portal hypertension, schistosomiasis Drug and toxin induced. Idiopathic PAH (with all other conditions / associations excluded)
Group 1′ and 1″ PH	*Pulmonary veno-occlusive disease (PVOD) and/or pulmonary capillary haemangiomatosis (PCH) (1′), related to small post-capillary occlusion* *Persistent pulmonary hypertension of the newborn (group 1″)*
Group 2, PH due to left-sided heart disease	Left ventricular systolic dysfunction Left ventricular diastolic dysfunction Valvular disease. Left heart inflow/outflow tract obstruction and congenital cardiomyopathies.
Group 3, PH due to lung diseases and/or hypoxia	Chronic obstructive pulmonary disease Interstitial lung disease Other pulmonary diseases with mixed restrictive and obstructive pattern Sleep-disordered breathing Alveolar hypoventilation disorders Chronic exposure to high altitude Developmental lung diseases
Group 4	Chronic thromboembolic pulmonary hypertension Other pulmonary artery occlusions (e.g. sarcoma)
Group 5, PH with unclear and/or multifactorial mechanisms	Haematological disorders Systemic disorders (e.g. sarcoidosis). Metabolic disorders (e.g. thyroid disorders). Others: tumoural obstruction, chronic renal failure, segmental PH

Note: BMPR, bone morphogenic protein receptor type II; CAV1, caveolin-1; ALK-1, activin receptor-like kinase-1; ENG, endoglin; KCNK3, potassium channel subfamily K member 3; HIV, human immunodeficiency virus; SLE, systemic lupus erythematosus; PAH, pulmonary arterial hypertension; PH, pulmonary hypertension.

Source: Adapted from Simonneau G, Gatzoulis MA, Adatia I, et al. Updated clinical classification of pulmonary hypertension. *J Am Coll Cardiol*. 2013;62(25 Suppl): D34–D41. Copyright 2013, with permission from The American College of Cardiology.

Table 45.3 Causes of pulmonary hypertension in ICU patients

Acute PH in ICU	Acute-on-chronic PH in ICU	ICU-specific iatrogenic causes
Acute pulmonary embolism Acute lung injury, sepsis	Pulmonary arterial hypertension (group 1 PH) or CTEPH (group 4): • Acute PAH exacerbation (due to hypoxia, sepsis/ARDS, PE, peri-operative, pregnancy-related, etc.). • Disease progression (no obvious precipitant).	Endothelial dysfunction related to cardiopulmonary bypass Drug-related increases in PVR (e.g. high-dose vasopressors; protamine).
Acute post-capillary PH (group 2): • Pulmonary venous hypertension due to LV dysfunction/failure with left atrial hypertension. • Acute MI, congestive cardiac failure, diastolic LV dysfunction, severe valvular heart disease (MR, MS).	Post-capillary (group 2) PH: any acute-on-chronic cause	Acute increase in PVR: Hypoxaemia, acidosis, hypercapnia, pain, laryngoscopy (sympathetic stimulation of pulmonary vascular alpha adrenoceptors).
Acute respiratory illness including pneumonia Often a combination of pathologies including OSA/OHS	PH due to other causes of pre-existing PH (groups 3–5) e.g. COPD, IPF, acute exacerbation	High Pplat or PEEP during IPPV causing small pulmonary vessel compression in high 'West zones' (also follows oedema).

Abbreviations: PAH, pulmonary arterial hypertension; PH, pulmonary hypertension; PVR, pulmonary vascular resistance; CTEPH, chronic thromboembolic pulmonary hypertension; P_{plat}, plateau pressure; PEEP, positive end-expiratory pressure; IPPV, intermittent positive-pressure ventilation; COPD, chronic obstructive pulmonary disease; ARDS, acute respiratory distress syndrome; IPF, interstitial pulmonary fibrosis; MI, myocardial infarction; MR, mitral regurgitation; MS, mitral stenosis; PE, pulmonary embolism; LV, left ventricular; OSA, obstructive sleep apnoea; OHS, obesity hypoventilation syndrome.

currently predominately focus on the underlying lung or heart disease in groups 2 and 3, respectively. Of note, this classification mostly applies to chronic stable PH.

Pulmonary Embolism

Massive and sub-massive pulmonary embolism (PE) are important causes of RV failure in ICU, in part due to mechanical obstruction of the pulmonary circulation, also hypoxaemia and local vasoconstrictor release (Chapter 43). The degree of angiographic obstruction correlates with severity: 5%–15% obstruction causes hypoxaemia; 25% obstruction causes PH; 35% obstruction or mPAP >30 mmHg results in an increase in right atrial pressure, and haemodynamic disturbance occurs with 50% obstruction.[3]

Acute Respiratory Distress Syndrome

Several factors contribute to PH in acute respiratory distress syndrome (ARDS), including vasoactive mediator imbalance, obstruction of the pulmonary microcirculation, later distal vascular muscularization, and true remodelling (Chapter 21).[4] RV dysfunction related to PH is seen in 7%–25% of patients with acute lung injury in recent years, with a fall from previously higher prevalence probably related to the widespread introduction of lung-protective ventilation strategies.[5] Patients with ARDS due to severe COVID-19 may develop PH and resulting RV dysfunction for several reasons including an increase in PVR due to immunothrombosis of the pulmonary microcirculation, local hypoxia, and lung parenchymal inflammation.

Pulmonary Hypertension Following Cardiothoracic Surgery

Pulmonary hypertension (PH) may follow corrective congenital cardiac surgery, valve (especially mitral) replacement surgery, heart transplantation surgery, and left ventricular assist device insertion. Predisposing factors include pre-existing PH, endothelial dysfunction related to cardiopulmonary bypass, positive-pressure and single-lung ventilation, and the effects of certain drugs that increase PVR or depress myocardial function.

PAH and CTEPH

In PAH, characteristic proliferative occlusive lesions occur in the vessel walls of pulmonary arteries and arterioles. Pulmonary veno-occlusive disease is a rare subgroup with additional occlusive remodelling in small pulmonary veins. About 20 years ago, PAH therapy was for symptomatic patients and life expectancy was short. Survival directly relates to RV failure. Treatment options have significantly advanced, yet overall 5-year survival remains 60%, although this is age and PH subgroup-dependent.[6] CTEPH is an important PH subgroup where occlusive vascular lesions follow a PE despite 3 months of anticoagulation and represents the only potentially curable form of PH, by pulmonary endarterectomy surgery.

ICU admission of patients with previously undiagnosed PAH or CTEPH is now rare. When admission to ICU or high dependency unit is required, mortality relating to RV failure in these patients is very high, especially in those with hypotension on admission, elevated (and rising) serum B-type natriuretic peptide, CRP, low sodium, or renal dysfunction.[7] Attempts at resuscitation are usually unsuccessful unless the precipitant is reversible.[8] Pregnancy, surgery, and anaesthesia are particularly high-risk scenarios and require careful haemodynamic monitoring following any procedure.

Pathophysiology of Right Ventricular Failure

A healthy pulmonary circulation is a 'high-flow–low-pressure system' which can tolerate large increases in blood flow by recruiting and dilating pulmonary vessels. In PH, increased RV wall tension increases end-diastolic volume and this volume overload may overwhelm the RV, leading to ventricular dysfunction and failure by ventricular interdependence,[9] reducing CO, as displacement of the intraventricular septum by the dilated RV impinges LV filling. As LV filling may depend on atrial contraction, atrial fibrillation and systemic vasodilators are tolerated poorly. Hypotension must be treated promptly or the pressure gradient between the aorta and RV required for right coronary artery perfusion will be reduced, precipitating RV ischaemia and worsening RV function.[10]

Clinically, acute or acute-on-chronic RV failure is characterized by a reduction in CO and an elevation in RV filling pressure, with signs including raised jugular venous pressure (with 'CV waves' due to tricuspid regurgitation (TR)), limb oedema, pulsatile hepatomegaly, renal, and gut dysfunction.

A 'PH crises' is defined by a hyper-acute rise in PVR, such that systemic and pulmonary pressures equalize, with the risk of RV ischaemia and rapid cardiovascular collapse.

Effects of Extracorporeal Circuits on Right Ventricular Function

Patients with severe acute respiratory failure may be supported by veno-venous (VV) extracorporeal membrane oxygenation (ECMO) (Chapter 22). In VV-ECMO, blood is drawn by a pump from a large vein passed through an artificial lung and returned to the venous system; thus, gas exchange is undertaken in a pre-pulmonary position. Since blood is removed and returned to the venous circulation, there is little haemodynamic consequence to this per se. PVR often falls as a consequence of the lungs receiving blood that is already well oxygenated and decarboxylated, but also due to a reduction in mechanical ventilation (e.g. lowering of positive end-expiratory pressure (PEEP) and plateau airway pressures) that is possible since the gas exchange needs of the patient are being fulfilled by the ECMO device. However, VV-ECMO does not influence the pulmonary process per se and indeed this may continue to progress, for example in patients with severe lung fibrosis awaiting transplantation.

In settings where there is associated cardiac dysfunction, patients may be supported with veno-arterial (VA) ECMO. In VA-ECMO, blood is pumped from the venous circulation, passed through an artificial lung and returned to the arterial system bypassing the heart and lungs. The consequences of very low or no pulmonary blood flow for prolonged periods are not known. It has been hypothesized however this may be at least in part responsible for the increased PVR that occurs following cardiopulmonary bypass for cardiac surgery.

Current Accepted Practice: Diagnosis and Management of PH in ICU

Diagnosis of PH in ICU

Signs of PH are often non-specific. Echocardiography is very useful, and invasive haemodynamic assessment remains the gold standard (Table 45.1). Remember that all the definitions of PH are in stable resting patients rather than in the ICU setting.

Invasive Haemodynamic Assessment and Monitoring

The onset of RV failure is suggested by a rising right atrial pressure and falling mean arterial pressure (with an associated tachycardia, rise in lactate, and worsening renal and liver function), so at the very least, arterial line and central venous pressure monitoring guide this. Use of the pulmonary artery (PA) catheter has fallen, but it can be useful in RV failure, where a rise in PVR would precede a fall in CO. PA catheters should not be used in patients with significant intra-cardiac shunts, and severe TR may affect thermodilution measurements. Other CO monitors using lithium dilution or pulsed contour analysis (LIDCO or PICCO, respectively) may be useful but have similar inaccuracy issues with marked TR.

Echocardiography

Transthoracic echocardiography can provide detailed right-heart assessment and suggest the aetiology of PH (e.g. LV dysfunction and shunts). Systolic PA pressure is estimated from the peak velocity of the tricuspid regurgitant jet by the simplified Bernoulli equation (peak pressure gradient of TR = 4 × TR velocity squared), added to the estimated right atrial pressure (RAP) to calculate RVSP, remembering that normal values increase with age, sex, and body mass index.[11] RV function is assessed by several methods including the tricuspid annular plane systolic excursion. A shortened acceleration time across the pulmonary valve less than 100 ms (pulmonary valve acceleration time) suggests the presence of high PVR. In ICU, images may be suboptimal due to body habitus, difficult positioning, and ventilatory support. An alternative is trans-oesophageal echocardiography, which requires sedation but allows continuous monitoring of RV function.

Management of PH in the ICU Patient

The aim of ICU management is to prevent and manage RV failure (Figure 45.1), and has also been reviewed in more detail.[12,13] Hypotension and arrhythmias should be treated promptly, and pre-existing pulmonary vasodilator therapies should not be stopped. Strategies include further reduction of RV afterload, optimization of ventilatory and fluid strategies, and support of the RV. Disease-specific therapies including anticoagulation and thrombolysis in PE are not covered in detail here (see chapter 43 for detailed coverage of this topic). Highlights of management are outlined below.

Oxygen Delivery

Aiming to maintain arterial saturations above 90% is reasonable in ICU patients with PH. Obstructive sleep apnoea and sleep-disordered breathing also frequently contribute to PH, which improves on treatment of the underlying condition. Nasal high-flow oxygen delivers high concentration oxygen with minimal airway pressure and is well tolerated.

Ventilation Strategies

Positive-pressure ventilation and PEEP can impair RV function by increasing airway plateau pressure (P_{plat}), due to compression of pulmonary vessels, and can also diminish venous return. On the other hand, insufficient PEEP may cause lung collapse and increased PVR. In ARDS with RV failure, the ideal ventilation strategy is to minimize P_{plat} and PEEP while adequately oxygenating and avoiding hypercapnia. In infants ventilated after cardiac surgery, increasing

PH and RV Failure in ICU

Monitoring (echo, CVP, arterial line)
Establish escalation plan
Are they on an active transplant list?
Consider CPR, palliative care

Exclude & treat reversible precipitants
Atrial arrhythmias
Ischaemia, infection, PE (do CTPA)
Exacerbation of underlying lung disease

AIRWAY/BREATHING
Avoid intubation/IPPV if possible. Optiflow well tolerated
Oxygen. Target SaO_2>95%, control pH and pCO_2 (NIV)
If ventilated, low tidal volume ventilation, maintain Pplat<30cmH_2O

CIRCULATION (steps 1–3 may be simultaneous)
1. Optimise RV preload
Diuretics usually needed. Aim CVP 10–12mmHg
Avoid volume overload. Haemofiltration (rarely)
2. Optimise RV contractility
Maintain MAP>65–70mmHg, crucial early step
Norepinephrine or low-dose vasopressin
Optimise cardiac output (low-dose dobutamine or milrinone)
3. Reduce RV afterload (IV/inhaled prostanoids; iNO if intubated)
IV or nebulised prostacyclin is optimum therapy in RV failure
Do not stop oral PAH therapies
May need to switch to IV sildenafil

If inadequate clinical response: consider VA-ECMO, surgical options

Figure 45.1 Algorithm for ICU management of PH and RV failure. Abbreviations: Echo, echocardiography; CVP, central venous pressure; PH, pulmonary hypertension; RV, right ventricular; IPPV, invasive positive-pressure ventilation; iNO, inhaled nitric oxide; IV, intravenous; ECMO, extracorporeal membrane oxygenation; PEEP, positive end-expiratory pressure; PE, pulmonary embolism; CTPA, computed tomography pulmonary angiogram; IV, intravenous; CPR, cardiopulmonary resuscitation; MAP, mean arterial pressure; CVP, central venous pressure; ICU, intensive care unit; VA-ECMO, veno-arterial extracorporeal membrane oxygenation.

pH from 7.44 to 7.48 using sodium bicarbonate reduced PVR and increased cardiac index without changing pCO_2,[14] and induction of alkalosis is recommended for acute management of PH crises in this population.[15]

Fluid Balance Management

Marked fluid retention with secondary hyperaldosteronism is characteristic of RV failure and often needs a combination of a furosemide infusion with an aldosterone antagonist (e.g. spironolactone) to normalize RV preload and contractility. Additional diuretics used include bendroflumethazide, or metolazone stat doses. If diuretics are unsuccessful, haemofiltration or renal replacement therapy may be needed.

Fluid balance must be titrated carefully. Fluid challenges may increase CO in those with restrictive physiology in the right ventricle, albeit at the expense of systemic venous hypertension. By contrast, failing dilated right ventricles often respond better to diuresis.

Pulmonary Vasodilators

Oral therapies including phosphodiesterase (PDE) type V inhibitors include sildenafil and tadalafil, which augment nitric oxide (NO) signalling, resulting in pulmonary vasodilation, attenuation of vascular remodelling, and improved RV function. Sildenafil (oral or IV) can be titrated to clinical response and systemic hypotension, and is usually well tolerated in ICU patients. Endothelin-1 is a potent vasoconstrictor and smooth muscle mitogen. Endothelin receptor antagonists including bosentan, ambrisentan, and macitentan are available orally. Prostanoids are potent short-acting pulmonary vasodilators and inhibitors of platelet activation and include epoprostenol and iloprost. Epoprostenol should be first-line therapy in PAH patients in RV failure. Side effects include hypotension, flushing, headache, jaw pain, and diarrhoea. Prostacyclins can increase bleeding (especially as issue in patients on ECMO), and their systemic administration may worsen ventilation perfusion (VQ) matching in the presence of parenchymal lung disease. Inhaled pulmonary vasodilators such as inhaled nitric oxide (NO) can be administered to ventilated patients to reduce PH and improves VQ matching, for example, following cardiac surgery, acute PE and ARDS. Sildenafil can limit rebound PH following NO withdrawal.

Inotropes and Vasopressors

Catecholamines and Vasopressin Analogues

Vasopressors include catecholamines (e.g. norepinephrine) and low-dose vasopressin, which cause systemic vasoconstriction (via alpha-adrenoceptors and V1 receptors, respectively), and should be used early to ensure adequate aortic root pressure and avoid RV ischaemia.[16] Dose-dependent inotropic effects are achieved through beta-adrenoceptor agonism by dopamine and dobutamine, balanced against increases in heart rate and systemic and pulmonary dilatation (beta-2 effects). Studies in acute PH models show that catecholamines (up to 0.5 mcg/kg/min norepinephrine; dopamine or dobutamine up to 10 mcg/kg/min) do not increase PVR (a theoretical risk due to alpha effects).[17] In RV failure in PH patients, dobutamine (often at 5 mcg/kg/min, peripherally) is often combined with norepinephrine (centrally) as a first-line vasopressor.

Inodilators

PDE3 inhibitors such as milrinone (intravenous or inhaled) have inodilating and pulmonary vasodilating effects, and are useful in PH and RV failure. Milrinone is often used in some centres in RV failure, inducing less tachycardia than catecholamines. Levosimendan improving contractility by increasing the sensitivity of cardiac myofilaments to calcium ions, and vasodilating via potassium channels and PDE3 inhibition is an attractive inodilator in RV failure.[18] Both milrinone and levosimendan can induce atrial arrhythmias and systemic vasodilatation, often requiring concurrent vasopressor use.

Surgical Interventions

Interventions may be considered in patients with severe PH and RV failure despite maximal medical therapy.

Atrial Septostomy

The creation of an interatrial shunt results in right-to-left flow decompressing the RV and improving left atrial filling, at the expense of oxygen saturations, and can improve haemodynamics in severe PAH and has a role as a bridge to transplantation although it is rarely used in the UK. Patients with severe RV failure (RAP > 20 mmHg) have high procedure-related mortality[19] although this may be reduced in experienced centres.[20]

Pulmonary Embolectomy and Pulmonary Endarterectomy Surgery

Pulmonary embolectomy may be considered in patients with acute massive central PE and where thrombolysis is contraindicated or has failed, with studies reporting 15% mortality and 80% 1-year survival.[21] Pulmonary endarterectomy for CTEPH involves careful dissection of organized fibrous tissue under cardiopulmonary bypass and deep hypothermic arrest, with ICU complications including persistent PH and RV failure, reperfusion pulmonary oedema (lung injury), and pulmonary haemorrhage. The use of low tidal volume ventilation strategies or methylprednisolone does not appear to reduce the incidence of lung injury in this population.[22,23]

Extracorporeal Devices

It is possible to support the failing RV mechanically. The goals of therapy dictate the appropriateness and best options for support. Supporting decompensated right-heart failure in the context of irreversible PH is only appropriate to bridge a patient to heart and/or lung transplantation. The use of support to bridge patients through the introduction of advanced therapies such as pulmonary vasodilators has not been tested. By contrast, many patients have been supported following cardiac surgery when the right heart is failing due to a multitude of reasons but including a reversible elevation in the PVR.

Support options include VA-ECMO or univentricular support with a percutaneous RV assist device such as the Impella RP (Abiomed) or Protek Duo cannula (Tandem Heart) attached to a centrifugal pump. The Protek Duo cannula is a dual lumen catheter that is placed via the internal jugular vein through the right ventricle and into the main PA. One lumen drains blood from the right ventricle/atrium while the other lumen allows blood to be returned to the tip, which is distal to the pulmonary valve. Finally, patients with PH have been bridged to transplantation after surgically placing an artificial membrane lung (for example Novalung) between the PA and left atrium; blood flows passively driven by the high PA pressures.[24] This is very difficult following the onset of significant RV failure. Extracorporeal support should be undertaken only at centres with specific governance arrangements to deliver these techniques safely.

Conclusions

PH and RV dysfunction are associated with high mortality in critical illness. Despite this, there is little trial data guiding the application of PH interventions in the critically ill. The acute changes in physiology faced by these patients in the ICU setting make large trials difficult to perform. Therefore, understanding of the pathophysiology of PAH and the ICU context is essential in understanding how to manage these patients. The development and use of pulmonary vasodilators, inotropes, and extracorporeal support systems should in theory improve outcomes, but further studies, however difficult to implement, are needed.

REFERENCES

1. Galie N, Humbert M, Vachiery J-L, et al. 2015 ESC/ERS Guidelines for the diagnosis and treatment of pulmonary hypertension. The Joint Task Force for the Diagnosis and Treatment of Pulmonary Hypertension of the European Society of Cardiology (ESC) and the European Respiratory Society (ERS). *Eur Respir J.* 2015;**46**(4):903–975.
2. Simonneau G, Gatzoulis MA, Adatia I, et al. Updated clinical classification of pulmonary hypertension. *J Am Coll Cardiol.* 2013;**62**(25 Suppl):D34–41.
3. McIntyre KM, Sasahara AA. Hemodynamic and ventricular responses to pulmonary embolism. *Prog Cardiovasc Dis.* 1974;**17**(3):175–190.
4. Snow RL, Davies P, Pontoppidan H, et al. Pulmonary vascular remodeling in adult respiratory distress syndrome. *Am Rev Respir Dis.* 1982;**126**(5):887–892.
5. Mekontso Dessap A, Boissier F, Charron C, et al. Acute cor pulmonale during protective ventilation for acute respiratory distress syndrome: Prevalence, predictors, and clinical impact. *Intensive Care Med.* 2016;**42**(5):862–870.
6. Ling Y, Johnson MK, Kiely DG, et al. Changing demographics, epidemiology, and survival of incident pulmonary arterial hypertension: Results from the pulmonary hypertension registry of the United Kingdom and Ireland. *Am J Respir Crit Care Med.* 2012;**186**(8):790–796.
7. Sztrymf B, Souza R, Bertoletti L, et al. Prognostic factors of acute heart failure in patients with pulmonary arterial hypertension. *Eur Respir J.* 2010;**35**(6):1286–1293.
8. Hoeper MM, Galie N, Murali S, et al. Outcome after cardiopulmonary resuscitation in patients with pulmonary arterial hypertension. *Am J Respir Crit Care Med.* 2002;**165**(3):341–344.
9. Jardin F, Dubourg O, Gueret P, et al. Quantitative two-dimensional echocardiography in massive pulmonary embolism: Emphasis on ventricular interdependence and leftward septal displacement. *J Am Coll Cardiol.* 1987;**10**(6):1201–1206.
10. Gibbons Kroeker CA, Adeeb S, Shrive NG, et al. Compression induced by RV pressure overload decreases regional coronary

blood flow in anesthetized dogs. *Am J Physiol Heart Circ Physiol.* 2006;**290**(6):H2432–2438.

11. McQuillan BM, Picard MH, Leavitt M, et al. Clinical correlates and reference intervals for pulmonary artery systolic pressure among echocardiographically normal subjects. *Circulation.* 2001;**104**(23):2797–2802.
12. Hoeper MM, Granton J. Intensive care unit management of patients with severe pulmonary hypertension and right heart failure. *Am J Respir Crit Care Med.* 2011;**184**(10):1114–1124.
13. Price LC, Wort SJ, Finney SJ, et al. Pulmonary vascular and right ventricular dysfunction in adult critical care: Current and emerging options for management: A systematic literature review. *Crit Care.* 2010;**14**(5):R169.
14. Chang AC, Zucker HA, Hickey PR, et al. Pulmonary vascular resistance in infants after cardiac surgery: Role of carbon dioxide and hydrogen ion. *Crit Care Med.* 1995;**23**(3):568–574.
15. Abman SH, Hansmann G, Archer SL, et al. Pediatric pulmonary hypertension: Guidelines from the American Heart Association and American Thoracic Society. *Circulation.* 2015;**132**(21):2037–2099.
16. Tayama E, Ueda T, Shojima T, et al. Arginine vasopressin is an ideal drug after cardiac surgery for the management of low systemic vascular resistant hypotension concomitant with pulmonary hypertension. *Interact Cardiovasc Thorac Surg.* 2007;**6**(6):715–719.
17. Kerbaul F, Rondelet B, Motte S, et al. Effects of norepinephrine and dobutamine on pressure load-induced right ventricular failure. *Crit Care Med.* 2004;**32**(4):1035–1040.
18. Kerbaul F, Rondelet B, Demester JP, et al. Effects of levosimendan versus dobutamine on pressure load-induced right ventricular failure. *Crit Care Med.* 2006;**34**(11): 2814–2819.
19. Rich S, Dodin E, McLaughlin VV. Usefulness of atrial septostomy as a treatment for primary pulmonary hypertension and guidelines for its application. *Am J Cardiol.* 1997;**80**(3):369–371.
20. Chiu JS, Zuckerman WA, Turner ME, et al. Balloon atrial septostomy in pulmonary arterial hypertension: Effect on survival and associated outcomes. *J Heart Lung Transplant.* 2015;**34**(3):376–380.
21. Leacche M, Unic D, Goldhaber SZ, et al. Modern surgical treatment of massive pulmonary embolism: Results in 47 consecutive patients after rapid diagnosis and aggressive surgical approach. *J Thorac Cardiovasc Surg.* 2005;**129**(5):1018–1023.
22. Bates DM, Fernandes TM, Duwe BV, et al. Efficacy of a low-tidal volume ventilation strategy to prevent reperfusion lung injury after pulmonary thromboendarterectomy. *Ann Am Thorac Soc.* 2015;**12**(10):1520–1527.
23. Kerr KM, Auger WR, Marsh JJ, et al. Efficacy of methylprednisolone in preventing lung injury following pulmonary thromboendarterectomy. *Chest.* 2012;**141**(1): 27–35.
24. Strueber M, Hoeper MM, Fischer S, et al. Bridge to thoracic organ transplantation in patients with pulmonary arterial hypertension using a pumpless lung assist device. *Am J Transplant.* 2009;**9**(4):853–857.

46

Organizing Pneumonia

Peter M George, Suveer Singh, and Felix Chua

KEY MESSAGES

- Although organizing pneumonia (OP) is an interstitial lung disease, it has unique imaging and histopathological hallmarks that distinguish it from other fibrosing lung diseases.
- It is often misdiagnosed for bacterial pneumonia sharing many clinical and radiological features, and so the diagnosis is often made once patients have not responded to antimicrobial therapy.
- OP can occur in the context of autoimmune conditions or pneumotoxic drugs but can also exist with no known trigger—cryptogenic organizing pneumonia.
- The key to a good outcome is an expedient diagnosis as the condition can be exquisitely responsive to corticosteroid therapy—the earlier this is initiated, the lower the chances of irreversible fibrotic lung disease.

CONTROVERSIES

- Viral infections including SARS-CoV-2 can lead to an organizing pneumonia pattern—the optimal longer treatment of COVID-related OP is yet to be determined but is the subject of ongoing research.

FURTHER RESEARCH

- More broadly, the role of steroids in post-acute respiratory distress syndrome (ARDS) OP remains an area of contention where further research is required.

Introduction

Organizing pneumonia (OP) is a clinicopathological entity with features that distinguish it from other consolidative and interstitial lung diseases (ILDs). Because it is commonly mistaken for bacterial pneumonia at presentation, a diagnosis of OP is often only made when antimicrobial therapy, including repeat treatment, has failed to produce clinical or radiological resolution. A lack of response to antimicrobials and in selected cases prompt responsiveness to corticosteroids are among the hallmarks of this condition. Although first proposed by Charcot as a chronic pneumonia in the 1870s, its early pathological description only emerged in the early 20th century with post-mortem findings of pneumonia that, instead of resolving, evolved into fibrosis. OP is defined histopathologically by the presence of intra-alveolar accumulation of loose connective tissues and cells including fibroblasts and a variable number of inflammatory cells.

Of the cases that come to the attention of healthcare professionals on the intensive care unit (ICU), OP can be distilled to the acute pulmonary presentations or complications of a systemic disorder such as connective tissue disease (CTD) or vasculitis, an idiopathic entity called 'acute fibrinous organizing pneumonia' (AFOP), or the injurious pulmonary reaction to drugs or pathogens. The pandemic caused by the severe acute respiratory syndrome coronavirus-2 (SARS-CoV-2) provides the latest example of infection-associated OP although the spectrum of lung abnormalities related to COVID-19, the disease caused by this virus, extends beyond OP and is extensively covered in a dedicated chapter (Chapter 35).

In conventional ILD practice, the term cryptogenic organizing pneumonia (COP) is widely used when a cause cannot be identified to explain the radiological presence of OP. Following its original description by Davison and colleagues in 1983,[1] more detailed characterization of its pathological features emerged, leading to the coining of the term 'bronchiolitis obliterans organizing pneumonia' (or BOOP) by Epler and co-workers.[2] COP and BOOP were used interchangeably and confusingly until 2002 when the former became the favoured term, in the hope of providing a unifying disease-directed framework for further studies.[3] While COP primarily affects the intra-alveolar spaces, its propensity to extend to the alveolar ducts and distal bronchioles during fibrotic progression justifies its inclusion within the ILD nomenclature. Overall, COP is not a common cause of OP encountered on the ICU.

Disease Associations of OP

Patients with underlying CTDs form the majority of patients with acute or acute-on-chronic ILD requiring ICU care.[4] The commonest CTDs to be implicated are the idiopathic inflammatory myositides (IIM), rheumatoid arthritis, systemic sclerosis, Sjögren's syndrome, and mixed CTD. IIM include polymyositis (PM), dermatomyositis (PM), and either PM or DM-predominant disease associated with antibodies against aminoacyl-tRNA synthetase—examples of the so-called 'anti-synthetase syndrome'.[5] Up to 30%–40% of patients with IIM develop ILD which can precede, follow, or present contemporaneously with muscle disease.[6,7] OP is a common pathological pattern in such cases, including in the small proportion of patients who present acutely with fulminant pulmonary disease manifesting as severe or even life-threatening respiratory failure. Among Japanese and Korean patients, OP appears to be more common than non-specific interstitial pneumonia (NSIP) in the setting of an acute ILD.[8,9]

Anti-Jo-1 antibody is the most commonly identified myositis-specific antibody (MSA), and its presence is the strongest predictor of ILD in IIM; the majority of anti-Jo-1-positive patients develop ILD.[10] Table 46.1 lists commonly associated auto-antibodies. Other notable MSAs include antibodies against PL7 and PL12.[11] Myositis-associated antibodies such as anti-PM/Scl-100 or anti-Ro52 antibody are more likely to be found in overlapping myositis syndromes where inflammatory muscle disease coexists with clinical manifestations that are more commonly associated with other CTDs such as Raynaud's phenomenon. The term 'clinically amyopathic dermatomyositis (CADM)' describes a subset of patients with dermatomyositis who do not have overt muscle disease but are nonetheless predisposed to severe and often highly progressive OP-predominant ILD and thus a high risk of needing critical care management.[12] The presence of serum anti-MDA5 antibody occurs in a subset of patients with CADM. As immunosuppressive therapies are commonly used in patients with CTDs, these patients are also at heightened risk of infection which needs to be excluded as a differential diagnosis following acute respiratory deterioration.

OP occurring in anti-neutrophil cytoplasmic antibody (ANCA)–associated pulmonary vasculitides such as granulomatosis with polyangiitis (GPA) is important to recognize for both its potential for rapid progression and potentially prompt response to treatment with cytotoxic immunosuppressants and biological therapies. In addition to OP, the characteristic 'mass-like' consolidative lesions of these disorders are frequently associated with ground-glass opacity (denoting alveolar haemorrhage) on a background of ANCA positivity. The presence of these findings can obviate the need for lung biopsy.

acute fibrinous organising pneumonia (AFOP) is a term used to describe a form of OP that may be misdiagnosed as infective pneumonia due to their clinical similarities including a short symptom history, fever, cough, and chest discomfort.[13,14] Two disease courses have been described, the first a fulminant presentation with rapid progression to severe respiratory failure and the second a subacute course with protracted dyspnoea and cough and prompt steroid responsiveness. Although AFOP may be associated with CTDs, infection, haematological malignancies, and inhalational injury, a clear predisposing factor is typically not identified. Its histological appearances are distinctive and include the presence of intra-alveolar deposits of 'fibrin balls' associated with type II pneumocyte hyperplasia. While a pathological pattern of OP predominates and may be closely associated with the fibrinous accumulation, the intervening interlobular septa are often spared. Additionally, the absence of hyaline membranes differentiates AFOP from diffuse alveolar damage (DAD), and a paucity of eosinophils distinguishes it from acute eosinophilic pneumonia. The use of CT alone without surgical lung biopsy may be insufficient to reach a definitive diagnosis of AFOP (Figures 46.1 and 46.2).

An increasing number of drugs are associated with a risk of developing iatrogenic OP (Table 46.2). Whereas agents such as nitrofurantoin and amiodarone are commonly cited, more recent examples of pneumotoxic drugs have included novel anti-cancer agents (Table 46.2). One common dilemma in managing drug-induced lung toxicity or disease is in establishing the degree of causal likelihood with the suspected offending agent. The situation is made more complex if the individual has been exposed to more than one drug or if the underlying condition for which the drugs were prescribed can itself give rise to pulmonary disease. An example in practice

Table 46.1 Auto-antibody profiles in conditions which manifest with OP

Disease associated with OP	Auto-antibody profile
Anti-synthetase syndrome	Commonest aminoacyl-tRNA synthetase antibodies Anti-Jo 1 Anti-PL 7 Anti-PL 12 Anti-OJ Anti-EJ
Myositis specific	Anti SRP Anti- MDA5 Anti-Mi-2
Myositis-associated overlap	ANA Anti-Ro/SSA Anti-PM-Scl Anti-Ku Anti-U2 snRNP

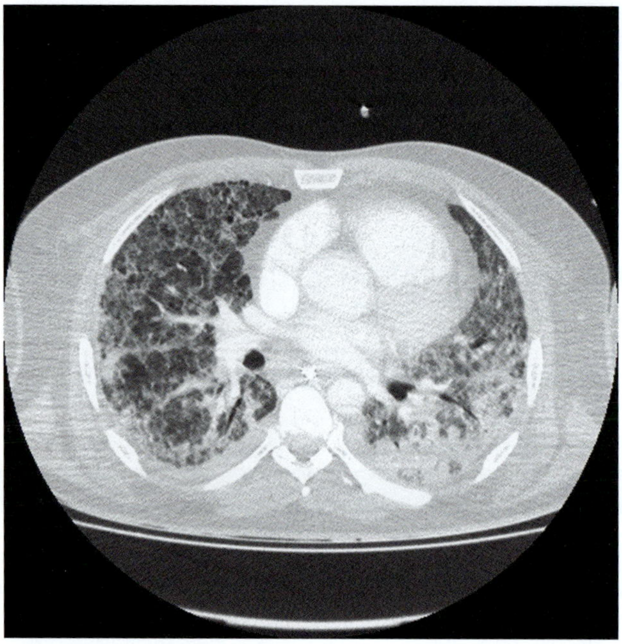

Figure 46.1 Axial CT image of acute fibrinous organising pneumonia (AFOP) showing diffuse ground-glass opacity and basal-dominant consolidation. These radiologic changes do not reliably differentiate AFOP from diffuse alveolar damage (DAD).

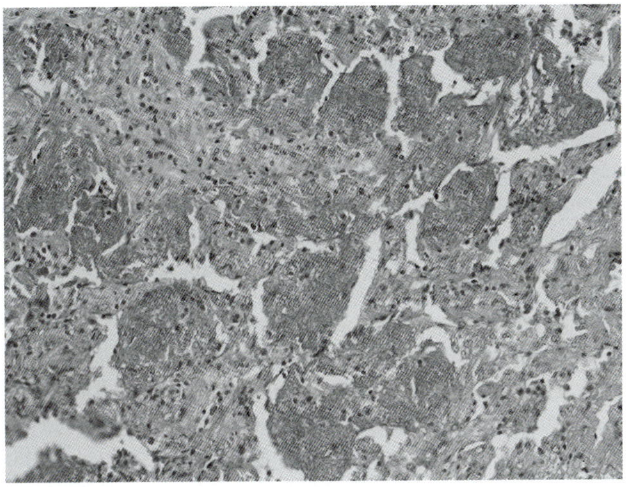

Figure 46.2 Photomicrograph of a Masson body composed of spindle-shaped fibroblasts in a loose matrix of immature connective tissue, typically forming intraluminal 'plugs' within alveolar ducts and sacs (200× magnification, H&E stain). See plate section.

is rheumatoid arthritis treated with methotrexate. In reality, RA-associated ILD is significantly more common than methotrexate-induced pneumonitis although the latter is raised as a concern far more often than its true prevalence justifies. In practice, drug-related OP is often concluded only when cessation of the culprit drug(s) is followed by clinical or radiological improvement.

OP can also develop as the sequelae of bacterial, viral, fungal, and parasitic infection. In such instances, unresolved pulmonary inflammation persists even after the infective process has been suppressed, allowing fibrinous exudates to accumulate and organize within the alveoli and prompting subsequent progression to OP.

Table 46.2 Commonly encountered associations with OP

Association	Examples
Connective tissue diseases	Idiopathic interstitial myositis (e.g. polymyositis, dermatomyositis, and the anti-synthetase syndrome) Rheumatoid arthritis Sjögren's syndrome Mixed connective tissue disease
Vasculitides	Granulomatosis with polyangiitis (GPA; Wegener's)
Drugs	Amiodarone Nitrofurantoin Methotrexate Interferon Chemotherapeutic drugs (e.g. oxaliplatin and immune checkpoint inhibitors such as PD-1 inhibitors like pembrolizumab and PD-L1 inhibitors like durvalumab)
Infections	SARS-CoV-2 *Streptococcus pneumonia* *Legionella pneumophila* *Mycoplasma pneumoniae* *Cryptococcus neoformans* *Pneumocystis jiroveci* *Influenzae* A and B *Mycobacterium tuberculosis* Human Immunodeficiency virus
Malignancy	Lung cancer
Transplant	Bone marrow transplant
Others	Radiotherapy, GORD, and aspiration

OP and more specifically AFOP can develop in transplanted lungs (Chapter 63) as a consequence of the same insults associated with bronchiolitis obliterans syndrome (BOS). BOS, the major pulmonary manifestation of lung or bone marrow transplant rejection and graft-versus-host disease, is characterized pathologically by constrictive bronchiolar narrowing that progresses steadily to severe fixed airflow obstruction. Lung transplant recipients who develop OP, although less common than BOS, also have a poor prognosis.[15] BOS is not to be confused with BOOP (bronchiolitis obliterans organizing pneumonia) which, as explained above, is now referred to as 'COP'.

Clinical Features of OP and Establishing a Diagnosis

Many patients with OP presenting acutely with respiratory failure suffer an exacerbation of pre-existing or chronic disease. However, de novo presentation of OP is not uncommon. By the extent of pulmonary involvement, the resulting hypoxaemia may be mild, moderate, or severe. Virtually all such patients will require, at some stage, either supplementary oxygen or some form of respiratory support. Whereas individuals with an established OP diagnosis may be difficult to manage, de novo presentations often pose the greatest diagnostic challenge, for example distinguishing post-infective from CTD-associated or drug-induced OP, particularly when some or all of these elements are present concomitantly. Moreover, the clinical features of OP may not be unique to its underlying cause except when distinctive extra-pulmonary manifestations are also present. In the acute setting including on the ICU, a number of diagnostic leads may have to be pursued simultaneously and in parallel with institution of an empiric therapeutic strategy.

Where possible, all patients with a potential diagnosis of OP should be questioned in detail and a thorough examination performed. Patients with infection-related OP, including COVID-19, will likely have a distinctive presentation. For others, the clinical history should focus on searching for pathological associations (Table 46.2). A focused line of enquiry should seek to identify previously undiagnosed CTD; potential clues might include a history of small joint arthralgia, skin rashes, Raynaud's phenomenon, proximal limb girdle weakness, or sicca symptoms. Urine should be analyzed by dipstick for haematuria or red cell casts on cytological examination to allude to or exclude vasculitis. Blood tests may identify an underlying infection, but leucocytosis per se and elevated C-reactive protein are not specific for infection and may be evident in acute flares of OP. A full autoimmune screen is mandatory and should include anti-nuclear antibody (ANA), antibodies against extractable nuclear antigen, ANCA, creatinine kinase (CK), and a full myositis panel including anti-MDA5. A raised CK might suggest the presence of myositis.

Radiological Features of OP

The classical and radiological appearance of OP is of multifocal peripheral consolidation, commonly with air bronchograms, associated

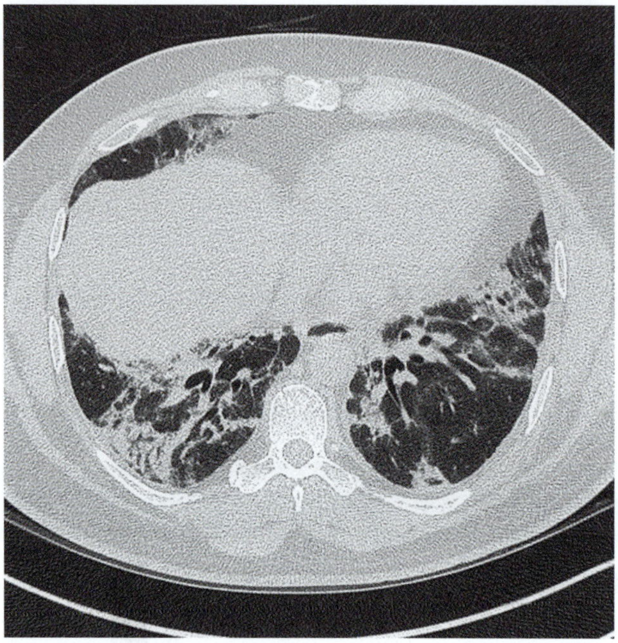

Figure 46.3 Axial CT image of OP in a patient with anti-Jo-1 antisynthetase syndrome, depicting dense patchy consolidation in peripheral and peribronchial locations.

by a variable quantity of ground-glass opacification (Figure 46.3). Although the patches of consolidation may change in location over weeks and affect any lobe, they commonly follow a lower zone predilection. 'Migration' of consolidative abnormalities and spontaneous resolution strongly favour OP as a diagnosis over the alternative of bacterial pneumonia. Other differentials include eosinophilic pneumonia and consolidative or mass-like pulmonary vasculitis. OP may also incorporate peribronchiolar (bronchocentric) consolidation that often 'runs into' denser areas peripherally.

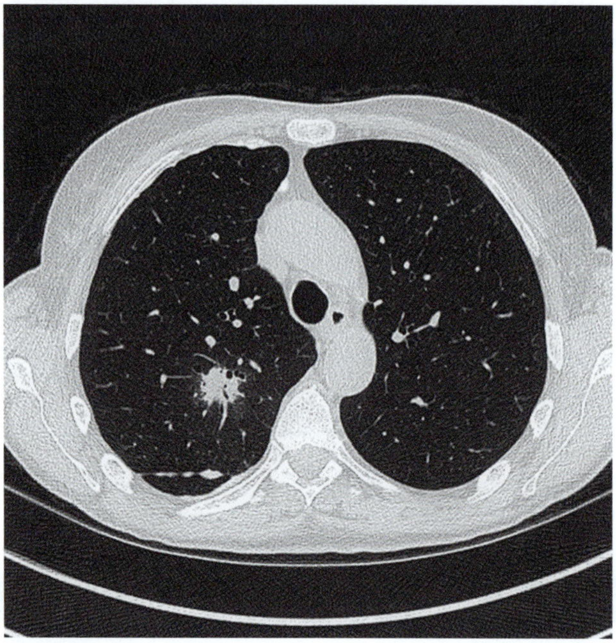

Figure 46.4 Nodular OP in the right upper lobe (cryptogenic organising pneumonia or COP).

A range of radiological features are recognized for OP depending on its pathological associations. For instance, COP may present as a focal mass or solitary nodule, often located in the upper lobes (Figure 46.4). Nodules may have an irregular or even spiculated outline and be multiple, ranging in diameter from under 5 mm to over 10 mm. Differentiating OP from lung cancer in this setting is challenging particularly as both entities can demonstrate moderate PET-FDG avidity. In other cases, the consolidation follows a perilobular pattern that highlights disease around the border of adjacent secondary pulmonary lobules. On certain CT sections, these appearances can look like 'arcades'. On the other hand, the reversed halo or 'Atoll sign' represents circumferential or crescentic consolidation with a central area of ground-glass opacity and unaffected lung (Figure 46.5). Although this sign was initially considered pathognomonic of COP, it has also been described in other conditions such as GPA and sarcoidosis. Where ground-glass opacification is associated with interlobular septal thickening, a 'crazy paving' appearance may emerge; this sign has been reported in OP related to bleomycin lung toxicity. Regardless of the initial OP pattern, the development of progressive fibrosis that is often evident as coarse basally predominant reticulation with traction bronchiectasis portends a poorer prognosis.

Pathological Features of OP

The development of OP involves an initial injury to the alveolar epithelium leading to an exuberant inflammatory response and leakage of plasma proteins into the alveolar spaces. These processes in turn promote aberrant coagulation, fibrogenic and fibrinolytic cascades, resulting in intraluminal fibrin deposition. A process of organization then predominates, characterized by intra-alveolar accumulation of buds of fibrous granulation tissue and matrix-producing fibroblasts within a connective tissue matrix. This is histologically recognized as the Masson body (Figure 46.6). The fibrous buds may propagate to other alveoli and 'incorporate' into the adjacent parenchymal interstitium to form expanding fibrous tissue.

Pure OP should be distinguished from DAD which clinically describes the non-specific reaction of the lung to a variety of toxic

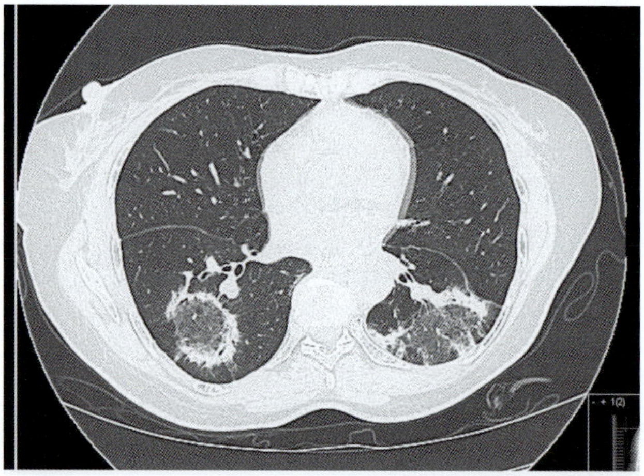

Figure 46.5 Axial CT image of the Atoll or 'reversed halo' sign (circular or partially circular consolidation surrounding an area of internal ground-glass opacity).

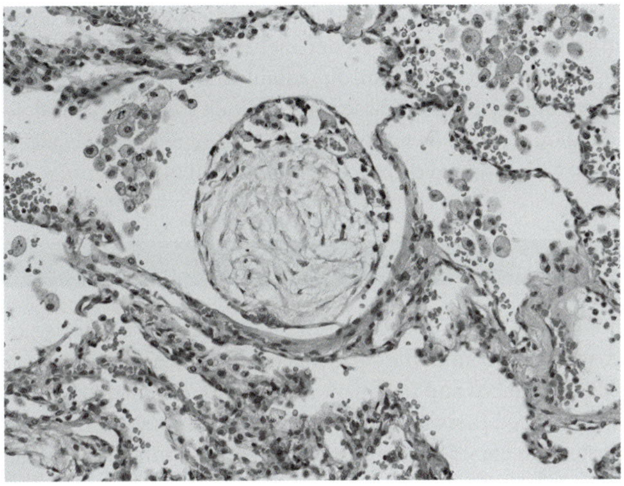

Figure 46.6 Photomicrograph of AFOP demonstrating intra-alveolar 'fibrin balls' and associated changes of organising pneumonia without obvious hyaline membrane formation (200× magnification, H&E stain). See plate section.

and inflammatory insults and histologically represents the sequelae of the acute respiratory distress syndrome (ARDS). The histologic appearance of DAD may vary depending on the timing of biopsy; in the acute phase, it is characterized by the presence of hyaline membranes, oedematous alveolar walls, damaged alveolar epithelial cells, and exposure of epithelial basement membranes, often with involvement of the endothelial cell layer. The organization phase may begin within a few days when the presence of organizing fibroblastic tissue within alveolar airspaces and the interstitium becomes prominent. Because DAD can take a clinical route that is different to OP despite some overlapping histological features, the ability to differentiate the two diagnoses clinically and radiologically may have important management implications. Bronchoscopy and bronchoalveolar lavage are important diagnostic tests in this context as they facilitate diagnosis of occult haemorrhage, exclusion of infection, and identification of coexisting inflammatory alveolitis which is typically confirmed with lymphocytosis on the cell differential.

Management of OP Encountered in the Intensive Care Unit

Prior to 2020, viral infection was a recognized but not common cause of OP. The pandemic caused by SARS-CoV-2 and the ensuing lung disease called 'COVID-19' have changed this axiomatic view. Patterns of OP or OP-like features are frequently encountered in such patients, including the development of dense peripheral consolidation in the lower lobes, accompanied peri-lobular abnormalities, and ground-glass opacification. As COVID-19 progresses, new areas of consolidation may appear including in less dependent areas and retain the recognizable features of OP (Figure 46.7). In a proportion of cases of pneumonic COVID-19, the severe consequences of lung injury fail to promptly resolve; instead, rapid fibroproliferative changes ensue and result in bronchial and bronchiolar distortion (such as tortuous traction), fissural irregularity, and coarse parenchymal reticulation. Although the potential for COVID-19 pneumonia to progress to chronic fibrosis is

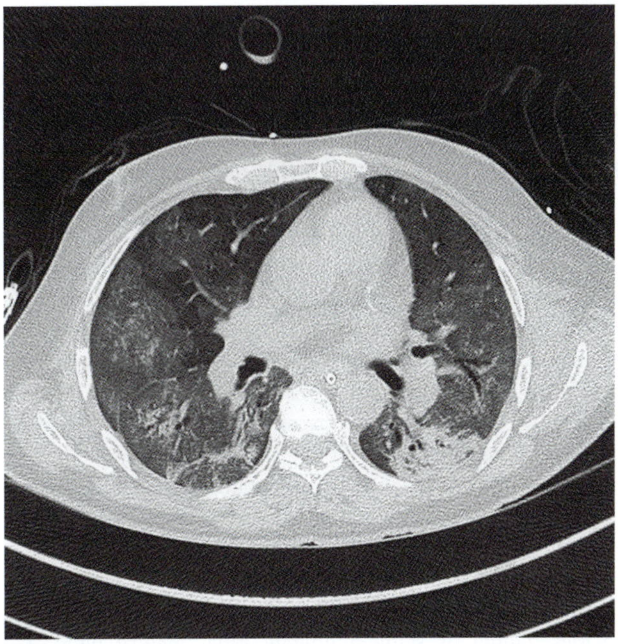

Figure 46.7 Axial CT image of a convalescing patient with COVID-19 pneumonia acquired 7 weeks following hospital admission showing patchy dense lower lobe OP-like changes on a background of ground-glass opacity.

acknowledged, the risk of progressive fibrotic sequelae has yet to be understood. At the time of writing, the evaluation of patients by fibrotic risk stratification is actively being studied. A discussion on COVID-19 is presented in Chapter 35.

The management of the critically unwell patient with respiratory failure in the context of a diffuse parenchymal lung disease prioritizes supportive measures concurrent with an exhaustive diagnostic search for 'probable cause', as outlined in preceding sections. Early imaging with CT allows clinicians and radiologists to narrow the differential diagnoses so that clinical management can be appropriately targeted. It is crucial to maintain a high index of suspicion for ILD with potential to progress rapidly to fulminant respiratory failure. Within this category, clinicians must consider the anti-synthetase/idiopathic myositis syndrome (classically but not exclusively the anti-Jo-1 phenotype), GPA and AFOP. The mainstay of treatment of OP is corticosteroids; indeed, one of the main characteristics of OP is its potential for rapid corticosteroid response. Given the clinical and radiological similarities between OP and bacterial pneumonia, treatment with corticosteroids may be briefly deferred in favour of parenterally administered broad-spectrum antimicrobials. However, a delay in commencing corticosteroid therapy can result in worsening hypoxaemia, progressive parenchymal changes, and the establishment of ARDS.

If commenced in a timely fashion, corticosteroids can result in a rapid clinical improvement with clearance of parenchymal changes. In the non-emergency setting, a starting prednisolone dose of 0.50–0.75 mg/kg daily or an equivalent dose of hydrocortisone may be used, taking into account the severity of disease, level of hypoxaemia, radiological interpretation, and comorbid issues. In mechanically ventilated patients, intravenous rescue therapy is mandated and agents with induction properties are often favoured. In this setting, first-line treatment is typically high-dose IV methylprednisolone administered over three consecutive days followed by IV hydrocortisone as continuing treatment.

Other immunomodulatory treatments may be required in severe disease—there is some evidence that these drugs can lead to improved outcomes in selected cases. Cyclophosphamide is an alkylating cytotoxic drug that is commonly used to treat patients with acute CTD-associated ILD. A total of six 'pulses' are usually administered, the first three doses at 2-weekly intervals to achieve a more rapid onset of action. Using this regimen, the earliest therapeutic effect would still not be expected for 4–6 weeks after treatment commencement. Oral cyclophosphamide has no role in the treatment of acute OP. Rituximab is an anti-CD20 monoclonal antibody which can deplete B cells for up to 6–9 months. Most of the data supporting it use comes from the vasculitis literature, but there is case series evidence of success with IV rituximab in patients with COP.[16] Intravenous immunoglobulin is a potent immunomodulatory treatment that can be a useful adjunct in severe OP although the evidence for this is still limited.

A pertinent clinical scenario is that of a mechanically ventilated patient, in a prolonged weaning state, with persisting radiological opacities, falling or stable moderate inflammatory biomarkers, and the presumption of no clinically active infection. Exclusion of infection is important prior to initiation of immunosuppressive therapy and a procalcitonin level within normal range (i.e. <0.5 ng/mL) may provide reassurance. Radiological separation between slow-to-resolve infective consolidation, ARDS, and OP is usually difficult in this situation, and lung biopsy via thoracotomy or the bronchoscopic route is often considered high risk. Some clinical questions that typically arise are 'what is the chance of the benefit of empirical steroid dosing?'; 'should higher or lower dose steroids be given?'; and 'when might a steroid response be anticipated?'.

While there are case series of lung biopsies in ventilated patients with non-resolving ARDS that demonstrate OP or other potentially steroid-responsive pathology, these are few. There is also a confirmation of the aphorism that the more severe the ARDS, the higher the chance of predominant DAD as the likely pathology by this mode. Nevertheless, the few studied patients who did have a steroid-responsive pathology diagnosed by open lung biopsy, without any prior strong predictors, have better outcomes.[17] A corollary is that CT surrogate features of fibroproliferation and established fibrosis, that is, traction bronchiectasis and bronchioloectasis, portend a worse prognosis despite steroids.[18]

The questions of timing and dosing present another challenge. A landmark randomized study of lower dose empirical steroids (2 mg/kg/d for 2 weeks and then 1 mg/kg/d for a further week) in non-resolving ARDS did not show a 60- or 180-day survival benefit. However, those given steroids after 14 days had higher mortality at both time points.[19] An earlier study of high-dose steroids (30 mg/kg × 4 doses of methylprednisolone) in the pre-protective lung ventilation era had not shown a survival benefit at 45 days but had much higher baseline mortality than post millennium outcomes.[20] There is some advocacy, and also disagreement, although not universally adopted in international guidelines, to reinstate lower dose steroids (i.e. 1–2 mg/kg/d for up to 14 days) in early ARDS due to benefits in ventilator free days and ICU stay, demonstrated at patient level meta-analyses.[21,22] While not directly referring to OP in this context, and contrasting the higher steroid doses used in clinically diagnosed OP, there appears to be an important distinction (albeit not a sharp dichotomy) here. Thus, the presence of OP (or significant elements of it) would favour higher steroid doses, as against non-resolving ARDS (assumed predominantly DAD), where lower dose steroids in the early phase of recognition should be considered. These should clearly be multi-disciplinary discussion associated decisions, with assumed clinical and radiological expertise.

Outcome

Generally, in the non-ICU setting, the prognosis of OP is good and, while it is common for patients to relapse when corticosteroid doses are reduced and treatment is discontinued, once treatment is re-commenced there is rapid improvement. However, as would be expected, outcomes are far worse for patients admitted to the ICU with OP. Patients who present with AFOP often have clinical outcomes akin to patients with ARDS. It has been shown that the presence of pulmonary hypertension, acute kidney injury, and traction bronchiectasis confer the worst prognosis when considering patients with ILD admitted to the ICU.[4] Other important poor prognostic factors are increasing age, the presence of shock, and a higher Sepsis-related Organ Failure Assessment score. Mortality rates are higher in those patients with acute-on-chronic idiopathic ILD exacerbation or drug-induced ILD as compared to CTD-associated ILD or acute idiopathic interstitial pneumonia which have better outcomes. When OP overlaps with acute interstitial pneumonia or ARDS, it has the poorest prognosis. Factors that appear to be associated with a poor outcome in COP include a predominantly reticular pattern on CT, a lack of lymphocytosis on broncho-alveolar lavage cell count, and established fibrosis on histological assessment.

REFERENCES

1. Davison AG, Heard BE, McAllister WA, et al. Cryptogenic organizing pneumonitis. *Q J Med.* 1983;**52**(207):382–394.
2. Epler GR, Colby TV, McLoud TC, et al. Bronchiolitis obliterans organizing pneumonia. *N Engl J Med.* 1985;**312**(3):152–158.
3. Society AT, Society ER. American Thoracic Society/European Respiratory Society International Multidisciplinary Consensus classification of the idiopathic interstitial pneumonias. *Am J Respir Crit Care Med.* 2002;**165**(2):277–304.
4. Zafrani L, Lemiale V, Lapidus N, et al. Acute respiratory failure in critically ill patients with interstitial lung disease. *PLoS One.* 2014;**9**(8):e104897.
5. Lundberg IE, Tjärnlund A, Bottai M, et al. 2017 European League Against Rheumatism/American College of Rheumatology classification criteria for adult and juvenile idiopathic inflammatory myopathies and their major subgroups. *Arthritis Rheumatol.* 2017;**69**(12):2271–2282.
6. Lilleker JB, Vencovsky J, Wang G, et al. The EuroMyositis registry: An international collaborative tool to facilitate myositis research. *Ann Rheum Dis.* 2018;**77**(1):30–39.
7. Chua F, Higton AM, Colebatch AN, et al. Idiopathic inflammatory myositis-associated interstitial lung disease: Ethnicity differences and lung function trends in a British cohort. *Rheumatology (Oxford).* 2012;**51**(10):1870–1876.
8. Fujisawa T, Hozumi H, Kono M, et al. Prognostic factors for myositis-associated interstitial lung disease. *PLoS One.* 2014;**9**(6):e98824.

9. Won Huh J, Soon Kim D, Keun Lee C, et al. Two distinct clinical types of interstitial lung disease associated with polymyositis-dermatomyositis. *Respir Med.* 2007;**101**(8):1761–1769.
10. Stone KB, Oddis CV, Fertig N, et al. Anti-Jo-1 antibody levels correlate with disease activity in idiopathic inflammatory myopathy. *Arthritis Rheum.* 2007;**56**(9):3125–3131.
11. Betteridge ZE, Gunawardena H, McHugh NJ. Novel autoantibodies and clinical phenotypes in adult and juvenile myositis. *Arthritis Res Ther.* 2011;**13**(2):209.
12. Lega JC, Reynaud Q, Belot A, et al. Idiopathic inflammatory myopathies and the lung. *Eur Respir Rev.* 2015;**24**(136):216–238.
13. Beasley MB, Franks TJ, Galvin JR, et al. Acute fibrinous and organizing pneumonia: A histological pattern of lung injury and possible variant of diffuse alveolar damage. *Arch Pathol Lab Med.* 2002;**126**(9):1064–1070.
14. Gomes R, Padrão E, Dabó H, et al. Acute fibrinous and organizing pneumonia: A report of 13 cases in a tertiary university hospital. *Medicine (Baltimore).* 2016;**95**(27):e4073.
15. Paraskeva M, McLean C, Ellis S, et al. Acute fibrinoid organizing pneumonia after lung transplantation. *Am J Respir Crit Care Med.* 2013;**187**(12):1360–1368.
16. Shitenberg D, Fruchter O, Fridel L, et al. Successful rituximab therapy in steroid-resistant, cryptogenic organizing pneumonia: A case series. *Respiration.* 2015;**90**(2):155–159.
17. Wong AK, Walkey AJ. Open lung biopsy among critically ill, mechanically ventilated patients. A metaanalysis. *Ann Am Thorac Soc.* 2015;**12**(8):1226–1230.
18. Gerard L, Bidoul T, Castanares-Zapatero D, et al. Open lung biopsy in nonresolving acute respiratory distress syndrome commonly identifies corticosteroid-sensitive pathologies, associated with better outcome. *Crit Care Med.* 2018;**46**(6):907–914.
19. Ichikado K, Muranaka H, Gushima Y, et al. Fibroproliferative changes on high-resolution CT in the acute respiratory distress syndrome predict mortality and ventilator dependency: A prospective observational cohort study. *BMJ Open.* 2012;**2**(2):e000545.
20. Steinberg KP, Hudson LD, Goodman RB, et al. Efficacy and safety of corticosteroids for persistent acute respiratory distress syndrome. *N Engl J Med.* 2006;**354**(16):1671–1684.
21. Bernard GR, Luce JM, Sprung CL, et al. High-dose corticosteroids in patients with the adult respiratory distress syndrome. *N Engl J Med.* 1987;**317**(25):1565–1570.
22. Meduri GU, Bridges L, Shih MC, et al. Prolonged glucocorticoid treatment is associated with improved ARDS outcomes: Analysis of individual patients' data from four randomized trials and trial-level meta-analysis of the updated literature. *Intensive Care Med.* 2016;**42**(5):829–840.

47

Interstitial Lung Disease

Philip L Molyneaux and Athol U Wells

KEY MESSAGES

- The management of interstitial lung disease (ILD) in critical care is complex and requires a multi-disciplinary approach to tailor therapy to the individual patient and specific disease process.
- The commonest presentation of ILD requiring critical care support is the acute deterioration in a patient with previously diagnosed ILD.
- Rapid identification and treatment of reversible courses of a deterioration is key (e.g. infection, cardiac decompensation, and pulmonary embolism).
- The outcomes of mechanical ventilation in patients with established ILD are generally poor and even worse with no identified trigger of deterioration.

CONTROVERSIES

- The decision to admit a patient with established ILD to critical care is often complex.
- The role of extra-corporeal membrane oxygenation (ECMO) and transplant off critical care for patients with ILD remains unclear.

FURTHER RESEARCH

- Development of biomarkers and algorithms to identify patients with ILD who are likely to benefit from critical care interventions.
- More work is needed to identify the optimal agents for and timing of immunomodulation.

Introduction

'Interstitial lung disease' (ILD) is an umbrella term for a number of conditions that range from acute, self-limited inflammatory conditions to inexorably progressive and ultimately fatal fibrotic lung diseases. It is this broad spectrum of disease that often causes confusion and uncertainty in discussions of the role of critical care in the management of ILD. However, there are specific conditions and scenarios where a timely intervention can be crucial, and these opportunities should not be missed. In this chapter, we review the common presentations of ILD in critical care, discuss the general management strategies and options available, highlight some of the areas of ongoing controversy, and summarize research needs.

Presentation

The two most common scenarios in which ILD patients present with acute respiratory failure requiring the input of critical care are (i) rapid deterioration of an established and previously diagnosed ILD, and (ii) an initial presentation of rapidly progressive disease.[1] Both scenarios present differing and unique challenges.

By far the more common of these scenarios is acute deterioration in a patient with previously diagnosed ILD, presenting with worsening oxygenation and new lung infiltrates, normally over a short time period. While the differential diagnosis always includes deterioration of the underlying disease, the more frequent (and often more easily treated) triggers such as infection, cardiac decompensation, and pulmonary embolism must be considered.

The presentation of an apparent de novo ILD associated with respiratory failure and diffuse lung infiltrates often has a sub-acute or indolent onset over weeks in a previously apparently healthy individual. In this situation, the clinical history and review of any prior imaging is crucial to establish that acute ILD is truly de novo, as distinct from progression of a long-standing but hitherto undiagnosed process. This distinction has significant impact upon both treatment and prognostication. The classical example of pre-existent ILD is the first presentation of idiopathic pulmonary fibrosis (IPF) as an acute exacerbation, with an additional insult resulting in loss of pulmonary reserve and, thus, an acute presentation of a chronic condition. The true de novo rapidly progressive ILDs are most frequently acute interstitial pneumonia or organizing pneumonia (Chapter 46), though alveolar haemorrhage and drug-induced lung disease should be considered, as should the other common disease processes such as infection and pulmonary oedema that can mimic ILD clinically and radiologically.[2] While the differential is wide, this is usually rapidly narrowed with investigations.

Investigations

In patients presenting with ILD and respiratory failure, there is often a window of opportunity during which investigations can be performed before ventilation is required. With input from an ILD multi-disciplinary team meeting, an inciting trigger can often be identified and the distinction between de novo and established but exacerbating ILD can often be made. This allows informed and timely decisions about escalation of care.

Reaching an accurate diagnosis is central to confident management, but a number of diagnostic challenges remain, given the marked physiological and biochemical overlap of the potential differentials in this patient population. Classical indices of infection (white blood cell count, erythrocyte sedimentation rate (ESR), and C-reactive protein (CRP)) lack sensitivity or specificity as all can be influenced by underlying systemic disease activity in some ILDs. While not common, lymphangitis carcinomatosis can be mistaken for acute ILD and occasionally tuberculosis and chronic fungal infections may mimic progressive ILD. Therefore, just as in ILD management, the multi-disciplinary team (MDT) has a central role in dissecting these diagnostic conundrums and directing therapy. Certain newer biomarkers such as the fungal serological marker beta-D-glucan, and bronchoalveolar galactomannan, or procalcitonin as an indicator of bacterial sepsis may be of additional value in this context.

Imaging

In most patients with known or suspected ILD deteriorating acutely, infection is the dominant differential diagnosis, with opportunistic infection a particular complication in patients already on immunosuppressive therapy. Cardiac decompensation, undiagnosed valvular disease, and pulmonary emboli also need to be excluded. Routine chest radiographs are rarely useful in this diagnostic pathway but can be used to gauge disease extent and/or progression from previous imaging. High-resolution computed tomography (HRCT), usually combined with CT pulmonary angiography, is normally the pivotal imaging investigation, providing a wealth of information, especially when combined with review of historical imaging.[3] Characteristic HRCT patterns are often pathognomonic for individual ILDs, negating the need for further diagnostic investigations. Specialist input from chest radiologists with an experience of ILD can often be diagnostically influential.

Microbiology

As in all critically unwell patients where infection is part of the differential, routine specimens should include blood cultures in febrile patients, sputum culture, Pneumococcal and Legionella urinary antigen testing, and a respiratory virus screen from a nasal swab or aspirate. In those patients on pre-existing immunosuppression, the exclusion of cytomegalovirus viremia and other atypical infections, such as *Pneumocystis jirovecii* pneumonia, is also appropriate. Newer culture-independent molecular microbial techniques often provide rapid diagnostic and antibiotic resistance information and are particularly useful in these cases.[4]

Bronchoscopy

In immunosuppressed patients presenting with new or worsening pulmonary infiltrates, bronchoscopy with bronchoalveolar lavage (BAL) can make a crucial contribution to the detection of opportunistic infection.[5] It is also an excellent tool to identify non-infective causes of diffuse alveolar shadowing such as alveolar haemorrhage and malignancy. BAL is usually well tolerated and safe in patients with ILD,[6] immunosuppressed patients, and in critically ill ventilated patients (Chapter 19).[7]

The decision to undertake bronchoscopy in the unwell but self-ventilating patient should be made on a case-by-case basis, with the risk of deterioration in respiratory mechanics and gas exchange a major consideration.[8] In high-risk patients, these procedures are often performed within critical care.

Biopsy

Transbronchial biopsy (TBB) and surgical lung biopsy (SLB) are both used in multi-disciplinary diagnostic pathways in ILD. Although invasive, they can be invaluable in the critically unwell patient when used correctly. The decision to undertake either procedure is a balance between diagnostic benefits and attendant risks, which can be significant for ventilated patients. When an empirical therapeutic option covers realistic diagnostic differentials or there is a historical diagnosis of pre-existing ILD, these tests are not normally recommended as they tend to provide limited additional clinical benefit.[9]

TBB is more frequently used in the immunocompromised patient, typically HIV, oncology, or post-transplant, presenting with de novo pulmonary infiltrates. In this patient population, TBB is much more diagnostically sensitive than BAL and serious complications are rare.[10] However, data regarding its use in patients with acute deteriorations of established ILD is less convincing and the risks of the procedure, including a 10%–25% prevalence of pneumothorax, generally outweighing potential benefits.

Surgical lung biopsies, either via a mini-thoracotomy or video-assisted thoracoscopy, are occasionally appropriate in a critically unwell patient with ILD. However, the significant morbidity and mortality associated with the procedure must be weighed up careful by the multi-disciplinary team. In experienced centres, the diagnostic yield can reach 100%, but in some studies the diagnostic yield does not exceed 50%, highlighting importance of careful decision-making processes.[11] The short-term mortality is around 10%, but up to a half of ventilated patients undergoing SLB will experience a complication, with persistent air leaks being the most significant. Patients at most risk of complications are often the exact population in which the procedure may have the highest diagnostic yield with immunosuppression, severe hypoxia, multi-organ failure, and older age all associated with a greater risk of complications.[12] Despite this, SLB can be useful, often by demonstrating the complete absence of reversible disease and allowing inappropriate support to be minimized. The emergence of transbronchial cryobiopsy offers a 'middle road' between TBB and SLB, with larger diagnostic samples. However, its place in the deteriorating patient remains to be elucidated.

Decisions to Admit

The likelihood of a successful outcome is the key consideration that informs decisions to admit patients with ILD to critical care for invasive ventilation. However, there is a limited evidence base upon which to make informed decisions, and the following guidance should be interpreted with this in mind. Although not always possible, irreversible disease should ideally be identified at the outset, usually by integrating imaging and clinical evaluation. By this means, the likely futility of invasive ventilation can be communicated to patients, family, and staff with understanding of the realistic limits of care, decisions not to intubate, and the institution of early palliation when appropriate.

In patients with pre-existing ILD, the underlying diagnosis is the most important single consideration when making these decisions. IPF is the most prevalent ILD and the disease envisaged by most clinicians when they think of ILD. It has a prognosis of only 3–4 years from diagnosis and an extremely high mortality in ventilated patients with acute exacerbations of IPF. Acute deteriorations in patients with IPF have a high mortality, whether due to infection, cardiac decompensation, or acute IPF exacerbations, with half of patients dead within the following 6 months whatever interventions are instituted.[13] Case series consistently demonstrate mortalities approaching 100% in intubated patients with established IPF, and this now largely precludes their admission to critical care.[14]

In ILD patients without IPF, previous longitudinal disease behaviour (is there evidence of pre-existing inexorable progression of disease?), the dominant radiological pattern (reversible vs irreversible disease), and responsiveness to previous ILD therapies contribute to the decision-making process. A disease process that is predominantly fibrotic, and has progressed despite therapy in a patient with severely impaired lung function, should be regarded as equivalent to IPF for decision-making purposes.[15]

When a patient with apparently de novo ILD requires critical care input, the threshold for intervention or admission is generally lower as there is normally a good pre-morbid physiologic baseline. However, as stressed earlier, evidence of pre-existing ILD should be sought based on a careful history and scrutiny of previous imaging.

Treatment Options

There is a dearth of high-quality evidence on which to base therapeutic decisions in the management of ILD in the critical care unit. Guidance is largely pragmatic, based on small observational studies, and heavily influenced by anecdotal experience. That being said, a few general interventions are almost always employed in an attempt to treat common triggers. The majority of patients receive early, effective empiric antimicrobial therapy. Invariably, broad-spectrum antibiotics, and often antifungals and antivirals, are commenced while investigations ensue and should be rationalized as more data become available.

Specific therapies for ILD aim to target inflammatory pathways and usually start with high-dose pulsed methylprednisolone, with the commonest regimen being a dose of 1 g given on three consecutive days. Pending assessment of the clinical and radiological response, a maintenance dose of between 0.5 and 1 mg/kg/day of prednisolone (or equivalent) is used. In responsive disease such as organizing pneumonia (Chapter 46), responsiveness is often evident within 5–7 days. At this point, corticosteroid therapy can be weaned to minimize complications and second-line therapies are considered. However, in severe disease, these so-called second-line therapies are often given concurrently with corticosteroids at first treatment as there is a short therapeutic window during which the patient is either free of infection or covered with empirical antimicrobials, during which vigorous immune modulation is feasible.

The most commonly used immunosuppressive agents are cyclophosphamide and rituximab. Intravenous cyclophosphamide, usually at a dose of 650 mg/m^2, offers obvious advantages because of a relatively rapid onset of action (often within 1 week), although it is relatively contraindicated in women of child-bearing age due to the risk of infertility. A further dose can be given as early as seven to 10 days later, white blood count nadir permitting, but it is normally repeated at 2 weeks. Rituximab has a slower onset of action but is considered to have a less toxic side effect profile than cyclophosphamide. Given the lack of robust evidence and the need for a longer duration of support than needed following high-dose steroid therapy (in order to evaluate responsiveness), the use of these agents should ideally be informed through multi-disciplinary discussion integrating ILD or rheumatologic expertise as sub-specialists in these fields, who routinely use both agents outside the critical care setting.

Ventilation, Extracorporeal Membrane Oxygenation (ECMO), and Transplant

When faced with a potentially reversible trigger, an unknown disease requiring investigation or isolated single organ failure, mechanical ventilation often seems an attractive option. However, it is often far from clear that weaning from mechanical ventilation will be possible, even with complete reversal of the acute process. Indeed, evidence from the largest systematic review confirms that mechanical ventilation is strongly associated with mortality, more so with IPF. For mixed-ILD, hypoxaemia and worse acute physiology and chronic health evaluation (APACHE) 2 score are additional poor prognostic factors.[16] Similar issues arise when considering the use of veno-venous ECMO despite the perception that there is a role for ECMO in carefully selected ILD patients where it buys time for immunosuppression to work while preventing injurious ventilatory damage (Chapter 22). More often than not, high flow oxygen, CPAP, or NIV is employed in an attempt to avert intubation. We strongly recommend that prior to these interventions, clear decisions should be made about potential escalation to invasive mechanical ventilation as these may influence an early decision that non-invasive ventilation is likely to fail and critical care intervention is appropriate.

Both invasive mechanical ventilation and ECMO are also seen as potential bridges to transplant for this patient population, but unfortunately transplantation during the acute episode is seldom practicable and less likely to be successful than transplantation of patients with chronic ILD. In a setting of irreversible ILD, with transplantation not achievable, prolonged ventilatory support can become 'a bridge to nowhere', highlighting the crucial importance of

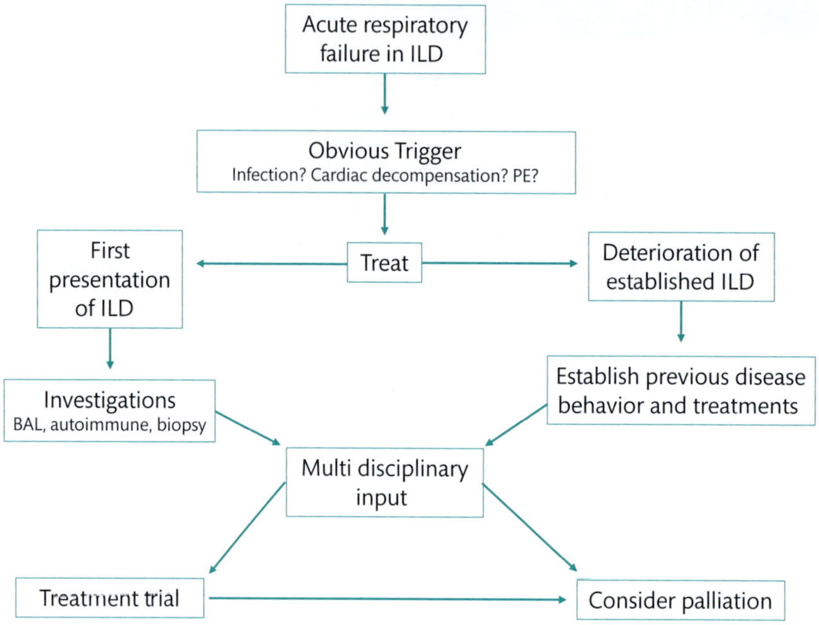

Figure 47.1 An algorithm for the management of patients with interstitial lung disease (ILD) presenting with acute respiratory failure.

multi-disciplinary evaluation as a basis for decision-making in the management of ILD in the critical care unit.[17]

End-of-life and Palliative Care

Despite frequently presenting with underlying treatable causes for their deterioration, patients with ILD requiring critical care input have a poor overall outlook unless there is careful selection of those in whom a good outcome can reasonably be hoped for.[18] Clear and realistic communication to patients, family, and staff is required at all steps of the journey to ensure that only appropriate interventions are undertaken. Ventilatory support allows time for interventions to work, but if there no realistic likelihood of responsiveness to therapy or it is clear that all possible interventions have failed, a switch to end-of-life care with palliation of symptoms as the sole focus is warranted, including the option of treatment withdrawal in the face of futility.[19] Palliative care team input is also appropriate before it is clear that further intervention is futile as this often helps family members to come to terms with the reality of the situation. The multi-disciplinary approach remains key here, integrating critical care and ILD experience with input from palliative care teams experienced in supporting the end of life for patients and families in critical care.[19]

An algorithm incorporating the main considerations of a decision tree is presented in Figure 47.1.

REFERENCES

1. Wells AU, Hirani N. Interstitial lung disease guideline. *Thorax.* 2008;**63**:v1–v58.
2. Kreuter M, Polke M, Walsh SLF, et al. Acute exacerbation of idiopathic pulmonary fibrosis: International survey and call for harmonisation. *Eur Respir J.* 2020;**55**:1901760.
3. Pesenti A, Tagliabue P, Patroniti N, et al. Computerised tomography scan imaging in acute respiratory distress syndrome. *Intensive Care Med.* 2001;**27**:631–639.
4. Pendleton KM, Erb-Downward JR, Bao Y, et al. Rapid pathogen identification in bacterial pneumonia using real-time metagenomics. *Am J Respir Crit Care Med.* 2017;**196**:1610–1612.
5. Stover DE, Zaman MB, Hajdu SI, et al. Bronchoalveolar lavage in the diagnosis of diffuse pulmonary infiltrates in the immunosuppressed host. *Ann Intern Med.* 1984;**101**:1–7.
6. Molyneaux PL, Smith JJ, Saunders P, et al. BAL is safe and well tolerated in individuals with idiopathic pulmonary fibrosis: An analysis of the PROFILE study. *Am J Respir Crit Care Med.* 2021;**203**:136–139.
7. Steinberg KP, Mitchell DR, Maunder RJ, et al. Safety of bronchoalveolar lavage in patients with adult respiratory distress syndrome. *Am Rev Respir Dis.* 1993;**148**:556–561.
8. Kamel T, Helms J, Janssen-Langenstein R, et al. Benefit-to-risk balance of bronchoalveolar lavage in the critically ill. A prospective, multicenter cohort study. *Intensive Care Med.* 2020;**46**:463–474.
9. Potter D, Pass HI, Brower S, et al. Prospective randomized study of open lung biopsy versus empirical antibiotic therapy for acute pneumonitis in nonneutropenic cancer patients. *Ann Thorac Surg.* 1985;**40**:422–428.
10. O'Brien JD, Ettinger NA, Shevlin D, et al. Safety and yield of transbronchial biopsy in mechanically ventilated patients. *Crit Care Med.* 1997;**25**:440–446.
11. Lim SY, Suh GY, Choi JC, et al. Usefulness of open lung biopsy in mechanically ventilated patients with undiagnosed diffuse pulmonary infiltrates: Influence of comorbidities and organ dysfunction. *Crit Care.* 2007;**11**:R93.
12. Poe RH, Wahl GW, Qazi R, et al. Predictors of mortality in the immunocompromised patient with pulmonary infiltrates. *Arch Intern Med.* 1986;**146**:1304–1308.

13. Collard HR, Ryerson CJ, Corte TJ, et al. Acute exacerbation of idiopathic pulmonary fibrosis an international working group report. *Am J Respir Crit Care Med.* 2016;**194**:265–275.
14. Blivet S, Philit F, Sab JM, et al. Outcome of patients with idiopathic pulmonary fibrosis admitted to the ICU for respiratory failure. *Chest.* 2001;**120**:209–212.
15. Flaherty KR, Wells AU, Cottin V, et al. Nintedanib in Progressive Fibrosing Interstitial Lung Diseases. *N Engl J Med.* 2019;**381**:1718–1727.
16. Huapaya JA, Wilfong EM, Harden CT, et al. Risk factors for mortality and mortality rates in interstitial lung disease patients in the intensive care unit. *Eur Respir Rev.* 2018;**27**:180061 [https://doi.org/10.1183/16000617.0061-2018].
17. Ali AA, Hartwig M, Lin S, et al. Bridging to lung transplant: What method and for whom? *Curr Respir Care Rep.* 2013;**2**:173–179.
18. Fumeaux T, Rothmeier C, Jolliet P. Outcome of mechanical ventilation for acute respiratory failure in patients with pulmonary fibrosis. *Intensive Care Med.* 2001;**27**: 1868–1874.
19. Mallick S. Outcome of patients with idiopathic pulmonary fibrosis (IPF) ventilated in intensive care unit. *Respir Med.* 2008;**102**:1355–1359.
20. Truog RD, Cist AF, Brackett SE, et al. Recommendations for end-of-life care in the intensive care unit: The Ethics Committee of the Society of Critical Care Medicine. *Crit Care Med.* 2001;**29**:2332–2348.

48

The Haematological Patient

Nilima Parry-Jones, Jack Parry-Jones, and Matthew P Wise

KEY MESSAGES

- Importance of early involvement of expert haematological and critical care physicians.
- Outcomes from critical illness are related more to reversibility of critical illness than underlying haematological diagnosis.
- Building an experienced multidisciplinary team involving radiology, microbiology, mycology, as well as haematology and critical care with regular morbidity and mortality meetings will benefit patients.

CONTROVERSIES

- A 'therapeutic trial' of critical care should be based upon careful multidisciplinary considerations.
- Should CAR-T therapies only be administered in a critical care environment?

FURTHER RESEARCH

- Critical care databases that track on long-term outcome for all patients with haematological malignancy.

Introduction

Severe sepsis and respiratory failure, frequently treatment-related, are common reasons for referral of patients with haematological malignancy to the intensive care unit (ICU).[1] Historical literature suggested poor ICU outcome for haemato-oncology patients, with up to 90% mortality, leading to the reluctance of some ICU clinicians to admit these patients. The American College of Critical Care Medicine, in their 1999 guideline, recommends 'Immediate Refusal of ICU admission'. More recent data, however, including that from the UK ICNARC (Intensive Care National Audit and Research Centre) database shows improved outcome, with 56.9% of haemato-oncology patients surviving to ICU discharge and 40.8% discharged home.[2] Possible contributors to improvement include better supportive care, less aggressive bone marrow transplant conditioning protocols, and earlier identification of the deteriorating patient with widespread use of track and trigger scoring systems.

Ward-based Assessment of the Critically Ill Haematology Patient

Haematology patients who develop critical illness require timely identification to enable prompt referral of those who may benefit from critical care. Duration of hospitalization prior to ICU admission is an independent predictor of adverse outcome in both solid tumour and haematology patients.[2,3] Among hospitalized patients with haematological malignancy, 7% develop critical illness, rising to 15.7% among recipients of a bone marrow transplant.[4,5]

Fifty-four per cent of patients with haematological malignancy admitted to critical care have severe sepsis as a diagnosis, and 55% require ventilation in the first 24 h.[2] Haematological malignancy increases the risk of sepsis, but can also abrogate some clinical features of systemic inflammation. There should be a high index of suspicion for infection causing critical illness, paying particular attention to the chest and in-dwelling devices: catheter-related blood stream infections are common; early line removal may be required.

Indications for ICU Referral, Information Required at Referral, and the Role of an 'ICU Trial'

The decision to admit a patient to ICU should involve direct discussion between senior clinicians from Haematology and Critical Care. Status of the underlying malignancy, prior treatment, pre-morbid performance status, patient wishes, previously agreed treatment limitations, and reversibility of the patient's current situation should be considered. Where it is not clear whether the patient will benefit from critical care, an 'ICU trial', a concept introduced by Lecuyer et al.,[6] may be appropriate: during a 3-year period, 188 patients scheduled for further cancer treatment or with good performance status were admitted to ICU without restriction, and the level of care reassessed in 103 patients who survived to day 5. It was not possible to distinguish survivors from non-survivors at admission, but requirement for ventilation, vasopressors, and renal replacement therapy, developing after day 3, was associated with a greater probability of death. Survival to hospital discharge was 21.8%.

Immunocompromise and Respiratory Failure

Immunocompromised patients may develop respiratory failure due to infectious or non-infectious causes, resulting in referral to critical care for respiratory support, help with diagnostic broncho-alveolar lavage (BAL) or facilitating imaging (Chapters 18 and 19). The differential diagnosis can be wide. A thorough history, review of previous treatment, and radiological investigations are important, particularly where fungal infection, including *Pneumocystis jirovecii* pneumonia (PJP), is being considered (Chapter 37). High-resolution CT of the chest reviewed by a radiologist with expertise in respiratory disease, microbiological analysis of the distal airways, and echocardiography are key along with consideration of drug toxicity and other non-infectious causes. Close, regular collaboration between senior haematology and critical care clinicians is essential. Infective aetiologies of respiratory failure may include reactivation of latent organisms and newly acquired infection. Duration of immune suppression and neutropenia and vaccination history are important considerations.

Infectious causes of respiratory failure include the following:

1. Community- and hospital-acquired bacterial pneumonia (Chapter 33): Duration of hospitalization and use of multiple antibiotic treatments increase risk of resistant organisms, including *Klebsiella*, *Enterobacter*, and *Pseudomonas* species. Knowledge of local patterns of infection and antibiotic resistance is important.
2. Viral pneumonia (Chapter 34): Influenza A and B, rhinovirus, coronavirus, and adenovirus may be circulating in the community. Reactivation, primary infection, or co-infection with cytomegalovirus (CMV), herpes simplex viruses, and varicella may occur. Selected haematology patients, for example stem cell transplant recipients, are normally monitored weekly for CMV by blood polymerase chain reaction assays.
3. Fungal pneumonia (Chapter 37): PJP infection is associated with immune compromise, particularly where T-cell function is impaired. Patients deemed at high risk of PJP normally receive cotrimoxazole prophylaxis, but breakthrough infection may occur. Aspergilloma or mycetoma may develop or increase in size during periods of immunocompromise, leading to haemoptysis and respiratory failure. Patients most at risk of invasive aspergillus infection undergo weekly fungal PCR blood test monitoring. Galactomannan can be measured in BAL and/or serum to aid diagnosis of invasive aspergillosis. Serum 1,3-beta-D-glucan is also useful. Results should be interpreted in corroboration with clinical picture and expert microbiology advice.
4. Reactivation of tuberculosis (Chapter 38).

Non-infective aetiologies of respiratory failure in the haematological patient include the following:

1. All-trans retinoic acid (ATRA) differentiation syndrome: Timely diagnosis and treatment of the rare acute myeloid leukaemia subtype; Acute promyelocytic leukaemia (APML) is a haematological emergency. Patients with APML require urgent (same-day) induction treatment with the differentiation agent ATRA. APML patients with presenting white cell count $>10 \times 10^9/L$ are at risk of ATRA differentiation syndrome, characterized by one or more of fever, unexplained weight gain, respiratory distress, interstitial pulmonary infiltrates, and pleural or pericardial effusions. Acute respiratory distress syndrome (Chapter 21) may develop, requiring non-invasive or invasive respiratory support. Temporary interruption of ATRA, intravenous dexamethasone, and diuretics may be required. APML can be associated with life-threatening coagulopathy, and blood products, including fibrinogen concentrate, platelets, or plasma may be urgently needed. After a high-risk period for mortality in the first 30 days, APML has an excellent long-term prognosis, with >70% long-term survivors.[7]
2. Leucocytosis: Primitive haematological cells (blasts) are hyperviscous. Patients presenting with high white count non-APML acute myeloid leukaemia ($>100 \times 10^9/L$) and occasionally patients with high count chronic myeloid leukaemia may present with respiratory symptoms caused by microvasculature occlusion by blast cells. Typical clinical symptoms from leucostasis include dyspnoea, hypoxia, headache, somnolence, and eventually coma. Urgent reduction of white cell count with cytoreductive chemotherapy such as hydroxycarbamide, and, in some cases, emergency leucopheresis, are required.[8]
3. Pulmonary oedema secondary to cardiac disease: A cumulative lifetime anthracycline dose equivalent to >500 mg/m^2 of Adriamycin is associated with increased risk of developing cardiomyopathy. Care is taken with treatment protocols not to exceed this limit, but idiosyncratic responses can occur.
4. Pulmonary oedema due to volume overload: It is important to assess volume status in conjunction with cardiac and renal function. A significant fluid volume load may be received as part of the chemotherapy treatment protocol or treatment for PJP with intravenous cotrimoxazole.
5. Primary respiratory disease: Organizing pneumonia (Chapter 46). New onset pulmonary fibrosis (Chapter 47) or pneumonitis may be consequent upon use of bleomycin or other treatments.
6. Haematological disease progression affecting the lung, pleura, or intra-thoracic lymph nodes.
7. Chimeric antigen receptor T-cell therapy (CAR-T therapy) and cytokine release syndrome (CRS):[9] CAR-T therapy is a rapidly developing therapeutic field (Chapter 49). CAR-T is an established treatment in selected cases of B-cell acute lymphoblastic leukaemia and relapsed diffuse large B-cell lymphoma, and expanding to other B-cell lymphomas, myeloma, and beyond.

Autologous T-cells are collected from the patient, and genetically modified in order that, when re-infused into the patient weeks later, they recognize as foreign and kill tumour cells. The CAR T-cell clone expands in vivo after re-infusion, and, in successful cases, circulating CAR T-cells persist. Currently available CAR-T products target the CD19 antigen or B-cell maturation antigen (CD269), both are expressed on B cells, with resultant increased immunosuppression after therapy. However, the indications for CAR-T therapy continue to expand and CAR-T products targeting other antigens are in development and will likely enter clinical use soon.

The majority of patients develop some degree of cytokine release syndrome (CRS) in the 24–48 h after CAR-T re-infusion, resulting in supra-physiological circulating cytokine levels, which may cause capillary leak. CRS is graded 1–4, according to clinical severity. Most cases are mild (grades 1 and 2), requiring only supportive care on the haematology ward. In severe CRS (grades 3 and 4), critical care involvement is required, for the treatment of hypoxia (high-flow nasal oxygen, non-invasive ventilation, or invasive ventilation), and/or hypotension requiring vasopressor support. In addition to cardiorespiratory support, tocilizumab, an anti-interleukin-6 monoclonal antibody may be given for grade 2 CRS, and, in more severe cases, where response to tocilizumab is poor, anakinra, an interleukin-1 receptor antagonist, may be employed along with steroids. CRS has a favourable outcome; patients warrant full escalation of critical care support.[9] Differential diagnosis of CRS should include the full gamut of infections, remembering that these patients are profoundly immunosuppressed and myelosuppressed. CAR-T therapy can also induce neurological complications known as Immune effector cell–associated neurotoxicity syndrome (ICANS) (see below).

8. Check point inhibitors: The programmed cell death-1 inhibitors, Nivolumab and Pembrolizumab, have recently been incorporated into treatment algorithms for relapsed Hodgkin lymphoma. A variety of haematological and non-haematological toxicities are seen, with respiratory toxicities relatively less common, but vigilance for and recognition of organ compromise is required.[10]

While sepsis accounts for more than half of critical care admissions, haematology patients frequently become unwell from non-sepsis complications of their underlying haematological disease or treatment. Examples of non-respiratory organ impairment include the following:

1. Acute kidney injury/renal failure: Use of nephrotoxic agents, hydronephrosis due to compression by large volume abdominal lymphadenopathy or, in myeloma patients, deposition of toxic free light chains in the renal tubules.
2. Tumour lysis syndrome (TLS) characterized by hyperuricaemia, hyperphosphataemia, hyperkalaemia, hypocalcaemia, and acute renal failure: Risk scoring systems help to identify patients at high risk and include those with aggressive, 'high-grade' lymphomas who have large tumour burden (mass > 10 cm), patients with Burkitt and Burkitt-like lymphomas, and patients with acute leukaemia who have white cell count $>100 \times 10^9$/L. Patients deemed at high risk of TLS normally receive the uric acid oxidase inhibitor, rasburicase, rather than allopurinol, for prophylaxis. Spontaneous tumour lysis may occur prior to any chemotherapy being given. Patients at high risk of TLS may be admitted to critical care for close monitoring. Preventative management may include intravenous hydration with loop diuretics employed where there is risk of fluid overload. Supportive care focuses on correction of the metabolic disturbances; hyperkalaemia being the commonest immediate threat to life, but severe hyperphosphataemia may result in long-term renal impairment and severe hypocalcaemia may need correction. Where metabolic disturbance is refractory to medical management, renal replacement therapy is indicated.
3. Metabolic disturbance: Development of severe hyponatraemia may complicate treatment with high-dose cyclophosphamide or bortezomib (Velcade).
4. Neurological complications, particularly seizure-related coma (GCS < 8/15), may be related to primary central nervous system (CNS) lymphoma, to secondary lymphomas spreading to CNS tissue, to metabolic complications, for example, hyponatraemia, or rarely due to direct drug toxicity, for example, methotrexate. Immune effector cell–associated neurotoxicity syndrome (ICANS), graded 1–4 according to clinical severity, may occur in up to 50% of CAR-T recipients following re-infusion of the genetically modified T-cells.[11] Grade 3–4 ICANS requires critical care input, and in grade 4 cases, tracheal intubation for airway protection and management of seizures may be necessary. ICANS tends to develop later than CRS, at 4–6 days, but they often coexist. Risk of ICANS peaks at 7–9 days after CAR-T re-infusion but can present several weeks later. Treatment is supportive, with use of tocilizumab, anakinra, and steroids (dexamethasone or methylprednisolone) in severe cases, to reduce cytokine levels and cerebral oedema. Urgent imaging is necessary, ideally MRI, but pragmatically usually CT. Response to treatment is very good and full escalation of care is warranted as in CRS.
5. Haemorrhage: Haematological malignancy and its treatment are often accompanied by bone marrow failure, requiring blood product support. APML has already been discussed, and APML patients are, in addition to bone marrow failure, at special risk of life-threatening coagulopathy, particularly in the first 30 days.

Special Blood Product Requirements

Some haemato-oncology patients have special blood product requirements, for example, for irradiated or CMV-screened blood products.[12] The hospital blood bank will normally be aware of an individual patient's requirements if they are being treated locally. Extra care should be taken for patients from outside the locality, whose special requirements may not be known. Early liaison with the haematologists and blood banks, before products are given, is advised.

Delivery of Chemotherapy on ICU

Patients with haematological malignancy sometimes present with critical illness at diagnosis, prior to any chemotherapy being given. In a critically ill patient suspected of having a high-grade lymphoma, it is important to obtain histology in order to plan correct treatment. A core biopsy may suffice. Rapidly growing lymphoid tumours may become briskly necrotic when steroids are administered, making subsequent definitive diagnosis difficult. It may, however, be reasonable to treat a critically ill patient with probable high-grade lymphoma with empiric high-dose steroids, for example, methylprednisolone 500–1000 mg daily for 2–3 days, while awaiting biopsy results. Occasionally, chemotherapy is initiated in ventilated patients, following discussion between senior clinicians in haematology and intensive care and next of kin.

Recognition of Futility and Role of Palliative Care

Despite improved outcome for critically ill patients with haematological malignancy, the result in up to 40% of cases is death.[2] Predicting the outcome of critical care support in some patients can be very difficult, and a trial of care may be the best option.[6] Scoring systems are poor at predicting outcome for individual patients. In the short term, reversibility of the critical illness aetiology is more important than the underlying haematological disease.

For some there will be a clear expectation of recovery from critical care, for example, in patients with CAR-T toxicity. Managing patient and family expectations prior to the development of critical illness is a key principle. Recognition and acceptance of futility, when therapy is delaying inevitable death, is important. Critical care is likely to be futile for a patient with poor performance status and where their haematological prognosis makes life-prolonging therapy unsuitable. Recognition of futility and end-of-life management are therefore core skills for both critical care physicians and haematologists. End-of-life management requires clear effective communication between the patient (where possible), next of kin, and clinical teams. A plan for treatment change to palliation and end-of-life care should be documented and may then follow a protocol.

REFERENCES

1. Wise MP, Barnes RA, Baudouin SV, et al. British Committee for Standards in Haematology. Guidelines on the management and admission to intensive care of critically ill adult patients with haematological malignancy in the UK. *Br J Haematol.* 2015;**171**:179–188.
2. Hampshire PA, Welch CA, McCrossan LA, et al. Admission factors associated with hospital mortality in patients with haematological malignancy admitted to UK adult, general critical care units: A secondary analysis of the ICNARC Case Mix Programme Database. *Crit Care.* 2009;**13**:R137.
3. Goldhill DR, McNarry AF, Hadjianastassiou VG, et al. The longer patients are in hospital before Intensive Care admission the higher their mortality. *Intensive Care Med.* 2004;**30**: 1908–1913.
4. Gordon AC, Oakervee HE, Kaya B, et al. Incidence and outcome of critical illness amongst hospitalised patients with haematological malignancy: A prospective observational study of ward and intensive care unit-based care. *Anaesthesia.* 2005;**60**:340–347.
5. Afessa B, Azoulay E. Critical care of the hematopoietic stem cell transplant recipient. *Crit Care Clin.* 2010;**26**:133–150.
6. Lecuyer L, Chevret S, Thiery G, et al. The ICU trial: A new admission policy for cancer patients requiring mechanical ventilation. *Crit Care Med.* 2007;**35**:808–814.
7. Montesinos P, Bergua JM, Vellenga E, et al. Differentiation syndrome in patients with acute promyelocytic leukemia treated with all-trans retinoic acid and anthracycline chemotherapy: Characteristics, outcome, and prognostic factors. *Blood.* 2009;**113**:775–783.
8. Kuo KH, Callum JL, Panzarella T, et al. A retrospective observational study of leucoreductive strategies to manage patients with acute myeloid leukaemia presenting with hyperleucocytosis. *Br J Haematol.* 2015;**168**:384–394.
9. Brudno JN, Kochenderfer JN. Recent advances in CAR T-cell toxicity: Mechanisms, manifestations and management. *Blood Rev.* 2019;**34**:45–55.
10. Delaunay M, Prévot G, Collot S, et al. Management of pulmonary toxicity associated with immune checkpoint inhibitors. *Eur Respir Rev.* 2019 6;**28**(154):190012.
11. Tallantyre EC, Evans NA, Parry-Jones J, et al. Neurological updates: Neurological complications of CAR-T therapy. *J Neurol.* 2021;**268**;1544–1554
12. Foukaneli T, Kerr P, Bolton-Maggs PHB, et al. BCSH Committee. Guidelines on the use of irradiated blood components. *Br J Haematol.* 2020; **191**:704–724.

49

Oncological Aspects of Respiratory Critical Care

Hemang Yadav, Alastair C Carr, and Philippe R Bauer

KEY MESSAGES

- Acute respiratory failure (ARF) is the commonest cause for intensive care unit (ICU) admission in patients with cancer and is often associated with poor prognosis.
- The causes of ARF can be divided into airway disorders, parenchymal lung disease, pulmonary vascular disorders, pleural disease, pericardial disease, and neurologic disorders.
- Given the often-guarded prognosis of respiratory failure in cancer patients, it is important to define goals of care early in the disease course.

CONTROVERSIES

- Airway stents are usually well tolerated, but obstruction or migration can occur and removal can be challenging. Optimal patient selection for stent placement remains clinically challenging.
- In the case of venous thromboembolism associated with advanced cancer, initiation and/or continuation of anticoagulation should take into account patients' values and preferences using a patient-centred approach.
- Although infection is the most frequent cause of acute respiratory distress syndrome (ARDS) in cancer patients, other causes are possible and are difficult to distinguish clinically from infection.

FURTHER RESEARCH

- Who are the oncological patients that would benefit the most from ICU admission?
- When should we implement extracorporeal membrane oxygenation (ECMO) for refractory hypoxaemia in patients with advanced cancers?

Introduction

Acute respiratory failure (ARF) is the commonest cause for intensive care unit (ICU) admission in patients with cancer and is typically associated with high morbidity and mortality. There is a myriad of causes of respiratory failure in patients with cancer (Table 49.1).

Airway Disease

Malignant airway obstruction may be either endobronchial or extrinsic. Primary pulmonary neoplasms are the most common cause of endobronchial malignant obstruction, and up to 30% of lung cancer patients will have airway obstruction at some point.[1] Other causes of malignant airway obstruction include oesophageal cancer, primary mediastinal tumours endobronchial pulmonary carcinoid tumours, and adenocystic carcinoma. Most solid organ tumours can also metastasize to the bronchial tree or to lymph nodes leading to extrinsic airway compression.

Airway obstruction may be central, upper, or lower. Central airway obstruction (CAO) is defined as obstruction of airflow in the trachea or mainstem bronchi. Upper airway obstruction is between the mouth and the trachea, including the nasopharynx and larynx. Lower airway obstruction is distal to the mainstem bronchi and is more typical with chronic obstructive pulmonary disease (COPD), asthma, and bronchiectasis.

The clinical features of central airway obstruction are non-specific, often subacute. The most common symptoms are dyspnoea, wheeze, cough, and haemoptysis and stridor. On examination, patients can have wheezing, which may be unilateral and monophonic if the lesion is distal to the carina. Patients with CAO can often be mistaken for an exacerbation of a lower airway disease such as COPD or asthma, leading to delayed recognition and diagnosis. Often malignant CAO is only diagnosed if there is unexplained recurrent (post-obstructive) pneumonia, a pre-existing suspicion of CAO due to known lung malignancy, or if a patient repeatedly fails to respond

Table 49.1 Causes of respiratory failure in oncological patients

Airway disorders	
Malignant airway obstruction	Endobronchial disease, extrinsic airway compression, and tracheoesophageal fistula
Post-obstructive pneumonia	
Pulmonary vascular disease	
Pulmonary thromboembolic disease	Deep venous thrombosis/pulmonary embolism
Tumour emboli	Tumour thrombotic microangiopathy/ lymphangitic carcinomatosis
Superior vena cava syndrome	
Pulmonary parenchymal disease	
Infective causes	Bacterial, viral, fungal, and atypical (mycobacterial, parasites)
Non-infective inflammatory causes	Radiation pneumonitis, chemotherapy-associated pneumonitis, aspiration pneumonitis, transfusion related lung-injury TRALI
Malignant causes	Lymphangitis carcinomatosis, diffuse non-lymphangitic metastatic disease, diffuse alveolar haemorrhage
Cardiogenic causes	Co-morbid ischaemic, valvular or myocardial disease, chemotherapy or radiation induced cardiac disease: cardiomyopathy, myocarditis, and coronary artery disease
Haemorrhage	Diffuse alveolar haemorrhage, focal pulmonary haemorrhage
Pleural/pericardial disease	
Malignant pleural effusion	
Trapped lung/lung entrapment	
Malignant pericardial effusion	
Neurological disorders	
Encephalopathy	Infectious
	Metabolic
Drug-induced	Opioid/narcotic use
Paraneoplastic disease	Lambert–Eaton syndrome

Source: Adapted from Colice GL, Curtis A, Deslauriers J, et al. Medical and surgical treatment of parapneumonic effusions: An evidence-based guideline. *Chest*. 2000;118(4):1158–1171. Copyright 2000, with permission from The American College of Chest Physicians.

to bronchodilator therapy for presumed lower airways disease. In some cases, CAO can present more acutely if there is acute bleeding or swelling of the obstructive lesion for any reason or if a foreign body compromises an already partially obstructed lumen.

In suspected CAO, patients should undergo computed tomography (CT). This can identify masses causing extrinsic compression, intraluminal defects suggestive of endobronchial disease, and post-obstructive lobar collapse and pneumonia. If the presentation is subacute, flow volume loops on pulmonary function testing can show characteristic features of airway obstruction (Figure 49.1).

If airway obstruction is acute, definitive management should focus on establishing a secure airway and proceeding to bronchoscopy (Chapter 19), without delay. The principles of airway management are outlined in Chapter 20 and do not differ in this setting. Bronchoscopy facilitates direct visualization of the obstruction and should be pursued after a definitive airway is secured. Bronchoscopy can assess the cause of CAO and plan an aetiology-specific intervention. The choice of intervention is primarily governed by the nature of the obstruction and the availability/experience. Irrespective of this, goals of treatment are airway patency and symptom palliation.

While flexible bronchoscopy is typically sufficient, rigid bronchoscopy is preferred for potentially unstable cases with high risk of bleeding. Ablative therapies include debridement, laser therapy, electrocautery, cryotherapy, argon plasma coagulation, and photodynamic therapy. Airway dilatation can be utilized for short stenoses but often does not have as persistent an effect in maintaining airway patency for malignant strictures compared to benign strictures.[2] Airway stents can be utilized to maintain airway patency.[3] Silicone stents are typically better tolerated than metal stents but require rigid bronchoscopy for placement.[4] Once placed, the patient requires daily maintenance nebulizer therapy and may additionally need periodic surveillance bronchoscopy to evaluate for re-occlusion due to granulation tissue or tumour growth, or stent migration.

Parenchymal Disease

Parenchymal lung disease is the most common cause of respiratory failure in patients with malignant disease (Table 49.1). Elucidating the precise disorder is necessary to direct treatment, aid prognostication, and, if appropriate, implement palliative measures.

Respiratory Support

As in other respiratory failure, patients may be too unstable to safely undergo imaging studies or bronchoscopy. In the immunocompromised cancer patient, intubation carries greater risk of worsening respiratory failure.[5] Alternatives to intubation, methods such as high flow supplemental oxygen or non-invasive ventilation (NIV) can be considered. However, failed trials of NIV and unnecessarily delaying intubation may lead to adverse outcomes when compared to early invasive ventilation.

Investigation for Respiratory Failure in Cancer Patients

In cancer patients, it can be difficult to distinguish infective from non-infective parenchymal disease. Focused history can provide clues for aetiology, especially drug and radiation exposures that may explain pneumonitis. The nature of infecting organisms is influenced by the relative suppression of cellular and humoral immune systems, in turn determined by the underlying malignancy and treatments employed. Importantly, the absence of fever or leucocytosis does not exclude infection.

CT can help characterize the nature, extent, and distribution of pathologies in the lungs and vasculature. Review by specialist thoracic radiologists familiar with subtle signs of radiation and infective and drug-related pneumonitis is recommended. Drug-related pneumonitis tends to be more central with peripheral sparing, radiation pneumonitis distributes to the field of irradiation, and infective pneumonitis has a more diffuse, widespread distribution.

Standard laboratory tests such as microbiological testing, complete blood counts, C-reactive protein, and procalcitonin may distinguish between infective and non-infective aetiologies. However, these markers may be elevated by the cancer itself, and infective

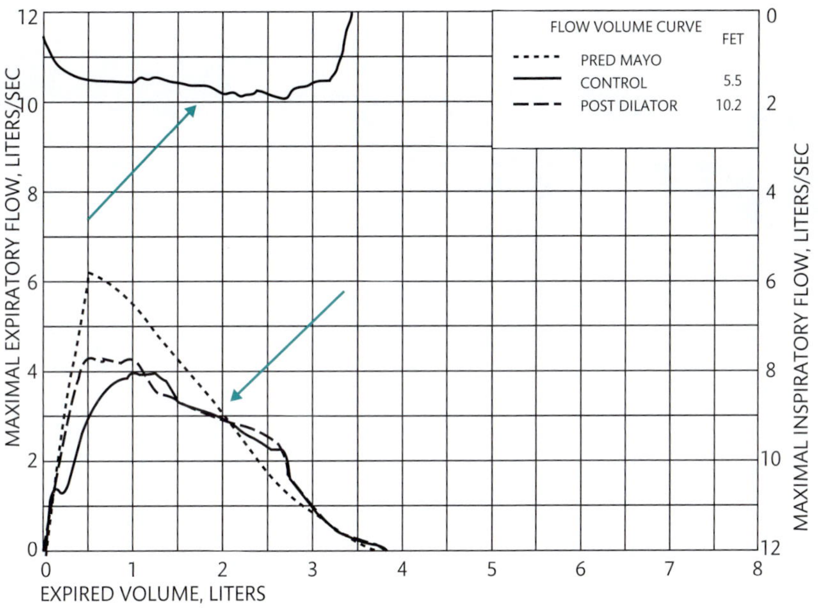

Figure 49.1 Flow volume loops for airway obstruction, showing a flattening of both inspiratory (top) and expiratory (bottom) flow volume curve.

and non-infective parenchymal disease may coexist. In this setting, empiric treatment of infection is typically initiated, and the determination of infection occurs post hoc after evaluating microbiology studies, as well as trends in the clinical course and trends in inflammatory markers.

Imaging can identify appropriate target for bronchoalveolar lavage (BAL).[3] Specimens are examined for micro-organisms, blood cells, and malignant cells (lymphangitis). Polymerase chain reaction amplification of nasopharyngeal aspirate and BAL samples may provide additional insights beyond standard microbiological testing. Immunocompromised cancer patients are more likely to develop respiratory failure from saprophyte organisms. Testing is increasingly available for organisms such as parainfluenza virus, coronavirus, rhinovirus, and metapneumovirus. Fungal organisms are more common in cancer patients, and fungal serology, urine antigen studies, and galactomannan-antigen testing on BAL can be helpful to identify these. Lastly, it is important to get sensitivity data on organisms identified since the high healthcare utilization in cancer patients and antibacterial and antifungal prophylaxis can all predispose to resistant organisms.

Other tests can be considered in specific situations. Wedged pulmonary arterial catheter blood sampling and cytology can be performed to assess for metastatic tumour emboli and lymphangitis carcinomatosis (Figure 49.2). Lung biopsy is occasionally indicated if diagnostic uncertainty remains and is particularly helpful in diagnosing some of the specific non-infective aetiologies outlined in Table 49.1.

Treatment of Parenchymal Lung Disease

Empiric broad-spectrum antimicrobial therapy including antiviral and antifungal therapy where appropriate (neutropenia >10 days duration, significant antibiotic exposure, recent steroids) is commonly started and adjusted as investigations yield results. Disease-specific therapies maybe indicated, for example, steroids, platelet support, and rVIIa in diffuse alveolar haemorrhage. Steroids are also routinely administered during the treatment of radiation pneumonitis and *Pneumocystis jiroveci* pneumonia. Use in other pneumonitis is generally held until infection has been excluded.

Mechanical respiratory support may be required. Supplemental oxygen is offered sparingly to minimize pulmonary hyperoxic injury while maintaining SpO_2 around 94%. In patients previously exposed to bleomycin, lower oxygen saturations (89%–92%) can be tolerated. Extracorporeal membrane oxygenation (Chapter 22) use in patients with cancer has been described in case series but historically has had poor outcomes. Only 4 (21%) of children survived in a 2006 case series. More recently, a 2014 case series of adults with haematological malignancies reported 50% (n = 7) survival to discharge[6], and 100% (n = 3) of the AV-ECMO and 36% (n = 4) of the VV-ECMO groups. ECMO may be appropriate if the prognosis of the malignant disease is potentially good. Further research is required.

Pleural/Pericardial Disease

Pleural effusions in cancer patients can be para malignant or malignant. Para malignant effusions occur where cytology-negative pleural fluid forms in the pleural space as an indirect effect of the cancer (e.g. bronchial obstruction or superior vena cava syndrome). Malignant pleural effusions are due to direct cancer involvement, and the pleural fluid cytology is positive for cancer cells (see also Chapter 52).

Malignant pleural effusions are most commonly diagnosed by pleural fluid cytology, which is positive in around 60% of cases. Of positive results, 65% are obtained on the initial sampling, with 27% and 5% obtained on the second and third samplings, respectively. A third sample does not increase the diagnostic yield further.[7]

Cancer patients should undergo diagnostic thoracentesis if the cause of the effusion is not known or if there is the possibility of infection in a known malignant effusion. Imaging features that

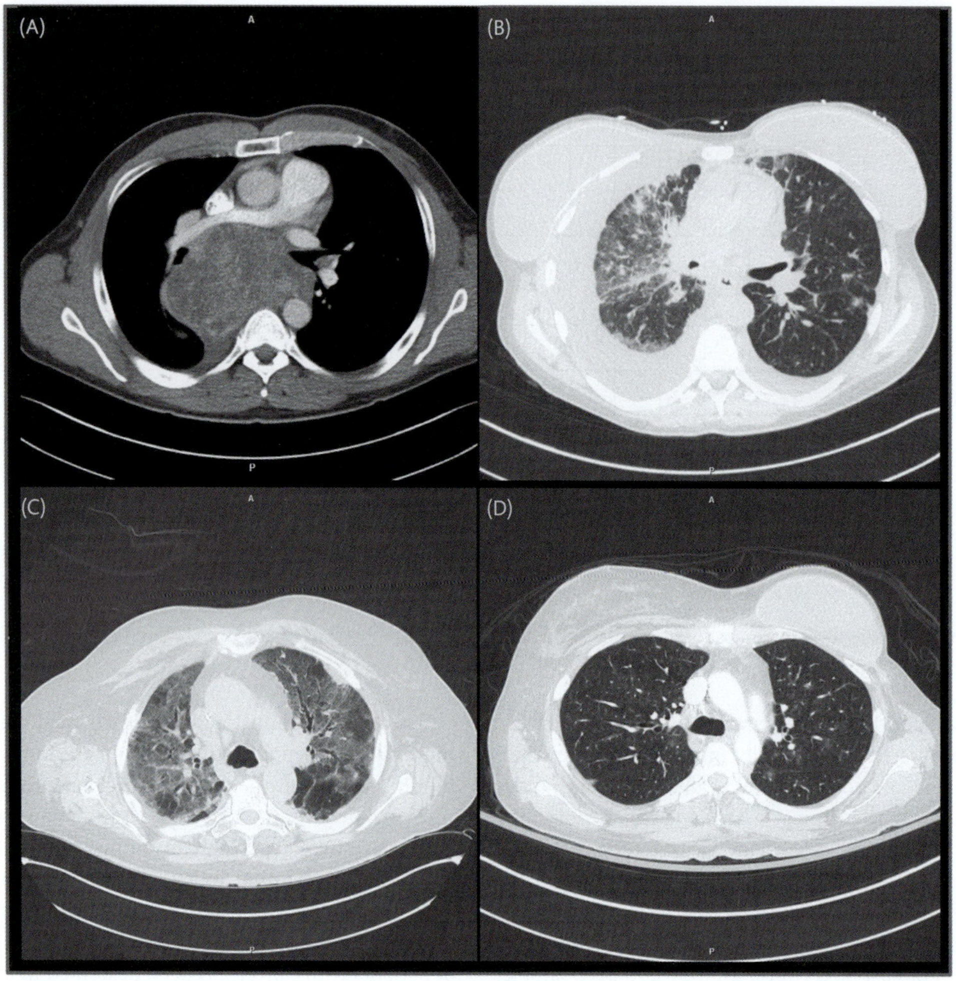

Figure 49.2 Computed tomography imaging of cancer patients in respiratory failure. (A) Top left: Solitary fibrous tumour of the middle mediastinal space causing extrinsic compression and large airway compression. (B) Top right: Lymphangitic carcinomatosis and malignant pleural effusion in a patient with lung cancer. (C) Bottom left: *Pneumocystis jirovecii* pneumonia in a patient receiving chemotherapy for widely metastatic small cell carcinoma of the prostate. (D) Bottom right: Tumour emboli syndrome. CT images show faint bilateral ground-glass opacities in a patient with metastatic breast cancer and hypoxemic respiratory failure. Ventilation perfusion scan was abnormal. The patient had elevated right heart pressures and ultimately underwent right heart catheterization. Cytology from wedged blood showed adenocarcinoma cells confirming tumour emboli syndrome.

favour diagnostic sampling are large size (>25 mm on decubitus film), loculations on ultrasound, and thickened parietal pleura on CT. Therapeutic thoracentesis should be performed if the effusion is large or symptomatic. Re-expansion pulmonary oedema (REPE) is rare complication of thoracentesis. This can be avoided performing pleural pressure manometry and terminating the procedure if the pressure drops below −20 cmH_2O. To reduce the risk of REPE, thoracentesis may be limited to 1.5 L, but this threshold is arbitrary.

Pleural effusions can be uncomplicated, complicated, or infected (empyema). Pleural fluid should be sent for cultures, pH (transported on ice and analyzed in a blood gas analyzer), and cell count with differential and chemistries (total protein, lactate dehydrogenase, and glucose).

An empyema is diagnosed by a positive pleural culture, but cultures may be negative if the patient has already received antibiotics or the causative organism is anaerobic. Empyema will require chest tube placement for adequate treatment. In general, a complicated parapneumonic effusion is more likely to require chest tube placement if the pH is less than 7.20 (Table 49.2).[8] Malignant pleural effusions often have features suggestive of a complicated effusion in pleural fluid studies (pH < 7.20, glucose < 60 mg/dL, and lactate dehydrogenase (LDH) greater than 1000 IU/L) in the absence of infection/pneumonia. Consequently, a coexistent complicated parapneumonic effusion should only be diagnosed in the setting of a compatible clinical picture.

In patients with empyema or complicated parapneumonic effusion where extensive loculations prevent adequate drainage, administration of intrapleural DNase coupled with fibrinolytic therapy has been shown to improve outcomes and reduce the need for surgical decortication.[9] The standard protocol using twice daily 10 mg intrapleural fibrinolytic therapy followed by 5 mg intrapleural DNase reduced total hospital stay by almost 7 days and substantially reduced the need for surgical intervention (odds ratio 0.17; 95% CI: 0.03–0.87). In a malignant pleural infection without coexistent infection, there is little data regarding the use of intrapleural lytic therapy, and current guidelines do not recommend its routine use.[10]

Table 49.2 Features suggestive of poor outcome in patients with parapneumonic effusions

Pleural space anatomy		Pleural fluid bacteriology		Pleural fluid chemistry	Category	Risk of poor outcome	Drainage
Minimal, free-flowing effusion (<10 mm on lateral decubitus)	AND	Culture and Gram stain results unknown	AND	pH unknown	1	Very low	No
Small to moderate free-flowing effusion (>10 mm and <1/2 hemithorax)	AND	Negative culture and Gram stain	AND	pH ≥ 7.20	2	Low	No
Large, free-flowing effusion (≥1/2 hemithorax) loculated effusion, or effusion with thickened parietal pleura	OR	Positive culture or Gram stain	OR	pH < 7.20	3	Moderate	Yes

Source: Adapted from the American College of Chest Physician's recommendations: Data from Colice GL, Curtis A, Deslauriers J, et al. Medical and surgical treatment of parapneumonic effusions: An evidence-based guideline. *Chest*. 2000;118(4):1158–1171. Copyright 2000.

In those patients with rapid re-accumulation where infection has been excluded, an indwelling pleural catheter (IPC) provides substantial symptomatic relief.[11] In randomized trials, IPCs have been shown to have similar efficacy to pleurodesis for the relief of dyspnoea, lung re-expansion, and quality of life.[12] As many as 70% of patients have spontaneous pleurodesis after 6 weeks.[13] While treatment of respiratory failure should not be delayed to facilitate IPC placement, it may be suitable to refer the patient for IPC placement in the critical care setting if the overall prognosis and goals of care are clear.

Pulmonary Vascular Disorders

Common pulmonary vascular disorders encountered in oncological malignancies include venous thromboembolism (VTE), pulmonary tumour embolism (or pulmonary tumour thrombotic microangiopathy), lymphangitic carcinomatosis, and superior vena cava syndrome.

Malignancy is associated with hypercoagulable state. VTE is frequent and may precede the diagnosis of cancer. Although the principles of treatment are the same as non-cancer patients, low molecular weight heparin (LMWH) is the preferred anticoagulant, associated with improved outcomes when compared to unfractionated heparin and warfarin.[10] Recent data suggests that direct oral anticoagulants may be a safe and effective alternative to LMWH in those wishing to avoid daily injections.[14] Duration of anticoagulation after a single event is typically indefinite in the setting of active malignancy.[11] Anticoagulation should not be given in the case of excessive risk of bleeding (e.g. critical thrombocytopenia). In that case, the placement of an inferior vena cava filter should be considered (see chapters 23 and 43).

Pulmonary tumour embolism and lymphangitic carcinomatosis are rare but portend a poor prognosis.[12] The former refers to the presence of cancer cells within the pulmonary vessels, whereas the later indicates the presence of cancer cells in the lymphatics. In both cases, dyspnoea and hypoxaemia are frequent. Pulmonary tumour embolism presents the same clinical picture than pulmonary embolism, but the CT pulmonary angiography is usually non-specific or apparently normal, although a tree-in-bud appearance may suggest the diagnosis (Figure 49.2). Pulmonary hypertension may be present and can be confirmed by right heart catheterization that will also allow blood capillary sampling for cytology. Ventilation–perfusion lung scanning is highly suggestive when showing multiple subsegmental perfusion defects with normal ventilation. Lymphangitic carcinomatosis is often suggested by the presence of thickened interlobular septae on CT in the absence of overt congestive heart failure (Figure 49.2). In both situations, aside from supportive measures, the mainstay of treatment is directed towards the underlying malignancy. There is no place for anticoagulation.

Superior vena cava syndrome can result from the extrinsic compression by the tumour, direct invasion or in situ thrombosis, especially with chronic indwelling catheters. Small cell lung cancer and lymphoma are frequently implicated. Dyspnoea, facial oedema, cyanosis, and venous distension are usually present. A chest radiograph will often detect the malignancy. Duplex ultrasonography and CT chest will confirm the diagnosis. Treatment depends on the severity, histology, and staging of the malignancy. In case of severe symptoms, the priority is the insertion of an endovascular stent, followed by radiation therapy with glucocorticoids or thrombolytic followed by anticoagulation in case of thrombus. Otherwise, staging and treatment of the underlying malignancy is the mainstay of treatment.[14]

Emerging Issues in the Respiratory Critical Care of Cancer Patients

COVID-19 and Cancer Patients

The global COVID-19 pandemic has had a substantial impact on patients with cancer, especially those with lung cancer and haematologic malignancies.[15] Patients with cancer may be more likely to get COVID-19, and those with cancer were more likely to have worse outcomes.[16] The scale of the COVID-19 pandemic also meant there was substantial strain on healthcare systems in regions with high disease burden. This resulted not only in compromised delivery of critical care in patients with COVID-19, but also reduced and delayed access to routine care, including oncological care, for patients without COVID-19 (see chapter 35).

Critical Care Aspects of Chimeric Antigen Receptor (CAR) T-cell Therapy

CAR-T therapy is a form of individualized autologous immunotherapy that represents an advanced treatment option for some patients with leukaemia and lymphoma (see Chapter 48). CAR-T therapy is associated with two unique syndromes that may require

ICU admission: cytokine release syndrome (CRS) and immune effector cell-associated neurotoxicity syndrome (ICANS).

CRS is a syndrome of excessive cytokine release from T-cells, macrophages, and endothelial cells seen in up to 50% of patients receiving CAR-T therapy. Although most cases are mild, associated only with fevers, arthralgias and myalgias, in its most severe form, CRS can be associated with distributive shock and multiorgan failure. If uncontrolled, patients may develop pulmonary oedema, renal failure, and cardiac dysfunction. As such, patients receiving CAR-T therapy must be hospitalized and closely monitored for CRS. Those patients who develop hypotension require vasopressor initiation, and those patients who develop hypoxaemia may require oxygenation or ventilatory support.

Severity of CRS is judged using a grading algorithm that takes into account the need for vasopressor support and supplemental oxygen.[17] Those with more severe CRS (requiring vasopressors or substantial oxygenation/ventilatory support) can be treated with glucocorticoids and targeted anti-cytokine therapy with tocilizumab.

ICANS is a neuropsychiatric syndrome associated with CAR-T therapy. Although it most commonly occurs in the days following CRS, it can also occur alongside CRS or independently in the absence of significant CRS. The key features of ICANS include encephalopathy, speech alterations and apraxia, impairment of fine motor skills, and hallucinations. The most severe end of ICANS is associated with life-threatening cerebral oedema, coma, and seizures.

Again, a grading system exists for assessing severity of ICANS, with seizures, unresponsiveness, and cerebral oedema all considered to be markers of severe disease.[17] Any patient with seizures, cerebral oedema, or unresponsiveness that only responds to tactile stimuli should be ideally monitored in an ICU setting. Patients with more severe ICANS are treated with corticosteroids and given seizure prophylaxis with levetiracetam.

Respiratory/Critical Care Issues Related to Checkpoint Inhibitor Therapy

Checkpoint inhibitor therapy are immunomodulatory antibodies that have substantially improved outcomes of patients with advanced solid organ and haematologic malignancies. The most common checkpoint inhibitors are those targeted against programmed cell death receptor 1 (PD-1; e.g. nivolumab and pembrolizumab), programmed cell death ligand 1 (PD-L1; e.g. atezolizumab), and cytotoxic T-lymphocyte-associated antigen 4 (CTLA-4, e.g. ipilimumab). Unlike conventional chemotherapy, the immunomodulatory nature of checkpoint inhibitor therapy means they are associated with a range of side effects collectively termed immune-related adverse events (irAEs). Checkpoint inhibitors are also uncommonly associated with radiation recall: a phenomenon where an acute inflammatory reaction occurs in previously irradiated areas of lung.[18]

The major respiratory irAE associated with checkpoint inhibitor therapy is pneumonitis.[19] The overall risk of pneumonitis after anti-PD1/PDL1 therapy is around 5%, and risk is increased when combined with anti-CTLA-4 therapy. The median time to diagnosis was around 3 months after initiation of therapy and is earlier in those treated with combination immunotherapy. Checkpoint inhibitor pneumonitis does not have any characteristic radiographic findings and has been associated with a range of CT findings including ground-glass opacities, increased interstitial markings, subpleural reticulation, interlobular septal thickening, and nodular infiltrates. Like other forms of drug-induced interstitial lung disease, the management of checkpoint inhibitor pneumonitis is focused on (i) cessation of the drug in all cases and (ii) a short course of systemic steroids in those with more severe disease. The major consequence of checkpoint inhibitor pneumonitis is often not the pulmonary disease but rather cancer progression as a result of no longer being able to checkpoint inhibitors alongside conventional chemotherapy.

Palliative Care and Advanced Care Planning

The final year of life generally involves disproportionately higher costs, disruption, and clinical interventions than its predecessors. This is especially true for patients dying during cancer treatment who may undergo surgery, radiotherapy, and chemotherapy in the hope of achieving remission or cure.[6]

Cancer patients' preferred place of death varies by country and culture. Despite a majority preference to die at home, most deaths occur in hospital. Patients' wishes may not be known by their treating physicians or unfulfilled owing to uncertainty as to their immediate prognosis when admitted. ICU intervention may reverse respiratory decline and afford opportunity for further oncology treatments, improving overall survival.

Key considerations when oncology patients present with respiratory failure include (i) providing appropriate respiratory support, (ii) rapidly diagnosing the cause of respiratory failure, (iii) treating reversible causes aggressively, and (iv) facilitating ongoing treatment of the underlying malignant process. In certain instances where respiratory failure is not due to active infection, reduced dose chemotherapy may be offered during respiratory support therapies.

Prior to ICU admission detailed discussions with the patient, their family and the referring team are recommended. The overall prognosis, the necessary performance status to allow future therapeutic interventions, and the current performance status should be understood. Cognitive dissonance may be encountered with unrealistic expectations of intensive care to improve performance status. Oncology teams may feel greater pressure to seek ICU intervention in cases of iatrogenic injury, for example, drug-induced pneumonitis.

Honesty about uncertainty in prognosis and understanding of patients' wishes in a spectrum of scenarios from rapid recovery through to development of multiorgan failure is useful. Many oncological treatments are life-prolonging rather than curative. Exploration of options around transitioning to palliative care as an alternative to ICU or within ICU if certain key events occur may be appropriate. Where feasible, patients may choose a high likelihood of a peaceful death at home with family or in the ICU or hospital ward.

REFERENCES

1. Noppen M, Meysman M, D'Haese J, et al. Interventional bronchoscopy: 5-year experience at the Academic Hospital of the Vrije Universiteit Brussel (AZ-VUB). *Acta Clin Belg.* 1997;**52**(6):371–380.

2. Noppen M, Schlesser M, Meysman M, et al. Bronchoscopic balloon dilatation in the combined management of postintubation stenosis of the trachea in adults. *Chest*. 1997;**112**(4):1136–1140.
3. Bolliger CT, Mathur PN, Beamis JF, et al. ERS/ATS statement on interventional pulmonology. European Respiratory Society/American Thoracic Society. *Eur Respir J*. 2002;**19**(2):356–373.
4. Ernst A, Silvestri GA, Johnstone D, et al. Interventional pulmonary procedures: Guidelines from the American College of Chest Physicians. *Chest*. 2003;**123**(5):1693–1717.
5. Bauer PR, Chevret S, Yadav H, et al. Diagnosis and outcome of acute respiratory failure in immunocompromised patients after bronchoscopy. *Eur Respir J*. 2019 Jul 25;**54**(1):1802442.
6. Wohlfarth P, Ullrich R, Staudinger T, et al. Extracorporeal membrane oxygenation in adult patients with hematologic malignancies and severe acute respiratory failure. *Crit Care*. 2014;**18**(1):R20.
7. Garcia LW, Ducatman BS, Wang HH. The value of multiple fluid specimens in the cytological diagnosis of malignancy. *Mod Pathol*. 1994;7(6):665–668.
8. Colice GL, Curtis A, Deslauriers J, et al. Medical and surgical treatment of parapneumonic effusions: An evidence-based guideline. *Chest*. 2000;118(4):1158–1171.
9. Rahman NM, Maskell NA, West A, et al. Intrapleural use of tissue plasminogen activator and DNase in pleural infection. *N Engl J Med*. 2011;**365**(6):518–526.
10. Roberts ME, Neville E, Berrisford RG, et al. Management of a malignant pleural effusion: British Thoracic Society Pleural Disease Guideline 2010. *Thorax*. 2010;**65**(Suppl 2):ii32–40.
11. Tremblay A, Michaud G. Single-center experience with 250 tunnelled pleural catheter insertions for malignant pleural effusion. *Chest*. 2006;**129**(2):362–368.
12. Davies HE, Mishra EK, Kahan BC, et al. Effect of an indwelling pleural catheter vs chest tube and talc pleurodesis for relieving dyspnea in patients with malignant pleural effusion: The TIME2 randomized controlled trial. JAMA. 2012;**307**(22):2383–2389.
13. Tremblay A, Mason C, Michaud G. Use of tunnelled catheters for malignant pleural effusions in patients fit for pleurodesis. *Eur Respir J*. 2007;**30**(4):759–762.
14. Agnelli G, Becattini C, Meyer G, et al. Apixaban for the treatment of venous thromboembolism associated with cancer. *N Engl J Med*. 2020;**382**(17):1599–1607.
15. Wang Q, Berger NA, Xu R. Analyses of risk, racial disparity, and outcomes among US patients with cancer and COVID-19 infection. JAMA Oncol. 2021 Feb 1;7(2):220–227.
16. Giannakoulis VG, Papoutsi E, Siempos, II. Effect of cancer on clinical outcomes of patients with COVID-19: A meta-analysis of patient data. *JCO Glob Oncol*. 2020;**6**:799–808.
17. Lee DW, Santomasso BD, Locke FL, et al. ASTCT consensus grading for cytokine release syndrome and neurologic toxicity associated with immune effector cells. *Biol Blood Marrow Transplant*. 2019;**25**(4):625–638.
18. Shibaki R, Akamatsu H, Fujimoto M, et al. Nivolumab induced radiation recall pneumonitis after two years of radiotherapy. *Ann Oncol*. 2017;**28**(6):1404–1405.
19. Naidoo J, Wang X, Woo KM, et al. Pneumonitis in patients treated with anti-programmed death-1/programmed death ligand 1 therapy. *J Clin Oncol*. 2017;**35**(7):709–717.

50

Sickle-cell Disease

Muriel Fartoukh, Guillaume Voiriot, Aude Gibelin, Julien Lopinto, and Armand Mekontso-Dessap

KEY MESSAGES

- Sickle-cell disease (SCD) is one of the most common autosomal recessive genetic disorders.
- Haemolysis and vaso-occlusive phenomena account for acute and chronic clinical manifestations of the disease.
- Among acute complications, the acute chest syndrome (ACS) is one of the leading causes of death.

CONTROVERSIES

- Does high-flow nasal oxygen (HFNO) improve outcomes in vaso-occlusive pain crisis (VOC) or ACS versus standards of care including non-invasive ventilation?
- Do oxygenation adjuncts for acute respiratory distress syndrome (ARDS) (i.e. inhaled nitric oxide) improve outcomes in ACS?
- Do extracorporeal carbon dioxide removal or membrane oxygenation improve outcomes in ARDS due to ACS?

FURTHER RESEARCH

- Studies to compare optimal antimicrobial strategies and the use of rapid diagnostic biomarkers (e.g. multiplex nucleic acid amplification assays and procalcitonin) for the treatment of ACS are needed.
- Potential therapeutic targets such as HbS polymerisation, erythrocyte sickling, oxidative damage and cell-based therapies, hold future promise.
- Clinical trials are needed for the management and monitoring of individuals with SCD to improve their survival and quality of life.

Introduction

Sickle-cell disease (SCD) is a pleiotropic genetic disorder caused by a mutation of haemoglobin, typically β6Glu>Val, known as 'sickle Hb', namely HbS.

Haemolysis and vaso-occlusive phenomena account for both acute and chronic clinical manifestations of the disease that are mainly related to the polymerization of deoxygenated HbS within the red blood cells (RBCs) and to the subsequent RBC sickling. Associated cellular changes are implicated within a complex network combining surface adhesion molecules expression, vascular endothelial cell activation, haemostasis activation, RBCs, leucocyte and platelet adhesion to the endothelial wall of postcapillary venules, ischaemia-reperfusion injury, and decreased nitric oxide bioavailability[1,2]—all of which contribute to multisystem vascular disease. The clinical spectrum of SCD may encompass extraordinarily diverse clinical phenotypes, among which the haemolytic (haemolysis and endothelial dysfunction) and vaso-occlusive (hyperviscosity and vaso-occlusion) phenotypes are the most characteristic.[1] Ballas et al. have suggested three main categories of clinical manifestations, that is, haematological complications, sickle-cell pain syndromes, and complications affecting major organs, in an attempt to standardize the definitions and the diagnostic criteria. Further to recommend the most appropriate management,[3] the diversity of clinical expression and the complex pathophysiology of the disease both emphasize the fact that every SCD individual cannot be treated exactly the same way. This chapter focuses on the acute clinical complications that may require intensive care unit (ICU) admission, especially vaso-occlusive pain crisis (VOC) and acute chest syndrome (ACS), by highlighting the key points of SCD pathophysiology at the clinical level.

Current Clinical Practice and Evidence Base

Acute Manifestations

The most common acute clinical manifestations of individuals with SCD are VOC and ACS. Acute pulmonary hypertension is common during VOC and ACS, and is a major cause of morbidity and mortality.

Other acute manifestations include acute exacerbations of anaemia (i.e. aplastic crisis, splenic sequestration, and hyperhaemolysis crisis), thrombotic thrombocytopenic purpura-like syndrome, acute stroke, acute renal failure, acute hepatic failure (hepatic

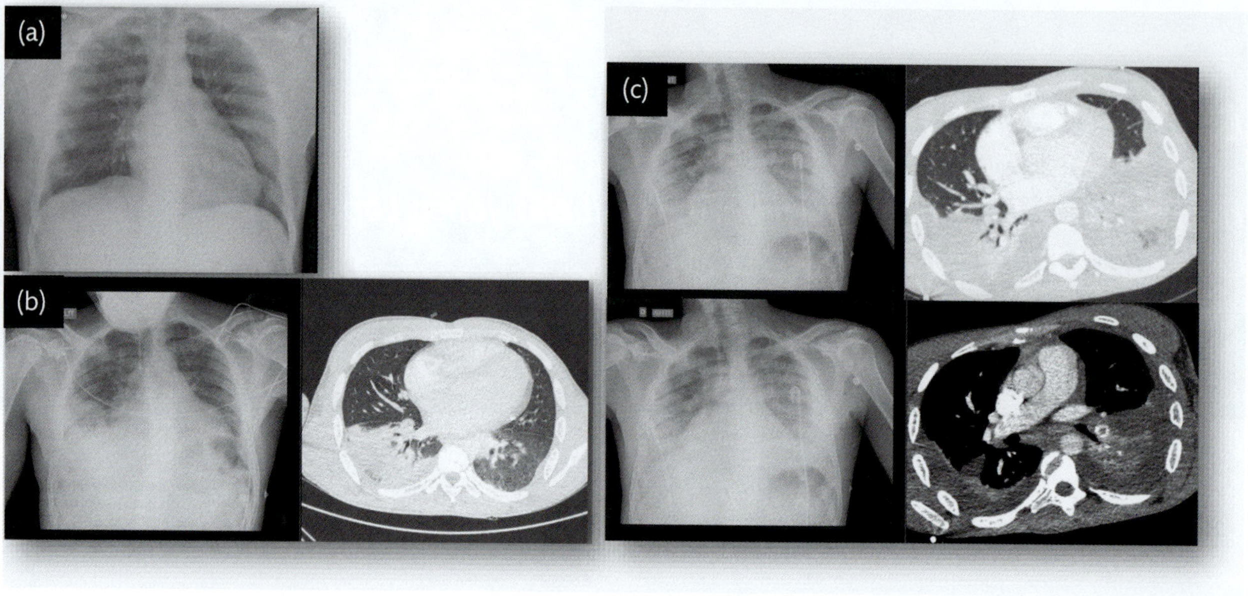

Figure 50.1 From vaso-occlusive crisis to the acute chest syndrome in sickle cell disease. A 25-year-old man with a history of homozygous sickle cell disease was referred to the ED with excruciating back and legs pain. Chest X-ray was normal (A). Three days later, he developed an acute chest syndrome (B). Despite hydration, supplemental oxygen, analgesia, and antibiotics, he was admitted to the ICU 2 days later for acute respiratory failure. High-resolution CT scan of the chest revealed bilateral alveolar consolidation with left pulmonary artery thrombosis (C). Abbreviations: ED, emergency department; SCD, sickle cell disease; ICU, intensive care unit; CT, computed tomography.

sequestration and acute intrahepatic cholestasis), and multisystem organ failure.[4] The range of acute manifestations depends on age; women are particularly at risk during pregnancy.

Worsening hypoxia, increasing respiratory rate, decreasing platelet count, decreasing haemoglobin concentration, multilobar involvement on chest X-ray, and neurological signs are markers of severity and should indicate prompt management and close monitoring in the ICU. SCD patients are at high mortal risk and in need of vital support when they are admitted to the ICU, especially those with a sustained drop in haemoglobin, acute respiratory distress, and acute kidney injury on ICU admission.[5]

The principles of management of acute clinical manifestation are mainly supportive. Recently published guidelines including the National Heart, Lung, and Blood Institute guidelines,[6] the British Committee for Standards in Haematology guidelines for ACS,[7] and the American Thoracic Society guidelines for pulmonary hypertension of SCD[8] may be helpful for clinical practice.

Vaso-occlusive crises are episodic and acute painful events that often have clear triggers in SCD individuals and represent the most common cause of hospitalization.[9] Deep muscle, periosteum, and bone marrow are the most often affected vascular beds. Pain may be very intense and indistinguishable to that of a bone fracture. VOCs should not be considered as trivial events as they may rapidly progress to refractory pain, bone infarct, and/or ACS. VOCs are treated with bed rest, hydration, warm packs, analgesics, and transfusion if necessary.

ACS is a lung injury syndrome with a complex pathophysiology that may involve infection, alveolar hypoventilation and atelectasis, bone infarcts-driven fat embolism, and in situ pulmonary artery thrombosis. ACS is the major critical acute complication, accounting for 70% of the ICU admissions, and is the primary cause of death in adult patients. ACS usually develops in 10%–20% hospitalized patients with VOC, after 2.5 days of hospitalization[5,10] (Figure 50.1). The main risk factors for ACS are young age, high steady-state haemoglobin and leucocyte count, and low foetal haemoglobin (HbF) concentration.[11] The diagnosis of ACS relies on the association of a clinical symptom or sign, for example, chest pain, fever, or dyspnoea usually characterized by rapid shallow breathing, with a new pulmonary infiltrate, typically a lower lobe consolidation in adults.[12] Bedside lung ultrasound outperforms chest radiograph.[13] Therapeutic management of ACS includes pain relief and respiratory support to increase oxygen carrying capacity and favour deeper breathing, and either simple or exchange transfusions depending on the severity of ACS and the haemoglobin level; the goal in severe cases is a reduction of HbS to less than 30% after exchange. Invasive mechanical ventilation is associated with increased morbidity and mortality.

Chronic Manifestations

Chronic complications may affect major organs, for example, brain, kidney, heart, lung, and bone, mainly in adults. They should be managed with prophylactic measures to decrease morbidity, according to the knowledge of the pathophysiology associated with SCD, that is, haemolysis and vaso-occlusion.

Physiology and Pharmacology of VOC and ACS

Some of the main principles of management of acute manifestations are discussed below.

Oxygenation

- *Goal objectives*: Improve alveolar oxygenation and alveolar ventilation; correct risk factors for acute cor pulmonale.

- *Clinical aims*: Closely monitor and maintain pulse oximetry above 95% or within 3% of patient' baseline value; alleviate right ventricle afterload.

SCD can be considered a model of ischaemia reperfusion. Sustained and intermittent hypoxaemia are common and may aggravate endothelial and platelet dysfunction, resulting in red cell adhesion and vascular dysfunction. Whatever the cause of ACS, there is a regional alveolar hypoxia, resulting in hypoxic pulmonary vasoconstriction, mechanical retention of sickle cells, and ventilation–perfusion mismatching.

Supplemental oxygen may partly reverse sickle cells trapping.

Respiratory physiotherapy may decrease ventilation–perfusion mismatching and improve alveolar oxygenation. Mandatory incentive spirometry in hospitalized paediatric patients with thoracic VOC is associated with a decrease in ACS occurrence and in transfusion for ACS.[14] Positive expiratory pressure may be useful in younger children. Conversely, despite physiological benefits (recruitment of collapsed lung, increase in functional residual capacity, and decrease in work of breathing), non-invasive ventilation is not associated with alveolar oxygenation improvement in adults with established mild-to-moderate ACS.[15] The place of high-flow nasal oxygen (HFNO) is unclear, with an ongoing randomised trial for the management of VOC and the prevention of secondary ACS (ClinicalTrials.gov Identifier: NCT03976180).

Invasive ventilation is indicated in patients with worsening respiratory failure despite optimal treatment, falling level of consciousness, or multiple organ failure. Most patients are managed with conventional mechanical ventilation. ARDS due to ACS is characterized by a major pulmonary vascular involvement, with pulmonary vascular dysfunction and acute cor pulmonale occurring in 100% and 80% of patients, respectively.[16] Close monitoring with echocardiography is mandatory especially in the most severe patients.[17] Prone positioning may be useful to alleviate right ventricle afterload.

Inhaled nitric oxide may ameliorate pulmonary hypertension and ventilation–perfusion mismatching, decrease alveolar inflammation, and protect against polymerization of sickle haemoglobin by increasing its affinity for oxygen. Inhaled nitric oxide (iNO) is associated with significant changes in pain scores in paediatric and adult SCD patients with VOC, but with no significant effect on time to VOC resolution.[18–20] The administration of 80 ppm iNO for 3 days did not reduce the rate of treatment failure in adults SCD patients with mild-to-moderate ACS, but a post hoc analysis suggested some benefit in hypoxaemic patients on or off mechanical ventilation.[21]

Extracorporeal membrane oxygenation may be useful in fulminant ARDS.[22]

Future trials exploring the potential role of iNO should select more severely ill patients with hypoxaemia and/or acute pulmonary hypertension. The usefulness of intravenous pulmonary vasodilators, extracorporeal carbon dioxide removal, or membrane oxygenation should also be assessed in this setting.

Blood Transfusions

- *Goal objectives*: Reduce haemolysis, HbS polymerization, and pulmonary ischaemia.
- *Clinical aims*: Maintain haemoglobin around 10 g/dL and decrease haemoglobin S below 30%–40%.

Aggressive chronic transfusion reduces the frequency of ACS and pain episodes.[23–25]

Despite the lack of RCT evidence, blood transfusion is effective and can be life-saving in acute conditions.[26] Two-thirds of patients with ACS will receive transfusions during hospitalization.[5] Clinical signs and symptoms, radiological involvement, and oxygenation parameters rapidly improve with early simple or exchange transfusions.[10,27,28] Simple transfusion and red cell exchange (erythrocytapheresis) are both safe and effective.[29,30] Simple top-up transfusion may be preferred in the case of Hb drop of 1.0 g/dL or more below the baseline value. Simple exsanguination or exchange transfusion may be preferred in patients with high haemoglobin level to reduce hyperviscosity. Indications for transfusion or exchange transfusion include patients with hypoxaemia (Figure 50.2), those with severe clinical features, or with evidence of progression despite initial symptomatic treatment: worsening hypoxaemia, increasing respiratory rate, decreasing platelet count or haemoglobin, multilobar chest X-ray involvement, and neurological signs.[31]

Blood should be sickle negative and completely matched for Rhesus (ABO-identical matching, including A1 status) and Kell. The aims are to maintain haemoglobin close to the baseline value whilst decreasing HbS below 30%–40% in the most severe cases.[6,7] A history of previous red cell antibodies should be sought, to avoid delayed haemolytic transfusion reaction (DHTR) that may be fatal.[32] Several risk factors of RBC allo-immunization have been identified, including an older age, female sex, and transfusion in the acute setting. DHTR may occur from 24 h to 21 days after a transfusion and should be considered in all patients with symptoms that appear or worsen within 21 days of an index transfusion.

Analgesia

- *Goal objectives*: Assess pain severity, relieve pain promptly and adequately monitor tolerance and side effects carefully, and involve specialist pain teams.
- *Clinical aims*: Pain control, deeper breathing, and fast rehabilitation.

Pain control is one of the mainstays in the management of sickle-cell patients. The pain severity and location should be assessed and monitored carefully, using pain analogue scoring scales. Patients with mild or moderate pain should be treated with non-opioid or weak opioid analgesia, including paracetamol (up to 4 g per day), nefopam (120 mg per day), and tramadol (200 mg per day). Patients with severe pain should always be offered opioid analgesia, using an initial titration (e.g. morphine intravenous bolus of 0.1 mg/kg, followed by 3 mg intravenous bolus every 5 min until a correct analgesia is obtained) (Figure 50.3). All patients with VOC and ACS should be given prompt and adequate pain relief. Multimodal analgesia including parenteral opioid-based patient-controlled analgesia is the modality of choice. However, adequate analgesia remains challenging in clinical practice, particularly because of hyperalgesia and opioid tolerance phenomena.

Paracetamol and non-steroidal anti-inflammatory drugs may be useful adjunct analgesics, especially for bone cortex pain.[33] Intravenous corticosteroids may shorten the duration of acute pain

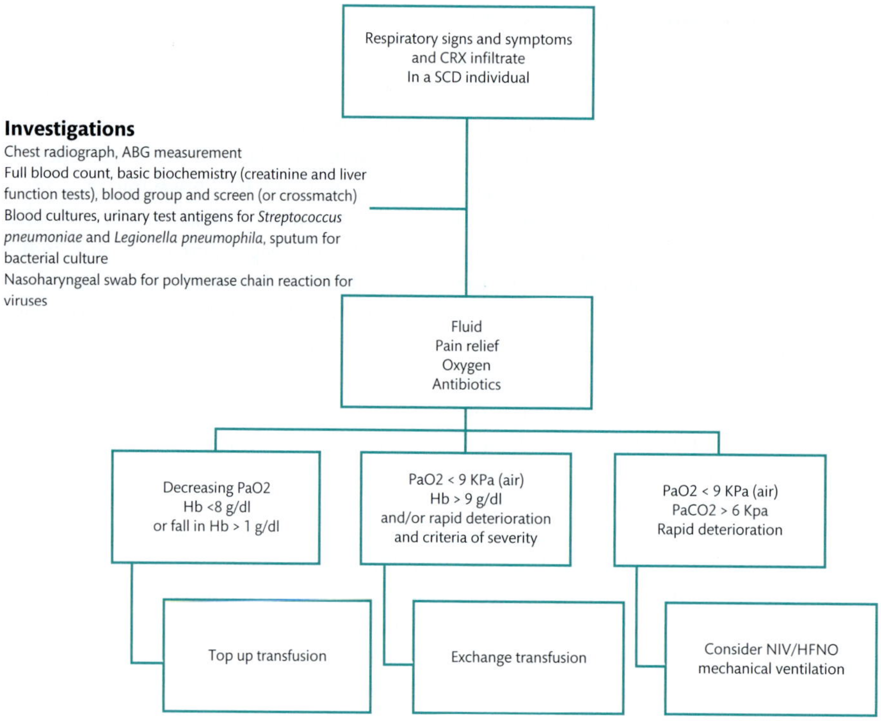

Figure 50.2 Suggested indications for transfusion in sickle cell disease adult individuals.

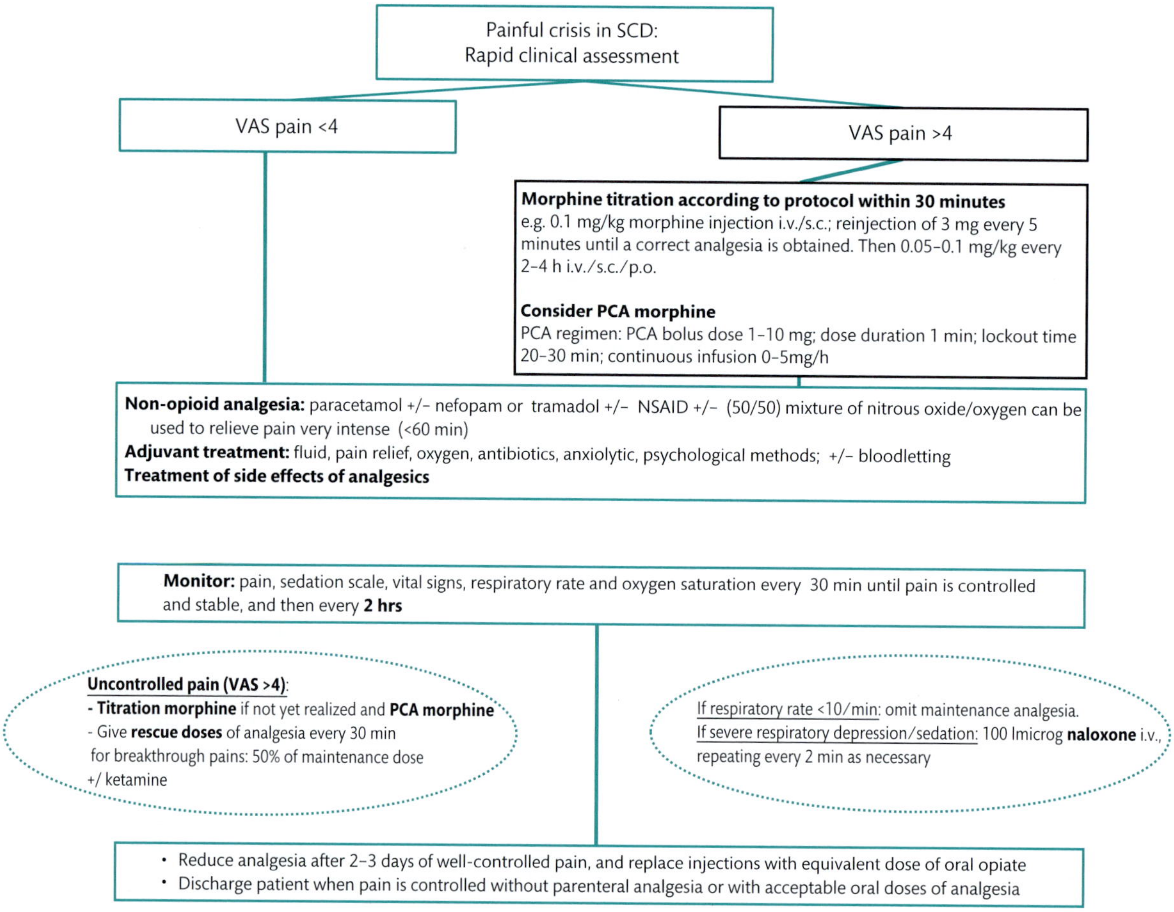

Figure 50.3 Suggested indications for analgesia in sickle cell disease adult individuals.

or ACS but should be avoided because of the high frequency of rebound pain and hospital re-admission.[34,35]

Hydroxycarbamide has no role in the management of an established acute painful episode.

Adjuvant treatment should be associated with the analgesics: hydration, supplemental oxygen and respiratory support, and anxiolytic (e.g. haloperidol and hydroxyzine). Tolerance and side effects of the analgesics should be anticipated, using laxatives (e.g. lactulose), antipruritics (e.g. hydroxyzine), and antiemetics (e.g. prochlorperazine). Respiratory rate, sedation scale, and other vital signs should be monitored carefully.

The use of non-pharmacological and psychological methods of pain management should be encouraged.

The role of ketamine and the use of other morphine derivatives (sufentanil) or techniques of regional anaesthesia should be assessed in uncontrolled acute pain, in combination with multimodal analgesia.

Antimicrobial Therapy

- *Goal objectives*: Use antibiotics with cover for atypical pathogens, even if blood and sputum cultures are negative.
- *Clinical aims*: Identify the microorganism; encourage measures to prevent infection.

There is an increased susceptibility to infection in sickle-cell individuals, especially associated with encapsulated bacterial pathogens. Infection may also induce a cascade of SCD-related pathophysiological changes. Altogether, infection is a significant contributor to morbidity and mortality in SCD, particularly in low–middle-income countries[36] although measures to prevent infection have contributed to improve survival and quality of life of sickle-cell individuals.

In the study by Vichinsky et al., micro-organisms were identified in 38% of ACS, using extensive microbiological investigations, including blood culture, sputum culture, nasopharyngeal swab for viral culture, and serology.[10] The prevalence of respiratory viruses and atypical bacteria was high.

Antimicrobial therapy is traditionally broad, combining a beta lactam and an antibiotic covering atypical bacteria, even if blood cultures and sputum cultures are negative (Table 50.1). Nasopharyngeal swab for viral testing should also be performed if clinically indicated, and anti-viral agents should be used in case of respiratory virus infection.[37]

Randomized clinical trial comparing different strategies for the treatment of ACS should be conducted.[38] The use of biomarkers as an aid for therapeutic decision, such as procalcitonin, should be assessed in this indication. An RCT of multiplex PCR and procalcitonin in this regard is ongoing (ClinicalTrials.gov Identifier: NCT03919266).

Controversies and Future Practice

New promising targets for therapeutic developments, entailing a thorough understanding of the pathophysiology of the disease, have emerged during the past decades (e.g. HbS polymerization and erythrocyte sickling, inflammatory vasculopathy, oxidative damage, cell-based therapies, and treatment of pain and iron overload).[39]

Table 50.1 Suggested antimicrobial regimen for ACS in SCD adult individuals (refer to local microbiology and infectious disease guidelines for specific differences from the suggested regimen)

Acute chest syndrome	
French recommendations[39]	Cefotaxime 1 g tds iv + spiramycin 1.5 MUI tds iv
	Penicillin-allergic Levofloxacin 500 mg bd po/iv
British recommendations[7]	Co-amoxiclav 1–2 g tds iv plus clarithromycin 500 mg bd iv/po Alternative regimen: Ceftriaxone 2 g od iv plus clarithromycin 500 mg bd iv/po
	Penicillin-allergic Ceftriaxone 2 g od iv plus clarithromycin 500 mg bd po/iv If true penicillin anaphylaxis: vancomycin 1 g bd iv plus clarithromycin 500 mg bd po/iv

Source: French recommendations: Data from Archer N, Galacteros F, Brugnara C. Clinical trials update in sickle cell anemia. *Am J Hematol.* 2015 Oct;90(10):934–950. British recommendations: Data from Howard J, Hart N, Roberts-Harewood M, et al. Guideline on the management of acute chest syndrome in sickle cell disease. *Br J Haematol.* 2015 May;169(4):492–505.

Clinical trials are needed for the management and the monitoring of individuals with SCD to improve their survival and quality of life. Recent guidelines[6–8] may be helpful for clinical practice.

REFERENCES

1. Gladwin MT, Vichinsky E. Pulmonary complications of sickle cell disease. *N Engl J Med.* 2008 Nov 20;**359**(21):2254–2265.
2. Noubouossie D, Key NS, Ataga KI. Coagulation abnormalities of sickle cell disease: Relationship with clinical outcomes and the effect of disease modifying therapies. *Blood Rev.* 2016 Jul;**30**(4):245–256.
3. Ballas SK, Lieff S, Benjamin LJ, et al. Definitions of the phenotypic manifestations of sickle cell disease. *Am J Hematol.* 2010 Jan;**85**(1):6–13.
4. Novelli EM, Gladwin MT. Crises in sickle cell disease. *Chest.* 2016 Apr;**149**(4):1082–1093.
5. Cecchini J, Lionnet F, Djibre M, et al. Outcomes of adult patients with sickle cell disease admitted to the ICU: A case series. *Crit Care Med.* 2014 Jul;**42**(7):1629–1639.
6. Yawn BP, Buchanan GR, Afenyi-Annan AN, et al. Management of sickle cell disease: Summary of the 2014 evidence-based report by expert panel members. *JAMA.* 2014 Sep 10;**312**(10):1033–1048.
7. Howard J, Hart N, Roberts-Harewood M, et al. Guideline on the management of acute chest syndrome in sickle cell disease. *Br J Haematol.* 2015 May;**169**(4):492–505.
8. Klings ES, Machado RF, Barst RJ, et al. An Official American Thoracic Society clinical practice guideline: Diagnosis, risk stratification, and management of pulmonary hypertension of sickle cell disease. *Am J Respir Crit Care Med.* 2014 Mar 15;**189**(6):727–740.
9. Ballas SK. Pathophysiology and principles of management of the many faces of the acute vaso-occlusive crisis in patients with sickle cell disease. *Eur J Haematol.* 2015 Aug;**95**(2):113–123.
10. Vichinsky EP, Neumayr LD, Earles AN, et al. Causes and outcomes of the acute chest syndrome in sickle cell disease. National Acute Chest Syndrome Study Group. *N Engl J Med.* 2000 Jun 22;**342**(25):1855–1865.

11. Castro O, Brambilla DJ, Thorington B, et al. The acute chest syndrome in sickle cell disease: Incidence and risk factors. The Cooperative Study of Sickle Cell Disease. *Blood.* 1994 Jul 15;**84**(2):643–649.
12. Mekontso-Dessap A, Deux JF, Habibi A, et al. Lung imaging during acute chest syndrome in sickle cell disease: Computed tomography patterns and diagnostic accuracy of bedside chest radiograph. *Thorax.* 2014 Feb;**69**(2):144–151.
13. Razazi K, Deux JF, de PN, et al. Bedside lung ultrasound during acute chest syndrome in sickle cell disease. *Medicine (Baltimore).* 2016 Feb;**95**(7):e2553.
14. Bellet PS, Kalinyak KA, Shukla R, et al. Incentive spirometry to prevent acute pulmonary complications in sickle cell diseases. *N Engl J Med.* 1995 Sep 14;**333**(11):699–703.
15. Fartoukh M, Lefort Y, Habibi A, et al. Early intermittent non-invasive ventilation for acute chest syndrome in adults with sickle cell disease: A pilot study. *Intensive Care Med.* 2010 Aug;**36**(8):1355–1362.
16. Cecchini J, Boissier F, Gibelin A, et al. Pulmonary vascular dysfunction and cor pulmonale during acute respiratory distress syndrome in sicklers. *Shock.* 2016 Oct;**46**(4):358–364.
17. Mekontso DA, Leon R, Habibi A, et al. Pulmonary hypertension and cor pulmonale during severe acute chest syndrome in sickle cell disease. *Am J Respir Crit Care Med.* 2008 Mar 15;**177**(6):646–653.
18. Gladwin MT, Kato GJ, Weiner D, et al. Nitric oxide for inhalation in the acute treatment of sickle cell pain crisis: A randomized controlled trial. *JAMA.* 2011 Mar 2;**305**(9):893–902.
19. Head CA, Swerdlow P, McDade WA, et al. Beneficial effects of nitric oxide breathing in adult patients with sickle cell crisis. *Am J Hematol.* 2010 Oct;**85**(10):800–802.
20. Weiner DL, Hibberd PL, Betit P, et al. Preliminary assessment of inhaled nitric oxide for acute vaso-occlusive crisis in pediatric patients with sickle cell disease. *JAMA.* 2003 Mar 5;**289**(9):1136–1142.
21. Maitre B, Djibre M, Katsahian S, et al. Inhaled nitric oxide for acute chest syndrome in adult sickle cell patients: A randomized controlled study. *Intensive Care Med.* 2015 Dec;**41**(12):2121–2129.
22. Medoff BD, Shepard JA, Smith RN, et al. Case records of the Massachusetts General Hospital. Case 17-2005. A 22-year-old woman with back and leg pain and respiratory failure. *N Engl J Med.* 2005 Jun 9;**352**(23):2425–2434.
23. Adams RJ, McKie VC, Hsu L, et al. Prevention of a first stroke by transfusions in children with sickle cell anemia and abnormal results on transcranial Doppler ultrasonography. *N Engl J Med.* 1998 Jul 2;**339**(1):5–11.
24. DeBaun MR, Gordon M, McKinstry RC, et al. Controlled trial of transfusions for silent cerebral infarcts in sickle cell anemia. *N Engl J Med.* 2014 Aug 21;**371**(8):699–710.
25. Miller ST, Wright E, Abboud M, et al. Impact of chronic transfusion on incidence of pain and acute chest syndrome during the Stroke Prevention Trial (STOP) in sickle-cell anemia. *J Pediatr.* 2001 Dec;**139**(6):785–789.
26. Alhashimi D, Fedorowicz Z, Alhashimi F, et al. Blood transfusions for treating acute chest syndrome in people with sickle cell disease. *Cochrane Database Syst Rev.* 2016;**8**:CD007843.
27. Emre U, Miller ST, Rao SP, et al. Alveolar-arterial oxygen gradient in acute chest syndrome of sickle cell disease. *J Pediatr.* 1993 Aug;**123**(2):272–275.
28. Emre U, Miller ST, Gutierez M, et al. Effect of transfusion in acute chest syndrome of sickle cell disease. *J Pediatr.* 1995 Dec;**127**(6):901–904.
29. Saylors RL, Watkins B, Saccente S, et al. Comparison of automated red cell exchange transfusion and simple transfusion for the treatment of children with sickle cell disease acute chest syndrome. *Pediatr Blood Cancer.* 2013 Dec 1;**60**(12):1952–1956.
30. Velasquez MP, Mariscalco MM, Goldstein SL, et al. Erythrocytapheresis in children with sickle cell disease and acute chest syndrome. *Pediatr Blood Cancer.* 2009 Dec 1;**53**(6):1060–1063.
31. Rees DC, Williams TN, Gladwin MT. Sickle-cell disease. *Lancet.* 2010 Dec 11;**376**(9757):2018–2031.
32. Habibi A, Mekontso-Dessap A, Guillaud C, et al. Delayed hemolytic transfusion reaction in adult sickle-cell disease: Presentations, outcomes and treatments of 99 referral center episodes. *Am J Hematol.* 2016 Oct;**91**(10):989–994.
33. Bartolucci P, El MT, Roudot-Thoraval F, et al. A randomized, controlled clinical trial of ketoprofen for sickle-cell disease vaso-occlusive crises in adults. *Blood.* 2009 Oct 29;**114**(18):3742–3747.
34. Bernini JC, Rogers ZR, Sandler ES, et al. Beneficial effect of intravenous dexamethasone in children with mild to moderately severe acute chest syndrome complicating sickle cell disease. *Blood.* 1998 Nov 1;**92**(9):3082–3089.
35. Platt OS. Sickle cell anemia as an inflammatory disease. *J Clin Invest.* 2000 Aug;**106**(3):337–338.
36. Booth C, Inusa B, Obaro SK. Infection in sickle cell disease: A review. *Int J Infect Dis.* 2010 Jan;**14**(1):e2–e12.
37. Lopinto J, Elabbadi A, Gibelin A. Infectious aetiologies of severe acute chest syndrome in sickle-cell adult patients, combining conventional microbiological tests and respiratory multiplex PCR. *Sci Rep.* 2021;**11**:4837.
38. Marti-Carvajal AJ, Conterno LO, Knight-Madden JM. Antibiotics for treating acute chest syndrome in people with sickle cell disease. *Cochrane Database Syst Rev.* 2019 Sep 18;**9**:CD006110.
39. Archer N, Galacteros F, Brugnara C. 2015 Clinical trials update in sickle cell anemia. *Am J Hematol.* 2015 Oct;**90**(10):934–950.

51

Neuromuscular Disease

Michael I Polkey

KEY MESSAGES

- Neuromuscular weakness should be considered when measured airway pressures and inspired oxygen fraction are low in a mechanically ventilated patient.
- Neuromuscular weakness is common in patients with prolonged intensive care unit (ICU) stays but may also be a cause of admission to ICU.
- Clues to pre-existing neuromuscular weakness may include prior orthopnoea, aspiration, dysarthria, or weakness of the limbs.
- Respiratory failure can be anticipated in patients with known neuromuscular disease using simple bedside measurements; depending on the underlying diagnosis, the identification of respiratory muscle weakness should prompt a discussion about advanced care planning.

CONTROVERSIES

- What should the role of long-term home tracheostomy ventilation be in chronic neuromuscular disease?

FURTHER RESEARCH

- What is the optimal therapeutic approach to expiratory muscle weakness?
- Is there any therapeutic role for diaphragm pacing in ICU-acquired diaphragm weakness?

Introduction

Weakness of skeletal muscle may diminish quality of life in numerous ways, but respiratory muscle (which is histologically and physiologically identical to other skeletal muscles) has a particular relevance to the need or otherwise for mechanical ventilation. In particular, adequate functioning of the inspiratory muscle pump is necessary to maintain blood gas homeostasis, while expiratory muscle weakness may also lead to difficulty expectorating and thus sputum clearance. Sputum expectoration is maximized when bulbar function is good; conversely, bulbar dysfunction is associated with aspiration of food and saliva.

Diverse neurological conditions may lead to respiratory difficulties and inevitably, when most severe, to a need for critical care. Physiologically, this is most straightforward where either muscle or lower motor neurons only are involved (e.g. in Guillain-Barré syndrome, GBS). The picture may be complex when there are coordination problems—for example, in Parkinson's disease, or where there is cognitive impairment as in the fronto-temporal variant of amyotrophic lateral sclerosis (ALS). Neurological disease also frequently develops as a complication of intensive care unit (ICU) care; generalized muscle weakness, termed ICU-acquired muscle weakness (ICUAW), occurs in the majority of patients with a prolonged ICU admission but does not in itself cause ventilator dependency, whereas acquired inspiratory muscle weakness does.

Physiology

Normal inspiration occurs by contraction of the diaphragm and other inspiratory muscles, and muscle shortening causes expansion of the thoracic cage and hence this causes the intrathoracic pressure to become increasingly sub-atmospheric, inspiratory airflow where the mouth is open (see also Chapter 2). Conversely, expiration is, at rest in normal humans, a passive process although the expiratory muscles are recruited during exercise and where there is respiratory distress. The respiratory muscles have a dual control; a direct corticospinal pathway exists which is used during voluntary manoeuvres, including tests of inspiratory muscle function. During normal spontaneous respiration, and especially during sleep, ventilation is controlled from the brainstem where it is very much influenced by chemical factors particularly hypoxia and hypercapnia. The brainstem drive to breath is reduced by sleep and the administration of various sedative, analgesic, and anaesthetic agents. The load on the respiratory system is also increased during sleep if there is narrowing of the upper airway as is the case in obstructive sleep apnoea,[1] which is increasing in prevalence as obesity becomes more common (Chapter 54). Aside from weakness, various physiological factors may diminish the functional outputs of the respiratory muscle pump:

(a) *Lung volume*: Hyperinflation reduces the proportion of the diaphragm's tension generation that is transmitted to the thoracic cavity and consequently the negative pressure that can be generated within it. This is seldom a problem in neuromuscular disease but may occur as a consequence of coexistent obstructive lung disease.
(b) *Fatigue*: It was at one time considered that fatigue (i.e. a transient and recoverable loss of tension generating capacity) of the respiratory muscles would contribute to weaning difficulty. However, the advent of phrenic nerve stimulation has enabled this hypothesis to be tested in vivo, and it transpires that, while diaphragm weakness is common in ICU patients with a prolonged admission,[2,3] fatigue itself does not develop during a weaning effort.[4]

Respiratory failure is the consequence of respiratory muscle weakness; since ventilation is maintained almost exclusively by the diaphragm during rapid eye movement (REM) sleep, hypoventilation is normally first evident during sleep (Figure 51.1), unless brainstem adaptation occurs, permitting activation of non-diaphragmatic muscles during REM.[5] As disease progresses, blunting of the hypercapnic respiratory drive occurs, and daytime hypercapnia ensues.[6]

Precipitating Diseases

Pre-existing Neurological Disease

An exhaustive list of neurological disease causing ventilator dependency is beyond the scope of this chapter, and it is more useful to consider conditions both as a function of their neurology, speed of onset, and potential for reversibility with therapy; more details may be found in ref. [7]. It is also important to consider regional differences; most notably envenomation is almost unheard of in the UK but can be a major public health problem in some countries.[8] An overview of neurological conditions causing respiratory failure is given in Table 51.1.

Acute weakness of muscle origin which is sufficiently profound to cause respiratory failure is uncommon in the context of severe multisystem illness but can occur with hypokalaemia, especially where there are co-morbidities. Conversely, type II respiratory failure is an almost inevitable consequence of muscular dystrophies[9]; however, in these cases, the diaphragm is seldom the first muscle involved. In current practice, respiratory muscle function is monitored ensuring non-invasive ventilatory support is initiated in a timely fashion as part of a holistic package of care (see Chapter 65). Adult onset Pompe's disease, however, commonly presents with the first symptoms arising in the respiratory system[10] and thus may first present to a respiratory physician although invasive ventilation in an undiagnosed patient for this reason is very unusual. Identification of Pompe's disease can easily be done with an α-glucosidase blood spot and is relevant since enzyme replacement therapy is now available.[11]

Semi-acute presentation of respiratory failure with either Lambert-Eaton syndrome (in association with underlying malignancy) or myasthenia gravis is well recognized. Numerous medicines can precipitate a myasthenic crisis in a patient receiving pyridostigmine therapy, and this should be considered whenever such a patient experiences unexpected deterioration.

GBS is perhaps the most common example of acute neuropathic respiratory failure; typically, weakness begins in the extremities but may ascend rapidly so close monitoring (see below) of respiratory muscle function is essential; nevertheless, respiratory muscle weakness in the absence of limb symptoms does not occur. Motor neurone disease (MND) progresses more slowly, but in 3% of cases MND presents with the first disease group involved being the diaphragm. Such patients may present to a chest physician and occasionally require intubation before a diagnosis is reached.[12]

Ventilator-induced Diaphragm Dysfunction (VIDD)

ICUAW is a well-recognized phenomenon that is now usually considered both a myopathy and a neuropathy[13,14]; patients with ICUAW have longer hospital stays and spend longer in ICU.[15] However, respiratory muscle involvement, VIDD, is to some extent a controversial area; it is relatively easy to obtain functional and histological evidence of diaphragm disease in animal models,

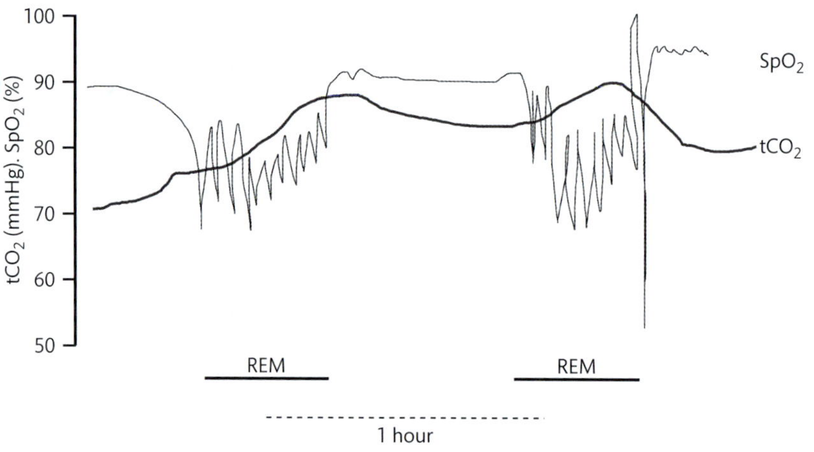

Figure 51.1 Representation of a recording from a patient showing arterial haemoglobin oxygen saturation (SaO_2) and transcutaneous carbon dioxide (tCO_2). Desaturation in REM sleep and hypercapnia are shown.
Image courtesy of Prof S Singh.

Table 51.1 Some neurological conditions associated with respiratory failure

	Muscle	Neuromuscular junction	Nerve	CNS (often associated with aspiration)
Acute (days)	Hypokalaemia Periodic paralysis	Myasthenic crisis	Guillain-Barré Acute polio Envenomation and toxins Organophosphates	Delirium Encephalitis
Chronic (weeks or months)	Muscular Dystrophies Polymyositis Pompe's disease Myotonic dystrophy	Myasthenia gravis Lambert-Eaton	Motor neurone disease Lyme disease IGG4 disease Prior polio Iatrogenic phrenic nerve damage Multifocal motor neuropathy Hereditary motor sensory neuropathy (Charcot-Marie-Tooth)	Parkinson's Dementia

Notes: Myotonic dystrophy has been placed in the muscle column because the respiratory effects are mainly mediated through muscle albeit with a central component although myotonic dystrophy is of course a multisystem disease.[27]

but such models may involve periods of controlled mechanical ventilation, and even very small amounts of spontaneous ventilation may attenuate the effect.[16] Further evidence supporting VIDD has been obtained from biopsy specimens obtained from humans, but it should be noted that these patients were brain dead and therefore effectively suffering an extreme form of denervation in addition to ICUAW. Moreover, in several studies, when diaphragm strength has been assessed by the effort-independent technique of magnetic nerve stimulation, the majority of patients have lower values than are observed in healthy adults.[2,3,17–19]

Identifying Respiratory Muscle Weakness

As noted above, respiratory muscle activity may be measured by electrical activity (electromyography, EMG), pressure measurement, or volume of air resulting from the activity. However, in practice, EMG, while of potential value for identifying the site of a neurophysiological defect, is of limited value in the day-to-day management of patients with neurological disease. This is because the techniques require specialist knowledge for accurate application but also because the outputs have a loose relationship with function.

Flow/volume measurements are widely used to assess respiratory muscle function, but of course are of little value where the patient is receiving continuous mechanical ventilation. The vital capacity (VC), however, is widely used to monitor patients with GBS and patients with chronic conditions such as ALS and the muscular dystrophies; the VC is possibly more valuable in GBS where a falling VC indicates respiratory muscle involvement and may be observed in a short space of time (a drop >30% is typically considered clinically relevant). However, in more slowly progressive disorders such as MND, the VC may not be a reliable guide to inspiratory muscle strength, perhaps because of the curvilinear shape of the pressure–volume curve of the lung.[20] Of note, in a pooled analysis of several ALS trials, intubation was required in a small but clinically significant number of patients with a VC greater than 50% predicted.[21]

Consequently, there is increasing interest in assessing inspiratory muscle strength as pressure. The background to this approach is the observation that oesophageal (i.e. pleural) pressure falls during a maximum inspiratory effort or indeed during a sniff. In the absence of glottic closure, this pressure may be measured in the upper airway as maximal inspiratory mouth pressure or maximal sniff nasal inspiratory pressure (SNIP). Sniff pressures are a more accurate predictor of hypercapnia[22] and survival[23] in MND than VC (Figure 51.2), and SNIP can now be easily measured using inexpensive handheld equipment. Airway pressure can also be measured in intubated or tracheostomized patients as negative inspiratory force (NIF) if the airway is transiently occluded, and many modern ICU ventilators offer this measurement as standard; however, the validity of the measurement relies on the subject making a maximal voluntary effort which is particularly hard to ensure in an ICU patient. Perhaps for this reason, NIF (as this manoeuvre is often termed) has wide interobserver variation in the ICU. In specialized centres, this may be overcome by measuring either the twitch transdiaphragmatic pressure (Tw Pdi) or mouth pressure (Tw Pmo) elicited by supramaximal magnetic stimulation of the phrenic nerves. A detailed description of this technique may be found elsewhere.[24]

Expiratory muscle function may be assessed as maximal static expiratory mouth pressure, cough gastric pressure, or cough peak flow[25]; a cough peak flow of 160 L/min or an MEP <40 cmH_2O has been recommended as a threshold below which the use of mechanical insufflation/exsufflation should be considered.[25] (Figure 51.3).

Management

The management of respiratory muscle weakness may be considered in the areas outlined below. However, in general, the management of the respiratory muscle weakness is the same as the management of the underlying condition (e.g. plasmapheresis in the case of Guillain-Barré); sadly, many of these conditions have no specific treatment, emphasizing the need for careful considerations of ceilings of care. Furthermore, while various anabolic drugs are in development, there is no medicine currently approved for use in this context.

General management principles may be considered as follows:

(a) Optimize nutrition and minimize other factors that may cause neurotoxicity (e.g. reduce use of neuromuscular blockade);

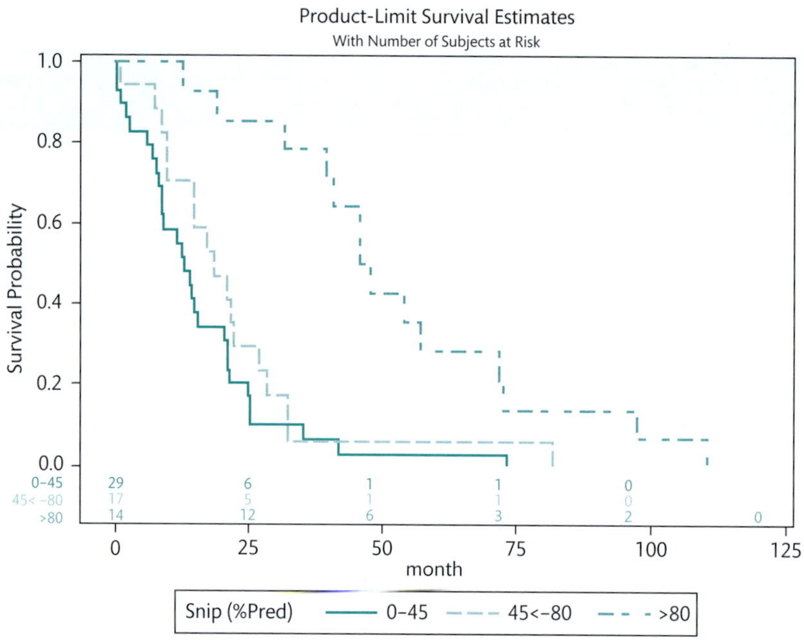

Figure 51.2 Kaplan Mier curves for survival of patients with ALS as a function of maximal sniff nasal inspiratory pressure.

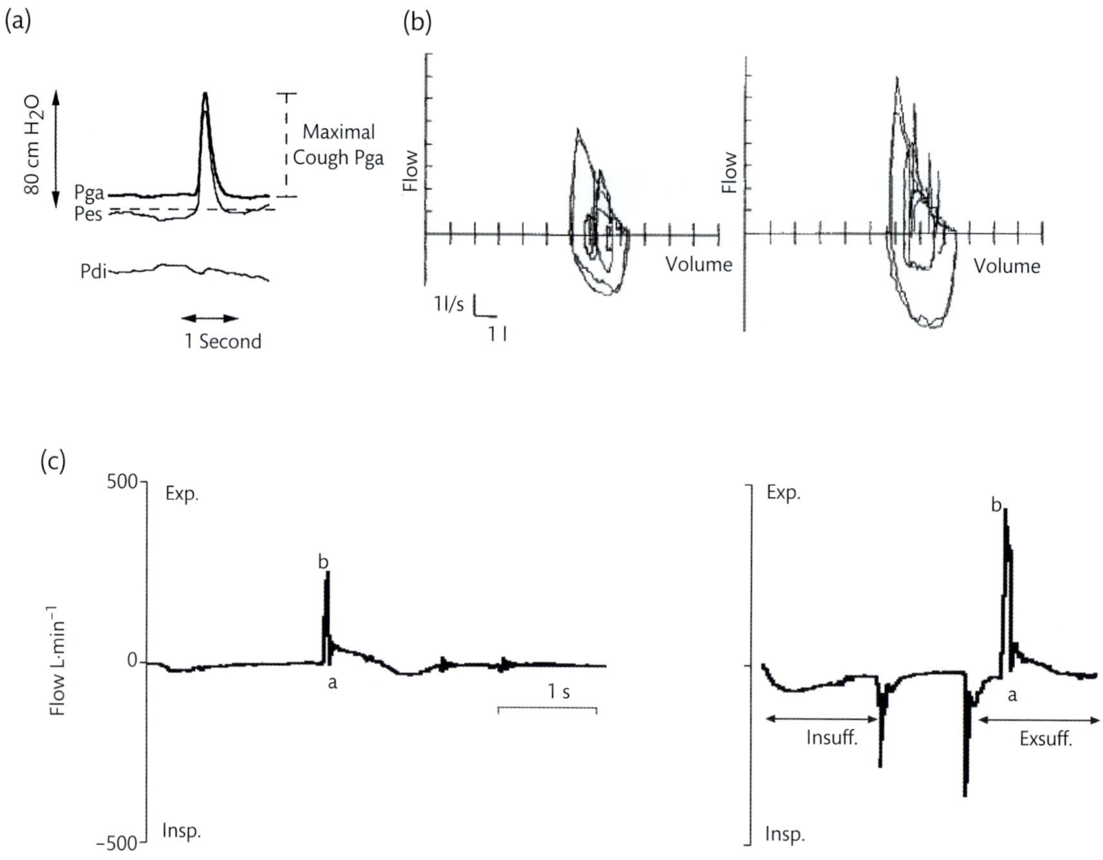

Figure 51.3 Cough in neuromuscular disease: (a) normal cough is associated with a sharp rise in gastric and oesophageal pressure which when strong enough is able to generate transient supramaximal flow; these flow transients are considered important for the shearing forces that contribute to transport of mucus up the bronchial tree. In (b), we see two patients with MND; the left hand one is unable to cough strongly enough to generate supramaximal flow but the right one is. The threshold for being able to do so is a cough gastric pressure >50 cmH_2O.

however, this practice is usual in modern ICUs, offering little additional scope for benefit.

(b) Allow as much spontaneous respiration as possible; even brief periods where the patient has to initiate respiration supported by pressure support or via neutrally adjusted ventilator assist (NAVA) might, based on animal data, attenuate VIDD compared to fully controlled ventilation.

(c) Make maximal use of insufflation–exsufflation and physiotherapy to facilitate adequate expectoration without the use of tracheostomy suction.

(d) Inspiratory muscle training may be considered, but the evidence for this technique is generally of poor quality, especially in the ICU.[26]

(e) Encourage mobilization on the ventilator with physiotherapy assistance.

(f) Reduce additional burdens on the respiratory muscle pump; beyond standard interventions (e.g. physiotherapy), one of the most overlooked problems is aspiration. In patients with pre-existing neuromuscular disease, a careful history should be taken for known aspiration prior to the index event or signs that it might have occurred (e.g. coughing after eating). While aspiration was not hitherto a feature of primary muscular dystrophies, it has become an increasing problem in patients whose longevity has been increased by non-invasive ventilation.

Outcomes, Prognosis, and Ceilings of Care

Patients with some conditions, most notably GBS, may make a full recovery, and therefore maximum effort and full ventilatory support is usually justified; although, even in this condition, a small proportion of patients retain substantial disability.

The most problematic area is where a patient with a known neuromuscular disease, for which there is no effective treatment, deteriorates. It is very helpful to discuss, in advance, what therapy the patient would like in such circumstances. The choice the patient makes will be influenced by cultural, regional, and often religious preferences and may also be influenced by what facilities are available to support home mechanical ventilation (Chapter 65), but the following considerations may prove helpful:

(a) If the patient was using non-invasive ventilation (NIV) only at night prior to the crisis occurring, with reasonable CO2 control, then they may prove weanable, particularly if there is an identifiable and reversible trigger for deterioration, but if not.

(b) The patient will usually have less respiratory reserve after intubation than before; therefore, except in the situation (a) above, it is likely they will require long-term tracheostomy ventilation (T-IPPV).

(c) This will likely (depending on the level of generalized neuromuscular weakness) increase their care requirements, which will make it more expensive to live at home; as a consequence, at least in the UK, this may in turn lead to a prolonged stay in a general ICU or transfer to a residential facility.

(d) T-IPPV does not treat the underlying condition; therefore, while it may increase longevity, the extra time 'earned' may be time spent with greater disability. In some conditions, notably MND, disease progression may make communication difficult.

Predicting the choice that a patient will make is difficult; it is, of course, good practice to involve friends or family close to the patient to support the patient during the discussion. In the author's experience, most patients appreciate the opportunity to have such a discussion in clinic. Tracheostomy seems to be more acceptable to patients with muscular dystrophies (where the patient will have had a lifetime experience of disability) than to adult patients who experience a rapid onset of symptoms, as with MND.

REFERENCES

1. Luo YM, Wu HD, Tang J, et al. Neural respiratory drive during apnoeic events in obstructive sleep apnoea. *Eur Resp J.* 2008;**31**(3):650–657.
2. Polkey MI, Duguet A, Luo Y et al. Anterior magnetic phrenic nerve stimulation: Laboratory and clinical evaluation. *Intensive Care Med.* 2000;**26**(8):1065–1075.
3. Supinski GS, Callahan LA. Diaphragm weakness in mechanically ventilated critically ill patients. *Crit Care.* 2013;**17**(3):R120.
4. Laghi F, Cattapan SE, Jubran A, et al. Is weaning failure caused by low-frequency fatigue of the diaphragm? *Am J Resp Crit Care Med.* 2003;**167**(2):120–127.
5. Bennett JR, Dunroy HM, Corfield DR, et al. Respiratory muscle activity during REM sleep in patients with diaphragm paralysis. *Neurology.* 2004;**62**(1):134–137.
6. Nickol AH, Hart N, Hopkinson NS, et al. Mechanisms of improvement of respiratory failure in patients with restrictive thoracic disease treated with non-invasive ventilation. *Thorax.* 2005;**60**(9):754–760.
7. Polkey MI, Lyall RA, Moxham J, Leigh PN. Respiratory aspects of neurological disease. *J Neurol Neurosurg Psych.* 1999;**66**:5–15.
8. Levine M, Ruha AM, Graeme K, et al. Toxicology in the ICU: Part 3: Natural toxins. *Chest.* 2011;**140**(5):1357–1370.
9. Simonds AK, Muntoni F, Heather S, Fielding S. Impact of nasal ventilation on survival in hypercapnic Duchenne muscular dystrophy. *Thorax.* 1998;**53**:949–952.
10. Engel AG. Acid maltase deficiency in adults: Studies in four cases of a syndrome which may mimic muscular dystrophy or other myopathies. *Brain.* 1970;**93**(3):599–616.
11. van der Ploeg AT, Clemens PR, Corzo D, Escolar DM, Florence J, Groeneveld GJ, et al. A randomized study of alglucosidase alfa in late-onset Pompe's disease. *N Engl J Med.* 2010;**362**(15):1396–1406.
12. Bradley MD, Orrell RW, Clarke J, et al. Outcome of ventilatory support for acute respiratory failure in motor neurone disease. *J Neurol Neurosurg Psych.* 2002;**72**(6):752–756.
13. Bloch S, Polkey MI, Griffiths M, Kemp P. Molecular mechanisms of intensive care unit-acquired weakness. *Eur Resp J.* 2012;**39**(4):1000–1011.
14. Polkey MI, Moxham J. Clinical aspects of respiratory muscle dysfunction in the critically ill. *Chest.* 2001;**119**(3):926–939.
15. De Jonghe B, Sharshar T, Lefaucheur JP, et al. Paresis acquired in the intensive care unit: A prospective multicenter study. *JAMA.* 2002;**288**(22):2859–2867.
16. Gayan-Ramirez G, Testelmans D, Maes K, et al. Intermittent spontaneous breathing protects the rat diaphragm from mechanical ventilation effects. *Crit Care Med.* 2005;**33**(12):2804–2809.
17. Watson AC, Hughes PD, Louise Harris M, et al. Measurement of twitch transdiaphragmatic, esophageal, and endotracheal tube pressure with bilateral anterolateral magnetic phrenic nerve

stimulation in patients in the intensive care unit. *Crit Care Med.* 2001;**29**(7):1325–31.
18. Mills GH, Ponte J, Hamnegard CH, et al. Tracheal tube pressure change during magnetic stimulation of the phrenic nerves as an indicator of diaphragm strength on the intensive care unit. *Br J Anaes.* 2001;**87**(6):876–884.
19. Demoule A, Jung B, Prodanovic H, et al. Diaphragm dysfunction on admission to the intensive care unit. Prevalence, risk factors, and prognostic impact—a prospective study. *Am J Respir Crit Care Med.* 2013;**188**(2):213–219.
20. De Troyer A, Borenstein S, Cordier R. Analysis of lung volume restriction in patients with respiratory muscle weakness. *Thorax.* 1980;**35**:603–610.
21. Gordon PH, Corcia P, Lacomblez L, et al. Defining survival as an outcome measure in amyotrophic lateral sclerosis. *Arch Neurol.* 2009;**66**(6):758–761.
22. Lyall RA, Donaldson N, Polkey MI, et al. Respiratory muscle strength and ventilatory failure in amyotrophic lateral sclerosis. *Brain.* 2001;**124**(Pt 10):2000–2013.
23. Polkey M, I., Lyall RA, Yang K, et al. Respiratory muscle strength as predictive biomarker for survival in amyotrophic lateral sclerosis. *Am J Respir Crit Care Med.* 2017;**195**(1):86–95.
24. Man WD, Moxham J, Polkey MI. Magnetic stimulation for the measurement of respiratory and skeletal muscle function. *Eur Resp J.* 2004;**24**(5):846–860.
25. Birnkrant DJ, Bushby KM, Amin RS, et al. The respiratory management of patients with Duchenne muscular dystrophy: A DMD care considerations working group specialty article. *Pediatr Pulmonol.* 2010;**45**(8):739–748.
26. Caruso P, Denari SD, Ruiz SA, et al. Inspiratory muscle training is ineffective in mechanically ventilated critically ill patients. *Clinics.* 2005;**60**(6):479–484.
27. Gilmartin JJ, Cooper BG, Griffiths CJ, et al. Breathing during sleep inpatients with myotonic dystrophy and non-myotonic respiratory muscle weakness. *Q J Med.* 1991;**285**:21–31.
28. Bye PT, Ellis ER, Issa FG, et al. Respiratory failure and sleep in neuromuscular disease. *Thorax.* 1990;**45**:241–247.
29. Polkey MI, Lyall RA, Green M, et al. Expiratory muscle function in amyotrophic lateral sclerosis. *Am J Respir Crit Care Med.* 1998;**158**:734–741.
30. Chatwin M, Ross E, Hart N, Nickol AH, Polkey MI, Simonds AK. Cough augmentation with mechanical insufflation/exsufflation in patients with neuromuscular weakness. *Eur Resp J.* 2003;**21**(3):502–508.

52

Pleural Disease

Fraser Brims and Edward TH Fysh

KEY MESSAGES

- Pleural effusion is common in patients admitted to intensive care.
- Intensive care-related pleural effusion is associated with significant morbidity and mortality.
- Without drainage, presumed clinical diagnoses of effusion aetiology are frequently inaccurate.
- Drainage of pleural effusion in the intensive care setting is safe if performed using ultrasound guidance. Use of ultrasound is recommended by international societies.
- Echogenic fluid and/or septation on thoracic ultrasound (TUS) can be used to predict exudative effusion, and complex septated effusion, in the right clinical context, can be highly suggestive of pleural infection.
- The clinical benefits of pleural effusion drainage as opposed to expectant management (while treating the presumed cause) are not well established.

CONTROVERSIES

- Should a pleural effusion be drained when its cause and the clinical impact are not immediately apparent? Many intensivists will adopt a watch-and-wait approach while optimizing fluid balance and treating other possible underlying causes. Observational data suggests that drainage can improve diagnostic accuracy and treatment options, oxygenation, and successful weaning from mechanical ventilation. This must be balanced against the risks of drainage complications. Not draining an effusion may also delay diagnosis of infection or postoperative complications.[1]
- What is the optimum size of a chest drain? There is evidence that small-bore (10–16 Fr) catheters have successful outcomes in most settings including mechanically ventilated, critically ill patients. Larger-bore catheters cause more pain, with impacts on sedo-analgesia and associated complications. If the small-bore catheter fails to achieve its goal, or there is a need for surgical pleural access, haemorrhage, or significant air leak, there remains a place for larger-bore catheters. However, in most indications, proponents of larger-bore drains now need to justify their reasoning with new evidence.

These controversies are elaborated on further below.

FURTHER RESEARCH

- Randomized studies are needed to guide clinical decision-making regarding drainage or expectant management of pleural effusion in the critically ill patient.[2] One such trial of drainage or expectant management in patients admitted to intensive care unit (ICU) with clinical equipoise is underway (ESODICE trial, ANZCTR no. ACTRN12620000519954). This will inform the design of other large clinical trials, powered to assess important clinical and patient-reported outcomes.
- Studies to guide a more targeted selection of patients likely to benefit from routine screening for pleural effusion are lacking, as the time taken to routinely screen every patient with thoracic ultrasound (TUS) needs to be balanced against the pre-test probability of the presence of a pleural effusion.
- A better understanding of the risks and benefits of drainage is needed, as are studies to offer algorithms for improved selection of those patients that will benefit from these procedures, as well as studies on thresholds of effusion size or gas exchange parameters that may confer advantage for drainage.
- Technological advances such as electrical impedance tomography (EIT) require further investigation into the utility of screening and monitoring for pleural effusion, as the ability to continuously, non-invasively monitor patients in an automated fashion may offer some advantages to intermittent, labour-intensive TUS use.

Introduction

Pleural effusions are common in patients admitted to the intensive care unit (ICU), with a prevalence of 62% in one series performing thoracic ultrasound (TUS) on 100 consecutive medical ICU patients.[2] The importance of focused training in pleural drainage procedures, and TUS to guide these procedures, is being advocated for in international guidelines.[3,4]

The majority of these effusions were small, and other series using clinical assessment and chest radiography report 3.1%–8.4% of patients admitted to the ICU develop a clinically significant pleural effusion.[1,5,6] Supine chest X-ray (CXR) can miss a significant proportion of pleural effusions compared to TUS, potentially explaining some of this variation in reported prevalence.[7]

Physiology of the Pleural Space

Fluid normally passes from systemic capillaries (and to a lesser extent pulmonary capillaries) into the pleural space at an estimated rate of 0.1 mL/kg/hour.[8] It then recirculates into the lymphatics through microscopic stomata in the parietal pleura, with the number of stomata and lymphatic inflow increasing along their cranial to caudal distribution (Figure 52.1). The lymphatic drainage of pleural fluid can increase up to 20-fold as fluid influx increases and is aided by the rhythmic changes in pleural pressure associated with spontaneous breathing. A pleural effusion represents excessive pleural fluid accumulation that results from either increased fluid release from the systemic circulation or decreased drainage through the parietal pleura or both.

One of the most frequent causes of pleural effusion in intensive care populations is heart failure/fluid overload (26%–35% of cases).[2,6] This results in increased movement of extravascular water across the visceral pleura into the pleural space. Proinflammatory conditions such as parapneumonic effusion (11%–43%) or malignancy (3%–14%) are also common. In this context, inflammation increases vascular permeability and fluid influx, and more cellular fluid with increased viscosity, reducing drainage from the pleural space. These inflammatory conditions usually require specific therapy beyond optimization of fluid balance and cardiac function and therefore must be investigated if clinically suspected. Light's criteria remain the best way of distinguishing transudative causes (heart failure, fluid overload, and atelectasis) from inflammatory or exudative causes of pleural effusion.

The incidence and causes of pleural effusions on ICU will vary dependent on the clinical setting, with the most common medical ICU causes including heart failure, fluid overload, atelectasis, parapneumonic effusion, empyema, and malignancy.[2,5] In the context of more specialized surgical ICUs, causes may be related to the conditions and surgery being performed. For instance, post-cardiac surgery pleural effusions are common with risk factors such as heart failure, arrhythmias, use of anticoagulants, use of topical hypothermia, and internal mammary grafts.

Clinical Impact of Pleural Effusion in the ICU

Pleural effusions in patients on ICU are associated with significant adverse clinical outcomes. Failure of oxygenation, prolonged mechanical ventilation, prolonged ICU stay, and increased mortality have all been reported to be associated with pleural effusions.[2,9–11] In patients who have undergone cardiac surgery, postoperative pleural effusion was one of the significant variables that independently predicted readmission to intensive care, and the presence of pleural effusion may be associated with increased mortality on ICU.[6]

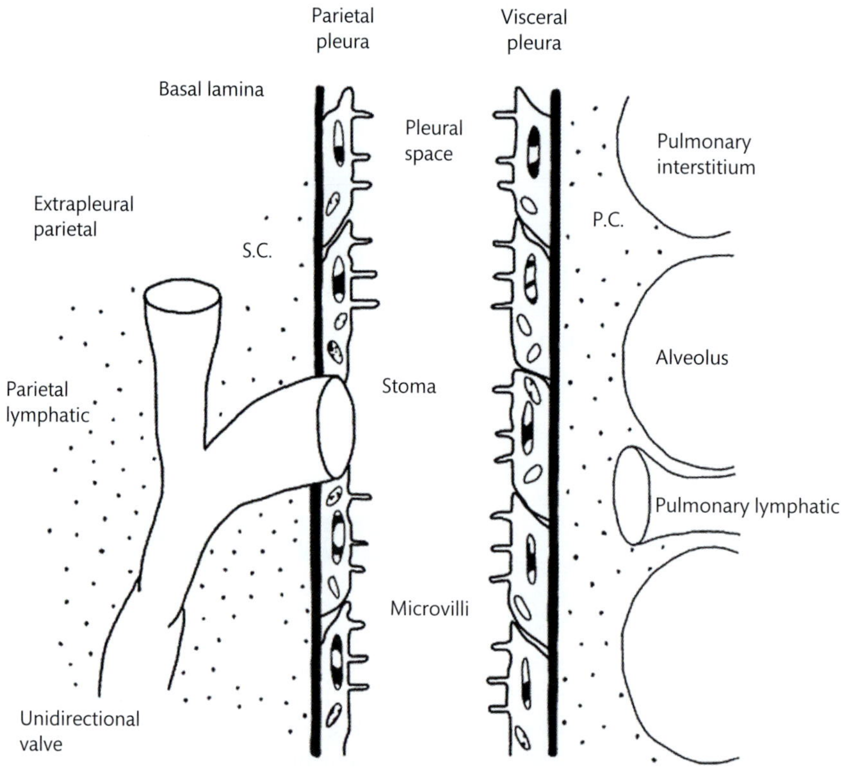

Figure 52.1 Structure and morphology of the pleural space. The pleural space is bordered by the parietal and the visceral pleura. The pleura is lined by mesothelial cells, which project out microvilli into the pleural space. The lymphatics are found both in the pulmonary interstitium as well as in the parietal interstitium. PC, pulmonary capillary; SC, systemic capillary.

Drainage of pleural fluid in patients with clinically significant pleural effusions has been shown to improve oxygenation and successful weaning from mechanical ventilation.[1,5, 9,12] A recent systematic review demonstrated the arterial oxygen tension (PaO_2)/fractional inspired oxygen (FiO_2) ratio before and after drainage increased by 23% (95% CI: 15%–31%).[13] Other retrospective studies have reported an increase in mortality following pleural drainage.[6] Selection bias is likely to have affected all of these studies, and randomized trials are required to inform clinical treatment guidelines.[8,14]

Screening for Pleural Effusion in the ICU

In the clinical setting, the presumed cause of pleural effusion according to clinical assessment alone is frequently wrong and is often changed significantly when pleural fluid analysis is undertaken.[1,5] Thus, an undiagnosed and/or large pleural effusion on ICU may directly impact upon clinical progress, particularly in the context of a parapneumonic effusion, pleural infection, or effusion due to malignancy which may have important implications for treatment and prognostication. Once detected, a pleural effusion should be regularly monitored as effusion volume and therefore clinical significance can change rapidly over time.

The times where screening for pleural effusion can have greatest impact are when:

- diagnostic assessments of the cause of pleural effusion are being made or re-evaluated;
- there is significant hypoxia (particularly when refractory to initial treatment);
- initiating ventilatory support for deteriorating respiratory function;
- there is delay or difficulty when weaning a patient from ventilatory support;
- there is pneumonia or sepsis of unknown cause and patients with underlying cancer with respiratory failure.

Clinical examination can be difficult in the intensive care population. Common factors that can impair examination include suboptimal patient positioning, uncooperative patients, obesity, presence of thoracoabdominal drains or dressings, or subcutaneous emphysema. The diagnostic accuracy of clinical assessment for pleural effusion in patients with acute respiratory distress syndrome (ARDS) in one study was found to be 61% compared to 47% for portable chest radiography and 93% for TUS, compared to chest computed tomography (CT) as gold standard.[15]

Upright posteroanterior CXRs require at least 200 mL of fluid for consistent recognition of pleural effusions and therefore have limitations in utility for screening ICU patients for pleural effusion, particularly with supine body position and with coexisting pulmonary pathology. For example, in chronic heart failure, CXR had a diagnostic accuracy for pleural effusion of 33% compared to clinical assessment of 56% and TUS of 91%.[16]

The International Consensus Conference on Lung Ultrasound has recommended that point-of-care TUS is 'more accurate than chest radiography and is as accurate as CT' for the detection of pleural effusion and has multiple benefits compared to CT imaging.[17] In the ICU setting, TUS was shown to be far superior to CXR for the detection of pleural effusion, with a sensitivity of 100% versus 65%, a specificity of 100% versus 81%, and a diagnostic accuracy of 100% versus 69%, respectively.[18] TUS can guide selection of the safest site for drainage,[19] be used to accurately estimate the volume of pleural effusion[20,21] and provide clinicians with pre-drainage information on the likely nature of the fluid. TUS therefore has become a key tool in the detection, diagnosis, and treatment of pleural effusion in intensive care and should be considered the optimal imaging method for routine assessment of patients with suspected pleural effusion.[3,4]

Electrical impedance tomography (EIT) is a new technique for non-invasive, real-time monitoring of the distribution of ventilation and alveolar recruitment in patients with respiratory failure and ARDS. EIT has been reported to be effective in detecting pleural effusions and indeed in showing effective lung reinflation after drainage.[22,23] However, TUS is still necessary for confirmation of the diagnosis of pleural effusion and guidance of drainage procedures. EIT, therefore, is unlikely to ever compete with TUS for diagnosing pleural effusion but may offer a role in ongoing assessment of patients with pleural effusions on ICU.

Determining the Need for Sampling or Draining Pleural Effusions

The decision of whether to drain pleural effusions in intensive care is frequently made without clear, evidence-based guidelines to support clinicians. Studies to date have mostly been observational, clinician choice studies that were not designed to rigorously question current dogma. There are certain indications that are undisputed such as pleural infection (Chapter 36) and haemothorax. The British Thoracic Society guidelines recommend sampling of an undiagnosed unilateral pleural effusion, suspected pleural infection, suspected malignant effusion, and bilateral effusions that do not have a clear cause and/or do not respond to attempts to treat the most likely underlying cause (heart failure, hypoalbuminaemia, etc.).[24] The recommendations are not strong, level C in the majority of cases, and the evidence behind them has not been tested in the intensive care setting.

The ultrasound appearances of pleural effusions can be very useful to guide clinicians in decision-making, for instance, echogenic fluid and/or septation on TUS can be used to predict exudative effusion and complex septated effusion in the right clinical context can be highly suggestive of pleural infection (Figure 52.2).[19] Pleural nodularity and thickening can also help in diagnosing malignant pleural effusion. However, anechoic, non-septated pleural effusion (the more common appearance) does not rule out an exudate and therefore caution should be employed if using the absence of these signs to negate the need for drainage (Figure 52.3).

The threshold of effusion size or volume above which patients will benefit from drainage is not clear, with observational studies and metanalyses demonstrating drainage of a 'clinically significant' pleural effusion can significantly improve oxygenation.[12–14] Respiratory mechanics can also be improved with drainage although the evidence that drainage may reduce time on ventilatory support is weak. Acknowledging the need for stronger evidence,

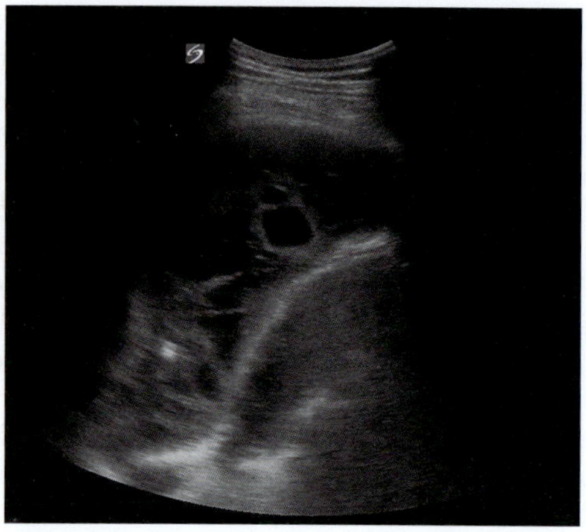

Figure 52.2 Hyperechoic, septated (loculated) pleural effusion diagnostic of exudative pleural effusion, in this case empyema.

pleural drainage should be considered in patients with significantly impaired oxygenation and/or ventilation, in the absence of contraindications.

The potential complications from pleural drainage procedures are vital in the assessment and consideration of a management plan. Complications include bleeding (~1%) pneumothorax (~3%), and visceral injury (~0.1%), which can be fatal, especially in a critically ill population (Figure 52.4).[25] However, pleural drainage can be done safely in mechanically ventilated patients, provided it is performed by properly trained clinicians.[12,21,25,26] The routine use of TUS is now recommended for all pleural drainage in both the American Thoracic Society and British Thoracic Society guidelines.[3,4]

Inaction or failure to investigate may also confer risk with the clinical (pre-procedure) diagnosis for the cause of pleural effusion frequently wrong, and harm from delay in drainage can be greater than the potential risk of the procedure(s). A protocol describing patient positioning, assessment for the absence of viscera from the drainage zone throughout the respiratory cycle, and a minimal safe depth of effusion (15 mm) has been proposed.[21]

All pleural procedures should ideally have pleural fluid testing of at least pH, protein, LDH, and glucose as well as microscopy, culture and sensitivity, and cytology with a differential cell count. The use of blood culture bottles for pleural fluid culture greatly increases the yield of microbiology testing, and at least 100 mL should be sent for cytology analysis if possible. If the volume of fluid drained is less than expected, a clinical decision as to which test is most important may need to be made, but it is strongly recommended that biochemical analysis using Light's criteria should be performed whenever the pleural fluid is analyzed.

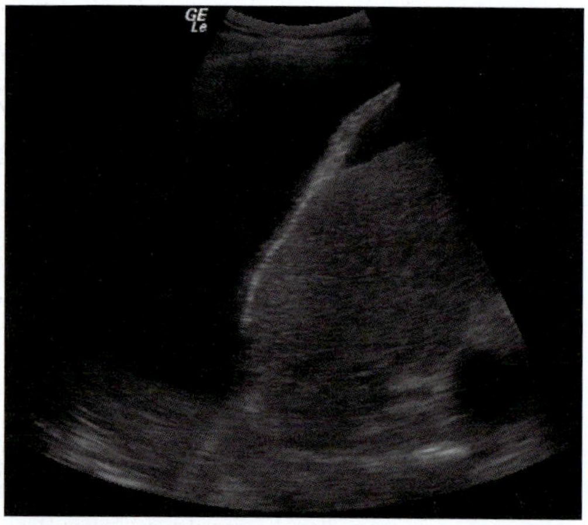

Figure 52.3 Large, anechoic pleural effusion in patient with hepatic hydrothorax and ascites. This appearance is consistent with, not diagnostic of, transudative pleural effusion.

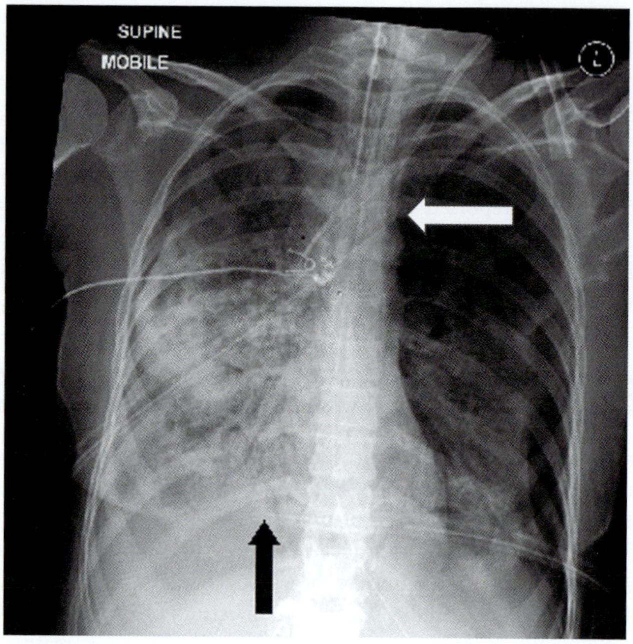

Figure 52.4 Chest radiograph from a 42-year-old lady with pneumonia and a right-sided parapneumonic effusion. A chest drain was inserted too far (white arrow), damaging her right lung, mediastinum, and left lung resulting in a right haemothorax and bilateral pneumothoraces. A left-sided chest drain was then inserted, again too far (black arrow). This punctured the inferior vena cava and liver. Unfortunately, this lady died from these complications.

Techniques and Types of Drain for Pleural Effusions in the ICU

Thoracentesis involves transient access of the pleural space using a large-bore cannula alone or a dedicated thoracentesis kit and generally involves the use of an access needle between 14 and 20 G in size (approximately 1–2 mm in external diameter). This allows short-term drainage of the pleural space, and while large volumes (1 L or more of fluid) can be drained, the equipment used is generally not designed to remain more than a matter of minutes in the pleural space. Pleural drain insertion involves the placement of a catheter into the pleural space which can be secured in place and allow controlled access to the pleural space for days. The size of the catheters in common use ranges from 6 to 34 Fr (2.0–11.3 mm external diameter).

Thoracentesis is generally considered for diagnostic pleural drainage, or in therapeutic drainage when the expected volume of pleural fluid is relatively low, the chance of reaccumulation of the fluid is considered low (or not a high priority) and there is no need for instillation of medications such as fibrinolytics or pleurodesing agents. The disadvantages of thoracentesis are that there are higher blockage and kinking rates of the cannula, reaccumulation of fluid is common on ICU, and instillation of intrapleural medications is not possible.

Evidence suggests that larger chest drains may have higher complication rates than thoracentesis with a systematic review reporting pneumothorax in 5.4% of 6509 cases of thoracentesis, as opposed to 9.4% of 1433 cases of chest drain insertion in non-trauma patients.[25] The rates of iatrogenic bleeding in these studies were 1.0% and 2.9%, respectively. It should be noted that this review included several studies where ultrasound was *not* used, and non-intensive care patients were also included. There is a wide selection of different size catheters for pleural drainage, all with differing lengths, numbers, and positions of fenestrations. Methods of insertion also vary, with blunt dissection and modified Seldinger techniques being the most common.[27] Training in both blunt dissection and modified Seldinger techniques is essential for trainees in the critical care specialties.

The optimal size of pleural drain is a controversial topic with a lack of quality data to guide decision-making. The only randomized study directly comparing 10 or 24 Fr catheters in patients with malignant pleural effusion was stopped early after only nine patients, as predefined end points in pain scores favouring the smaller drains had already been reached. Intuitively, the larger the drain size, the more tissue trauma and pain insertion will cause. Large-bore drains (typically defined as >16 Fr) should therefore be used only when there is a sound reason for doing so with studies demonstrating the efficacy of smaller-bore drains to drain viscous fluid such as pus. Further, the MIST-2 trial confirmed the safety and efficacy of fibrinolytic therapy in combination with DNase to break down septations and reduce the fluid viscosity.[28] Guidelines now recommend the initial use of small-bore drains for pleural infection.[4]

The situations where large-bore drains may have benefit over smaller-bore ones are iatrogenic or traumatic haemothorax (where the volume and/or rate of bleeding may influence decisions for surgery or radiological embolization and there is risk of clotting/blockage of a small-bore tube) and when there is a need for a larger hole in the parietal pleura, such as traumatic hydropneumothorax (as ultrasound is not able to image the pleural space due to the presence of air and a finger sweep technique is required to ensure safe pleural access). In this circumstance, the insertion of a small-bore tube through a large pleural defect can result in subcutaneous emphysema particularly in patients requiring positive pressure ventilation. This principle also holds for when a large-bore access port has been, or is going to be, required for thoracoscopy.

Conclusion

Pleural effusions commonly develop in patients requiring intensive care, and they are associated with significant morbidity and mortality. It is vital that clinicians working in the critical care specialties have a thorough knowledge of the potential aetiologies and potential impacts of pleural effusion. This must include the indications for pleural effusion sampling and drainage and treatment, using ultrasound (or other imaging) guidance as appropriate. Further research is required to fill vital knowledge gaps in the optimal selection of critically ill patients with pleural effusions for intervention.

REFERENCES

1. Fysh ETH, Smallbone P, Mattock N, et al. Clinically significant pleural effusion in intensive care: A prospective multicenter cohort study. *Crit Care Explor*. 2020;**2**(1):e0070.
2. Mattison LE, Coppage L, Alderman DF, et al. Pleural effusions in the medical ICU: Prevalence, causes, and clinical implications. *Chest*. 1997;**111**(4):1018–1023.
3. Feller-Kopman DJ, Reddy CB, DeCamp MM, et al. Management of malignant pleural effusions. An official ATS/STS/STR clinical practice guideline. *Am J Respir Crit Care Med*. 2018;**198**(7):839–849.
4. Havelock T, Teoh R, Laws D. BTS guidelines for pleural procedures—pleural aspiration, chest drain insertion and thoracic ultrasound. *Thorax*. 2010;**65**:i61–i76.
5. Fartoukh M, Azoulay E, Galliot R, et al. Clinically documented pleural effusions in medical ICU patients: How useful is routine thoracentesis? *Chest*. 2002;**121**(1):178–184.
6. Bateman M, Alkhatib A, John T, et al. Pleural effusion outcomes in intensive care: Analysis of a large clinical database. *J Intensive Care Med*. 2020;**35**(1):48–54.
7. Gryminski J, Krakowka P, Lypacewicz G. The diagnosis of pleural effusion by ultrasonic and radiologic techniques. *Chest*. 1976;**70**(1):33–37.
8. Walden A, Jones Q, Matsa R, et al. Pleural effusions on the intensive care unit; hidden morbidity with therapeutic potential. *Respirology*. 2013;**18**(2):246–254.
9. Brims FJH, Davies MG, Elia A, et al. The effects of pleural fluid drainage on respiratory function in mechanically ventilated patients after cardiac surgery. *BMJ Open Respir Res*. 2015;**2**(1):e000080.
10. Koga Y, Kaneda K, Mizuguchi I, et al. Extent of pleural effusion on chest radiograph is associated with failure of high-flow nasal cannula oxygen therapy. *J Crit Care*. 2016;**32**:165–9.
11. Razazi K, Thille AW, Carteaux G, et al. Effects of pleural effusion drainage on oxygenation, respiratory mechanics, and hemodynamics in mechanically ventilated patients. *Ann Am Thorac Soc*. 2014;**11**(7):1018–1024.
12. Goligher E, Leis J, Fowler R, et al. Utility and safety of draining pleural effusions in mechanically ventilated patients: A systematic review and meta-analysis. *Crit. Care*. 2011;**15**(1):R46.
13. Mattock N, Fysh E. Pleural drainage and oxygenation in intensive care: Review and meta-analysis. *Respirology*. 2019;**24(supp 1)**:54
14. Vetrugno L, Bignami E, Orso D, et al. Utility of pleural effusion drainage in the ICU: An updated systematic review and META-analysis. *J Crit Care*. 2019;**52**:22–32.
15. Lichtenstein D, Goldstein I, Mourgeon E, et al. Comparative diagnostic performances of auscultation, chest radiography, and lung ultrasonography in acute respiratory distress syndrome. *Anesthesiology*. 2004;**100**(1):9–15.
16. Kataoka H, Takada S. The role of thoracic ultrasonography for evaluation of patients with decompensated chronic heart failure. *J Am Coll Cardiol*. 2000;**35**(6):1638–1646.
17. Volpicelli G, Elbarbary M, Blaivas M, et al. International evidence-based recommendations for point-of-care lung ultrasound. *Intensive Care Med*. 2012;**38**(4):577–591.

18. Xirouchaki N, Magkanas E, Vaporidi K, et al. Lung ultrasound in critically ill patients: Comparison with bedside chest radiography. *Intensive Care Med*. 2011;**37**(9):1488–1493.
19. Yang PC, Luh KT, Chang DB, et al. Value of sonography in determining the nature of pleural effusion: Analysis of 320 cases. *Am J Roentgenol*. 1992;**159**(1):29–33.
20. Balik M, Plasil P, Waldauf P, et al. Ultrasound estimation of volume of pleural fluid in mechanically ventilated patients. *Intensive Care Med*. 2006;**32**:318–321.
21. Lichtenstein D, Hulot JS, Rabiller A, et al. Feasibility and safety of ultrasound-aided thoracentesis in mechanically ventilated patients. *Intensive Care Med*. 1999;**25**(9):955–958.
22. Becher T, Bußmeyer M, Lautenschläger I, et al. Characteristic pattern of pleural effusion in electrical impedance tomography images of critically ill patients. *Br J Anaesth*. 2018;**120**(6):1219–1228.
23. Rara A, Roubik K, Tyll T. Effects of pleural effusion drainage in the mechanically ventilated patient as monitored by electrical impedance tomography and end-expiratory lung volume: A pilot study. *J Crit Care*. 2020;**59**:76–80.
24. Maskell NA, Butland RJA. BTS guidelines for the investigation of a unilateral pleural effusion in adults. *Thorax*. 2003;**58**(Suppl 2):ii8–ii17.
25. Wrightson JM, Fysh E, Maskell NA, et al. Risk reduction in pleural procedures: Sonography, simulation and supervision. *Curr Opin Pulm Med*. 2010;**16**(4):340–350.
26. Mayo P, Goltz H, Tafreshi M, et al. Safety of ultrasound-guided thoracentesis in patients receiving mechanical ventilation. *Chest*. 2004;**125**:1059–1062.
27. Fysh ET, Smith NA, Lee YC. Optimal chest drain size: The rise of the small-bore pleural catheter. *Semin Respir Crit Care Med*. 2010;**31**(6):760–768.
28. Rahman NM, Maskell NA, West A, et al. Intrapleural use of tissue plasminogen activator and DNase in pleural infection. *N Engl J Med*. 2011;**365**(0):518–526.

53

Chest Wall Disease and Post-thoracic Surgery

Thomas Kiss and Marcelo Gama de Abreu

KEY MESSAGES

- Kyphoscoliosis is characterized by diminished chest wall compliance and impaired respiratory mechanics and can be complicated by interstitial lung disease, sleep apnoea, spontaneous pneumothorax, and secondary infection.
- Pleural effusions can be managed by drainage but volume drained does not correlate well with improvements in gas exchange or breathlessness.
- Open and video-assisted thoracoscopic surgical (VATS) pleural decortications are effective procedures in the treatment of pleural empyema.
- Ankylosing spondylitis is associated with restrictive pulmonary function but patients seldom complain of respiratory symptoms. Although incurable, it can respond well to biological therapy and rehabilitation.
- Congenital chest wall conditions include pectus carinatum and pectus excavatum, the latter is more commonly associated with cardiopulmonary impairment.

CONTROVERSIES

- Surgical outcome for patients with adolescent idiopathic scoliosis is generally favourable but not for adults. When, if ever, is there an indication for elective chest wall surgery in adults?

FURTHER RESEARCH

- The impact of newer therapeutic biological agents for ankylosing spondylitis on chest wall and other pulmonary complications.

Introduction

Chest wall diseases, including mechanical and neuromuscular disorders, may have profound effects on the respiratory system due to impairment of the ability to breathe and maintain adequate gas exchange. In this chapter, we address the main congenital and acquired entities as listed below:

- kyphoscoliosis,
- chest wall infections including pleural effusion and thoracic fibrosis,
- ankylosing spondylitis (AS),
- congenital deformities including pectus excavatum and carinatum, and
- chest trauma and flail chest.

Kyphoscoliosis

Definition

'Kyphoscoliosis' is a generic term that includes a spectrum of deformities ranging from kyphosis to scoliosis. Most instances are combinations of the two, with one or the other predominating. The degree of scoliosis is generally expressed in terms of the angle formed by the converging limbs of the curve as visualized on an X-ray of the spine (Cobb angle). 'Kyphosis' is generally used to designate any posterior angulation of the spine. Most kyphoscolioses are idiopathic (80%), beginning already in childhood, while others are secondary to underlying illnesses[1,2].

Cardiopulmonary Function

The relationship between lung volume and height can be estimated from different formulae, for example, those from Baldwin et al[2]. Usually, growth in vertical height parallels general body development. Unfortunately, this premise does not apply to individuals with kyphoscoliosis. In those patients, standing height should be substituted by arm span for predicting normal lung volume values[2].

Kyphoscoliosis is characterized by reduced chest wall compliance and impaired respiratory mechanics, leading to progressive hypoventilation, hypercapnia, and chronic respiratory failure[3].

It has been shown that thoracic scoliosis is associated with decreased pulmonary function.

Kyphoscoliotic patients usually show a restrictive pattern of pulmonary function, with decreased total lung capacity, vital capacity, and residual volume. The vital capacity is far more seriously affected than the residual volume. Lung compliance eventually decreases due to progressive atelectasis and air trapping, a consequence of breathing at low lung volumes. Additionally, chest wall compliance decreases with age, further increasing work of breathing and risk of respiratory muscle fatigue in elderly patients. Dead space fraction may be increased, and alveolar hypoventilation may ensue with resultant hypercapnia. As a result of persistent hypoxaemia, pulmonary hypertension with *cor pulmonale* can develop[3].

Treatment

Medical therapy for respiratory dysfunction due to kyphoscoliosis includes non-invasive ventilation (NIV). It has been shown that intermittent positive-pressure ventilation therapy during the night improves daytime oxygenation, respiratory muscle performance, and hypoventilation-based symptoms in patients with severe kyphoscoliosis. Furthermore, a physical rehabilitation programme for 4 months has shown to improve forced expiratory vital capacity, inspiratory capacity, forced expiratory volume in one second (FEV1), expiratory reserve volume, and performance assessed by 6-min walk test. The programme consisted of stretching and low energetic-demand aerobic exercises, such as slow and progressive walks as well as aerobic exercises on a treadmill or stationary bicycle. One single centre intensive care study evaluated acute and chronic respiratory failure management in kyphoscoliotic patients[1]. All included patients were hypercapnic, and 88% of patients were both hypercapnic and hypoxemic. The primary reasons for acute respiratory failure were *cor pulmonale* and sepsis, with pneumonia the primary cause of sepsis. NIV failure patients had a higher mortality rate than initially intubated patients which may be attributed to delayed intubation due to a minimal improvement of arterial blood gas values after the first hour of NIV treatment. The authors concluded that in the presence of sepsis NIV failure may result, and the authors strongly discourage the use of NIV in the case of septic shock.

In the presence of established kyphoscoliosis in adults, surgery is of questionable benefit and carries a significant complication rate. Outcome for patients with adolescent idiopathic scoliosis is generally good[4]. Adolescent idiopathic scoliosis is scoliosis with Cobb angle ≥10°, age of onset ≥10 years, and no underlying aetiology. Indications for consultation of an orthopaedic surgeon for adolescent idiopathic scoliosis include Cobb angle >20° and rapid progression of Cobb angle ≥5°. Options for the treatment of adolescent idiopathic scoliosis include observation, bracing, and surgery[4]. Management is individualized according to the magnitude of the Cobb angle, remaining growth potential, best estimate of risk for progression, and patient and family preferences (Figure 53.1).

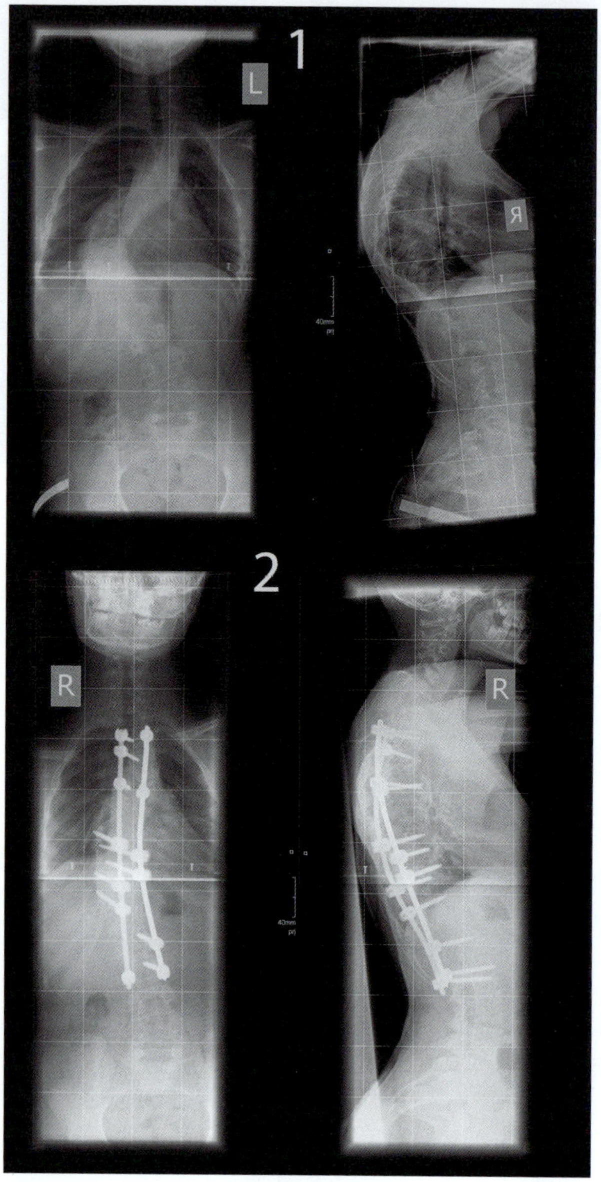

Figure 53.1 Radiographic image of a 13-year-old girl (141 cm and 39 kg) with thoracolumbar kyphoscoliosis and systemic sclerosis: 5 days before (1) and 3 months after (2) surgery. The Cobb angle was 90° before and 30° after surgery. Echocardiography of the heart revealed no pathologic values. She showed no clinical signs of a significantly impaired lung function.

Chest Wall Infections Including Pleural Effusion and Fibrothorax

Definition

The pleural space may be infected by several ways, among others, direct distribution of pathogens through the alveolar air space, rupture of a subpleural tuberculous cavity, haematogenous dissemination, penetration of pathogens through the skin barrier from open chest trauma, or translocation of intra-abdominal infections across the diaphragm (Chapter 36)[5].

Fibrothorax results from fibrosis of the visceral pleura surrounding the lung and is clinically manifested by decreased respiratory excursion and restrictive pulmonary physiology[6].

Pleural fibrosis may be the consequence of empyema, organized haemorrhagic effusion, tuberculous effusion, or asbestos-related pleural disease and can manifest itself as discrete localized lesions or diffuse pleural thickening and fibrosis. Although fibrothorax is the result of underlying pleural or pulmonary disease, the physiologic manifestations are similar to those seen in chest wall disorders[6].

Pleural effusions are characterized by excess fluid accumulation in the pleural cavity. Effusions may impair breathing by limiting the expansion of the lungs. Pleural effusions are common in the critically ill, occurring in over 60% of patients in some series. Their occurrence is multifactorial and include heart failure, pneumonia, hypoalbuminemia, intravenous fluid administration, atelectasis, and positive-pressure ventilation[7] (see chapter 52 for more details on pleural diseases).

Cardiopulmonary Function

The limitation in chest wall movement due to fibrothorax results in a restrictive ventilatory defect on pulmonary function testing, similar to other diseases that result in decreased chest wall compliance. Fibrothorax can result in a characteristic, abrupt cessation of flow at end-inspiration. Hypercapnia from alveolar hypoventilation can develop as a consequence of lung entrapment, and perfusion to the affected hemithorax appears to be reduced out of proportion to the drop in ventilation[6].

Pleural effusions do not appear to alter chest wall elastance or resistance. No evidence links abnormal gas exchange caused by pleural effusions to the symptom of breathlessness[8].

Although thoracentesis can improve the FEV1, vital capacity and lung volumes, the magnitudes of increase are highly variable and often do not correlate with the volume of fluid drained.

Improvements in gas exchange after thoracentesis are more consistently found at 24 h rather than immediately the procedure, and hypoxemia has been shown to worsen up to 2 h after thoracentesis. In mechanically ventilated patients, improvements in PaO_2/FiO_2 have been associated with the volume drained and the increase in end-expiratory lung volume. In general, small or moderate effusions do not cause major haemodynamic changes. Even in mechanically ventilated patients, drainage of effusions does not significantly alter cardiac output, blood pressure, or catecholamine dose requirements. Large effusions do not usually reduce cardiac output at rest but can limit its rise during exercise.

Treatment

The surgical removal of a restrictive layer of fibrous tissue overlying the lung, chest wall, and diaphragm is called 'decortication'[9], which aims to allow the lung to re-expand. Decortication is frequently necessary when other minor interventions (e.g. chest tube) have not resulted in clearance of the infection or haemothorax[9,10].

Open and video-assisted thoracoscopic surgical (VATS) pleural decortications are effective procedures in the treatment of pleural empyema in the fibrinopurulent stage. Early referral for surgery gives a better chance of success in VATS pleural decortications[9,10].

Open pleural decortication is an effective alternative, when VATS pleural decortications cannot be performed due to an obliterated pleural space. The results after decortication are often dependent from postoperative motivation of the patient with a special focus on respiratory physiotherapy. Decortication in general has a good outcome in young people.

If infected pleural fluid becomes loculated and resistant to drainage with a single chest tube, intrapleural administration of a fibrinolytic agent may facilitate empyema drainage by dissolving fibrous adhesions. However, empyema formation will require surgical intervention for optimal management. Complex parapneumonic effusions without signs of infection may be treated with intrapleural tissue plasminogen activator and deoxyribonuclease only and can consequently reduce the need for surgery. Non-septated effusions may be treated with insertion of small diameter pig tail catheters while surgical intervention should be requested in cases where this approach fails. Antibiotic therapy for parapneumonic effusions should be in line with current local guidelines. In case of empyema, anaerobic coverage should be included[10].

Ankylosing Spondylitis

Definition

Spondyloarthropathies are a group of inflammatory arthritis that consist of AS, reactive arthritis, arthritis/spondylitis associated with psoriasis, and arthritis/spondylitis associated with inflammatory bowel diseases[11]. The association with human leukocyte antigen (HLA)-B27, peripheral joint involvement predominantly of the lower extremities, sacroiliitis, spondylitis, enthesitis, dactylitis, uveitis, enteric mucosal lesions, and skin lesions are the shared manifestations of the diseases. The HLA-B27 status is extremely relevant to the early diagnosis of spondyloarthropathies. In the population at large, 5%–10% of individuals are HLA-B27-positive, versus 80%–95% of patients with AS. AS is the most common and most typical form of spondyloarthropathies and usually affects young men. A patient can be classified as having definite AS if at least one clinical criterion (inflammatory back pain, limitation of lumbar spine, or limitation of chest expansion) and radiologic criterion (bilaterally grade 2 or unilateral grade 3–4 sacroiliitis) are fulfilled[11].

Cardiopulmonary Function

Patients with AS rarely complain of respiratory symptoms or functional impairment unless there is coexistent cardiovascular or respiratory disease. For most patients, the pain, stiffness, and fatigue associated with the disease is the most limiting factor[12,13].

Several studies showed significantly impaired pulmonary function in the AS patients compared to controls and reference data, and demonstrated a clear relationship between reduced spinal mobility and restrictive pulmonary function. Pulmonary function test results showed reduced FEV1 and forced vital capacity (FVC) and increased FEV1/FVC[12].

A systematic review examined pulmonary abnormalities on high-resolution computed tomography in patients with AS[14]. The most commonly found changes were pleural thickening (52%), parenchymal bands (45%) and interlobular septal thickening (30%). Apical fibrosis was seen in 7% and was prominent in patients with greater duration of disease[14]. Furthermore, interstitial lung disease, sleep apnoea, spontaneous pneumothorax, and secondary infection are well-known pulmonary complications. Relative preservation of lung volumes has been attributed to increased abdominal excursion of the diaphragm, fixation of the thorax at greater lung volumes, and preservation of chest wall symmetry and rib excursion. The functional residual capacity and residual volume are normal or increased due to fixation of the rib cage, leading to a higher resting position of the chest wall. Gas exchange, airflow, and lung compliance are usually normal. Maximal inspiratory pressure and maximal expiratory pressure may be mildly reduced.

Cardiac dysfunction (aortitis, aortic valve diseases, conduction disturbances, cardiomyopathy, and ischaemic heart disease) are well known and commonly reported extra-articular manifestations.

Treatment

Although not curable, AS is one of the most rehabilitable of all the chronic rheumatic diseases[15]. Less than 10% develop relentlessly crippling disease. Treatment of AS is primarily preventive and supportive and focuses on pain and inflammation control and maintenance of maximum skeletal mobility to prevent deformities[16]. Regular exercise such as aerobic fitness should ameliorate loss of muscular strength and endurance. It may take years of therapy with tumour necrosis factor-alpha antagonists to slow radiographic progression of the spinal disease.

Congenital Deformities

Definition

The two most familiar and most common chest wall abnormalities are *pectus excavatum* (also called 'funnel chest', 'trichterbrust', or 'thorax en entonnoir') and *pectus carinatum*. There are, however, several other less well known but more problematic malformations including Poland's syndrome, sternal defects, and vertebral and rib abnormalities including asphyxiating thoracic dystrophy and rib dysplasia[17].

Pectus excavatum accounts for >90% of all congenital chest wall abnormalities. It is estimated to occur in approximately 1 of every 300 live births predominantly affecting white males. The presence of pectus excavatum is usually evident during the first year of life, and the deformity becomes more severe during rapid skeletal growth. In contrast, *pectus carinatum* may remain undiagnosed until the late adolescence.

Pectus excavatum is occasionally concomitant with other anomalies, such as Marfan syndrome or scoliosis (Figure 53.2). About 66% of Marfan patients have either *pectus excavatum* or *carinatum*. The documentation of the severity of *pectus excavatum* may be objectivized by computed tomographic scan and by calculating the Haller index, which is performed by dividing the distance at the widest point of the inner chest by that between the sternum and the vertebral column[17,18].

Pectus carinatum (keel chest) is a deformity of the chest characterized by a protrusion of the anterior chest wall with a greater variation than that which occurs in pectus excavatum deformities. The most common variety consists of anterior displacement of the sternal gladiolus with the appropriate cartilages in tow. In severe forms, there is also a narrowing of the transverse diameter of the chest, which seems to further exaggerate the anomaly.

Cardiopulmonary Function

Pectus excavatum patients typically present with decreased physical condition, pain, and recurrent episodes of common cold. Relative to the severity of the anomaly, the sterno-vertebral space is narrowed with the heart shifting into the hemithorax. Pulmonary expansion can be limited accordingly. The diminished anteroposterior diameter of the chest may hinder the filling of the right atrium and, if patients with *pectus excavatum* are stressed, limited cardiac output may prevent to endure the intense exercise. Evaluation of pulmonary function has demonstrated that children and adolescents have a restrictive defect with low normal total lung capacity and vital capacity measurements. Infants and young children generally have no symptoms, but the condition often worsens during adolescence. On deep inspiration, the deformity is usually accentuated.

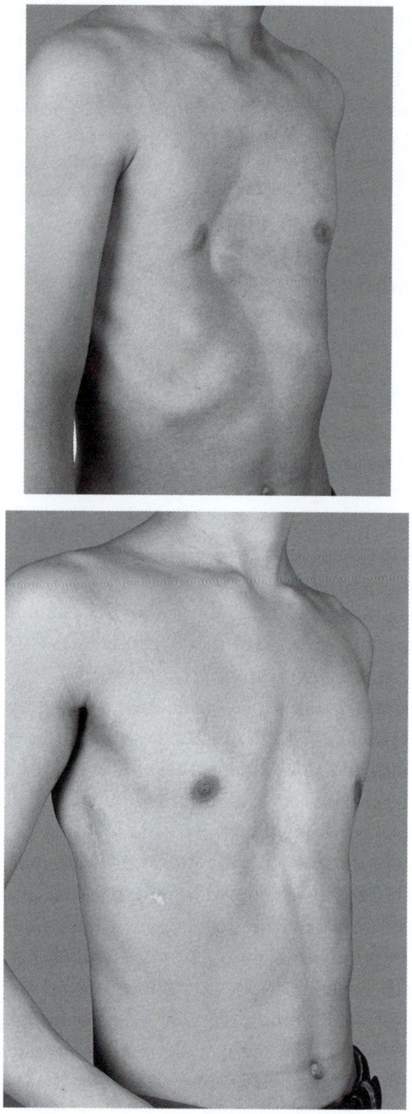

Figure 53.2 Photography of a 14-year-old boy (48 kg and 169 cm) with pectus excavatum: 7 months before (left side) and 1 year after surgery. The lateral chest scar is visible after the Nuss procedure.

Echocardiographic and magnetic resonance imaging (MRI) studies have demonstrated the occurrence of mitral valve prolapse in conjunction with *pectus excavatum* leading to an often-heard systolic murmur, and this has been attributed to anterior compression on the mitral valve annulus.

Although a restricted respiratory pattern has been observed in *pectus carinatum* patients, symptoms are usually rare until early adulthood. Cardiopulmonary effects and concomitant scoliosis are seen less often than in pectus excavatum. It is assumed that ventilation is limited as a result of a fixed chest wall leading to increased residual lung volumes (Figure 53.3).

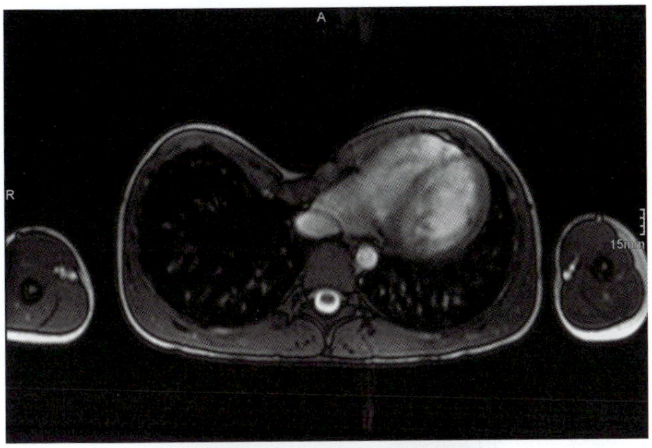

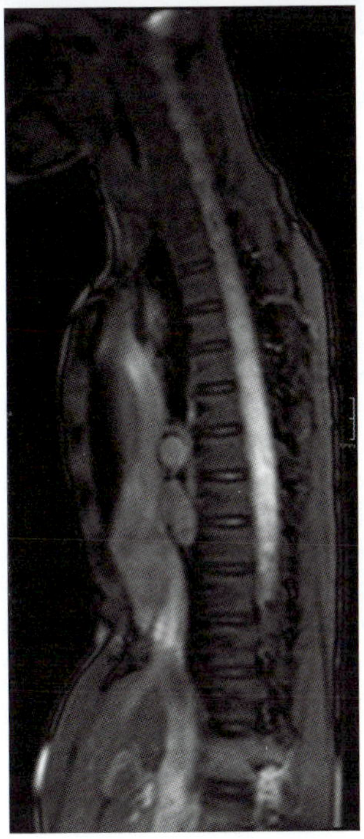

Figure 53.3 Corresponding magnetic resonance imaging: transversal (upper) and sagittal (lower) planes. Although the heart is dislocated to the left side, echocardiography revealed no significant pathologies. The shortest distance between sternum and anterior edge of the spine is 2.2 cm and Haller index 10.5.

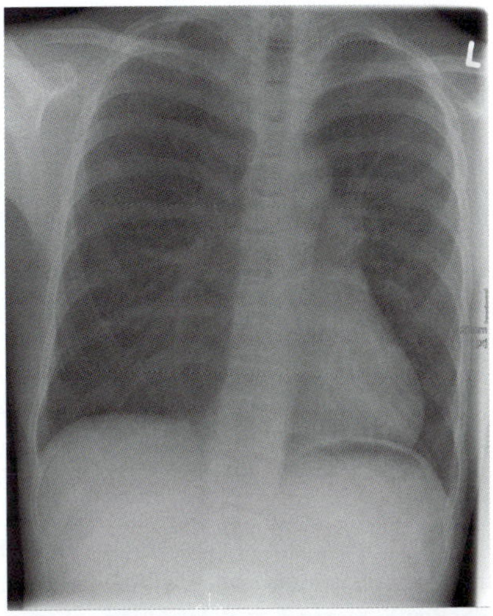

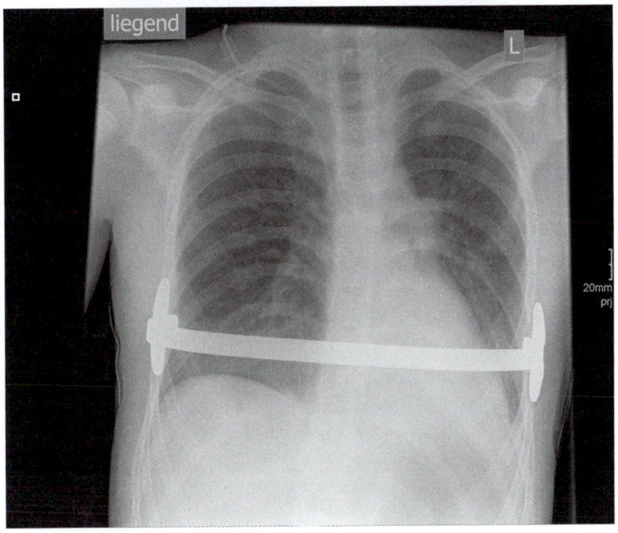

Figure 53.4 Imaging before and after the Nuss procedure for pectus excavatum. The corresponding chest X-ray 1 day before and 4 days after minimal invasive surgery (Nuss procedure). A concave stainless-steel bar has been placed under the sternum through lateral chest incisions. The lung function test showed normal values. The boy complained of stress-induced dyspnoea and suffered from his physical appearance. Lung function testing revealed aside from lung hyperinflation no restrictive or obstructive pathologies (vital capacity 3.14 L, forced expiratory volume in one second 2.58 L, and peak expiratory flow 333 L per minute).

Treatment

Nuss and colleagues shifted the paradigm in *pectus excavatum* surgery during the 1990s with publication of their results using minimally invasive techniques[19]. The Nuss repair, which has become widely accepted, comprises lateral chest incisions and the insertion of a retrosternal steel bar to elevate the sternum without the need for cartilage resection. The ideal age for surgery is just before puberty because, at that age, the chest is still very formable, the steel bar is in place during pubertal growth, the recovery time is short, and the incidence of recurrence is low (Figure 53.4). The number of patients presenting for repair has increased significantly. The long-term results have shown good outcome, and patient satisfaction studies have shown similar results.

Both surgical and nonoperative treatments are available to patients seeking correction of their pectus carinatum deformity. Modern operative techniques have evolved from the descriptions of Ravitch in 1960 and Welch in 1973[20]. As an alternative to surgery, external bracing techniques can significantly improve pectus carinatum deformities. The obvious advantage of external compression braces is the prevention of perioperative pain and morbidity. Current protocols, however, recommend wearing these braces for up to 23 h per day for prolonged periods of time. Therefore, the outcomes are dependent on the motivation and compliance of the typically young patients.

Amongst the commonest causes of chest wall pathology in the ICU is trauma, arising from blunt or penetrating injury. This topic is dealt with in detail in chapter 55.

In conclusion, chest wall pathology may arise from a number of different insults, and may impair cardiopulmonary function. Management of chest wall disease in ICU requires close liaison between intensivists, thoracic surgeons and other specialist teams such as respiratory medicine and rheumatology depending on the underlying causes.

REFERENCES

1. Adiguzel N, Karakurt Z, Güngör G, et al. Management of kyphoscoliosis patients with respiratory failure in the intensive care unit and during long term follow up. *Multidiscip Respir Med*. 2012;7(1):30.
2. Baldwin, ED, Cournand A, Richards DW. Pulmonary insufficiency; physiological classification, clinical methods of analysis, standard values in normal subjects. *Medicine (Baltimore)*. 1948;**27**(3):243–278.
3. Bergofsky EH, Turino GM, Fishman AP. Cardiorespiratory failure in kyphoscoliosis. *Medicine (Baltimore)*. 1959;**38**:263–317.
4. Lonner BS, Ren Y, Yaszay B, et al. Evolution of Surgery for adolescent idiopathic scoliosis over 20 years: have outcomes improved? *Spine* (Phila Pa 1976) 2018;**43**:402.
5. Hage CA, Abdul-Mohammed K, Antony VB. Pathogenesis of pleural infection. *Respirology*. 2004;**9**(1):12–15.
6. Huggins JT, Sahn SA. Causes and management of pleural fibrosis. *Respirology*. 2004;**9**(4):441–447.
7. Azoulay E. Pleural effusions in the intensive care unit. *Curr Opin Pulm Med*. 2003 Jul;**9**(4):291–297.
8. Thomas R, Jenkins S, Eastwood PR, et al. Physiology of breathlessness associated with pleural effusions. *Curr Opin Pulm Med*. 2015;**21**(4):338–345.
9. Petro W, Maassen W, Greschuchna D, et al. Regional and global lung function in unilateral fibrothorax after conservative therapy and decortication. *Thorac Cardiovasc Surg*. 1982;**30**(3): 137–141.
10. Godfrey MS, Bramley KT, Detterbeck F. Medical and Surgical Management of Empyema. *Semin Respir Crit Care Med*. 2019 Jun;**40**(3):361–374.
11. Akgul O, Ozgocmen S. Classification criteria for spondyloarthropathies. *World J Orthop*. 2011;**2**(12):107–115.
12. Berdal G, Halvorsen S, van der Heijde D, et al. Restrictive pulmonary function is more prevalent in patients with ankylosing spondylitis than in matched population controls and is associated with impaired spinal mobility: A comparative study. *Arthritis Res Ther*. 2012;**14**(1):R19.
13. Cho H, Kim T, Kim TH, et al. Spinal mobility, vertebral squaring, pulmonary function, pain, fatigue, and quality of life in patients with ankylosing spondylitis. *Ann Rehabil Med*. 2013;**37**(5):675–682.
14. El Maghraoui A, Dehhaoui M. Prevalence and characteristics of lung involvement on high resolution computed tomography in patients with ankylosing spondylitis: a systematic review. *Pulm Med*. 2012;**2012**:965956.
15. Millner JR, Barron JS, Beinke KM, et al. Exercise for ankylosing spondylitis: An evidence-based consensus statement. *Semin Arthritis Rheum*. 2016 Feb;**45**(4):411–427.
16. Ward MM, Deodhar A, Gensler LS, et al. 2019 Update of the American College of Rheumatology/Spondylitis Association of America/Spondyloarthritis Research and Treatment Network Recommendations for the Treatment of Ankylosing Spondylitis and Nonradiographic Axial Spondyloarthritis. *Arthritis Rheumatol*. 2019 Oct;**71**(10):1599–1613.
17. Duncan Phillips J, Hoover JD. Chest wall deformities and congenital lung lesions: what the general/thoracic surgeon should know. *Surg Clin North Am*. 2022 Oct;**102**(5): 883–911.
18. Shamberger RC. Congenital chest wall deformities. *Curr Probl Surg*. 1996;**33**(6):469–542.
19. Nuss D. Minimally invasive surgical repair of pectus excavatum. *Semin Pediatr Surg*. 2008;**17**(3):209–217.
20. Robicsek F, Watts LT, Fokin AA. Surgical repair of pectus excavatum and carinatum. *Semin Thorac Cardiovasc Surg*. 2009;**21**(1):64–75.

54

Obesity

Audrey de Jong and Samir Jaber

KEY MESSAGES

- Obese patients are at increased risk of atelectasis and pulmonary complications when admitted to the intensive care unit (ICU).
- A difficult airway should be anticipated in obese patients about to undergo intubation with necessary measures to reduce the risks.
- Obstructive sleep apnoea, obesity hypoventilation, and other co-morbidities should be suspected, investigated, and treated in the obese patient admitted to ICU.
- Higher levels of positive end-expiratory pressure (PEEP) may be appropriate in ventilated obese patients.

CONTROVERSIES

- Does high-flow nasal cannula (HFNC)–delivered oxygen offer the same effects in the obese critically ill patient as PEEP by continuous positive airway pressure (CPAP) or non-invasive ventilation (NIV)?
- The optimal level of PEEP in obese patients and the best means to titrate PEEP are still unknown. How should transpulmonary pressure and optimal PEEP be measured routinely?
- How is the 'obesity paradox' of survival benefit with acute respiratory distress syndrome (ARDS) explained?

FURTHER RESEARCH

- How to most accurately and effectively assess and adjust transpulmonary pressures, 'optimal' PEEP in the ventilated and non-ventilated patients.
- The utility of practical oesophageal pressure monitoring during mechanical ventilation. How to optimize the volume–pressure relationship in the obese, critically ill, ventilated patient.
- The role of electrical impedance tomography (EIT) and other developing non-invasive bedside technologies to track safe and unsafe lung recruitment in obese patients during mechanical ventilation.

Introduction

In obese patients, the negative effects of thoracic wall weight and abdominal fat mass on pulmonary compliance, leading to decreased functional residual capacity (FRC) and arterial oxygenation, are exacerbated by a supine position and further worsened after general anaesthesia and mechanical ventilation. Atelectasis formation is therefore increased in the obese patient compared to the non-obese patient and is one of the main causes of hypoxaemia and pulmonary infections during and after mechanical ventilation. Duration of mechanical ventilation and length of stay are increased in obese patients in ICU. Moreover, obese patients often present with co-morbidities such as obstructive sleep apnoea syndrome (OSA) or obesity hypoventilation syndrome (defined as a combination of obesity (Body mass index (BMI) ≥ 30 kg/m^2), daytime hypercapnia ($PaCO_2 > 45$ mmHg), and disordered breathing during sleep[1]).

Appropriate respiratory management of obese patients, taking into account physiology and co-morbidities, is challenging for the intensivist and some recommendations for management are summarized in Figure 54.1.

Current Accepted Practice

Non-invasive Respiratory Management

In the case of acute respiratory failure, especially in the perioperative setting, non-invasive ventilation (NIV) is of particular interest in obese patients. Moderate-to-high levels of positive end-expiratory pressure (PEEP) can be used to prevent atelectasis. High-flow nasal cannula oxygen (HFNC) devices help administer a high flow of humidified and warmed oxygen and provide a moderate level of PEEP.

Airway Management

The risk of difficult mask ventilation and/or intubation must be anticipated in obese patients. The intubation procedure in a morbidly obese patient should be considered as potentially difficult, and adequate preparation should occur, according to an algorithm for difficult airways. Videolaryngoscopes may be helpful as first-use devices in obese patients, and their use should be offered early as adjuncts in case of identifiable risk factors for difficult intubation.

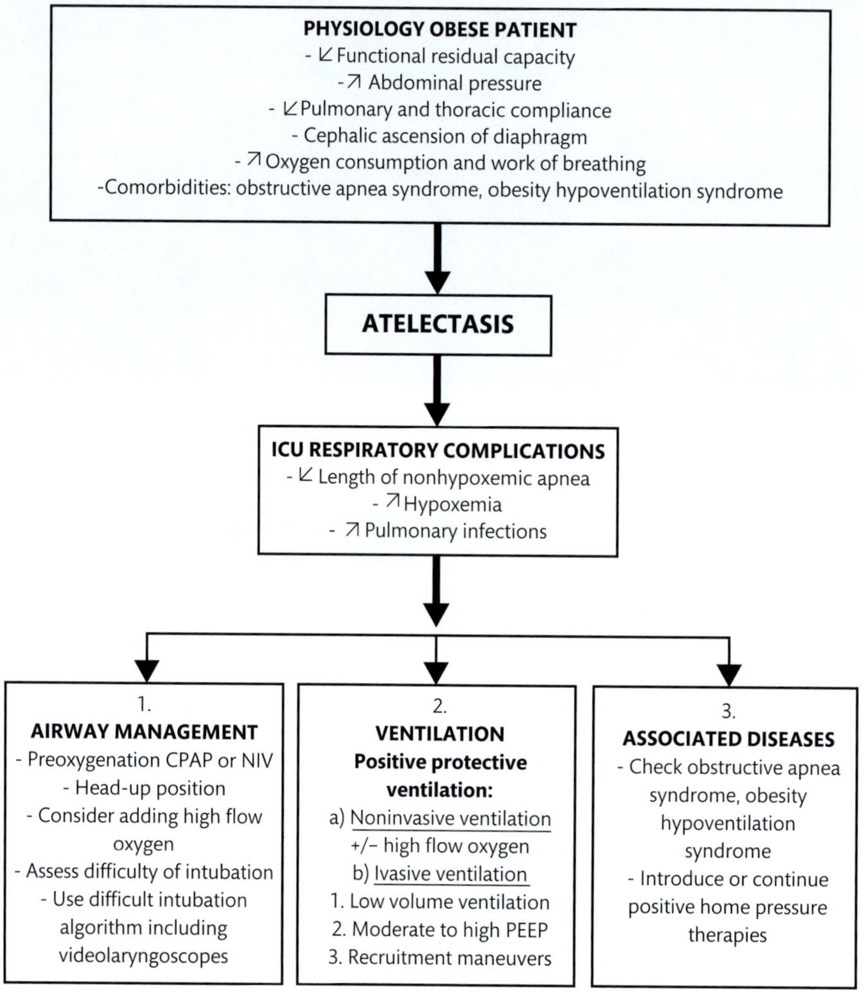

Figure 54.1 Key points of respiratory critical care management of obese patients. ICU, intensive care unit; CPAP, continuous positive airway pressure; NIV, non-invasive ventilation.

The main risk factors of difficult intubation in obese, critically ill patients are an elevated Mallampati score, reduced cervical mobility, and the presence of OSA.[2]

During the intubation procedure, preoxygenation using NIV in head-up position can improve expired oxygen fraction compared to classic bag-mask ventilation, with improved PaO_2, and decreased atelectasis (see Chapter 20).[3]

Mechanical Ventilation

In obese as in non-obese patients, lung-protective ventilation (low tidal volume (TV) + PEEP + recruitment manoeuvres) should be applied. The optimal recommended TV is between 6 and 8 mL/kg ideal body weight (IBW). An easier-to-remember formula for the calculation of IBW is: IBW (kg) = height (cm) − 100 for men and height (cm) − 110 for women. Recommended PEEP levels are higher than in the non-obese patient, aiming for at least 10 cmH_2O,[4] although with due attention to the potential side hemodynamic effects such as decreased oxygenation and arterial hypotension arising from compromised venous return. To open collapsed alveoli, recruitment manoeuvres should be used, transitorily increasing the transpulmonary pressure.[4] Because of the increased production of carbon dioxide, the respiratory rate may need to be increased. No ventilatory mode has proven its superiority in obese patients.

If acute respiratory distress syndrome (ARDS) develops in the obese patient, the prone position is an evidence-based and effective treatment when implemented by a trained team.[5]

Weaning from Mechanical Ventilation

T-piece and pressure support (PS) ventilation 0 and PEEP 0 cmH_2O tests were recently found to be the best weaning tests in critically ill obese patients.[6]

Specificities of Acute on Chronic Respiratory Failure

Positive airway pressure therapies should be implemented in ICU and continued at home. Identification of sleep-related breathing disorders, including obesity hypoventilation syndrome, should be followed up by a specialist after the ICU discharge, ideally in the setting of a multi-disciplinary bariatric programme.

Specificities of Perioperative Management

To decrease the risk of respiratory failure following extubation in a perioperative setting, a postoperative analgesia strategy avoiding opioids where possible, oxygenation by continuous positive airway pressure (CPAP) or NIV, careful patient positioning avoiding supine position, and monitoring have proven their efficacy. CPAP or NIV must be resumed as soon as possible after extubation and into the postoperative period.[7]

Evidence Base

Non-invasive Respiratory Management

NIV may be applied in an acute respiratory failure to avoid intubation in obese patients,[8] although it should not delay intubation if indicated. In hypercapnic obese patients, higher ventilatory pressures for longer periods of time may be required to reduce the $PaCO_2$ to within the normal range.

Airway Management

Obesity, if combined with OSA, is a risk factor for difficult intubation and difficult mask ventilation. Thus, elevated Mallampati score, reduced cervical mobility, and the presence of an OSA were associated with difficult intubation in obese patients.[2]

Following preoxygenation, there is a reduction of the non-hypoxic apnoea time (length of apnoea following the anaesthetic induction during which the patient has no oxygen desaturation) in obese patients.[9] A preoxygenation of 5 min with NIV, combining PS and PEEP, allows quicker attainment of exhaled fractional oxygenation (FeO_2) >90%.[3] The use of NIV can limit the decrease of lung volume and so improve oxygenation when compared to conventional face mask preoxygenation.[4]

Mechanical Ventilation

In obese patients with ARDS, low tidal volume ventilation (TV, 6 mL/kg) and moderate-to-high PEEP is beneficial.[10] In the perioperative setting, IMPROVE, a multicentre, randomized, double-blinded study, in patients with moderate risk of postoperative pulmonary complications showed that protective ventilation reduced complications from 27.5% to 10.5% and the length of hospitalization by 2 days.[11] In the randomized European study PROVHILO, which included patients at risk of postoperative pulmonary complications after abdominal surgery, there were significantly more haemodynamic failures in the group with high PEEP (12 cmH_2O) and TV of 8 mL/kg than in the group with low PEEP (2 cmH_2O) and TV of 8 mL/kg, without differences on pulmonary complications.[12] These two large randomized studies are complementary in interpretation: while the first showed the usefulness of protective ventilation to decrease pulmonary and extrapulmonary postoperative complications, the second study warns against the haemodynamic dangers of excessive levels of PEEP for all patients, in particular when high PEEP is not combined with low TV. Obese patients, particularly at risk of atelectasis, given their decreased FRC, are all the more sensitive to atelectasis and lack of PEEP. In several studies, the respiratory mechanics and alveolar recruitment are significantly improved by the application of PEEP (demonstrated by an improvement in compliance and a decrease in inspiratory resistance), as is the gas exchange.[13]

Some recommend a controlled pressure mode of ventilation because the decelerating flow pattern might allow a better distribution of the flow in the alveoli. However, studies comparing the two ventilatory modes (i.e. controlled flow or controlled pressure) report contradictory data.[14] In practice, the advantages and disadvantages of each mode must be known with the physician selecting the mode they are most familiar and comfortable with, mitigating the known downsides of each.

Prone positioning in obese patients with ARDS tends to improve PaO_2/FiO_2 ratio more than in the non-obese patient and is not associated with a greater rate of complications.[5]

Weaning from Mechanical Ventilation and Extubation

A recent physiological study specifically investigated the inspiratory effort during weaning of mechanical ventilation in a population of critically ill morbidly obese patients. The main result of this study was that, for obese patients, T-piece and PSV 0 + PEEP 0 cmH_2O weaning tests were the tests that best predicted post-extubation inspiratory effort and work of breathing.[6]

Specificities of Perioperative Management and Acute on Chronic Respiratory Failure

The prophylactic application of NIV after extubation allows decreased risk of acute respiratory failure by 16% and length of stay.[15,7] Moreover, in obese hypercapnic patients, the use of NIV following extubation is associated with decreased mortality.[16] A randomized controlled trial performed in morbidly obese patients after bariatric surgery found an improvement in ventilatory function when CPAP was immediately implemented after extubation compared to CPAP introduction 30 min after extubation.[17]

Physiology and Pharmacology

Even before respiratory failure and anaesthesia for mechanical ventilation, oxygenation decreases with greater weight. Oxygen consumption and work of breathing are increased in obese patients.[18] Obese patients have a higher CO_2 production due to their increased oxygen consumption and increased of work of breathing, and is compounded when co-morbid obesity hypoventilation syndrome is present and reduces ventilation.[19]

Pelosi et al. compared the postoperative course of 10 obese subjects with 10 non-obese subjects receiving sedatives and neuromuscular blockers. They found that obese patients had decreased pulmonary and thoracic compliance, a reduction of FRC and an increased work of breathing, compared to non-obese patients.[20] They are therefore prone to atelectasis, a risk factor for pulmonary infection.

Transpulmonary pressure (the difference between alveolar pressure and pleural pressure) is different from transthoracic pressure (the difference between pleural pressure and atmospheric pressure). Indeed, ventilation-induced lung injury is related to excessive transpulmonary pressure. Elevated ventilatory pressures can reflect an elevated transthoracic pressure even when the transpulmonary pressure is normal.

Controversies and Future Practice

Some uncertainties regarding the management of obese patients remain. The optimal level of PEEP in the obese patient and the best means to titrate PEEP are still unknown. Some obese patients may benefit from higher levels of PEEP. Evaluating trans-diaphragmatic pressure seems crucial to determining the maximum pressure minimizing alveolar damage, taking into consideration that plateau pressure is both related to transthoracic and trans-alveolar pressures.

In the same way, the best recruitment manoeuvre has not been determined in the obese patient. Levels of pressure needed to open the alveoli seem to be higher than in the non-obese patient, mostly due to the increased transthoracic pressure. Ongoing studies are examining the optimal type of recruitment manoeuvre. The reference method is an expiratory pause with a PEEP level of 40 cmH_2O for 40 s, but many alternatives exist: progressive increase of PEEP until 20 cmH_2O with a constant TV within 35 cmH_2O of plateau pressure (staircase) or progressive increase of the TV.[21] The ideal frequency for recruitment manoeuvres has still not been determined.

HFNC is of considerable potential in obese patients, both for preoxygenation of obese patients, including apnoeic oxygenation, and for oxygenation in case of acute respiratory failure. HFNC delivers continuously humidified and warmed oxygen through nasal cannula, with an adjustable FiO_2. The flow administered can reach 60 L/min with a 100% FiO_2.[22] A moderate level of PEEP has been provided with this device[22] when the patient breaths with a closed mouth. A recent study comparing standard facial mask, CPAP, or HFNC for preoxygenation in 33 patients found that the median levels of arterial pressure in oxygen (PaO_2) were comparable between the three groups. However, other studies are being performed to better assess HFNC as a means of preoxygenation in these patients. Between sessions of NIV or CPAP, HFNC has not been assessed in the obese patient but can be considered.

Finally, while obesity contributes to many diseases and is associated with higher all-causes of mortality in the general population, obesity and mortality in ICU are inversely associated.[23] In particular, obese ARDS patients, in whom diaphragmatic function is challenging, have a lower mortality risk when compared to non-obese patients.[5] Studies exploring this 'obesity paradox' are ongoing.[24]

REFERENCES

1. Pepin JL, Timsit JF, Tamisier R, et al. Prevention and care of respiratory failure in obese patients. *Lancet Respir. Med.* 2016;**4**(5):407–418.
2. De Jong A, Molinari N, Pouzeratte Y, et al. Difficult intubation in obese patients: Incidence, risk factors, and complications in the operating theatre and in intensive care units. *Br J Anaesth.* 2015;**114**(2):297–306.
3. Delay JM, Sebbane M, Jung B, et al. The effectiveness of non-invasive positive pressure ventilation to enhance preoxygenation in morbidly obese patients: A randomized controlled study. *Anesth Analg.* 2008;**107**(5):1707–13.
4. Futier E, Constantin JM, Pelosi P, et al. Noninvasive ventilation and alveolar recruitment maneuver improve respiratory function during and after intubation of morbidly obese patients: A randomized controlled study. *Anesthesiology.* 2011;**114**(6):1354–1363.
5. De Jong A, Molinari N, Sebbane M, et al. Feasibility and effectiveness of prone position in morbidly obese patients with ARDS: A case-control clinical study. *Chest.* 2013;**143**(6):1554–1561.
6. Mahul M, Jung B, Galia F, et al. Spontaneous breathing trial and post-extubation work of breathing in morbidly obese critically ill patients. *Crit Care.* 2016;**20**(1):346.
7. Jaber S, Chanques G, Jung B. Postoperative noninvasive ventilation. *Anesthesiology.* 2010;**112**(2):453–461.
8. Jaber S, Michelet P, Chanques G. Role of non-invasive ventilation (NIV) in the perioperative period. *Best Pract Res Clin Anaesthesiol.* 2010;**24**(2):253–265.
9. De Jong A, Futier E, Millot A, et al. How to preoxygenate in operative room: Healthy subjects and situations 'at risk'. *Ann Fr Anesth Reanim.* 2014;**33**(7–8):457–461.
10. Petrucci N, De Feo C. Lung protective ventilation strategy for the acute respiratory distress syndrome. *Cochrane Database Syst Rev.* 2013;**2013**(2):CD003844.
11. Futier E, Constantin JM, Paugam-Burtz C, et al. A trial of intraoperative low-tidal-volume ventilation in abdominal surgery. *N Engl J Med.* 2013;**369**(5):428–437.
12. Hemmes SN, Gama de Abreu M, Pelosi P, et al. High versus low positive end-expiratory pressure during general anaesthesia for open abdominal surgery (PROVHILO trial): A multicentre randomised controlled trial. *Lancet.* 2014;**384**(9942):495–503.
13. Pelosi P, Croci M, Ravagnan I, et al. The effects of body mass on lung volumes, respiratory mechanics, and gas exchange during general anesthesia. *Anesth Analg.* 1998;**87**(3):654–660.
14. Aldenkortt M, Lysakowski C, Elia N, et al. Ventilation strategies in obese patients undergoing surgery: A quantitative systematic review and meta-analysis. *Br J Anaesth.* 2012;**109**(4):493–502.
15. Jaber S, De Jong A, Castagnoli A, et al. Non-invasive ventilation after surgery. *Ann Fr Anesth Reanim.* 2014;**33**(7–8):487–491.
16. El-Solh AA, Aquilina A, Pineda L, et al. Noninvasive ventilation for prevention of post-extubation respiratory failure in obese patients. *Eur Respir J.* 2006;**28**(3):588–595.
17. Neligan PJ, Malhotra G, Fraser M, et al. Continuous positive airway pressure via the Boussignac system immediately after extubation improves lung function in morbidly obese patients with obstructive sleep apnea undergoing laparoscopic bariatric surgery. *Anesthesiology.* 2009;**110**(4):878–884.
18. Kress JP, Pohlman AS, Alverdy J, et al. The impact of morbid obesity on oxygen cost of breathing (VO(2RESP)) at rest. *Am J Respir Crit Care Med.* 1999;**160**(3):883–886.
19. Pepin JL, Borel JC, Janssens JP. Obesity hypoventilation syndrome: An underdiagnosed and undertreated condition. *Am J Respir Crit Care Med.* 2012 Dec 15;**186**(12):1205–1207.
20. Pelosi P, Croci M, Ravagnan I, et al. Total respiratory system, lung, and chest wall mechanics in sedated-paralyzed post-operative morbidly obese patients. *Chest.* 1996;**109**(1):144–151.
21. Constantin J-M, Jaber S, Futier E, et al. Respiratory effects of different recruitment maneuvers in acute respiratory distress syndrome. *Crit. Care.* 2008;**12**(2):R50.
22. Chanques G, Riboulet F, Molinari N, et al. Comparison of three high flow oxygen therapy delivery devices: A clinical physiological cross-over study. *Minerva Anestesiol.* 2013;**79**(12):1344–1355.
23. Oliveros H, Villamor E. Obesity and mortality in critically ill adults: A systematic review and meta-analysis. *Obesity.* 2008;**16**(3):515–521.
24. De Jong A, Jung B, Chanques G, et al. Obesity and mortality in critically ill patients: Another case of the Simpson paradox? *Chest.* 2012;**141**(6):1637–1638.

55

Trauma

Timothy E Scott and Christopher MR Satur

KEY MESSAGES

- Improved pre-hospital care is increasing the frequency and severity of casualties with traumatic chest injuries being treated in the intensive care unit (ICU).
- Trauma is increasingly seen in the elderly population who require a lower threshold for admission to intensive care.
- Surgical fixation of major thoracic wall injuries reduces mortality.
- Several mechanisms of injury may coexist in a particular patient.
- Regional neuronal blockade and structured analgesic protocols improve survival.

CONTROVERSIES

- Chest wall reconstruction is increasingly undertaken in trauma centres in the absence of evidence from randomized controlled studies.

FURTHER RESEARCH

- Good quality data describing optimal chest wall reconstruction following chest wall trauma is required.

Introduction

Thoracic trauma constitutes one-third of trauma-related hospital admissions and accounts for one-quarter of trauma-related mortality. It is second only to head injury as the most frequent cause of trauma-related death.

Effective management of chest trauma requires a detailed understanding of the mechanisms of injury and an understanding of patterns of injury to the chest wall and cardiovascular and pulmonary systems. The complexity of injury that may accompany thoracic trauma requires measured balance between conservative and interventional treatment to achieve best outcomes. This is exemplified by the case for the management of pulmonary injuries that may be multifactorial in aetiology, management of which may affect survival. It is the adept medical team that is able to balance competing priorities of protective lung ventilation, mitigation of the inflammatory response, and timely surgical intervention when indicated.

Traumatic injury of the chest is broadly divided into blunt or penetrating injury. Penetrating injury is further divided into high energy transfer (e.g. rifle bullet) or low energy transfer (e.g. stab wound or minor fragmentation injury). Exposure to explosive blast over-pressure represents a unique form of chest injury seen most often in military conflict but also as a result of peacetime industrial accidents and terrorist attacks.

Traumatic chest injury may be complicated by either inhalation of toxins or irritants such as cyanide or phosgene (poisoning, see Chapter 62). The major principles for the treatment of thoracic injury are supportive care with judicious application of mechanical ventilation, chest drainage as required, and early surgical management of skeletal and intrathoracic injuries. Nutritional support, careful attention to fluid balance, and an appropriate thromboprophylaxis strategy are an equally integral part of the therapeutic pathway.

Penetrating Chest Injury

The energy imparted on tissue by a penetrating object is a function of its mass (m) and the square of its velocity (v) (kinetic energy = $(1/2)mv^2$). Rifle bullets travel at speeds measured in thousands of m s^{-1} and are considered high-velocity objects, with the potential to cause significant energy transfer on passing through human tissue. Most of the resulting injury from a penetrating rifle bullet results from cavitation of the tissue that surrounds a bullet trajectory, due to dissipation of energy, rather than direct mechanical damage. Bullets from pistols, travelling at <600 m s^{-1}, and stab injuries are considered low velocity and result in much less energy transfer to lung parenchyma. Low-energy penetrating wounds lateral to the midclavicular line are less likely to cause mediastinal injury and life-threatening haemorrhage. The majority of low-energy penetrating injuries to the chest can be adequately managed conservatively by the insertion of an intercostal chest drain. Such injuries result in surgical intervention and ventilatory support in approximately 5% of adult cases rising to 20% in the paediatric population.

Significant injury to the lung parenchyma may require surgical repair or resection. Smaller lacerating injuries may be managed by direct repair or resection of limited areas of lung tissue. Injury to larger areas of lung tissues or injury of hilar structures such as the main bronchus or trachea occurs infrequently. Management may extend from direct repair of perforated airways or vascular structures to resection of a major pulmonary lobes though an extremely rare event. It is worth noting that resection or repair lines on lung or bronchus are prone barotrauma during supported ventilation, and surgical strategy should consider reinforced techniques of repair. Definitive surgery for high-energy-transfer wounds will require a period of time to allow the full extent of tissue damage to demarcate.

Blunt Injury and Flail Chest

In the UK, falls are responsible for 40% of thoracic trauma with an equal proportion arising from low-level (<2 m) and high-level (>2 m) falls. Low-level falls are most common in older patients. Blunt injury resulting from assault or cattle or horse trampling can cause severe chest wall disruption and lung injury. Such crush injuries generate a unique pattern of devitalized lung injury that may require debridement once demarcated and when global physiology allows. The chest wall disruption caused includes flail chest that may compromise respiratory and cardiac function and is often associated with haemothorax and pneumothorax.

Definition of flail chest has evolved from a simplistic, rib centric approach to considering the chest wall to be a cylindrical system comprising of the ribs, sternum, clavicles, and vertebral column.[1,2] Four categories of flail chest, as a modification of the original definition,[1,2] are described (Figure 55.1). Type A flail (38%) consists of sternal, clavicular, and bilateral peri-sternal rib fractures. Type A flail injuries often result from high-speed road traffic collisions. Type B flail (36%) chests are a unilateral injury consisting of anterior rib fractures usually resulting from a low-level fall or seatbelt injury. Type C flail (19%) consists of peri-scapula rib fractures and vertebral transverse process fractures resulting from a high-speed impact to the shoulder. Type D flail (6%) results from a significant crush injury leading to bilateral rib fractures in parallel to the vertebral column that may also have unstable fractures. A flail chest injury may cause paradoxical movement of a segment of the chest wall and if large enough will compromise gas exchange in the underlying lung. Large flail segments, and in particular those that cross the midline, may impair spontaneous respiration sufficiently to require mechanical ventilation.[2]

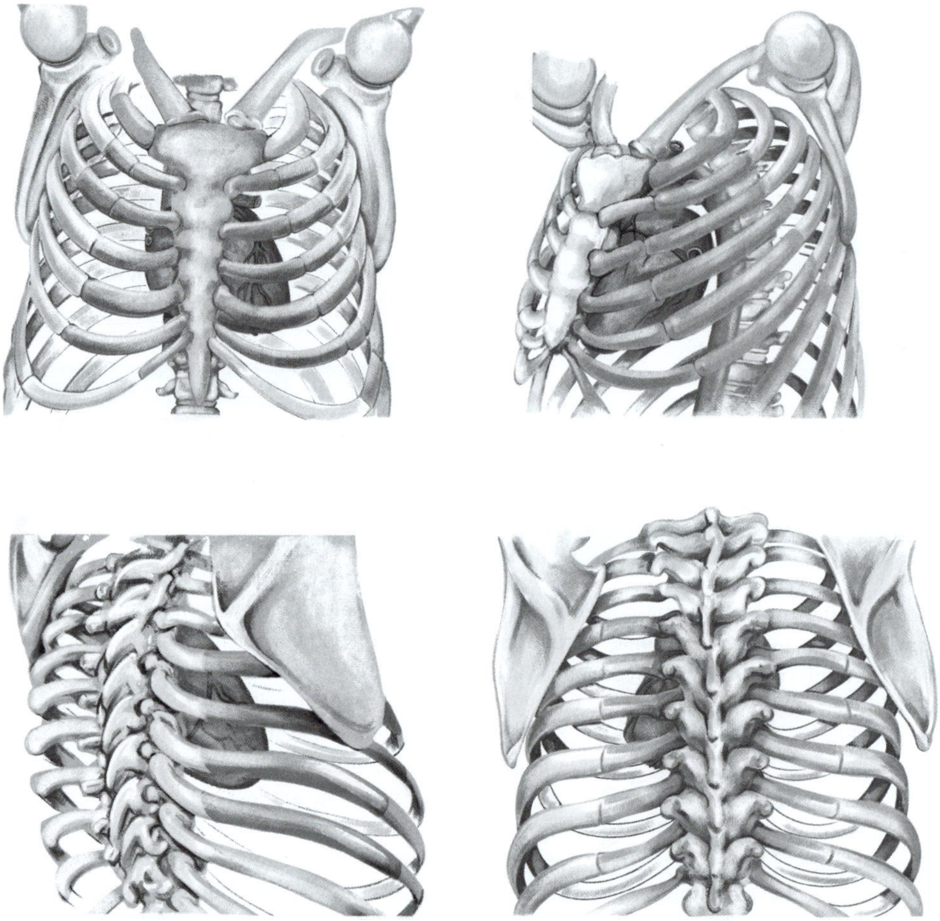

Figure 55.1 Flail chest classification. Type A: bilateral peri-sternal and clavicular fractures; type B: unilateral anterior fractures; type C: peri-scapular and transverse process fractures; type D: bilateral rib fractures adjacent to the spinal column.

Surgical stabilization of T2–T10 rib fractures, either unilaterally or bilaterally, associated with fixation of sternal, clavicular, and vertebral fractures, performed within 14 days of injury results in earlier weaning from mechanical ventilation, reduced intensive care unit (ICU) length of stay, reduced pneumonia and tracheostomy rate, and improved lung function.[3,4,5] Internal reduction and stabilization of rib or other bony structures aims to restore mechanical competency and chest volume, and decrease the risk of secondary complications arising from lung contusion and compromised ventilation associated with paradoxical movement.

Simple pneumothoraces occupying 20% or less of the ipsilateral lung volume in a spontaneously breathing patient can be observed. Positive pressure ventilation increases the possibility of converting larger pneumothoraces to a tension pneumothorax, and while close observation remains a viable approach, drainage of all but very small pneumothoraces should be considered (see Chapter 56). Haemothorax results from injury to the lung parenchyma, the heart or mediastinal structures, intercostal vessels, the diaphragm, liver, or spleen. While haemodynamic instability or the acute drainage of 1500 mL or more mandates urgent surgical evaluation and possible intervention, the majority of cases of haemothorax can be managed with tube thoracotomy. Retained haematoma or empyema are longer-term complications requiring surgery.

Chest drains should be inserted under ultrasound guidance. The mid-axillary line above the nipple level offers the easiest and safest location for surgical access. Chest drains can be removed once the lung is fully inflated, when bubbling in the underwater seal has ceased for more than 24 h, and are draining less than 200 mL of minimally blood stained or serosanguinous fluid in 24 h.

Good analgesia is fundamental to the care of these patients. Epidural analgesia does not reduce mortality, ICU, and hospital length of stay when compared to standard opioid regimes.[6] Epidural catheters insertion is contraindicated in coagulopathic patients but remain a useful analgesic option in selected cases. More recently, the serratus anterior plane block (SAPB) is proving to be a safe and effective option for treating rib fracture pain. Insertion of the SAPB catheter does not require difficult patient positioning and represents much less of a bleeding risk.[7] In the intermediate and longer terms, neuropathic pain frequently complicates this type of injury (particularly in younger patients) that may require analgesic adjuncts such as gabapentin and lidocaine patches.

Blast Injury and Behind Armour Blunt Trauma (BABT)

Blast exposure can cause chest injury by a variety of mechanisms (Table 55.1), any combination of which may coexist within any particular casualty. Fragmentation (secondary) injury is the most common injury pattern seen following explosions. Primary blast lung injury (PBLI) results from the interaction of the explosive's supersonic shock wave with lung tissue and is defined as 'radiological and clinical evidence of acute lung injury occurring within 12 h of exposure and not due to secondary or tertiary injury'.[8] The energy from an explosion dissipates in an inverse cube relationship with the 'stand-off' distance from its epicentre making the injury relatively uncommon in open-air environments. Reflected shock waves are however directly additive and so the presence of reflecting surfaces greatly increases the energy transfer to victims. The incidence of PBLI therefore increases significantly with closer proximity to an explosion and also when an explosion occurs within a confined space such as a bus or underground train.[9] It is a disease characterized by intra-parenchymal haemorrhage, laceration, and pneumothoraces.[10] PBLI is a frequent finding at autopsy in non-survivors following explosive events with air embolism regarded as being the fatal event. Patients present with respiratory distress and may suffer haemoptysis. In survivors, it is normally clinically apparent on arrival at hospital, but presentation of milder cases may be delayed. Patients who remain asymptomatic at 6 h, post-blast exposure can be discharged from close observation. Patients respond well to conventional mechanical ventilation and can expect to make a good recovery of lung function on discharge from hospital.[11]

Table 55.1 Nomenclature of blast injury

Primary injury	Results from exposure to an explosive shock wave
Secondary injury	Either a primary or secondary fragmentation injury from energized bomb material or loose environmental material, respectively
Tertiary injury	Results from movement of larger objects including the casualty themselves and building collapse as a result of the blast wind
Quaternary injury	Includes exposure to toxic substances including radiation or poisonous gases

Note: Several or all types of injuries may coexist in a casualty.

Source: Adapted from Scott TE, Haque M, Kirkman E, et al. Primary blast lung injury—A review. *Br J Anaes.* 2017;118(3):311–316. Copyright 2017, with permission from The Board of Management and Trustees of the British Journal of Anaesthesia.

BABT results from rapid deformation of the chest wall and shock wave generation as rigid body armour is struck by a high-velocity projectile. It is predominantly a contusional injury of varying severity though laceration of mediastinal structures occur that have resulted in fatalities.[12,13]

Extra-thoracic Injury Affecting the Lungs

The entire cardiac output traverses the lung parenchyma that is a highly vascular and friable capillary bed. The lungs are therefore particularly susceptible to the systemic effects of extra-thoracic injury. In the following section, we consider the pulmonary effects of long bone fractures and managing a patient with central nervous system injury.

Approximately 10% of adult patients suffering significant bony injury (pelvic, femoral, and tibial fractures) will develop fat embolism syndrome (FES).[14] It is occasionally seen following severe burns, hepatic injury, and can complicate orthopaedic intra-medullary nailing. FES consists of a constellation of respiratory, haematological, neurological, and cutaneous manifestations,[14] which is fatal in 7%–10% of cases.[15] In the absence of a universally accepted definition and diagnostic tool, the diagnosis remains clinical, made often by exclusion but aided by both a variety of eponymous criteria

Table 55.2 Gurd's fat embolism syndrome (FES) diagnostic criteria

Major criteria	Minor criteria	Laboratory criteria
Petechial rash	Heart rate >120 bpm	Macroglobulinemia
Respiratory compromise	Temperature >39.4 •C	50% decrease in platelet count
Neurological compromise	Jaundice	ESR >71 mm/h
	Renal compromise	20% decrease in haemoglobin
	Retinal signs	

Note: One major criterion and four other features are required to make the diagnosis. This composition has been varied by other authors.

Source: Reproduced from Gurd AR, Wilson RI. The fat embolism syndrome. *J Bone Joint Surg Br*. 1974;56B:408–416.

including Gurd's (Table 55.2) or Lindeque's criteria[16] (namely a femoral or tibial fracture combined with at least one of arterial PaO_2 of <8 kPa on room air, $PaCO_2$ of >7.3 kPa or pH <7.3, and respiratory rate of >30 or respiratory distress). Lindeque's criteria are arguably more objective than Gurd's, in that they relate to defined thresholds of respiratory physiological abnormality. However, Lindeque's criteria are non-specific, with hypoxia, impaired gas exchange, and respiratory distress potentially arising from a range of different pathologies in a patient suffering major trauma. While a petechial rash in the distribution of the internal carotid and subclavian arteries (neck, axilla, upper arms, and oral mucosa) is regarded as pathognomonic for the condition, none of these criteria have been formally validated, are not universally recognized, and diagnosis remains a clinical one based on an integrated assessment of the patient with high index of suspicion.

FES most commonly presents with respiratory compromise and neurological deterioration. The onset of symptoms is over 12–36 h post injury[17,18] (including surgical insult) but can present acutely with profound cardio-respiratory collapse, cor pulmonale, and sudden death. Respiratory symptoms and signs can include tachypnoea, haemoptysis, and hypoxaemic respiratory failure culminating in adult respiratory distress syndrome (ARDS, see Chapter 21) and the requirement for mechanical ventilation. Confusion, deteriorating level of consciousness, and seizures all may herald the neurological component of the syndrome. The presence of a patent foramen ovale will allow the systemic component of the disease to develop in the absence of respiratory symptoms.[19]

Fundoscopy will demonstrate exudates or small haemorrhages in approximately 50% of cases. Fat globules in the urine are a commonly seen, but non-specific finding. Hypocalcaemia may develop as a result of chelation with increased levels of free fatty acids. Derangement in coagulation studies will reflect the underlying severity of the condition and can evolve to the extent of disseminated intravascular coagulation in fulminant cases. In the presence of significant lung injury, intra-medullary nailing of long bone fractures should be delayed. Both neurological and respiratory symptoms resolve over the course of the subsequent week or so.

Head injury is common in traumatized patients. Such patients have impaired cerebral metabolic homeostasis that is so tightly regulated in health. In the absence of functioning homeostatic mechanisms, the intensive care clinician must physiologically support the brain by maintaining its perfusing pressure, oxygen and carbon dioxide tensions, and blood glucose levels within prescribed ranges.[20] This is achieved by maintaining mean arterial pressure at some 65 mmHg above intracranial pressure (ICP). The same considerations are thought to apply to swelling around spinal cord injury. To this end, patients must be fluid resuscitated to normovolaemia after which vasopressors should be introduced as required to maintain the target mean arterial pressure (MAP). Utilizing hypertonic crystalloid fluids to achieve this will also help manage cerebral and pulmonary oedema.

The management priority remains ensuring adequate gas exchange and so positive end-expiratory pressure (PEEP) should be applied as required and is unlikely to adversely affect ICP.[20,21] Nursing the patient in the head-up position will aid both ventilation and a reduction in ICP. Similarly, pharmacological muscular paralysis will reduce both ventilatory pressures and ICP.[20] Deeply sedated patients do not require cervical collars, which may impair cerebral venous drainage and so should be removed. Likewise, alternatives to jugular venous access should be considered. Should a high-resolution computed tomography scan of the cervical and thoracolumbar spine demonstrate no bone injury, then a sedated or otherwise obtunded patient can be regarded as having had their spine radiologically cleared and can be mobilized as required by nursing staff.[22]

Elderly Trauma

Elderly patients account for approximately 20% of trauma admissions. This proportion will increase in the future as this population continue to form a larger part of the overall demographic.[23] Pre-existing medical conditions and reduced physiological reserve mean that elderly traumatized patients will require close monitoring and organ support at a lower level of injury than is required in younger patients. Patients over the age of 65 suffer double the mortality for blunt injury compared to matched younger victims, and survivors have longer intensive care and hospital stays. Predictably, quality of life and personal independence following discharge from hospital also compare poorly to younger survivors. The use of an older person specific trauma unit can reduce morbidity and length of hospital stay.[24]

Ventilatory Support

Patients with chest injury require low tidal volume (LTV) mechanical ventilation as prescribed by the Acute Respiratory Distress Syndrome Network Working Group (ARDSnet) described in Chapter 21. Patients who have undergone a non-anatomical lung resection or have a broncho-pleural air leak will need a more conservative application of PEEP than might normally be considered. In circumstances where significant amounts of lung tissue have been removed, and in particular if the remaining tissue is damaged, post-operative extra-corporeal membrane oxygenation may be required (see Chapter 22.3). Avoiding unnecessary fluid administration will help prevent pulmonary and other tissue oedema. Prone positioning is a useful strategy in this group of patients and will improve oxygenation reduce pulmonary morbidity and duration of ventilation, and may also reduce mortality.[25,26] Interest is growing in airway pressure release ventilation as an alternative to LTV ventilation,[27] though evidence for its use in the trauma population is currently being sought. Applying low-level suction to chest drains does not speed up the resolution of air leaks and is not helpful.[28]

REFERENCES

1. Sillar W. The crushed chest, management of the flail anterior segment. *J Bone Joint Surg*. 1964;**43B**:738–745.
2. D'Abreu AL. Thoracic injuries: A critical review. *J Bone Joint Surg*. 1964;**46B**:581–597.
3. MS Chereuvu, R Chubsey, M Blagojevic-Bucknall, CMR Satur. Chest wall reconstruction reduces hospital mortality following major chest wall trauma: a retrospective cohort study. *Ann R Coll Surg Engl*. 2023;**000**:1–12.
4. Tanaka H, Yukioka T, Yamaguti Y, et al. Surgical stabilization of internal pneumatic stabilization? A prospective randomized study of management of severe flail chest patients. *J Trauma*. 2002;**52**:727–733.
5. Marasco SF, Davies AR, Cooper J, et al. Prospective randomized controlled trial of operative rib fixation in traumatic flail chest. *J Am Coll Surg*. 2013;**216**:924–932.
6. Carrier FM, Turgeon AF, Nicole PC, et al. Effect of epidural analgesia in patients with traumatic rib fractures: A systematic review and meta-analysis of randomized controlled trials. *Can J Anaes*. 2009;**56**:230–242.
7. May L, Hillermann C, Patil, S. Rib fracture management. *BJA Education*. 2016; **16**:26–32.
8. Mackenzie I, Tunicliffe B, Clasper J, et al. What the intensive care doctor needs to know about blast-related lung injury. *J Intensive Care Soc*. 2013;**14**:303–312.
9. Pizov R, Oppenheim-Eden A, Matot I, et al. Blast lung injury from an explosion on a civilian bus. *Chest*. 1999;**115**:165–172.
10. Scott TE, Haque M, Kirkman E, et al. Primary blast lung injury—a review. *Br J Anaes*. 2017;**118**:311–316.
11. Scott TE, Johnston AM, Keene DD, et al. Primary blast lung injury: The UK military experience. *Military Med*. 2020;**185**:e568–e572.
12. Cannon L. Behind armour blunt trauma—an emerging problem. *J R Army Med Corps*. 2001;**147**:87–96.
13. Carr DJ, Horsfall I, Malbon C. Is behind armour blunt trauma a real threat to users of body armour? A systematic review. *J R Army Med Corps*. 2016;**162**:8–11.
14. Fabian TC, Hoots A, Stanford DS, et al. Fat embolism syndrome: Prospective evaluation in 92 fracture patients. *Crit Care Med*. 1990;**18**:42–46.
15. Mellor A, Soni N. Fat embolism. *Anaesthesia*. 2001;**56**:145–154.
16. Lindeque BG, Schoeman HS, Dommisse GF, et al. Fat embolism syndrome: a double blind therapeutic study. *J Bone Joint Surg Br*. 1987;**69**:128–131.
17. Bulger EM Smith DG, Maier RV, et al. Fat embolism syndrome. A 10-year review. *Arch Surg*. 1997;**132**:435–439.
18. Sevitt S. The significance and pathology of fat embolism. *Ann Clin Res*. 1977;**9**:173–180.
19. Scopa M, Magatti M, Rossitto P. Neurologic symptoms in fat embolism: A case report. *J Trauma*. 1994;**36**:906–908.
20. Dinsmore J. Traumatic brain injury: An evidence-based review of management. *Contin Educ Anaesth Crit Care Pain*. 2013;**13**:189–195.
21. Mascia L, Grasso S, Fiore T, et al. Cerebro-pulmonary interactions during the application of low levels of positive end-expiratory pressure. *Intensive Care Med*. 2005;**31**: 373–379.
22. Scott TE, Coates PJB, Davies SR, et al. Clearing the spine in the unconscious trauma patient: An update. *J Intensive Care Soc*. 2012;**15**:113–116.
23. Keller JM, Sciadini MF, Sinclair E, et al. Geriatric trauma: Demographics, injuries, and mortality. *J Orthop Trauma*. 2012;**26**:e161–e165.
24. Mangram AJ, Mitchell CD, Shifflette VK, et al. Geriatric trauma service: A one-year experience. *J Trauma Acute Care Surg*. 2012;**72**:119–122.
25. Davis JW Lemaster DM, Moore EC, et al. Prone ventilation in trauma or surgical patients with acute lung injury and adult respiratory distress syndrome: Is it beneficial? *J Trauma*. 2007;**62**:1201–1206.
26. Voggenreiter G, Aufmkolk M, Stiletto RJ, et al. Prone positioning improves oxygenation in post-traumatic lung injury—a prospective randomized trial. *J Trauma*. 2005;**59**:333–343.
27. Roy S, Habashi N, Sadowitz B, et al. Early airway pressure release ventilation prevents ARDS—a novel preventative approach to lung injury. *Shock*. 2013;**39**(1):28–38.
28. Alphonso N, Tan C, Utley M, et al. A prospective randomized controlled trial of suction versus non-suction to the under-water seal drains following lung resection. *Eur J Cardiothorac Surg*. 2005;**27**:391–394.
29. Gurd AR, Wilson RI. The fat embolism syndrome. *J Bone Joint Surg Br*. 1974;**56B**:408–416.

56

Pneumothorax and Air Leaks

Giorgio Della Rocca and Luigi Vetrugno

KEY MESSAGES

- A lung-protective ventilation strategy should be adopted to reduce the incidence of barotrauma and bio-trauma.
- The increased use of ultrasound for the most common procedures, that is, central venous catheterization, thoracentesis, and lung biopsy, has led to a decrease in the incidence of iatrogenic pneumothorax in critically ill patients.
- The widespread use of lung ultrasound may improve the bedside diagnosis of pneumothorax.
- Small chest drains have been shown to be useful and less invasive in the treatment of pneumothorax.

CONTROVERSIES

- No clear guidelines are presently available for the treatment of traumatic and iatrogenic pneumothorax in the critical care setting.
- The best practice for the treatment of small pneumothoraces before the initiation of mechanical ventilation still needs to be determined; studies involving larger patient numbers (than those currently available) are required.
- A recent study revealed that contralateral tracheal deviation and jugular venous distension, typically taught in medical schools to be classic signs of tension pneumothorax, were actually found to be uncommon.
- No consensus exists regarding the treatment of air leaks; thus, surgeons are required to make decisions largely based on their own experience.

FURTHER RESEARCH

- In the context of the critical care unit, guidelines to facilitate the prompt recognition of pneumothorax and recommend the best timing of treatment remain to be identified. A consensus view on how to treat air leaks is also lacking. The new endobronchial valves, which offer mini-invasive systems, seem to provide a promising solution to the challenge of treating air leaks; however, large-scale trials are still required.

Introduction

Pneumothorax is a potentially life-threatening condition requiring prompt recognition and management in critically ill patients. Previous studies have reported its incidence to range between 4% and 15%[1]; however, more recent work indicates a lower incidence, probably due to the introduction of lung-protective ventilation strategies[2] and the increased use of ultrasound (US) guidance in the most common procedures.[3] Conversely, the widespread use of point-of-care US has also brought about an improvement in the bedside diagnosis of the pneumothorax[4] and its semi-quantitative evaluation, and provides a useful instrument for the positioning of chest tube drains in the treatment of this condition.[5]

Pneumothorax Classification

Pneumothorax can be classified as spontaneous, traumatic, or iatrogenic. Spontaneous pneumothorax (Figure 56.1) is more frequent in the emergency department, predominantly occurring in young, otherwise healthy individuals. It presents a significant global burden with an estimated incidence of 18–28/100,000 men and 1.2–6/100,000 women annually.[6] Spontaneous pneumothorax is sub-classified into primary and secondary. In primary pneumothorax, there is no apparent underlying lung disease, while coexisting lung disease is present in secondary pneumothorax—most commonly chronic obstruction pulmonary disease since the decline of tuberculosis in high-income countries.[6] Traumatic and iatrogenic pneumothorax, on the other hand, are the most frequent forms presenting in the intensive care unit (ICU).[1,7] Traumatic pneumothorax is usually secondary to a blunt chest trauma with rib fractures and/or penetrating weapon wounds, occurring in up to 60% of polytrauma cases[8]; while iatrogenic pneumothorax is related to invasive procedures, including central venous catheterization, thoracentesis, or pleural biopsy, or may occur in patients receiving mechanical ventilation with excessive tidal volume and/or high airway pressures. With regard to iatrogenic pneumothorax, one study has demonstrated a reduction in its incidence from 8% in the 1980s to 3% as assessed at the time of investigation 10 years ago.[7] In this study, the cumulative incidences of iatrogenic pneumothorax over 30 days were ascribed to

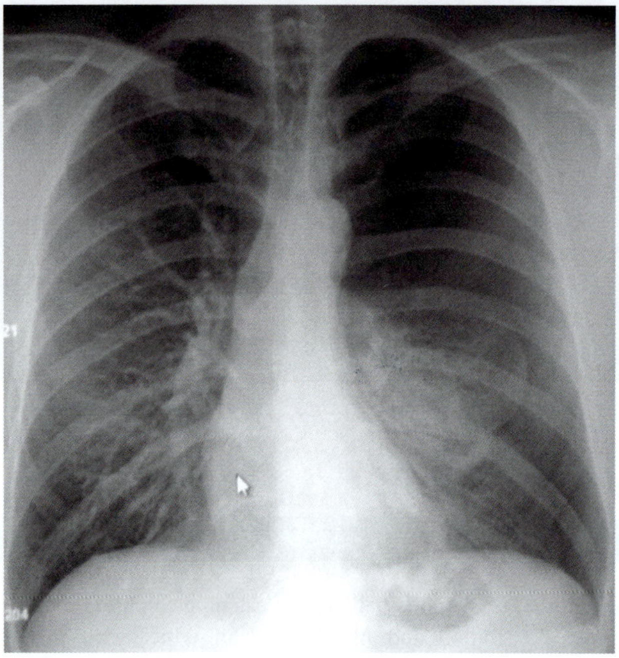

Figure 56.1 Left spontaneous pneumothorax.

the following: 1.3% secondary to ventilation, 0.9% secondary to central venous catheterization, and 0.7% after thoracentesis.[7] It is likely that this downwards trend in pneumothorax incidence has since continued, reaching levels as low as 0.1% for internal jugular vein cannulation under US.

Pneumothorax in Practice

In clinical practice, the pathophysiological mechanism underlying pneumothorax is extremely important. For example, pneumothorax is classified as '*open*' if there is a continuous transfer of air across the lung, the pleural space, and the chest wall, as may occur in the case of an open chest wall injury, or '*closed*', in the absence of chest wall damage, if the transfer of air across the air leak occurs in one direction only, that is, air enters the pleural space during inspiration but is unable to leave the pleural cavity, leading to lung collapse.[6,8] This mechanism is known as a 'one-way-valve' effect and, if unrecognized and left untreated, can lead to respiratory failure and cardiovascular collapse due to decreased venous return and a shift of the mediastinum with cardiac arrest. The development of tension in the pleural space gives rise to '*tension*' pneumothorax, generated by the build-up of a pressure gradient between intrapleural pressure and alveolar pressure. Mechanical ventilation can increase the air flow through the 'valve', allowing more air to pass per unit of time. The incidence of tension pneumothorax is not well established, reported ranges vary from 5.4% in major trauma patients in pre-hospital settings to between 1.1% and 3.8% in the ICU.[9] Its diagnosis is difficult as it can present with different signs and symptoms, depending on the respiratory condition of the patient. In the recent COVID19 pandemic, various centres have reported an apparent increase in pneumothorax among both ICU and non-ICU patients.[10]

Air Leak

Air leaks are described as any extrusion of air outside the tracheal–bronchial tree or through the lung, or even through the upper airways. In the first case, the tracheal–bronchial–pleural fistula communicates between the tracheal–bronchial tree and the pleural space, leading to pneumothorax or pneumomediastinum, or both. The nature of the air leak is of great importance, and pneumothorax in trauma and iatrogenic patients are less likely to settle spontaneously.[11] The magnitude of the leak is also crucial: small air leaks may heal quickly and spontaneously over a few days, especially if the patient can be weaned onto spontaneous ventilation. Conversely, larger leaks from the lung or a major bronchus will not settle by themselves and require surgery. In the ICU, one of the major problems is the loss of the delivered tidal volume with persistent lung collapse and difficulty ventilating the patient. Mechanical ventilation has been correlated with the formation of air leaks caused by barotrauma (excessive airway pressure) in patients with reduced lung compliance, usually those with acute respiratory distress syndrome (ARDS). The major factors associated with barotrauma include a peak inspiratory pressure equal or above 40 cmH_2O and the use of positive end-expiratory pressure. Thus, the following advice remains valid today despite being proposed 30 years ago: 'ensure the restoration of mechanical ventilation while being able to face any resulting complications, such as the immediate drainage of a barotrauma-induced pneumothorax'.[12] In a recent report, pneumothorax occurred in just 4.0% of patients with early ARDS treated with neuromuscular blockers compared with 11.7% of patients in the control group.[13] Interestingly, before the development of pneumothorax, none of these patients had an elevated plateau pressure that necessitated changes in the mechanical-ventilation settings; this leads us to suggest that the underlying mechanism involved is more likely due to bio-trauma rather than barotrauma. Nevertheless, 'protective lung ventilation', achieved by reducing tidal volume to a maximum of 6–8 mL/kg of ideal body weight, certainly reduces both types of damage[12–14] (ARDS, see Chapter 21).

Signs and Symptoms

The classic symptoms of pneumothorax include acute thoracic pain, shortness of breath, tachypnoea, tachycardia, and hypoxia; the following signs may also be indicative of pneumothorax: a reduction in lung expansion, diminished breath sounds, and cyanosis. These signs and symptoms are potentially concealed in critically ill, sedated, ventilated patients, and the only features may be an increase in the alveolar–arterial oxygen gradient and acute respiratory alkalosis.[11] In many cases, the diagnosis can be confirmed by standard chest X-ray. One of the most frequent signs of suspected pneumothorax in ventilated patients is subcutaneous emphysema of the chest wall, detected by palpation. Palpation elicits a characteristic feeling that is best described as the sensation of 'fresh snow under the fingers'.

Tension pneumothorax in spontaneously breathing patients may present shortness of breath, tachypnoea, respiratory distress, hypoxaemia, and ipsilateral decreased air entry that develops in a relatively delayed fashion[15]; moreover, chest X-rays are commonly available before thoracic decompression is performed. It has also been shown that contralateral tracheal deviation and jugular venous distension, typically taught in medical school as classic signs of tension pneumothorax, are actually uncommon.[15] In contrast, these above-mentioned signs and symptoms of pneumothorax will not be present in patients receiving mechanical ventilation. In these cases, clinicians should be prepared to perform an urgent thoracic decompression, even in the absence of chest radiographic confirmation of pneumothorax, if the patient presents with sudden cardiac arrest and tension pneumothorax is suspected.

Pneumomediastinum or Mediastinal Emphysema

This pathophysiological process, first described by Macklin as 'the transport of air along sheaths of pulmonic blood vessels from alveoli to mediastinum', can be schematized as follows: 'alveolar ruptures, air dissection along bronchovascular sheaths, and its spreading into the mediastinum'.[16] Pneumomediastinum may also arise from the upper airways and the mechanisms involved are the same as described for pneumothorax: trauma, asthma crises, mechanical ventilation, and Valsalva manoeuvres. Pneumomediastinum rarely originates from oesophageal or tracheal injuries.[17] It may present itself with a typical 'Hamman's sign' or 'Hammond's crunch', a crunching, rasping sound, synchronous with the heartbeat, heard over the precordium and produced by the heart beating against air-filled tissues. Except in rare cases of tension pneumomediastinum, it is not a life-threatening condition and does not require any treatment[11,16] (Figure 56.2).

Occult Pneumothorax

Cases of pneumothorax that are not identified by standard chest X-ray, but are instead detected by computed tomography scan, can be defined as 'occult' X-ray pneumothorax.[18] The incidence of occult pneumothorax in trauma patients is generally reported to be between 2% and 10%[19] although an incidence as high as 15% has also been reported.[20] The pathophysiological mechanism results in air in the pleural space that tends to accumulate in the least dependent area of the chest (air goes up, while fluids go down); indeed, it has been shown that the location of occult pneumothorax is apical in 57%, basal in 41%, anterior in 84%, lateral in 24%, and medial in 27%, but never posterior (0%).[21] The air is not detected on supine chest X-rays, giving rise to a false-negative result for pneumothorax.[22] The failure to recognize occult pneumothorax can be very dangerous because it may become enlarged, particularly in mechanically ventilated patients, leading to tension with hemodynamic instability.[19]

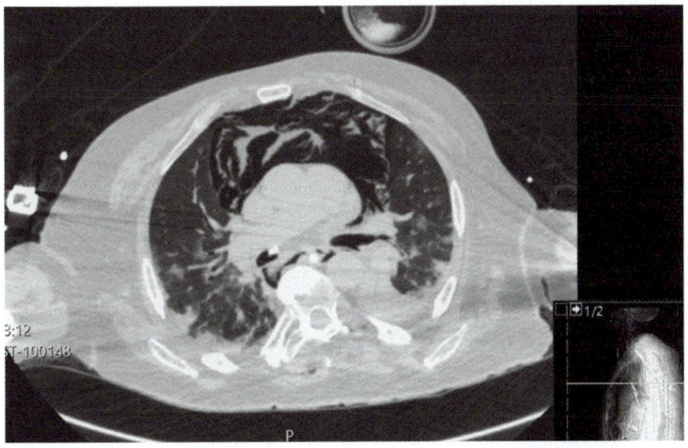

Figure 56.2 Pneumomediastinum in a patient experiencing a severe asthmatic crisis.

Reproduced from Wali A, et al. Pneumomediastinum following intubation in COVID-19 patients: a case series. *Anaesthesia* 2020; 75, 8: 1076–81, with permission from the Association of Anaesthetists and Wiley.

Lung Ultrasound

Lung ultrasound has become a valuable diagnostic tool that allows for the rapid assessment of lung and pleural diseases.[4–5] Briefly, the presence of 'lung sliding' is able to rule out pneumothorax, while the 'lung point' sign can be taken as a strong indication of pneumothorax, as illustrated in Figure 56.3; a more complete algorithm is available elsewhere[5]; an in-depth discussion of lung US is beyond the scope of this chapter. In cases of occult pneumothorax, lung US has been shown to be superior to supine chest X-ray with a sensitivity and a specificity of 92% and 99.4%, respectively, and an accuracy of 98.6%[22]; the same study revealed a sensitivity of 52% and a specificity of 100% for supine chest X-ray. However, it should also be emphasized that, in cases of thoracic trauma with tissue emphysema, air prevents the transmission of US and thus inhibits detection of the lung sliding phenomenon and other sonographic signs; as a consequence, US is no longer a valuable tool in such cases.

Treatment

At least three guidelines exist for the treatment of spontaneous pneumothorax,[23,24] while no specific guidelines have been published for the treatment of traumatic and iatrogenic pneumothorax. A general consensus exists among experts that the volume of pneumothorax should be a determining factor in the decision as to whether a chest tube should be inserted or whether conservative treatment is required. Pneumothoraces can be classified according to their relative size: small, moderate, and large. In general, small spontaneous, traumatic, and iatrogenic pneumothorax may resolve themselves without the need for treatment and require monitoring only. Moderately sized spontaneous, iatrogenic, and traumatic pneumothorax may initially be treated by needle aspiration. However, as stated above, in critically ill trauma patients, a standard treatment approach may not be suitable. The residual lung, as a result of lung contusion or due to a pre-existing chronic pulmonary disease or an early ventilation-associated pneumonia, may be unable to provide adequate functional parenchyma, irrespective of pneumothorax size.[3] Furthermore, pneumothorax may be bilateral in trauma patients, and thus the sum of its effects must be considered. In such cases, the choice of treatment is largely determined by the specific symptoms and hemodynamic compromise. It goes

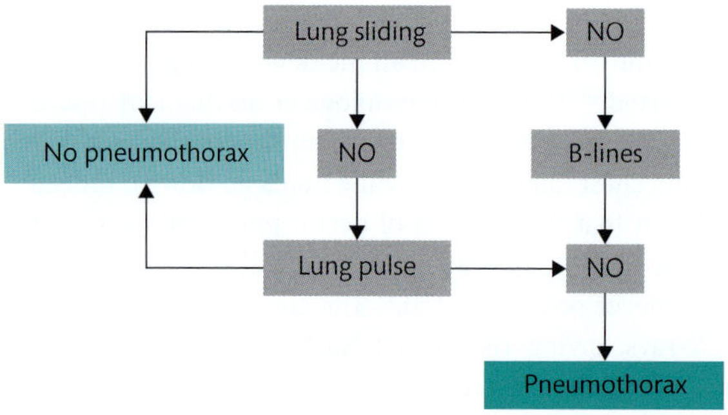

Figure 56.3 Flow diagram for rule-in or rule-out pneumothorax with lung ultrasound.

without saying that large pneumothorax should be treated with a chest tube. In the ICU and the operating theatre, it is important to consider whether any small pneumothoraces exist and whether they require draining before the initiation of mechanical ventilation. In the Advanced Trauma Life Support guidelines (produced by the American College of Surgeons), drainage is recommended before anaesthesia or transportation (within or outside the hospital, including air transportation).[25] However, overall consensus regarding these guidelines is ambiguous. The Eastern Association for Surgery of Trauma Practice Guidelines for the management of haemothorax and occult pneumothorax[8] state that '*occult pneumothorax may be observed in a stable patient regardless of positive pressure ventilation*'. Some physicians are in favour of chest drainage, while others recommend close observation only, since complications after drainage may occur in up to 15% of patients and a suboptimal tube thoracostomy position may result in as many as 15%.[26] It has been shown that only very small anterior pneumothoraces are observed with a high success rate (81%).[18] While it has been suggested that ventilated patients with pneumothorax managed only by close observation developed a high rate of complications, these results were not confirmed in a prospective randomized study.[27] The low sample numbers of the above-mentioned studies remain problematic for their interpretation, and thus debate on the best treatment strategies for pneumothorax continues.

In the case that insertion of a chest drain is required, the British Thoracic Society recommends that it is inserted within the 'triangle of safety', as illustrated in Figure 56.4. This area, bordered by the lateral edge of the latissimus dorsi and the lateral border of the pectoralis major muscle, and superior to the horizontal level of the fifth intercostal space, minimizes the risk to underlying structures and avoids damage to muscle and breast tissue. For apical pneumothorax, the second intercostal space in the mid-clavicular line is sometimes chosen. However, this route may lead to mammary arterial injury and bleeding. Once again, US may be helpful in non-urgent situations and help avoid further complication. Traditionally, large-bore chest tubes (24–32 F) have been used for pneumothorax, but, more recently, smaller-bore tubes (<14 F) using the modified Seldinger technique have been shown to be as effective as the bigger ones with fewer related complications.[28–30] The risk of serious complications associated with small-bore catheters is low with a frequency of injury of 0.2% and a malpositioning rate of 0.6%.[29] Both types of drain can be attached to a water seal device and can be left in place until the lung expands against the chest wall and the air leak resolves. If the lung fails to re-expand, suction should be applied to the water seal device. Positive pressure ventilation could result in maintaining the air leak open; where possible, the optimal strategy for small leaks is to wean the patient from ventilation to facilitate sealing of the leak. Assuming that air leakage has stopped, a pneumothorax will gradually resolve as the air is reabsorbed into pulmonary capillaries; oxygen supplementation could increase this absorption.

Once again, no consensus exists about the treatment of air leaks in traumatic and iatrogenic pneumothorax. In patients with persistent air leaks and pneumothorax, the use of suction through chest drains has been advocated with the scope of increasing the air flow out through the drain in the hope that visceral and parietal shouldering may close the aperture.[30] A negative pressure of -10 to -20 cmH_2O is normally recommended.[28] However, following drainage of a pneumothorax, the early application of suction should be avoided due to the increased risk of re-expansion pulmonary oedema.[28–30] Expert opinion states that a persistent air leak on day 3 post injury should prompt a video-assisted thoracoscopic surgery (VATS) evaluation.[11] Finally, endobronchial valve devices are currently being evaluated for their use in the treatment of air leaks. This technology represents promising treatment for patients with air leaks for whom the usual treatments have not worked and for those unable to undergo surgery.[31]

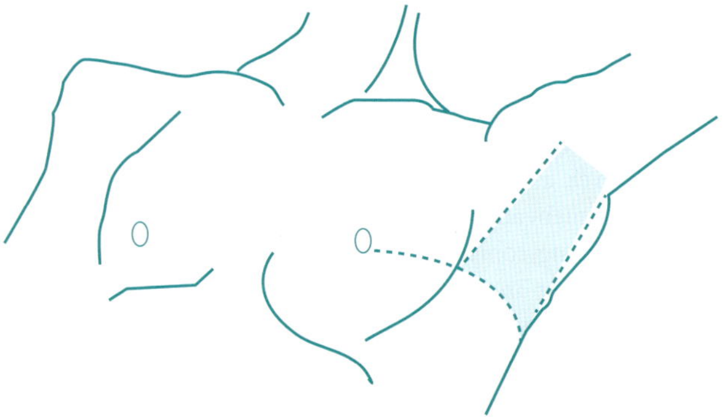

Figure 56.4 The 'triangle of safety'. This area is bordered by the lateral edge of the latissimus dorsi and the lateral border of the pectoralis major muscle and is superior to the horizontal level of the fifth intercostal.

REFERENCES

1. Yarmus L, Feller-Kopman D. Pneumothorax in the critically ill patient. *Chest*. 2012; **141**(4):1098–1105.
2. Miller MP, Sagy M. Pressure characteristics of mechanical ventilation and incidence of pneumothorax before and after the implementation of protective lung strategies in the management of pediatric patients with severe ARDS. *Chest*. 2008;**134**(5):969–973.
3. Frankel HL, Kirkpatrick AW, Elbarbary M, et al. Guidelines for the appropriate use of bedside general and cardiac ultrasonography in the evaluation of critically ill patients—part I: General ultrasonography. *Crit Care Med*. 2015;**43**(11):2479–2502.
4. Barbara DW. Images in anesthesiology: Bedside lung ultrasonography: A tool for rapid assessment of pneumothorax. *Anesthesiology*. 2015;**122**(4):921.
5. Volpicelli G. Sonographic diagnosis of pneumothorax. *Intensive Care Med*. 2011;**37**(2):224–232.

6. MacDuff A, Arnold A, Harvey J. BTS Pleural Disease Guideline Group. Management of spontaneous pneumothorax: British Thoracic Society Pleural Disease Guideline 2010. *Thorax*. 2010;**65**(Suppl 2):ii18–31.
7. de Lassence A, Timsit JF, Tafflet M, et al. Pneumothorax in the intensive care unit: Incidence, risk factors, and outcome. *Anesthesiology*. 2006;**104**(1):5–13.
8. Mowery NT, Gunter OL, Collier BR, et al. Practice management guidelines for management of hemothorax and occult pneumothorax. *J Trauma*. 2011;**70**(2):510–518.
9. Ludwig J, Kienzle GD. Pneumothorax in a large autopsy population. A study of 77 cases. *Am J Clin Pathol*. 1978;70(1):24–26.
10. Martinelli AW, Ingle T, Newman J et al. COVID-19 and pneumothorax: A multicentre retrospective case series. *Eur Respir J*. 2020;**56**:2002697.
11. Paramasivam E, Bodenham A. Air leaks, pneumothorax, and chest drains. *Contin Educ Anaesth Crit Care Pain*. 2008;**8**(6):204–209.
12. Terragni P, Ranieri VM, Brazzi L. Novel approaches to minimize ventilator-induced lung injury. *Curr Opin Crit Care*. 2015;**21**(1):20–25.
13. Papazian L, Forel J-M, Arnaud Gacouin A, et al. Neuromuscular blockers in early acute respiratory distress syndrome. *N Engl J Med*. 2010;**363**:1107–1116.
14. The Acute Respiratory Distress Syndrome Network. Ventilation with lower tidal volumes as compared with traditional tidal volumes for acute lung injury and the acute respiratory distress syndrome. *N Engl J Med*. 2000;**342**(18):1301–1308.
15. Roberts DJ, Leigh-Smith S, Faris PD, et al. Clinical presentation of patients with tension pneumothorax: A systematic review. *Ann Surg*. 2015;**261**(6):1068–1078.
16. Macklin CC. Transport of air along sheaths of pulmonic blood vessels from alveoli to mediastinum: Clinical implications. *Arch Intern Med*. 1939;**64**:913–926.
17. Wintermark M, Schnyder P. The Macklin effect: A frequent etiology for pneumomediastinum in severe blunt chest trauma. *Chest*. 2001;**120**(2):543–547.
18. Wolfman NT, Myers WS, Glauser SJ, et al. Validity of CT classification on management of occult pneumothorax: A prospective study. *Am J Roentgenol*. 1998;**171**:1317–1320.
19. Moore FO, Goslar PW, Coimbra R, et al. Blunt traumatic occult pneumothorax: Is observation safe? Results of a prospective, AAST multicenter study. *J Trauma*. 2011;**70**(5):1019–1023.
20. Ball CG, Kirkpatrick AW, Laupland KB, et al. Incidence, risk factors, and outcomes for occult pneumothoraces in victims of major trauma. *J Trauma*. 2005;**59**(4):917–925.
21. Ball CG, Kirkpatrick AW, Laupland KB, et al. Factors related to the failure of radiographic recognition of occult posttraumatic pneumothoraces. *Am J Surg*. 2005;**189**(5):541–546.
22. Soldati G, Testa A, Sher S, et al. Occult traumatic pneumothorax: Diagnostic accuracy of lung ultrasonography in the emergency department. *Chest*. 2008;**133**(1):204–211.
23. Baumann MH, Strange C, Heffner JE, et al. Management of spontaneous pneumothorax: An American College of Chest Physicians Delphi consensus statement. *Chest*. 2001;**119**:590–602.
24. De Leyn P, Lismonde M, Ninana V, et al. Guidelines Belgian Society of Pulmonology. Guidelines on the management of spontaneous pneumothorax. *Acta Chir Belg*. 2005:**105**;265–267.
25. American College of Surgeons Committee on Trauma. Advanced Trauma Life Support (ATLS): Ninth Edition. Chicago, IL: American College of Surgeons. *J Trauma Acute Care Surg*. 2013;**74**(5):1363–1366.
26. Kirkpatrick AW, Rizoli S, Ouellet JF, et al. Occult pneumothoraces in critical care: A prospective multicenter randomized controlled trial of pleural drainage for mechanically ventilated trauma patients with occult pneumothoraces. *J Trauma Acute Care Surg*. 2013;**74**(3):747–754.
27. Brasel KJ, Stafford RE, Weigelt JA, et al. Treatment of occult pneumothoraces from blunt trauma. *J Trauma*. 1999;**46**:987–990.
28. Havelock T, Teoh R, Laws D, et al. BTS Pleural Disease Guideline Group Pleural procedures and thoracic ultrasound: British Thoracic Society pleural disease guideline. *Thorax*. 2010;**65**(Suppl 2):61–76.
29. Lin YC, Tu CY, Liang SJ, et al. Pigtail catheter for the management of pneumothorax in mechanically ventilated patients. *Am J Emerg Med*. 2010;**28**(4):466–471.
30. Cerfolio RJ, Bryant AS, Singh S, et al. The management of chest tubes in patients with a pneumothorax and an air leak after pulmonary resection. *Chest*. 2005;**128**(2):816–820.
31. National Institute for Clinical Excellence Interventional Procedures Programme. Interventional procedure overview of insertion of endobronchial air valves for persistent air leaks. IP 1025 [IPG448] 27 March 2013. https://www.nice.org.uk/guidance/ipg448/evidence/overview-438804829

57

The Obstetric Patient

Timothy Crozier

KEY MESSAGES

- The need for intensive care unit (ICU) admission in the obstetric population is uncommon but important.
- Pregnancy is associated with specific physiological changes that affect both diagnostic and management aspects of care. These changes persist into the postpartum period.
- There is a higher incidence of failed intubation in both the obstetric population and the ICU population.
- Care should be taken with patient positioning (use of lateral tilt to avoid aorto-caval compression), choice of imaging studies, and prescribing.
- In general terms, respiratory management of the obstetric ICU patient should largely mirror that of the non-pregnant patient.
- Multi-disciplinary management and close involvement of an obstetrician is essential.
- Pregnancy is a pro-coagulable state, and deep venous thrombosis (DVT) prophylaxis in ICU is extremely important.

CONTROVERSIES

- Evidence for precise physiological target setting in the pregnant patient is scarce.
- The timing and utility of obstetric delivery in the setting of maternal critical illness/severe respiratory failure is unclear.

FURTHER RESEARCH

- Long-term outcome studies of women and children after an ICU admission in pregnancy are required.
- Should ventilatory management aim to mimic the normal respiratory alkalosis of pregnancy?

Introduction

Obstetric patients comprise a small but important subset of intensive care patients. The term 'obstetric patient' applies to women that are currently pregnant or within 6 weeks post-delivery. Most women admitted to the intensive care unit (ICU) are postpartum.[1] Outcomes in the obstetric intensive care population are generally good as these women are usually young and relatively healthy. However, new reproductive technologies are enabling women of more advanced age to conceive, and other medical advances have allowed many more women with severe coexistent medical diseases such as cystic fibrosis to reach childbearing age and start families. Congenital heart disease (especially cyanotic conditions) and pulmonary hypertension are associated with very significantly increased maternal and foetal risk in pregnancy.[2] Severe obesity (Chapter 54) is an increasing factor in the obstetric population and has been associated with increased maternal morbidity and adverse neonatal outcomes.[3,4]

Acute respiratory failure requiring intensive care admission may be due to a number of insults (Box 57.1). Asthma has been implicated as a contributor to maternal deaths,[5] and pregnancy increases complications in community-acquired pneumonia.[6] Influenza pneumonia during the 2009/2010 H1N1 pandemic severely and preferentially affected pregnant women.[5,7] Severe pulmonary oedema may be the result of pre-eclampsia, cardiac disease, or intravenous fluid therapy. Acute respiratory distress syndrome (ARDS) may be caused by a number of insults (Chapter 21), including pregnancy-specific causes such as pre-eclampsia.[8] Severe maternal hypoxia and cardiorespiratory collapse may occur with amniotic fluid embolism (AFE) or pulmonary embolus (Chapter 43).

In addition to the conditions described above, respiratory issues or the need for mechanical ventilation may complicate another illness process and lead to a maternal ICU admission.

Although the majority of obstetric ICU admissions occur in the postpartum period, this chapter largely addresses issues involved in the care of the pregnant patient. It should be remembered that physiological changes of pregnancy persist into the postpartum period and that 'obstetric' conditions such as eclampsia may occur for the first time following delivery.

Aspects of 'General Care' in the Obstetric ICU Patient

In general terms and in most cases, best care of the mother will also constitute best care for the foetus. Physiological changes during pregnancy and the presence of this 'second patient' can make both diagnostic and management decision-making difficult. Optimal management of the critically ill pregnant woman in ICU is also

Box 57.1 Respiratory critical care in obstetrics: respiratory conditions requiring ICU care

Asthma (Chapter 42)
Pneumonia (bacterial/viral/other) (Chapters 32–35)
Aspiration pneumonitis
Pulmonary oedema (cardiogenic or non-cardiogenic)
Pre-eclampsia
Amniotic fluid embolism
Pulmonary embolism (Chapter 43)
ARDS (Chapter 21)
Neuromuscular weakness, including post-anaesthesia (Chapter 51)
Pulmonary hypertension (Chapter 45)
Chronic lung disease, including cystic fibrosis
Other: trauma, immersion injury, inhalational injury, etc. (Chapters 55, 60, and 61)

difficult because of a lack of high-quality evidence. Current ICU practice generally relies upon extrapolation of evidence from the non-pregnant population; these strategies may be modified to allow for the physiological changes seen in normal pregnancy and for the protection of the foetus. Certain general care aspects should be kept in mind when looking after these women. These are outlined in Box 57.2. Care of these women requires a multi-disciplinary approach, and the close involvement of an obstetrician is mandatory.

Respiratory System Changes in Pregnancy

Pregnancy leads to increased mucosal vascularity (oedema and hyperaemia) in the upper airway.[10] As pregnancy proceeds, the gravid uterus displaces the diaphragm upwards with subsequent rib flaring. Expiratory reserve volume, residual volume, and functional residual capacity (FRC) are reduced by 15%–20% at term.[11] There is some reduction in total respiratory compliance in the third trimester although lung compliance is not altered in pregnancy.[12] Pregnancy results in an increase in minute ventilation. Minute ventilation increases by up to 40%–50% at term with an increase in tidal volume (hyperpnoea) rather than respiratory rate being responsible.[13] This is thought to be hormonally mediated via progesterone.

Box 57.2 General care aspects to consider when caring for the obstetric ICU patient

Avoidance of supine positioning
Supine posture results in aorto-caval compression by the gravid uterus causing hypotension and possible circulatory collapse. Lateral tilt should ideally be maintained at all times
Care with medication prescribing
Care with radiology use (follow applicable local guidelines[9])
Thrombo-prophylaxis (pregnancy is a pro-coagulant state)
Increased nutrition requirements
Physiological changes of pregnancy may confound assessment
Physiological targets should consider both maternal and foetal needs
Foetal monitoring/assessment of foetal viability/consideration and planning for delivery
Close involvement of an obstetrician
Postpartum care: perineum care/breast care and lactation issues/baby contact
Involvement of midwifery staff

There is a resultant respiratory alkalosis with the normal $PaCO_2$ in pregnancy sitting between 28 and 32 mmHg (3.7–4.3 kPa), with a compensatory metabolic acidosis resulting in a bicarbonate level of 18–21 mEq/L.[12]

Airway Management and Intubation

Management of the obstetric airway is frequently difficult, and requires forward planning and appropriate skills and staffing (Chapter 20). Late pregnancy is associated with increased mucosal oedema of the airway and increased bleeding risk from instrumentation, as well as reduced FRC from superior displacement of the diaphragm. This results in more rapid desaturation during apnoea and hypoventilation, and reduced lower oesophageal sphincter pressure and increased intra-abdominal pressure contribute to an increased risk of aspiration. These factors are exacerbated in obesity.[11]

Rapid sequence induction is the technique of choice in pregnancy.[11,14] Given the higher incidence of failed intubation in both the obstetric population and the ICU in general,[15] intubation should be performed by the most experienced and expert practitioners available. Guidelines have been published in the United Kingdom on difficult and failed intubation in obstetrics with algorithms dealing with safe induction, failed intubation, and the 'can't intubate, can't oxygenate' scenario[16] (Chapter 20).

Sedation and Muscle Relaxants

ICU sedation should be approached in largely the same manner as the non-pregnant population (Chapter 25). One multinational observational study showed that opiates, benzodiazepines, and propofol are all routinely used.[17] Muscle relaxants do not cross the placenta in significant amounts and should be used for same indications as in the non-pregnant population. Dexmedetomidine has been used in the anaesthetic setting,[18] but good ICU data is lacking. It should be noted that there is a lack of robust data regarding foetal outcomes following periods of prolonged maternal sedation in the ICU setting.

Oxygenation and Ventilation

A number of factors need consideration when setting ventilator parameters and physiological targets in the pregnant patient. The utero-placental circulation is sensitive to carbon dioxide (CO_2) levels, with hyperventilation/severe *hypo*carbia and alkalosis, in particular, causing uterine vasoconstriction and subsequent placental hypoperfusion. Significant *hyper*carbia also causes foetal acidosis. Maternal hypoxia causes uterine vasoconstriction with subsequent foetal hypoxia and acidosis. There is no good evidence to suggest a 'safe' maternal oxygenation target, but a pO_2 of 70 mmHg (9 kPa) has been suggested.[19] Observational data and experience suggest that lower oxygenation levels (>88%–90% SpO_2) are tolerated in practice,[17] but outcome data is lacking.

As noted above, pregnant women develop a mild respiratory alkalosis, with pCO_2 levels around 30 mmHg (4 kPa) (27–34 mmHg (3.7–4.3 kPa), to allow placental CO_2 excretion).[12] It is currently unknown as to whether mechanical ventilation targets should aim to mimic this; however, the potential worsening of maternal lung damage through injurious mechanical ventilation makes ruthless targeting of this low pCO_2 unjustifiable. In addition, other conditions such as traumatic brain injury may make this level of sustained hypocapnia impractical or frankly contraindicated from a maternal management perspective. In the case of maternal lung pathology such as ARDS (Chapter 21), targeting a normal (non-pregnant) CO_2 level or higher is established practice, and observational data suggests that strict targeting of this lower CO_2 is not routinely performed even in women without significant lung injury.[17] If permissive hypercapnia is required, then mild/moderate hypercarbia ($pCO_2 < 60$ mmHg (8 kPa)) has been recommended in pregnancy.[12]

No specific mode of ventilation is recommended in pregnancy. Ventilator settings and parameters should try to follow evidence for the non-pregnant population, being mindful of the additional factors of utero-placental flow and blood gas indices as described.

Circulatory Support in Respiratory Critical Care

Normal pregnancy is a hyperdynamic state with an increase in blood volume[20] and cardiac output, often with an accompanying fall in blood pressure due to reduced systemic vascular resistance.[21] The utero-placental circulation does not auto-regulate like other tissue beds,[22] and maternal shock from any cause results in foetal hypoxia and acidosis. Maternal acidosis, hypoxia, and alkalosis cause constriction of the uterine artery with foetal acidosis, and cardiovascular collapse causes severe foetal injury or death within minutes. In women with respiratory failure, echocardiography should be performed early to rule out structural heart disease or systolic heart failure. Isolated right ventricular dilatation/failure may be seen in pulmonary hypertension (Chapter 45) or pulmonary or AFE. Left or biventricular systolic failure may be due to myocarditis, peripartum cardiomyopathy, AFE, or other pathology. Diastolic dysfunction with increased left ventricular mass is frequently seen in pre-eclampsia.[23] Iatrogenic pulmonary oedema is a considerable risk in pregnancy[24] and particularly in pre-eclampsia. Loop diuretics such as frusemide should be used for volume overload although in general diuretics should be cautiously used in pregnancy. Persistent hypotension requires vasoactive support. There is little or no evidence to guide blood pressure targets in the pregnant ICU patient; however, an initial mean arterial pressure target of ≥65 mmHg is reasonable. Aims may be titrated depending on end-organ (including placental) function. There is minimal evidence as to choice of agent: dobutamine and adrenaline are commonly used inotropes, whereas noradrenaline is the initial vasopressor of choice.

Critical Care of Specific Respiratory Conditions in Pregnancy

In general, care of specific respiratory disorders in the critically ill obstetric patient should follow usual (non-pregnant) practice. Some specific points are made here.

Asthma

Critical care treatment of severe acute exacerbations of asthma in pregnancy is similar to that in the non-pregnant patient. Appropriate glucocorticoid therapy should *not* be withheld due to pregnancy. Interpretation of blood gases should always take into account expected changes in pregnancy with particular attention to rising carbon dioxide levels (see Chapter 42).

Viral Pneumonia

After the H1N1 pandemic of 2009/2010, awareness of the possibility of influenza pneumonia in pregnancy has increased. Oseltamivir should be given to all pregnant women with acute respiratory failure until influenza is excluded (see Chapter 34). There is evidence that pregnant women may be at increased risk of severe COVID-19 compared to non-pregnant women, and although data is limited regarding use of therapies, corticosteroids (dexamethasone or prednisolone) are recommended if indicated. Decisions regarding other therapies such as tocilizumab and remdesivir should be taken with an expert multi-disciplinary team or wider maternal medicine network. Antivirals such as Molnupiravir and Lopinavir/ritonavir and agents such as baracitinib should not be used.[25] (See chapter 35).

ARDS

A multitude of obstetric or non-obstetric insults may cause ARDS.[8] As discussed, ventilation strategies should mirror those in the non-obstetric population. Rescue therapies such as inhaled nitric oxide, prone positioning, and extracorporeal support have all been applied in the obstetric population (see Chapter 21).[7,26]

Deep Venous Thrombosis and Pulmonary Embolism (PE)

Pregnancy is a high-risk state for venous thromboembolism. American Thoracic Society Guidelines for the evaluation of suspected PE in pregnancy are available.[27] Both V/Q and CT pulmonary angiography can be used for the diagnosis of PE,[27,28] depending on clinical circumstances. In addition, echocardiography is safe, quick to obtain, and provides useful information. Low-molecular-weight heparin is preferred for thrombo-prophylaxis and treatment in pregnancy[29] although unfractionated heparin and/or inferior vena cava filters may be used if bleeding risk is high or if delivery is considered imminent or likely. A multi-disciplinary approach with obstetric and haematology input is required. Supportive treatment essentially mirrors that of the non-pregnant patient and is discussed in Chapter 43. Radiological clot retrieval techniques, open surgical thrombectomy, and intravenous thrombolytic therapies[30] have all been used in pregnancy (see Chapter 43).

Obstetric Conditions Causing Respiratory Failure/Compromise

Pre-eclampsia and the Hypertensive Disorders of Pregnancy

Pre-eclampsia is a disease characterized by maternal hypertension (>140/90 mmHg) and proteinuria. It occurs after 20 weeks gestation and may progress to seizures (eclampsia), multi-organ failure (especially hepatic and renal failure), and maternal and foetal death. Pre-eclampsia is recognized as a cause of ARDS,[8] and women with this condition are at high risk of pulmonary oedema as a result of cardiac factors[23] and abnormal lung permeability and endothelial dysfunction.[31] Treatment involves supportive ICU care, a restrictive fluid strategy, aggressive blood pressure control, magnesium sulphate for prevention of eclampsia, and careful timing of delivery.

Amniotic Fluid Embolism

Amniotic fluid embolism (AFE) is a rare but devastating condition that occurs during pregnancy and delivery. Amniotic fluid enters the maternal circulation, causing hypotension, acute hypoxemic respiratory failure, and disseminated intravascular coagulation. Most women present with rapid cardiorespiratory collapse. Acute pulmonary hypertension and right and subsequently left ventricular failure lead to severe hypoxemia and cardiogenic shock with pulmonary oedema a frequent complication. The diagnosis is made on clinical grounds and requires exclusion of other catastrophes such as anaphylaxis and massive PE. Treatment involves early and aggressive maternal resuscitation and ongoing supportive care with rapid decision-making regarding delivery if the woman is undelivered. Rescue therapies such as inhaled nitric oxide and extracorporeal circulatory support have been successfully used. The Society of Maternal-Fetal Medicine has recently released evidence-based guidelines surrounding diagnosis and management.[32] In the case of maternal arrest from AFE or any other cause, management should largely mirror that of the non-obstetric population with some important modifications.[33] These include performing cardiopulmonary resuscitation in the supine position with manual lateral displacement of the uterus and performing urgent caesarean section primarily for maternal benefit (resuscitative hysterotomy) if no recovery after 4 min of resuscitation. Guidelines for cardiac arrest in pregnancy are available online.

Foetal Monitoring and Delivery

Management of the pregnant ICU patient generally follows the premise that best care of the mother creates the best chance of a successful pregnancy outcome, and that continuation of preterm pregnancy is preferable to extreme prematurity or the maternal risks of delivery. However, occasionally maternal or foetal factors render continuation of the pregnancy risky or impossible. In late pregnancy, it might be expected that delivery may improve maternal lung compliance and oxygenation; however, evidence for a consistent significant maternal benefit is lacking.[12] Foetal monitoring can be helpful in decision-making and should be undertaken by obstetrics staff experienced with critically ill women. Maternal factors such as heavy sedation may make interpretation difficult, and there is very limited evidence to guide practice. Decision-making surrounding delivery or termination is complex and requires multi-disciplinary input. Early detailed evaluation should be undertaken even if the risk of early delivery appears low with a crisis plan ready for immediate implementation if required.

REFERENCES

1. Pollock W, Rose L, Dennis CL. Pregnant and postpartum admissions to the intensive care unit: A systematic review. *Intensive Care Med.* 2010;**36**:1465–1474.
2. Yucel E, DeFaria Yeh D. Pregnancy in women with congenital heart disease. *Curr Treat Options Cardiovasc Med.* 2017;**19**:73.
3. McKeating A, Maguire PJ, Daly N, et al. Trends in maternal obesity in a large university hospital 2009–2013. *Acta Obstet Gynecol Scand.* 2015;**94**:969–975.
4. Gunatilake RP, Perlow JH. Obesity and pregnancy: Clinical management of the obese gravida. *Am J Obstet Gynecol.* 2011;**204**:106–119.
5. Knight MK, Bocklehurst S, Neilson P, et al. (eds), on behalf of MBRRACE-UK. Saving Lives, Improving Mothers' Care—lessons learned to inform future maternity care from the UK and Ireland Confidential Enquiries into Maternal Deaths and Morbidity 2009–12: Oxford: National Perinatal Epidemiology Unit, University of Oxford; 2014.
6. Goodnight WH, Soper DE. Pneumonia in pregnancy. *Crit Care Med.* 2005;**33**:S390–S397.
7. Knight M, Pierce M, Seppelt I, et al. Critical illness with AH1N1v influenza in pregnancy: A comparison of two population-based cohorts. *Brit J Obstet Gynaec.* 2011;**118**:232–239.
8. Cole DE, Taylor TL, McCullough DM, et al. Acute respiratory distress syndrome in pregnancy. *Crit Care Med.* 2005;**33**:S269–S78.
9. Austin LM, Frush DP. Compendium of national guidelines for imaging the pregnant patient. *AJR Am J Roentgenol.* 2011;**197**:W737–746.
10. Toppozada H, Michaels L, Toppozada M, et al. The human respiratory nasal mucosa in pregnancy. An electron microscopic and histochemical study. *J Laryngol Otol.* 1982;**96**:613–626.
11. Soens MA, Birnbach DJ, Ranasinghe JS, et al. Obstetric anesthesia for the obese and morbidly obese patient: An ounce of prevention is worth more than a pound of treatment. *Acta Anaesthesiol Scand.* 2008;**52**:6–19.
12. Lapinsky SE. Acute respiratory failure in pregnancy. *Obstetric Med.* 2015;**8**(3):126–132.
13. Elkus R, Popovich J, Jr. Respiratory physiology in pregnancy. *Clin Chest Med.* 1992;**13**:555–565.
14. Nejdlova M, Johnson T. Anaesthesia for non-obstetric procedures during pregnancy. *Contin Edu Anaes Crit Care Pain.* 2012;**12**:203–206.
15. Cook TM, MacDougall-Davis SR. Complications and failure of airway management. *Br J Anaesth.* 2012;**109**(Suppl 1):i68–i85.
16. Mushambi MC, Kinsella SM, Popat M, et al. Obstetric Anaesthetists' Association and Difficult Airway Society guidelines for the management of difficult and failed tracheal intubation in obstetrics. *Anaesthesia.* 2015;**70**:1286–1306.
17. Lapinsky SE, Rojas-Suarez JA, Crozier TM, et al. Mechanical ventilation in critically-ill pregnant women: A case series. *Int J Obstet Anesth.* 2015;**24**:323–328.
18. Nair A, Sriprakash K. Dexmedetomidine in pregnancy: Review of literature and possible use. *J Obstet Anaes Crit Care.* 2013;3:3–6.
19. Meschia G. Fetal oxygenation and maternal ventilation. *Clin Chest Med.* 2011;**32**:15–19.
20. Yeomans ER, Gilstrap LC. Physiologic changes in pregnancy and their impact on critical care. *Crit Care Med.* 2005;**33**:S256–S258.
21. Carbillon L, Uzan M Fau-Uzan S, Uzan S. Pregnancy, vascular tone, and maternal hemodynamics: A crucial adaptation. *Obstet Gynecol Surv.* 2000;**55**:574–581.
22. Chau A, Tsen LC. Fetal optimization during maternal sepsis: Relevance and response of the obstetric anesthesiologist. *Curr Opin Anaesthesiol.* 2014;**27**:259–266.
23. Melchiorre K, Sutherland GR, Baltabaeva A, et al. Maternal cardiac dysfunction and remodeling in women with preeclampsia at term. *Hypertension.* 2011;**57**:85–93.
24. Dennis AT, Solnordal CB. Acute pulmonary oedema in pregnant women. *Anaesthesia.* 2012;**67**:646–659.
25. Royal College of Obstetricians and Gynaecologists. Coronavirus (COVID-19) infection in pregnancy: information for healthcare professionals. Version 16, December 2022. Available from https://www.rcog.org.uk/media/ftzilsfj/2022-12-15-coronavirus-covid-19-infection-in-pregnancy-v16.pdf
26. Grasselli G, Bombino M, Patroniti N, et al. Use of extracorporeal respiratory support during pregnancy: A case report and literature review. *ASAIO J.* 2012;**58**:281–284.
27. Leung AN, Bull TM, Jaeschke R, et al. An Official American Thoracic Society/Society of Thoracic Radiology Clinical Practice Guideline: Evaluation of suspected pulmonary embolism in pregnancy. *Am J Resp Crit Care Med.* 2011;**184**:1200–1208.
28. McLintock C, Brighton T, Chunilal S, et al. Recommendations for the diagnosis and treatment of deep venous thrombosis and

pulmonary embolism in pregnancy and the postpartum period. *Aust N Z J Obstet Gynaecol.* 2012;**52**:14–22.
29. Marshall AL. Diagnosis, treatment, and prevention of venous thromboembolism in pregnancy. *Postgrad Med.* 2014;**126**:25–34.
30. Martillotti G, Boehlen F, Robert-Ebadi H, et al. Treatment options for severe pulmonary embolism during pregnancy and the postpartum period: A systematic review. *J Thromb Haemost.* 2017;**15**:1942–1950.
31. Roberts JM, Redman CW. Pre-eclampsia: More than pregnancy-induced hypertension. *Lancet.* 1993;**341**:1447–1451.
32. Society for Maternal-Fetal Medicine (SMFM), Pacheco LD, Saade G, et al. Amniotic fluid embolism: Diagnosis and management. *Am J Obstet Gynecol.* 2016;**215**:B16–24.
33. Jeejeebhoy FMZC, Lipman SCB, Joglar J, et al. Cardiac arrest in pregnancy: A scientific statement from the American Heart Association. *Circulation.* 2015;**132**:1747–1773.

58

Transfusion

Markus Honickel, Oliver Grottke, and Rolf Rossaint

KEY MESSAGES

- Transfusion-associated adverse events (TAEs) may be acute or delayed, immune or non-immune mediated, with certain predisposing and potential second hit factors for TRALI.
- Transfusion of blood products may seriously impact the respiratory system predominantly through transfusion-related acute lung injury (TRALI) or transfusion-associated circulatory overload (TACO).
- TRALI and TACO are distinguishable by clinical, physiological, and laboratory features but not radiology.
- Secondary effects of TAEs include anaphylactic dyspnoea and pneumonia.

CONTROVERSIES

Regarding the interrelation of transfusion and the respiratory system, controversies persist concerning the following:

- Transfusion triggers and thresholds
- Storage-related impairments of blood products
- Ratios of blood products in cases of bleeding
- Pathophysiology of TRALI and TACO
- Specific diagnostic markers
- Therapy of post-transfusion oedema

FURTHER RESEARCH

- Development of cultured blood cells from induced pluripotent stem cells to reduce TAE.
- New pharmacologic agents (i.e. TRPV4 antagonists) to trigger clearance of pulmonary oedema.

Introduction

Transfusion involves the administration of blood products, including corpuscular elements, plasma, and plasma-derived proteins. Transfusion compensates for loss of blood components in severe anaemia. In patients with impaired respiratory function, sufficient oxygen-carrying capacity is essential for oxygen delivery. Under conditions of acute bleeding, transfusion of platelets and coagulation factors may also be necessary.[1]

Each blood product transfused carries a potential risk of adverse events. Transfusion reactions affecting the respiratory system, although infrequent, may be particularly severe and potentially life-threatening. Transfusion-related acute lung injury (TRALI) and transfusion-associated circulatory overload (TACO) accounted for 55% of all fatal transfusion reactions reported to the United States Food and Drug Administration between 2016 and 2020.[2] Anaphylactic dyspnoea (Chapter 59) and pneumonia (Chapter 33) could also develop due to transfusion. Due to their respiratory prominence, this chapter focuses on TRALI and TACO whilst giving an overview of patient blood management (PBM).

Currently Accepted Practice

Red Blood Cells (RBCs)

RBCs are derived from fresh whole blood or processed via cell separation. Transfusion of RBCs has been shown to increase oxygen-carrying capacity and to avoid anaemic hypoxaemia. For safe transfusion of RBCs, the donor blood group antigens must be compatible with those of the recipient (Table 58.1), and fertile Rhesus-negative (dd) women should not receive Rhesus-positive (DD, Dd) blood, except in an emergency. Such transfusions of donor–recipient-compatible RBCs are necessary and safe as long as their donor–recipient compatibility is appropriately checked. Despite controversies regarding transfusion thresholds in patients with cardiac disease or bleeding, restrictive strategies appear to be associated with better patient outcomes, and avoidable transfusions are an independent predictor of death and multi-organ failure.[3] Patients in septic shock did not benefit from liberal RBC transfusion regimes, and a similar mortality was observed between both groups.[4] Even in elderly patients (>50 years) with either cardiovascular disease or known risk factors for cardiovascular disease, a liberal transfusion regime was not favourable after follow-up for 3 years.[5] Frequently used restrictive transfusion thresholds range from 7 to 8 g/dL. Although storage time of RBCs alters their physiological properties, the clinical impact of RBC storage remains a matter of debate.[3]

Table 58.1 Compatibility of the ABO system for RBC transfusion (1.1) and plasma transfusion (1.2)

1.1 red blood cell transfusion		Recipient			
		A	B	AB	0
Donor	A	++	–	+	–
	B	–	++	+	–
	AB	–	–	++	–
	0	+	+	+	++
1.2 plasma transfusion		**Recipient**			
		A	B	AB	0
Donor	A	++	–	–	+
	B	–	++	–	+
	AB	+	+	++	+
	0	–	–	–	++

Note: ++ indicates a matching transfusion; + indicates a compatible transfusion; and – indicates a mismatch. Note type AB plasma is rare in European donor banks, and its use should be limited to type AB recipients.

The implementation of PBM reduces avoidable transfusions.[6] PBM is based on four main objectives: (1) management of anaemia, (2) treatment of potential coagulopathy, (3) conservation of blood, and (4) an individualized approach. These main objectives of RBC transfusion can be applied to the transfusion of any blood product.

Plasma

Plasma is obtained from individual donors via apheresis or is pooled from several donors. Plasma transfusion is used to treat coagulopathy in bleeding patients with significant acquired coagulation factor deficiency or to address coagulation factor deficiencies not amenable to individual factor correction (e.g. Factor V, XI deficiency). In general, plasma is administered in an ABO-matching manner, except in an emergency, in which ABO-compatible plasma might be accepted (Table 58.2). There is controversy concerning the use of plasma in bleeding patients with respect to the transfusion volume and the ratio of plasma to other blood products (e.g. administration of RBCs:FFP:platelets at a fixed 1:1:1 ratio).[7] There has been a shift from an empirical coagulation therapy towards a goal-directed, individualized approach with using recombinant or lyophilized coagulation factor concentrates. Owing to the drawbacks of plasma use (e.g. low concentration of coagulation factors, TACO, TRALI, and citrate intoxication), a more restrictive and more careful consideration of plasma substitution might be required. However, plasma use is steadily increasing.

Table 58.2 Acute and delayed transfusion-associated adverse events

Transfusion-associated adverse events	
Acute	• Acute haemolytic transfusion reaction • Non-haemolytic febrile transfusion reaction* • Bacterial contamination (platelets) and septic transfusion reaction • Anaphylactic reaction • Hypotensive transfusion reaction • TRALI • TACO • Transfusion associated dyspnoea (TAD)**
Delayed	• Delayed haemolytic transfusion reaction • Transfusion-associated graft-versus-host disease • Transmission of bacteria, viruses, or parasites • Post-transfusion purpura (rare)
Additional transfusion-associated adverse events	• Transfusion-related immune modulation*

Note: Delayed onset of transfusion reactions with respiratory features is also possible.
*Rare in leucocyte-depleted blood products.
**TAD is a diagnosis by exclusion with unknown pathophysiology and with milder clinical outcomes than TRALI and TACO.

Platelet Concentrates

Platelet concentrates are obtained via apheresis or can be pooled from several donors. Quarantine storage of platelets is impossible and, as a result, the risk of infectious disease transmission is increased. Platelets are transfused for prophylactic purposes (e.g. for chronic thrombocytopenia) or to compensate for bleeding-associated losses. Despite limited evidence from clinical trials, transfusion thresholds have been defined, ranging from $<50 \times 10^3/\mu L$ as a prophylactic treatment for non-bleeding patients to $<100 \times 10^3/\mu L$ for patients with massive bleeding or traumatic brain injury.[1] Platelet transfusion should be blood group compatible when possible.

Transfusion-Associated Adverse Events

Transfusion-associated adverse events (TAEs) are defined as an undesirable response or effect in a patient that is temporally associated with the administration of blood or blood components. The adverse events with greatest risk are non-infectious complications. TAEs differ according to the type and volume of blood products and are classified into acute and delayed adverse events (Table 58.2). If TAEs are suspected, standardized measures include (1) discontinuation of the transfusion, (2) immediate report of the incident to the blood bank, (3) storage of the transfused material, and (4) laboratory analysis to identify the aetiology of the adverse event.

Prophylaxis of TRALI

Prophylaxis of TRALI could be based on exclusion of multiparous, previously transplanted or transfused donors, who may be suspected to carry pre-formed human leucocyte or human neutrophil antibodies (HLA and HNA).[8,9] The incidence of TRALI has been reduced by approximately two-thirds due to plasma donor pre-selection (e.g. male-only selection or antibody screening).[9] Additionally, leucoreduction and use of pooled plasma with diluted antibody titres each reduce the incidence of TRALI. No cases of TRALI have been reported using pooled solvent–detergent–plasma.[9] Outcome may also be improved by an increased awareness of factors predisposing patients for TRALI (Table 58.3).

Prophylaxis of TACO

Prophylaxis of TACO may be considered for patients with predisposing risk factors (Table 58.3); in these patients, a positive fluid balance should be avoided.[10] Furthermore, the transfusion rate and the overall volume of infused fluids administered prior to transfusion could be associated with the development of TACO.[11] Omitting any avoidable transfusions and applying restrictive fluid regimes ($\leq$2–4 mL kg^{-1} h^{-1}) might prevent TACO.[10–12] Haemodynamic monitoring facilitates early detection of circulatory overload and

Table 58.3 Recipient risk factors for the development of TRALI (3.1) and TACO (3.2)[11,12,23]

(1) Risk factors predisposing patients to TRALI ('first hit')	
Age	Mechanical ventilation
(Acute) renal failure	Elevated transfusion requirements
Major surgery	SIRS/sepsis (elevated CRP levels)
Chronic alcohol abuse	Smoking
(2) Risk factors predisposing patients to TACO	
Age >60 years	Female gender
(Chronic) renal failure	Cardiac or pulmonary impairment
Ethnicity (white)	Anaemia

adoption of corrective actions,[13] such as reducing the transfusion rate. The incidence of TACO can also be reduced by abstaining from volume-intensive plasma transfusion in favour of coagulation factor concentrates in bleeding patients.[14] Timely decisions can be supported by surveillance systems and algorithms to identify risk factors and onset of TRALI and TACO.[10]

Differential Diagnosis between TRALI and TACO

Differential diagnosis between TRALI and TACO starts with a brief review of associated risk factors (Table 58.3) and an exclusion of alternative causes of pulmonary oedema. TRALI and TACO are characterized by common and divergent symptoms (Table 58.4) and manifest within 6 h after transfusion.[9,11] Potential hybrid forms of TRALI and TACO, displaying clinical features and biomarkers of both syndromes, have been observed.[11] For both syndromes, chest X-ray shows signs of pulmonary oedema, but, specifically for TACO, pleural effusions or an enlarged silhouette of the heart may be present.[10] Additionally, echocardiography may reveal cardiac dysfunction, confirming the cardiogenic aetiology of oedema.[15] Further, TRALI might be distinguished from TACO by the absence of signs of circulatory overload, such as normal central venous pressure and normal pulmonary capillary wedge pressure.

Assays of interleukin levels can support clinical decisions because IL-6 and IL-8 are primarily elevated in TRALI, but IL-10 is primarily elevated in TACO[11] although these interleukins may also be elevated in a wide range of other illnesses encountered in the critically ill patient. Decreased counts of white blood cells and thrombocytes are commonly observed in patients with TRALI. Although brain natriuretic peptide (BNP) and NT-proBNP are more commonly elevated in patients with TACO, the specificity of these biomarkers is moderate.[10,11] The presence of HLA and HNA antibodies confirms the diagnosis of TRALI, but this assay is time intensive and has no direct influence on the therapy provided.

Treatment of TRALI

Treatment of TRALI is non-specific and is largely supportive.[9] Mild forms of TRALI may respond to supplemental oxygen therapy. Severe forms of TRALI may require mechanical ventilation (70%–90%), preferably with a low tidal volume and intensive care unit support.[9,16] In some cases, circulatory stabilization with catecholamines is necessary. In patients with TRALI, maintaining normovolaemia avoids concomitant circulatory overload.[9]

Treatment of TACO

Treatment of TACO is based on strategies addressing cardiogenic pulmonary oedema. Haemodynamic monitoring should at a minimum include oxygen saturation, cardiac monitoring, and assessment of fluid balance.[10] In patients with TACO, further volume load should be avoided, the transfusion rate should be reduced, and the indications for transfusion should be re-evaluated. Patients benefit from placement in an upright position and oxygen supplementation. Depending on the severity of TACO, positive pressure ventilation preserves sufficient oxygenation. Non-invasive positive pressure and ventilatory support ameliorates outcome in less severe cases,[10,17] whereas endotracheal intubation is necessary in severe cases.[18] Lung-protective ventilation (using a low tidal volume) reduces mortality and pulmonary injury.[19] Administration of vasodilators (nitrates or angiotensin converting enzyme (ACE) inhibitors) appears to be beneficial to patients with pulmonary oedema.[20] Diuretics probably optimize fluid balance,[10] but contraindications for diuretics should be considered. In cases of renal impairment, renal replacement therapies could help to reduce circulatory overload.[10]

Evidence Base

The currently available evidence supports the use of the following measures to ameliorate the effects of transfusion and associated respiratory impairments:

- PBM
- Restrictive transfusion regimes
- Leucoreduction of blood products
- Pre-selection of donors to prevent TRALI
- Lung-protective ventilation for TRALI and TACO

Frequently applied measures whose efficacy remains under debate are summarized in the section titled 'Controversies'.

Physiology and Pharmacology

Pathophysiology of Transfusion-Related Pulmonary Oedema in Patients with TRALI or TACO

The underlying oedema in patients with TRALI is synonymously referred to as 'non-cardiogenic' or 'increased-permeability' oedema, which is differentiated from the 'cardiogenic', 'hydrostatic', or 'hemodynamic' oedema in patients with TACO. Nevertheless, these two syndromes present with common clinical symptoms (Table 58.4).

Pathophysiology of TRALI

The definitions of TRALI are based on the occurrence of non-cardiogenic pulmonary oedema within 6 h of transfusion of blood products. TRALI can be categorized into antibody-mediated TRALI (~80%) and non-antibody-mediated TRALI (~20%), both of which are collectively termed 'possible' TRALI or TRALI Type II if other risk factors for acute respiratory distress syndrome (ARDS) are present.[15,21] Consequently, TRALI evolves via different, partly connected, pathways[15,21] with similar final mechanisms of

Table 58.4 Differential diagnosis between TRALI and TACO[11,12]

	TRALI	TACO
	Common symptoms	
Auscultation	Crackles	
Respiration	Dyspnoea	
Oxygen saturation	Hypoxia	
Chest radiography	Pulmonary oedema with bilateral diffuse infiltrates	
	Divergent symptoms and laboratory markers	
Blood pressure	Hypotension	Hypertension
Body temperature	Fever	No specific changes
Left ventricular function	Normal	Normal to decreased
Chest radiography	(see common symptoms)	Pleural effusions/enlarged silhouette of the heart
Pulmonary capillary wedge pressure	Normal	Elevated
Pro-inflammatory cytokines	Elevated IL6 and IL8 levels	Elevated IL10 levels
White blood cell count	Leucopenia	No specific changes
Platelet count	Thrombocytopenia	No specific changes
Brain natriuretic peptide (BNP) and NT-proBNP	Not elevated	Elevated
Expectorate	Exudates	Transudates
Efficacy of diuretics	None	Marked
Circulatory load	No specific changes	Positive

Note: Clinical features could overlap, and both entities could present with less distinctive symptoms. Other reasons for ARDS must be excluded prior to a diagnosis of TRALI or TACO.

lung injury. The interplay of transfusion with predispositions for TRALI is reflected by different models of the onset of TRALI. The least sophisticated two-hit model might be the most convenient in clinical practice: a first hit (Table 58.3) predisposes an individual for the onset of TRALI, and a subsequent second hit is provided by transfusion factors.[9,22] The second hit is derived from either donor antibodies to recipient antigens (HLA and HNA) or, in non-antibody-mediated TRALI, biologic response modifiers (e.g. bioactive lipids, sCD40L, or cell debris).[9,15] Because healthy individuals can develop TRALI without a 'first hit', other models, including the threshold and sufficient-cause models of TRALI onset, have been proposed.[22]

The final common mechanism of TRALI is pulmonary oedema with capillary leakage due to inflammatory disruption of the endothelial and epithelial basement membranes.[9] This oedema can be caused by different inflammatory mechanisms such as neutrophil-primed inflammation (HLA class I and HNA), antibody-dependent direct cell destruction, monocyte activity (HLA class II), endothelial activation (HLA class I), platelet-triggered formation of neutrophil extracellular traps (NETs), complement pathway signalling, and currently unknown mechanisms or a combination of these triggers.[15,21]

Pathophysiology of TACO

Under physiologic conditions, fluid balance exists between fluid filtration from the pulmonary capillaries caused by hydrostatic pressure to the interstitium, colloid osmotic pressure of the pulmonary capillaries, and lymphatic drainage. This equilibrium prevents fluid from crossing the alveolar-capillary basement membrane.[10,20] In TACO, the volume transfused exceeds the circulatory capacity of the patient, and acute hydrostatic pulmonary oedema develops. Whenever the hydrostatic pressure in the pulmonary capillaries increases, the wall tension and transmural filtration exceed the colloid osmotic pressure.[20] Simultaneously, due to an increase in systemic venous pressure, lymphatic drainage is impaired, a critical threshold of the former equilibrium is reached, and fluid accumulates in the interstitium and subsequently alveoli.[10,20] In patients with predisposing factors (Table 58.2), even a moderate increase in blood volume after transfusion can trigger TACO.[10]

Future Practice

Current research includes the development of cultured blood cells from induced pluripotent stem cells, which are less likely to induce adverse events. Modulating C-reactive protein (CRP) levels prior to transfusion might reduce the risk for TRALI.[15] New pharmacologic agents (i.e. transient receptor ion permeable potential vanilloid receptor, TRPV4 antagonists) might trigger the active clearance of pulmonary oedema.[20] Microbead-based assays might refine antibody diagnostics,[21] and the search for adequate biomarkers to distinguish TRALI and TACO is ongoing.[10,11] New vasodilators (clevidipine and serelaxin) might further augment the current therapeutic options for TACO.[20] Finally, ventricular assist devices might play a more prominent role in the treatment of TACO in the future.[20]

REFERENCES

1. Spahn DR, Bouillon B, Cerny V, et al. The European guideline on management of major bleeding and coagulopathy following trauma, Fifth edition. *Crit Care.* 2019;**23**(1):98.
2. Fatalities Reported to FDA Following Blood Collection and Transfusion. Annual Summary for Fiscal Year 2020:available from https://www.fda.gov/vaccines-blood-biologics/report-problem-center-biologics-evaluation-research/transfusiondonation-fatalities; Accessed 27.02.2023.
3. Shah A, Stanworth SJ, McKechnie S. Evidence and triggers for the transfusion of blood and blood products. *Anaesthesia.* 2015;**70**(Suppl 1):10–19.
4. Holst LB, Haase N, Wetterslev J, et al. Lower versus higher hemoglobin threshold for transfusion in septic shock. *N Engl J Med.* 2014;**371**(15):1381–1391.
5. Carson JL, Sieber F, Cook DR, et al. Liberal versus restrictive blood transfusion strategy: 3-year survival and cause of death results from the FOCUS randomised controlled trial. *Lancet.* 2015;**385**(9974):1183–1189.
6. Meybohm P, Richards T, Isbister J, et al. Patient blood management bundles to facilitate implementation. *Transfus Med Rev.* 2017;**31**(1):62–71.
7. Kelly JM, Callum JL, Rizoli SB. 1:1-warranted or wasteful? Even when appropriate, high ratio transfusion protocols are costly: Early transition to individualized care benefits patients and transfusion services. *Expert Rev Hematol.* 2013;**6**(6):631–633.
8. Rogers TS, Fung MK, Harm SK. Recent advances in preventing adverse reactions to transfusion. *F1000Res.* 2015 Dec 17;**4**:F1000 Faculty Rev-1469.
9. Vlaar AP, Juffermans NP. Transfusion-related acute lung injury: A clinical review. *Lancet.* 2013;**382**(9896):984–994.
10. Roubinian NH, Murphy EL. Transfusion-associated circulatory overload (TACO): Prevention, management, and patient outcomes. *Int J Clin Transfus Med.* 2015;**3**:17–28.
11. Roubinian NH, Looney MR, Kor DJ, et al. Cytokines and clinical predictors in distinguishing pulmonary transfusion reactions. *Transfusion.* 2015;**55**(8):1838–1846.
12. Li G, Rachmale S, Kojicic M, et al. Incidence and transfusion risk factors for transfusion-associated circulatory overload among medical intensive care unit patients. *Transfusion.* 2011;**51**(2):338–343.
13. Lieberman L, Maskens C, Cserti-Gazdewich C, et al. A retrospective review of patient factors, transfusion practices, and outcomes in patients with transfusion-associated circulatory overload. *Transfus Med Rev.* 2013;**27**(4):206–212.
14. Sarode R, Milling TJ Jr, Refaai MA, et al. Efficacy and safety of a 4-factor prothrombin complex concentrate in patients on vitamin K antagonists presenting with major bleeding: A randomized, plasma-controlled, phase IIIb study. *Circulation.* 2013;**128**(11):1234–1243.
15. Semple JW, Rebetz J, Kapur R. Transfusion-associated circulatory overload and transfusion-related acute lung injury. *Blood.* 2019;**133**(17):1840–1853.
16. The Acute Respiratory Distress Syndrome Network, Brower RG, Matthay MA, et al. Ventilation with lower tidal Volumes as compared with traditional tidal Volumes for acute lung injury and the acute respiratory distress syndrome. *N Engl J Med.* 2000;**342**(18):1301–1308.
17. Peter JV, Moran JL, Phillips-Hughes J, Graham P, Bersten AD. Effect of non-invasive positive pressure ventilation (NIPPV) on mortality in patients with acute cardiogenic pulmonary oedema: A meta-analysis. *Lancet.* 2006;**367**(9517):1155–1163.
18. Shirakabe A, Hata N, Yokoyama S, et al. Predicting the success of noninvasive positive pressure ventilation in emergency room for patients with acute heart failure. *J Cardiol.* 2011;**57**(1):107–114.
19. Serpa Neto A, Cardoso SO, Manetta JA, et al. Association between use of lung-protective ventilation with lower tidal Volumes and clinical outcomes among patients without acute respiratory distress syndrome: A meta-analysis. *JAMA.* 2012;**308**(16):1651–1659.
20. Clark AL, Cleland JG. Causes and treatment of oedema in patients with heart failure. *Nat Rev Cardiol.* 2013;**10**(3):156–170.
21. Vlaar AP, Toy P, Fung M, et al. A consensus redefinition of transfusion-related acute lung injury. *Transfusion.* 2019;**59**(7):2465–2476.
22. Middelburg RA, van der Bom JG. Transfusion-related acute lung injury not a two-hit, but a multicausal model. *Transfusion.* 2015;**55**(5):953–960.
23. Maślanka K, Uhrynowska M, Łopacz P, et al. Analysis of leucocyte antibodies, cytokines, lysophospholipids and cell microparticles in blood components implicated in post-transfusion reactions with dyspnoea. *Vox Sang.* 2015;**108**(1):27–36.

59

Anaphylaxis

Jasmeet Soar, Fiona Moghaddas, and Stephen M Robinson

KEY MESSAGES

- Anaphylaxis admissions to the intensive care unit are uncommon and the mortality is 5%–10%.
- Adrenaline and supportive treatment based on an Airway Breathing Circulation Disability Exposure (ABCDE) approach are the key immediate interventions.
- A raised serum mast cell tryptase at the time of the reaction can help confirm the diagnosis. A normal serum mast cell tryptase does not exclude anaphylaxis.
- Patients with suspected anaphylaxis should be referred to a specialist allergy clinic to help identify the trigger and avoid future reactions.

CONTROVERSIES

- The role of steroids and antihistamines for the initial treatment of anaphylaxis.
- How early should intramuscular adrenaline be given—very early during the first onset of symptoms or only in those who develop life-threatening features.

FURTHER RESEARCH

- The emergency nature of anaphylaxis makes randomized controlled trials difficult. In addition, there is a lack of equipoise for interventions such as adrenaline which has become the standard of care. A registry of anaphylaxis events may provide useful observational data. Further studies are required to establish sensitive and specific diagnostic tools, especially in light of newly described mechanisms of anaphylaxis.

Introduction

Anaphylaxis-related critical care admissions are very uncommon and few result in death.[1] About 60% of intensive care admissions are patients with suspected anaphylaxis during anaesthesia and surgery or related to inpatient medications. Out-of-hospital cases of suspected anaphylaxis are usually managed successfully in the pre-hospital or emergency department setting. Angioedema cases with airway compromise may be admitted, but very few of these will be due to anaphylaxis. Isolated angioedema can be idiopathic, drug related, or (very rarely) due to inherited C1-esterase inhibitor deficiency.

Definition of Anaphylaxis

A precise definition of anaphylaxis is not important for emergency treatment. Anaphylaxis is a serious systemic hypersensitivity reaction that is usually rapid in onset and may cause death.[2] It is characterized by rapidly developing life-threatening airway and/or breathing and/or circulation problems usually associated with skin and mucosal changes.[3] Urticaria with or without angioedema are relatively benign, and common emergency department presentations which, when they occur in isolation, are not anaphylaxis.

Pathophysiology

Anaphylaxis can be triggered by immunological mechanisms (classically immunoglobulin (Ig)E medicated, or Coombes and Gell type 1 hypersensitivity) or non-immunological mechanisms (e.g. non-steroidal anti-inflammatory drugs (NSAIDs) directly interfere with arachidonic acid metabolism). Both mechanisms cause degranulation of granulocytes such as mast cells and basophils releasing pro-inflammatory and vasoactive agents including histamine, prostaglandins, leukotrienes, platelet-activating factor, nitric oxide, and eosinophil and neutrophil chemotactic factors. These cause increased vascular permeability with swelling, vasodilation, hypotension, cardiovascular collapse, bronchospasm, and wheeze. Mast cell tryptase (MCT), another released factor, has a longer half-life compared with other factors such as histamine, and its detection in serum helps support the diagnosis of anaphylaxis.

More recently, activation of the Mas-related G-protein-coupled receptor member X2 receptor by drugs such as neuromuscular blocking agents (NMBAs), opioids, and some antibiotics leading to non-IgE-mediated mast cell degranulation, has been described.[4] Furthermore, IgG-mediated neutrophil degranulation in cases of anaphylaxis to NMBAs where skin prick testing, specific IgE, and MCTs were non-contributory have been reported.[5]

Epidemiology

Anaphylaxis affects about 1 in 300 of the European population at some stage in their lives with an incidence of 1.5–7.9 per 100,000 person-years.[6] Anaphylaxis is caused by a broad range of triggers including food, drugs, and stinging insects. Food is the commonest trigger in children and younger adults, and drugs the commonest in older adults.[7] Nuts and certain drugs (muscle relaxants, antibiotics, and NSAIDs) cause most reactions.

Very few people die of anaphylaxis. The estimated case-fatality rate for hospital admissions is 0.5%–1%.[7] Over the period 2005–2009, there were 81 paediatric and 1269 adult admissions with anaphylaxis admitted to UK critical care units, and survival to unit discharge was 95% for children and survival to hospital discharge was 92% for adults.[1] In a US study of 38,695 patients seen in the emergency department for anaphylaxis, 4431 (11.5%) were admitted, 2057 (5.3%) were admitted to the intensive care unit (ICU), and 567 (1.5%) required tracheal intubation. From a case series, fatal food reactions cause respiratory arrest typically after 30–35 min; insect stings cause collapse from shock after 10–15 min; and deaths caused by intravenous (IV) medication occur most commonly within 5 min. Most deaths occurred withing the first 2 h, 8% deaths occurred after 2 h, 3% after 4 h, and 2.5% after 6 h.[8]

The risk of death is increased in those with pre-existing poorly controlled asthma. Asthma and anaphylaxis often coexist and share some similar features. In particular, poorly controlled asthma is associated with increased recurrence and severity of anaphylaxis. Those with cardiovascular co-morbidities also have an increased risk of critical illness, and death as the ability to compensate for the acute physiological derangement is impaired. The Sixth National Audit Project of the Royal College of Anaesthetists (NAP6) observed an increased risk of death from perioperative anaphylaxis when there was prolonged hypotension, in patients who were older, obese, had coronary artery disease, or multiple co-morbidities, or in patients taking beta-blockers or angiotensin-converting enzyme inhibitors.[9] It is, however, difficult to separate the role of medications from the associated co-morbidities. There was no association with asthma in this perioperative study, but no meaningful comparison can be made to non-operative anaphylaxis. The ability to give 100% inspired oxygen and manage bronchospasm early during anaesthesia may help prevent the life-threatening effects of hypoxaemia.

Recognition of Anaphylaxis

Anaphylaxis is the likely diagnosis if a patient who is exposed to a trigger (allergen) develops a sudden illness (usually within minutes) with rapidly developing life-threatening airway and breathing and/or circulatory problems usually associated with skin and mucosal changes. Hypotension can reduce or delay skin changes. Urticaria was not noted in the 10 fatalities in the NAP6 study and was present in less than 10% of the cardiac arrests. Table 59.1 provides specific criteria from the European Academy of Allergy and Clinical Immunology's (EAACI) Taskforce on Anaphylaxis.[10]

Initial Treatment of Anaphylaxis

The initial treatment of anaphylaxis consists of a rapid assessment and early use of intramuscular adrenaline (0.5 mg in adults). The evidence supporting specific interventions for the treatment of anaphylaxis is limited.[11] An Airway, Breathing Circulation, Disability, Exposure (ABCDE) approach to recognize and treat anaphylaxis is recommended with the early use of adrenaline. All patients who have suspected anaphylaxis should be monitored as soon as possible. Specific issues to consider are outlined below.

Patient Positioning

Patients with anaphylaxis can have severe postural hypotension and are at risk of cardiac arrest if made to sit up or stand up. All patients should be placed in a comfortable position, and sudden movement should be avoided. Patients with airway and breathing problems may prefer to sit up as this will make breathing easier. Lying flat with or without leg elevation is helpful for patients with a low blood pressure.

Table 59.1 Diagnostic criteria for anaphylaxis

Anaphylaxis is highly likely when any one of the following three criteria is fulfilled:			
1. Acute onset of an illness (minutes to several hours) with involvement of the skin, mucosal tissue, or both (e.g. generalized hives, pruritus or flushing, and swollen lips–tongue–uvula) *and at least one of the following*:			
a. Respiratory compromise (e.g. dyspnoea, wheeze–bronchospasm, stridor, reduced peak expiratory flow (PEF), and hypoxaemia)		b. Reduced blood pressure (BP) or associated symptoms of end-organ dysfunction (e.g. hypotonia (collapse), syncope, and incontinence)	
2. Two or more of the following that occur rapidly after exposure to a likely allergen for that patient (minutes to several hours):			
a. Involvement of the skin–mucosal tissue (e.g. generalized hives, itch flush, and swollen lips–tongue–uvula)	b. Respiratory compromise (e.g. dyspnoea, wheeze–bronchospasm, stridor, reduced PEF, and hypoxaemia)	c. Reduced BP or associated symptoms (e.g. hypotonia (collapse), syncope, and incontinence)	d. Persistent gastrointestinal symptoms (e.g. crampy abdominal pain and vomiting)
3. Reduced BP after exposure to known allergen for that patient (minutes to several hours):			
a. Infants and children: low systolic BP (age specific) or >30% decrease in systolic BP		b. Adults: systolic BP of <90 mmHg or >30% decrease from that person's baseline	

Source: Reproduced from Muraro A, Roberts G, Worm M, et al. Anaphylaxis: Guidelines from the European Academy of Allergy and Clinical Immunology. *Allergy*. 69(8):1026–1045, Copyright 2014, European Academy of Allergy and Clinical Immunology (EAACI).

Remove the Trigger if Possible

Stop any drug suspected of causing anaphylaxis. Remove the stinger after a bee sting. Early removal is more important than the method of removal. Do not delay definitive treatment if removing the trigger is not feasible.

Cardiorespiratory Arrest Following Anaphylaxis

Start cardiopulmonary resuscitation (CPR) immediately and follow current guidelines. Prolonged CPR may be necessary. Rescuers should ensure that help is on its way as early advanced life support is essential.

Evidence from the NAP6 study showed patients with a very low blood pressure (<50 mmHg), but who did not have a cardiac arrest were managed less well than other patients in terms of speed of treatment, administration of adrenaline, and CPR when indicated. The recommendation is to start CPR promptly if there is no pulse palpable.[12] Pulseless electric activity was the commonest electrocardiogram (ECG) presentation of cardiac arrest under anaesthesia in 34 out of 40 cases often preceded by bradycardia. The four episodes of ventricular fibrillation/pulseless ventricular tachycardia were preceded by a tachycardia.

Adrenaline (Epinephrine)

Adrenaline (epinephrine) is the most important drug for the treatment of anaphylaxis. Delayed administration of adrenaline increases the risk of a fatal outcome with pre-hospital administration associated with lower hospitalization rates than first dose administration in the emergency department.[13] Although there are no randomized controlled trials, early adrenaline is a logical treatment of breathing and circulation problems associated with anaphylaxis. Its alpha-receptor agonist effects reverse peripheral vasodilation and reduce oedema, and its beta-agonist effects are bronchodilator and inotropic. In addition, activation of beta-2 adrenergic receptors on mast cells suppresses mast cell degranulation inhibiting the fundamental pathological process.

In most settings, rescuers should use intramuscular adrenaline as there is a greater margin of safety, does not require IV access, and is much easier to learn. Intramuscular adrenaline can be repeated after 5 min if there is no improvement. The best site for injection is the anterolateral aspect of the middle third of the thigh. Most reactions respond to a single dose of adrenaline, 10% require more than one dose, and about 2% require three or more doses.

If repeated adrenaline doses are needed, start an IV adrenaline infusion. IV adrenaline should be used in monitored settings by those experienced in the use and titration of vasopressors. Adjustment of the adrenaline infusion will be required to avoid excessive doses that can lead to life-threatening hypertension, tachycardia, arrhythmias, and myocardial ischaemia.

Antihistamines

Antihistamines are no longer part of the initial treatment of anaphylaxis and should not be used first line or as monotherapy. The main benefit is for the symptomatic treatment of urticaria and angioedema. Non-sedating oral antihistamines (e.g. cetirizine, fexofenadine, and loratadine) may be given following stabilization, in preference to chlorphenamine, which can cause sedation and hypotension.

Corticosteroids

Corticosteroids are no longer part of the initial treatment of anaphylaxis. There is no evidence they help prevent or shorten protracted reactions. A recent observation study showed a risk adjusted (including for severity of reaction) increase in intensive care admission for those patients given steroids.[14,15] They may be given to help treat wheeze if asthma symptoms persist after adrenaline use, and for severe urticaria and angioedema. Steroids may also be considered as part of shock treatment when the need for vasopressor support is persisting or increasing.

Specific Critical Care Interventions for Anaphylaxis

Patients with refractory anaphylaxis do not improve or continue to deteriorate despite initial treatment with two doses of adrenaline (Figure 59.1).

Airway and Breathing

Airway Obstruction

Anaphylaxis can cause airway swelling and obstruction. This will make airway and ventilation interventions (e.g. bag-mask ventilation, tracheal intubation, and cricothyroidotomy) difficult. Get expert airway help and follow current difficult airway guidelines for emergency airway management. In practice, only a small proportion require specific airway interventions. In one case series, only 3.3% of patients with angioedema required tracheal intubation and 0.3% a surgical airway.[16]

Oxygen

Oxygen should initially be given at the highest feasible inspired oxygen concentration and then titrated to achieve an oxygen saturation of 94%–98%.

Bronchodilators

The first-line treatment for respiratory symptoms including wheeze caused by anaphylaxis is adrenaline. Consider bronchodilator therapy with salbutamol, ipratropium, or aminophylline according to current guidelines for acute asthma as a second-line therapy.

Ventilation

Pulmonary oedema and inflammation can occur in severe anaphylaxis requiring ventilation. Standard measures to decrease lung water and protect the lungs should be followed. In patients with bronchospasm, ventilator settings aimed at avoiding barotrauma will be required. In practice, a 6 mL kg^{-1} tidal volume, a respiratory rate of 10–14 breaths min^{-1}, tolerating hypercapnia, a low positive end expiratory pressure (PEEP) setting, and aiming to maintain a plateau pressure less than 30 cmH_2O will usually suffice until the bronchospasm resolves.[17]

Circulation

Intravenous Fluid Therapy

Anaphylaxis can cause rapid severe hypovolaemia. An observational study estimated the increase in tissue permeability caused

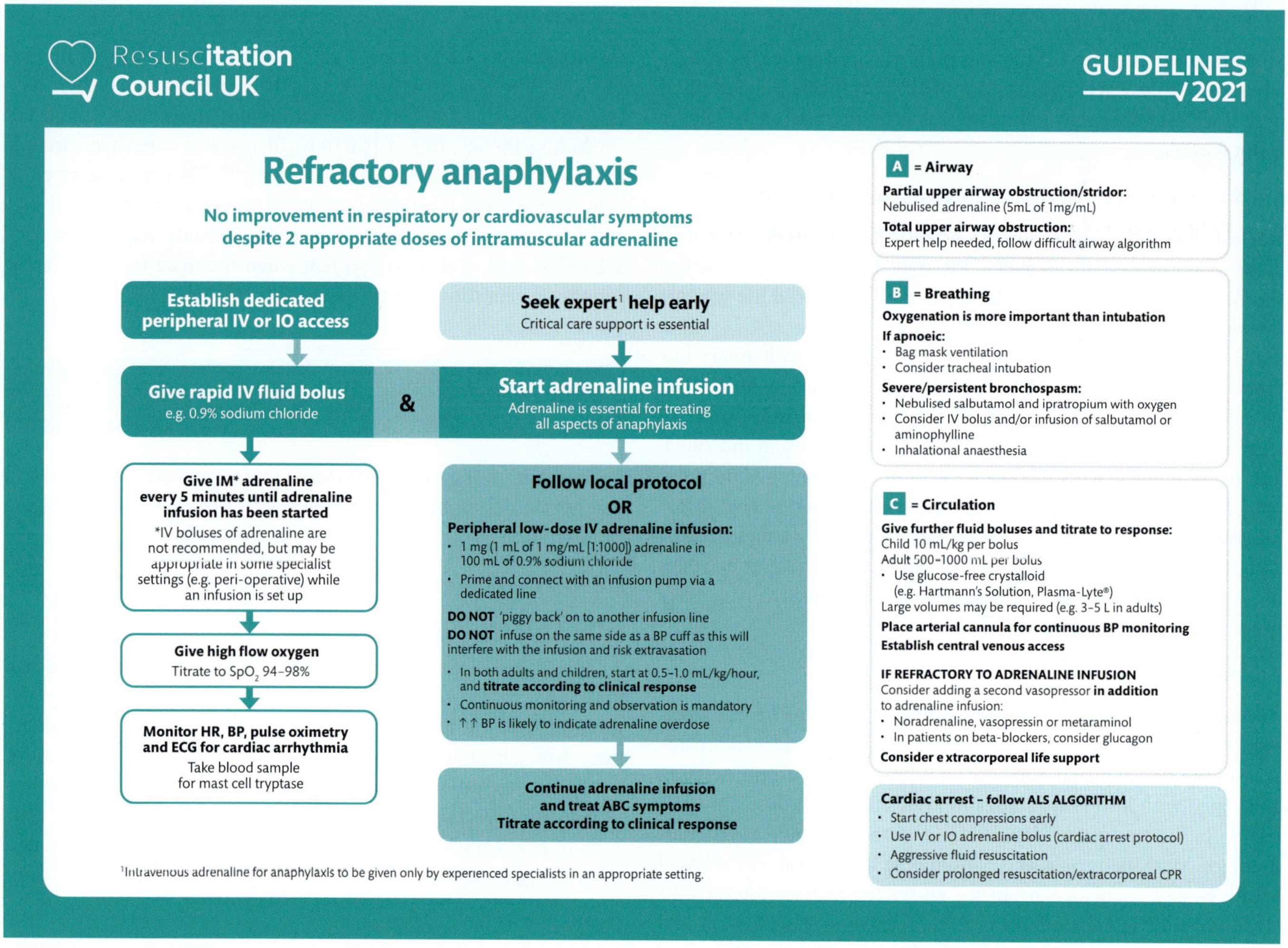

Figure 59.1 The refractory anaphylaxis algorithm.
Reproduced with permission of the Resuscitation Council UK.

by anaphylaxis was associated with a loss of about one-third of the plasma volume over 10 min in some patients.[18] Give rapid intravenous fluid challenges (500–1000 mL in an adult) and monitor the response; give further doses as necessary and large volumes may be required. Consider colloid infusion as a cause in a patient receiving a colloid at the time of onset of anaphylaxis and stop the infusion.

Further Vasopressor Therapy

Adrenaline is the first-line vasopressor for the treatment of anaphylaxis. Other vasopressors and inotropes (noradrenaline, vasopressin, terlipressin metaraminol, methoxamine, enoximone, and glucagon) may have a role in the treatment of persistent shock despite resuscitation with adrenaline and fluids. However, evidence for the use of these second-line agents is restricted to case reports and series.

Extracorporeal Life Support

In settings where it is feasible, consider mechanical circulatory or respiratory support with extracorporeal life support techniques for severe anaphylaxis. Specifically, veno-veno (VV) extracorporeal membrane oxygenation (ECMO) can be used in severe respiratory failure or veno-arterial (VA)-ECMO to support the circulation.

Acute Coronary Syndromes

Acute coronary syndromes can be associated with anaphylaxis ('Kounis syndrome').[19] Three variants are described; type I is defined as chest pain during a reaction caused by coronary artery spasm—this may resolve with treatment of the anaphylaxis but may require coronary vasodilator therapy; type II occurs in patients with pre-existing ischaemic heart disease in whom the reaction causes an acute myocardial infarction; type III occurs in patients who have coronary artery stent thrombosis associated with an allergic reaction. In addition to treating the acute coronary syndrome, there needs to be a carefully considered approach that balances the risks of treating life-threatening anaphylaxis with adrenaline and worsening myocardial ischaemia.

Coagulopathy

Coagulopathy can occur with anaphylaxis, and anaphylaxis can be associated with disseminated intravascular coagulation in some cases. Coagulation should therefore be monitored and corrected if necessary.

Investigations and Follow-up

Mast Cell Tryptase

MCT is a specific test to help confirm a diagnosis of anaphylaxis. In anaphylaxis, mast cell degranulation may lead to an increase in blood tryptase concentrations. Tryptase concentrations in the blood may not increase significantly until 30 min or more after the onset of symptoms, and peak 1–2 h after onset.[20] The half-life of tryptase is approximately 2 h, and concentrations may be back to normal within 6–8 h, so timing of any blood samples is very important. The time of onset of the anaphylaxis is the time when symptoms were first noticed.

(a) *Minimum*: One sample as soon as possible and certainly within 1–2 h after the start of symptoms.

(b) *Ideally*: Three timed samples:
- Initial sample as soon as feasible after resuscitation has started—do not delay resuscitation to take sample.
- Second sample at 1–2 h after the start of symptoms.
- Third sample either at 24 h or in convalescence (e.g. in a follow-up allergy clinic). This provides baseline tryptase levels—some individuals have an elevated baseline level.

Serial samples have better specificity and sensitivity than a single measurement in the confirmation of anaphylaxis; however, negative predictive values remain poor. There is international consensus that changes in tryptase defined as $>(1.2 \times \text{baseline}) + 2$ can be used to determine a significant change even when individual measurements are within the normal range with a specificity of 91% and a positive predictive value of 98%.[21]

Biphasic Reactions

Biphasic reactions occur in about 5% of cases, but it is not clear whether some of these cases are due to insufficient initial treatment.[22,23] They are more common when there has been a severe initial reaction or the need for more than one dose of intramuscular adrenaline. There is, however, no reliable way of predicting who will have a biphasic reaction. A systematic review showed that a period of observation of 6–12 h would capture most cases of a biphasic reaction.[24]

Adrenaline Auto-injectors

These should be given to patients before hospital discharge when the suspected allergen is difficult to avoid (e.g. food allergy or unknown cause). Patients, parents, or carers should be trained in both when and how to use the auto-injector device at the time of prescribing. The prescribing of two epinephrine devices is recommended to remove the risk of the first pen failing or the possibility of requiring a second dose.

Allergy Clinic Referral

All patients presenting with anaphylaxis should be referred to an allergy clinic to identify the cause, and thereby reduce the risk of future reactions and to prepare the patient to manage future episodes themselves. Allergy clinics should be provided with all the relevant clinical information by the referring team. For example, if anaphylaxis occurs during anaesthesia, a copy of the anaesthetic chart and a list of possible triggers should be provided.

REFERENCES

1. Gibbison B, Sheikh A, McShane P, et al. Anaphylaxis admissions to UK critical care units between 2005 and 2009. *Anaesthesia.* 2012;**67**(8):833–839.
2. Cardona V, Ansotegui IJ, Ebisawa M, et al. World allergy organization anaphylaxis guidance 2020. *World Allergy Organ J.* 2020;**13**(10):100472.
3. Soar J, Pumphrey R, Cant A, et al. Emergency treatment of anaphylactic reactions—guidelines for healthcare providers. *Resuscitation.* 2008;**77**(2):157–169.
4. McNeil BD, Pundir P, Meeker S, et al. Identification of a mast-cell-specific receptor crucial for pseudo-allergic drug reactions. *Nature.* 2015;**519**(7542):237–241.
5. Jönsson F, de Chaisemartin L, Granger V, et al. An IgG-induced neutrophil activation pathway contributes to human drug-induced anaphylaxis. *Science Transl Med.* 2019;**11**(500):eaat1479.
6. Panesar SS, Javad S, de Silva D, et al. The epidemiology of anaphylaxis in Europe: A systematic review. *Allergy.* 2013;**68**(11):1353–1361.
7. Turner PJ, Campbell DE, Motosue MS, et al. Global trends in anaphylaxis epidemiology and clinical implications. *J Allergy Clin Immunol Pract.* 2020;**8**(4):1169–1176.
8. Turner PJ, Gowland MH, Sharma V, et al. Increase in anaphylaxis-related hospitalizations but no increase in fatalities: An analysis of United Kingdom national anaphylaxis data, 1992–2012. *J Allergy Clin Immunol.* 2015;**135**(4):956–963 e1.
9. Harper NJN, Cook TM, Garcez T, et al. Anaesthesia, surgery, and life-threatening allergic reactions: Epidemiology and clinical features of perioperative anaphylaxis in the 6th National Audit Project (NAP6). *Br J Anaesth.* 2018;**121**(1):159–171.
10. Muraro A, Roberts G, Worm M, et al. Anaphylaxis: Guidelines from the European Academy of Allergy and Clinical Immunology. *Allergy.* 2014;**69**(8):1026–1045.
11. Dodd A, Hughes A, Sargant N, et al. Evidence Update for the treatment of Anaphylaxis. *Resuscitation.* 2021 Apr 23;**163**:86–96.
12. Harper NJN, Nolan JP, Soar J, et al. Why chest compressions should start when systolic arterial blood pressure is below 50 mm Hg in the anaesthetised patient. *Br J Anaesth.* 2020;**124**(3):234–238.
13. Fleming JT, Clark S, Camargo CA, Jr, et al. Early treatment of food-induced anaphylaxis with epinephrine is associated with a lower risk of hospitalization. *J Allergy Clin Immunol Pract.* 2015;**3**(1):57–62.
14. Gabrielli S, Clarke A, Morris J, et al. Evaluation of prehospital management in a Canadian Emergency Department Anaphylaxis Cohort. *J Allergy Clin Immunol Pract.* 2019;**7**(7):2232–2238 e3.
15. Campbell DE. Anaphylaxis management: Time to re-evaluate the role of corticosteroids. *J Allergy Clin Immunol Pract.* 2019;**7**(7):2239–2240.
16. Tai S, Mascaro M, Goldstein NA. Angioedema: A review of 367 episodes presenting to three tertiary care hospitals. *Ann Otol Rhinol Laryngol.* 2010;**119**(12):836–841.
17. Leatherman J. Mechanical ventilation for severe asthma. *Chest.* 2015;**147**(6):1671–1680.
18. Fisher MM. Clinical observations on the pathophysiology and treatment of anaphylactic cardiovascular collapse. *Anaesth Intensive Care.* 1986;**14**(1):17–21.
19. Fassio F, Losappio L, Antolin-Amerigo D, et al. Kounis syndrome: A concise review with focus on management. *Eur J Intern Med.* 2016;**30**:7–10.

20. Schwartz LB. Diagnostic value of tryptase in anaphylaxis and mastocytosis. *Immunol Allergy Clin North Am.* 2006;**26**(3):451–463.
21. Passia E, Jandus P. Using baseline and peak serum tryptase levels to diagnose anaphylaxis: A review. *Clin Rev Allergy Immunol.* 2020;**58**(3):366–376.
22. Lee S, Bellolio MF, Hess EP, et al. Time of onset and predictors of biphasic anaphylactic reactions: A systematic review and meta-analysis. *J Allergy Clin Immunol Pract.* 2015;**3**(3):408–416.e1–2.
23. Kraft M, Scherer Hofmeier K, Ruëff F, et al. Risk factors and characteristics of biphasic anaphylaxis. *J Allergy Clin Immunol Pract.* 2020;8(10):3388–3395.e6.
24. Kim TH, Yoon SH, Hong H, et al. Duration of observation for detecting a biphasic reaction in anaphylaxis: A meta-analysis. *Int Arch Allergy Immunol.* 2019;**179**(1):31–36.

60

Aspiration and Drowning

Simone Bazurro, Andrea Carsetti, and Greg McAnulty

KEY MESSAGES

- *Drowning* is defined as a process resulting in primary respiratory impairment from submersion/immersion in a liquid medium.
- The primary injury from drowning is due to hypoxia.
- Cardiac arrest is usually a secondary event.
- Patient outcome depends on the duration of hypoxia.
- Oxygenation, ventilation, and perfusion should be restored as soon as possible.

CONTROVERSIES

- The role of and effect of antibiotics after non-fatal drowning. Currently, no evidence base favouring that but limited quality evidence.

FURTHER RESEARCH

- Can public awareness campaigns and public health interventions reduce the frequency of drowning episodes globally.

Introduction

Drowning is a serious event that often affects the younger population with the longest life expectancy. Every year, more than 380,000 people worldwide die by drowning, making it the third leading cause of accidental death (after road accidents and falls). About 28,000 fatal drownings occur every year in Europe, with an average rate of about 35 deaths per million inhabitants/year. Eastern Europe is the area with the highest risk, with Belarus, Latvia, Lithuania, Russia, and Ukraine having higher mortality rates. In these nations, cold water temperatures, high alcohol consumption, and difficulty implementing rapid intervention services are factors that contribute to high mortality rates.

In around 40% of cases, victims are unable to get back to dry land despite an ability to swim. This may be because of currents, wind or rocks, and other obstacles. In open water, waves are a significant hazard. The morphology of waves is dependent on interactions with the seabed. Waves break in shallow water; the steeper the seabed the closer the waves break to shore. These breakers are important as they collect and transfer vast amounts of water forming 'water piles'. Breakers cause a 'raising wave', which corresponds to 'a downwards wave' in the area where the water is removed. As water goes back, it carries floating objects, including swimmers, with it, with return currents reaching up to 9 km/h. Breaking waves are the dominant risk for open-water bathers, trapping and exhausting swimmers, and thus drowning them.

Drowning has a characteristic course with a series of successive stages through which people who can swim are progressively transformed into non-swimmers, and the victim gradually losing their ability to stay afloat. Drowning rarely manifests as it does in the classic Hollywood scene, where a novice swimmer shakes his arms desperately trying to be noticed before drowning. Drowning occurs silently. Experienced free divers suffering syncope due to hypoxia after hyperventilation, swimmers caught by tides and waves, and unattended children near stretches of water are often the protagonists of these sad events.

The International Liaison Committee on Resuscitation (ILCOR) defines drowning as a process resulting in primary respiratory impairment from submersion/immersion in a liquid medium. Implicit in this definition is that a liquid/air interface is present at the entrance of the victim's airway, preventing the victim from breathing air.[1] Table 60.1 shows the phases and causes of drowning.

Pathophysiology

The most important factors that contribute to mortality and morbidity are hypoxaemia, acidosis, and the effects that follow. Central nervous system damage can be caused by hypoxia during drowning or as a result of subsequent arrhythmia, lung injury, reperfusion injury, or multiorgan failure. The presence of water in the oral cavity and at the laryngeal level causes laryngospasm, airway obstruction, hypoxia, and hypercapnia. As the partial pressure of arterial oxygen falls, laryngospasm resolves, and the victim draws water into the lungs, thus worsening hypoxaemia. Soon after, bradycardia occurs, followed by cardiac arrest. Therefore, it is essential to note that cardiac arrest occurs as a consequence of hypoxia, and hypoxaemia correction is crucial to obtain return of spontaneous circulation.[2]

Table 60.1 Phases of drowning (left-hand column) and causes of drowning (right-hand column)

Drowning phases	Causes of drowning
1. Panic	Swallowing of water
2. Inability to breathe	Fatigue
3. Decrease of floating power	Inability to cope with and manage the current
4. Physical exhaustion	Hypothermia
5. Drowning	Injuries
6. Cardiac arrest	Loss of consciousness
	Entanglement in submerged plants

Fresh water is hypotonic compared to plasma and quickly spreads into the vessels, increasing blood volume and decreasing the concentration of electrolytes. It also causes the loss of surfactant with alveolar collapse, atelectasis, decreased lung compliance, and mismatch in ventilation/perfusion. Salt water, which is hyperosmolar, increases the osmotic gradient that draws fluid into the alveoli, dilutes the surfactant (washout), decreases the blood volume, and increases the concentration of electrolytes. These alterations lead to a reduction in lung compliance, and the alveolar-capillary membrane is directly damaged with severe hypoxia and non-cardiogenic pulmonary oedema develops. Despite these pathophysiological effects, several studies have shown that the tonicity of the inhaled liquid does not produce clinically important differences. This is likely because a drowned patient ingests about 3–4 mL/kg of water, but at least 22 mL/kg is required to produce important electrolyte imbalances. In 10%–15% of cases, laryngospasm with glottic closure persists, preventing water aspiration, and 80%–90% of these patients can be successfully resuscitated.

Clinical Presentation

Drowning outcomes are fatal or non-fatal. In non-fatal drowning, the process of respiratory impairment is stopped before death. The Non-fatal Drowning Categorization Framework (NDCF), proposed by the World Health Organization,[3] categorizes non-fatal drowning along two dimensions: the severity of respiratory impairment immediately after the drowning process stopped, and the morbidity category at the time when non-fatal drowning information is gathered (Table 60.2).

The victims of drowning by submersion are at risk of developing acute respiratory distress syndrome (ARDS). Although no randomized controlled trials have been conducted in this particular group of patients, it seems reasonable to apply a protective ventilation strategy that has been shown to improve survival in patients with ARDS arising from other causes (see Chapter 21), namely:

- limiting airway pressures and low tidal volume;
- PEEP higher than 5 cmH_2O.

The severity of lung injury ranges from mild, self-limiting disease to cases of refractory hypoxaemia. The irritation of airways due to inhalation of water and particulate matter produces cough and bronchospasm. Cough should be treated aggressively as it can precipitate severe dyspnoea. The drugs of choice are inhaled beta-agonists. In more severe cases, the extracorporeal membrane oxygenation (ECMO) has been used with some success. ECMO was safe and effective when used in patients in cardiac arrest or developing ARDS after drowning, and it may be used as a resuscitation strategy in patients with heart or lung failure unresponsive to conventional ventilation therapy.[4] Although the development of pneumonia is common after drowning, antibiotic prophylaxis is not effective. However, it could be considered after submersion in grossly contaminated water such as sewage. Broad-spectrum antibiotics should be administered if signs of infection develop later.[5] If the patient is exposed to water contaminated with rat's urine, there is a risk of developing leptospirosis, and doxycycline is the antibiotic of choice in this disease.

Pre-hospital Management

The victim of drowning must be removed safely from water as quickly as possible. The incidence of cervical spine injuries is very low (0.5%).[6] Cervical spine immobilization is not recommended except in the presence of specific signs or if the dynamics of the immersion raise a suspicion of cervical injury. A misplaced cervical collar may cause airway obstruction in unconscious patients. Treatment of hypoxia is the primary goal of first aid:

- In shallow water, perform five ventilations as soon as possible.
- In deep water, perform 10–15 breaths per minute.

Table 60.2 Non-fatal Drowning Categorization Framework (NDCF)

Severity of respiratory impairment after the drowning process stopped		
(1) Mild impairment	**(2) Moderate impairment**	**(3) Severe impairment**
• Breathing • Involuntary distressed coughing and • Fully alert	• Difficulty breathing and/or • Disoriented but conscious	• Not breathing and/or • Unconscious
Morbidity category (based upon any decline from previous functional capacity) at the time of measurement		
(A) No morbidity	**(B) Some morbidity**	**(C) Severe morbidity**
• No decline	• Some decline	• Severe decline

Source: Reproduced with permission from the World Health Organization from Clarification and Categorization of Non-fatal Drowning. https://www.who.int/publications/m/item/clarification-and-categorization-of-non-fatal-drowning.

- If <5 min from the shore, continue ventilations until reaching the shore.
- If >5 min from the shore, perform additional ventilation in place for a minute and then transport to shore as fast as possible without further attempts.[7]

Chest compressions are ineffective in the water as the victim must be placed on a hard surface. In the majority of cases, victims of drowning develop cardiac arrest following hypoxia. In these patients, cardiopulmonary resuscitation with chest compressions alone is probably less effective and should be avoided. Rescue ventilations require very high pressure of insufflation to be effective and can be difficult to perform with the presence of water in the airway. However, every effort should be made to continue ventilation until the arrival of the medical team. The regurgitation of gastric contents and the aspiration of water during resuscitation are very common events.[8] Abdominal thrusts should generally be avoided as they can cause regurgitation of gastric contents and other life-threatening injuries. If regurgitation completely prevents ventilation, the victim must be turned on their side and the regurgitated material must be removed by direct aspiration. Care should be taken if you suspect a spinal cord injury, but this should not prevent or delay rescue operations such as opening the airway, artificial ventilation, and chest compressions.

For spontaneously breathing patients

- high-flow oxygen via face mask with reservoir should be administered;
- when initial treatment is ineffective, positive pressure ventilation should be initiated.[9]

Early tracheal intubation and controlled ventilation should be considered for patients with a reduced level of consciousness or those unresponsive to initial management. After correct positioning of the tracheal tube, the fraction of inspired oxygen should be adjusted to achieve a SaO_2 of 94%–98%. PEEP should be set initially between 5 and 10 cmH_2O, but higher values (15–20 cmH_2O) may be needed in severe hypoxaemia.[10] Supraglottic airway devices have a limited role because of the high levels of pressure needed to overcome reduced lung compliance.

In assessing the victim of drowning, differentiation between respiratory arrest and cardiac arrest is particularly important. During cardiac arrest, any delay in starting chest compressions reduces survival. ILCOR states that recognition of gasping from the initial spontaneous respiratory efforts of a victim in recovery after a drowning is very difficult, and pulse palpation as the sole indicator of the presence or absence of a cardiac arrest is unreliable.[11] Where available, ECG, end-tidal CO_2, and echocardiography can be used to confirm cardiac arrest. Victims of drowning following prolonged immersion can become hypovolemic because of the hydrostatic pressure on the body, and IV fluids may be required to correct hypovolemia.

Hypothermia after immersion:

- *Primary*: Submersion in icy water (<5 °C) with rapid decrease in core temperature may have a protective role against anoxic injury.
- *Secondary*: Due to prolonged submersion and consequent heat loss through evaporation during resuscitation attempts. If body temperature is <30 °C:

Table 60.3 Grade of drowning by clinical features as suggested by Szpilman

Grade	Clinical findings	Mortality rate (%)
1	Normal pulmonary auscultation +/− cough	0
2	Crackles in some lung fields	0.6
3	Crackles in all fields without hypotension	5.2
4	Crackles in all fields with hypotension	19.4
5	Respiratory arrest without cardiac arrest	44
6	Cardiopulmonary arrest	93

Source: Reprinted from Szpilman D. Near-drowning and drowning classification: A proposal to stratify mortality based on the analysis of 1,831 cases. *Chest*. 1997;112(3):660-665. Copyright 1997, with permission from the American College of Chest Physicians.

- Limit defibrillation attempts to three shock and postpone IV drugs administration until the core temperature is higher than 30 °C.

ILCOR suggests that the victims be warmed to achieve a core temperature of 32-34 °C, taking care to avoid hyperthermia (>37 °C) during the subsequent period of intensive care.

Outcomes

Szpilman[12] proposed the following classification based on the analysis of 1831 cases of drowned patients over the age of 19 years in Brazil. Outcome depends by several factors. Szpilman proposed a grading scheme with associated mortality risk (Table 60.3). Negative prognostic factors include the following:

- GCS ≤5
- Time of immersion >5 min
- CPR started with delay
- pH <7
- Water temperature >10 °C
- Asystole at arrival in hospital

Withdrawal of Resuscitation Efforts

Resuscitation should be continued until there is evidence that attempts are useless, or if timely evacuation to medical facility is not possible. Several cases of survived patients with intact neurological status even after immersion for more than 60 min have been reported in the literature. However, the majority of these cases concerned children submerged in icy water.

REFERENCES

1. Idris AH, Berg RA, Bierens J, et al. Recommended guidelines for uniform reporting of data from drowning: The 'Utstein style'. *Resuscitation*. 2003;**59**:45–57.
2. Layon AJ, Modell JH. Drowning: Update 2009. *Anesthesiology*. 2009;**110**:1390–1401.
3. Clarification and Categorization of Non-fatal Drowning. World Health Organisation. March 14th 2019. https://www.who.int/

publications/m/item/clarification-and-categorization-of-non-fatal-drowning
4. Kim KI, Lee WY, Kim HS, et al. Extracorporeal membrane oxygenation in near-drowning patients with cardiac or pulmonary failure. *Scand J Trauma Resusc Emerg Med.* 2014;**12**;22:77.
5. Ellis G. Towards evidence based emergency medicine: Best BETs from the Manchester Royal Infirmary. BET 1: Prophylactic antibiotic use to prevent Weil's disease after immersion in water. *Emerg Med J.* 2011;**28**:1074–1075.
6. Watson RS, Cummings P, Quan L, et al. Cervical spine injures among submersion victims. *J Trauma.* 2001; **51**:658–662.
7. Szpilman D, Soares M. In-water resuscitation—is it worthwhile? *Resuscitation* 2004;**63**:25–31.
8. Manolios N, Mackie I. Drowning and near-drowning on Australian beaches patrolled by life-savers: A 10-year study, 1973–1983. *Med J Aust.* 1988;**148**:165–167, 70–71.
9. Modell JH, Calderwood HW, Ruiz BC, et al. Effects of ventilatory patterns on arterial oxygenation after near-drowning in sea water. *Anesthesiology.* 1974;**40**:376–384.
10. Moran I, Zavala E, Fernandez R, et al. Recruitment manoeuvres in acute lung injury/acute respiratory distress syndrome. *Eur Respir J Suppl.* 2003;**42**: 37s–42s.
11. Sayre MR, Koster RW, Botha M, et al. Adult basic life support chapter collaborators. Part 5: Adult basic life support: 2010 International Consensus on Cardiopulmonary Resuscitation and Emergency Cardiovascular Care Science With Treatment Recommendations. *Circulation.* 2010;**122**:S298–324.
12. Szpilman D. Near-drowning and drowning classification: A proposal to stratify mortality based on the analysis of 1,831 cases. *Chest.* 1997;**112**(3):660–665.

61

Burns Inhalation Injury

Sabri Soussi, Matthieu Legrand, and Suveer Singh

KEY MESSAGES

- Smoke inhalation should be highly suspected in a flame injury.
- Early administration of 100% oxygen and early intubation if airway at risk.
- Early bronchoscopic diagnosis, grading, and therapeutic washout.
- Utilize lung-protective ventilation strategies and proning position in acute respiratory distress syndrome (ARDS).
- Use of antidote hydroxycobalamin in the case of severe cyanide poisoning.
- Adapt fluid therapy to physiologic targets to avoid both under- and over-resuscitation.
- Nebulized heparin 5–10,000 units and *N*-acetylcysteine 3 mL of 20% 4-hourly, when the diagnosis is made. Bronchodilation may also be of benefit.

CONTROVERSIES

- Use of extracorporeal membrane oxygenation (ECMO) in adult critically ill burn patients has limited evidence, but severe ARDS criteria remain an indication.
- In severe carbon monoxide intoxication, the value of hyperbaric oxygen to reduce brain carbon monoxide (CO) build-up and poor neurologic outcomes remains uncertain.
- Fluid management strategy remains controversial (including the use of albumin); in particular, determining the optimal fluid requirements at different timepoints following burns injury and subsequent critical illness.

FURTHER RESEARCH

- The role of inhaled or systemic antioxidants, and other modulators of the activated inflammatory/coagulation pathways, which may attenuate the reactive oxygen species associated pulmonary damage.
- Repositories of burn inhalation bronchoscopic images to further evaluate and inform more accurate and practical composite prognostic indicators of inhalation injury would be of clinical value.

Introduction

Inhalation injury is an independent risk factor of mortality and morbidity in burn injury.[1–3] Furthermore, it is associated with increased risk of pneumonia, acute respiratory distress syndrome (ARDS), and haemodynamic instability.[4,5] Smoke inhalation injury is a non-specific term that refers to damage caused by thermal injury, chemical irritation of the respiratory tract, systemic toxicity mainly due to carbon monoxide (CO), and cyanide or any combination of these.[6] This review focuses on early evaluation and management of burned adult patients with inhalation injury, understanding of current pathophysiology, treatment options, and future therapeutic strategies.

Epidemiology

The incidence of inhalation injury ranges from 2% to 30% of intensive care unit (ICU) admissions after burn injury, mainly in patients with thermal injury from fires and explosions.[7] Risk factors are low socio-economic status, winter season, and lack of smoke detectors. Furthermore, mortality can increase by 20% in the presence of inhalation injury alone and 60% when both inhalation injury and pneumonia are present.[8] The association of inhalation injury and pneumonia with worse outcomes (mortality) was found to be independent and additive in an early landmark study.[9] Moreover, this has led to modification of burn-specific outcome predictive tools, such as the Baux score, to incorporate the additional influence of inhalation injury[10] (Figure 61.1). Smoke inhalation injury can lead to respiratory complications, such as pneumonia, lobar collapse, and ARDS, with increased ventilator and hospital days. Survivors may be left with residual pulmonary and functional abnormalities at follow-up.[11] Adults over 65 years of age have a notably higher mortality from burns, most likely associated with increased comorbidities and reduced physiological reserve and frailty.[12]

Pathophysiology

Inhalation injury mechanisms consist of (1) direct heat injury to upper airway from inhalation of hot steam and/or gases;

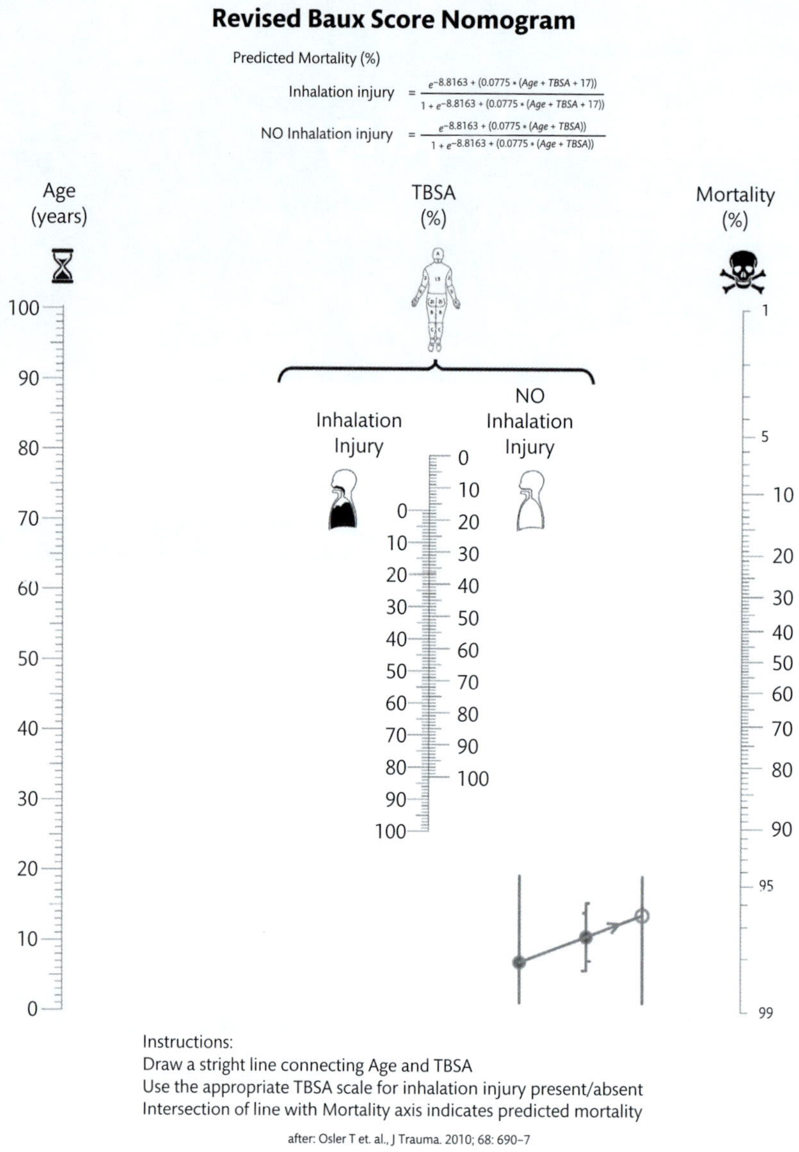

Figure 61.1 Modified Baux Score.

Reprinted from *Burns*, 41(1), Williams DJ and Walker JD, A nomogram for calculation of the Revised Baux Score, pp. 85–90. Copyright 2015, with permission from the International Society for Burn Injuries. After Osler T et al., *J Trauma*. 2010; 68: 690-7.

(2) chemical injury mainly related to carbonaceous particles (soot) to the epithelium of the trachea and bronchi, and alveolar epithelial and endothelial damage due to inhalation of the toxic products or thermal transmission from the fire; and (3) tissue hypoxia related to impairment of oxygen delivery processes or oxygen utilization by inhalation of CO and hydrogen cyanide (HCN), respectively.[13,14]

Injury to the upper airways usually leads to swelling with oedema, erythema, and ulceration. In these conditions, the patient may develop airway obstruction with inspiratory stridor, hoarse voice and dyspnoea, oedema of face, pharynx, glottis, and larynx, which continue to develop over the first 24–36 h post-injury and usually resolve in 3–6 days. Upper airway oedema is exacerbated by fluid administration during the resuscitation phase and perpetuated by so-called fluid creep of overexuberant fluid maintenance after the first 48 h. The degree of inhalation injury is dependent on such factors as inhaled components, exposure burden, host response, and co-morbidities.

Tracheobronchial and alveolar injury is mainly related to the effect of chemical irritants. Smoke from a house fire contains combustion products that vary depending on the materials. The main smoke containing irritants are nitrogen oxides from fabric, aldehydes from wood and paper (e.g. acrolein), and halogen acids and sulphur dioxide from rubber. Combustion of plastics produces CO, dioxins, and cyanide. Chemical exposure leads to alteration of mucociliary clearance of bacteria and mucosal debris[13] through denuding of the epithelium. Distally, there is impairment of surfactant production and a local cascade of inflammatory mediators including neuropeptides such as substance P and calcitonin gene-related peptide as well as nitric oxide synthase and reactive oxygen species (ROS). These produce sloughing, bronchoconstriction, increased pulmonary vascular permeability, and exudative leak. Notably higher release of pulmonary inflammatory cytokines is identifiable in inhalation injury compared with sepsis.[14] As a result, bronchospasm, obstruction of airways, bronchiolitis, microatelectasis, protein airway cast formation, and/or pneumonia ensue. Furthermore, the ROS and inflammatory cytokines can cause loss of hypoxic pulmonary vasoconstriction and activation of intravascular coagulation. A combination of these processes can lead to intrapulmonary shunt, ventilation/perfusion mismatch, and potentially ARDS.

CO intoxication causes tissue hypoxia through a series of processes. First, it acts by binding tightly to haemoglobin displacing oxygen. CO has a 200–250-fold higher affinity than oxygen to the same binding sites on haemoglobin. Second, CO intoxication induces a shift of the oxyhaemoglobin dissociation curve to the left and reduces oxygen delivery to tissues. Finally, mitochondrial cytochrome c oxidase function is directly altered by CO, impairing cellular utilization of oxygen. Carboxyhaemoglobin (COHb) levels higher than 10%–20% are toxic (headache, nausea, and vomiting) and those exceeding 50%–60% can leads to confusion, seizures, coma, cardio-respiratory depression, and death. The half-life of COHb is 4 h when breathing room air and is reduced to 40–60 min when breathing 100% oxygen (see chapter 62).

HCN is a toxic gas related to the burning of nitrogenous materials, present in plastics such as poly-vinyl chloride. HCN intoxication should be suspected in the case of smoke inhalation with metabolic acidosis and *hyperlactacidemia*, without alteration of oxygen delivery alteration. The primary effect of HCN is a blocking of the mitochondrial respiration chain resulting in cytotoxic hypoxia. In this condition, the inhibition of cytochrome c oxidase is related to the high affinity of HCN to heme a3 of the enzyme. The effect is a structural change, reduced activity of the enzyme, and aerobic utilization switches to the anaerobic pathway with an increase in lactate production resulting in metabolic acidosis. The presence of CO and cyanide has a synergistic effect causing tissue dysoxia[15] (see chapter 62).

Diagnosis of Inhalation Injury

A diagnosis of inhalation injury is based on a history of fire and smoke exposure in an enclosed space associated with impaired consciousness. Physical and biological findings including facial or neck burns, singed nasal and/or facial hair, carbonaceous sputum, changes in voice, stridor, hypoxia, wheezing, and increased COHb levels are supplementary information to support the diagnosis. Fibreoptic bronchoscopy (FOB) within the first 24 h is the gold standard to confirm the diagnosis, assess the severity of inhalation injury, and prognosticate.[6,16] It may reveal carbonaceous debris, erythema, oedema, or ulceration. Of note, severe vasoconstriction from hypovolaemia may mask significant injury initially in the absence of soot. Apart from this exception, bronchoscopy has a high accuracy in confirming the diagnosis of established inhalation injury. Furthermore, the abbreviated injury score grading scale (0–4) for inhalation injury on bronchoscopy, first proposed by Endorf and Gamelli, has been shown to be correlated with worse outcomes (Figure 61.2).[5,15,17] While Endorf's study of 80 patients demonstrated increased mortality (particularly more severe grades 2–4), others have not demonstrated increased mortality although have shown more ventilator days, ICU days, or increased chance of ARDS amongst those with more severe grades.[18–20] Hassan et al. demonstrated increased mortality as the severity of bronchoscopically diagnosed inhalation injury increased.[21]

The main limitation of FOB is the lack of routine access to or its sensitivity for assessment of the distal airways, respiratory bronchioles, and alveoli, where the parenchymal injury associated with acute respiratory failure is thought to occur. Indeed, there is no good correlation with the grade of inhalation injury and ARDS in burn injury. This is likely due to the variable distal effects of the less soluble inhaled injurious gaseous agents, which bypass the upper airways.[22] Moreover, bronchoscopy is not usually able to assess the distal airways, and this may explain some of the discordance between bronchoscopic findings and parenchymal disease as can be noted by thickened airway walls or ground glass on computed tomography (CT).

Other modalities than bronchoscopy or CT also described to confirm inhalation injury and assess its severity include radionuclide imaging with ^{133}xenon, or pulmonary function testing. A grading radiology CT score assessing the extent of normality increased interstitial markings, ground glass, or consolidation on axial slices within 24 h of inhalation injury correlated with a composite of pneumonia/ARDS or death. Together with bronchoscopic grading, it also increased the likelihood of clinically significant inhalation injury 12.7-fold.[23] It has not, however, been widely adopted. Indeed, these non-bronchoscopic modalities lack sensitivity, and their optimal timing is a subject of debate.[6]

Management Strategies

There is no specific therapeutic intervention for inhalation injury. Treatment is based on supportive respiratory care: early and serial bronchoscopic pulmonary lavage is very effective in clearing soot, slough, and debris. It is associated with better outcomes such as reduced ventilator and hospital days in those with moderate-sized TBSA 30%–59%, pneumonia and inhalation injury, but no statistical survival benefit, from the National Burns Repository data.[24]

Indications for Tracheal Intubation

Special early attention must be given to the airway evaluation and management. There are many potential indications for early airway control in severely burn patients:

- Respiratory failure
- Symptoms of airway obstruction
- Severe CO and/or HCN intoxication
- Extensive burns to the head and neck
- Altered consciousness
- Haemodynamic instability
- Extensive burns >40% total body surface area

Not all patients who have smoke inhalation require tracheal intubation. However, early/prophylactic intubation can be lifesaving in patients with a high risk of facial and upper airway oedema related to thermal injury mainly in the case of large volume of fluid resuscitation. Indeed, the study of Venus et al. suggests that prophylactic intubation can decrease pulmonary-related mortality in patients with inhalation injury.[25] Rapid sequence or awake fibreoptic

Grade	Severity	Endobronchial features	Image
0	**No inhalation injury**	Absence of carbonaceous deposits, erythema, oedema, bronchorrhoea or obstruction	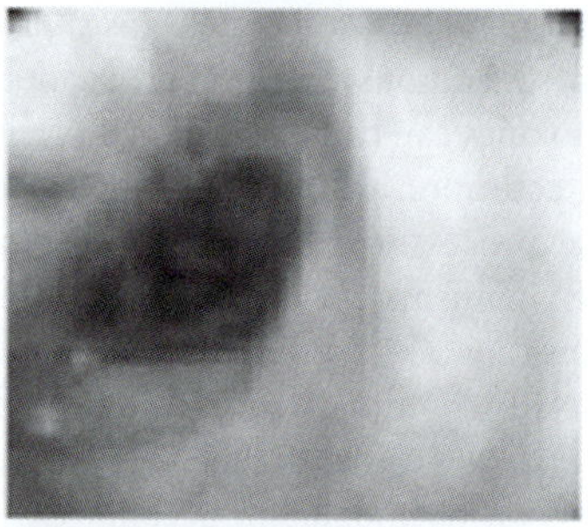
I	**Mild injury**	Minor or patchy areas of erythema, carbonaceous deposits in proximal or distal bronchi (any or combination)	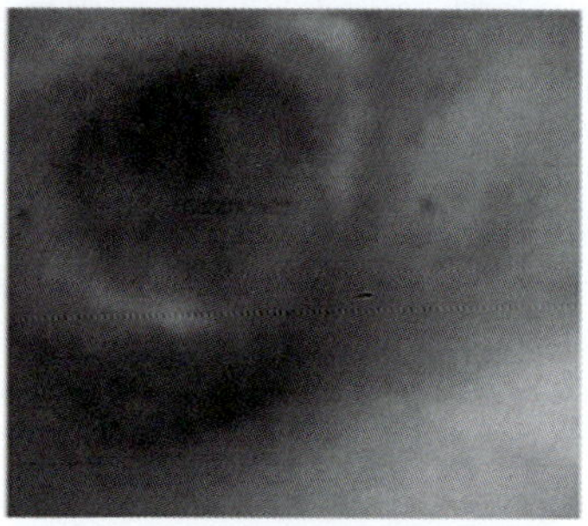
II	**Moderate injury**	Moderate degree of erythema, carbonaceous deposits, bronchorrhoea, with or without compromise of the bronchi (any or combination)	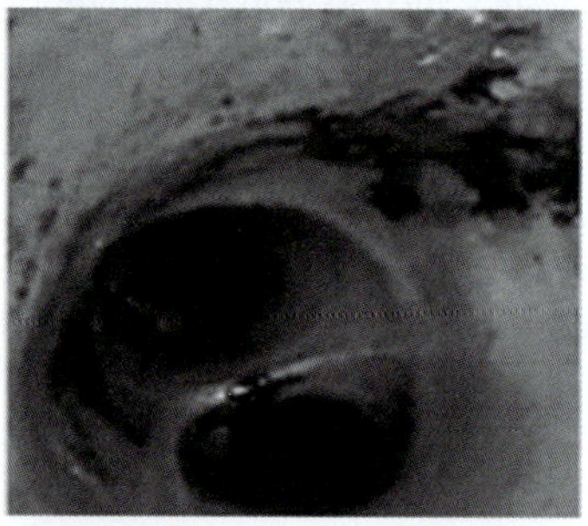
III	**Severe injury**	Severe inflammation with friability, copious carbonaceous deposits, bronchorrhoea, bronchial obstruction (any or combination)	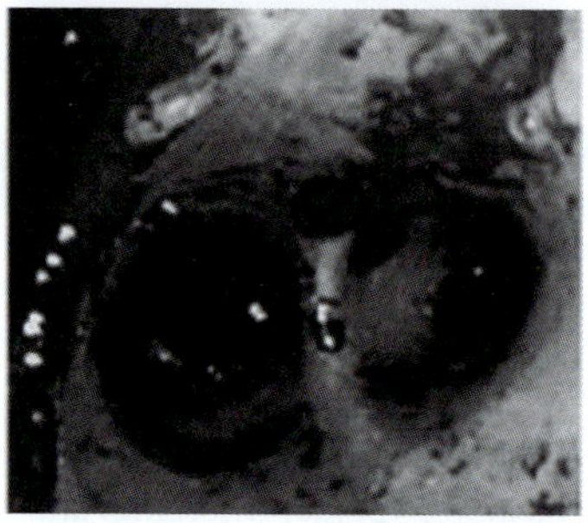
IV	**Massive injury**	Evidence of mucosal sloughing, necrosis, endoluminal obliteration (any or combination)	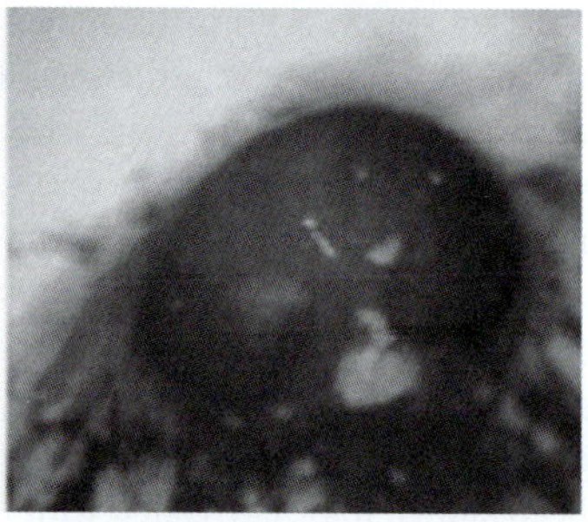

Figure 61.2 Abbreviated injury score. See plate section.

Reproduced from Singh S. Bronchoscopy in Intensive care. In: Herth F, Shah PL, Gompelmann D, eds. *Interventional Pulmonology* (ERS Monograph). Copyright European Respiratory Society, 2017; pp. 000–000 [https://doi.org/10.1183/2312508X.10002517].

intubation have to be considered for anaesthesia induction by an experienced clinician as part of a planned difficult airway protocol. Suxamethonium (associated with a hypnotic) can be used safely in the first 48 h after a major burn injury; or alternatively, rocuronium if available. In the patients requiring prolonged mechanical ventilation and/or multiple anaesthetics for surgical procedures, tracheostomy is proposed. This may be delayed for several days if the anterior neck skin has been involved. If not deemed suitable for percutaneous tracheostomy insertion, it may be performed in theatre by a surgical approach or often a hybrid approach of surgical tissue dissection and bleeding control to the pretracheal fascia, followed by a percutaneous Seldinger style tracheostomy insertion thereafter. In the absence or clear evidence of the benefit of early tracheostomy in severely burned patients, the risk of complications should be balanced with a significant benefit in each case.

Respiratory Support

In the case of full thickness circumferential chest burn with restricted chest movements and high inspiratory pressures, a thoracic escharotomy is urgently required. Furthermore, there is no ideal respiratory support strategy for the patient with inhalation injury. Consensus guidelines for mechanical ventilation in ARDS patients are extrapolated to burn patients with inhalation injury.[26] Lung-protective ventilation strategy (low tidal volumes ≤6 mL/kg and plateau pressures <30 cmH_2O), permissive hypercapnia (with a pH >7.2–7.25), and an optimized positive end expiratory pressure (PEEP) are now adopted by most of the burn centres to reduce ventilator-induced injury. However, these setting limits can prove challenging in patients with airway fibrin casts, chest wall thermal injury, and large fluid resuscitation volumes due to a combination of increased airways resistance and reduced thoracic compliance. Conventional mechanical ventilation, either volume or pressure controlled, is most commonly adopted. Some authors have suggested that the prophylactic use of high-frequency percussive ventilation (HFPV), developed by Dr Forrest Bird in the 1980s, allows gas exchange at lower inspiratory pressures and may improve the clearance of sloughed respiratory mucosa and plugs.[27–29] A randomized controlled study suggested that HFPV is associated with higher PaO_2/FiO_2 ratios on days 0 and 3 without a significant increase in ventilator-free days compared to patients ventilated conventionally with low tidal volume. There was a reduced incidence of pneumonia but no survival difference.[30] Nevertheless, a recent systematic review evaluating the decreased incidence of ventilator-associated pneumonia in burn patients with inhalation injuries who are on HFPV compared to those on volume control ventilation was inconclusive.[31] Airway pressure release ventilation (APRV), a pressure-controlled time-cycled ventilation mode, with higher mean airway pressures due to prolonged inspiration:expiration time, has been evaluated in a prospective experimental studies. In a model of ARDS caused by severe smoke inhalation in swine, APRV-treated animals developed ARDS faster than conventional mechanical ventilation-treated animals, showing a lower PaO_2/FiO_2 ratio in the first 24 h after injury, which equilibrated at 48 h. No survival difference was seen between APRV and conventional mechanical ventilation in this series.[32] Non-ventilator therapies to consider for inhalation injury include prone positioning. Hale et al. showed that prone positioning improves oxygenation in burn patients with severe ARDS and was safely implemented in a burn ICU.[33]

Inhalation Protocol

Aerosolized heparin is used in many centres to decrease the formation of fibrin casts, which contribute to obstruction of the airways following inhalation injury. The main mechanism of heparin is an activation of antithrombin III, leading to thrombin inactivation, so decreasing airway fibrin cast formation.

Inhaled *N*-acetylcysteine (NAC) has also been used as a mucolytic agent, with antioxidant properties, that could decrease airway cast formation. NAC contains a thiol group enabling a strong reducing capacity that breaks the disulphide bonds that give stability to the mucoprotein network within mucus.[34]

The combination of inhaled heparin (5000 iu) and acetylcysteine (3 mL of 20%) was used in a paediatric inhalation injury population 4-hourly for up to 7 days and showed an improvement in reintubation rates and survival outcomes when compared with a historical control group.[35] In a recent systematic review, inhaled anticoagulation regimens, which included heparin, heparinoids, antithrombin, and fibrinolytics, in both pre-clinical and clinical studies, were evaluated. In some pre-clinical and clinical studies, inhaled anticoagulants were associated with a favourable effect on survival.[36] Unfortunately the planned HEPBURN trial of heparin proved unfeasible.[37] However, a recent retrospective study demonstrated a reduction in ventilator days for those given higher dose heparin 10,000 units qds for 7 days.[38] Finally, inhaled irritants and NAC itself can induce bronchospasm, which can be managed using β2-adrenergic agonists such as albuterol and salbutamol. However, not all burn centres have universally adopted these inhalation treatment protocols.[28]

Fluid Management

In the case of inhalation injury, up to 40% higher fluid requirements for the same size burn are observed within 48 h. This should be balanced with the risks of pulmonary and peripheral oedema. Inadequate fluid administration early on can exacerbate the effects of inhalation injury and alter oxygenation. Regardless of which formula is used, it should serve only as a guideline for the very initial resuscitation. Thereafter, fluid resuscitation should be titrated to achieve physiologic endpoints (cardiac output, mean arterial pressure, central venous saturations, urine output, base deficit, and lactate kinetics).[39,40] Other strategies to reduce fluid administration include the use of vasopressors mainly in vasoplegic patients and albumin administration in severely burned patients.[41,42] A key concern is to prevent under fluid resuscitation early on in the knowledge that severe burn injury patients are generally in very high cardiac output states, often tolerating lower mean arterial pressures without compromise of end organ perfusion (i.e. renal function through urine output).

Extracorporeal Membrane Oxygenation (ECMO)

The use of veno-venous ECMO in inhalation injury has not been formally studied in randomized clinical trials. However, it is an accepted and established means of rescue ventilatory therapy in this group of patients as with others who develop severe refractory acute respiratory failure.[43] The current literature is based on insufficient studies and patient numbers with a limited level of evidence.[44] Of that, there was a trend to higher survival in those receiving ECMO therapy. The other main findings in this review are that survivors had shorter average run times (<200 h) versus non-survivors (>200 h) and no difference in mortality between patients with PaO_2/FiO_2 ratios above or below 60 at ECMO initiation. Surgical logistic factors for patients on ECMO are manageable as the circuits can now be run without the need for anticoagulation, albeit requiring earlier circuit changes. An important factor is that a major predictor for survival, that being early surgical wound debridement, should not be compromised or overly delayed by the requirements for ECMO support. This requires careful early discussion and coordination between the burn surgical team, intensive care, and ECMO service providers. Co-location of services is desirable, but mobility of burn surgical teams during the ECMO run may be another factor in situations where this is not possible. More published clinical data is required prior to future definitive recommendations.

Potential Future Therapeutic Strategies

Much progress has been made in understanding the molecular pathophysiology of inhalation injury. Further research is ongoing about the use of antioxidants. There is emerging evidence that inhaled vitamin E (γ-tocopherol) and hydrogen sulphide may have therapeutic benefits in inhalation-related lung injury.[45] In view of the very high CO_2 production in burn patients, together with the desire to ventilate protectively, another area for future investigation is the early use of extracorporeal CO_2 removal (ECCO2R) for the treatment of ARDS due to smoke inhalation and burns.[46] Further clinical trials are needed to assess these novel therapeutic interventions in inhalation injury. Consideration of burn trauma patients as a priori subgroups within planned ventilator support trials (i.e. ECMO, ECCO2R, prone positioning, etc.) may be an approach to pursue.

Systemic Toxicity from Carbon Monoxide and/or Hydrogen Cyanide

In CO intoxication, early symptoms include headache, nausea, vomiting, and lowered mental status. Diagnosis requires direct measurement of COHb by arterial oximetry or pulse CO oximetry. The administration of high-flow oxygen via a non-rebreathing mask can be sufficient, but in severe cases (coma, myocardial ischaemia significant acidosis, and initial COHb levels >30%) intubation and ventilation with $FiO_2 = 1$ is required. Hyperbaric oxygen is proposed to treat the neurological effects CO poisoning, through increased clearance, in the case of severe neurologic signs and/or pregnancy with COHb levels >15%, but there is no consensus on the indications, treatment parameters, or outcome benefits.[47] Moreover, logistical factors have limited the utilization of hyperbaric oxygen.

In the emergency setting, HCN intoxication is based on a presumptive clinical diagnosis. As HCN levels are not easily available, the following suggest cyanide poisoning:

- Lactate >8–10 mmol/L
- Elevated anion gap acidosis
- Reduced arteriovenous oxygen gradient

In the case of severe toxicity (seizures, coma, arrhythmias, myocardial ischaemia, and cardiovascular collapse), tracheal intubation, ventilation with $FiO_2 = 1$, and administration of an antidote is required as soon as possible. The most commonly used antidote is hydroxocobalamin (Cyanokit), which is given intravenously over 15 min at the dose of 5 g, and may be repeated one time in patients with severe toxicity or poor clinical response (70 mg/kg for paediatric patients). Hydroxocobalamin turns the urine and skin purple. More severe side effects are described, such as hydroxocobalamin-associated acute kidney injury due to oxalate nephropathy.[48] Cyanokit is being suggested and indeed used prophylactically in higher total burn surface area (TBSA) burns with inhalation injury.

Complications and Outcomes

Inhalation injury is an independent predictor of mortality in burns. Respiratory complications are responsible for over three-quarter deaths. Carbon monoxide poisoning is a strong association. Of 769 patients with smoke-inhalation-related acute lung injury identified across 68 US burn centres, in-hospital mortality rate was 26%. Among those who also had severe burns (>20% TBSA), it was 50%. Higher age and early vasopressor use were further strong negative predictors of outcomes[49] (Table 61.1).

The most frequent complication following inhalation injury is respiratory tract infection.[50] In the study of Shirani et al., with almost 1000 burn patients, 35% had inhalation injury. Of these patients, 38% had subsequent pneumonia. Among the patients without inhalation injury, pneumonia occurred in 8.8% of cases. Inhalation injury alone increased mortality by a maximum of 20% and pneumonia by a maximum of 40%, with a maximum increase of approximately 60% when both were present.[9] Furthermore, ventilator-associated infective complications worsen outcomes compared with the absence of ventilator-associated events in inhalation injury.[11]

About 20%–30% of patients with inhalation injury suffer from acute airway obstruction related to supraglottic oedema.[25,28] Peak oedema is usually around 24 h post-burn trauma and decreases over the following days. Delayed consequences of prolonged intubation include subglottic stenosis. Complications associated with tracheostomies include tracheal ulcerations, tracheitis, and bleeding.[6] Other complications associated with inhalation injury are vocal cord fixation or fusion, dysphonia, endobronchial polyps, bronchiectasis, and bronchiolitis obliterans.[51] In order to identify these complications, long-term post-ICU follow-up, including pulmonary function testing, chest imaging, and bronchoscopy (if indicated), is advisable.

Conclusion

Inhalation injury refers to damage to the respiratory tract and/or lung parenchyma by heat, smoke, or chemical irritants. Inhalation injury also causes systemic toxicity by toxic gases (CO and HCN being the most notable). It is associated with increased mortality in critically ill burn patients. Bronchoscopy confirms diagnosis, defines the severity, and aids therapeutic airway clearance.[52] Treatment of inhalation injury is mainly supportive: Securing a definitive airway early, protective mechanical ventilation, airway clearance strategies, surveillance for pulmonary infection, inhalation strategies of 4-hourly inhaled heparin, and NAC plus bronchodilators.[53] Post-recovery respiratory sequelae require follow-up. Future therapeutic strategies may address the complex pathophysiology that involves control of the inflammatory, oxidative stress, and coagulation pathways and their effects on the respiratory tract at the molecular level.[54]

Table 61.1 Strategies for inhalation injury

Issue	Standard of care	Further options
Diagnosis	Clinical history and examination	Bronchoscopy, CT scan, and radionuclide scan
Carbon monoxide poisoning	100% oxygen for >6 h (normocarbic)	Hyperbaric oxygen
Cyanide exposure	Fluid resuscitation and hydroxycobalamin	Empirical hydroxycobalamin in high-TBSA burns and inhalation injury
Indication for intubation	Overt or imminent upper airway obstruction, hoarse voice stridor, poor gas exchange, and reduced conscious level	Anticipation of upper airway obstruction, when fluid resuscitation occurs, planned patient transfer, and worsening neurology
Ventilation strategy	Protective lung volume ventilation; consider prone if ARDS	High-frequency percussive ventilation; consider ECMO if severe ARDS
Pulmonary clearance	Cough, physiotherapy and adjuncts, and bronchoscopic lavage	Serial therapeutic bronchoscopic lavage
Inhaled therapies	None	Nebulized heparin 5–10,000 units 4 hourly; NAC 3 mL of 20% 4 hourly; bronchodilator salbutamol—all together
Empirical therapies	None	Corticosteroids +/− antibiotics (no evidence base for benefit)

REFERENCES

1. Rehberg S, Maybauer MO, Enkhbaatar P, et al. Pathophysiology, management and treatment of smoke inhalation injury. *Expert Rev Respir Med*. 2009;**3**:283–297.
2. Mackie DP, Spoelder EJ, Paauw RJ, et al. Mechanical ventilation and fluid retention in burn patients. *J Trauma*. 2009;**67**:1233–1238.
3. McCall JE, Cahill TJ. Respiratory care of the burn patient. *J Burn Care Rehabil*. 2005; **26**:200–206.
4. Dries DJ, Endorf FW. Inhalation injury: Epidemiology, pathology, treatment strategies. *Scand J Trauma Resusc Emerg Med*. 2013;**21**:31.
5. Endorf FW, Gamelli RL. Inhalation injury, pulmonary perturbations, and fluid resuscitation. *J Burn Care Res*. 2007;**28**:80–83.
6. Walker PF, Buehner MF, Wood LA, et al. Diagnosis and management of inhalation injury: An updated review. *Crit Care*. 2015 Oct 28;**19**:351.
7. Clark WR, Bonaventura M, Myers W. Smoke inhalation and airway management at a regional burn unit: 1974–1983. Part I: Diagnosis and consequences of smoke inhalation. *J Burn Care Rehabil*. 1989;**10**:52–62.
8. Pruitt Jr., BA, Erickson DR, Morris A. Progressive pulmonary insufficiency and other pulmonary complications of thermal injury. *J Trauma*. 1975;**15**:369–379.
9. Shirani KZ, Pruitt BA Jr., Mason AD Jr. The influence of inhalation injury and pneumonia on burn mortality. *Ann Surg*. 1987;**205**(1):82–87. doi:10.1097/00000658-198701000-00015
10. Williams DJ, Walker JD. A nomogram for calculation of the Revised Baux Score. *Burns*. 2015;**41**:85–90.
11. Younan D, Griffin R, Zaky A, et al. Burn patients with infection-related ventilator associated complications have worse outcomes compared to those without ventilator associated events. *Am J Surg*. 2018 Apr;**215**(4):678–681. doi:10.1016/j.amjsurg.2017.10.034. Epub 2017 Oct 31. PubMed PMID: 29126595.
12. Porro LJ, Demling RH, Pierira CT, et al. Care of the geriatric patient. In: Herndon DN, ed. *Total Burn Care*. 4th ed. Elsevier, Amsterdam; 2009:415.
13. Dries DJ, Endorf FW. Inhalation injury: Epidemiology, pathology, treatment strategies. *Scand J Trauma Resusc Emerg Med*. 2013 Apr 19;**21**:31.
14. Singh S, Grover V, Christie L, et al. A comparative study of bronchoscopic microsample probe versus bronchoalveolar lavage in patients with burns-related inhalational injury, acute lung injury and chronic stable lung disease. *Respiration*. 2015;**89**(1):19–26. doi:10.1159/000368367. Epub 2015 Jan 6. PubMed PMID: 25573649.
15. Rehberg S, Maybauer MO, Enkhbaatar P, et al. Pathophysiology, management and treatment of smoke inhalation injury. *Expert Rev Respir Med*. 2009;**3**:283–297.
16. You K, Yang HT, Kym D, et al. Inhalation injury in burn patients: Establishing the link between diagnosis and prognosis. *Burns*. 2014;**40**(8):1470.
17. Ching JA, Ching YH, Shivers SC, et al. An analysis of inhalation injury diagnostic methods and patient outcomes. *J Burn Care Res*. 2016;**37**(1):e27–32.
18. Albright JM, Davis CS, Bird MD, et al. The acute pulmonary inflammatory response to the graded severity of smoke inhalation injury. *Crit Care Med*. 2012;**40**(4):1113–1121.
19. Mosier MJ, Pham TN, Park DR, et al. Predictive value of bronchoscopy in assessing the severity of inhalation injury. *J Burn Care Res*. 2012; **33**:65–73.
20. Spano S, Hanna S, Li Z, et al. Does bronchoscopic evaluation of inhalation injury severity predict outcome? *J Burn Care Res*. 2016 Jan-Feb;**37**(1):1–11.
21. Hassan Z, Wong JK, Bush J, et al. Assessing the severity of inhalation injuries in adults. *Burns*. 2010;**36**(2):212–216.
22. Singh S, Handy JM. The respiratory insult in burns injury. *Curr Anaesth Crit Care*. **19**:264–268.
23. Oh JS, Chung KK, Allen A, et al. Admission chest CT complements fiberoptic bronchoscopy in prediction of adverse outcomes in thermally injured patients. *J Burn Care Res*. 2012;**33**(4):532–538.
24. Carr J, Phillips BD, Bowling WM. The utility of bronchoscopy after inhalational injury complicated by pneumonia in burn patients: Results from the National Burn Repository. *J Burn Care Res*. 2009;**30**:967–974.
25. Venus B, Matsuda T, Copiozo JB, et al. Prophylactic intubation and continuous positive airway pressure in the management of inhalation injury in burn victims. *Crit Care Med*. 1981;**9**:519–523.
26. Mackie DP, Spoelder EJ, Paauw RJ, et al. Mechanical ventilation and fluid retention in burn patients. J Trauma. 2009;**67**:1233–1238; discussion 1238.

27. Mlcak RP, Suman OE, Herndon DN. Respiratory management of inhalation injury. *Burns*. 2007;**33**:2–13.
28. Sheridan RL. Fire-related inhalation injury. *N Engl J Med*. 2016;**375**:464–469.
29. Cioffi WG, Graves TA, McManus WF, et al. High-frequency percussive ventilation in patients with inhalation injury. *J Trauma*. 1989;**29**:350–354.
30. Chung KK, Wolf SE, Renz EM, et al. High-frequency percussive ventilation and low tidal volume ventilation in burns: A randomized controlled trial. *Crit Care Med*. 2010;**38**(**10**):1970–1977.
31. Al Ashry HS, Mansour G, Kalil AC, et al. Incidence of ventilator associated pneumonia in burn patients with inhalation injury treated with high-frequency percussive ventilation versus volume control ventilation: A systematic review. *Burns*. 2016;**42**:1193.
32. Batchinsky AI, Burkett SE, Zanders TB, et al. Comparison of airway pressure release ventilation to conventional mechanical ventilation in the early management of smoke inhalation injury in swine. *Crit Care Med*. 2011;**39**:2314–2321.
33. Hale DF, Cannon JW, Batchinsky AI, et al. Prone positioning improves oxygenation in adult burn patients with severe acute respiratory distress syndrome. *J Trauma Acute Care Surg*. 2012;**72**:1634–1639.
34. Mlcak RP. Respiratory care. In: Herndon DN, ed. *Total Burn Care*, 4th ed. Elsevier, Amsterdam; 2009.
35. Desai MH, Mlcak R, Richardson J, et al. Reduction in mortality in pediatric patients with inhalation injury with aerosolized heparin/N-acetylcystine therapy. *J Burn Care Rehabil*. 1998;**19**:210–212.
36. Miller AC, Elamin EM, Suffredini AF. Inhaled anticoagulation regimens for the treatment of smoke inhalation-associated acute lung injury: A systematic review. *Crit Care Med*. 2014;**42**:413–419.
37. Glas GJ, Muller J, Binnekade JM, et al. HEPBURN—investigating the efficacy and safety of nebulized heparin versus placebo in burn patients with inhalation trauma: Study protocol for a multi-center randomized controlled trial. *Trials*. 2014;**15**:91. Epub 2014 3 25.
38. McIntire AM, Harris SA, Whitten JA, et al. Outcomes Following the Use of Nebulized Heparin for Inhalation Injury (HIHI Study). *J Burn Care Res*. 2017;**38**(1):45–52.
39. Berger MM, Que YA. A protocol guided by transpulmonary thermodilution and lactate levels for resuscitation of patients with severe burns. *Crit Care*. 2013;**17**:195.
40. Salehi SH, As'adi K, Mousavi J. Comparison of the outcome of burn patients using acute-phase plasma base deficit. *Ann Burns Fire Disasters*. 2011;**24**(4):203–208.
41. Arlati S, Storti E, Pradella V, et al. Decreased fluid volume to reduce organ damage: A new approach to burn shock resuscitation? A preliminary study. *Resuscitation*. 2007;**72**:371–378.
42. Park SH, Hemmila MR, Wahl WL. Early albumin use improves mortality in difficult to resuscitate burn patients. *J Trauma Acute Care Surg*. 2012;**73**:1294–1297.
43. Combes A, Hajage D, Capellier G, et al. Extracorporeal membrane oxygenation for severe acute respiratory distress syndrome. *N Engl J Med*. 2018;**378**:1965–1975. doi:10.1056/NEJMoa1800385
44. Asmussen S, Maybauer DM, Fraser JF, et al. Extracorporeal membrane oxygenation in burn and smoke inhalation injury. *Burns*. 2013;**39**:429–435.
45. Yamamoto Y, Sousse LE, Enkhbaatar P, et al. γ-tocopherol nebulization decreases oxidative stress, arginase activity, and collagen deposition after burn and smoke inhalation in the ovine model. *Shock*. 2012; **38**(6):671–676.
46. Kreyer S, Scaravilli V, Linden K, et al. Early utilization of extracorporeal CO2 removal for treatment of acute respiratory distress syndrome due to smoke inhalation and burns in sheep. *Shock*. 2016;**45**(1):65–72.
47. Buckley NA, Juurlink DN, Isbister G, et al. Hyperbaric oxygen for carbon monoxide poisoning. *Cochrane Database Syst Rev*. 2011;**4**:CD002041.
48. Legrand M, Michel T, Daudon M, et al. PRONOBURN Study Group. Risk of oxalate nephropathy with the use of cyanide antidote hydroxocobalamin in critically ill burn patients. *Intensive Care Med*. 2016; **42**(6):1080–1081.
49. Kadri SS, Miller AC, Hohmann S, et al. US Critical Illness and Injury Trials Group: Smoke Inhalation-associated Acute Lung Injury (SI-ALI) Investigators (USCIIT-SI-ALI). Risk Factors for In-Hospital Mortality in Smoke Inhalation-Associated Acute Lung Injury: Data From 68 United States Hospitals. *Chest*. 2016;**150**(6):1260. Epub 2016 Jun 15.
50. Pruitt Jr BA, Erickson DR, Morris A. Progressive pulmonary insufficiency and other pulmonary complications of thermal injury. *J Trauma*. 1975;**15**:369–379.
51. Slutzker AD, Kinn R, Said SI. Bronchiectasis and progressive respiratory failure following smoke inhalation. *Chest*. 1989;**95**(6):1349.
52. Singh S. Bronchoscopy in intensive care. In: Herth F, Shah PL, Gompelmann D, eds. *Interventional Pulmonology (ERS Monograph)*. Sheffield, European Respiratory Society; 2017:29–48.
53. Walker, PF, Buehner MF, Wood LA, et al. Diagnosis and management of inhalation injury: An updated review. *Crit Care*. 2015;**19**:351.
54. O'Dea KP, Porter JR, Tirlapur N, et al. Circulating microvesicles are elevated acutely following major burns injury and associated with clinical severity. *PLoS One*. 2016 Dec 9;**11**(12):e0167801.

62

Poisoning

Omender Singh, Suneel Kumar Garg, and Deven Juneja

KEY MESSAGES

- Critical care physicians routinely manage poisoning and drug overdose. Clinical scenarios may vary from unknown poisoning, drug overdose, to toxin exposure. It may arise from suicidal, accidental, and sometimes as a chemical weapon exposure or iatrogenic drug errors and toxicities.
- Respiratory failure is a common complication of poisoning and overdose. It is more likely to develop in patients with limited pulmonary reserve. Poisoning and overdose may cause respiratory failure by compromising respiratory pump function and/or by causing direct injury to the lung parenchyma. Respiratory failure may also develop from central nervous system depression due to drug overdose or poisoning.
- In poisonings associated with respiratory failure, arterial blood gas (ABG) should always be performed with co-oximetry.
- Supportive care remains the mainstay of treatment but may need to be modified in certain poisoning and overdose where oxygen therapy may aggravate toxicity. Where specific antidotes exist, they may have a dramatic effect on respiratory failure. Decontamination and aggressive supportive measures remain the main focus of treatment.
- Poisoning and overdose-induced respiratory failure is complex and needs understanding of the mechanism responsible for respiratory failure, which may result in better outcomes.

CONTROVERSIES

- Activated charcoal is of most value in the awake patient, within <30–60 min of known ingestion of toxins (e.g. paracetamol, aspirin, metformin, citalopram, venlafaxine, digoxin, etc.). However, its use beyond that is controversial. It should not be completely dismissed later but used based upon the clinical status, projected risks, and potential benefit.
- The timing of use of digoxin-specific antibodies in chronic digoxin overdose (i.e. inadvertent) and outcomes (despite demonstrable reduction in digoxin levels).

FURTHER RESEARCH

- International strategies to support studies (and newer designs like adaptive platforms) into common or less common toxins/poisonings through pre-clinical and real-world clinical studies.
- Improved public health awareness of poisons/toxins risks in low and middle income nations and access to antidotes as part of the broader public health strategy.

Introduction

Poisoning and overdose can present with various clinical manifestations including respiratory failure. Clinical scenarios may vary from drug overdose, poisoning, and suicidal to environmental exposure by various routes.[1] Exposure by the inhalational route is of growing concern particularly as a route for chemical weapons. In cases of unknown poisoning and drug overdose, respiratory failure may be the only clue to the diagnosis at the time of presentation. Poisoning and overdose may acutely precipitate respiratory failure by compromising respiratory function and/or by causing lung injury.

The response to ingestion depends on the time of ingestion or exposure, quantity or dose, route, duration, concentration, and the type of poison. Such responses may lead to single-organ dysfunction (e.g. inhalational lung injury) or multi-organ dysfunction (best described by the toxidrome) (Table 62.1).[1]

The prognosis and clinical course of recovery of patients with respiratory failure due to poisoning significantly depends on the quality of the care delivered within the first few hours from pre-hospital through the emergency department to the intensive care unit (ICU), if required. In most cases, the poison or drug leading to respiratory failure may be identified by careful history, physical examination, and appropriate laboratory tests. Clinicians taking care of patients should have access to expertise in the interpretation of complex analytical toxicology.[2] All efforts should be made to identify the poison or drug as, in some cases, appropriate antidote, if given early, can prevent further deterioration and may be lifesaving. Physicians should also consider all measures to minimize the absorption or exposure to the poison or drug and utilize available measures to enhance elimination of poison or drug from the body. This chapter discusses general issues of poisoning management and then covers four common respiratory scenarios where specific antidotes exist (namely respiratory depressants, carbon monoxide (CO) poisoning, methaemoglobinemia, and cyanide toxicity).

Table 62.1 Identification of suspected toxin based on toxidrome (clinical manifestations)

Manifestations	Toxin
Drowsiness with hypoventilation	Primarily central nervous system (CNS) depressants
Rapid onset of breathlessness with rapid recovery if removed from site of exposure	Simple asphyxiants
Acute onset of tearing, eye burning, and nasal and throat irritation, with or without coughing, stridor, or wheezing	Water-soluble irritant
Subacute or chronic symptoms of chest tightness, decreased exercise tolerance or wheezes, and finding of rales or rhonchi	Water-insoluble irritant
Acute lung injury with hypoxia or pulmonary oedema	Direct pulmonary toxin
Cyanosis unresponsive to supplemental oxygen with a SpO_2 reading of a mid-80% saturation	Methaemoglobinemia
Absence of cyanosis, but the presence of prominent CNS manifestation	Carbon monoxide poisoning
Rapid onset of metabolic acidosis with cardiac and CNS symptoms, particularly in the presence of similar measured oxygen saturations of mixed venous and arterial blood gas	Mitochondrial toxin
Hypertension, hyperthermia, bronchospasm and wheezing, tachycardia, mydriasis, acute psychosis, and delirium	Sympathomimetics

Pulmonary Physiology and Response to Injury

Human beings have an efficient engineered system of gas exchange (Chapters 2 and 3) that can be disrupted in several ways, including by poisoning that directly suppress the nervous system and predispose the patients to life-threatening respiratory failure. Respiratory failure can also be caused by agents causing direct and indirect pulmonary injury.

Direct lung injury is caused by acute exposure to inhalants, and it may cause respiratory complications ranging from mild irritation to death by asphyxiation. Indirect lung injury may be caused by commonly used cardiovascular drugs, that is, anti-arrhythmic and anti-hypertensive agents.

Specific pharmacological agents with pulmonary toxicity include amiodarone that can cause an acute interstitial pneumonitis, which may lead to refractory and even fatal hypoxaemia if not rapidly discontinued and steroid treatment initiated.[3] Angiotensin converting enzyme (ACE) inhibitors are generally associated with mild symptoms like chronic dry cough, but in common with beta-blockers may cause bronchospasm and breathlessness. Anti-inflammatory agents like acetylsalicylic acid may lead to pulmonary complications including aggravation of asthma and non-cardiogenic pulmonary oedema. Some anti-cancer chemotherapeutic agents, that is, bleomycin and busulfan, may lead to pulmonary infiltrates and acute interstitial pneumonitis, which may cause severe hypoxaemia and can be fatal if unrecognized and offending drug is not discontinued. Bleomycin is particularly challenging as the toxicity is exacerbated by increased oxygen concentrations. Further details of specific respiratory toxicities are set out in Tables 62.2–62.4.

Table 62.2 Poisons and drugs causing respiratory depression and failure

Poison/drug	Comments
Alcohol Barbiturate Benzodiazepine Botulinum toxin Carbamate Cyclic Antidepressant Opioid Organophosphorus-agriculture insecticide, sarin gas, tabun gas, and soman gas Sedative-hypnotic	Poisons and drug overdose causing respiratory failure altered mental status, bradycardia and, hypotension Diagnosis is generally made on history of abuse, supportive clinical findings, and appropriate laboratory examinations ABG may reveal type-1, type-2, or mixed respiratory failure depending on the poison and overdose Some agents have specific antidotes, that is, flumazenil for benzodiazepine, naloxone for opioid, and pralidoxime for organophosphorus poisoning

Table 62.3 Agents causing direct pulmonary injury

Simple asphyxiants	Comments
Heavier than air Argon Butane Carbon dioxide Ethane Methyl isocyanate Natural gases Propane **Lighter than air** Acetylene Ethylene Methane Neon Nitrogen	Simple asphyxiants are inert gases or vapours; occupational exposures and fires may cause tissue hypoxia by displacing oxygen in inspired air when present in high concentrations Manifestations of mild toxicity include headache, dizziness, nausea, and vomiting, dyspnoea, altered sensorium, cardiac dysrhythmia, syncope, seizure, and even death can occur in severe toxicity Diagnosis is based on a consistent history, group victims, clinical features, and rapid resolution of symptoms on removal of patients away from exposure Hypoxaemia must be corrected quickly to avoid hypoxic brain injury and myocardial ischaemia; rescuers should take care not to enter an oxygen-deficient environment to ensure that they do not become secondary victims
Respiratory irritants	**Comments**
High solubility Ammonia Chlorine Formaldehyde Sulphur dioxide **Low solubility** Hydrogen sulphide Nitrogen mustards Oxides of nitrogen Phosgene sulphur mustards	Agents causing varied extent of injury in upper and lower airways leading to respiratory failure
Direct airway injury	**Comments**
Corrosives Hydrocarbons	Toxicity may range from mild respiratory distress to severe respiratory failure requiring oxygen and mechanical ventilation

Table 62.4 Agents causing indirect pulmonary injury

Chemical asphyxiants	Comments
Inhibiting oxygen transport	Interfere with oxygen transport, causing tissue hypoxia and development of lactic acidosis Treatment is high-flow oxygen and specific antidote if available
Carbon monoxide (CO)	
Hydrogen sulphide	
Methaemoglobin (MetHb) inducer	
Oxides of nitrogen	
Inhibiting cellular oxygen utilization	Inhibit cellular oxygen utilization by affecting cellular mitochondrial system leading to tissue hypoxia and lactic acidosis Treatment is high-flow oxygen and specific antidote if available
Acrylonitrile	
Cyanide	
Phosphine	
Cardiogenic pulmonary oedema	**Comments**
Aluminium phosphide	Diagnosis is made by history of ingestion, clinical examination, chest X-ray, and echocardiography Haemodynamic monitoring will reveal high right heart pressures and low cardiac output Treatment is usually supportive with oxygen, diuretic, and mechanical ventilation when indicated
Amphotericin B	
Anti-arrhythmic	
β-Blockers	
Bleomycin	
Carbamazepine	
Cocaine	
Cyclic antidepressant	
Sulfasalazine	
Tetracycline	
Non-cardiogenic pulmonary oedema	**Comments**
β-Adrenergic agonists	Diagnosis is made by history of ingestion, clinical examination, chest X-ray, and echocardiography Haemodynamic monitoring will reveal normal or high right heart pressures and normal cardiac output Treatment includes oxygen and supportive and mechanical ventilation when indicated
Cocaine	
Cyclophosphamide	
Ethylene glycol	
Heroin	
Hydrochlorothiazide	
Hydrocarbons	
Iodinated radio-contrast agents	
Inhalation injury	
Methadone and meprobamate	
Methotrexate	
Opioids	
Paraquat	
Phenobarbitone	
Propoxyphene	
Phosgene	
Sulfasalazine	
Salicylates	
Tocolytic agents	

(*continued*)

Table 62.4 Continued

Bronchospasm	Comments
ACE inhibitors	Mechanism includes inhibition of the cyclooxygenase enzyme by aspirin and cough by ACE inhibitors Treatment is usually discontinuation of the offending drug, oxygen, supportive care, and bronchodilators
Acetylsalicylic acid	
Amiodarone	
Amphotericin B	
β-Blockers	
Cocaine	
Dipyridamole	
Heroin	
Inhaled pentamidine	
Nitrofurantoin	
Organophosphate	
Penicillamine	
Sulfasalazine	
Alveolar haemorrhage	**Comments**
Amiodarone	Life-threatening disorder manifested with or without haemoptysis, low haemoglobin, diffuse pulmonary infiltrate, and type-1 respiratory failure A detailed history including drugs and physical examination help to establish the aetiology of alveolar haemorrhage; chest X-ray, CT chest, and broncho-alveolar lavage are usually diagnostic; management consists of withdrawal of offending drug, oxygen, supportive care, ventilatory support, and steroids
Anticoagulants and antiplatelets	
Chemotherapeutic agents (cyclophosphamide, mitomycin C, and cytarabine)	
Cocaine	
Nitrofurantoin	
Penicillamine	
Drug-induced pleural disease	**Comments**
ACE inhibitors	Uncommon entity and manifestations include pleural effusion, pneumothorax, or pleural thickening; a detailed drug history and the relationship between symptom onset after initiation of offending agent can help to make a diagnosis Radiology including chest X-ray and CT scan is helpful to differentiate between pleural disorders; pleural fluid examination is of utmost importance as the presence of marked eosinophilia is suggestive of drug-induced pleural effusion Management consists of oxygen, supportive care, and withdrawal of offending drug
Amiodarone	
Bleomycin	
Carmustine	
Cocaine	
Cyclophosphamide	
Hydralazine	
Methotrexate	
Nitrofurantoin	
Phenytoin	
Procainamide	
Procarbazine	
Retinoic acid	
Interstitial lung disease (ILD)	**Comments**
Antimicrobial agents (amphotericin B, isoniazid, nitrofurantoin, and sulfasalazine)	Not very common and usually a diagnosis of exclusion Treatment includes discontinuation of the offending drug, oxygen, and supportive care; steroids may be beneficial in some causes of ILD; most of the patients improve with symptomatic care and withdrawal of offending drug
Anti-inflammatory agents (aspirin, NSAIDS, and methotrexate)	
Biological agents (rituximab, bevacizumab, and TNF-α blockers)	
Cardiovascular agents (ACE inhibitors, amiodarone, β-blockers, statins, and hydrochlorothiazide)	
Chemotherapeutic agents (azathioprine, bleomycin, busulfan, chlorambucil, cyclophosphamide, hydroxyurea, and paclitaxel)	
Miscellaneous (bromocriptine, carbamazepine, and phenytoin)	

Approach to the Poisoned Patient

History, physical examination, and treatment often occur simultaneously and are integral part of making diagnosis and management of poisoning. History should include information about type of toxin or drug, time (acute vs chronic) and place of exposure, quantity taken, and route of administration (ingestion, inhalation, intravenous, and intramuscular). Efforts should be made to understand whether the nature of the poisoning was accidental, suicidal, therapeutic, via mass exposure, or chemical warfare. A history of psychiatric illness or previous poisoning should be sought. Poisoning patients may be unreliable in terms of providing accurate information, particularly in cases of attempted suicide or illicit drug abuse.[4] Family members, friends, and family physician may provide vital collateral information in identifying the toxin.

All efforts should be made to identify the toxidrome and subsequently the offending toxin.

Laboratory evaluation should include immediate arterial blood gas (ABG) with co-oximetry (to detect altered haemoglobins; carboxyhaemoglobin (COHb), cyanohaemoglobin (HbCN), and methhaemoglobin (MetHb)). An ABG will reveal the severity of hypoxaemia and type of respiratory failure. It will also be useful to identify ‘three gaps of toxicology’: the anion gap, the osmolar gap, and the arterial oxygen saturation gap. If any gap is increased, then toxic ingestion should be suspected. An arterial oxygen saturation gap is defined by a >5% difference between the saturation of oxygen in ABG and saturation measured by pulse oximetry. It is seen in CO poisoning and methaemoglobinemia. Hydrogen sulphide and cyanide interfere with cellular utilization of oxygen leading to abnormally high venous oxygen saturation.

Urine toxicology screen should be done routinely.[5] Serum toxin levels should be performed depending upon clinical suspicion of drug overdose and toxin. Identification of the suspected toxin is crucial in definite management, that is, administering a specific antidote. Additional laboratory tests and radiological investigation are guided by the suspected drug or toxin and physiological condition.

All patients suspected of significant poisoning or drug overdose should be admitted to the hospital with close supervision for at least 24 h. For apparently asymptomatic or paucisymptomatic patients toxicology services can advise on duration of required observation based on the toxin and suspected ingested amount. Supportive measures include management of airway, support of breathing and circulation, and prevention of harms from coma, but may need to be modified in certain poisonings and overdoses. For instance, oxygen therapy may actually aggravate toxicity in certain situations such as paraquat, diquat, and chlorine gas poisoning. Although tracheal intubation has a key role in protecting the airway, in cases of short-acting sedative overdose such as gamma-hydroxybutyrate (GHB), it should only be used if rapid awakening does not occur.[6]

Various methods of decontamination exist, including gastric emptying (gastric lavage, activated charcoal, or whole bowel irrigation), forced diuresis, extracorporeal removal of toxin, and specific antidote. Gastric lavage and activated charcoal can be administered in cases of ingestion of potentially life-threatening amount of poison within 60 min of exposure, only if benefits outweigh the risk of aspiration.[7] Activated charcoal should be given as soon as possible after gastric lavage.[8]

Antidote therapy should be limited to poisonings caused by life-threatening overdose and only when clinically indicated. In war-affected zones with the possibility of chemical nerve agents such as sarin gas, it is advisable to provide auto-injector of pralidoxime (reactivates anticholinesterases) to the victims which should be self-administered intramuscularly immediately after the exposure. Civilian practitioners should also be aware of nerve toxin poisoning, and several high-profile assassination attempts have used these agents, as have terrorist attacks. For instance, Novichok is now a well-known such agent, for which recognizing the cholinergic signs, providing support, atropine, and the pralidoxime (or equivalent) early are essential for survival.

Patients with severe toxicity can be supported with continuous veno-venous hemodiafiltration along with charcoal hemoperfusion, if indicated.[9] Veno-venous extracorporeal membrane oxygenation (ECMO) can be considered for refractory hypoxaemia and veno-arterial ECMO for refractory shock with reversible cardiotoxicity. ECMO is not a substitute to standard management of poisoning, and if used this should be alongside conventional toxin elimination treatments.

Figure 62.1 illustrates the modified Airway, Breathing, Circulation, Disability, Exposure (ABCDE) approach to poisoning, and Table 62.5 gives indications for ICU admission.

Specific Management

Specific antidotes are listed in Table 62.6

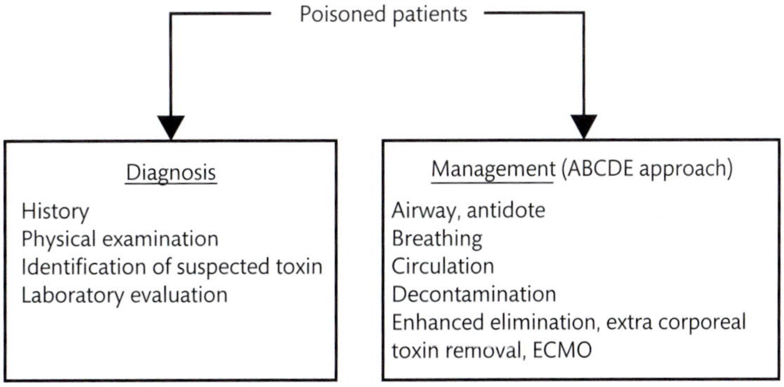

Figure 62.1 Approach to poisoning-induced respiratory failure.

Table 62.5 Criteria for ICU admission

Respiratory depression (pCO_2 > 45 mmHg)
Severe/refractory hypoxaemia
Pulmonary oedema induced by drugs or toxin inhalation (acute respiratory distress syndrome)
Shock
Cardiac arrhythmias
Reduced consciousness/inability to protect the airway (Glasgow coma score < 12)
Seizures
Worsening metabolic acidosis
Severe electrolyte abnormalities
Need for continuous infusion of antidote and its monitoring
Need for dialysis or hemoperfusion
Need for extracorporeal membrane oxygenation (ECMO)
Requirement for exchange transfusion

Respiratory Suppressants

Flumazenil, a specific antidote, is available for benzodiazepines; however, its use is restricted to acute overdose without chronic use as it may precipitate acute withdrawal and seizures in chronic users.[10] The recommended initial dose of flumazenil is 0.2 mg intravenous over 30 s followed by 0.3 mg over 30 s if the desired clinical effect is not seen within 30 s; followed by 0.5 mg over 30 s at 1 min intervals as needed to a total dose of 3 mg. There is no additional benefit of flumazenil dosed beyond 3 mg. Flumazenil can also be given by continuous infusion (0.1–0.5 mg/h).

Naloxone is a specific opioid antagonist, and it reverses opioid-induced sedation, hypotension, and respiratory depression.[11] The initial dose is 0.4 mg intravenous or 0.8 mg intramuscular or subcutaneously. An additional dose of 1–2 mg can be administered intravenously if naloxone does not produce a clinical response after 2–3 min. Total dose of naloxone should not go beyond 6–10 mg, and if patient is showing lack of response to this dose, one can exclude opioid overdose.[12] Continuous infusion of naloxone starting at 2/3rds of the dose required to reinstate effective ventilation per hour can be used for longer-acting opioids.

Table 62.6 Antidotes

Toxin	Antidote/intervention
Benzodiazepine	Flumazenil
Opioid	Naloxone
Organophosphates/carbamates/sarin	Atropine and pralidoxime
Tri-cyclic antidepressant	Sodium bicarbonate and alpha-agonist
Carbon monoxide	100% oxygen and hyperbaric oxygen
Cyanide	Nitrites, thiosulfate, and hydroxocobalamin
Coumarin derivatives	Vitamin K1, FFP, and prothrombin complex
Antiplatelets	Platelet transfusion
β-Blockers	Glucagon, calcium, and insulin
Calcium channel blocker	Calcium, glucagon, and insulin

Table 62.7 CarboxyHb levels and clinical manifestations

CarboxyHb levels (%)	Symptoms
1–2	No symptoms can be found in normal persons
5–10	Slight loss of concentration Normal levels in smokers without any symptoms
10–20	'Flu-like' symptoms
30–40	Fatigue, severe headache, angina, and myocardial infarction even in young and otherwise healthy persons
40–50	Confusion and loss of consciousness
60–70	Coma, seizures, and cardiovascular collapse, leading to death
>70	Usually rapidly fatal

Carbon Monoxide Poisoning

CO has very high haemoglobin binding affinity relative to oxygen. COHb interferes with offloading of oxygen in tissues by shifting the oxyhaemoglobin dissociation curve to the left. It decreases blood oxygen-carrying capacity and oxyhaemoglobin saturation, thus leaving the patient at risk of tissue hypoxaemia, notably the cardiac and cerebral tissues that have high oxygen consumption. The key to the pathogenicity of CO is its propensity to attach itself to the ferrous (Fe^{3+}) in the heme prosthetic group of haemoproteins, which includes haemoglobin, myoglobin, and some intracellular enzymes (cytochromes, P-450).

Clinical symptoms do not always correlate with carboxyHb levels. Patients with CO poisoning can present with vague symptoms, which may not initially be attributed to CO poisoning and may mimic other illnesses (Table 62.7).

Diagnosis is based on history, clinical features, and potential for group poisoning. Pulse oximetry is unreliable in detecting COHb because it cannot distinguish carboxyhaemoglobin from oxyhaemoglobin and so will often show falsely normal saturations. ABG with co-oximetry is diagnostic, showing hypoxaemia, elevated carboxy-haemoglobin levels, and metabolic acidosis. Arterial oxygen saturation (SaO_2) will be low as most of the blood gas machines calculate SaO_2 from PaO_2. False SpO_2 levels may be misleading with increase in carboxyHb. Newer devices may overcome these limitations and they can be used to screen for CO poisoning.[13] Patients with suspected CO poisoning can be screened by analysis of venous blood as venous COHb levels accurately predict arterial blood levels.

All patients should be removed from the site of exposure and administered high concentration oxygen irrespective of pulse oximetry. Elective intubation should be performed in the case of fire with smoke inhalation. Breathing 100% oxygen reduces the half-life of COHb from 5 to 6 h on room air to 40–90 min. Although the use of hyperbaric oxygen (HBO) remains controversial, it further reduces the half-life of COHb to 15–30 min. HBO should be considered in patients with life-threatening exposure, those who do not improve with conventional treatment, and patients with co-morbidities, for example, pregnancy and coronary artery disease.

Table 62.8 MetHb levels and clinical manifestations

MetHb levels (%)	Symptoms
3–5	Slight discoloration (e.g., pale, grey, and blue) of the skin
15–20	Cyanosis though patients may be relatively asymptomatic
25–50	Headache, dyspnoea, syncope, weakness, confusion, palpitations, and chest pain
50–70	Abnormal cardiac rhythms, altered mental status, delirium, seizures, coma, and profound acidosis
>70	Usually fatal

Methaemoglobinemia

Poisoning and overdose causing methaemoglobinemia include industrial toxins, that is, organic and inorganic nitrates, dapsone, and industrial/household agents such as aniline dyes,[14] nitrobenzene, naphthalene (moth balls), and nitroethane (nail polish remover). In the ICU setting, methaemoglobinaemia may arise from therapies used in the unit, including nitric oxide (NO) for mechanical ventilation in ARDS, sodium nitroprusside, and local anaesthetic agents such as benzocaine.

In acute methaemoglobinemia, which is usually acquired, a history of exposure to MetHb inducers can be vital in establishing the diagnosis. Occupational history is particularly important as a large proportion of patients with severe methaemoglobinemia have access to offending substances at the workplace, for example, aniline dyes.[14]

Patients usually present with shortness of breath and cyanosis typically non-responsive to oxygen. Symptoms are proportional to the methaemoglobin level and include skin colour changes, blood colour changes (chocolate coloured venous blood),[14] and neurologic and cardiac symptoms. Levels higher than 70% are usually fatal (Table 62.8).

ABG with co-oximetry is usually diagnostic. Pulse oximetry is not reliable as it typically plateaus in mid-80% (80%–85%) saturation. However, newer-generation pulse oximeters may correlate with co-oximetry.[15]

Initial care includes administration of high concentration oxygen and removal of offending substance. Investigations should be undertaken to rule out cardiac, pulmonary, and other causes of cyanosis. After acute exposure to an oxidizing agent, it is advisable to treat patients with methaemoglobin levels of 20% or higher. This threshold should be reduced to 10% if there is significant co-morbidity especially in the presence of end-organ dysfunction.

Methylene blue is the primary emergency treatment for symptomatic methaemoglobinemia (Figure 62.2). It is available as a 1% solution (10 mg/mL) and should be given in dose of 1–2 mg/kg (up to a maximum of 50 mg in adults) and diluted in saline over 3–5 min. Methylene blue may be repeated at a dose of 1 mg/kg every 30–60 min to control symptoms with close monitoring of methaemoglobin levels. Dosage more than 7.5 mg/kg can, itself, cause methaemoglobinemia in susceptible patients.

HBO and exchange transfusion may be an option for patients where methylene blue is contraindicated, for instance in glucose-6-phosphate dehydrogenase deficiency where it may cause haemolysis or when methylene blue is ineffective.

Cyanide (CN-) Poisoning

CN– belongs to the group of chemical asphyxiants, which inhibits aerobic metabolism and oxygen utilization leading to tissue hypoxaemia. It reversibly binds to cytochrome oxidase and inhibits the last step of mitochondrial oxidative phosphorylation. It is found in a variety of synthetic and natural substances in gases and liquid and solid forms, for example, plastics, glue removers, wool, silks, nylons, and various seeds and plants. Poisoning with cyanide may include accidental, homicidal, and industrial exposure.

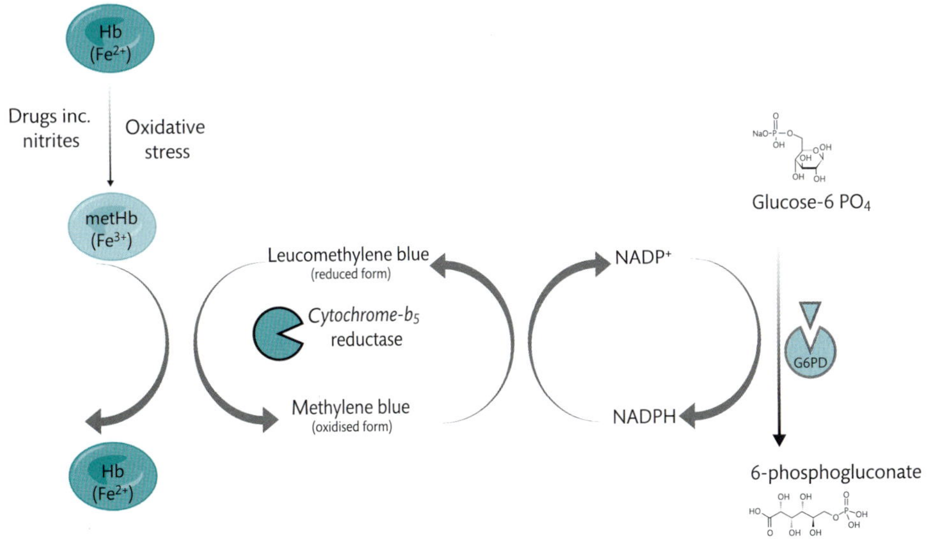

Figure 62.2 Mechanism of action of methylene blue in treating methaemoglobinaemia. Methylene blue acts as electron exchange shuttle, allowing reduced nicotinamide adenine dinucleotide phosphate (NADPH) to exchange electrons with methaemoglobin (MetHb, Fe^{3+}) to reform ferrous (Fe^{2+}) haemoglobin (Hb). NADPH is generated by glucose-6-phosphate dehydrogenase (G6DP), deficiency of which increases risk of methaemoglobinaemia. Under physiological conditions, cytochrome-b5 reductase reduces MetHb to Hb.
Diagram by A Conway Morris created with BioRender.com.

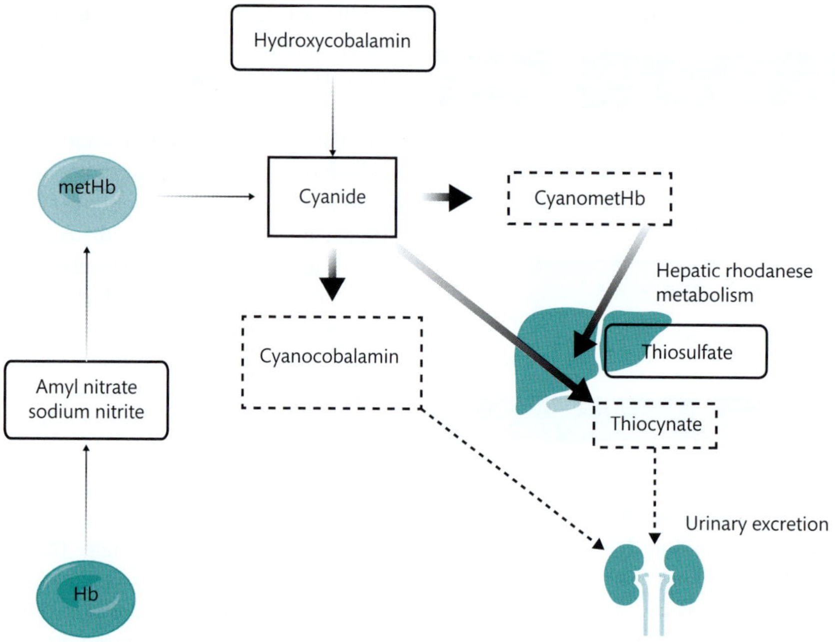

Figure 62.3 Treatment of cyanide poisoning. Nitrates convert haemoglobin (Hb) into methaemoglobin (MetHb) that binds to cyanide, removing it from cytochrome oxidase and preventing cellular hypoxia. Thiosulfate donates sulphur ions to allow rhodanase conversion of cyanide to thiocyanate that is excreted renally. Hydroxocobalamin (vitamin B12) is converted to cyanocobalamin that is harmless and can be excreted renally. Hashed boxes indicate metabolites of cyanide and rounded boxes indicate therapeutics.
Diagram by A Conway Morris created with BioRender.com.

Rapid onset of coma, seizures, and cardiopulmonary dysfunction are highly suggestive of CN– poisoning. Cyanosis is uncommon.

The diagnosis of cyanide poisoning is classically made on history of exposure, clinical suspicion, often in the setting of smoke inhalation injury, where combined carbon monoxide and cyanide toxicity occurs. ABG and venous blood gas analysis is characterized by normal PaO_2, very high venous SaO_2, decreased arteriovenous oxygen difference (<10%), high anion gap metabolic acidosis, and hyperlactatemia.[16] ECG is non-specific and may shows sinus bradycardia or tachycardia, AV block, ST-T changes, and tachyarrhythmias.

Treatment of CN– poisoning begins with identification and treatment of life-threatening problems. Survival depends on prompt and successful CPR. Treatment includes high concentration of oxygen,[16] supportive care, and specific antidotes, that is, amyl nitrite, sodium nitrite, and sodium thiosulfate (Figure 62.3). 100% oxygen enhances effects of nitrites and thiosulfate. Amyl nitrite is used 0.3 mL as inhalation by crushing the ampoule contents poured onto gauze and placed in front of patient's mouth or endotracheal tube, if patient intubated, to inhale over 15–30 s repeated until IV sodium nitrite is available. IV sodium nitrite is used at a dose of 300 mg or 10 mg/kg over 2–5 min. Sodium thiosulfate is used at 12.5 g intravenously over 10 min. It acts synergistically to accelerate the detoxification of CN– to thiocyanate. Hydroxocobalamin is used at a dose of 70 mg/kg (usually 5 g) infusion over 15 min.

Summary

Poisoning can lead to respiratory failure via a number of mechanisms. Beyond supportive care, the key to management is the identification of the toxin and administration of appropriate antidotes and decontamination treatments. Where available, local and national poison information services can greatly assist the management of these conditions.

REFERENCES

1. Singh O, Javeri Y, Juneja D, et al. Profile and outcome of patients with acute toxicity admitted in intensive care unit: Experiences from a major corporate hospital in urban India. *Indian J Anaesth.* 2011;**55**:370–374.
2. Kulling P, Persson H, Singh O, Nasa P, Junega D. Role of the intensive care unit in the management of the poisoned patient. *Med Toxicol.* 1986;**1**:375–386.
3. Mathru M, McDaniel LB. *Primum non nocere.* Is the therapy worse than the disease? *Chest.* 1994;**105**:1634–1636.
4. Singh O, Nasa P, Juneja D. General poisoning management. In: Chawla R, Todi S, eds. *ICU Protocols, A Stepwise Approach.* 2nd ed. Springer: Berlin, 2020;151–158.
5. Kellerman AL, Fihn SD, LoGerfo JP, et al. Impact of drug screening in suspected overdose. *Ann Emerg Med.* 1987;**16**:1206.
6. O'Connell T, Kaye L, Plosay JJ. 3d Gamma-hydroxybutyrate (GHB): A newer drug of abuse. *Am Fam Phys.* 2000;**62**:2478–2483.
7. Vale JA. American Academy of Clinical Toxicology, European Association of Poison Control Centres and Clinical Toxicologists. Position Statement: Gastric lavage. *J Toxicol Clin Toxicol.* 1997;**35**:711.
8. Chyka PA, Seger D. Position Statement: Single-dose activated charcoal. American Academy of Clinical Toxicology, European Association of Poisons Centres and Clinical Toxicologists. *J Toxicol Clin Toxicol.* 1997;**35**:721.

9. Nasa P, Singh A, Juneja D, et al. Continuous venovenous hemodiafiltration along with charcoal hemoperfusion for the management of life-threatening lercanidipine and amlodipine overdose. *Saudi J Kidney Dis Transpla.* 2014;**25**:1255–1258.
10. Longmire AW, Seger DL. Topics in clinical pharmacology: Flumazenil, a benzodiazepine antagonist. *Am J Med Sci.* 1993;**306**:49.
11. Handal KA, Schauben JL, Salamone FR. Naloxone. *Ann Emerg Med.* 1983;**12**:438.
12. Albertson TE, Dawson A, de Latorre F, et al. Tox-ACLS: Toxicologic oriented advanced cardiac life support. *Ann Emerg Med.* 2001;**37**:S78.
13. Chee KJ, Nilson D, Partridge R, et al. Finding needles in a haystack: A case series of carbon monoxide poisoning detected using new technology in the emergency department. *Clin Toxicol.* 2008;**46**:461–469.
14. Donnelly GB, Randlett MS. Methemoglobinemia. *N Engl J Med.* 2000;**343**:337.
15. Feiner JR, Bickler PE. Improved accuracy of methemoglobin detection by pulse CO-oximetry during hypoxia. *Anesth Analg.* 2010;**111**:1160–1167.
16. Taitelman U. Acute cyanide poisoning. In: Hall JB, Schmidt GA, Wood LDH, eds. *Principles of Critical Care.* McGraw-Hill: New York; 1992: p.2125.

63

Lung Transplantation

Thomas Bein and Michael Pfeifer

KEY MESSAGES

- Lung transplantation (LT) is a promising and effective option in selected end-stage lung diseases (chronic obstructive pulmonary disease, septic or fibrotic lung disease, and pulmonary arterial hypertension).
- Intraoperative as well as post-transplant intensive care management is characterized by specific, expert-driven support (mechanical ventilation and haemodynamic and pharmacologic management) to avoid or reduce typical complications in the early period (infection, rejection, ischaemia-reperfusion injury, and early graft dysfunction).
- The survival rate following LT is ≈50% after 5 years. Successful long-term outcome is strongly associated with a balanced immunosuppression, a careful infection prophylaxis, and the avoidance of chronic allograft dysfunction. Pathophysiology of chronic allograft dysfunction is not well understood but is an important cause of poor late outcomes.

CONTROVERSIES

- The allocation and acceptance of organs and the evaluation of transplant candidates in times of organ shortage.
- Intraoperative and/or early post-transplant measures (lung-protective ventilation, positive end-expiratory pressure, strict or liberal transfusion strategy, and anti-inflammatory pharmacologic intervention) to reduce the incidence of early or chronic graft dysfunction.
- The role of extracorporeal lung support systems as bridge to transplant to improve outcome.
- LT following COVID ARDS has been published in small case series internationally. However, it is rare, most frequently declined, subject to highly specific criteria and currently not considered a conventional indication.

FURTHER RESEARCH

- Extracorporeal membrane oxygenation as alternative to mechanical ventilation for bridging patients to transplantation—prospective randomized studies. Pathophysiologic bases of early and chronic graft dysfunction—experimental animal studies. Ex vivo perfusion in human donor lungs—feasibility and outcome studies.

Indications and Evaluation of Lung Transplant Candidates

Lung transplantation (LT) has been established as a standard of care to treat end-stage pulmonary diseases although an increasing number of patients with chronic lung disorders stay in contrast to worldwide organ shortage which may hinder the more extended use of such a promising measure. Recent advances in operative techniques as well as significant improvements in the immunosuppressive management have led to better survival rates, but the careful evaluation of candidates is of particular importance for the success of LT.

The following broad indication groups for LT were selected by the International Society for Heart and Lung Transplantation (ISHLT[1]):

- Obstructive lung disease, especially chronic obstructive pulmonary disease (COPD).
- Septic lung disease, for example, cystic fibrosis.
- Fibrotic lung disease (interstitial pulmonary fibrosis).
- Vascular lung disease (pulmonary arterial hypertension).

Further selection criteria include limited life expectancy, limitations in daily life activity, adequate cardiac function and general comorbidity, nutritional status, potential for rehabilitation, appropriate age, an effective social support system, and adherence to medical therapy. A careful evaluation in each individual patient is necessary to estimate potential contraindications (previous malignancy, psychiatric disorders, lack of family support or other social networks, and active chronic infections). As infective lung diseases are part of indications for LT, they create a special challenge in these patients in terms of careful identification and eradication of common or uncommon pathogens (mycobacteria or multi-resistant bacteria, aspergillus, and chronic viral infections). In LT candidates presenting with a 'septic lung', bilateral transplantation is the only option, since leaving a septic part after LT is not advisable.

Similarly, the evaluation and allocation of donor lungs is part of a careful concept including the use of a 'lung allocation score' (USA), which has been adopted in several other countries.[2] The evaluation of an offered donor lung includes chest X-ray, organ size matching, bronchoscopy, and some clinical functional assessments (gas exchange capacity and compliance of the respiratory system). The technique of ex vivo lung perfusion aimed at evaluation of lung quality from donation after circulatory death is currently discussed.[3] In various experimental animal studies and some human observational investigations, ex vivo lung perfusion has proved its value as an efficient tool to increase donor utilization. For the definite assessment of safety aspects and effects on transplant outcome, further large studies are required.

The Role of Extracorporeal Lung Support in LT Candidates

Critically ill patients with decompensated respiratory function and thus needing LT were traditionally provided with orotracheal intubation and mechanical ventilation. In a propensity analysis of a large data cohort,[4] it was found that patients on mechanical ventilation awaiting LT had a lower 12-month post-transplant survival rate (62%) compared to patients who received no ventilation support prior to LT (79%). The rapid development in extracorporeal lung support (ECLS) systems in recent years regarding the technical improvement, the reduction in complication rates, and the general ease of use has led to an increasing interest in the application of ECLS as a 'bridge to transplant' in critically ill candidates. Fuehner et al.[5] reported on the use of extracorporeal membrane oxygenation (ECMO) in patients awaiting LT who were awake and spontaneously breathing ('awake ECMO concept') as an alternative to mechanical ventilation due to terminal respiratory or cardiopulmonary failure. In a retrospective, single-centre, intention-to-treat analysis, the investigators could demonstrate a survival 6 months after LT that was better in the awake ECMO group (80%) compared with a historical control group of patients (50%) treated with conventional mechanical ventilation. In a recent systematic review regarding the current evidence how ECLS influences a patient's outcome after LT,[6] 14 retrospective studies including 441 patients were used for a final analysis. The results from prospective randomized studies were not available, and there was a paucity of high-quality data and a significant heterogeneity among studies since, in most of the studies, patients awaiting LT received ECMO *and* mechanical ventilation. In conclusion, the hypothesis remains unproven that the use of ECLS as an alternative to mechanical ventilation will improve outcome. However, ECLS might present a therapeutic option for individual patients after careful evaluation by an inter-disciplinary, experienced team weighing benefit versus harm.

Surgical Approach and Perioperative Management

Surgical Approach

Based on pre-transplant evaluation, the appropriate surgical approach maybe single-lung, bilateral-lung, bilateral lobar, or heart–lung transplantation.[7] For example, bilateral orthotopic lung transplantation (BOLT) is the preferred strategy in cystic fibrosis or severe pulmonary hypertension and in patients presenting with lower perioperative risk, while single-lung transplantation (SOLT) is favoured in higher risk patients (increased age, comorbidities, and frailty). A bilateral anterolateral thoracotomy (4th intercostal space) in conjunction with sternotomy is routinely performed for BOLT, while in SOLT patients receive a one-sided anterolateral incision on the same anatomical level. In larger allograft size discrepancies between donor and recipient, a donor lung can be downsized anatomically (implantation of a lower or upper lobe). In recent data analysis,[8] it was seen that BOLT is associated with prolonged survival compared to SOLT. The quality of the airway anastomoses is of crucial importance for the prevention of postoperative complications and for the healing process. The evolution of microsurgery techniques and improved suture material and techniques has helped to reduce airway complications (necrosis, dehiscence, stenosis, and malacia). In situations of complex vascular abnormalities, specific surgical measures like a simultaneously performed allograft of the right ventricular outflow tract might be necessary. The intraoperative use of extracorporeal lung circulation support is addressed below.

Intraoperative and Anaesthetic Management

The main goals of intraoperative anaesthetic management are the stabilization of the cardiopulmonary system, the prevention of allograft-related complications, and the prevention of alterations of other organ systems.[9] A strategy of a strict intraoperative lung protection is included in a 'bundle' of anaesthetic procedures (Table 63.1). Mechanical ventilation should follow a low-tidal-volume strategy, combined with a relatively high respiratory frequency and moderate positive end-expiratory pressure (PEEP). Transoesophageal echo examinations allow continuous assessment of (right) ventricular function and early detection of cardiac dysfunction or haemodynamic collapse. Acute pulmonary artery hypertension can be counteracted by pulmonary vasodilators like milrinone or inhaled nitric oxide. A special management is required for the period of single-lung ventilation, which might be characterized by an increase in intrapulmonary shunt, hypoxaemia, and haemodynamic instability.

In situations of continuous instability—despite maximal vasoactive and mechanical ventilation support—initiation of cardiopulmonary bypass (CPB) or ECMO must be considered. ECMO is of increasing interest in the scenario of LT. The pre-transplant indication for ECMO is a bridging to transplantation.[5] The a priori intraoperative use of ECMO in critical cardiopulmonary constellations has replaced CPB in many centres. A retrospective comparison of outcome parameters between lung transplant recipients who were bridged with extracorporeal life support and those who underwent CPB[10] has shown significant advances for the ECMO group in terms of early outcome parameters (duration of mechanical ventilation, length of stay at the ICU, and blood product transfusion requirement), but mortality was not different between ECMO and CPB groups. The indications for the *intraoperative* implementation of ECMO are the following[11]:

- *Start of surgical approach*: Respiratory/haemodynamic instability despite nitric oxide inhalation or other pharmacologic strategies to control pulmonary artery hypertension.
- *Lung transplantation*: Inability to tolerate pulmonary artery clamping or single-lung ventilation.
- *Ventilation/reperfusion of the newly implanted graft*: New or continuing haemodynamic instability or severe impairment of pulmonary gas exchange.

Table 63.1 A 'bundle' of intraoperative anaesthetic procedures during lung transplantation

Aim	Measure	Comment
Lung protection	Low-tidal-volume ventilation	Allow permissive hypercapnia but avoid decompensated acidosis
Continuous assessment of ventricular function and pulmonary artery pressures	• Placement of a transoesophageal echo probe • Pulmonary artery catheterization	• Early detection and correction of massive pulmonary hypertension and/or ventricular failure • In severe cardiac dysfunction: consider cardiopulmonary bypass or ECMO
Cardiovascular stabilization	• Continuous arterial blood pressure • Frequent arterial blood gases	A balance of inotropic and vasoactive agents
Avoid primary graft dysfunction	• Low-tidal-volume ventilation • Moderate positive end-expiratory pressure	Consider intraoperative inhalation of nitric oxide
Avoid ischaemia-reperfusion injury	• Balanced volume replacement • Avoid hypervolemia	Avoid intraoperative colloid administration

Source: Adapted from Castillo M. Anesthetic management for lung transplantation. *Curr Opin Anesthesiol*. 2011;24:32–36. Copyright 2011, Wolters Kluwer.

The decision whether to use veno-venous ECMO or veno-arterial ECMO depends on the severity of respiratory and/or cardiovascular impairment. Most reports on the intraoperative use of ECMO refer to (retrospective) cohort analyses, and prospective randomized data on benefit/harm aspects among ECMO use during LT is not available. Furthermore, the specific use and management of ECMO or CPB is predominantly associated with a 'centre philosophy' and less with evidence-based medicine. For the use of ECMO circuit, often percutaneous cannulation of two large vessels ('dual' cannulation: veno-venous or veno-arterial) is preferred, while experienced centres may apply specific strategies by cannulation of three large vessels ('triple' cannulation: veno-veno-arterial or veno-arterial-venous) for complex situations.[12] A bicaval dual-lumen cannula requires only one large access and allows for parallel input and output (bi-caval catheter is illustrated in Figure 63.1). In the post-transplant period, such a cannula system might facilitate the patient's mobilization or ambulation.

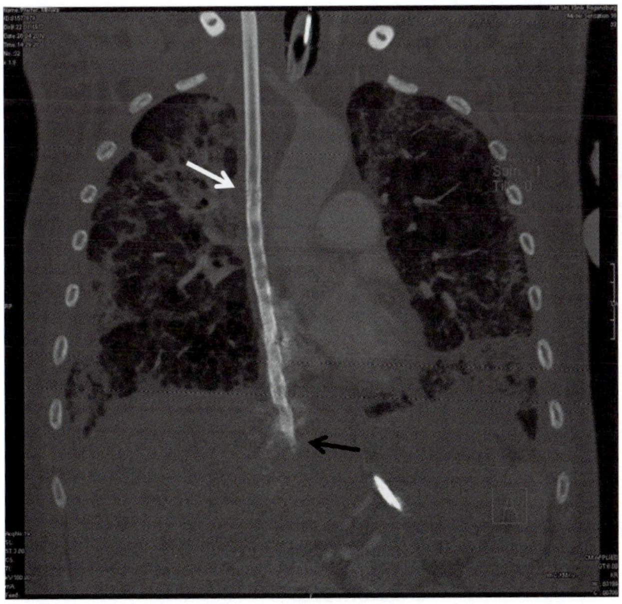

Figure 63.1 Chest imaging of a patient suffering from severe post-transplant pneumonia. A bicaval dual lumen cannula was placed for extracorporeal lung support. The arrows indicate blood suctioning (black arrow) and re-infusion (white arrow).

Early Postoperative Period

The successful management of the early post-transplant period is critical in determining the outcome for the recipient. The initiation of immunosuppression, a strategy of balanced volume replacement, monitoring of wounds and drains, early liberation from mechanical ventilation combined with mobilization and physiotherapy, and infection prevention or treatment are the responsibility of experienced intensive care physicians in the context of daily inter-disciplinary rounds.[13] A key issue for the early postoperative days is the identification and prompt management of acute allograft injury following transplantation (Table 63.2). The main causes are fluid overload/cardiac dysfunction, acute infection, (hyper-)acute rejection, ischaemia-reperfusion injury or primary graft dysfunction, or airway anastomose associated complications.[14] An algorithm for a differential diagnosis of early allograft failure is given in Figure 63.2. Blood gases, lab values, and imaging techniques are the first steps to identify the severity of graft failure. Further advanced measures (echo/pulmonary artery catheter, bronchoscopic examination, and alveolar lavage) allow for differentiation and specific therapy of the respiratory failure.

Immunosuppression

The immunosuppression regimen in lung transplant recipients is characterized by a fragile balance between rejection and infection.[15] During transplantation, a high load of immunosuppressive agents is necessary to be followed by a steady-state strategy with a certain tapering over time, but lifelong pharmacologic immunosuppression is required. The currently employed classes of immunosuppressive drugs are as follows[15]:

- Polyclonal anti-lymphocyte antibody preparations (e.g., thymoglobulin) → 'traditional' part of induction therapy.
- Monoclonal anti-lymphocyte antibody preparation (e.g. OKT3) → rarely used for induction.
- Anti-cytokine receptor antibodies (e.g. basiliximab) → most commonly used for induction.

Table 63.2 Important causes of acute allograft injury after lung transplantation

Pathophysiology	Diagnosis	Therapy	Comment
Fluid overload/cardiac dysfunction	• Chest X-ray: infiltrations • Echo: ventricular function ↓ • Pulmonary artery pressure ↑	• Negative fluid balance • Inotropes/levosimendan • Inhaled nitric oxide	In refractory cases: consider ECMO
Acute infection	• Chest X-ray: lobar or diffuse consolidation, cavitation, and nodules • Laboratory: inflammation parameters • Bronchoalveolar lavage	• Targeted antibiotic, antiviral, and/or antifungal therapy	Preventive antimicrobial therapy is started intraoperatively
Acute rejection	• Chest X-ray: ground-glass opacities and interlobular septal thickening • Blood gas: hypoxaemia • Transbronchial biopsy/ bronchoscopy: lymphocytic bronchiolitis • Monitor anti-HLA-antibodies	• Steroid pulses (methylprednisolone 500 mg) • In severe cases: consider antithymocyte antibodies	Antibody mediated rejection: specific protocol!
Ischaemia-reperfusion injury	• Chest X-ray: perihilar haze and peribronchiolar thickening	• Lung-protective ventilation • In refractory cases: consider ECMO	*Prevention*: • Perioperative protective ventilation • Fibrinolysis • Surfactant • Ex vivo perfusion
Primary graft dysfunction	• Blood gas: hypoxaemia • Ventilator: lung compliance ↓ • Chest X-ray: infiltration and oedema • Pulmonary artery pressure ↑ • Chest CT: diffuse pulmonary oedema	• Lung-protective ventilation • Nitric oxide inhalation	• 'diagnosis of exclusion' • In refractory cases: consider ECMO
Complications associated with airway anastomoses: necrosis, dehiscence, stenosis, and malacia	• Chest X-ray: regional infiltration • Bronchoscopy: visible damage of anastomosis • Chest CT scan with multiplanar reconstructions: identification and amount of the leakage	• Endoscopic application of stents or fibrin glue • Surgical revision	Early detection and prompt correction of airway complications improve the outcome!

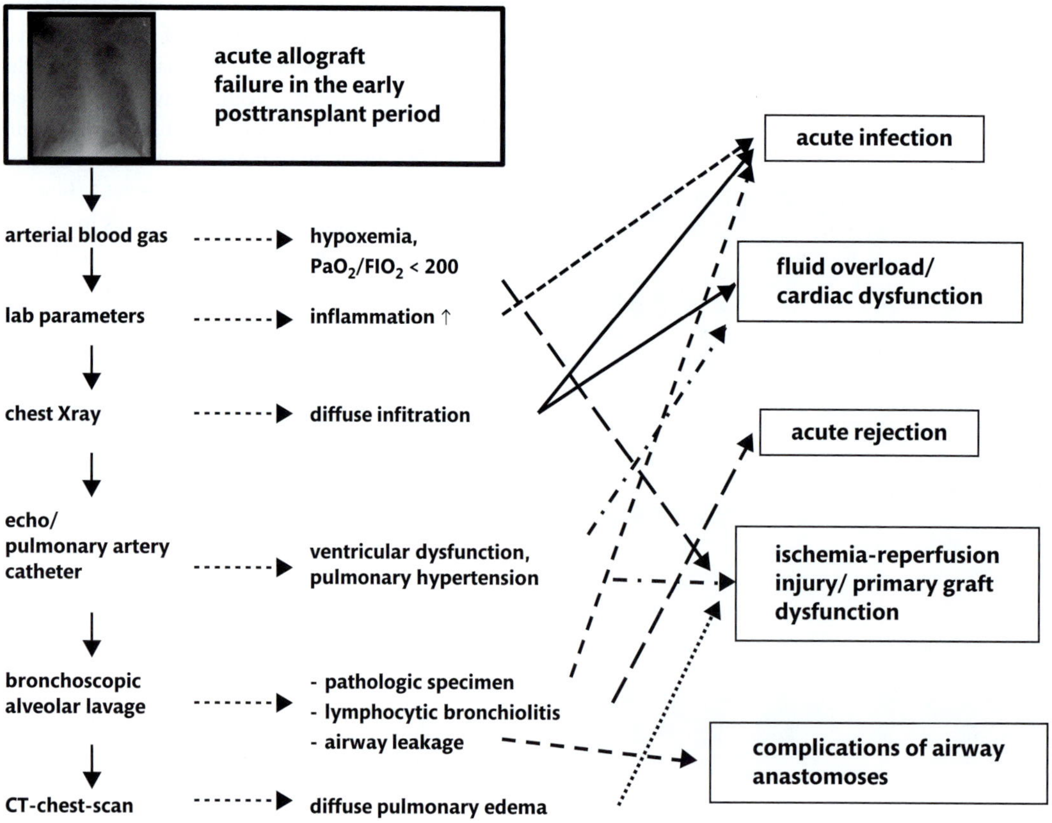

Figure 63.2 An algorithm for a differential diagnosis of early allograft failure.

- Calcineurin inhibitors (e.g. cyclosporine A, tacrolimus) → commonly used for steady state in a combination with other agents.
- Corticosteroids (e.g. methylprednisolone) → important drug for induction, maintenance, and rejection therapy.
- Antimetabolites (e.g. mycophenolic acid) → for long-term use together with calcineurin inhibitors.
- mTOR inhibitors (e.g. sirolimus) → increasingly used after LT but severe side effects possible.

Induction of immunosuppression is predominantly performed by intravenous antibody therapy targeting activated host lymphocytes. The steady-state maintenance immunosuppression is based in most centres on a triple regimen: a calcineurin inhibitor composed with an anti-metabolite agent and corticosteroids. The specific choice of these compounds may differ from centre to centre. For long-term anti-rejection therapy, low-dose corticosteroids often are combined with a calcineurin inhibitor or an anti-metabolite. For acute rejection episodes, intravenous steroid pulses (e.g. methylprednisolone 500 mg/d for 3 days) are recommended, while in chronic rejection no evidence-based recommendation is given, and the use of mTOR inhibitors was found to be effective by some observational studies. Multicentre prospective randomized trials are urgently needed to compare and assess combinations of immunosuppressant drugs in lung transplant recipients, and further insights into lung transplant immunobiology and an improved immune monitoring might help to find a 'tailored' (antibody) therapy regimen for the individual patient.[16]

Post-transplant and Long-term Management

Infections—Evaluation, Prophylaxis, and Therapy

Infectious complications are main causes of death after LT, during the early as well as the late post-transplant period. Large epidemiologic data on infections are rare; in a retrospective analysis of 51 lung transplant recipients,[17] the main sources of infections were pulmonary (60%), the aetiology was predominantly bacterial in 48%, viruses (especially *cytomegalovirus*) in 35%, and fungal infections (predominantly *Aspergillus*) in 13%. The infection-related mortality in this cohort was 6%. Infections are not only contributors to mortality, but they might have a significant influence on chronic allograft dysfunction.[18] In the management of lung transplant recipients, prophylaxis strategies play an important role in the early post-transplant period, and they have to be guided by careful infection monitoring and control (sputum and blood cultures, endotracheal suctioning, and urine probes). The post-transplant prophylaxis includes antimicrobial, antiviral (cytomegalovirus: dependent on serostatus), and antifungal agents. The specific strategy of infection prophylaxis is often modified in experienced centres with a high number of transplantations, and some topics, for example, the application of antifungal prophylaxis is a matter of controversial debate.[19] The antimicrobial therapy of manifest infections depends on the identification and source of a pathologic specimen, and it is guided by a benefit/harm consideration of the choice of the drug, the dose, the application mode, and a possible combination therapy. A recent analysis from South Korea[20] found that multidrug-resistant bacterial infections increase mortality in the early period. Respiratory virus infections mostly developed 6 months after transplantation.

Long-term Immunosuppression

The pulmonary parenchyma is characterized by a marked immunogenicity requiring for high immunosuppression, especially in the immediate post-transplant period. After induction of immunosuppression, a tapered-down triple regimen will be maintained lifelong.[15] The triple regimen is composed of a calcineurin inhibitor (cyclosporine A or tacrolimus), an anti-metabolite agent (e.g. mycophenolate mofetil), and steroids (e.g., prednisolone). Currently, novel classes of immunosuppressive agents (mTOR inhibitors) are being evaluated in prospective studies.

Chronic Allograft Dysfunction

The survival rate following LT is ≈50% after 5 years,[8] and chronic lung allograft dysfunction contributes markedly to the limitations of long-term success. The term *chronic allograft dysfunction* is a unifying term for various and heterogeneous conditions that may—in part—influence each other and which are not fully understood yet.[21] The probability of developing this syndrome by 5 years was reported to be around 50%. The bronchiolitis obliterans syndrome (BOS) was seen as the main manifestation of chronic allograft dysfunction, and late infections or chronic rejection were easily associated with these entities. Traditionally *chronic allograft dysfunction* includes the following:

- Bronchiolitis obliterans syndrome
- Restrictive allograft syndrome
- Chronic rejection
- Diffuse alveolar damage
- Late infections

Meanwhile, the immune mechanisms involved in chronic allograft rejection are partly identified[21] by detecting innate or adaptive immune reactions induced by the environment or by the graft itself. Perspectives of therapeutic interventions among the syndrome of chronic allograft dysfunction are limited since it remains irreversible and unpredictable so far.

Long-term Outcome

Longitudinal multidimensional investigations in survivors after LT regarding health-related quality of life (HrQoL) or physical and cognitive functioning are rare. The main categories for the assessment of HrQoL were psychosocial factors (depression and anxiety), physical functioning (daily activities and grade of mobility), or specific items (BOS, dyspnoea, and chronic pain). In a systematic review of 73 studies among HrQoL,[22] it was found in general that HrQoL improves substantially within the first year after LT, but longer-period results are scarce. In the analyzed studies, it was consistently observed that the following items were associated with a significant poorer HrQoL:

- Presence of bronchiolitis obliterans syndrome
- Adverse effects of immunosuppression
- Dyspnoea
- Chronic pain
- Perceived risk of graft rejection and burden on relationships

In pre- and post-transplant comparisons of HrQoL, it was found that LT is associated with a sustained increase in quality of life,[23] especially in physical health and functioning. The impact of a specific early post-transplant programme including physical rehabilitation, early self-care behavioural interventions,[24] psychosocial stabilization and integration, a frequent visit and support by healthcare workers, or other targeted interventions have to be investigated systematically in the coming years.

REFERENCES

1. Christie JD, Edwards LB, Kucheryavaya AY, et al. International Society of Heart and Lung Transplantation. The Registry of the International Society for Heart and Lung Transplantation: 29th adult lung and heart–lung transplant report-2012. *J Heart Lung Transplant*. 2012;**31**:1073–1086.
2. Egan TM. The lung allocation score goes global. *Am J Transplant*. 2014;**14**:1234–1235.
3. Sanchez PG, Mackowick KM, Kon ZN. Current state of ex-vivo lung perfusion. *Curr Opin Organ Transplant*. 2016;**21**:258–266.
4. Mason DP, Thuita L, Nowicki ER, et al. Should lung transplantation be performed for patients on mechanical respiratory support? The US experience. *J Thorac Cardiovasc Surg*. 2010;**139**:765–773.
5. Fuehner T, Kuehn C, Hadem J, et al. Extracorporeal membrane oxygenation in awake patients as bridge to lung transplantation. *Am J Respir Crit Care Med*. 2012;**185**:763–768.
6. Chiumello D, Coppola S, Froio S, et al. Extracorporeal life support as bridge to lung transplantation: A systematic review. *Crit Care*. 2015;**19**:19.
7. Gray AL, Mulvihill MS, Hartwig MG. Lung transplantation at Duke. *J Thorac Dis*. 2016;**8**:E185–196.
8. Yeung JC, Keshavjee S. Overview of clinical lung transplantation. *Cold Spring Harb Perspect Med*. 2014;**4**:a015628.
9. Castillo M. Anesthetic management for lung transplantation. *Curr Opin Anaesthesiol*. 2011;**24**:32–36.
10. Machuca TN, Collaud S, Mercier O, et al. Outcomes of intraoperative extracorporeal membrane oxygenation versus cardiopulmonary bypass for lung transplantation. *J Thorac Cardiovasc Surg*. 2015;**149**:1152–1157.
11. Ius F, Sommer W, Tudorache I, et al. Five-year experience with intraoperative extracorporeal membrane oxygenation in lung transplantation: Indications and midterm results. *J Heart Lung Transplant*. 2016;**35**:49–58.
12. Napp LC, Kühn C, Hoeper MM, et al. Cannulation strategies for percutaneous extracorporeal membrane oxygenation in adults. *Clin Res Cardiol*. 2016;**105**:283–296.
13. Schuurmans MM, Benden C, Inci I. Practical approach to early postoperative management of lung transplant recipients. *Swiss Med Wkly*. 2013;**143**:w13773.
14. Anile M, Diso D, Rendina EA, et al. Airway anastomosis for lung transplantation. *J Thorac Dis*. 2016;**8**(Suppl 2):S197–203.
15. Korom S, Boehler A, Weder W. Immunosuppressive therapy in lung transplantation: State of the art. *Eur J Cardiothorac Surg*. 2009;**35**:1045–1055.
16. Afshar K. Future direction of immunosuppression in lung transplantation. *Curr Opin Organ Transplant*. 2014;**19**:583–590.
17. Parada MT, Alba A, Sepúlveda C. Early and late infections in lung transplantation patients. *Transplant Proc*. 2010;**42**: 333–335.
18. Martin-Gandul C, Mueller NJ, Pascual M, et al. The impact of infection on chronic allograft dysfunction and allograft survival after solid organ transplantation. *Am J Transplant*. 2015;**15**:3024–3040.
19. Patel TS, Eschenauer GA, Stuckey LJ, et al. Antifungal prophylaxis in lung transplant recipients. *Transplantation*. 2016;**100**:1815–1826.
20. Yun JH, Lee SO, Jo KW, et al. Infections after lung transplantation: Time of occurrence, sites, and microbiologic etiologies. *Korean J Intern Med*. 2015;**30**:506–514.
21. Royer PJ, Olivera-Botello G, Koutsokera A, et al. SysCLAD consortium. Chronic lung allograft dysfunction: A systems review of mechanisms. *Transplantation*. 2016 ;**100**:1803–1814.
22. Singer JP, Chen J, Blanc PD, et al. A thematic analysis of quality of life in lung transplant: The existing evidence and implications for future directions. *Am J Transplant*. 2013;**13**:839–850.
23. Singer JP, Singer LG. Quality of life in lung transplantation. *Semin Respir Crit Care Med*. 2013;**34**:421–430.
24. Osadnik CR, Rodrigues FM, Camillo CA, et al. Principles of rehabilitation and reactivation. *Respiration*. 2015;**89**:2–11.

PART 10

Weaning and Long-term Ventilation

64

Liberation from Mechanical Ventilation

Patrick B Murphy, Andrew Jones, and Luigi Camporota

KEY MESSAGES

- A structured approach to simple weaning utilizing readiness testing, sedation holds, and spontaneous breathing trials is recommended.
- Weaning is not always limited by respiratory system load–capacity-drive, and therefore weaning failure requires a multi-system assessment to identify the barrier to progress.
- Patients undergoing prolonged mechanical ventilation should have a systematic review from a specialist multi-disciplinary team with experience of complex weaning to produce a bespoke weaning plan.
- Specialist weaning centres should be involved in management of complex weaning patients as they are associated with improved clinical outcomes and cost-effective delivery of care.

CONTROVERSIES

- The adoption of weaning predictors to guide weaning strategy and extubation.
- Avoiding intubation or early tracheostomy in patients with neuromuscular disease by the use of dedicated secretion management with mechanical insufflation–exsufflation and non-invasive ventilation (NIV).

FURTHER RESEARCH

- Validation of the role of high-flow humidified oxygen systems and NIV combinations following extubation or decannulation in specific patient cohorts.
- Long-term outcomes of patients weaned following prolonged mechanical ventilation and subsequent healthcare utilization.

Introduction

Endotracheal intubation and invasive mechanical ventilation are associated with significant morbidity with the risks rising with duration of mechanical ventilation.[1,2] The process of weaning and subsequent liberation from mechanical ventilation is therefore a vital step in patient management within critical care. Although the majority of patients undergo simple weaning, the minority who undergo prolonged (>21 days) weaning consume a significant quantity of critical care resources.[3]

Discontinuation of mechanical ventilation is a two-phase process consisting of the evaluation of readiness to wean (through readiness testing) and weaning itself (discontinuation or liberation). Readiness testing is the evaluation of objective criteria to determine whether a patient might be able to successfully and safely be liberated from the ventilator, while weaning may involve either an immediate switch from full ventilatory support to a period of breathing without assistance from the ventilator or a gradual reduction in the amount of ventilator support.[4] It is useful to distinguish weaning, in which the reduction of assistance given to the patient aims to achieve liberation from the ventilator, from titration, which is a process aimed at optimizing the level of support in patients not yet deemed suitable for liberation from mechanical ventilation.

Types of Weaning

Patients can be categorized into three groups in relation to the time taken to achieve liberation from mechanical ventilation[5–8]:

(1) *Simple weaning* (~60% patients): Patients who can be extubated after the first weaning test (spontaneous breathing trial, SBT). The main clinical goal is the identification of readiness to wean through a systematic screening strategy that avoids delays in extubation.
(2) *Difficult weaning* (30%–40% of patients): Patients who require up to three SBTs (or 7 days) to be successfully extubated. The reasons for failed weaning have to be identified and corrected. The pathophysiology of weaning failure should be understood for the optimal management of the patient.
(3) *Complex weaning* (6%–15% of patients): This term applies to patients who exceed the limits of difficult weaning and is often associated with prolonged mechanical ventilation >7 days.

Regardless of the time required to achieve liberation, the accepted extubation failure rate is 10%–20%. A re-intubation rate <5%–10% may indicate a too conservative approach to extubation that may lead to delayed liberation in some patients. On the contrary, a re-intubation rate >20%–30% may indicate premature extubations.

Stages of Weaning

Management of liberation (simple weaning stage) is illustrated in Figure 64.1, and the management of patients with difficult and prolonged weaning is illustrated in Figure 64.2.

Stage 1 (pre-weaning) is a stage when the main aim is the treatment of the underlying condition and weaning or liberation is not considered or desirable. Titration of ventilation is still possible (see above).

Stage 2 (suspicion) is the period of diagnostic triggering, the time when a physician begins to think that their patient might have a reasonable probability of coming off the ventilator.

Stage 3 is the time of measuring and interpreting daily weaning predictors.

Stage 4 is the time of decreasing ventilator support (abruptly through a SBT or gradually via the process of weaning).

Stage 5 is extubation.

Stage 6 is the use of non-invasive ventilation (NIV) and/or high-flow nasal oxygen after extubation.

Stage 7 is re-intubation.

Failure to appreciate stage 2 probably leads to the greatest delay in weaning.[5,6]

Readiness Testing: Clinical Assessment

Readiness testing has the dual purpose of identifying patients who are ready to be liberated from mechanical ventilation and thus avoiding extubation delays but also to identify patients who are unable to be liberated, thereby avoiding the risks of premature extubation. Clinicians have been consistently shown to underestimate patients' ability to breathe without ventilatory support with many patients being extubated on the day of first readiness testing and 50% of self-extubations not requiring re-intubation.[9,10] Furthermore, readiness testing should not be regarded as an absolute prerequisite for weaning as many patients not satisfying these criteria can be successfully weaned.[11] Criteria for readiness testing are provided in Box 64.1.

Patients who fulfil the readiness to wean criteria, if not already receiving pressure support (PS) ventilation, can be started on a trial of PS. The level of PS will be titrated to patient comfort to achieve tidal volumes of 6–8 mL kg^{-1} ideal body weight and a respiratory rate <30 breaths min^{-1}. The patient can also be considered for a spontaneous breathing trial (SBT) that is discussed below.

Readiness Testing: Weaning Predictors

Weaning predictors and indices were developed to identify those patients who have passed readiness testing and have a high chance of successful weaning and low chance of weaning failure. They are based on single or composite scores of respiratory physiological measurements, and a selection of tests is provided in Table 64.1.

Weaning indices should be evaluated before the SBT, which functions as a diagnostic test to determine the probability of successful extubation. Although many weaning predictors exist, few are used routinely within critical care, particularly those which require specialist equipment to obtain. The rapid shallow breathing index (RSBI) is the most commonly performed as it benefits from being simple to measure and has an acceptable performance.[12] The RSBI can be influenced by a number of parameters such as PS, PEEP, or recent clinical intervention, for example, tracheal suctioning, and should therefore be measured without ventilator support, that is, with the ventilator set to a PS and PEEP of 0.[13–15] Weaning predictors have arisen as many clinicians remain concerned regarding moving to weaning phase based on readiness testing alone. However, this fear seems unfounded as those that fail an SBT are not harmed in the process.[16] Rather, evidence suggests that automatic progression to an SBT upon satisfying readiness testing may reduce weaning time in comparison to the addition of a weaning predictor.[17] However, weaning predictors can be particularly useful in situations in which the decision to liberate from mechanical ventilation is problematic and to identify whether respiratory insufficiency is the underlying cause of weaning failure.

Weaning Test: Spontaneous Awakening and Breathing Trials Spontaneous Awakening Trial (SAT)—Daily Interruption of Sedatives

A prerequisite of progression to an SBT is that the patient needs to be awake and aware and daily sedation holds have been shown to support weaning in critical care.[22] An SAT involves establishing a time and a safe opportunity to interrupt or reduce all sedatives and analgesics used for sedation; this excludes analgesics needed for active pain that should continue. This daily sedation hold is the first part of readiness testing with patients safely progressing to an SBT if they meet the objective criteria. If patients fail an SAT, sedatives should be restarted at half the previous dose and then titrated to achieve patient comfort.[6–8,23] An SAT will need to be adapted for each patient by the critical care team based on individual patient requirements with close observation required during testing to detect agitation, distress, and prevent accidental extubation.

Spontaneous Breathing Trial

An SBT refers to a time during which a patient breathes through the endotracheal tube (ETT) either without any or with minimal ventilator support (e.g. a low level of PS, automatic tube compensation

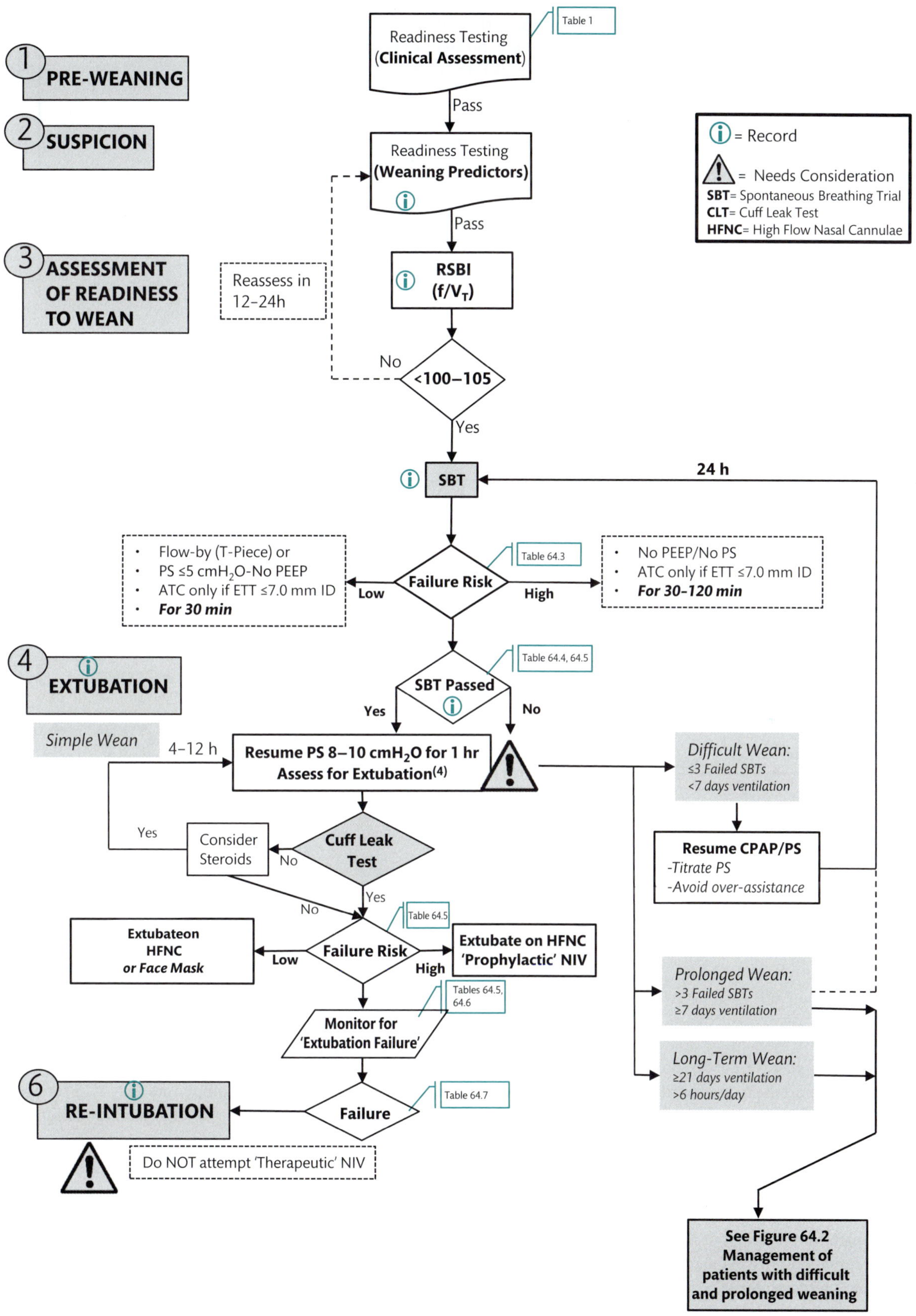

Figure 64.1 Management of liberation (simple weaning stage).

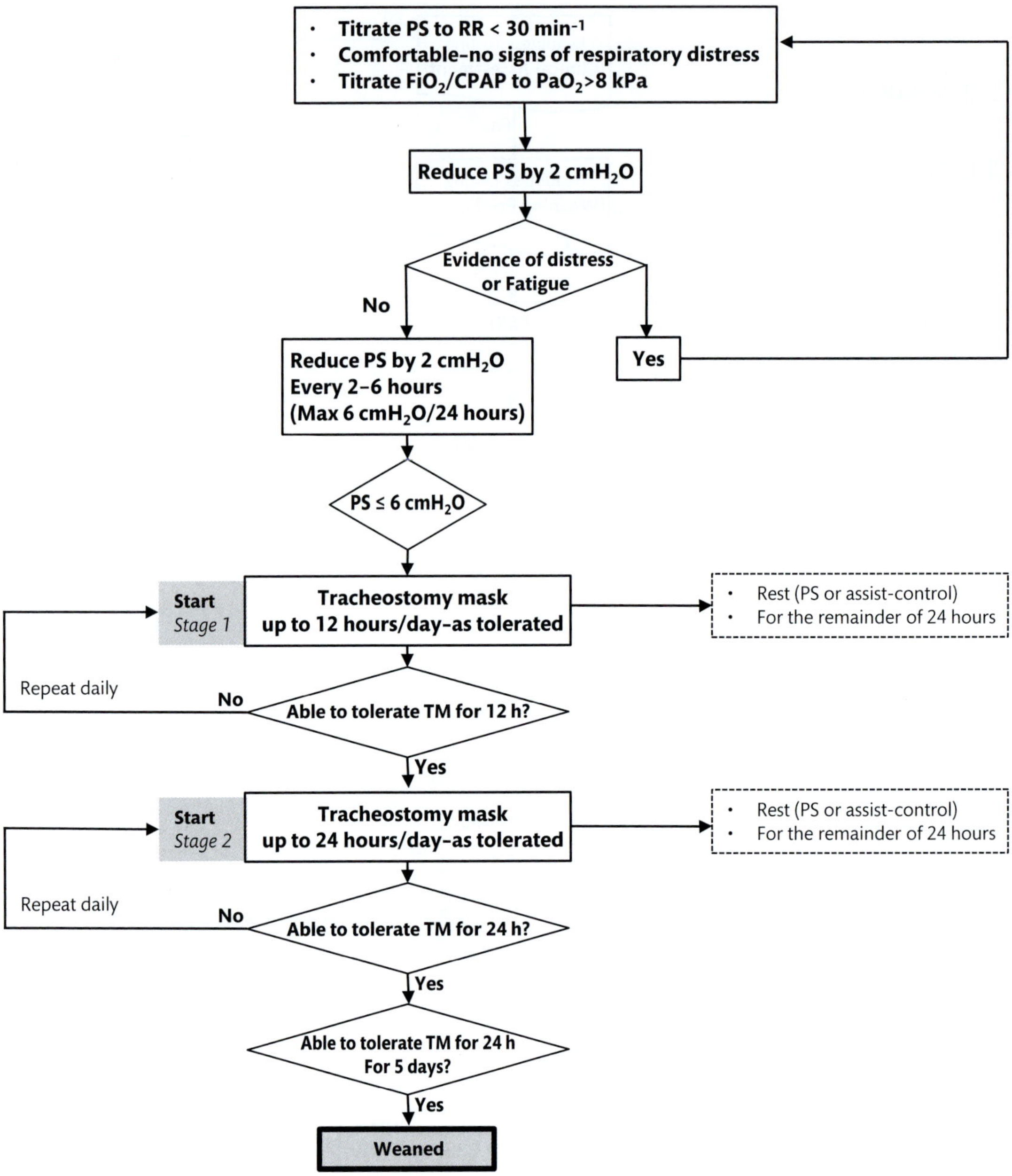

Figure 64.2 Management of patients with difficult and prolonged weaning.

(ATC), or continuous positive airway pressure (CPAP)). There is strong evidence to support the recommendation of an SBT as the initial liberation strategy for patients with acute respiratory failure.[24–26] The SBT provides objective criteria to determine if patients can be successfully extubated.[26] A 'T-piece test' (usually performed in 'flow-by' mode on the ventilator) accurately replicates the work of breathing required from the patient after extubation and constitutes a reliable assessment of the ability of an intubated patient to maintain sufficient ventilation once extubated. By contrast, adding even low PS levels may lead to underestimation of the risk of extubation failure in some patients.[5,27,28] PS is commonly believed to be needed to overcome the resistance of the ETT, but these beliefs fail to account for the increased resistance of the inflamed upper airways following extubation so that the work of breathing following extubation is often greater than during the weaning process.[29] In other words, post-extubation work of breathing is best approximated by an SBT without assistance or tube compensation.[5,7,8,30] Therefore, a low-PS SBT may underestimate the risk of extubation failure, especially if the prevalence of extubation failure is high (e.g. in patients under prolonged mechanical ventilation or having intensive care unit (ICU)-acquired polyneuromyopathy), while low PS (5 cmH_2O) may be used in patients at low risk of failure. ATC can be added if the internal diameter of the ETT is ≤7 mm, which significantly increases work of breathing during the SBT. Similarly, maintaining PEEP during the SBT may increase the rate of extubation failures as PEEP may mask worsening in LV function.[7] Eliciting the patient's subjective impression about the ability to breathe unassisted at the end of the weaning test has been shown to improve the predictive value of the weaning test.[31] The use of repeat SBT within 24 h has not been shown to improve weaning and may induce fatigue

Box 64.1 Readiness testing: clinical assessment

Conditions that must be satisfied before commencing the liberation process

- Improvement or resolution of the underlying cause of acute respiratory failure
- Patient cooperative and pain free
- Able to sustain spontaneous breathing
- Able to cough with minimal secretions (defined as the need for suctioning less frequently than 2 hourly)
- PEEP ≤8 cmH_2O, pressure support ≤8–10 cmH_2O; FiO_2 ≤0.4 with SaO_2 >90% and a PaO_2 >8–9 kPa; PaO_2/FiO_2 >20–26.6 kPa
- Stable hemodynamics; no or minimal vasopressor support
- No uncorrected metabolic abnormalities
- Fluid balance optimized
- Consider measuring NT-proBNP for patients with left ventricular dysfunction—this may guide fluid management
- Tympanic temperature between 36 and 38 •C
- No relevant electrolyte disorder and consider optimal haemoglobin level

that can take over 24 h to recover and so should be avoided.[32] The SBT should last at least 30 min and may be increased up to 120 min in patients considered to be a higher risk of re-intubation (Box 64.2).[8,33,34] The SBT is considered to have failed if the clinician determines significant clinical instability has been induced or if any of the objective criteria listed in are Box 64.3 are breached. The role of NIV to facilitate extubation of patients who fail an SBT has been investigated in small works previously. Although this strategy appears promising in reducing mortality, ventilator-associated pneumonia (VAP), duration of mechanical ventilation, and the need for tracheostomy, without an increased rate of re-intubation,[35] this approach is not currently recommended in common practice and did not demonstrate earlier liberation from mechanical ventilation (4.3 d vs 4.5 d) in the randomized 'Breathe' study.[36]

Box 64.2 Risk factors associated with high risk of extubation failure

- Age >65 years or underlying chronic cardiorespiratory disease
- COPD*
- Heart failure/left ventricular dysfunction*
- OSA/obesity*
- Low PImax*
- $PaCO_2$ >6.5 kPa*
- Neuromuscular disorders*
- Positive fluid balance
- Ventilation >6 days

*These patients may benefit from 'prophylactic' NIV immediately post-extubation if SBT is successful.[37–43]

Extubation

The absence of air leakage when the ETT cuff is deflated is a marker of upper airway obstruction. The amount of air leakage can be quantified using a cuff-leak test (CLT). CLT measures the difference between the inspiratory tidal volume (V_ti) and the expired tidal volume

Table 64.1 Weaning indices that predict successful ventilator discontinuation

Indices	Cut-off value	Ref.	AUC
Rapid shallow breathing index (RSBI) = f/V_t	<105 breaths min^{-1} L^{-1}	(12)	0.89
$P_{0.1}$	<−5.0 cmH_2O*	(18)	0.93
PImax	<−30 cmH_2O (i.e. the more negative the better) Or >−15 cmH_2O**	(12)	0.61
$P_{0.1}$/PImax	<0.09–0.14	(18, 19)	0.99
$P_{0.1} \times f/V_t$	<270 cmH_2O/breaths min^{-1} L^{-1} Or <450 cmH_2O/breaths min^{-1} L^{-1}	(20, 21)	0.81
IWI (integrative weaning index) $(C_{RS} \times SaO_2)/(f/V_t)$	>25 mL cmH_2O^{-1} $breaths^{-1}$ min^{-1} L^{-1}	(21)	0.96

f: respiratory rate; V_t: tidal volume; $P_{0.1}$: airway occlusion pressure at 100 ms; PImax: maximum inspiratory pressure; SaO_2: oxyhaemoglobin saturation in arterial blood; C_{RS}: static respiratory system compliance; IWI: integrative weaning index; AUC: area under the (ROC) curve.

*A $P_{0.1}$ value = 3.5 cmH_2O corresponds to a respiratory effort of approximately 0.75 J/L. Respiratory effort values lower than 0.75 J/L are considered predictive of successful weaning from MV.

**A low PImax is a valuable parameter because patients who present with extreme inspiratory muscle weakness (MIP < −15 cmH_2O) will probably be unable to breathe spontaneously.

Box 64.3 SBT failure criteria

The new onset of any one of the following:

Physiological assessment:

- Heart rate >20% of baseline or >140 beats min^{-1}
- Systolic BP >20% of baseline or >180 mmHg or <90 mmHg
- Cardiac arrhythmias
- Respiratory rate >50% of baseline value or >35 min^{-1}
- Respiratory rate (min)/tidal volume (L) >105 min^{-1} L^{-1}

Arterial blood gases:

- PaO_2 <8 kPa on FiO_2 >0.5 or (SpO_2 < 90%)
- $PaCO_2$ >6.5 kPa or increase by >1 kPa
- pH <7.32 or fall by >0.07 units

Clinical assessment:

- Agitation and anxiety
- Depressed mental status
- Sweating/clammy
- Cyanosis
- Increased respiratory effort (accessory muscles, facial distress, and dyspnoea)

Additional measures—if possible:

- At the beginning and at the end of an SBT, ask the patient the following question: *'do you feel able to breathe without the help of the machine?'**
- Measure $ScvO_2$ if available before and at the end of the SBT**

*Patients who report confidence in the ability to breathe without assistance have an odds ratio for extubation success of 9.22 (3.74–22.42).[31]

**A decrease in $ScvO_2$ >4.5% post SBT could be a marker of worsening of cardiac function.[44]

Box 64.4 How to perform a cuff-leak test

Cuff-leak test is performed in the following method[47]:

- Switch patient to volume assist/control (volume A/C) V_t = 8 mL kg^{-1}
- Measure difference between inspiratory and expiratory tidal volumes (V_ti – V_te) for six consecutive breaths with cuff inflated
- Measure difference between inspiratory and expiratory tidal volumes (V_ti – V_te) for six consecutive breaths with cuff deflated
- Reinflate cuff
- Return patient to CPAP/PS

Extubation failure is pragmatically defined as the need for re-intubation within 48 h (72 h if NIV is used). Clinical criteria that indicate extubation failure and the need for re-intubation are provided in Box 64.5.

Source: Data from Ochoa ME, Marin Mdel C, Frutos-Vivar F, et al. Cuff-leak test for the diagnosis of upper airway obstruction in adults: A systematic review and meta-analysis. *Intensive Care Med.* 2009 Jul;35(7):1171–1179.

(V_te) in assist-control volume mode after balloon cuff deflation, see Box 64.4 for a description of the method of performing a CLT.[7,45,46] A low cuff-leak volume (<110–130 mL) before extubation may indicate a high risk of upper airway obstruction post-extubation.[7,45,46] Although the absence of air leak is a good predictor of upper airway obstruction, the presence of a detectable leak does not rule out upper airway oedema.[47] The CLT is useful because steroid therapy at 4–12 h before extubation seems to reduce the incidence of stridor and the rate of re-intubation.[48] The risk to benefit ratio of steroids in patients with negative CLT results seems to favour steroid administration.[7,48–52] The absence of both an audible cough and a cuff leak indicates that the patient is 10 times more likely to develop post-extubation stridor.[53] A reasonable approach may be a routine CLT before extubation followed by steroid administration when this test is negative particularly in patients who had received mechanical ventilation for >6 days.[7] It is important to consider that the CLT can be falsely negative (i.e. no air leak measured) if the ETT to laryngeal size ratio is >45% (Laryngeal size can be determined using the following equation: antero-postero (A-P) diameter (mm) = (33.9 × height (m)) – 33.7).[54] Box 64.5 summarises the indications for immediate reintubation following attempted extubation.

Failure to Wean: Practical Approach

Difficulties in weaning patients from mechanical ventilation contribute to significant bed occupancy within ICU. A systematic approach to physiological, clinical, psychological, and organizational factors that influence weaning should be adopted. Common causes and suggested approaches to weaning failure are outlined in Table 64.2 with focus on complex weaning patients, which assumes resolution of the initial insult leading to critical illness (see below for details). Patients who have progressed through simple to difficult weaning should be considered for tracheostomy. The timing of tracheostomy insertion remains controversial and although prolonged endotracheal intubation is known to be associated with significant complications, tracheostomy insertion itself poses a risk and may delay weaning in certain patient groups. While early data indicated a benefit from early tracheostomy formation,[55] it has not been shown in subsequent systematic reviews or meta-analyses that early (<10 days) tracheostomy insertion produces improved clinical outcomes compared to delayed (>10 days) tracheostomy insertion.[56,57] However, the majority of units in the Europe perform tracheostomies in patients who have failed to wean within the first 2 weeks post intubation.[58,59] Clinical predictors for prolonged mechanical ventilation are not highly accurate.[60] Moreover, case-specific alternative strategies may be important, such as high-risk neuromuscular patients, in whom aggressive secretion management with mechanical insufflation–exsufflation and extubation onto non-invasive ventilation are recommended.[61] The combination of high-flow nasal oxygen and NIV in those patients with higher risk (i.e. COPD, heart failure, high secretion load, and obesity) of re-intubation is better than HFNO alone at reducing re-intubation (*high wean*).[62]

Box 64.5 Major clinical events that prompted immediate re-intubation (one criterion needed)

- Respiratory or cardiac arrest
- Respiratory distress (SpO_2 <90%, respiratory rate >35/min with visible accessory muscle recruitment or thoraco-abdominal paradoxical breathing despite administration of O_2 and NIV)
- Persistent inability to remove respiratory secretions
- Upper airway obstruction with stridor and/or triage
- Hemodynamic instability (severe arterial hypotension with need for vasoactive drugs)
- Neurologic deterioration (loss of consciousness or psychomotor agitation)

Physiological

The need for prolonged mechanical ventilation should prompt detailed assessment for barriers to the weaning process. The need for physiological dependence on mechanical ventilation is due to persisting imbalance in the load–capacity–drive relationship of the respiratory system. Detailed evaluation of the factors influencing this pivotal relationship should occur to identify reversible causes in this complex patient group.

Respiratory Muscle Load

Chronic respiratory morbidity such as that caused by COPD and asthma contributes to increased work of breathing that can limit patients' ability to wean from mechanical ventilation. Increased airway resistance contributing to airflow limitation and subsequent dynamic hyperinflation acts detrimentally on pulmonary mechanics in weaning patients, and therefore optimal bronchodilation should be maintained in these patients. Patients with obesity have increased work of breathing due to reduced chest wall compliance, and this is exaggerated in patients with obesity-related respiratory failure.[63,64] Similarly patients with chest wall deformity have reduced chest wall compliance adding to respiratory muscle load.[65]

Respiratory Muscle Capacity

Respiratory muscle weakness is associated with prolonged mechanical ventilation and extubation failure. The clinical significance of ventilator-induced diaphragm dysfunction (VIDD) is debated as it has been largely documented in animal models or in less favoured modes of ventilation.[66] Although respiratory muscle weakness can be demonstrated within unselected critically ill patients, diaphragm

Table 64.2 Common causes of weaning failure and proposed solutions[111]

	Possible causes	Suggested approach
Simple weaning	• Delayed awakening due to accumulation of sedative drugs • Lack of screening for risk • Excessive level of ventilatory assist • Lack of systematic discussion about readiness and extubation during rounds • Reduced staffing levels	• Review of sedation • Establish a target sedation score • Daily 'sedation holds' (i.e. stop or halve sedatives) if patient oversedated[22,23] • Identification during the safety briefing • Document weaning plan • Standardize and document weaning readiness measurements • Avoid excessive ventilator assistance
Difficult weaning	• Accumulation of sedative drugs • Fluid overload • Left heart failure • Respiratory muscle weakness (myopathy) • Excessive workload due to infection, secretions, unresolved sepsis, etc.	• Review of sedation • Establish a target sedation score • Physiotherapy and secretion management • Document weaning plan during the ward round • Weaning readiness measurements • Echo • Measurement of NT-ProBNP[74,75,109,110] • Optimization of haemodynamics[111] • Address underlying condition • Review readiness criteria parameters and consider SBT every 24 h
Prolonged weaning	• Severe chronic heart failure • Severe chronic respiratory insufficiency • Respiratory muscle weakness • Depression • Poor sleep quality and delirium • Persistence of underlying condition • Recurring sepsis • Neurological dysfunction	• Consider tracheostomy • Measurement of NT-ProBNP[72,73,107,108] • Optimization of haemodynamics and fluid balance[109,110] • Optimization of cardiac failure • Address underlying condition • Arrange MDT involvement including physiotherapy, pharmacist, dieticians, neurology, etc. • Correct metabolic alkalosis

Source: Reprinted from Frutos-Vivar F, Ferguson ND, Esteban A, et al. Risk factors for extubation failure in patients following a successful spontaneous breathing trial. *Chest*. 2006 Dec;130(6):1664–1671. Copyright 2006, with permission from the American College of Chest Physicians.

fatigue does not appear to be a causative factor in weaning failure.[67,68] Furthermore, care needs to be taken while weaning as the principal treatment for respiratory muscle fatigue is rest. It is therefore slightly paradoxical that inspiratory muscle training has been pursued as a therapeutic intervention in weaning—again, with equivocal results,[69,70] although the small sample sizes of the studies make definitive statements difficult. In addition, pre-existing myopathies and muscular dystrophies may complicate critical illness in patients within ICU or may be diagnosed following presentation with acute respiratory failure to critical care. Such conditions are often associated with both inspiratory and expiratory muscle weakness meaning weaning strategies need to be coupled with aggressive secretion management. Mechanical insufflation–exsufflation devices have been shown to improve physiological cough peak flows and reduce duration of secretion management sessions in patients with neuromuscular disorders.[71,72] They have also been used successfully to avoid the need for tracheostomy formation in critically ill patients with neuromuscular disease.[60]

Respiratory Muscle Drive

Patients with chronic hypercapnic respiratory failure are most appropriately ventilated to their 'usual' CO_2 threshold to ensure adequate drive to breathe when weaning ventilator support or during SBTs. Patients with chronic respiratory failure who present to the ICU should be ventilated to normalize pH with careful adjustment of ventilator support based on daytime triggering of ventilation and work of breathing to assess respiratory drive. A number of acute conditions, Guillan-Barré, poliomyelitis, spinal cord injury, and transverse myelitis, as well as chronic conditions such as motor neurone disease and myasthenia gravis, result in reduced neural respiratory drive to the respiratory muscles. These patients are likely to undergo prolonged mechanical ventilation or complex weaning with bespoke comprehensive weaning and rehabilitation packages required.

Cardiac

Some ventilator-dependent patients have significant cardiac disease that contributes to their failure to wean.[73] Positive end-expiratory pressure provides cardiac support, and its withdrawal can induce cardiac ischaemia and cardiac dysfunction. Patients with evidence of either cardiac ischaemia or dysfunction following SBTs are more likely to fail weaning attempts. This can be assessed using changes in $ScvO_2$ before and after weaning attempts, with a fall in $ScvO_2$ due to failure to appropriately increase cardiac output in response to weaning being associated with weaning failure.[44] In addition, B-type natriuretic peptide (BNP) levels prior to an SBT indicate volume overload and increased risk of weaning failure; this increased risk can be mitigated by appropriate diuretic therapy; as would be expected, BNP-driven diuretic therapy is most successful in patients with left ventricular dysfunction.[74,75] Optimization of cardiac status with coronary intervention or optimization of medical management can assist with weaning in these cases. The use of the inotrope levosimendan may have additional benefits on respiratory muscle function with early evidence that it enhances diaphragm contractility.[76]

Clinical

Nutrition

The optimal nutritional strategy for patients with critical illness remains unclear with equivocal data on short-term outcomes from trophic or full feeding.[77,78] However, difference in patient population and thus clinical phenotype can in part explain these differences. Further clouding the situation on feeding strategy is that the optimal calorie intake required for critically ill patients is unclear, with risks associated with over-feeding and under-feeding.[79,80] Adequate early feeding during critical illness appears particularly important in those patients going on to suffer prolonged mechanical ventilation.[81] Replacement of trace elements such as magnesium has been shown to enhance respiratory muscle function, but a clear clinical effect in the weaning population is lacking.[82,83]

Physical Rehabilitation

Critical illness is associated with an initial catabolic phase that drives acute muscle loss.[84] This muscle loss can progress to ICU-acquired weakness that is highly prevalent in patients undergoing prolonged weaning[85] and is a marker of risk for prolonged weaning.[86] Although simple bedside screening tests have been applied previously these are unreliable and have poor predictive value for clinical outcomes.[87] Patients undergoing prolonged mechanical ventilation and complex weaning have often had lengthy periods of critical illness and as such significant muscle loss. This peripheral muscle weakness is associated with respiratory muscle weakness and as such physical reconditioning is a vital part of the weaning process.[88,89] The use of early physical rehabilitation in ICU improves functional and clinical outcomes including weaning, although the seminal study was based on a multimodal intervention that included sedation holds and thus the exact contribution of physical rehab is hard to confirm.[90] However, there remains substantial perceived and actual barriers to early mobilization of critically ill patients and this is not yet a prevalent practice.[91,92]

Ventilator-associated Pneumonia Prevention

Recurrent episodes of VAP are associated with PMV and increased weaning duration. Many of the steps already described are vital in the process of tackling VAP such as minimizing sedation, appropriate move towards tracheostomy, and cuff down trials to promote bulbar function. It is also vital to ensure good oral hygiene is maintained to limit pathogenic bacterial load within the mouth that may be translocated to the lungs during critical illness. The use of anti-septic mouthwash has been demonstrated as superior to both selective oral decontamination or standard oral hygiene in reducing the incidence of VAP although this is not consistently used.[93,94] Furthermore, although contradictory study results are published, the use of ETTs with sub-glottic suction to aid the removal of supra-cuff secretions has been shown to reduce VAP and improve clinical outcomes in patients with an expected ventilation time of >48–72 h.[95] The use of sub-glottic suction tracheostomy tubes has less available evidence but should be considered in those with poor bulbar function undergoing PMV.[96]

Psychological

Patients who have survived critical illness have significant levels of psychological morbidity,[97,98] which can impact on the engagement needed to progress with complex weaning. Direct engagement with patients by the use of biofeedback techniques has been shown to have promise in difficult and prolonged weaning patients.[99,100]

Organizational

A lack of a systematic approach to weaning without daily consideration of both sedation holds, and readiness testing contributes to weaning delay. While these factors can be addressed by weaning protocols or even automated weaning, these have not been shown to be superior to care when provided in tertiary centres that aim for bespoke patient care plans.[101] Patients with complex weaning who have sufficiently recovered from other aspects of critical illness may be managed within specialist weaning units with a focus on multi-disciplinary approach to weaning and rehabilitation. The use of such units is associated with considerable success in liberating complex patients from mechanical ventilation and has been shown to be cost-effective.[102–104] However, it must be acknowledged that the long-term outcomes for these patients remains poor, with less than 1 in 3 being discharged home and approximately 1 in 4 dying during the weaning phase.[105] The appropriate identification of complex weaning patients within ICU and where available, the use of regional specialist weaning centres allows optimization of bed capacity within ICU and improves outcomes.[106]

Failure to Wean: Long-term Follow-up

Despite the use of dedicated specialist centres, some long-term survivors of critical illness are unable to be decannulated and liberated from mechanical ventilation.[102] These patients may be fully ventilated via tracheostomy, ventilated at night only with daytime self-ventilating via tracheostomy or transitioned to NIV, which may be all daytime or night-time only. The long-term prognosis for these patients is an approximate 50% 1 year mortality; this reflects both the severity of underlying disease as well as the risks of ongoing mechanical ventilation.[103,107] The complexity of care required for these patients' means that of those unable to be decannulated the majority will stay within care institutions, although they may be able to be stepped down from weaning centres to specialist community long-term care facilities.[108] The cost of providing this care is large, the quality of life for the patient limited with additional impacts on the caregivers, and so detailed discussions with patients, caregivers, and family are required prior to embarking on this pathway.

REFERENCES

1. Esteban A, Anzueto A, Frutos F, et al. Characteristics and outcomes in adult patients receiving mechanical ventilation: A 28-day international study. *JAMA*. 2002 Jan 16;**287**(3):345–355.
2. Epstein SK, Ciubotaru RL, Wong JB. Effect of failed extubation on the outcome of mechanical ventilation. *Chest*. 1997 Jul;**112**(1):186–192.
3. Lone NI, Walsh TS. Prolonged mechanical ventilation in critically ill patients: Epidemiology, outcomes and modelling the potential cost consequences of establishing a regional weaning unit. *Crit Care*. 2011;**15**(2):R102.
4. Slutsky AS. Mechanical ventilation. American College of Chest Physicians' Consensus Conference. Chest. 1993 Dec;**104**(6):1833–1859.
5. Boles JM, Bion J, Connors A, et al. Weaning from mechanical ventilation. *Eur Respir J*. 2007 May;**29**(5):1033–1056.

6. Tobin MJ, Laghi F, Jubran A. Ventilatory failure, ventilator support, and ventilator weaning. *Compr Physiol.* 2012 Oct;**2**(4):2871–2921.
7. Thille AW, Richard JC, Brochard L. The decision to extubate in the intensive care unit. *Am J Respir Crit Care Med.* 2013 Jun 15;**187**(12):1294–1302.
8. Perren A, Brochard L. Managing the apparent and hidden difficulties of weaning from mechanical ventilation. *Intensive Care Med.* 2013 Nov;**39**(11):1885–1895.
9. Brochard L, Rauss A, Benito S, et al. Comparison of three methods of gradual withdrawal from ventilatory support during weaning from mechanical ventilation. *Am J Respir Crit Care Med.* 1994 Oct;**150**(4):896–903.
10. Epstein SK, Nevins ML, Chung J. Effect of unplanned extubation on outcome of mechanical ventilation. *Am J Respir Crit Care Med.* 2000 Jun;**161**(6):1912–1916.
11. Ely EW, Baker AM, Evans GW, et al. The prognostic significance of passing a daily screen of weaning parameters. *Intensive Care Med.* 1999 Jun;**25**(6):581–587.
12. Yang KL, Tobin MJ. A prospective study of indexes predicting the outcome of trials of weaning from mechanical ventilation. *N Engl J Med.* 1991 May 23;**324**(21):1445–1450.
13. El-Khatib MF, Zeineldine SM, Jamaleddine GW. Effect of pressure support ventilation and positive end expiratory pressure on the rapid shallow breathing index in intensive care unit patients. *Intensive Care Med.* 2008 Mar;**34**(3):505–510.
14. Seymour CW, Cross BJ, Cooke CR, et al. Physiologic impact of closed-system endotracheal suctioning in spontaneously breathing patients receiving mechanical ventilation. *Respir Care.* 2009 Mar;**54**(3):367–374.
15. Desai NR, Myers L, Simeone F. Comparison of 3 different methods used to measure the rapid shallow breathing index. *J Crit Care.* 2012 Aug;**27**(4):418 e1–6.
16. Ely EW, Bennett PA, Bowton DL, et al. Large scale implementation of a respiratory therapist-driven protocol for ventilator weaning. *Am J Respir Crit Care Med.* 1999 Feb;**159**(2): 439–446.
17. Tanios MA, Nevins ML, Hendra KP, et al. A randomized, controlled trial of the role of weaning predictors in clinical decision making. *Crit Care Med.* 2006 Oct;**34**(10):2530–2535.
18. Capdevila XJ, Perrigault PF, Perey PJ, et al. Occlusion pressure and its ratio to maximum inspiratory pressure are useful predictors for successful extubation following T-piece weaning trial. *Chest.* 1995 Aug;**108**(2):482–489.
19. Nemer SN, Barbas CS, Caldeira JB, et al. Evaluation of maximal inspiratory pressure, tracheal airway occlusion pressure, and its ratio in the weaning outcome. *J Crit Care.* 2009 Sep;**24**(3):441–446.
20. Sassoon CS, Mahutte CK. Airway occlusion pressure and breathing pattern as predictors of weaning outcome. *Am Rev Respir Dis.* 1993 Oct;**148**(4 Pt 1):860–866.
21. Nemer SN, Barbas CS, Caldeira JB, et al. A new integrative weaning index of discontinuation from mechanical ventilation. *Crit Care.* 2009;**13**(5):R152.
22. Kress JP, Pohlman AS, O'Connor MF, et al. Daily interruption of sedative infusions in critically ill patients undergoing mechanical ventilation. *N Engl J Med.* 2000 May 18;**342**(20):1471–1477.
23. Girard TD, Kress JP, Fuchs BD, et al. Efficacy and safety of a paired sedation and ventilator weaning protocol for mechanically ventilated patients in intensive care (Awakening and Breathing Controlled trial): A randomised controlled trial. *Lancet.* 2008 Jan 12;**371**(9607):126–134.
24. Ely EW, Baker AM, Dunagan DP, et al. Effect on the duration of mechanical ventilation of identifying patients capable of breathing spontaneously. *N Engl J Med.* 1996 Dec 19;**335**(25):1864–1869.
25. Esteban A, Ferguson ND, Meade MO, et al. Evolution of mechanical ventilation in response to clinical research. *Am J Respir Crit Care Med.* 2008 Jan 15;**177**(2):170–177.
26. Esteban A, Frutos F, Tobin MJ, et al. A comparison of four methods of weaning patients from mechanical ventilation. Spanish Lung Failure Collaborative Group. *N Engl J Med.* 1995 Feb 9;**332**(6):345–350.
27. Hess DR, MacIntyre NR. Ventilator discontinuation: Why are we still weaning? *Am J Respir Crit Care Med.* 2011 Aug 15;**184**(4):392–394.
28. Haas CF, Loik PS. Ventilator discontinuation protocols. *Respir Care.* 2012 Oct;**57**(10):1649–1662.
29. Mehta S, Nelson DL, Klinger JR, et al. Prediction of post-extubation work of breathing. *Crit Care Med.* 2000 May;**28**(5):1341–1346.
30. Straus C, Louis B, Isabey D, et al. Contribution of the endotracheal tube and the upper airway to breathing workload. *Am J Respir Crit Care Med.* 1998 Jan;**157**(1):23–30.
31. Perren A, Previsdomini M, Llamas M, et al. Patients' prediction of extubation success. *Intensive Care Med.* 2010 Dec;**36**(12):2045–2052.
32. Laghi F, D'Alfonso N, Tobin MJ. Pattern of recovery from diaphragmatic fatigue over 24 hours. *J Appl Physiol* (1985). 1995 Aug;**79**(2):539–546.
33. Vallverdu I, Calaf N, Subirana M, et al. Clinical characteristics, respiratory functional parameters, and outcome of a two-hour T-piece trial in patients weaning from mechanical ventilation. *Am J Respir Crit Care Med.* 1998 Dec;**158**(6):1855–1862.
34. Vitacca M, Vianello A, Colombo D, et al. Comparison of two methods for weaning patients with chronic obstructive pulmonary disease requiring mechanical ventilation for more than 15 days. *Am J Respir Crit Care Med.* 2001 Jul 15;**164**(2):225–230.
35. Burns KE, Meade MO, Premji A, Adhikari NK. Noninvasive positive-pressure ventilation as a weaning strategy for intubated adults with respiratory failure. *Cochrane Database Syst Rev.* 2013 Dec;**2013**(12):CD004127.
36. Perkins GD, Mistry D, Gates S, et al; Breathe Collaborators. Effect of protocolized weaning with early extubation to noninvasive ventilation vs invasive weaning on time to liberation from mechanical ventilation among patients with respiratory failure: The breathe randomized clinical trial. *JAMA.* 2018 Nov 13;**320**(18):1881–1888. doi: 10.1001/jama.2018.13763. PMID: 30347090; PMCID: PMC6248131.
37. Girault C, Bubenheim M, Abroug F, et al. Noninvasive ventilation and weaning in patients with chronic hypercapnic respiratory failure: A randomized multicenter trial. *Am J Respir Crit Care Med.* 2011 Sep 15;**184**(6):672–679.
38. Burns KE, Meade MO, Premji A, et al. Noninvasive ventilation as a weaning strategy for mechanical ventilation in adults with respiratory failure: A Cochrane systematic review. *Can. Med. Assoc. J.* 2014 Feb 18;**186**(3):E112–122.
39. Ornico SR, Lobo SM, Sanches HS, et al. Noninvasive ventilation immediately after extubation improves weaning outcome after acute respiratory failure: A randomized controlled trial. *Crit Care.* 2013 Mar 4;**17**(2):R39.
40. Nava S, Gregoretti C, Fanfulla F, et al. Noninvasive ventilation to prevent respiratory failure after extubation in high-risk patients. *Crit Care Med.* 2005 Nov;**33**(11):2465–2470.

41. Ferrer M, Valencia M, Nicolas JM, et al. Early noninvasive ventilation averts extubation failure in patients at risk: A randomized trial. *Am J Respir Crit Care Med*. 2006 Jan 15;**173**(2):164–170.
42. Nava S, Ambrosino N, Clini E, et al. Noninvasive mechanical ventilation in the weaning of patients with respiratory failure due to chronic obstructive pulmonary disease. A randomized, controlled trial. *Ann Intern Med*. 1998 May 1;**128**(9):721–728.
43. Vaschetto R, Turucz E, Dellapiazza F, et al. Noninvasive ventilation after early extubation in patients recovering from hypoxemic acute respiratory failure: A single-centre feasibility study. *Intensive Care Med*. 2012 Oct;**38**(10):1599–1606.
44. Jubran A, Mathru M, Dries D, et al. Continuous recordings of mixed venous oxygen saturation during weaning from mechanical ventilation and the ramifications thereof. *Am J Respir Crit Care Med*. 1998 Dec;**158**(6):1763–1769.
45. Miller RL, Cole RP. Association between reduced cuff leak volume and postextubation stridor. *Chest*. 1996 Oct;**110**(4):1035–1040.
46. Jaber S, Chanques G, Matecki S, et al. Post-extubation stridor in intensive care unit patients. Risk factors evaluation and importance of the cuff-leak test. *Intensive Care Med*. 2003 Jan;**29**(1):69–74.
47. Ochoa ME, Marin Mdel C, Frutos-Vivar F, et al. Cuff-leak test for the diagnosis of upper airway obstruction in adults: A systematic review and meta-analysis. *Intensive Care Med*. 2009 Jul;**35**(7):1171–1179.
48. Francois B, Bellissant E, Gissot V, et al. 12-h pretreatment with methylprednisolone versus placebo for prevention of postextubation laryngeal oedema: A randomised double-blind trial. *Lancet*. 2007 Mar 31;**369**(9567):1083–1089.
49. Jaber S, Jung B, Chanques G, et al. Effects of steroids on reintubation and post-extubation stridor in adults: Meta-analysis of randomised controlled trials. *Crit Care*. 2009;**13**(2):R49.
50. Fan T, Wang G, Mao B, et al. Prophylactic administration of parenteral steroids for preventing airway complications after extubation in adults: Meta-analysis of randomised placebo controlled trials. *BMJ*. 2008;**337**:a1841.
51. Markovitz BP, Randolph AG, Khemani RG. Corticosteroids for the prevention and treatment of post-extubation stridor in neonates, children and adults. *Cochrane Database Syst Rev*. 2008 Apr;**2008**(2):CD001000.
52. McCaffrey J, Farrell C, Whiting P, et al. Corticosteroids to prevent extubation failure: A systematic review and meta-analysis. *Intensive Care Med*. 2009 Jun;**35**(6):977–986.
53. Maury E, Guglielminotti J, Alzieu M, et al. How to identify patients with no risk for postextubation stridor? *J Crit Care*. 2004 Mar;**19**(1):23–28.
54. Higenbottam T, Payne J. Glottis narrowing in lung disease. *Am Rev Respir Dis*. 1982 Jun;**125**(6):746–750.
55. Terragni PP, Antonelli M, Fumagalli R, et al. Early vs late tracheotomy for prevention of pneumonia in mechanically ventilated adult ICU patients: A randomized controlled trial. *JAMA*. 2010 Apr 21;**303**(15):1483–1489.
56. Siempos, II, Ntaidou TK, Filippidis FT, et al. Effect of early versus late or no tracheostomy on mortality and pneumonia of critically ill patients receiving mechanical ventilation: A systematic review and meta-analysis. *Lancet Respir Med*. 2015 Feb;**3**(2):150–158.
57. Gomes Silva BN, Andriolo RB, Saconato H, et al. Early versus late tracheostomy for critically ill patients. *Cochrane Database Syst Rev*. 2012;**3**:CD007271.
58. Krishnan K, Elliot SC, Mallick A. The current practice of tracheostomy in the United Kingdom: A postal survey. *Anaesthesia*. 2005 Apr;**60**(4):360–364.
59. Kluge S, Baumann HJ, Maier C, et al. Tracheostomy in the intensive care unit: A nationwide survey. *Anesth Analg*. 2008 Nov;**107**(5):1639–1643.
60. Young D, Harrison DA, Cuthbertson BH, et al. Effect of early vs late tracheostomy placement on survival in patients receiving mechanical ventilation: The TracMan randomized trial. *JAMA*. 2013 May 22;**309**(20):2121–2129.
61. Bach JR, Sinquee DM, Saporito LR, et al. Efficacy of mechanical insufflation–exsufflation in extubating unweanable subjects with restrictive pulmonary disorders. *Respir Care*. 2015 Apr;**60**(4):477–483.
62. Thille AW, Muller G, Gacouin A, et al. REVA research network. High-flow nasal cannula oxygen therapy alone or with non-invasive ventilation during the weaning period after extubation in ICU: The prospective randomised controlled HIGH-WEAN protocol. *BMJ Open*. 2018 Sep 5;**8**(9):e023772. doi: 10.1136/bmjopen-2018-023772. PMID: 30185583; PMCID: PMC6129104.
63. Rubinstein I, Zamel N, DuBarry L, et al. Airflow limitation in morbidly obese, nonsmoking men. *Ann Intern Med*. 1990 Jun 1;**112**(11):828–832.
64. Sharp JT, Henry JP, Sweany SK, et al. The total work of breathing in normal and obese men. *J Clin Invest*. 1964 Apr;**43**:728–739.
65. Nickol AH, Hart N, Hopkinson NS, et al. Mechanisms of improvement of respiratory failure in patients with restrictive thoracic disease treated with non-invasive ventilation. *Thorax*. 2005 September 1;**60**(9):754–760.
66. Yang L, Luo J, Bourdon J, et al. Controlled mechanical ventilation leads to remodeling of the rat diaphragm. *Am J Respir Crit Care Med*. 2002 Oct 15;**166**(8):1135–1140.
67. Watson AC, Hughes PD, Louise Harris M, et al. Measurement of twitch transdiaphragmatic, esophageal, and endotracheal tube pressure with bilateral anterolateral magnetic phrenic nerve stimulation in patients in the intensive care unit. *Crit Care Med*. 2001 Jul;**29**(7):1325–1331.
68. Laghi F, Cattapan SE, Jubran A, et al. Is weaning failure caused by low-frequency fatigue of the diaphragm? *Am J Respir Crit Care Med*. 2003 Jan 15;**167**(2):120–127.
69. Martin AD, Smith BK, Davenport PD, et al. Inspiratory muscle strength training improves weaning outcome in failure to wean patients: A randomized trial. *Crit Care*. 2011;**15**(2):R84.
70. Caruso P, Denari SD, Ruiz SA, et al. Inspiratory muscle training is ineffective in mechanically ventilated critically ill patients. *Clinics (Sao Paulo)*. 2005 Dec;**60**(6):479–484.
71. Chatwin M, Simonds AK. The addition of mechanical insufflation/exsufflation shortens airway-clearance sessions in neuromuscular patients with chest infection. *Respir Care*. 2009 Nov;**54**(11):1473–1479.
72. Chatwin M, Ross E, Hart N, et al. Cough augmentation with mechanical insufflation/exsufflation in patients with neuromuscular weakness. *Eur Respir J*. 2003;**21**(3):502–508.
73. Lemaire F, Teboul JL, Cinotti L, et al. Acute left ventricular dysfunction during unsuccessful weaning from mechanical ventilation. *Anesthesiology*. 1988 Aug;**69**(2):171–179.
74. Mekontso-Dessap A, de Prost N, Girou E, et al. B-type natriuretic peptide and weaning from mechanical ventilation. *Intensive Care Med*. 2006 Oct;**32**(10):1529–1536.
75. Mekontso Dessap A, Roche-Campo F, Kouatchet A, et al. Natriuretic peptide-driven fluid management during ventilator

weaning: A randomized controlled trial. *Am J Respir Crit Care Med*. 2012 Dec 15;**186**(12):1256–1263.
76. Doorduin J, Sinderby CA, Beck J, et al. The calcium sensitizer levosimendan improves human diaphragm function. *Am J Respir Crit Care Med*. 2012 Jan 1;**185**(1):90–95.
77. Arabi YM, Tamim HM, Dhar GS, et al. Permissive underfeeding and intensive insulin therapy in critically ill patients: A randomized controlled trial. *Am J Clin Nutr*. 2011 Mar;**93**(3):569–577.
78. Needham DM, Dinglas VD, Bienvenu OJ, et al. One year outcomes in patients with acute lung injury randomised to initial trophic or full enteral feeding: Prospective follow-up of EDEN randomised trial. *BMJ*. 2013;**346**:f1532.
79. Krishnan JA, Parce PB, Martinez A, et al. Caloric intake in medical ICU patients: Consistency of care with guidelines and relationship to clinical outcomes. *Chest*. 2003 Jul;**124**(1):297–305.
80. Faisy C, Lerolle N, Dachraoui F, et al. Impact of energy deficit calculated by a predictive method on outcome in medical patients requiring prolonged acute mechanical ventilation. *Br J Nutr*. 2009 Apr;**101**(7):1079–1087.
81. Wei X, Day AG, Ouellette-Kuntz H, et al. The association between nutritional adequacy and long-term outcomes in critically ill patients requiring prolonged mechanical ventilation: A multicenter cohort study. *Crit Care Med*. 2015 Aug;**43**(8):1569–1579.
82. Dhingra S, Solven F, Wilson A, et al. Hypomagnesemia and respiratory muscle power. *Am Rev Respir Dis*. 1984 Mar;**129**(3):497–498.
83. Johnson D, Gallagher C, Cavanaugh M, et al. The lack of effect of routine magnesium administration on respiratory function in mechanically ventilated patients. *Chest*. 1993 Aug;**104**(2):536–541.
84. Puthucheary ZA, Rawal J, McPhail M, et al. Acute skeletal muscle wasting in critical illness. *JAMA*. 2013 Oct 16;**310**(15):1591–1600.
85. De Jonghe B, Sharshar T, Lefaucheur JP, et al. Paresis acquired in the intensive care unit: A prospective multicenter study. *JAMA*. 2002 Dec 11;**288**(22):2859–2867.
86. De Jonghe B, Bastuji-Garin S, Sharshar T, et al. Does ICU-acquired paresis lengthen weaning from mechanical ventilation? *Intensive Care Med*. 2004 Jun;**30**(6):1117–1121.
87. Connolly BA, Jones GD, Curtis AA, et al. Clinical predictive value of manual muscle strength testing during critical illness: An observational cohort study. *Crit Care*. 2013;**17**(5):R229.
88. Chiang LL, Wang LY, Wu CP, et al. Effects of physical training on functional status in patients with prolonged mechanical ventilation. *Phys Ther*. 2006 Sep;**86**(9):1271–1281.
89. De Jonghe B, Bastuji-Garin S, Durand MC, et al. Respiratory weakness is associated with limb weakness and delayed weaning in critical illness. *Crit Care Med*. 2007 Sep;**35**(9):2007–2015.
90. Schweickert WD, Pohlman MC, Pohlman AS, et al. Early physical and occupational therapy in mechanically ventilated, critically ill patients: A randomised controlled trial. *Lancet*. 2009 May 30;**373**(9678):1874–1882.
91. Nydahl P, Ruhl AP, Bartoszek G, et al. Early mobilization of mechanically ventilated patients: A 1-day point-prevalence study in Germany. *Crit Care Med*. 2014 May;**42**(5):1178–1186.
92. Berney SC, Harrold M, Webb SA, et al. Intensive care unit mobility practices in Australia and New Zealand: A point prevalence study. *Crit Care Resusc*. 2013 Dec;**15**(4):260–265.
93. Labeau SO, Van de Vyver K, Brusselaers N, et al. Prevention of ventilator-associated pneumonia with oral antiseptics: A systematic review and meta-analysis. *Lancet Infect Dis*. 2011 Nov;**11**(11):845–854.
94. Price R, MacLennan G, Glen J. Selective digestive or oropharyngeal decontamination and topical oropharyngeal chlorhexidine for prevention of death in general intensive care: Systematic review and network meta-analysis. *BMJ*. 2014;**348**:g2197.
95. Muscedere J, Rewa O, McKechnie K, et al. Subglottic secretion drainage for the prevention of ventilator-associated pneumonia: A systematic review and meta-analysis. *Crit Care Med*. 2011 Aug;**39**(8):1985–91.
96. Ledgerwood LG, Salgado MD, Black H, et al. Tracheotomy tubes with suction above the cuff reduce the rate of ventilator-associated pneumonia in intensive care unit patients. *Ann Otol Rhinol Laryngol*. 2013 Jan;**122**(1):3–8.
97. Chatila W, Kreimer DT, Criner GJ. Quality of life in survivors of prolonged mechanical ventilatory support. *Crit Care Med*. 2001 Apr;**29**(4):737–742.
98. Jubran A, Lawm G, Kelly J, et al. Depressive disorders during weaning from prolonged mechanical ventilation. *Intensive Care Med*. 2010 May;**36**(5):828–835.
99. Corson JA, Grant JL, Moulton DP, et al. Use of biofeedback in weaning paralyzed patients from respirators. *Chest*. 1979 Nov;**76**(5):543–545.
100. Holliday JE, Hyers TM. The reduction of weaning time from mechanical ventilation using tidal volume and relaxation biofeedback. *Am Rev Respir Dis*. 1990 May;**141**(5 Pt 1):1214–1220.
101. Blackwood B, Alderdice F, Burns K, et al. Use of weaning protocols for reducing duration of mechanical ventilation in critically ill adult patients: Cochrane systematic review and meta-analysis. *BMJ*. 2011;**342**:c7237.
102. Scheinhorn DJ, Hassenpflug MS, Votto JJ, et al. Post-ICU mechanical ventilation at 23 long-term care hospitals: A multicenter outcomes study. *Chest*. 2007 Jan;**131**(1): 85–93.
103. Pilcher DV, Bailey MJ, Treacher DF, et al. Outcomes, cost and long term survival of patients referred to a regional weaning centre. *Thorax*. 2005 Mar;**60**(3):187–192.
104. Schonhofer B, Euteneuer S, Nava S, et al. Survival of mechanically ventilated patients admitted to a specialised weaning centre. *Intensive Care Med*. 2002 Jul;**28**(7):908–916.
105. Scheinhorn DJ, Hassenpflug MS, Votto JJ, et al. Ventilator-dependent survivors of catastrophic illness transferred to 23 long-term care hospitals for weaning from prolonged mechanical ventilation. *Chest*. 2007 Jan;**131**(1):76–84.
106. Heffner JE. A wake-up call in the intensive care unit. *N Engl J Med*. 2000 May 18;**342**(20):1520–1522.
107. Kahn JM, Benson NM, Appleby D, et al. Long-term acute care hospital utilization after critical illness. *JAMA*. 2010 Jun 9;**303**(22):2253–2259.
108. Wise MP, Hart N, Davidson C, et al. Home mechanical ventilation. *BMJ*. 2011;**342**:d1687.
109. Mekontso Dessap A, Katsahian S, Roche-Campo F, et al. Ventilator-associated pneumonia during weaning from mechanical ventilation: Role of fluid management. *Chest*. 2014 Jul;**146**(1):58–65.
110. Ouanes-Besbes L, Dachraoui F, Ouanes I, et al. NT-proBNP levels at spontaneous breathing trial help in the prediction of post-extubation respiratory distress. *Intensive Care Med*. 2012 May;**38**(5):788–795.
111. Frutos-Vivar F, Ferguson ND, Esteban A, et al. Risk factors for extubation failure in patients following a successful spontaneous breathing trial. *Chest*. 2006 Dec;**130**(6):1664–1671.

65

Home Mechanical Ventilation

Rachel D'Oliveiro and Michael Davies

KEY MESSAGES

- Home mechanical ventilation (HMV) services have undergone significant expansion in the last few decades, driven by use of non-invasive ventilation (NIV).
- NIV improves survival and quality of life for patients with respiratory failure associated with progressive neuromuscular disorders. Such patients should be referred to HMV services before the onset of respiratory failure.
- The expansion in HMV services is associated, at least in part, by the increased use of NIV for patients with obesity-related respiratory failure.
- Current evidence strongly supports the role of NIV to treat patients with hypercapnic chronic obstructive pulmonary disease (COPD), especially if still hypercapnic following acute NIV.

CONTROVERSIES

- Ensuring the 'right' treatment for the 'right' patient: There is a strong evidence base to support the use of NIV for specific conditions. Real life is less clear-cut however, and outside of clinical trials patients present with multiple co-morbid conditions making the evidence less generalizable to the individual patient. Advances in ventilator and monitoring technology are appealing though should be supported by evidence of patient benefit before they are introduced into routine practice.
- How to ensure that HMV services and their local referral networks are organized to ensure equitable and consistent provision of HMV.

FURTHER RESEARCH

- Establishing optimal care pathways, including the role of telemonitoring.
- Establishing which modes of ventilation provide benefit to which particular patient groups.

Introduction

Use of long-term home mechanical ventilation (HMV) to support the breathing of patients with chronic hypercapnic respiratory failure has a long history. Early negative pressure tank ventilators first appeared in the 19th century though were rarely used. Poliomyelitis epidemics in the early part of the 20th century created a demand for respiratory support and stimulated the development of the 'iron lung' (see Chapter 1). In 1952, demand for ventilators outstripped capacity during a poliomyelitis epidemic in Copenhagen. With emerging evidence supporting the use of positive pressure ventilation, the Copenhagen group established large numbers of patients on invasive ventilation via tracheostomy with medical students providing continuous manual ventilation in shifts. Survival rates improved compared to negative pressure techniques, leading to the development of modern intensive care services and greater reassurance around the feasibility of long-term positive pressure ventilation.

However, long-term ventilation via tracheostomy remained an impractical option. Negative pressure techniques therefore continued for the small number of patients treated. The 1980s saw the emergence of non-invasive positive pressure ventilation (commonly referred to as NIV) to support patients with acute exacerbations of chronic lung or neuromuscular disease, typically used intermittently during sleep. Its greater effectiveness and convenience led to NIV becoming the standard mode of HMV and a significant expansion in the number of individuals treated with long-term respiratory support (see Chapter 8 for further details on NIV ventilators and Chapter 9 for acute NIV use).

Services have grown and evolved, and the evidence base and indications for NIV have expanded. Advances in ventilator and monitoring technologies have led to newer ways of working. While poliovirus contributed to the start of HMV, the most recent pandemic due to SARS-CoV-2 has accelerated a pre-existing trend towards simplifying HMV treatment pathways, including ambulatory set-ups and more remote monitoring.

Current Accepted Practice

Patient Presentation

The nature and severity of the underlying respiratory disorder, along with co-morbidities, influence patient presentation with chronic hypercapnic respiratory failure. Before starting HMV, the clinician must consider all these factors alongside the wishes of the patient. Shared decision-making is critical for treatment success.

Some conditions, such as Duchenne muscular dystrophy (DMD) and motor neurone disease (MND), confer a definite future risk of hypercapnic respiratory failure. National guidance, in the United Kingdom, recommends referral to a specialized HMV centre before respiratory symptoms start. Serial assessment of function helps determine the optimal time to start HMV and provides the opportunity for patient involvement in decision-making from an early stage.

In contrast, for others the need for HMV may only become clear during an acute admission. For example, acute NIV may be lifesaving for selected patients with chronic obstructive pulmonary disease (COPD). On recovery, many patients will wean from acute NIV, whereas others show a continued requirement for NIV and convert to HMV during the admission. A further group may wean initially from acute NIV and then deteriorate again within weeks.

Symptoms and Signs of Chronic Hypercapnic Respiratory Failure

A detailed history provides vital information about the severity and speed of progression of ventilatory failure. Symptoms of alveolar hypoventilation include early morning headache, sleep disturbance, and excessive daytime sleepiness. Onset may be insidious and symptoms vague, leading to difficulties in recognizing chronic hypercapnic respiratory failure. Examination should include an assessment of the respiratory pump, including chest-wall inspection for skeletal deformity. Inspection of chest wall and abdominal movement during tidal breathing can provide helpful information; paradoxical inward movement of the abdomen during inspiration suggests significant diaphragm weakness. Patients with neuromuscular disease may recruit accessory respiratory muscles to compensate for loss of diaphragmatic function. Rarely, as inspiratory muscle weakness progresses, respiratory alternans may occur in which the diaphragm and accessory muscles contract during alternate breaths. Severe airflow obstruction may also cause inwards movement of the intercostal spaces and ribcage during inspiration.

Indications for NIV

Studies demonstrate significant international heterogeneity in the prevalence and indications for HMV. As the evidence base evolves, more patients are being treated with improved recognition of benefit.

Neuromuscular Disease

Progressive neuromuscular diseases such as MND and DMD typically cause hypercapnic respiratory failure due to loss of respiratory muscle capacity. Overnight use of NIV can mitigate this risk and improve quality of life, particularly for those with less severe bulbar dysfunction. With disease progression, some patients may become increasingly dependent on NIV during the daytime, leading to 24-h dependence (see Chapter 51).

Motor Neurone Disease

MND results in hypercapnic respiratory failure for most patients although the rate of decline is variable; life expectancy is 3 years from symptom onset although 10% of patients survive more than 10 years. Urgent indications for NIV include daytime hypercapnia ($PaCO_2 > 6$ kPa), new onset orthopnoea, and symptomatic nocturnal hypoventilation.

Since respiratory failure is a predictable consequence of MND, UK national guidance recommends referral to a specialist HMV team. Respiratory function should be monitored alongside open discussions with the patient (and carers) about the potential future role for NIV, including likely benefits and implications. Careful monitoring is recommended with routine clinical follow-up at three-monthly intervals or sooner if symptoms are of concern. Monitoring via oxygen saturations alone is falsely reassuring, as SpO_2 94% may be achieved despite coexistent hypercapnia for patients with hypoventilation in the absence of parenchymal lung disease. Lung function is helpful, especially trends. Absolute measures such as vital capacity lower than 50% of predicted values can provide additional support towards a trial of NIV.

NIV does not alter disease progression but can provide improved respiratory reserve and resilience from respiratory infections. Worsening respiratory failure leads to an increased NIV requirement such that use during wakefulness may become necessary. Some patients cannot tolerate NIV; in this circumstance, a palliative approach predominates in the UK. International experience differs with some countries providing home ventilation via tracheostomy for a larger proportion of patients with MND.

NIV can stop at any stage if the patient no longer wants to continue with it. In addition, advance directives help to frame patient wishes about treatment of an acute decline. At the end of life, epidemiological data shows that NIV does not complicate the dying process. Active withdrawal of NIV at patient request is rarely required.

Duchenne Muscular Dystrophy

Patients with DMD typically require wheelchairs by the age of 10 years, and untreated the average age of death is 17–19 years old. Besides assisted ventilation, factors that improve outcomes for such patients include use of corticosteroids while still ambulant, successful spinal surgery to correct scoliosis and specialized multidisciplinary care.

As with MND, proactive surveillance of respiratory function is recommended. Patients with DMD and their carers (typically parents) usually adapt well to NIV and continue to derive benefit into complete ventilator-dependence, retaining a good quality of life.

On its emergence, NIV superseded invasive ventilation via tracheostomy (T-IMV); however, complete NIV-dependence may prompt consideration of T-IMV despite preservation of bulbar function. There is no gold standard of care although preservation of the ability to communicate is vital in maintaining quality of life. NIV combined with intensive secretion clearance such as cough assist provides similar survival outcomes to T-IMV and provides effective care for some. Conversion to T-IMV may be more appropriate for others, with cuff deflated during wakefulness to allow speech.

International data supports a coordinated, individualized approach delivered by a dedicated multi-disciplinary team. As survival improves, an increasing proportion of patients develop significant co-morbidities such as cardiomyopathy. Services are therefore evolving to meet the changing and complex needs of these patients.

Other Neuromuscular Conditions

MND and DMD provide templates for the management of other neuromuscular conditions if adapted for the relative risk of progression to respiratory failure. There is also some variability within individual conditions; for example, the respiratory risk for patients with myotonic dystrophy may differ with the severity of the underlying genetic abnormality. Patients with other forms of myopathy may also require ventilation. As for the more progressive conditions, serial assessment of function can provide insight and guide future monitoring plans.

Extra-pulmonary Restrictive Disease

Chest-wall Deformity

Significant deformity of the chest wall from conditions such as congenital scoliosis, post-poliomyelitis scoliosis, and post-thoracoplasty may cause severe impairment to lung function. With reduced respiratory reserve, respiratory failure may then occur in the setting of age-related decline in lung function or in the presence of other co-morbid conditions, such as COPD or obesity. Prognosis is poor if left untreated. Given the benefits of NIV, surveillance should be considered for patients with non-paralytic scoliosis and reduced respiratory reserve (see Chapter 53).

Chest-wall deformity was previously the most common indication for HMV though represents a reducing proportion of new patients. Thoracoplasty for tuberculosis (TB) became unnecessary with the emergence of streptomycin in the 1950s, and there will now be few patients alive who underwent thoracoplasty in the pre-streptomycin era. Furthermore, patients with congenital scoliosis now benefit from more effective care such as spinal surgery at an earlier stage, reducing the long-term adverse impact on lung function.

Obesity-related Respiratory Failure

Obesity hypoventilation syndrome (OHS) is characterized by the presence of hypercapnic respiratory failure in the presence of obesity (body mass index greater than 30 kg/m^2) and in the absence of any other cause for respiratory failure. A diagnosis of OHS therefore requires the clinician to exclude other respiratory co-morbidities. In the presence of other conditions such as COPD, obesity may then contribute to the development of respiratory failure (see Chapter 54).

Obesity impedes ventilatory function by several mechanisms, including increased elastic load due to extra-thoracic restriction. Hypercapnia is more likely if vital capacity is less than 2.5 L. Abnormal respiratory drive is also observed in some patients although it remains unclear whether this is cause or effect. Finally, over 90% of patients with OHS have coexistent obstructive sleep apnoea syndrome, possibly via inadequate ventilation between apnoeic episodes.

Treatment of OHS with positive pressure therapy may include continuous positive airway pressure (CPAP) or NIV. Both forms of therapy have evidence to support their use though it remains uncertain whether one modality is superior. CPAP therapy is simpler and cheaper and may be used successfully for patients with severe obstructive sleep apnoea but only mild hypercapnia. NIV is usually reserved for patients with more severe hypercapnia.

Parenchymal Lung Diseases

Chronic Obstructive Pulmonary Disease

For patients admitted with acute hypercapnic exacerbations of COPD, treatment with acute NIV reduces hospital mortality by 50%, reduces the need for intubation, and reduces the overall length of stay (see Chapter 41).[1] As described in the following section, the use of HMV in COPD is an evolving field. Current indications include

- persistent hypercapnia ($PaCO_2$ > 7 kPa) 2–4 weeks after resolution of acidaemia in patients who have required acute NIV,
- uncontrolled or worsening hypercapnia in patients who require long-term oxygen therapy, and
- stable, significantly hypercapnic COPD.

COPD is not a single condition, but rather a series of overlapping phenotypes. Some phenotypes may be more likely to benefit from ventilation than others. For example, patients with a combination of COPD and obesity appear more likely to tolerate and benefit from acute NIV. Undiagnosed coexistent sleep disordered breathing may contribute towards the case for HMV.

Evidence Base

Neuromuscular Disease

Early case series demonstrated that NIV improved arterial blood gas tensions and symptoms of hypoventilation, including headache, insomnia, and excessive somnolence. Robust randomized controlled trial (RCT) evidence to support the role of NIV in MND was provided via a UK multicentre study in 2006.[2] NIV use in the setting of respiratory failure was associated with a significant improvement in quality of life and survival compared to the control group, for whom median survival was only 2 weeks in the setting of daytime hypercapnia. Uptake of HMV via NIV increased and is now the standard of care for patients who develop respiratory failure secondary to MND. The RCT showed no significant survival advantage for patients with significant bulbar dysfunction though bulbar dysfunction is not a contraindication in clinical practice. Inpatient titration may increase the likelihood of successful NIV initiation for such patients.[3]

NIV is only one aspect of respiratory support for patients with generalized neuromuscular disorders characterized by significant respiratory muscle weakness. Cough assistance, gastrostomy, and tracheostomy are important considerations with respect to likelihood of benefit and timing. Coordinated multi-disciplinary care is essential.[4] Use of T-IMV in MND shows significant international variation and likely reflects cultural differences in approach and adequacy of health and social care infrastructure.

Diaphragm pacing represents a further option to support breathing, and pilot studies suggested benefit for patients with MND. However, a subsequent RCT was terminated early due to a mortality excess for patients treated with diaphragm pacing.[5] It appears unlikely that diaphragm pacing will provide benefit for patients with MND although it can provide periods off the ventilator for patients with high spinal-cord lesions.

Use of NIV has transformed outcomes for patients with DMD, alongside other improvements in care such as multi-disciplinary clinics and scoliosis surgery.[6] Proactive monitoring is recommended with NIV introduced when there is evidence of nocturnal hypoventilation.[7] In a UK study, NIV was required during sleep alone for approximately 5 years after starting it, with increasing daytime NIV requirement developing later, including use of mouthpiece ventilation.[8] T-IMV may be considered in the event of complete dependence though an individualized approach is recommended. Coordinated multi-disciplinary care is essential,[9] including management of cardiac problems,[10] optimized cough clearance, and nutrition support.

Extra-pulmonary Restrictive Disease

Chest-wall Deformity

There are no RCTs although early uncontrolled studies showed longer survival for patients with scoliosis who were treated with NIV compared to oxygen therapy. This was despite a higher level of pre-treatment hypercapnia for those treated with NIV.

Obesity-related Respiratory Failure

Obesity Hypoventilation Syndrome (OHS) is now the most common indication for NIV. The majority of such patients have severe obstructive sleep apnoea.[11] Other co-morbid conditions often contribute to the development of respiratory failure, leading to difficulties in designing clinical trials that isolate the effect of obesity alone. Nevertheless, current data shows that NIV improves quality of life and survival if compared to lifestyle measures alone.[12] In this study, NIV was compared to CPAP therapy and lifestyle modification alone in 221 patients with obesity-related respiratory failure. NIV and CPAP were superior to lifestyle modification alone for sleep quality and reduction in hypercapnia. Significant weight loss was associated with NIV use, but not CPAP or lifestyle modification.

Weight loss remains crucial to successful treatment in OHS. After starting NIV, a clinical programme of rehabilitation and dietary modification resulted in an additional 10 kg weight loss, improved quality of life, and improved lung function when compared to usual care.[13] Use of CPAP has been associated with weight gain in some studies[14] though further research is required.

Parenchymal Lung Diseases

Chronic Obstructive Pulmonary Disease

Early studies exploring the role of HMV for patients with COPD were limited by poor study design, inadequate correction of ventilation, and suboptimal NIV compliance. However, more recent studies have addressed these issues and a robust evidence base is emerging.

For patients who present following an acute admission, Murphy et al. recruited patients who had been hospitalized for acute hypercapnic COPD requiring NIV.[15] They compared HMV via NIV to home oxygen therapy in those who remained hypercapnic ($PaCO_2$ > 7 kPa) 2–4 weeks after resolution of the acidaemia. They found a 51% reduction in the risk of death or hospital readmission in the group treated with NIV. This translated to a need to treat six patients to avoid one hospital admission or death in 12 months. Exacerbations were reduced by 34% if treated with NIV. Average compliance to NIV was 7.6 h per night at 12 months. The positive results of this trial reinforce the importance of early follow-up and screening for all patients hospitalized with hypercapnic COPD and treated with acute NIV.

Within this acute on chronic cohort, there may be subgroups more likely to benefit from HMV. These include patients with co-existent obesity; in a series exploring outcomes for patients with COPD treated with acute NIV, one-third of patients had significant obesity and experienced fewer acute hospital admissions at 1 year.

In addition, patients who experience frequent exacerbations requiring acute NIV also benefit from the provision of HMV. UK national audit data shows higher treatment success rates for patients treated with acute NIV on more than one occasion. If a patient remains hypercapnic 2–4 weeks after acute NIV, the evidence strongly supports the use of HMV.[15]

HMV has also been assessed in patients with stable hypercapnic COPD. In a multicentre study comparing NIV and long-term oxygen therapy (LTOT) to LTOT alone, McEvoy and colleagues found that HMV improved survival over a 2-year period of follow-up, but did not improve arterial blood gas tensions and worsened measures of quality of life.[16] However, this study used suboptimal NIV inspiratory positive airway pressure (IPAP) settings (average 12.9 cmH_2O) such that no differences in ventilation (change in $PaCO_2$) were identified between the NIV group and the control group. In a separate study, Kohnlein et al. used higher IPAP settings (average 21.6 cmH_2O) when comparing NIV and LTOT.[17] They found that those in the NIV group experienced a significant improvement in survival, blood gas tensions, exercise tolerance, and measures of quality of life. Notably, both studies found it difficult to recruit patients with stable hypercapnic COPD, perhaps suggesting that patient identification for HMV is more challenging compared to the post-acute NIV group.

In summary, current data supports a beneficial role for NIV in selected patients with persistent hypercapnia after acute NIV, and in patients with stable hypercapnic COPD provided that sufficient respiratory support is used to improve carbon dioxide tensions. If used correctly, then HMV improves survival, exercise tolerance, and quality of life if compared to standard therapy.

Physiology and Pharmacology

Physiology of Respiratory Failure

The purpose of the respiratory system is to move and exchange gases between the blood and atmosphere through the processes of ventilation, diffusion, and perfusion. In this way, arterial partial pressures of oxygen and carbon dioxide are maintained within set limits to permit aerobic oxidation in the tissues and preserve normal blood pH. The respiratory system comprises the respiratory muscle pump to facilitate gas flow and ventilation, and the lungs to carry out gas exchange. Respiratory failure occurs when the demands on the respiratory system exceed its capacity, resulting in impaired exchange of oxygen and carbon dioxide.

Type 1 respiratory failure (or hypoxaemic hypoxia) is characterized by arterial hypoxaemia without hypercapnia. It is caused by V/Q mismatching, shunt, impaired diffusion, and hypoventilation. In contrast, type 2 respiratory failure (or ventilatory failure) is characterized by arterial hypercapnia and hypoxaemia, and occurs as a result of alveolar hypoventilation. Arterial carbon dioxide is inversely proportional to alveolar ventilation:

$$P_aCO_2 = K\frac{\dot{V}_{CO_2}}{\dot{V}_A}$$

The alveolar gas equation demonstrates how alveolar hypoventilation causes both hypercapnia and hypoxaemia, as a result of increased $PaCO_2$:

$$P_AO_2 = F_iO_2(P_B - P_{SVP\ water}) - \frac{P_aCO_2}{R}$$

Key

K = constant (0.015 kPa or 863 mmHg)
$\dot{V}CO_2$ = rate of carbon dioxide (CO_2) production
$\dot{V}_A$ = alveolar ventilation
P_AO_2 = alveolar partial pressure of oxygen
F_iO_2 = fraction of inspired oxygen
P_B = atmospheric pressure (101.325 kPa or 760 mmHg at sea level)
$P_{SVP\ water}$ = saturated vapour pressure of water (6.3 kPa or 47 mmHg at 37 °C)
R = respiratory quotient (usually taken as 0.8)

The respiratory muscle pump consists of the inspiratory muscles (diaphragm and extra-diaphragmatic accessory muscles) and expiratory muscles (predominantly the abdominal wall muscles) in combination with central respiratory drive originating from the brainstem. To maintain adequate alveolar ventilation, the load applied cannot exceed capacity (see Figure 65.1).

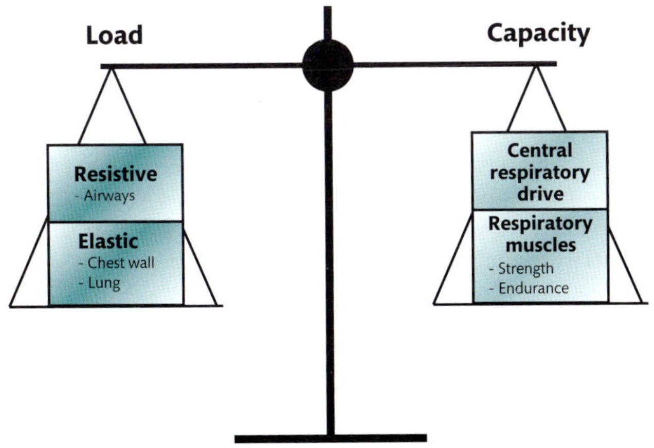

Figure 65.1 The balance of load and capacity. To maintain adequate alveolar ventilation, the sum of resistive and elastic loads must not exceed the capacity of the respiratory muscle pump and central respiratory drive.

Respiratory capacity depends on muscle strength and endurance and the generation of an adequate central drive to breathe. Respiratory muscle weakness may occur at the level of the motor neurone (e.g. MND and poliomyelitis), the neuromuscular junction (e.g. myasthenia gravis), or the muscle itself (e.g. muscular dystrophies). In addition, parenchymal diseases of the lung such as emphysema may lead to insufficient alveolar surface area for gas exchange and hence respiratory failure.

Respiratory load consists of the force needed to overcome the *elastic forces* of the lung parenchyma and chest wall, as well as the *resistive force* of the airways. This may increase in the context of chest-wall deformities, suboptimal alignment of the respiratory muscles (e.g. kyphoscoliosis), morbid obesity, severe sleep apnoea, and obstructive lung disease.

Respiration changes during sleep and is affected by a number of other normal physiological changes including a decrease in metabolic rate and cerebral blood flow. Minute ventilation is reduced by approximately 15% in normal subjects and varies according to sleep stage. During rapid eye movement (REM) sleep, the activity of all respiratory muscles is reduced except for the diaphragms, parasternal intercostal muscles, and strap muscles of the upper respiratory tract. In health, sufficient capacity remains to maintain ventilation and gas exchange during sleep. However, co-morbid conditions that impair respiratory capacity or increase load may tip the balance into insufficient ventilation during sleep, resulting in REM-related hypercapnia and eventually daytime hypercapnia. In such circumstances, using a ventilator to support breathing during sleep may help to maintain normal gas exchange despite insufficient native ventilation. For most conditions, using a ventilator during 6–8 h of sleep is sufficient to maintain stable gas exchange during wakefulness.

How Do Ventilators Work?

The purpose of a ventilator is to move a sufficient volume of gas into the lungs to maintain alveolar ventilation, and therefore normal levels of oxygen and carbon dioxide. An ideal ventilator should be able to deliver this volume while being comfortable for the patient and simple to operate.

NIV utilizes an open circuit (see Figure 65.2) in which leaks can occur and reduce the volume of gas reaching the lungs. As a result, HMV has largely evolved using ventilators that are pressure-targeted rather than volume-targeted. Provided that the resistance of the airways and lung compliance remains constant, higher delivered pressures result in greater volumes. Setting a pressure target also reduces the impact of circuit leaks, that is, leak compensation.

Ventilator Modes

For pressure-targeted ventilators, an expiratory positive airway pressure (EPAP) is set to prevent upper airway closure and also to allow exhaled gases to exit via the exhalation port and prevent rebreathing. An IPAP is set at a higher level than the EPAP to provide a pressure gradient (IPAP-EPAP) and increase tidal volumes. Ventilators also provide a back-up respiratory rate.

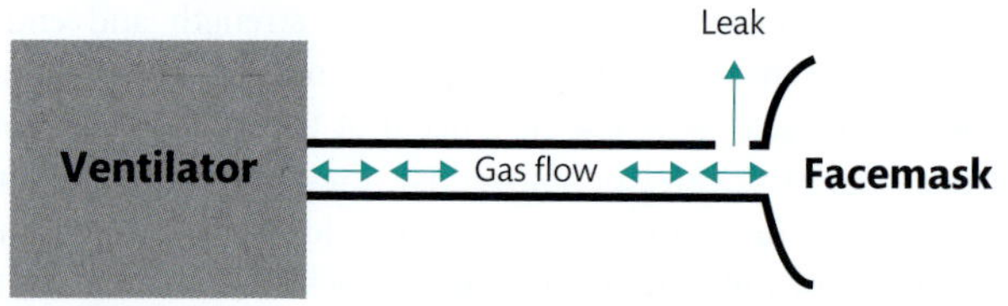

Figure 65.2 A schematic of a simplified single limb NIV circuit with intentional leak, otherwise known as a vented respiratory circuit. The ventilator delivers positive-pressure breaths to the patient via the ventilator tubing and facemask. Exhalation occurs through one or more openings in the mask or ventilator tubing.

Pressure control mode is pressure-targeted, with a set (controlled) duration of inspiration in which a decelerating inspiratory flow rate achieves the target pressure. The back-up rate often becomes the respiratory rate during sleep, meaning that the patient is now ventilated rather than simply supported. For patients with COPD treated with HMV, pressure-controlled ventilation is associated with improved quality of life compared to simple pressure support mode. This is likely achieved via a reduction in spontaneously triggered breaths with more even and effective ventilation during sleep.[18]

Pressure support mode provides support to the patient's own breathing cycle. The patient triggers the ventilator to deliver a pressure-augmented breath, which stops when the inspiratory flow falls below a set percentage of the peak value, usually 25%. Unlike pressure-controlled ventilation, the patient controls the duration of inspiration.

New modes of ventilation have emerged, largely designed to reduce any disadvantages of providing ventilation by targeting either volume or pressure alone. An example of a hybrid mode of ventilation is average volume-assured pressure support (AVAPS), which uses an algorithm to incrementally adjust the delivered IPAP until the targeted (set) tidal volume is reached.

New Patient Set-up for Home Ventilation

For most current patients, pressure control or pressure support ventilation is used. The ventilator is adjusted during a period of adaptation and optimization. This may occur manually although newer ventilators can automate this process to some extent.

Optimization of ventilator settings to ensure that the patient and ventilator are working in synchrony is a vital aspect of care. It requires practical experience and close attention to trigger settings. Ventilators may be triggered by changes in flow or pressure and function to provide a breath as soon as it is desired. During wakefulness, patient triggering helps to maintain the sensation of control over the ventilator. During sleep, the aim is to provide effective ventilation with maximal rest for the respiratory muscles.

Patients treated with HMV may be supported by a range of interfaces, including nasal masks, nasal pillows, and full face masks. The large variety of masks available reflects the fact that there is no perfect interface for NIV. In the acute setting, a full face mask (covering the nose and mouth) is most appropriate as the majority of individuals with respiratory distress breathe through the mouth. In the home setting, the most appropriate interface is one that maximizes patient comfort taking into account whether they breathe through the mouth or nose when sleeping.

Ongoing Care

The successful use of long-term, nocturnal NIV is dependent upon multiple healthcare and patient-related factors. The clinical team delivering care must have significant expertise to ensure that mask fit and ventilator settings are appropriate for the individual patient. Effective treatment initiation is important for successful ongoing delivery of NIV.

Equally important for a successful home NIV service is continuation of care into the home environment. Discharge home with a new form of treatment such as NIV can be daunting for patients, especially if it is commenced during a prolonged acute admission. Patient and carer education are vital. Prior to discharge home, the patient or carer must demonstrate competence in the use of their ventilator. While this is generally very straightforward, it is important to assume nothing during training and to recognize this as a practical skill that must be mastered. Many centres use a formal checklist of competencies and may provide the patient with an action plan to troubleshoot common problems though ready access to the HMV centre is essential.

Controversies and Future Practice

What does the future hold for HMV? With increasing experience and indications, attention turns to different ventilatory strategies and novel ways of improving patient outcomes.

New Indications

As we have already discussed, there is a reasonable evidence base to support the use of NIV for specific conditions. Real life is less clear-cut however, and outside of clinical trials patients present with multiple co-morbid conditions making the evidence less generalizable to the individual patient. NIV is a complex therapy and not a small undertaking for patients or their carers; before starting this treatment, one needs to be convinced that benefit will be achieved. The use of NIV in patients with heart failure is a current area of controversy. Adaptive servoventilation (ASV) is a mode of ventilation that was developed to counter the impact of Cheynes Stokes respiration, a form of central sleep apnoea classically seen in heart failure. Despite initial promise, a multicentre study was stopped early after showing higher rates of cardiovascular and all-cause mortality for patients with chronic heart failure who were treated with ASV.

Newer Modes of Ventilation

Newer modes of ventilation such as volume-assured pressure support have made their way into clinical practice and offer the comfort of pressure supported modes combined with the reassurance of guaranteed minute ventilation. Evidence to date suggests that AVAPS is as effective as pressure-targeted ventilation with respect to improvements in gas exchange, daytime somnolence, and quality of life. However, there are no convincing improvements in patient compliance to ventilation, frequency of hospitalizations, or long-term survival. Careful optimization of ventilator settings is probably more important than the mode itself although it is feasible that a greater degree of automation could reduce the time needed to achieve this. This could have a positive impact on length of stay for patients who start NIV on an inpatient basis.

Reducing Variation of Access to HMV

To date, HMV services in the UK have evolved in an uncontrolled manner via local commissioning. This has led to quite significant variations in the staffing and infrastructure of individual centres. Some centres provide all aspects of complex HMV, including weaning from prolonged invasive ventilation, whereas others do not. Some regions have developed a network approach to facilitate access for complex patients whilst also providing more local HMV services for more stable patients with fewer care needs. Complex HMV services are included within NHS England's Specialized Respiratory Clinical Reference Group and there are accepted service specifications, though the degree to which services may be delegated to regional bodies is currently under review. If implemented, such specifications could provide standards for care and reduce regional variation.

Furthermore, there is an increasing population of children and young adults treated with long-term ventilation at home. Advances in care and increasing use of HMV have resulted in a growing number of patients transitioning into adult services. This presents a new set of challenges to healthcare providers who support patients, carers, and families during the process. For young adults receiving long-term ventilation, this encompasses changes in ventilator set-up to more complex issues such as the provision of funding for ongoing care and equipment. Adjusting to adult infrastructure may also take some time as the separation of adult services means that patients may require several specialist appointments instead of one.

Patients are vulnerable during the transition process, and risk gaps in provision of health and social care or at worst being lost to services entirely. Considerable planning and coordination are needed from an early stage to guard against this; although one size does not fit all in terms of models of care, measures such as written transition plans, health passports, and joint clinics help to bridge the gap. As the population of patients receiving HMV evolves, so must healthcare delivery.

Telemonitoring and Optimal Treatment Pathways

As demands on healthcare increase, so does interest in treating patients outside the hospital environment. Telemedicine and telemonitoring have been shown to reduce readmissions, but not mortality, in patients with heart failure. There is however limited experience in patients treated with HMV although the ability to access data remotely is of interest. In principle, earlier detection of problems such as reduced minute ventilation, increased leak, or falling SpO_2 enables prompt adjustment in treatment. Studies to date have varied in their complexity and provided mixed results. Outcomes for patients in the actively monitoring arms of such studies have ranged from a decrease in hospitalizations[19] to an increase in home visits and hospitalization.[20]

The COVID-19 pandemic has placed healthcare systems under extreme pressure, and this was particularly the case for HMV services. In the UK at least, ICU bed capacity and staffing is a significant constraint. Many HMV inpatient beds and teams were deployed towards the efforts to manage critically ill patients with COVID-19 pneumonitis. With pathway simplification, the avoidance of hospital admission, and infection prevention and control as increasingly important considerations, numerous services moved to a more ambulatory approach to starting HMV. Simple telemonitoring in the initial part of therapy has been adopted by many. Though borne out of necessity for some, emerging data indicates that starting HMV on an ambulatory basis is just as effective as inpatient titration for selected patients and is associated with reduced costs.

Currently, there are more questions than answers though the trend is towards fewer hospital visits. What parameters should we measure? How might we achieve this? Is more intensive monitoring of physiological parameters more effective than clinical vigilance of the patient and treating team? When introducing any new technology, we must ensure that it reduces disease burden on patients and carers as opposed to creating new anxieties. Consideration must also be given to data security and reliability of its transmission as well as what legal principles would apply. The role of telemonitoring in patients requiring home ventilation is evolving, but there is more work to be done before this becomes the norm.

Conclusions and Key Messages

HMV services have undergone significant expansion in the last few decades driven by use of NIV.

Patients who may benefit from HMV vary in their complexity of care requirements. Services should be configured to ensure that they can match the needs of the patients they treat. Simpler HMV, such as nocturnal support for most patients with obesity-related respiratory failure, may be delivered safely by most centres. In contrast, providing safe care for patients with complex clinical issues requires significant service infrastructure. In the UK at least, there is geographical variation in referral pathways to HMV services for patients who have required acute NIV. Improving and simplifying access for HMV for patients who are likely to benefit is a current priority.

For patients with neuromuscular disorders, NIV improves survival and quality of life. Proactive monitoring improves the uptake of NIV and helps to determine the correct time for it to start.

The most significant growth in HMV services has been in its use for patients with obesity-related respiratory failure. NIV or CPAP may benefit though emerging evidence suggests that NIV is preferred. There is a need for a coordinated approach such that weight loss and physical rehabilitation are supported.

Current evidence strongly supports the role of NIV to treat patients with hypercapnic COPD, especially if still hypercapnic following acute NIV.

REFERENCES

1. Plant PK, Owen JL, Elliott MW. Early use of non-invasive ventilation for acute exacerbations of chronic obstructive pulmonary disease on general respiratory wards: A multicentre randomised controlled trial. *Lancet*. 2000:355:1931–1935.
2. Bourke SC, Tomlinson M, Williams TL, et al. Effects of non-invasive ventilation on survival and quality of life in patients with amyotrophic lateral sclerosis: A randomised controlled trial. *Lancet Neurol*. 2006;5:140–147.
3. Farrero E, Prats E, Povedano M, et al. Survival in amyotrophic lateral sclerosis with home mechanical ventilation: The impact of systematic respiratory assessment and bulbar involvement. *Chest*. 2005;127:2132–2138.
4. Traynor BJ, Alexander M, Corr B, et al. Effect of a multidisciplinary amyotrophic lateral sclerosis (ALS) clinic on ALS survival: A population based study, 1996–2000. *J Neurol Neurosurg Psychiatry*. 2003;74:1258–1261.
5. DiPALS Writing Committee. Safety and efficacy of diaphragm pacing in patients with respiratory insufficiency due to amyotrophic lateral sclerosis (DiPALS): A multicentre, open-label, randomised controlled trial. *Lancet Neurol*. 2015;14:883–892.
6. Eagle M, Baudouin SV, Chandler C, et al. Survival in Duchenne muscular dystrophy: Improvements in life expectancy since 1967 and the impact of home nocturnal ventilation. *Neuromuscul Disord*. 2002;12:926–929.
7. Hull J, Aniapravan R, Chan E, et al. British Thoracic Society guideline for respiratory management of children with neuromuscular weakness. *Thorax*. 2012;67:i1–i40.
8. Simonds AK, Muntoni F, Heather S, et al. Impact of nasal ventilation on survival in hypercapnic Duchenne muscular dystrophy. *Thorax*. 1998;53:949–952.
9. Bushby K, Bourke J, Bullock R, et al. The multidisciplinary management of Duchenne muscular dystrophy. *Curr Paediatr*. 2005;15:292–300.
10. Duboc D, Meune C, Lerebours G, et al. Effect of perindopril on the onset and progression of left ventricular dysfunction in Duchenne muscular dystrophy. *J Am Coll Cardiol*. 2005;45:855–857.
11. Pépin J-L, Timsit J-F, Tamisier R, et al. Prevention and care of respiratory failure in obese patients. *Lancet Respir Med*. 2016;4:407–418.
12. Masa JF, Corral J, Alonso ML, et al. Efficacy of different treatment alternatives for obesity hypoventilation syndrome. Pickwick study. *Am J Respir Crit Care Med*. 2015:192;86–95.
13. Mandal S, Suh E, Harding R, et al. Nutrition and Exercise Rehabilitation in Obesity hypoventilation syndrome (NERO): A pilot randomised controlled trial. *Thorax*. 2018;73:62–69.
14. Drager LF, Brunoni AR, Jenner R, et al. Effects of CPAP on body weight in patients with obstructive sleep apnoea: A meta-analysis of randomised trials. *Thorax*. 2014;70:1–7.
15. Murphy PB, Rehal S, Arbane G, et al. Effect of home noninvasive ventilation with oxygen therapy vs oxygen therapy alone on hospital readmission or death after an acute COPD exacerbation: A randomized clinical trial. *JAMA*. 2017;31:2177–2186.
16. McEvoy RD, Pierce RJ, Hillman D, et al. Nocturnal non-invasive nasal ventilation in stable hypercapnic COPD: A randomised controlled trial. *Thorax*. 2009;64:561–566.
17. Köhnlein T, Windisch W, Köhler D, et al. Non-invasive positive pressure ventilation for the treatment of severe stable chronic obstructive pulmonary disease: A prospective, multicentre, randomised, controlled clinical trial. *Lancet Respir Med*. 2014;2:698–705.
18. Dreher M, Storre JH, Schmoor C, et al. High-intensity versus low-intensity non-invasive ventilation in patients with stable hypercapnic COPD: A randomised crossover trial. *Thorax*. 2010:65;303–308.
19. Vitacca M, Bianchi L, Guerra A, et al. Tele-assistance in chronic respiratory failure patients: A randomised clinical trial. *Eur Respir J*. 2009;33:411–418.
20. Chatwin M, Hawkins G, Panicchia L, et al. Randomised crossover trial of telemonitoring in chronic respiratory patients (TeleCRAFT trial). *Thorax*. 2016;71:305–311.

Index

For the benefit of digital users, indexed terms that span two pages (e.g., 52–53) may, on occasion, appear on only one of those pages.

Tables, figures, and boxes are indicated by *t*, *f*, and *b* following the page number